W9-AZG-639

CANCER IN THE NERVOUS SYSTEM

SECOND EDITION

Preface

The first edition of *Cancer in the Nervous System* was created to fill a need I became aware of after moving from The University of California at San Francisco to The University of Texas M. D. Anderson Cancer Center in 1988. It became clear quite quickly that neuro-oncology was so broadly multidisciplinary that no one person could expect to be "expert" in all the diverse fields that impinge on the nervous system and psyche. Indeed, the clinical practice of neuro-oncology has always been a humbling experience. Those practicing neuro-oncology had to have a background or understanding of cancer biology, neurology, neurosurgery, pathology, radiology, radiation therapy, medical oncology, psychiatry, neuropsychology, pharmacology, pain and symptom management, and rehabilitative medicine. It was also clear that no freestanding textbook of general oncology, neurology, neurosurgery, radiation therapy, or internal medicine provided a sufficient singular reference.

Because of the complexity of the nervous system and the uncommonness of many conditions that affect it, becoming expert or even accomplished in some of these areas would require years of clinical practice. As such, neuro-oncology presents a tremendous challenge to generalists in medicine, to physicians practicing away from major medical centers and in Third World countries, to trainees, as well as to many specialists who are not overly familiar with cancer or diseases of the nervous system. I believed when the first edition of *Cancer in the Nervous System* was conceived that these physicians would benefit from a single-source textbook that dealt with pleiotropic effects of cancer on the central nervous system (CNS). To make reading easier for such a diverse audience, we eliminated almost all jargon and abbreviations from the text and also hoped to increase the appeal of this book to other caregivers in nursing, psychology, and rehabilitative medicine.

Our task for this text was expansive: to represent the many fields and specialty practices that provide for those cancer patients whose disease or treatment affects the nervous system or psyche. To achieve that task, we cover the diagnosis and multimodality treatment of primary CNS tumors and secondary metastases to the CNS; the epidemiology of CNS cancers; current molecular and genetic knowledge associated with the development of the most common primary CNS tumors; neurologic syndromes that occur secondary to certain cancers; the neurotoxicity of cancer treatment; psychiatric problems of cancer patients and treatment approaches; cancer-related pain and its treatment; diagnostic imaging; and a new chapter on rehabilitation of cancer patients. For most of our chapters on tumors in the first edition, we used team-writing to bring together opinions from experts in neurology, neurosurgery, radiation oncology, and pathology. In both editions, when these "specialists" had different opinions, I exercised editorial prerogative, hoping to provide a clear path for the reader. Because therapy and clinical management are constantly moving targets for some diseases, we provide a road map rather than a cookbook. We believe the varied presentations inherent to specific disease entities and efficacious approaches for their management are the mainstays of proper and innovative care and will provide a solid base to which the reader will be able to integrate new approaches and treatments when they occur.

I and the rest of the authors hope that this book helps to provide the best care for patients and alleviates some of the anxiety that physicians have when seeking the best course of management for their patients with cancer of the central nervous system.

Houston, Texas V.A.L.

Acknowledgments

While I had contemplated creating a book like this for several years, it was the encouragement of my wife Ellen that got the process moving and her final typing that brought the first edition of *Cancer in the Nervous System* to completion. The second edition, however, would not have been possible without the assistance of Joann Aaron, whose editorial skill, intellectual curiosity, and tenacity helped turn my dream into a reality. I wish also to thank my administrative assistant, Mary Moncrief, for her organizational skill in sending the second edition on its way and helping to find time for me to work on the greatly revised second edition. I also owe a great debt to those authors who found time and energy to work with us to create extensively revised and new chapters for the second edition of what we all believe is an outstanding and helpful textbook.

CONTENTS

CONTRIBUTORS

Jeffrey C. Allen, M.D.
Professor, Division of Neuro-Oncology
Department of Neurology
Beth Israel Medical Center
New York, NY

Joann Ater, M.D.
Associate Professor
Department of Pediatrics
The University of Texas M. D. Anderson Cancer Center
Houston, TX

Mitchel S. Berger, M.D.
Professor and Chairman
Department of Neurological Surgery
University of California San Francisco
San Francisco, CA

Susan M. Blaney, M.D.
Associate Professor, Department of Pediatrics
Hematology-Oncology Section
Baylor College of Medicine
Texas Children's Cancer Center
Houston, TX

Lisa Bomgaars, M.D.
Assistant Professor, Department of Pediatrics
Hematology-Oncology Section
Baylor College of Medicine
Texas Children's Cancer Center
Houston, TX

Melissa L. Bondy, Ph.D.
Associate Professor
Department of Epidemiology
The University of Texas M. D. Anderson Cancer Center
Houston, TX

Jeffrey Bruce, M.D.
Associate Professor
Department of Neurological Surgery
College of Physicians and Surgeons
Columbia University
New York, NY

Janet M. Bruner, M.D.
Professor and Chairman, Department of Pathology
The University of Texas M. D. Anderson Cancer Center
Houston, TX

Marc C. Chamberlain, M.D.
Professor, Departments of Neurology & Neurosurgery
USC/Norris Comprehensive Cancer Center
Los Angeles, CA

Eric L. Chang, M.D.
Assistant Professor
Department of Radiation Oncology
The University of Texas M. D. Anderson Cancer Center
Houston, TX

Mikhail Chernov, M.D.
Neurosurgeon
Department of Surgical Neuro-Oncology
Senior Research Assistant
Russian Polenov
Neurosurgical Institute
St. Petersburg, Russia

Lisa M. DeAngelis, M.D.
Chairman, Department of Neurology
Memorial Sloan-Kettering Cancer Center
Professor, Department of Neurology
Cornell University
New York, NY

Franco DeMonte, M.D.
Associate Professor
Department of Neurosurgery
The University of Texas M. D. Anderson Cancer Center
Houston, TX

Randa El-Zein M.B., Ch.B., Ph.D.
Assistant Professor
Department of Epidemiology
The University of Texas M. D. Anderson Cancer Center
Houston, TX

Jonathan L. Finlay, M.B., Ch.B.
Director of Neuro-Oncology and
Pediatric Oncology Programs
New York University Medical Center
Hassenfeld Children's Center
New York, NY

Alexandra Flowers, M.D.
Assistant Professor
Department of Neurology and Neuro-Oncology
Hartford Hospital
Assistant Professor,
University of Connecticut School of Medicine
Hartford, CT

Arthur Forman, M.D.
Associate Professor
Department of Neuro-Oncology
The University of Texas M. D. Anderson Cancer Center
Houston, TX

Henry S. Friedman, M.D.
Professor, Department of Pediatrics
Associate Professor, Department of Surgery
Associate Professor, Department of Medicine
Duke University Medical Center
Durham, NC

Gregory N. Fuller, M.D., Ph.D.
Associate Professor
Department of Pathology, Section of Neuropathology
The University of Texas M. D. Anderson Cancer Center
Houston, TX

Theresa A. Gillis, M.D.
Associate Professor and
Chief, Section of Physical Medicine and Rehabilitation
The University of Texas M. D. Anderson Cancer Center
Houston, TX

Ziya L. Gokaslan, M.D.
Associate Professor, Department of Neurosurgery
The University of Texas M. D. Anderson Cancer Center
Houston, TX

Ying Guo, M.D.
Assistant Professor
Department of Physical Medicine and Rehabilitation
The University of Texas M. D. Anderson Cancer Center
Houston, TX

C. Stratton Hill, Jr., M.D.
Professor Emeritus
Department of Neuro-Oncology
The University of Texas M. D. Anderson Cancer Center
Houston, TX

Edward F. Jackson, Ph.D.
Associate Professor
Department of Diagnostic Radiology
The University of Texas M. D. Anderson Cancer Center
Houston, TX

Kurt A. Jaeckle, M.D.
Professor, Departments of Neurology and Medicine
Mayo Clinic Jacksonville
Jacksonville, FL

C. David James, Ph.D.
Professor, Department of Experimental Pathology
Mayo Clinic
Rochester, MN

Robert B. Jenkins, M.D., Ph.D.
Professor, Department of Laboratory Medicine and Pathology
Mayo Clinic
Rochester, MN

Anne E. Kayl, Ph.D.
Instructor
Department of Neuro-Oncology
The University of Texas M. D. Anderson Cancer Center
Houston, TX

E. Edmund Kim, M.D.
Professor, Department of Nuclear Medicine
The University of Texas M. D. Anderson Cancer Center
Houston, TX

Ashok J. Kumar, M.D.
Professor, Department of Radiology, Section of Neuroradiology
The University of Texas M. D. Anderson Cancer Center
Houston, Texas

Larry E. Kun, M.D.
Professor and Chairman
Department of Radiation Oncology
Professor, Department of Pediatrics
St. Jude Children's Research Hospital
Memphis, TN

Lara J. Kunschner, M.D.
Assistant Professor
Department of Neurology
Allegheny Neurological Association
Pittsburgh, PA

Lauren Langford, M.D.
Associate Professor,
Department of Pathology, Section of Neuropathology
The University of Texas M. D. Anderson Cancer Center
Houston, TX

Normand J. Laperriere, M.D.
Associate Professor
Department of Radiation Oncology
University of Toronto
Princess Margaret Hospital
Toronto, Ontario

Edward Laws, Jr., M.D.
Professor, Department of Neurosurgery
Professor, Department of Internal Medicine
University of Virginia School of Medicine
Charlottesville, VA

Adrian W. Laxton, M.A.
University of Toronto
Faculty of Medicine
Toronto, Ontario

Norman E. Leeds, M.D.
Professor, Department of Radiology, Section of Neuroradiology
The University of Texas M. D. Anderson Cancer Center
Houston, TX

Steven A. Leibel, M.D.
Professor and Chairman
Department of Radiation Oncology
Memorial Sloan-Kettering Cancer Center
New York, NY

Victor A. Levin, M.D.
Professor, Department of Neuro-Oncology
The University of Texas M. D. Anderson Cancer Center
Houston, TX

D. Andrew Loblaw, M.D.
Assistant Professor,
Department of Radiation Oncology
Toronto-Sunnybrook Regional Cancer Centre
Toronto, Ontario

Eric Marmor, M.D.
Resident, Department of Neurosurgery
Jewish General Hospital
Montreal, Quebec

Mary Jane Massie, M.D.
Professor
Department of Clinical Psychiatry
Cornell University Medical College
New York, NY

Ian E. McCutcheon, M.D.
Associate Professor, Department of Neurosurgery
The University of Texas M. D. Anderson Cancer Center
Houston, TX

Michael W. McDermott, M.D.
Associate Professor and Vice Chairman
Department of Neurological Surgery
University of California San Francisco
San Francisco, CA

Christina A. Meyers, Ph.D.
Associate Professor
Department of Neuro-Oncology
The University of Texas M. D. Anderson Cancer Center
Houston, TX

Ann Yuriko Minn, M.S.
Research Assistant
Department of Neurology
Stanford University Medical Center
Stanford, CA

Roger J. Packer, M.D.
Professor, Departments of Neurology and Pediatrics
George Washington University School of Medicine
Clinical Professor, Department of Neurosurgery
University of Virginia School of Medicine
Chairman, Department of Neurology
Children's National Medical Center
Washington, DC

Steven D. Passik, Ph.D.
Director, Oncology Symptom Control and Research
Community Cancer Care, Inc.
Clinical Professor of Psychiatry
Indiana University School of Medicine
Indianapolis, IN

Richard G. Perrin, M.D.
Associate Professor, Department of Surgery,
Division of Neurosurgery
University of Toronto Faculty of Medicine
Head, Division of Neurosurgery,
The Wellesley Hospital
Toronto, Ontario

David G. Poplack, M.D.
Professor, Department of Pediatrics and Head, Hematology-Oncology Section
Baylor College of Medicine
Director, Texas Children's Cancer Center, Texas Children's Hospital
Houston, TX

Alfredo Quinones-Hinosa, M.D.
Resident, Department of Neurological Surgery
University of California San Francisco
San Francisco, CA

Suresh K. Reddy, M.D.
Assistant Professor
Department of Chronic Pain
The University of Texas M. D. Anderson Cancer Center
Houston, TX

Lisa R. Rogers, D.O.
Associate Professor, Department of Neurology
Wayne State University School of Medicine
Detroit, MI

Raymond Sawaya, M.D.
Professor and Chairman, Department of Neurosurgery
The University of Texas M. D. Anderson Cancer Center
Houston, TX

Justin S. Smith, M.D., Ph.D.
Resident, Department of Neurological Surgery
University of California San Francisco
San Francisco, CA

Nancy J. Tarbell, M.D.
Professor, Department of Radiation Oncology
Harvard Medical School
Massachusetts General Hospital
Boston, MA

Alan D. Valentine, M.D.
Associate Professor
Department of Psychiatry
The University of Texas M. D. Anderson Cancer Center
Houston, TX

Rena Vassilopoulou-Sellin, M.D.
Professor
Department of Endocrine Neoplasia and Hormonal Diseases
The University of Texas M. D. Anderson Cancer Center
Houston, TX

Charles B. Wilson, M.D.
Professor
Department of Neurological Surgery
University of California San Francisco
San Francisco, CA

Franklin C. Wong, M.D., Ph.D., J.D.
Associate Professor
Department of Nuclear Medicine
The University of Texas M. D. Anderson Cancer Center
Houston, TX

Margaret Wrensch, Ph.D.
Adjunct Professor
Department of Epidemiology & Biostatistics
University of California San Francisco
San Francisco, CA

Rajesh Yadav, M.D.
Assistant Professor
Department of Physical Medicine and Rehabilitation
The University of Texas M. D. Anderson Cancer Center
Houston, TX

W. K. Alfred Yung, M.D.
Professor and Chairman
Department of Neuro-Oncology
The University of Texas M. D. Anderson Cancer Center
Houston, TX

Part I

Diagnostic Imaging

1

Diagnostic Imaging

NORMAN E. LEEDS, ASHOK J. KUMAR, AND EDWARD F. JACKSON

Magnetic resonance imaging (MRI) performed with and without intravenous (IV) contrast material is the technique of choice for imaging abnormalities of the brain in patients with cancer of the central nervous system (CNS). The technique provides an excellent depiction of anatomic detail in multiple planes and reveals pathologic abnormalities to advantage. The use of an IV contrast medium results in tissue opacification. The major reason for using an IV contrast medium is that it creates a visual distinction between normal brain capillaries and lesions caused by a breakdown in the blood–brain barrier (BBB) or by tumor endothelial cells; these lesions might be present but would otherwise remain invisible. In addition to MRI's visualization of anatomic detail and its ability to detect the presence of pathologic abnormalities, its other advantages are visualization of vascular detail; capability for producing high-resolution images; and use of thin slices to improve anatomic detail, fat saturation for improved tissue visualization, and fast spin-echo and spoiled grass sequences to reduce imaging time. Other techniques for imaging arteries and veins may be added to provide additional anatomic information. Thus, the wide range of pulse sequences and techniques available with MRI make it the ideal imaging technique for most cases.

Computed tomography (CT) still has a role in the evaluation of a patient's CNS cancer. The CT scans are sometimes useful to obtain optimum information on calcification, bony abnormalities, acute hemorrhage, and subarachnoid hemorrhage. Computed tomography is also an excellent modality for examining uncooperative or mobile patients and seriously ill patients with monitoring equipment and for evaluating subarachnoid spaces and sulci to demonstrate cortical or cerebellar involution.

Magnetic resonance imaging is also advantageous for visualizing the bony structure of the spine, particularly marrow spaces and intraspinal contents, including leptomeninges, pia arachnoid, spinal cord, nerve roots, and ganglia. Use of an IV contrast medium heightens the sensitivity in diagnosis. Magnetic resonance imaging is the technique of choice for demonstrating disease metastatic to osseous structures because it reveals metastasis even when findings from plain roentgenograms of the bone and bone scan are negative. This is possible because MRI visualizes marrow space where metastases can localize, demonstrates seeding of the leptomeninges or pia arachnoid, and may reveal metastases to the spinal cord. Of particular benefit to patients with cord compression, MRI demonstrates to advantage the presence of single or multiple lesions, the site of bony involvement, the extradural component, and the extent of disease, which allows planning of the appropriate therapeutic approach. Thus, by replacing myelography with MRI for lesions affecting the spinal cord, tumor extent and tissue components can be identified within the neoplasm.

Computed tomography scans demonstrate osseous structures to advantage but are not very useful for evaluating intraspinal contents except when contrast medium is introduced into the spinal canal (CT myelography). It is an excellent technique for demonstrating intraspinal pathology, for example, extradural, intradural extramedullary, and intramedullary masses.

Computed tomography myelography will not, however, permit visualization of intraspinal tissue changes except for calcification, fat, or hemorrhage or the presence of a cavity within the central canal (syrinx). Computed tomography or CT myelography is thus a secondary diagnostic option that can be used to obtain complementary information when necessary. CT myelography may be the examination of choice for patients suspected of having cord compression who are unable to undergo MRI.

An MRI examination should not be used for patients who have a pacemaker, paramagnetic aneurysm clips, metal within the orbit, or other paramagnetic devices installed for purposes such as tympanoplasty. The risk that MRI poses to the fetus, especially during the first trimester of pregnancy, is unknown. Most physicians believe, however, that the risk is certainly not as great as that from X-rays; thus, depending on the perceived risk/benefit ratio, MRI may be performed in this setting. The referring physician must recommend this procedure and discuss it with the patient. A signed consent form should be obtained to ensure that the patient has been properly informed of potential risks. After the first trimester, the risk to the fetus appears to diminish. Nevertheless, the risk/benefit ratio should be explained to the patient, although the probable risks are significantly lessened.

Approximately 10% of CNS cancer patients are claustrophobic, and these patients may need to be sedated before the examination can be performed. The sedative may be sublingual lorazepam in milder cases at a dose of 1.0 to 1.5 mg, depending on patient size, and IV diazepam at a dose of 3 to 5 mg in more severe cases.

This chapter discusses the basic imaging features of brain and spinal cord tumors and is oriented toward the nonspecialist. For a more detailed presentation, the reader is referred to the articles cited in the references.

IMAGING OF PRIMARY BRAIN TUMORS

Cerebral Infiltrating Astrocytomas

Cerebral infiltrating astrocytomas vary from low-grade astrocytomas to high-grade malignant glioblas-

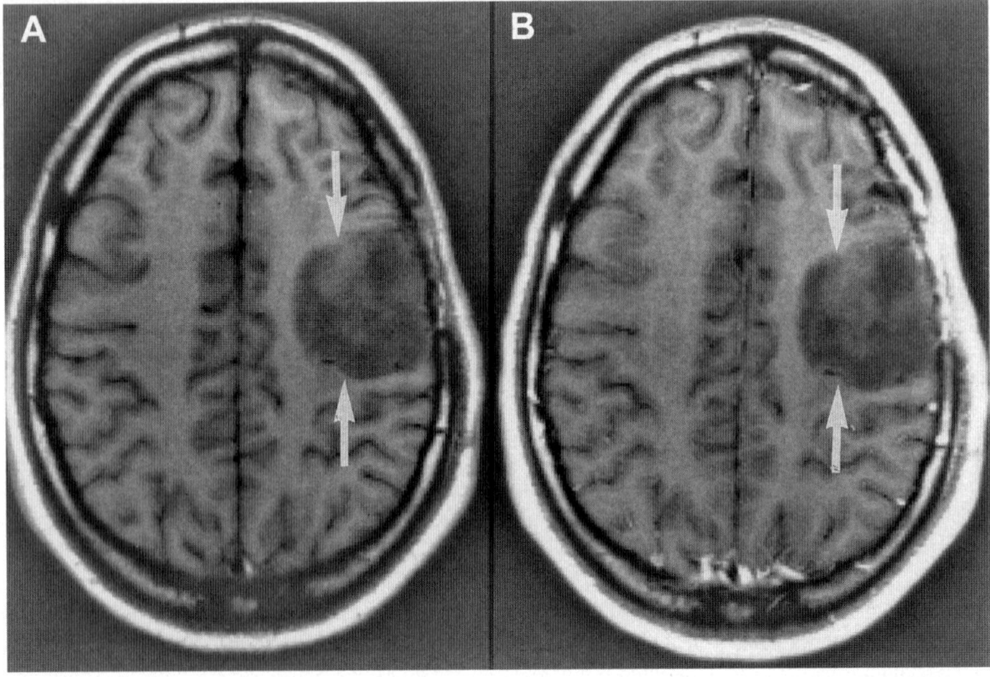

Figure 1–1. Low-grade nonenhancing astrocytoma. Pre-contrast **(A)** and post-contrast **(B)** axial MRI images show a nonenhancing tumor (arrows).

toma multiforme. Computed axial tomography and MRI can usually, but not invariably, predict histologic staging of astrocytomas. Low-grade gliomas tend to be nonenhancing to minimally enhancing tumors following the administration of IV contrast material (Fig. 1–1), whereas glioblastoma multiforme shows high-grade heterogeneous enhancement with variable zones of necrosis (Fig. 1–2). Anaplastic astrocytomas, which are graded at an intermediate level, reveal variable degrees of contrast enhancement without necrosis. Brain tumors not only produce multiple neurologic deficits but can also result in symptoms secondary to brain herniations. Occurrences of brain herniations are secondary to occurrences of intracranial masses and associated vasogenic edema within the white matter (Fig. 1–2). MRI, with its multiplanar capability, can easily assess the degree of various types of herniation associated with cerebral tumors (Fig. 1–2). It is important to recognize herniation early because immediate therapy may be necessary to reduce the effect of the mass. The use of glucocorticoids and/or osmotic agents (e.g., mannitol or glycerol) minimizes the degree of edema; likewise, emergency surgical debulking of the tumor may be necessary. Despite aggressive therapy, glioblastoma multiforme can grow like a wildfire, spreading into the ventricular system and subarachnoid space and even metastasizing to the spinal cord

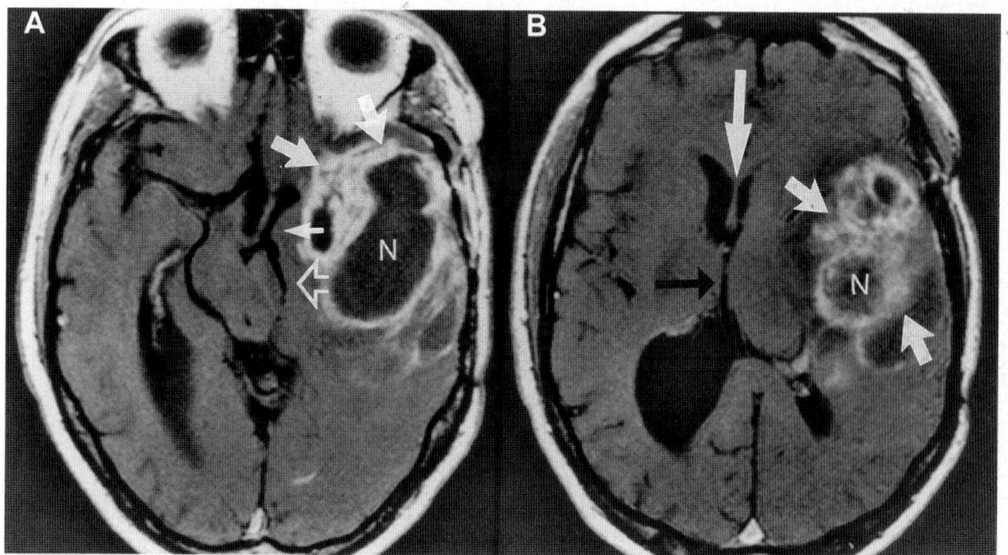

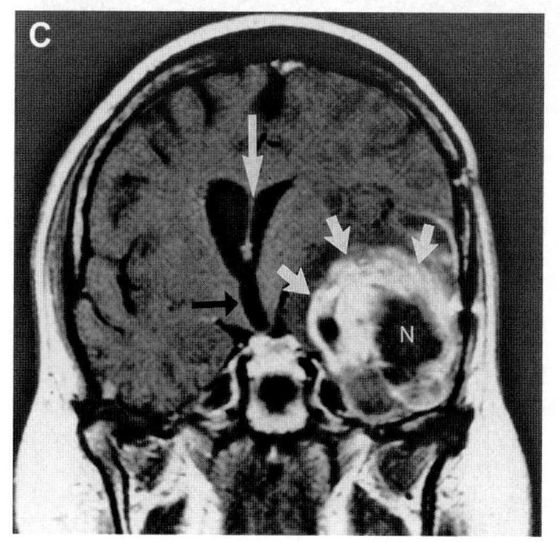

Figure 1–2. Glioblastoma multiforme. Post-contrast axial **(A, B)** and coronal **(C)** MRI images. Irregular, thick, nodular, peripherally enhancing mass (smaller white arrows in A, B, C) occupying the temporal lobe with areas of central necrosis (N in A, B, C) is a typical feature of glioblastoma. The tumor and the vasogenic edema resulted in marked subfalcine herniation as noted by a contralateral shift of the septum pellucidum (large white arrows in B and C) and the third ventricle (black arrows in B and C). There is also uncal (small white arrow in A) and hippocampal herniation (open white arrow in A) with midbrain compression.

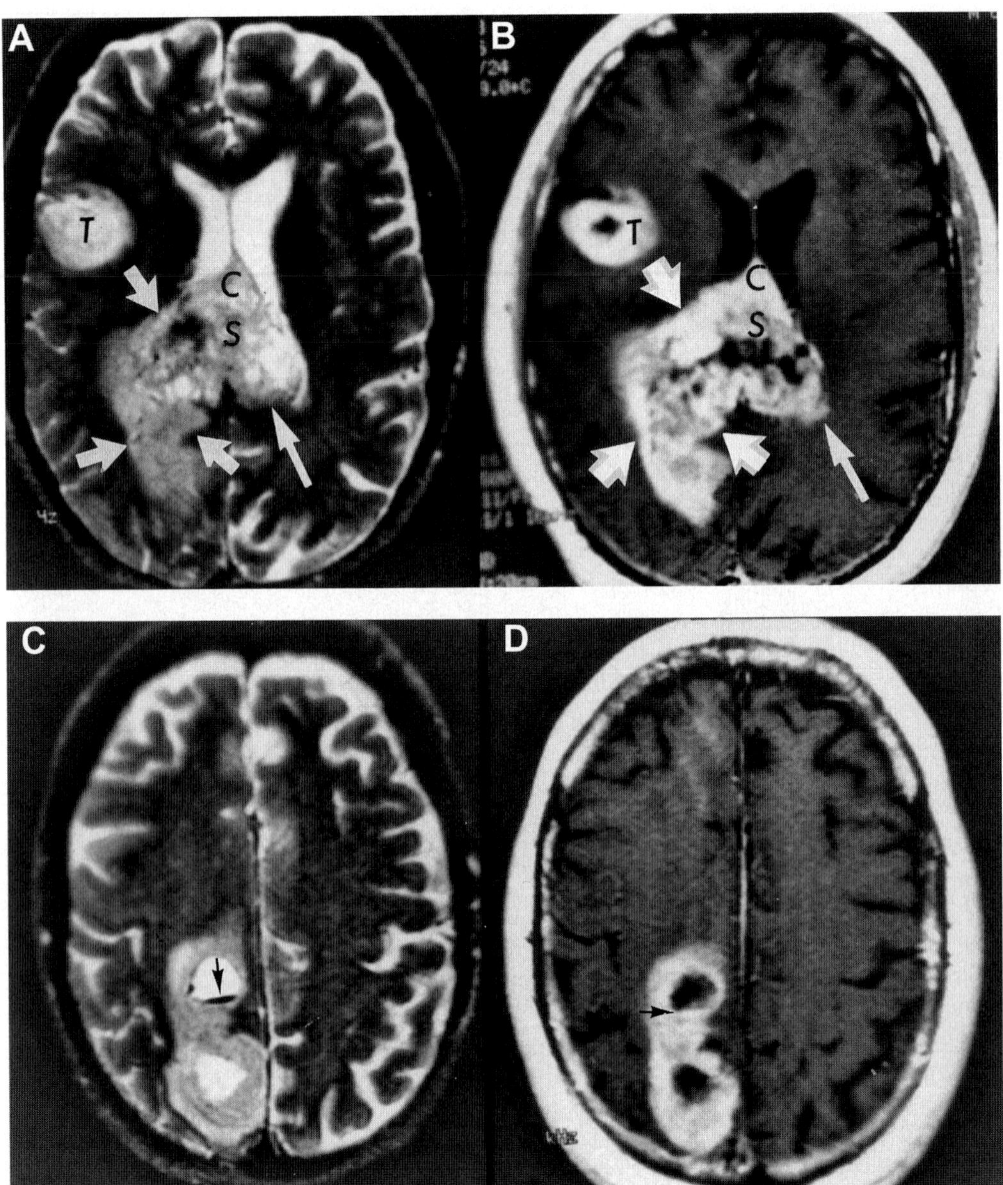

Figure 1–3. Patient with multifocal glioblastoma multiforme. **(A)** T_2-weighted image reveals heterogeneous hyperintensity extending in butterfly fashion from the right parieto-occipital region across the splenium (S) and corpus callosum (C) to the left hemispheres (arrows). Hypointense (dark) foci within the lesion represent intratumoral hemorrhage. A second right frontal focus (T) is seen that probably has transcortical connections to the other lesion despite not being observed. **(B)** Post-contrast T_1-weighted image shows enhancement of the two lesions with a focus of hypointensity within the right frontal convexity lesion not seen in A that represents a focus of necrosis. The hypointense foci within the butterfly lesion probably represent either hemorrhage, as in A, and/or necrotic foci. **(C)** T_2-weighted image through centrum semiovale reveals superior extent of right-sided tumor, which is of heterogeneous hyperintensity with evidence of two round lesions. The more anterior lesion has a fluid level representing a hemorrhagic cavity with sediment that is hypointense (black arrow) with the remainder hyperintense (bright) fluid. The more posterior lesion is round and hyperintense and represents a cystic focus. **(D)** Axial T_1-weighted image post-contrast shows contrast enhancement of the lesion except for the two round foci observed in C that are now hypointense and represent foci of necrosis, with the more anterior hypodense lesion showing reversal of densities from C with sediment now bright (arrow).

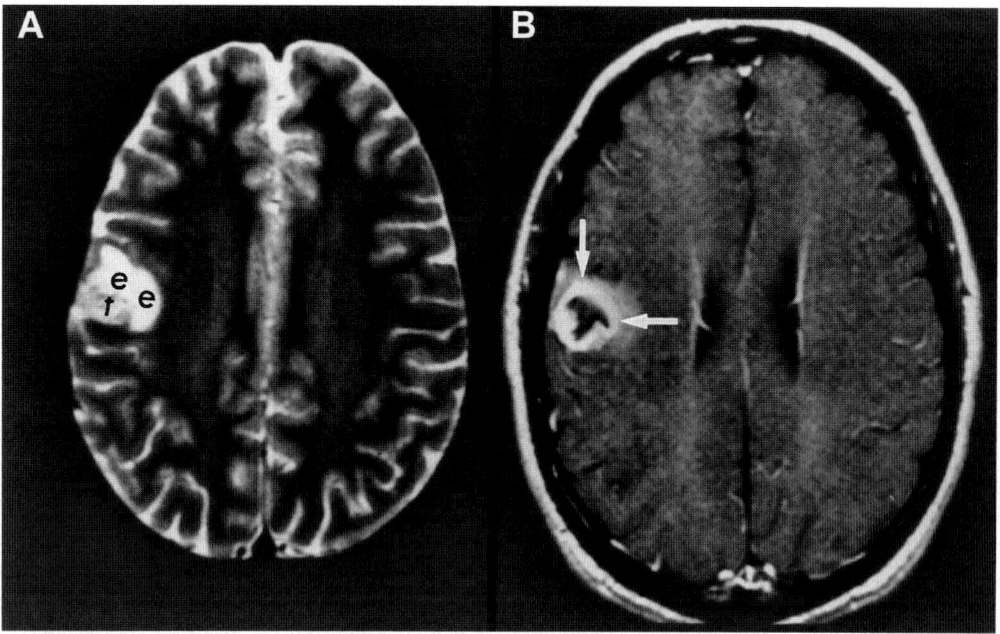

Figure 1–4. Patient with glioblastoma multiforme peripherally situated that looks like metastasis. **(A)** T_2-weighted image reveals peripheral lesion of heterogeneous intensity (t) with surrounding edema (e). **(B)** T_1-weighted image post-contrast shows enhancing peripheral zone (arrows) with central necrosis (hypointensity within tumor).

and spinal subarachnoid space in a relatively short period of time (Choucair et al., 1986; Kyritsis et al., 1993).

When an anaplastic astrocytoma or glioblastoma originates in the corpus callosum, it can extend across the midline to involve the opposite cerebral hemisphere, forming a "butterfly" pattern (Fig. 1–3). Both anaplastic astrocytoma and glioblastoma multiforme can be multifocal in origin (Kyritsis et al., 1993) (Fig. 1–3). Glioblastomas are rarely circumscribed, but on occasion may mimic a metastatic tumor (Fig. 1–4).

Oligodendrogliomas

Oligodendrogliomas are low-grade glial tumors and have a prognosis similar to that of astrocytomas. Oligodendrogliomas are usually slow-growing tumors that elicit chronic symptoms, and patients most often present with seizures. The presence of calcification is a characteristic feature of oligodendrogliomas. Computed tomography is more sensitive than MRI for detecting calcifications. Calcification in a tumor is a useful indicator of the benign nature of the malignant neoplasm. Oligodendrogliomas are sharply demarcated on a cortical surface and show only minimal, if any, enhancement with contrast. As in astrocytomas, various grades may be observed, depending on the degree of anaplasia, vascular endothelial proliferation, and necrosis.

Pilocytic Astrocytomas

Pilocytic astrocytomas are well defined and have a cystic or multicystic component. They usually occur in the suprasellar region, arising from the optic apparatus, and in the posterior fossa. Pilocytic astrocytomas are relatively benign and extremely slow growing. They may be easily removed, depending on their location, because of the presence of a distinct capsule. Thus, they have a relatively favorable prognosis, particularly when located in anatomic areas such as the vermis and the cerebellar hemispheres. Magnetic resonance imaging is more sensitive than CT in differentiating solid from cystic components of pilocytic astrocytomas.

Optic Chiasm and Hypothalamic Astrocytomas

Optic chiasm gliomas are seen most frequently in children and young adults and can occur in association with neurofibromatosis type 1. They are usually low-grade neoplasms that spread along the visual pathways. Hypothalamic gliomas behave more aggressively and produce symptoms earlier, such as diabetes insipidus, inappropriate antidiuretic hormone secretion, or disturbances of temperature, appetite, or metabolism. Frequently, both the optic apparatus and the hypothalamus are affected, and determining the site of origin is difficult.

The specific anatomic structural involvement of optic chiasma/hypothalamic regions by tumor can be best demonstrated by MRI of the sagittal and coronal planes (Fig. 1–5). The tumors are often enhanced with IV contrast medium.

Brain Stem Astrocytoma

Brain stem astrocytomas are more common in children but also occur in adults. Patients usually present with projectile vomiting, ataxia, and multiple cranial nerve palsies. Magnetic resonance imaging is the modality of choice for diagnosing brain stem gliomas, and it can easily detect early tumoral involvement of brain stem and outline the extent of tumor spread. These tumors are known to infiltrate the midbrain, pons, medulla, and upper cervical cord. Grossly enlarged brain stem gliomas can be easily depicted in sagittal views (Fig. 1–6). Brain stem gliomas show variable enhancement with contrast. Magnetic resonance imaging is superior to CT in its ability to clearly differentiate cystic and solid tumor components (Fig. 1–6). A surgical decompression of a cyst can often aid in relieving symptoms caused by compression of vital structures by tumor.

Poorly Differentiated Tumors of Neuronal Cell Origin

Medulloblastomas are tumors that occur in children second in frequency to astrocytomas. They are highly cellular and locally invasive and are best represented in sagittal and axial views of MRI scans. They are characteristically located in the region of the posterior roof of the fourth ventricle. Medulloblastomas are intensely enhanced by IV contrast (Fig. 1–7). These tumors rarely calcify and often seed into the subarachnoid space, ventricular system, and spinal canal.

Intraventricular Tumors

Choroid Plexus Papillomas

Choroid plexus papillomas, which are usually seen in children, originate from the choroid plexus of the lateral ventricles and the fourth ventricle. They account for less than 1% of all intracranial neoplasms.

Magnetic resonance imaging can easily demonstrate the intraventricular location of the mass. Choroid plexus papillomas intensively enhance with IV contrast and are highly vascular. Even when they arise posteriorly in the lateral ventricles with no apparent obstruction, a disproportionate degree of hydrocephalus develops because of overproduction of cerebrospinal fluid (CSF), which is a characteristic feature of choroid plexus papilloma.

Ependymomas

Ependymomas represent about 5% of all primary intracranial gliomas, occurring most frequently in children. They originate from the ependymal lining of the ventricular cavity and are located in the fourth, third, and lateral ventricles. Ependymomas are slow-growing malignant tumors that grow by expansion and infiltration. Ventricular and subarachnoid seeding is common. Magnetic resonance imaging can demonstrate the intraventricular location of the mass (Fig. 1–8). Characteristic imaging features of ependymomas include an intraventricular location, intense enhancement with contrast, and calcification. Ependymomas arising within the fourth ventricular cavity often extend through the foramen of Luschka region into the cerebellopontine angle regions.

Colloid Cysts

Colloid cysts are rare benign tumors that originate from primitive neuroepithelium of the roof of the anterior third ventricle. These tumors are classically located in the foramen of Monro region. Colloid cysts may have a stalk and can cause intermittent hydrocephalus, giving rise to intermittent fainting episodes. Because of the initial location of the mass, tumors as

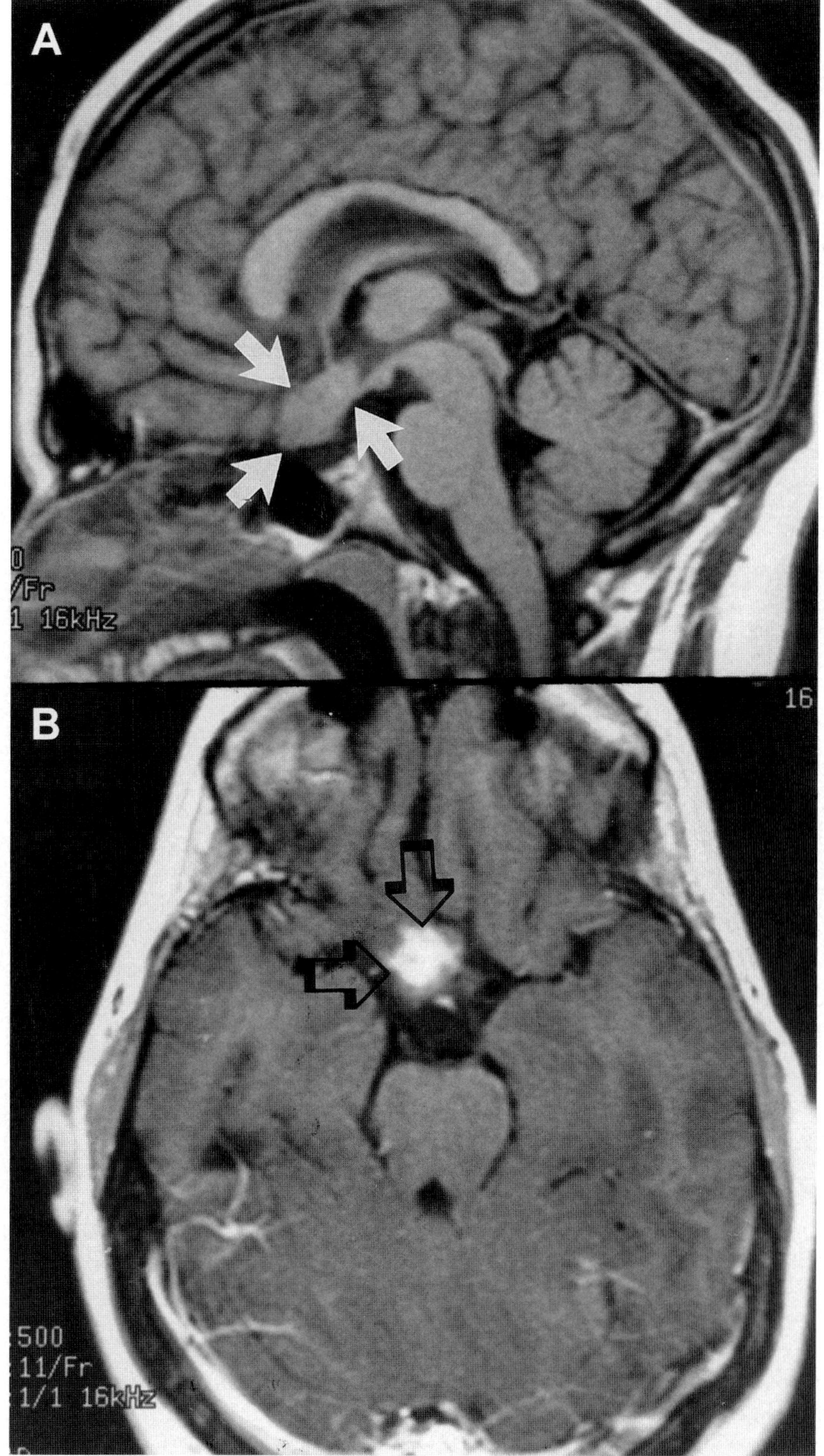

Figure 1–5. Optic chiasma glioma in a patient with neurofibromatosis. Mass involving the optic chiasma (arrows) is clearly shown in a sagittal non-contrast T_1-weighted image of the brain **(A).** Post-contrast axial T_1-weighted image **(B)** reveals contrast enhancement (open arrows), a feature of optic chiasma glioma.

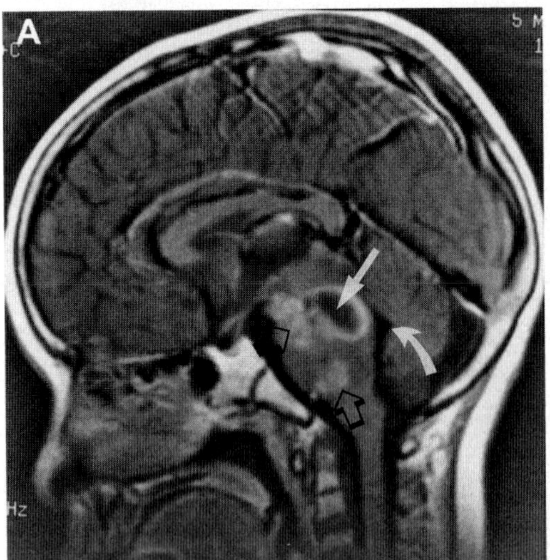

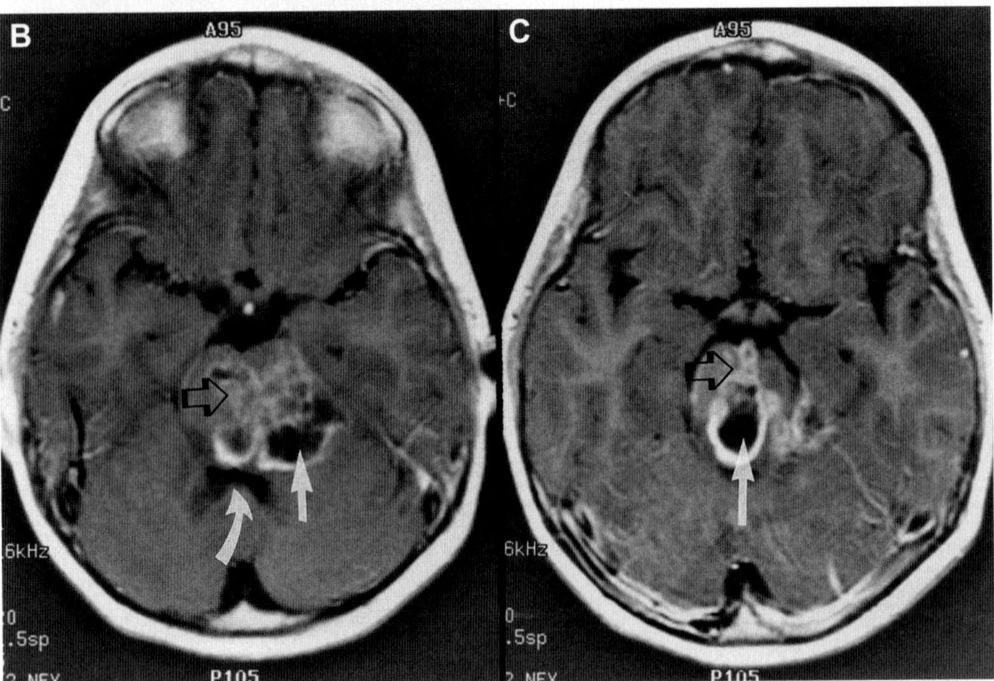

Figure 1–6. Brain stem astrocytoma. Post-contrast sagittal **(A)** and post-contrast axial MRI scans at the mid **(B)** and upper **(C)** pons. The brain stem is markedly expanded by solid (open arrows) and cystic (white arrows) components of tumor. The IV ventricle (curved arrows in A and B) is displaced posteriorly by the brain stem tumor.

small as 1 cm can cause obstructive hydrocephalus. A well-defined nonenhancing mass in the foramen of Monro region should favor the diagnosis of colloid cyst. The diagnosis can be readily made with either CT or MRI.

Subependymal Giant Cell Astrocytomas

Subependymal giant cell astrocytomas involving the lateral ventricles characteristically occur in patients with tuberous sclerosis. These are relatively benign

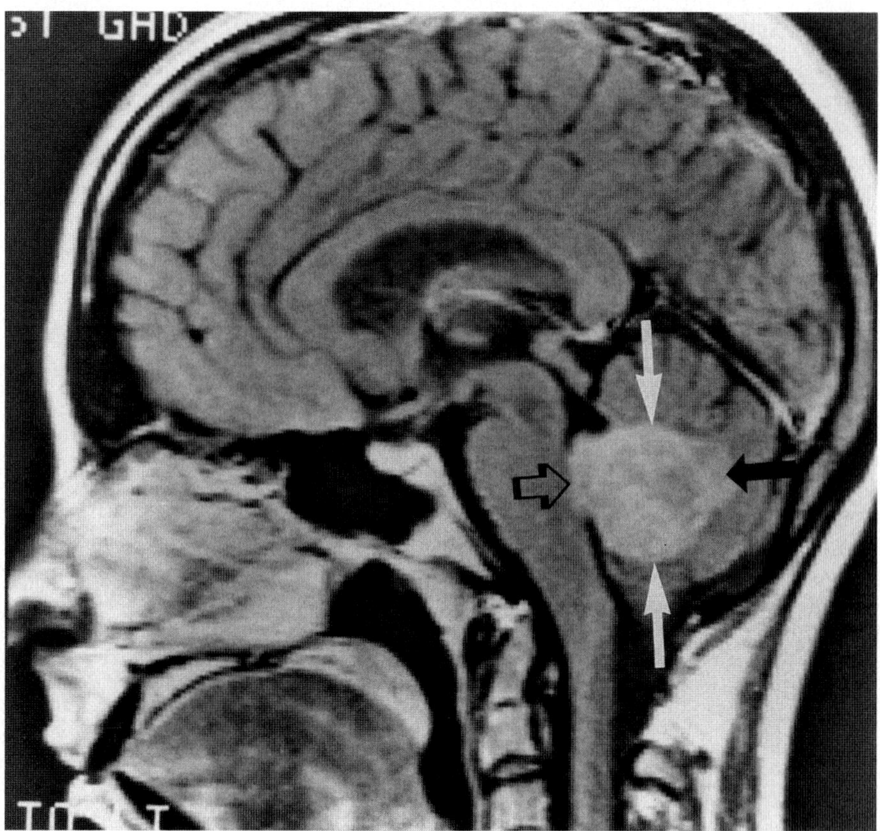

Figure 1–7. Medulloblastoma. Post-contrast sagittal MRI scan shows the tumor located along the posterior roof of the fourth ventricle (white arrows) with extension to vermian (black arrow) and fourth ventricular (open arrow) areas. The location of the mass and the intense tumoral enhancement are characteristic features of medulloblastoma.

tumors occurring particularly in and around the foramen of Monro region, anterior third ventricle, and frontal horns. These tumors are recognized by their location, intense enhancement on post-contrast CT or MRI examinations, and the presence of calcification (Fig. 1–9).

Intrasellar and Suprasellar Tumors

Chromophobe Adenoma

Chromophobe adenomas are the most common intrasellar tumors. They cause the sella to swell into a balloon shape, and they can grow in all directions. Suprasellar extension of the tumor can result in optic nerve and optic chiasma compression, which can cause visual-field defects. The tumors can be easily diagnosed by MRI examination of the pituitary gland and are best seen in sagittal and coronal planes as soft tissue masses within the sella turcica. Intravenous contrast often results in inhomogeneous enhancement of pituitary tumors (Fig. 1–10).

Other symptoms may develop as a result of hemorrhage or pituitary apoplexy (acute hemorrhage into a pituitary tumor) and may require immediate evaluation to determine the need for surgery. Magnetic resonance imaging is quite sensitive in detecting a hemorrhage into the tumor. When chromophobe adenomas are less than 10 mm in size, they are called *pituitary microadenomas.* Acromegaly and Cushing's syndrome are often caused by microadenomas. Magnetic resonance imaging can detect such tumors as small as 3 mm.

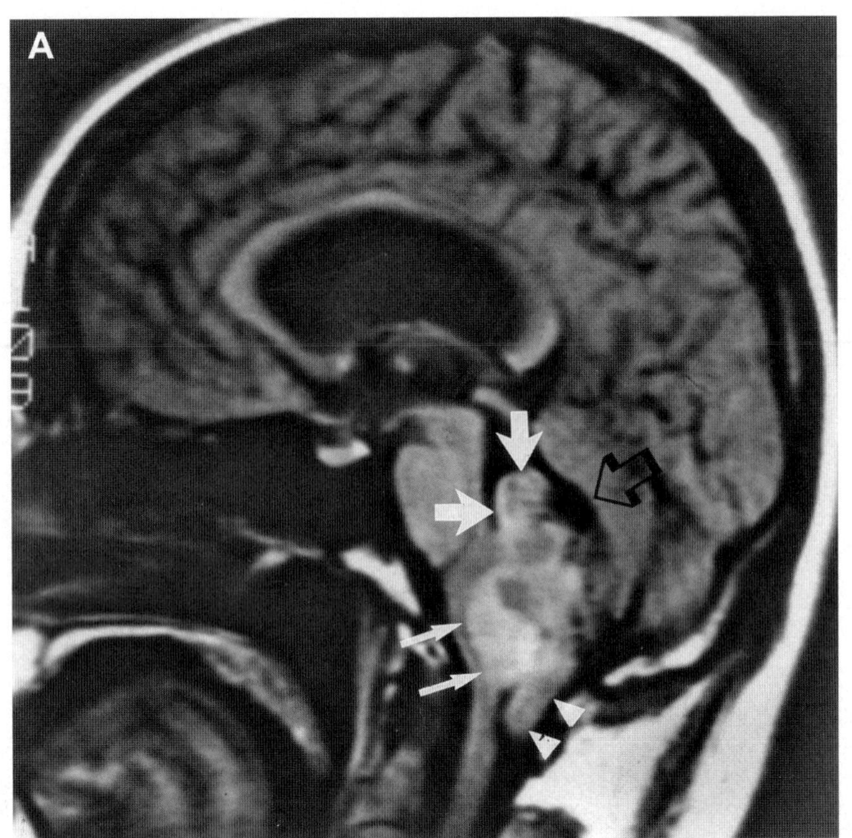
A

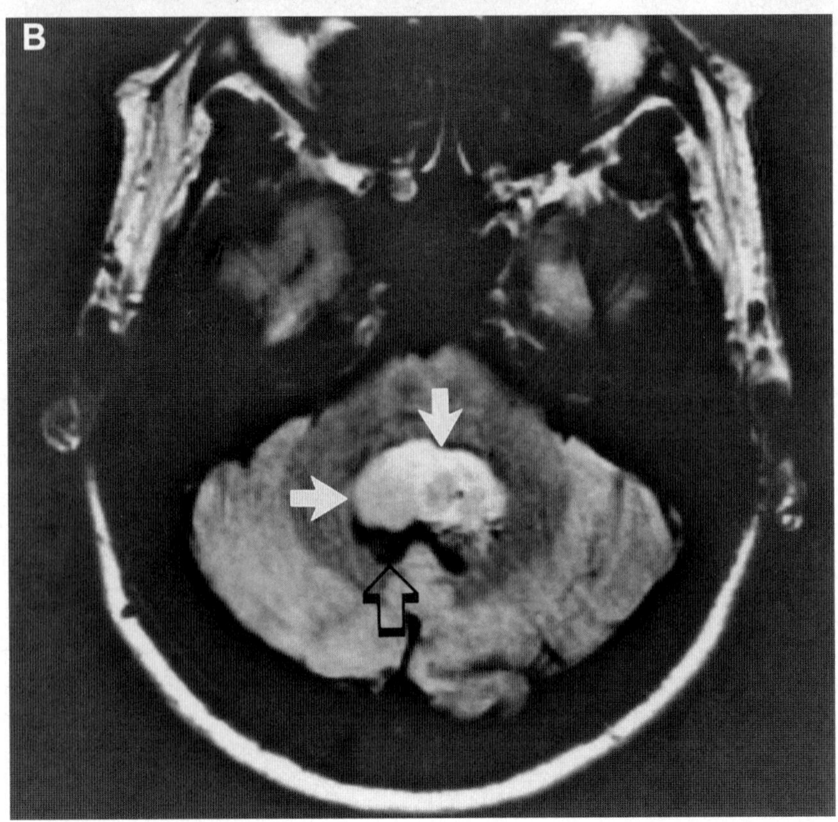
B

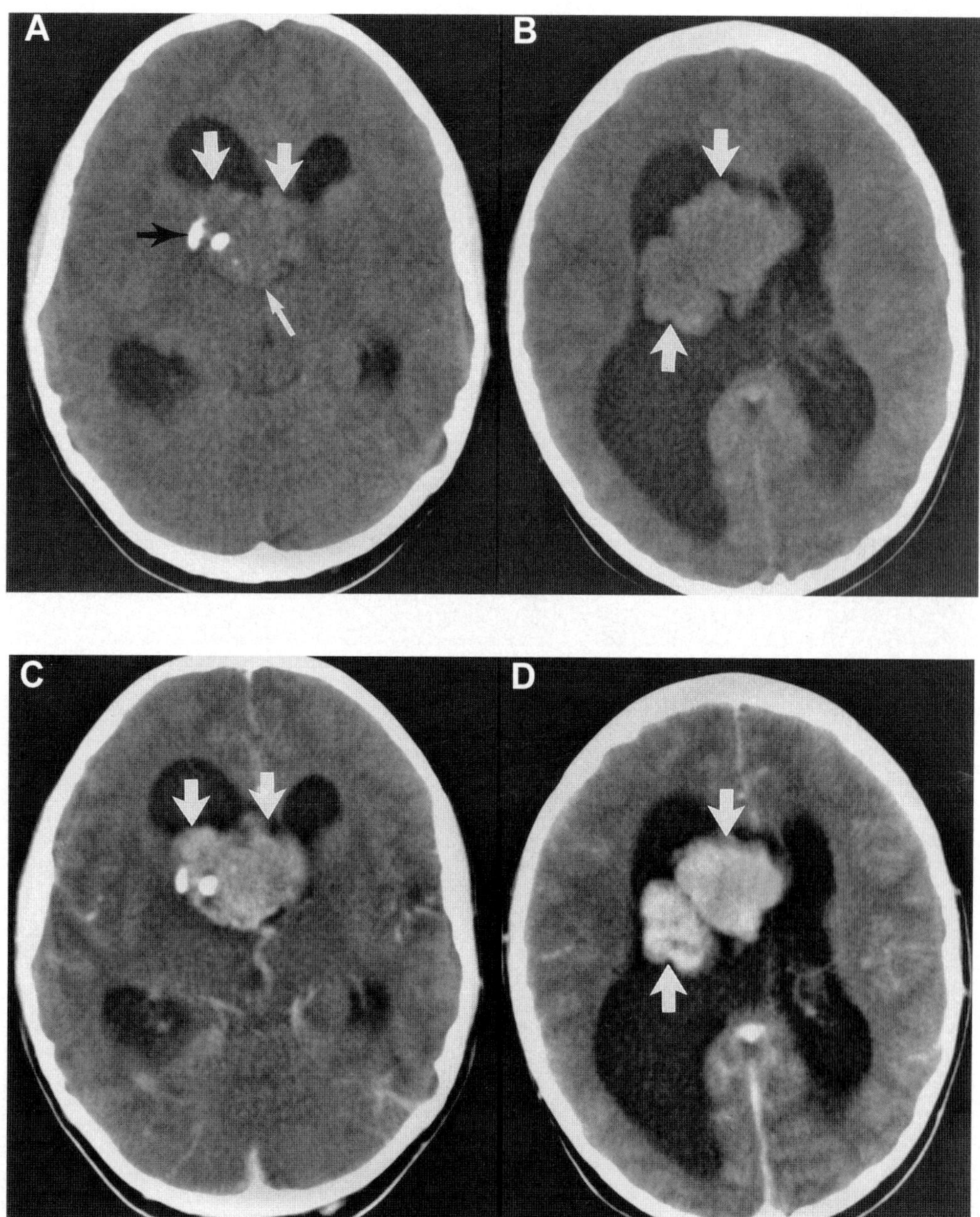

Figure 1–9. An 11-year-old boy with tuberous sclerosis and with intraventricular masses (subependymal giant cell astrocytoma). **(A,B)** Non-contrast CT of the brain. Dense mass with calcifications (black arrow in A) is shown occupying the frontal horns and body of lateral ventricles (arrows) extending down to the foramen of Monro region (small arrow in A). **(C,D)** Intravenous contrast CT of the brain. Enhancing features of the tumor (arrows) are revealed in post-contrast images.

Figure 1–8. Ependymoma of the fourth ventricle. Post-contrast sagittal **(A)** and axial **(B)** MRI views. Intraventricular enhancing mass (large arrows) with invasion of medulla (small arrows in A) is clearly depicted by MRI. The mass has produced a tonsillar herniation (arrowheads in A). The fourth ventricle (open arrow) is expanded by the mass.

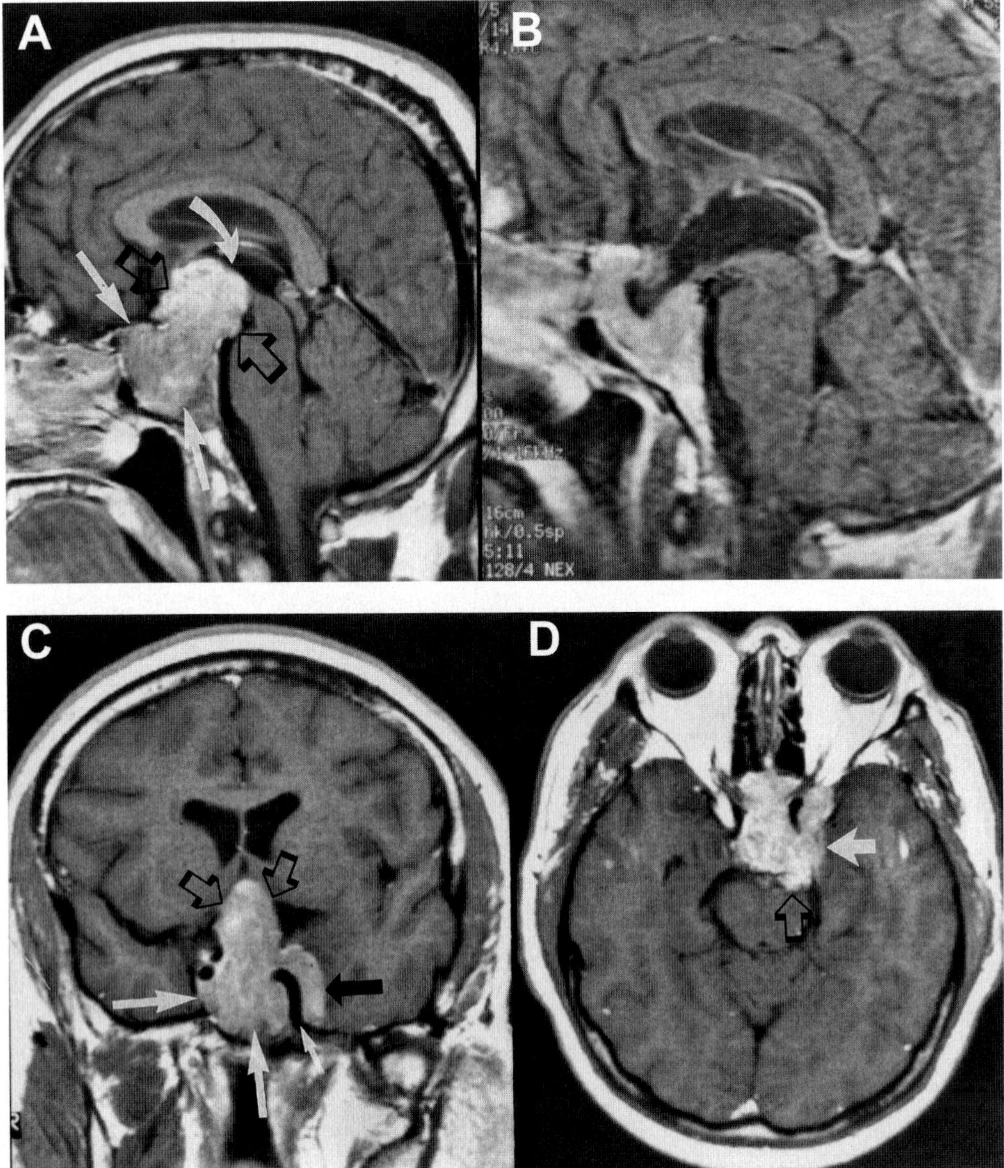

Figure 1–10. Pituitary adenoma (prolactinoma). Post-contrast sagittal MRI scans, pre-bromocriptine **(A)** and post-bromocriptine **(B)** therapy. There is a very large intrasellar mass (arrows) with a suprasellar extension (open arrows) compressing the optic chiasma and anterior third ventricle (curved arrow) as shown in A. A dramatic decrease in suprasellar and intrasellar tumor followed bromocriptine therapy (B). Post-contrast coronal MRI of the pituitary (before therapy; **C**) reveals the intrasellar mass (large white arrows) and the suprasellar extension (open arrows). The tumor extension to the cavernous sinus (black arrow) and the relationship of the tumor to the internal carotid artery (small arrow) are best demonstrated in this projection. Post-contrast axial MRI of the brain (before therapy; **D**) shows the parasellar (arrow) and posterior fossa (open arrow) extension of the tumor.

Craniopharyngiomas

Craniopharyngiomas originate from the epithelial remnants of Rathke's pouch at the junction of the infundibulum and the pituitary gland. They are the most common suprasellar tumors in young children. They can also occur in adults in the fifth decade of life. Characteristic imaging features of craniopharyngioma include suprasellar location, tumor containing solid and cystic components, and calcifications. Calcifications occur in 80% of childhood craniopharyngiomas. Solid portions of the tumor enhance with IV contrast medium.

Pineal Region Tumors

Pineal region tumors are uncommon neoplasms that account for less than 1% of all intracranial tumors. Tumors that occur in this location include germ cell tumors (germinoma, choriocarcinoma, teratoma) and pineal parenchymal tumors (pinealoblastoma, pinealocytoma).

Germinomas

Germinomas are the least differentiated germ cell tumor, occurring predominantly in men (boys and young adult men) and accounting for 50% of all pineal region tumors. Features of these tumors are calcifications and intense enhancement with IV contrast. Germinomas are readily diagnosed by CT or MRI examination (Fig. 1–11). The diagnosis of germinoma is important therapeutically because the tumor is extremely sensitive to radiation and can "melt away" with radiotherapy. Subependymal spread as well as leptomeningeal seeding may occur with germinomas.

Pinealoblastomas and Pinealocytomas

Pinealoblastomas and pinealocytomas are embryonal tumors that arise from neuroepithelial cells of the pineal gland. Pinealoblastoma is a highly aggressive, infiltrative tumor composed of poorly differentiating cells. They occur in children and have a poor prognosis due to subarachnoid metastatic tumor seeding. Pinealocytomas occur in adults. They are well defined, less infiltrative, and less cellular than pinealoblastomas.

Tumors of the Cranial Nerves

Vestibular Schwannomas

Vestibular schwannomas are also called *acoustic neurinoma* and are the most common cranial nerve sheath neoplasm. Vestibular schwannomas, the most commonly occurring cerebellopontine angle tumors, originate from the VIIIth cranial nerve. Sensorineural hearing loss and dizziness are the most common presenting complaints. Magnetic resonance imaging can differentiate acoustic nerve sheath tumors from other masses that may occur in this location, such as meningioma, arachnoid cysts, and epidermoid tumors. Tumors as small as 3 to 4 mm that arise within the internal auditory canal (intracanalicular tumors)

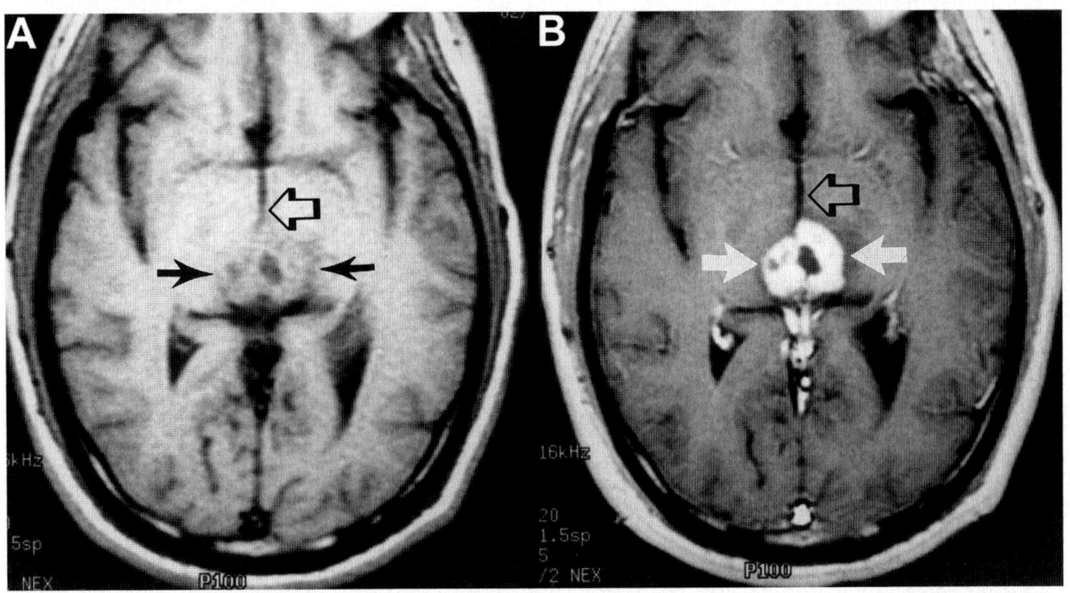

Figure 1–11. Pineal mass (germinoma). Pre-contrast **(A)** and post-contrast **(B)** MRI scans reveal enhancing posterior third ventricular and pineal region mass (arrows) produced by pathologically proven germinoma. Open arrows in A and B point to the anterior portion of the third ventricle.

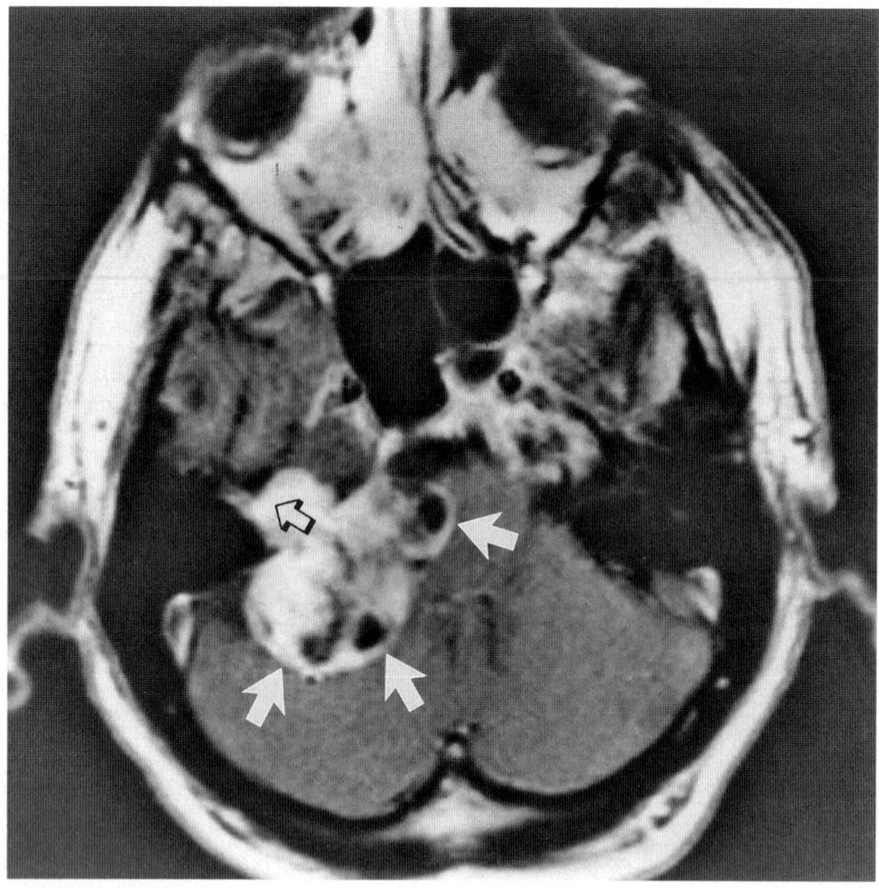

Figure 1–12. Vestibular schwannoma. Post-contrast axial MRI scan shows an enhancing right cerebellopontine angle, partially cystic, mass (arrows) with extension into internal auditory canal (open arrow) in a patient with hearing loss.

can be recognized by MRI due to their contrast-enhancing features (Fig. 1–12). Large acoustic nerve sheath tumors may give rise to symptoms related to brain stem compression.

Trigeminal Schwannoma

Trigeminal schwannomas are recognized by their location in the region of the trigeminal ganglion and its major branches. They occur in and around the region of petrous apex and in the parasellar region, presenting in a dumbbell-like fashion in both the posterior and middle fossae. Trigeminal nerve irritation by tumors can give rise to tic douloureux. Trigeminal neurinoma can be readily diagnosed by CT or MRI examinations by their enhancing features and their location along the path of the trigeminal nerve and its branches (Fig. 1–13).

Tumors of the Reticuloendothelial System

Primary lymphoma of the brain is rare, occurring in less than 1% of intracranial tumors and usually in individuals in the fifth and sixth decades of life. Primary CNS lymphomas occur in the basal ganglia, hypothalamus, corpus callosum, septum pellucidum, and paraventricular regions. Following injection of an IV contrast medium, the tumors show intense homogeneous enhancement on CT and MRI scans (Fig. 1–14). Cerebral lymphomas are radiosensitive tumors and can disappear after radiotherapy. In some

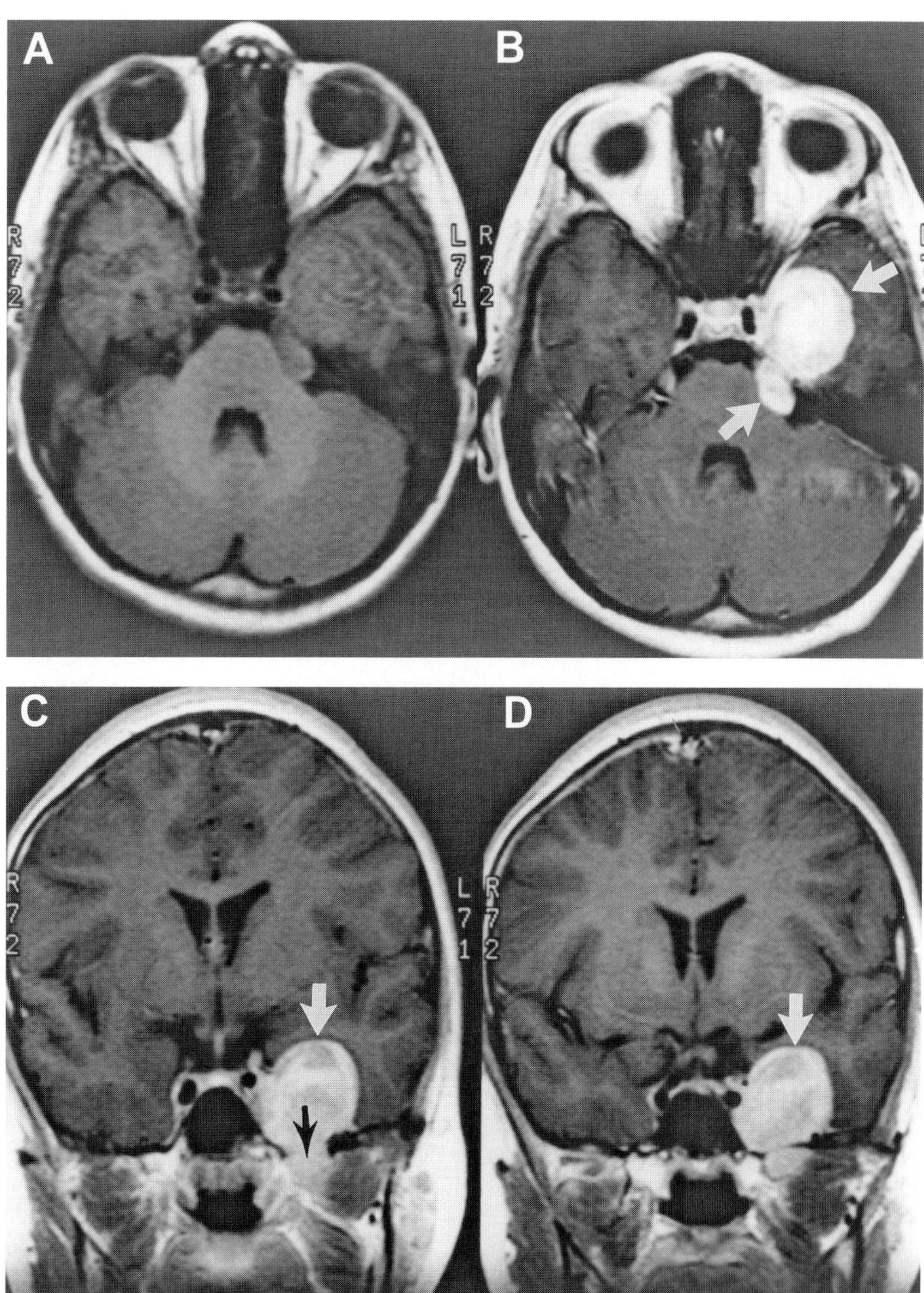

Figure 1–13. Trigeminal schwannoma. Pre-contrast axial **(A)**, post-contrast axial **(B)**, and coronal **(C,D)** MRI scans. A well-defined enhancing mass (arrows in B, C, and D) is seen along the course of the trigeminal nerve. A small portion of the tumor projects below the skull base enlarging the foramen ovale (black arrow in C).

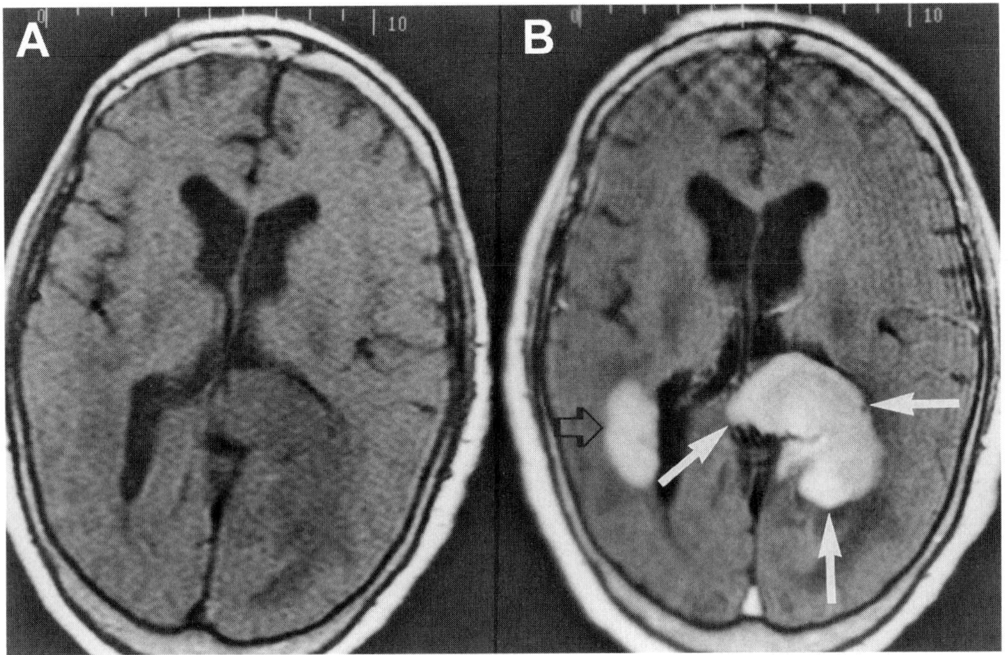

Figure 1–14. Primary lymphoma of the brain. Non-contrast **(A)** and post-contrast **(B)** MRI scans at the level of the lateral ventricles. An enhancing mass involving the splenium of the corpus callosum (arrows) and right paraventricular region (open arrow) is shown. The location of the mass and the homogeneous enhancement of tumor are commonly seen in lymphoma.

instances, glucocorticoids alone are sufficient to reverse the vascular permeability of the tumor and lyse tumor cells. Imaging features of metastatic lymphoma of the brain secondary to systemic lymphoma are similar to those of primary lymphoma, and calvarial and meningeal involvements are frequently observed.

Tumors of Developmental Origin

Lipoma, epidermoid tumors, dermoid tumors, and teratomas are tumors of developmental origin that may occur intracranially, collectively accounting for about 1% of all intracranial tumors.

Epidermoid Tumors

Epidermoid tumors result from the inclusion of ectodermal elements during closure of the neural tube between the third and fifth weeks of gestation. They commonly occur in the cerebellopontine angle cisterns, in the suprasellar region, and within the ventricles, pineal region, and spinal canal. Epidermoid tumors are nonenhancing on CT and MRI examination but may reveal slight signal increase on proton-weighted and T_2-weighted images (Fig. 1–15). Epidermoid tumors in the cerebellopontine angle region can cause irritation of the trigeminal nerve, and patients may present with tic douloureux.

Dermoid Tumors

Dermoid tumors are infrequently occurring lesions that result from inclusion of epithelial cells and skin appendages (e.g., hair follicles, sebaceous glands, and sweat glands) during closure of the neural tube. They occur within the midline and often contain calcifications and fatty tissue. These tumors can rupture, with spillage of fatty contents into the ventricular cavity and subarachnoid spaces (Fig. 1–16).

Teratomas

Teratomas contain elements of ectodermal, endodermal, and mesodermal germ cells. They are rare and occur in the pineal, anterior third ventricular, and sellar regions.

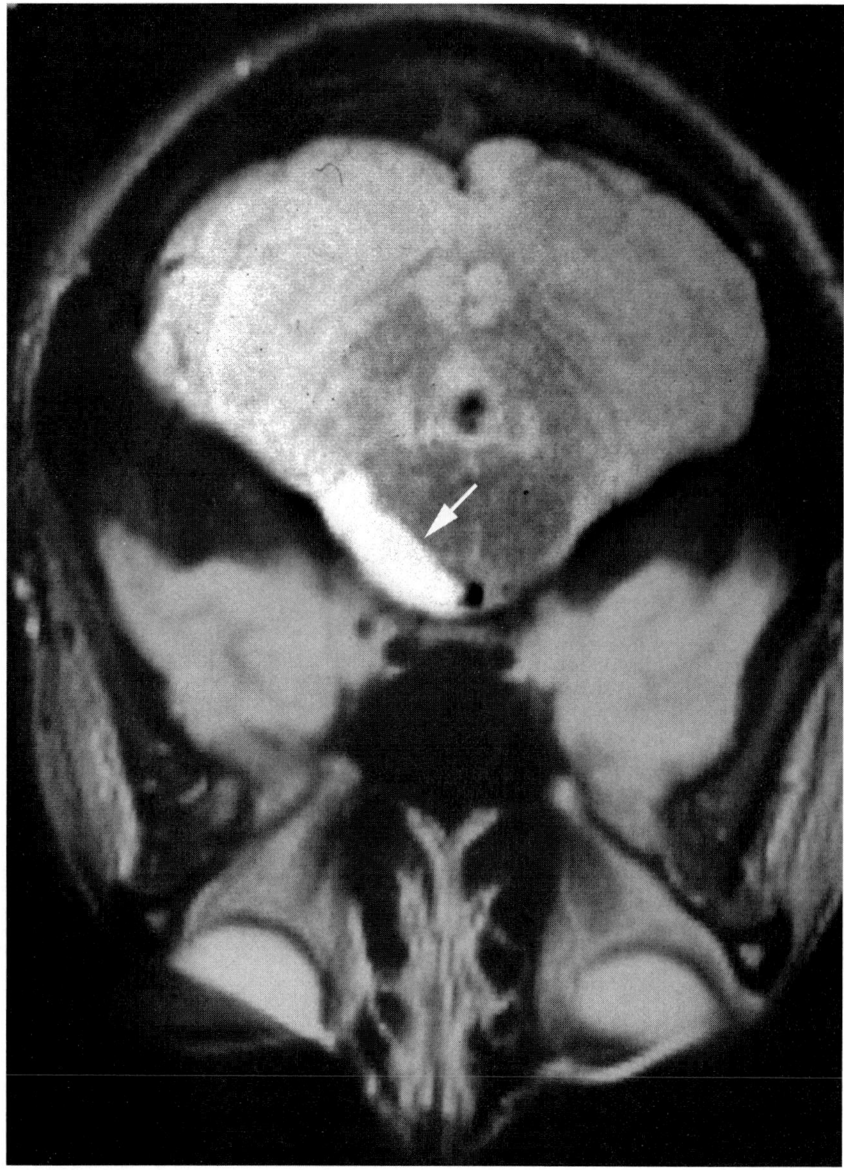

Figure 1–15. Epidermoid tumor. The tumor is in the left cerebellopontine angle region in a patient presenting with acute tic douloureux. Proton-weighted MRI scan reveals hyperintense mass (arrow).

Lipomas

Lipomas are fatty tissue tumors that are considered an incidental finding and are located in the quadrigeminal plate cistern (Fig. 1–17), suprasellar cistern, and cerebellopontine angle cisterns. The fatty tissue has a unique signal characteristic, as demonstrated by MRI examination, and thus can be easily distinguished from other tumors.

Tumors of Blood Vessel Origin

Hemangioblastomas

Hemangioblastomas contain proliferative blood vessels or hemangioblasts and occur in the third and fourth decades of life. They often have cystic and solid components with a mural nodule. Magnetic resonance imaging can clearly identify the cystic component of tumor and the solid mural nodule that are

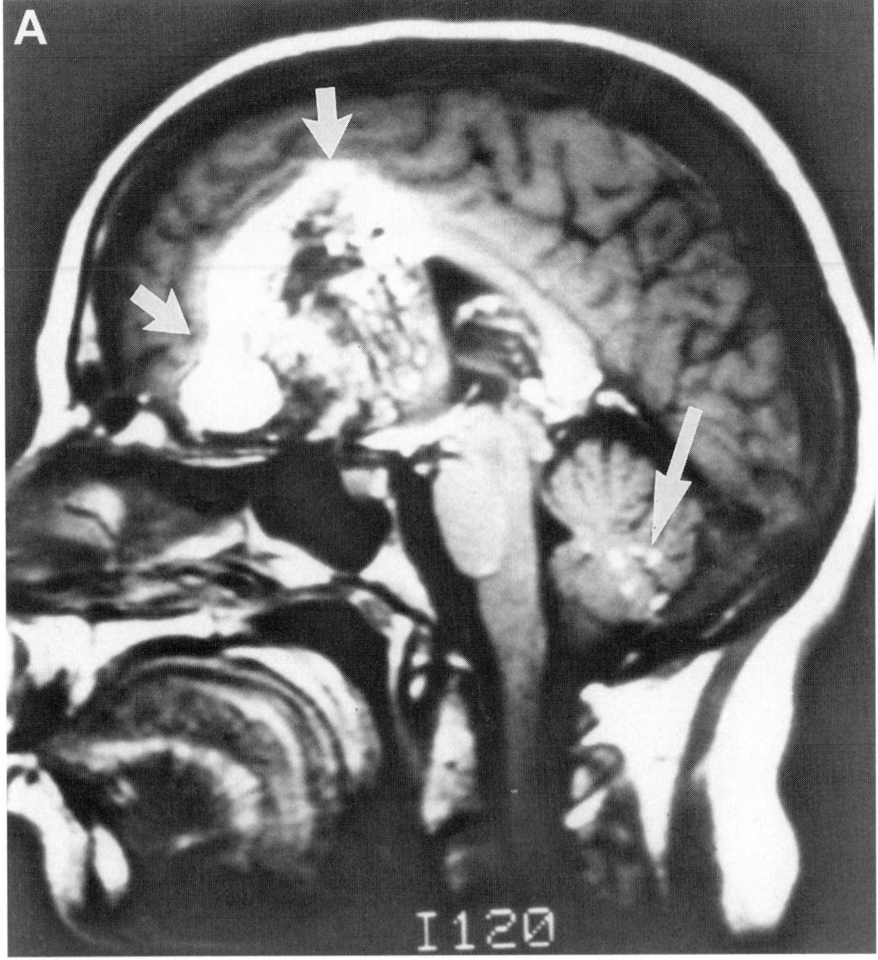

Figure 1–16. Dermoid cyst. Sagittal T_1-weighted images of the brain **(A,B)**. Huge frontal lobe dermoid cyst (arrows) with fatty tumor rupturing into the ventricular cavity with fat-CSF level (fat, small white arrow; CSF, black arrow in B) and into the subarachnoid space of the posterior fossa (large arrow in A). (*continued*)

enhanced strikingly with a contrast medium. Hemangioblastomas are highly vascular tumors, and a vascular nodule can be readily identified by angiography. Hemangioblastomas may be observed in younger patients with von Hippel-Lindau disease, a familial disorder that is composed of angiomatosis retinae and pancreatic cysts and that can result in renal cell carcinoma. Hemangioblastomas often occur as multiple lesions. Cerebral angiography may be required to confirm their diagnosis even if only a solitary lesion has been identified on CT or MRI examination.

Cavernous Angiomas

Cavernous angiomas can present as an intracranial mass and may mimic a neoplasm. These lesions often contain blood, and MRI signal characteristics are able to differentiate old blood from new areas of hemorrhage. These malformations also contain calcifications. Unlike primary gliomas and metastases, cavernous angiomas do not grow rapidly, and follow-up examinations may be useful in differentiating cavernous angiomas from neoplasms. They also do not

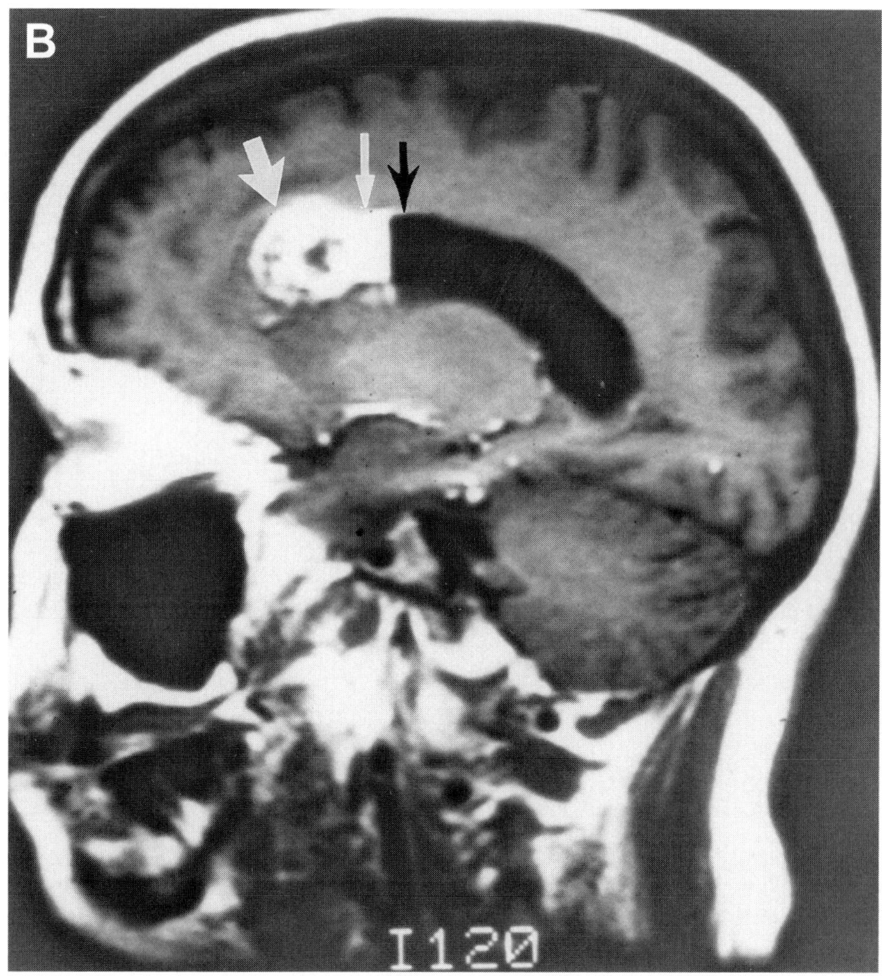

Figure 1–16. (*Continued*)

usually show contrast enhancement and frequently occur as multiple lesions.

Tumors of Mesodermal Origin

Meningiomas

Meningiomas account for 15% of all intracranial tumors and are the most common type of extra-axial benign neoplasm. They originate from the dura or arachnoid and occur in middle-aged adults. The tumors grow slowly and may be present for years before symptoms are evident. Meningiomas commonly occur in the parasaggital region; over the cortex, sphenoid wings, parasellar region, and cerebellopontine angle; and from the tentorium.

Meningiomas can be easily recognized on CT scans. In non-contrast CT, meningiomas appear dense, and in post-contrast images, intense enhancement is evident. The tumors also frequently contain calcification and induce reactive hyperostosis of adjacent bone, which is a characteristic feature of meningioma. Magnetic resonance imaging is also sensitive in detecting meningiomas (Fig. 1–18). The extra-axial nature of the meningioma can be easily depicted by MRI examination. Meningiomas are highly vascular and demonstrate homogeneous tumor blush on angiography. A meningeal reaction (meningeal tag) is often observed and may be secondary to tumor involvement or a reaction to the presence of the neoplasm.

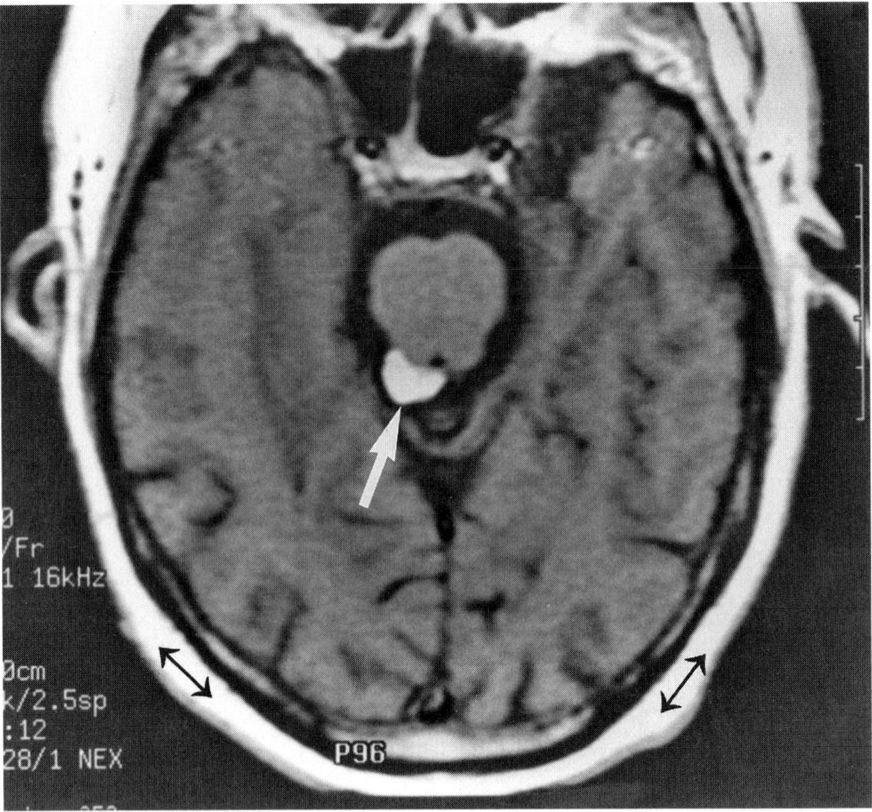

Figure 1–17. An incidental lipoma of the brain. Non-contrast axial MRI of the brain at the level of the midbrain. A bright signal intensity mass (arrow) is seen posterior to the midbrain within the quadrigeminal plate cistern, producing no mass effect. Note that the signal intensity of the mass is similar to that in subcutaneous fatty tissue of the calvarium (arrow) in this T_1-weighted pulse sequence. The mass also behaved like the signal intensity of fat in a T_2-weighted pulse sequence. The lesion did not enhance with contrast.

IMAGING OF SPINAL CORD TUMORS

Intramedullary Primary Tumors

Astrocytomas

Astrocytomas represent 40% of spinal cord neoplasms. Astrocytomas in the spinal cord are often less malignant than those that occur within the brain. Small cord astrocytomas occur most often in patients between 30 and 40 years of age. The usual clinical symptoms are spasticity, stiffness in the legs, sensory changes, and urinary incontinence.

Magnetic resonance imaging is extremely sensitive in the detection of primary spinal cord neoplasms. Combined sagittal and axial post-contrast images with gadopentetic acid clearly outline the intramedullary location of the tumor, which is enhanced following administration of an IV contrast medium (Fig. 1–19). Magnetic resonance imaging is also useful in differentiating the solid from the cystic components of this tumor. These neoplasms are often infiltrating with poorly defined margins. In addition, cystic components are common above, below, or within the neoplasm. Approximately 75% of the lesions occur at the thoracic and cervical levels. Lumbar lesions are uncommon.

Ependymomas

Ependymomas are slow-growing, benign neoplasms that arise from the ependymal cells in the central canal or in ependymal rests that are present in the filium terminale. Ependymomas represent 60% to 70% of spinal cord tumors. They typically occur between the third and sixth decades of life. They are fre-

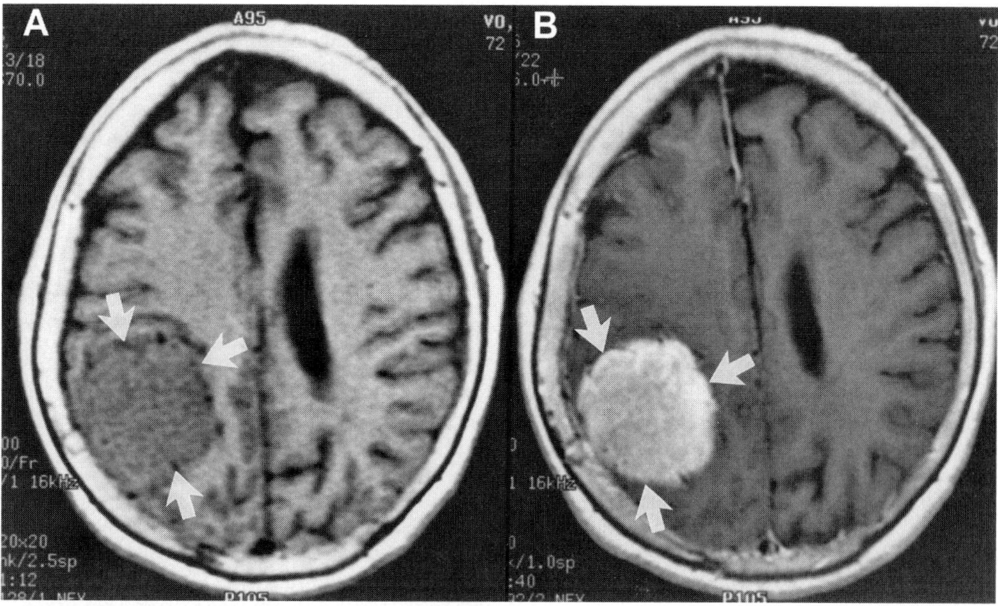

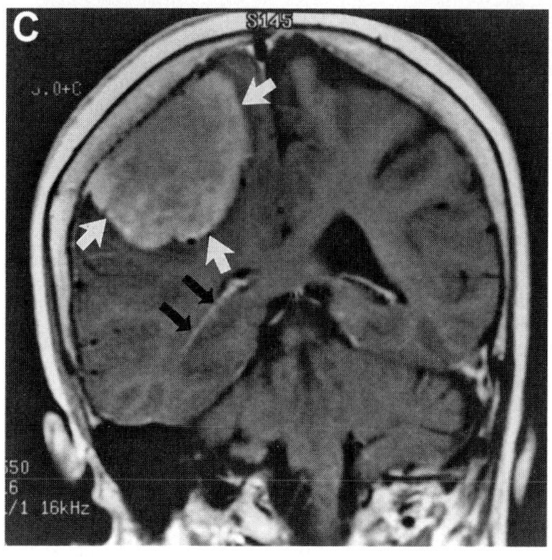

Figure 1–18. Meningioma. Pre-contrast axial MRI **(A)** demonstrates a large mass (arrows) occupying the right parietal high-convexity region. The tumor lights up like a bulb in post-contrast images (arrows in B), a characteristic feature of meningioma. Post-contrast coronal images **(C)** further reveal the extra-axial location of the mass (white arrows) with its broad base touching the inner table of the calvarium and compressing the adjacent lateral ventricle (black arrows).

quently well circumscribed, surgically resectable, and potentially curable. Ependymomas may occur anywhere in the spinal cord. Sixty percent commonly occur within the cauda equina or filium terminale. Contrast-enhanced MRI scans clearly outline these tumors (Fig. 1–20).

Hemangioblastomas

Hemangioblastoma, as described previously, is a benign tumor that originates from endothelial cells. The tumor, composed of a dense network of capillary and sinus channels, may present as a solitary lesion or as multiple tumors and is associated with von Hippel-Lindau disease in young patients. Patients with this disorder have angiomatosis retinae and pancreatic cysts and may develop renal cell carcinoma. Hemangioblastomas characteristically have a cystic component with a mural nodule. Magnetic resonance imaging is useful in identifying the cystic component of the tumor and the mural nodule, which intensely enhances with contrast.

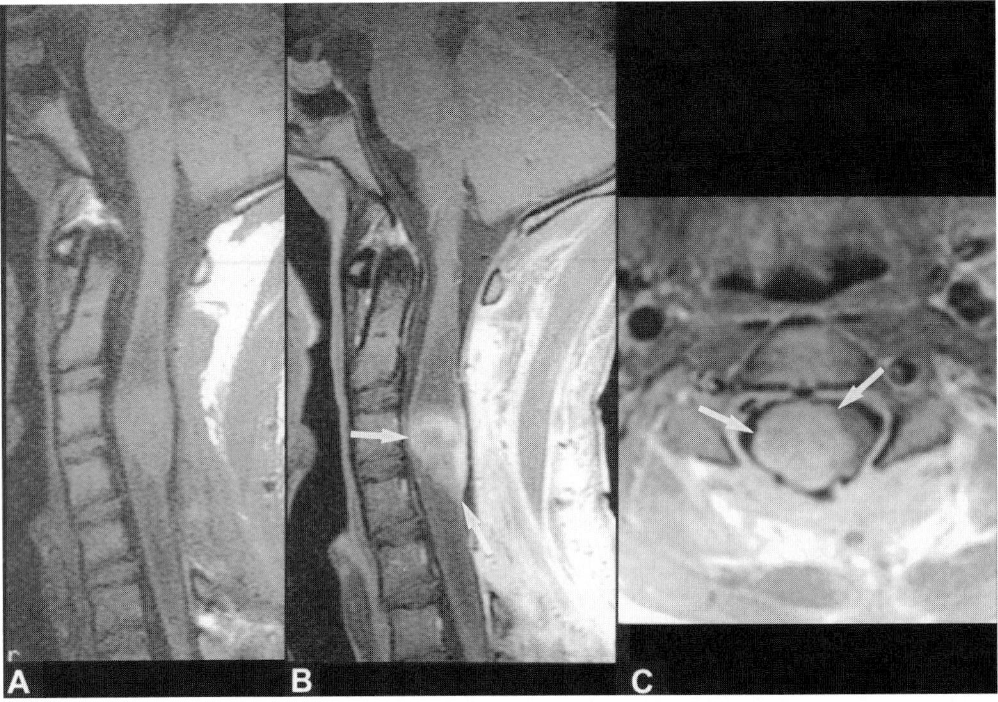

Figure 1–19. Astrocytoma of the cervical cord. Pre-contrast **(A)** and post-contrast **(B)** sagittal and axial **(C)** T_1-weighted images of the cervical cord show enhancing intramedullary tumor (arrows in B and C).

Intramedullary Spinal Cord Metastasis

Metastasis to the spinal cord is a rare occurrence, observed in 1% to 3% of patients with tumors. Common systemic tumors are lung and breast cancers. Melanoma and lymphoma can also metastasize to the spinal cord. Tumors metastasize to the spinal cord via the hematogenous route and by leptomeningeal tumor spread with penetration into the spinal cord. Leptomeningeal tumors are pathologically characterized by sheets of tumor cells coating the leptomeninges (Fig. 1–21). The clinical presentation includes backache, plexopathy, myelopathy, and cranial nerve defects. The most common primary CNS tumors are glioblastoma multiforme, ependymoma, and medulloblastoma. Dissemination is typically via the subarachnoid space and, less often, via the central canal.

Post-contrast MRI scans reveal solitary and multiple metastatic sites that are seen as enhancing nodules or linear bands reflecting pial involvement (Fig. 1–22). Leptomeningeal tumor infiltration is readily recognized in the entire subarachnoid space, although it is more common in the lumbar area. Infiltration is identified by the presence of enhancing tumor nodules, matting, and irregular nodular thickening of nerve roots.

Intradural Extramedullary Tumors

Meningiomas

Meningiomas occur most commonly in females and in adults, with a peak incidence at 45 years. They often occur in the thoracic spinal canal. On post-contrast MRI scans, meningiomas are clearly visualized as a homogeneously enhancing intradural mass that is usually situated dorsally. The extent of cord compression by these tumors can be readily evaluated through MRI scanning.

Schwannomas

Schwannomas (neurinomas) are benign nerve sheath tumors that usually originate from the sensory nerve roots. Neurinomas predominantly occur in males. Intraspinal neurinomas can protrude into the

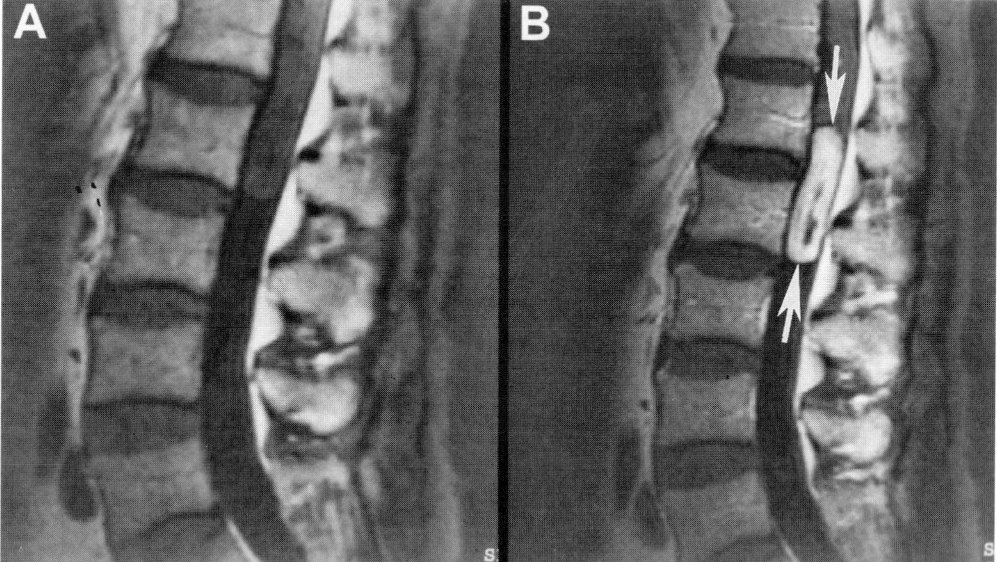

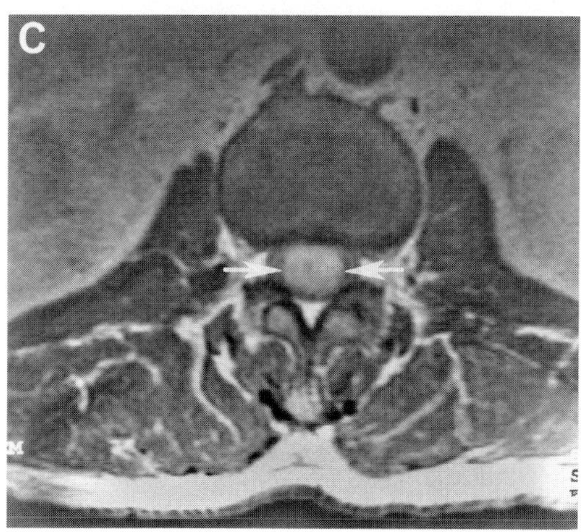

Figure 1–20. Ependymoma. Post-contrast sagittal **(A)** and axial **(B)** images of the lumbar spinal cord. An enhancing mass (arrows) is seen in the upper lumbar subarachnoid space. Axial images reveal the central location of the mass (arrows in B), favoring the diagnosis of ependymoma. The tumor is only faintly visible in the non-contrast image **(C)**.

paraspinal region through an enlarged neural foramen, and the tumors often take on a dumbbell-like shape. On post-contrast MRI, neurinomas appear as a well-defined, intradural enhancing mass.

Neurofibromatosis

Multiple cranial and spinal nerve neurofibromas are associated with neurofibromatosis type 1 (Fig. 1–23). Astrocytomas and ependymomas can also occur in neurofibromatosis. Neurofibroma can undergo malignant degeneration into neurofibrosarcoma.

Congenital Tumors

Teratomas, epidermoid tumors, and dermoid tumors are congenital tumors that arise within the spinal cord. Teratomas, although rare, may be readily diagnosed by MRI, which can distinguish various components of the tumor, fat, bone, and teeth. A fatty mass combined with solid and cystic components of tumor, particularly located in the sacro-coccygeal region, are classic characteristics of teratomas. These tumors may be seen at birth. Magnetic resonance imaging can distinguish various components of the tumor.

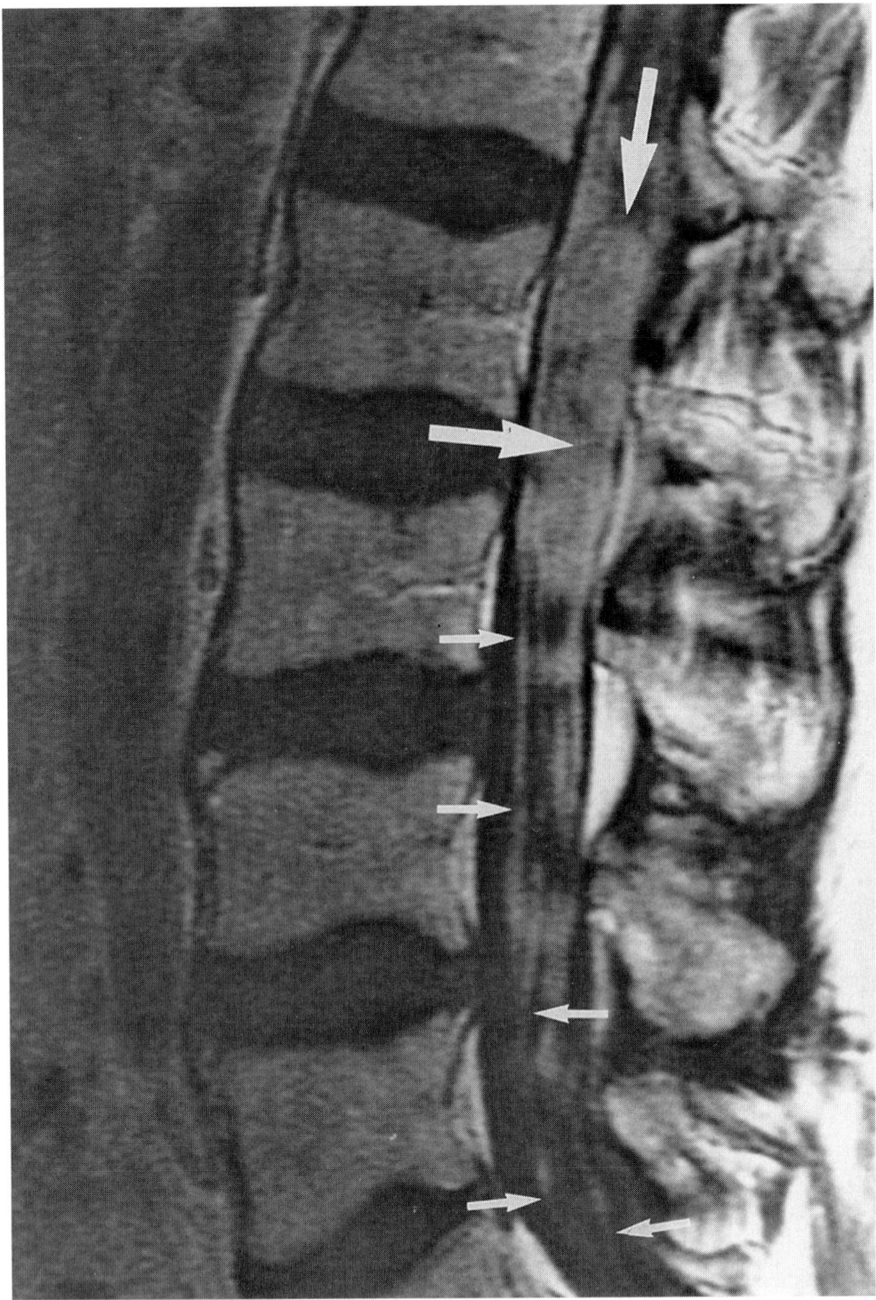

Figure 1–21. Melanoma with leptomeningeal metastatic tumor infiltration of the lumbar nerve roots. Post-contrast sagittal MRI scan shows that the lumbar subarachnoid space is filled with metastatic tumor (arrows). Lumbar nerve roots are markedly thickened with nodular enhancement (small arrows), indicating tumor infiltration.

IMAGING OF BRAIN METASTASES

Metastatic tumor growth, as in most neoplasms, depends on angiogenesis, which is the development of new blood vessels. Blood and Zetter (1990) found that secondary tumors will grow only 1 to 2 mm if no angiogenesis is present. When Frank et al. (1987) injected VX2 rabbit carcinoma cells into the internal carotid artery of rabbits, 93% developed metastases; ocular metastases appeared in 86% of animals, with

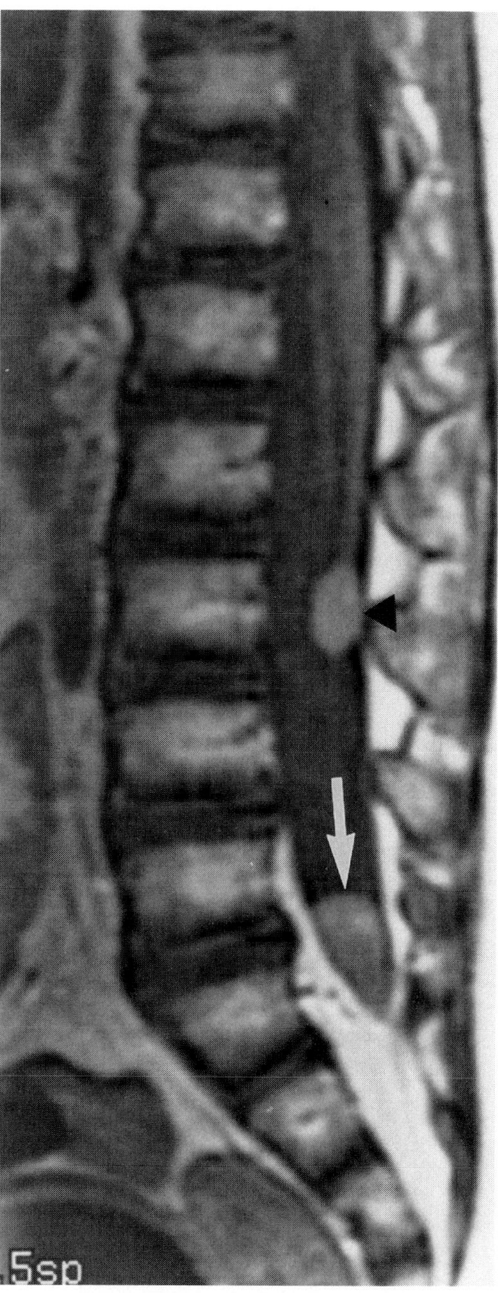

Figure 1–22. Medulloblastoma with dropped metastasis to the lumbar subarachnoid space. Post-contrast sagittal T_1-weighted images of the spine reveal dropped metastasis to the caudal end of the lumbar subarachnoid space (arrow) and at the L3 level (arrowhead).

anterior chamber involvement observed by the third day. These tumors were as large as 6 mm in diameter and demonstrated contrast enhancement after administration of IV gadopentetic acid, evidence that tumor endothelial cells were leakier than the blood–brain or blood–ocular barriers.

Either delaying the time between injection and scan or increasing the amount of contrast medium administered can enhance the appearance of a tumor on a CT scan. Davis et al. (1991) demonstrated that double doses delayed contrast infusion and that CT scans detected more lesions and provided additional information in 67% of cases examined.

Similar approaches in MRI have also yielded better detection of brain metastases. Yuh et al. (1992) examined 51 patients with MRI immediately after the administration of gadoteridol (Squibb, Princeton, NJ) in single and triple doses. No adverse effects were observed. In 10 of 27 cases examined with the triple-dose technique, improved lesion conspicuity and new lesion detection resulted in alterations to these patients' therapeutic regimens. Schorner et al. (1986) demonstrated the advantages of delaying imaging after IV contrast infusion during MRI by up to 68.5 minutes and found optimum imaging between 8.5 and 30 minutes after injection. Under these conditions, perifocal edema was minimally enhanced and was often visually less intense than normal brain, whereas necrosis was characterized by a slow, continuous increase in signal intensity, with maximum intensity reached toward the end of the examination but still continuing to rise. This effect probably reflects changes in variable tumor capillary permeability.

Sze et al. (1990) recommended that the MRI of the patient suspected of metastases should first include a pre-contrast axial short TR scan to determine if bone lesions or hemorrhage are present. Intravenous contrast should then be administered, followed by long TR scans and then by a short TR scan to demonstrate the presence of abnormal accumulations of contrast enhancement.

Elster and Chen (1992), in a study of patients with systemic cancer, demonstrated that nonenhancing white matter lesions have little chance of being a metastatic focus. Heier and Zimmerman (1992), in their comment on the Elster and Chen paper, are in general agreement with the caveat; however, they also concluded that white matter lesions without contrast enhancement that are localized, sharply defined, in proximity to subcortical U fibers, and have neurologic symptoms could be metastatic lesions.

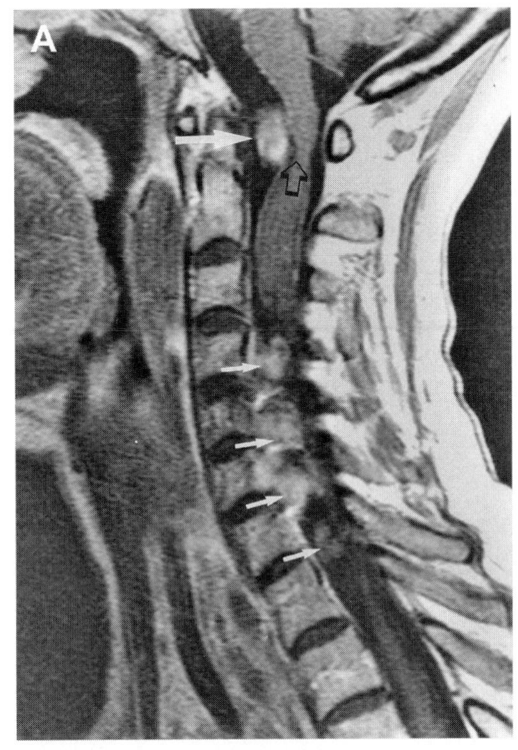

Figure 1–23. Plexiform neurofibromatosis involving the cervical and thoracic spinal canal in a patient with neurofibromatosis. **(A)** Post-contrast sagittal T_1-weighted image of the cervical spine reveals an intradural neurofibroma (large white arrows) at the C1–C2 level, causing cervical cord compression (open arrow). Multiple neurofibromas are also seen at the C4, C5, C6, and C7 levels (small white arrows). **(B)** Pre-contrast axial T_1-weighted image at the C1–C2 level reveals a bilateral dumbbell-shaped neurofibroma with intraspinal (large white arrows) and extraspinal (black arrows) components passing through and enlarging the neural foramen (arrowheads). Note that the spinal cord (open arrows) is being squeezed on either side by bilateral neurofibromas. **(C)** Post-contrast sagittal T_1-weighted image of the thoracic spine reveals neurofibromas originating from the nerve roots at levels T11 and T12 (arrows). (*continued*)

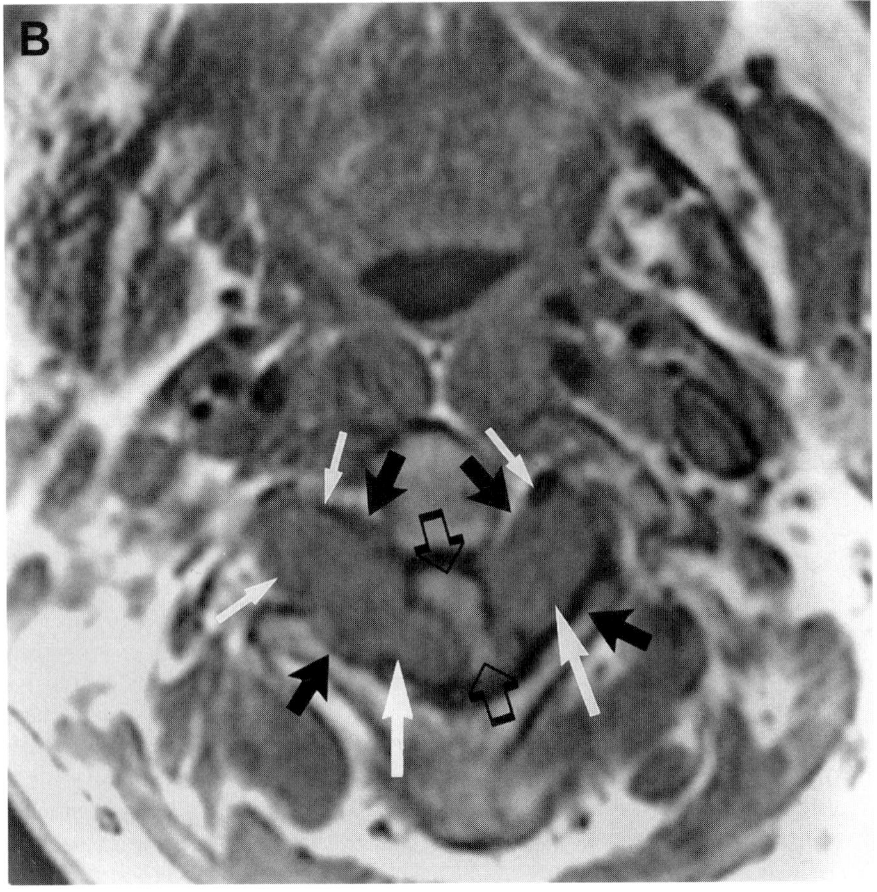

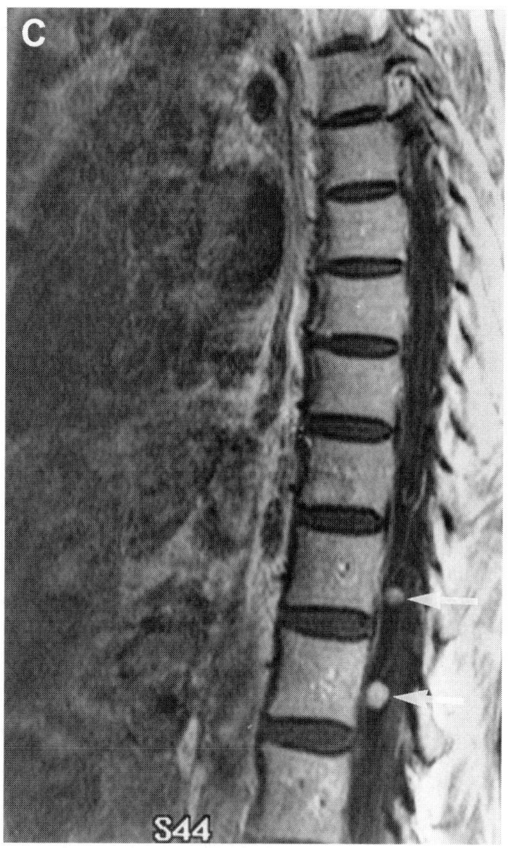

Figure 1–23. *(Continued)*

Presentation of Metastases

Tumors that metastasize to the brain have myriad appearances. They are often visualized as multiple metastatic foci of different sizes located on the meningeal surface in proximity to the subcortical U fibers or at the corticomedullary junction, with variable amounts of surrounding edema (Fig. 1–24). Lesions are solitary in as many as 50% of cases (Fig. 1–25). Intratumoral hemorrhage is observed, particularly in patients with melanoma (Fig. 1–26) and germ cell tumors (Fig. 1–27). In some instances, these hemorrhagic lesions must be distinguished from cavernous angiomas (Fig. 1–26). The edema pattern, according to Cowley (1983), migrates along short- and long-association bundles. The corpus callosum, although a major white matter tract, tends to be resistant because of a variation in makeup unless directly affected.

Leptomeningeal metastasis indicates involvement of the subarachnoid space. The outer border of the subarachnoid space is formed by the arachnoid mater. The inner border represents pia mater that is closely applied to the surface of the brain and the accompanying sulci. Leptomeningeal spread of metastases may occur in systemic neoplasms in either localized or diffuse patterns (Fig. 1–28). These lesions have to be distinguished from infections, stroke, and postoperative occurrences with meningeal enhancement following shunt procedures, multiple lumbar punctures, and the presence of postural hypotension. Infective lesions often appear identical to leptomeningeal metastasis, so a history may be helpful. Because cancer patients are often immunocompromised, however, infections as well as neoplastic spread may develop. In stroke patients, differential features include gyral prominence on T_2-weighted images and enhancement patterns with visualization of affected arteries in the region early in the disease course. In another group of patients, lesions principally affect the dura mater and are usually unchanging.

Solitary nonmetastatic lesions, including inflammatory lesions, granulomas, and glioblastoma multiforme, may appear similar to metastatic lesions (Fig. 1–4), whereas multiple lesions on occasion may not be metastatic but rather are inflammatory, granuloma multifocal, or multicentric glioblastomas (Fig. 1–3). The presence of multicentric glioblastoma multiforme indicates that the tumor arises from separate sites of origin, whereas multifocal glioblastoma multiforme indicates that a communication exists between the multiple lesions. Calvarial metastases may be visualized on pre- and post-contrast imaging studies (Fig. 1–29). Cerebral abscess, glioblastoma multiforme, or metastasis may present on CT or MRI as a ring lesion. A simple ring lesion will usually be a metastasis or an abscess, but a complex ring lesion is usually a glioblastoma multiforme (Figs. 1–2 and 1–3).

Triple-dose examinations may be indicated for patients with solitary lesions who have negative single-dose studies but a positive history (Fig. 1–30) to exclude the presence of more lesions or to confirm whether a questionable lesion is a tumor (Yuh et al., 1992).

METASTASIS TO THE SPINE AND EPIDURAL TUMORS

Disease that is metastatic to vertebral bodies is usually blood borne. In pelvic neoplasms, the transport of tumor cells via the lumbar spine is secondary to

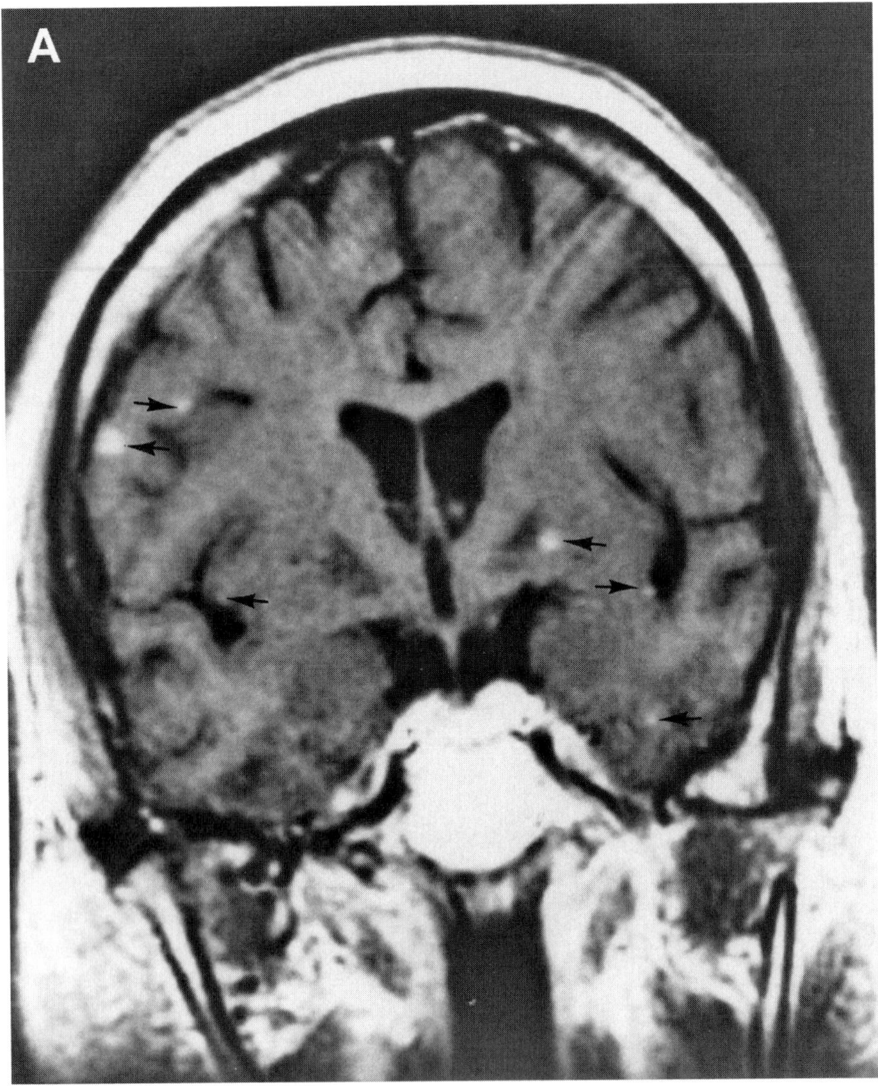

Figure 1–24. Multiple melanoma metastases. Post-contrast coronal T_1-weighted images **(A,B)** reveal multiple metastases of variable size (arrows). *(continued)*

transport via Batson's venous plexus. The spinal canal is involved secondarily, with epidural tumor producing spinal cord compression. Magnetic resonance imaging is very sensitive in detecting spinal vertebral body metastasis, including the presence of an epidural component and the degree of spinal cord compression. Primary tumors of the bone affecting the spinal canal are rare; however, tumors such as chordoma (Fig. 1–31) and aneurysmal bone cysts can produce expansile destructive changes in the bone, giving rise to epidural tumors with subsequent spinal cord compression. The entire spinal column can be easily studied without invasive procedures. Thus, MRI has proved to be the imaging modality of choice when dealing with patients who present with symptoms of acute spinal cord compression.

Carcinomas of the breast, lung, kidney, and prostate most commonly metastasize to the spine. Others include sarcomas, neuroblastomas, and melanomas. Most metastatic tumors are destructive (os-

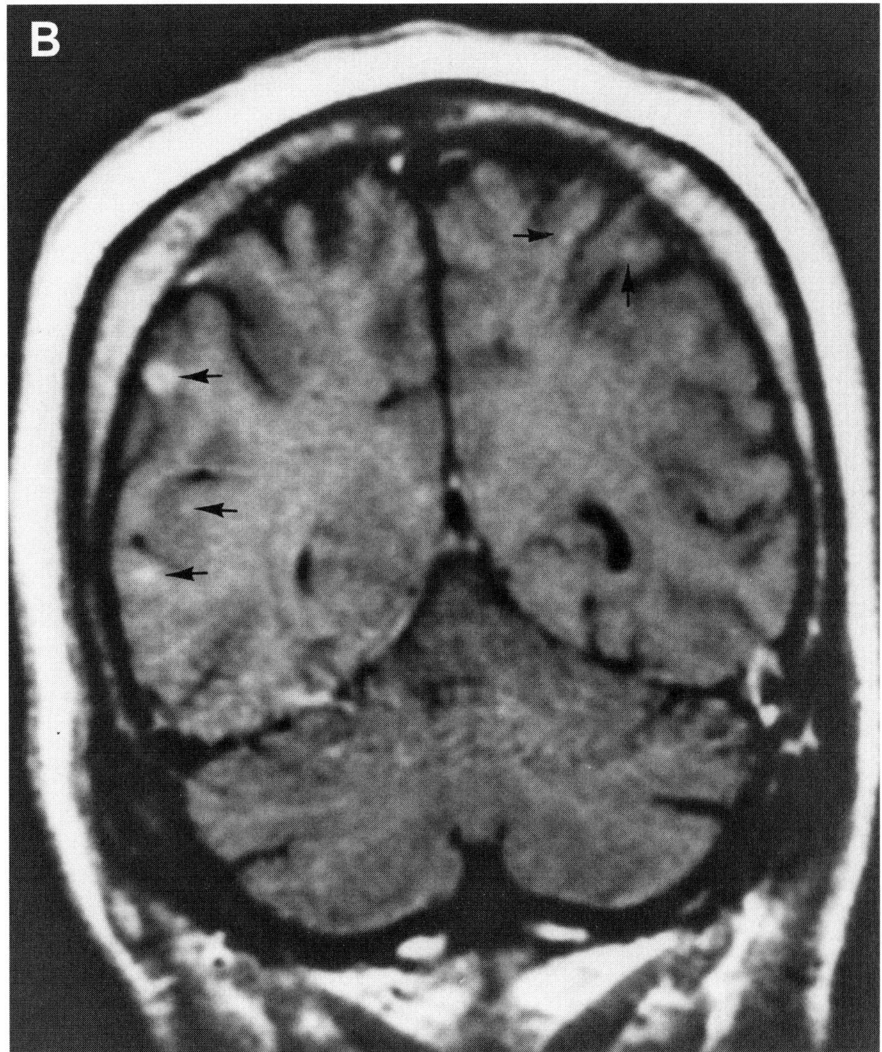

Figure 1–24. (*Continued*)

teolytic) in nature (Fig. 1–32). Common osteoblastic metastases are prostate and breast (Fig. 1–33). Because it demonstrates marrow replacement, MRI is more sensitive than ^{99m}Technetium bone scanning in detecting early bone marrow metastasis before destructive changes take place.

Lymphoma readily infiltrates the vertebral marrow cavity, and the replacement of marrow by tumor cells can be easily diagnosed using MRI scans. Lymphoma can also infiltrate the epidural space, spinal cord, and roots (Fig. 1–34). A characteristic feature of epidural lymphoma is the long extent of the tumor.

Multiple myeloma comprises approximately 34% of malignant bone tumors, with a peak incidence at 50 to 70 years of age. Malignant proliferation of plasma cells in the bone marrow of the spine results in tumor replacement of normal marrow. The involved vertebral body may show localized masses and pathologic fracture. The presence of epidural tumor and spinal cord compression may be best evaluated through MRI. Early identification of vertebral body involvement by myeloma may permit prevention of many neurologic sequelae by directing the early institution of radiotherapy or chemotherapy.

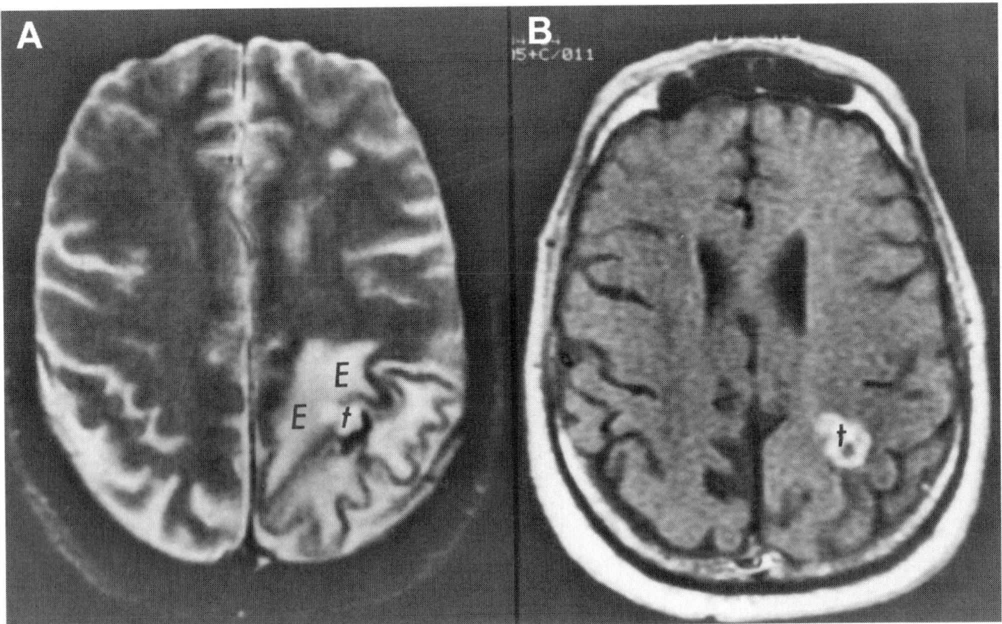

Figure 1–25. Solitary metastasis in a patient with non–small cell lung cancer. An axial T_2-weighted image **(A)** reveals multilobulated tumor *(t)* with surrounding edema *(E)*. The post-contrast axial T_1-weighted image **(B)** reveals a focal multilobular-enhancing lesion with a central low-intensity zone representing necrosis.

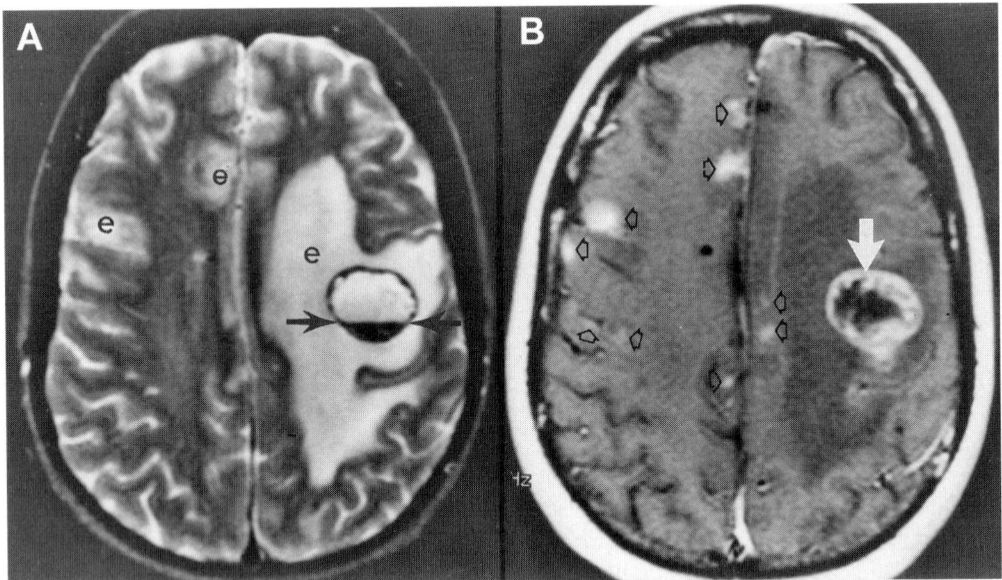

Figure 1–26. Multiple melanoma metastases with hemorrhage and leptomeningeal metastases. **(A)** Axial T_2-weighted image reveals multiple foci of edema of variable size (e) also with hemorrhagic metastasis and fluid level (black arrows). **(B)** Post-contrast axial T_1-weighted image at almost the same level with parenchymal metastases (white arrow) and leptomeningeal metastases (open arrows). **(C)** Axial T_2-weighted image at the ventricular level demonstrates multiple foci of edema (e) as well as a focus of heterogeneous signal intensity on the left with both hyperintensity and hypointensity in the region of the basal ganglia–paraventricular region (black arrowhead) and a paraventricular focus on the right (black arrowhead). **(D)** Post-contrast axial T_1-weighted image at the ventricular level reveals diffuse leptomeningeal disease involving arachnoid and pia mater (open arrows) and also arising from the ependyma of the lateral ventricles (closed arrows). *(continued)*

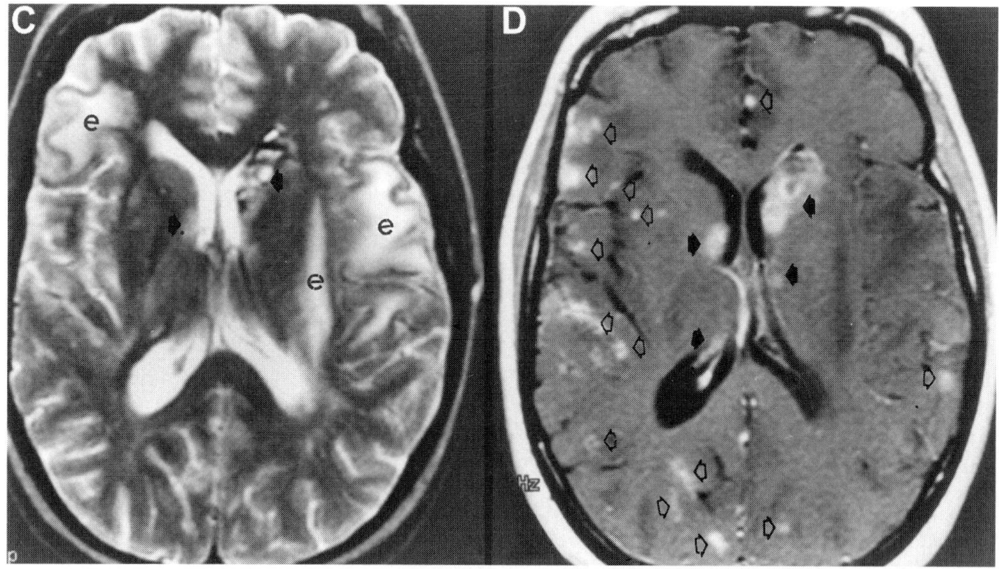

Figure 1–26. (*Continued*)

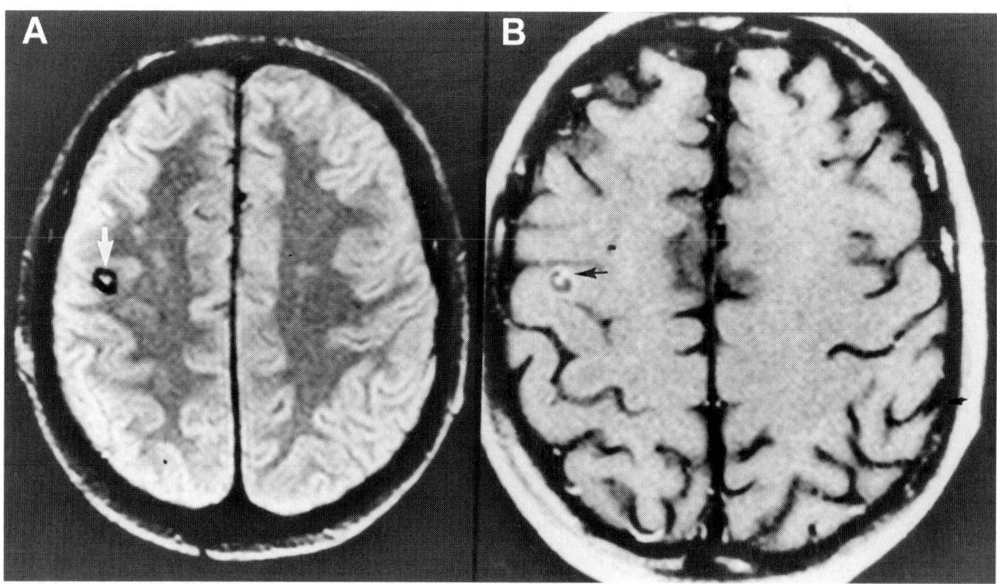

Figure 1–27. A patient with a metastatic germ cell tumor. Proton density-weighted image at the level of the centrum semiovale **(A)** reveals a target lesion with a hypointense black rim (arrow) and a central hyperintensity. This image raised the possibility of a cavernous angioma. **(B)** The post-contrast T_1-weighted image reveals contrast enhancement medially and superiorly (arrow). The hypointense margin is less distinct, although the central hypointensity is unchanged. The contrast enhancement favors the diagnosis of hemorrhagic metastases rather than cavernous angioma.

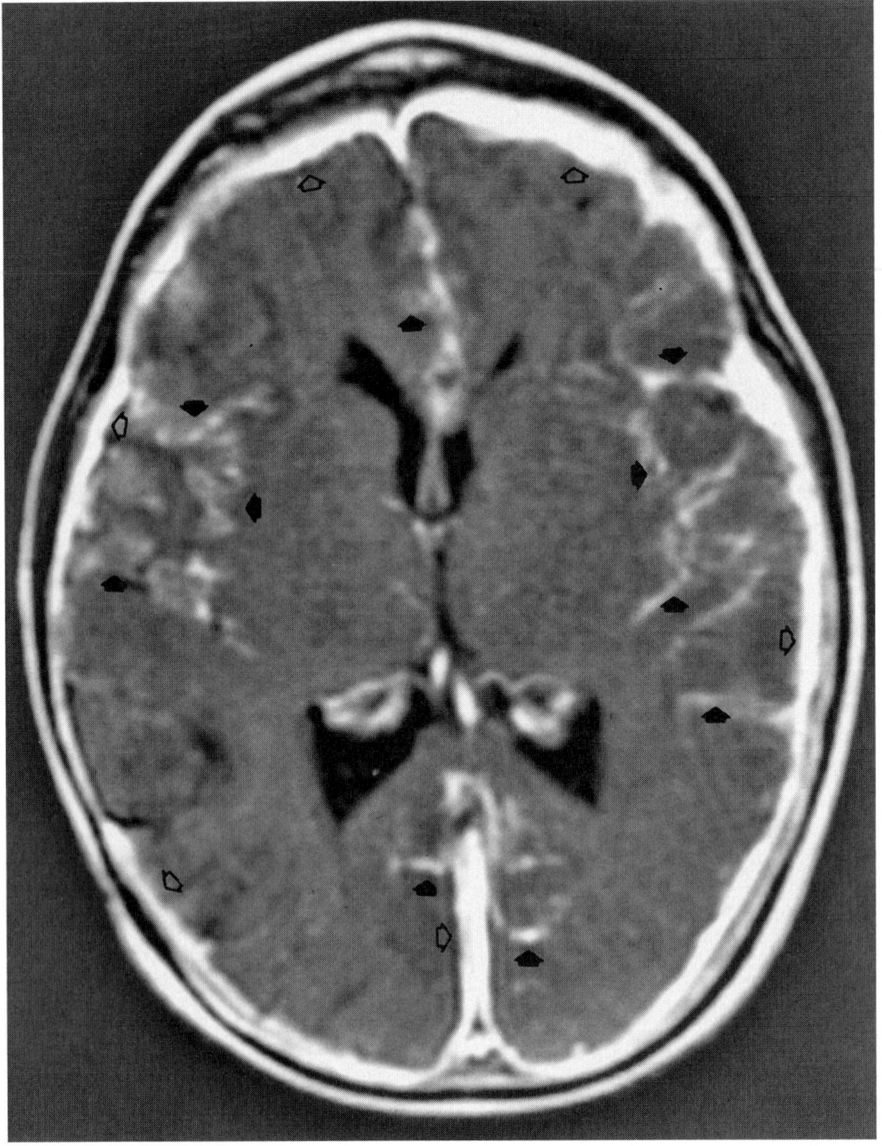

Figure 1–28. Child with medulloblastoma and leptomeningeal seeding. Post-contrast T_1-weighted image reveals diffuse, dural–arachnoid (open arrows) and pial enhancement (black arrows).

PLEXOPATHY

Patients with CNS malignant tumors can present with symptoms similar to those that occur with nerve root compression. The most common cause of neuralgia in these patients is the coexisting herniated disc in the cervical or lumbar region. Magnetic resonance imaging can clearly distinguish nerve root compression caused by a herniated disc (Fig. 1–35) from nerve root infiltration by malignant tumors (Fig. 1–21).

Magnetic resonance imaging is also sensitive in detecting lesions affecting nerve roots outside the spinal canal, such as brachial plexus (Fig. 1–36) and lumbosacral plexus. Lesions that can give rise to brachial plexus neuralgia are Pancoast tumors, metastatic lymphadenopathy, malignant spinal tumors, radiation fibrosis, and benign tumors such as nerve sheath tumors.

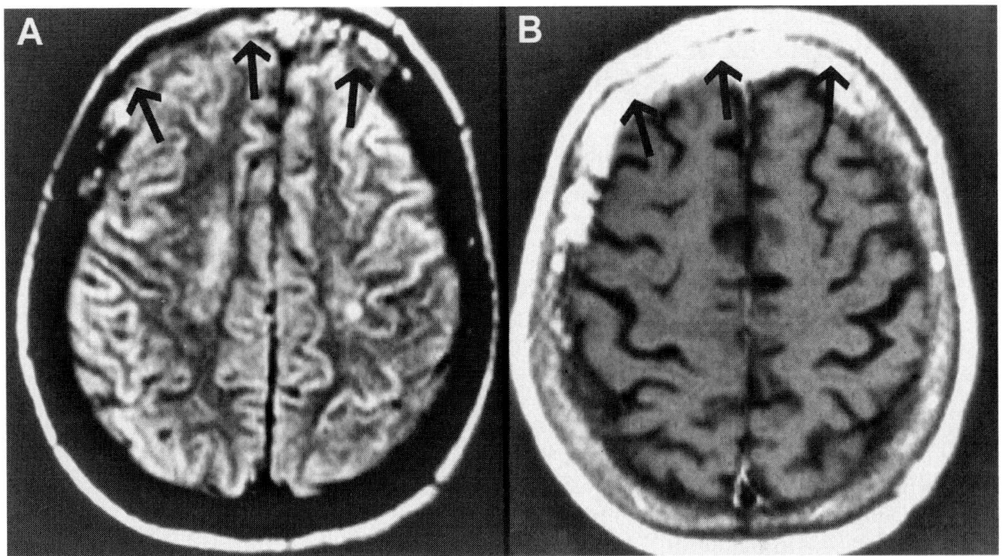

Figure 1–29. Calvarial metastases in a patient with breast cancer. **(A)** Axial proton density-weighted image shows extensive hyperintensity within frontal bone due to metastases (arrows), whereas uninvolved calvarium is hypointense (black). **(B)** The post-contrast axial T_1-weighted image shows contrast enhancement of the diffuse calvarial metastatic lesion (arrows) compared with the remainder of the calvarium, which shows heterogeneous hyperintensity reflecting marrow replacement by fat.

IMAGING OF RADIATION DAMAGE

Basis for Radiation Changes

Radiation damage to the CNS has been observed with increasing frequency because of treatment sequencing hyperfractionation, the use of radiation doses over 60 Gy, more older patients receiving radiation, adjunctive chemotherapy given during and after radiotherapy, and the increased duration of patient survival (Kyritsis et al., 1993; Fike et al., 1984; Ball et al., 1992; Burger and Boyko, 1991). Effects from radiation may be divided into early, early delayed, and delayed reactions (Hoffman et al., 1979; Fike et al., 1984; Ball et al., 1992; Burger and Boyko, 1991; Castel and Caille, 1989).

Early reactions are caused by acute or subacute effects that persist as long as 6 weeks after therapy. These reactions may follow conservative radiation treatment and leave no lingering effects, although in rare cases permanent sequelae or death may result. In early reactions a transient vasodilatation occurs with a breakdown of the BBB and development of vasogenic edema (Fike et al., 1984; Ball et al., 1992; Burger and Boyko, 1991; Castel and Caille, 1989).

In patients with early delayed injury, capillary vasodilatation, capillary permeability and breakdown of the BBB, vasogenic edema, and demyelination may develop, but may be transient (Hoffman et al., 1979; Ball et al., 1992; Burger and Boyko, 1991). The risk period is generally considered to be 4 to 18 weeks after the completion of irradiation (Hoffman et al., 1979).

A delayed reaction can occur months to more than a decade following treatment. In patients with delayed injury, severe changes occur, which tend to be permanent. Among these are vascular endothelial injury with infarction and white matter changes, including focal or diffuse demyelination or necrosis (Ball et al., 1992). The mechanisms that contribute to the resultant brain damage are incompletely understood, but likely include alterations of fibrinolytic enzymes, direct injury to white matter, direct damage to glial cells, immune mechanisms, and vascular-related effects.

Authors disagree about which pathologic changes occur first. Although one factor might be more important than another, it is most probable that a combination of changes occur simultaneously as a reactive cascade of events. Vascular changes are obviously important because they result in ischemia, infarction,

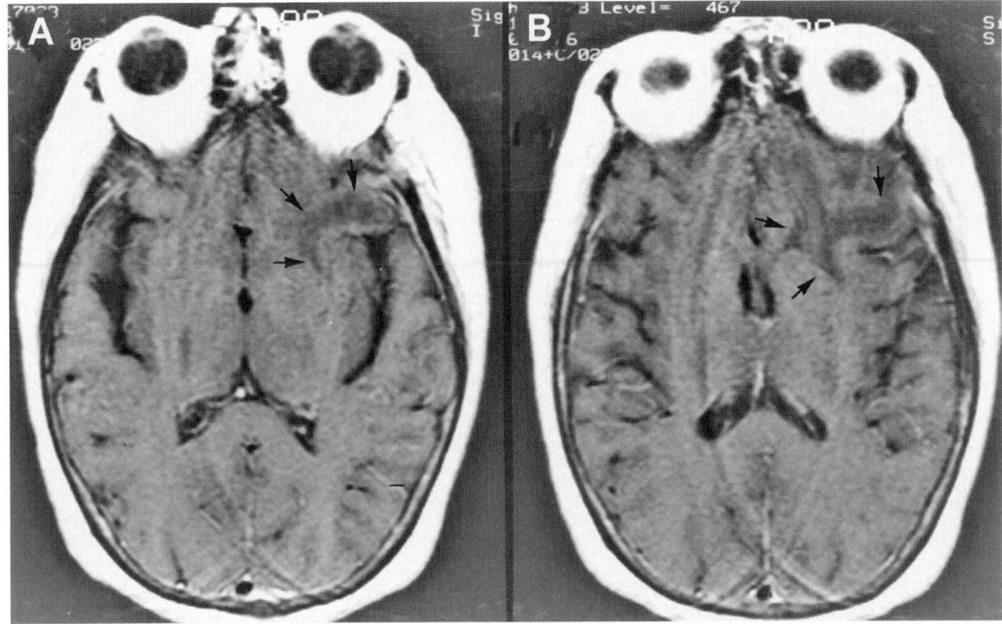

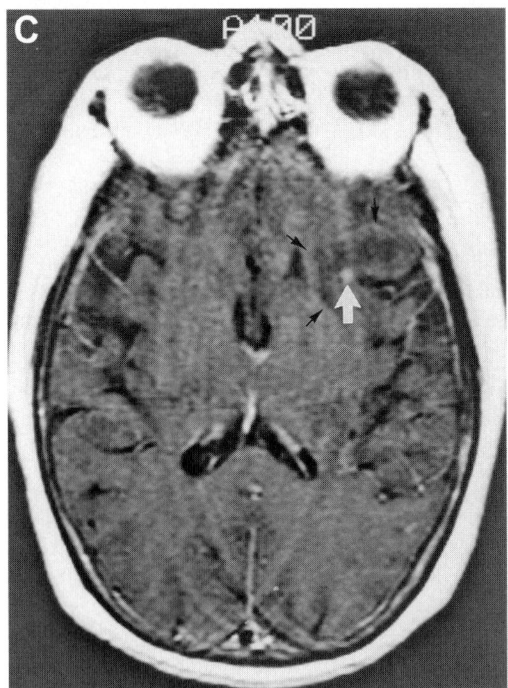

Figure 1–30. Triple-dose contrast agent demonstrates a metastatic focus. **(A,B)** Axial T_1-weighted images after a single dose of contrast material reveals, on two slices 6.5 mm apart, no evidence of enhancing lesion, although an edematous focus is present (arrows). **(C)** T_1-weighted image after a triple dose of contrast material at the same level as in B now demonstrates a single metastatic focus (white arrow). Black arrows point to edema surrounding the tiny metastatic focus.

and edema. Positron emission tomography (PET) studies demonstrate significant effects on metabolic activity (Doyle et al., 1987; Valk and Dillon, 1991). Oligodendrocytes, which have a large composition of myelin, are damaged early (Fike et al., 1984). Myelin is hydrophobic, and its loss is associated with increased extracellular fluid (Fike et al., 1984). Direct injury to cerebral tissue causes structural changes that result in decreased brain volume (Ball et al., 1992).

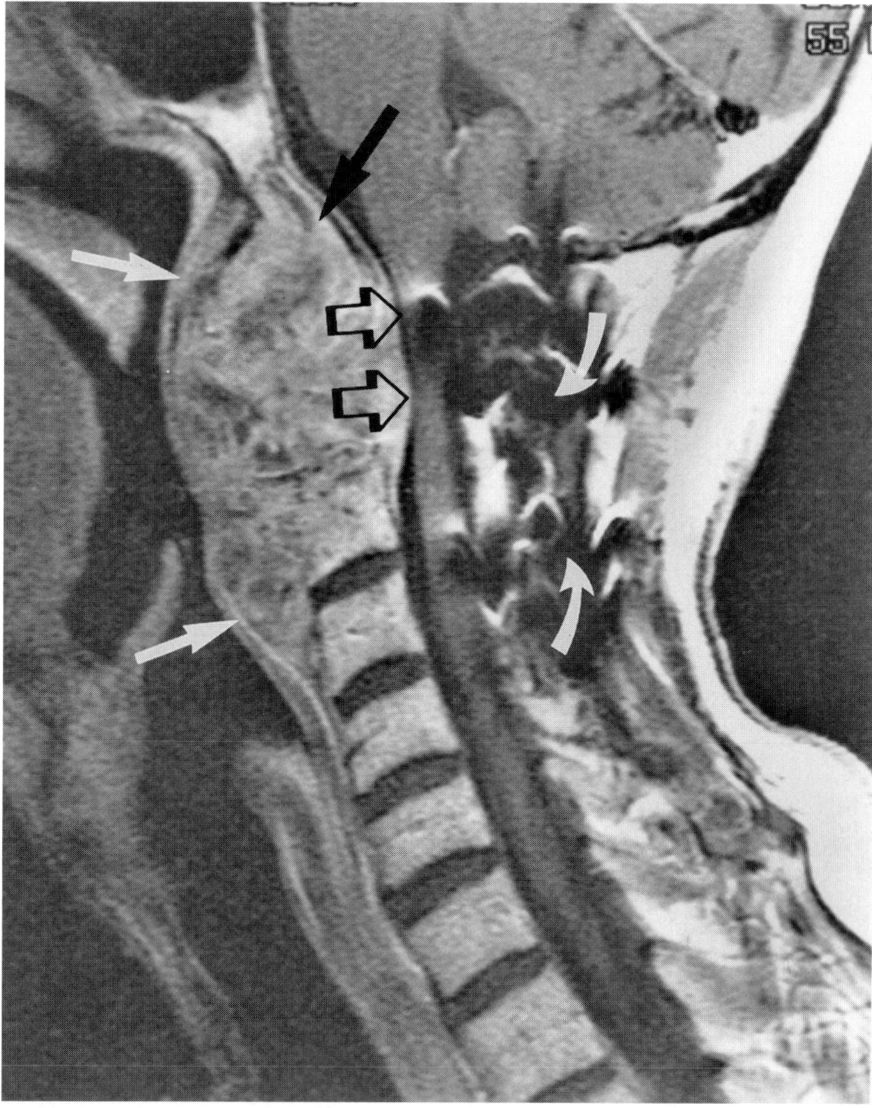

Figure 1–31. Chordoma involving the clivus (black arrow), C1, and C2 vertebral bodies. The chordoma is associated with a large epidural tumor (black arrow), producing cervical cord compression (open arrows). There is also a prevertebral soft tissue tumor (white arrows). Curved white arrows point to artifacts created by surgical clips.

Radiation-Induced Damage to the Brain

Magnetic resonance imaging is far more sensitive than CT in detecting radiation-induced damage to the brain. The severe form of radiation-induced damage to the brain is radiation necrosis, the end result of perivascular coagulative necrosis affecting the white matter. As would be expected, radiation necrosis occurs most commonly at the site of maximum radiation delivery in the immediate vicinity of the tumor site and surrounding the surgical cavity of a partially or totally resected tumor (Fig. 1–37). Radiation necrosis can resemble recurrent tumor on MR or CT imaging because of the following shared characteristics: *(1)* origin at or close to the original tumor site, *(2)* contrast enhancement, *(3)* growth over time, *(4)* edema, and *(5)* exertion of mass effect.

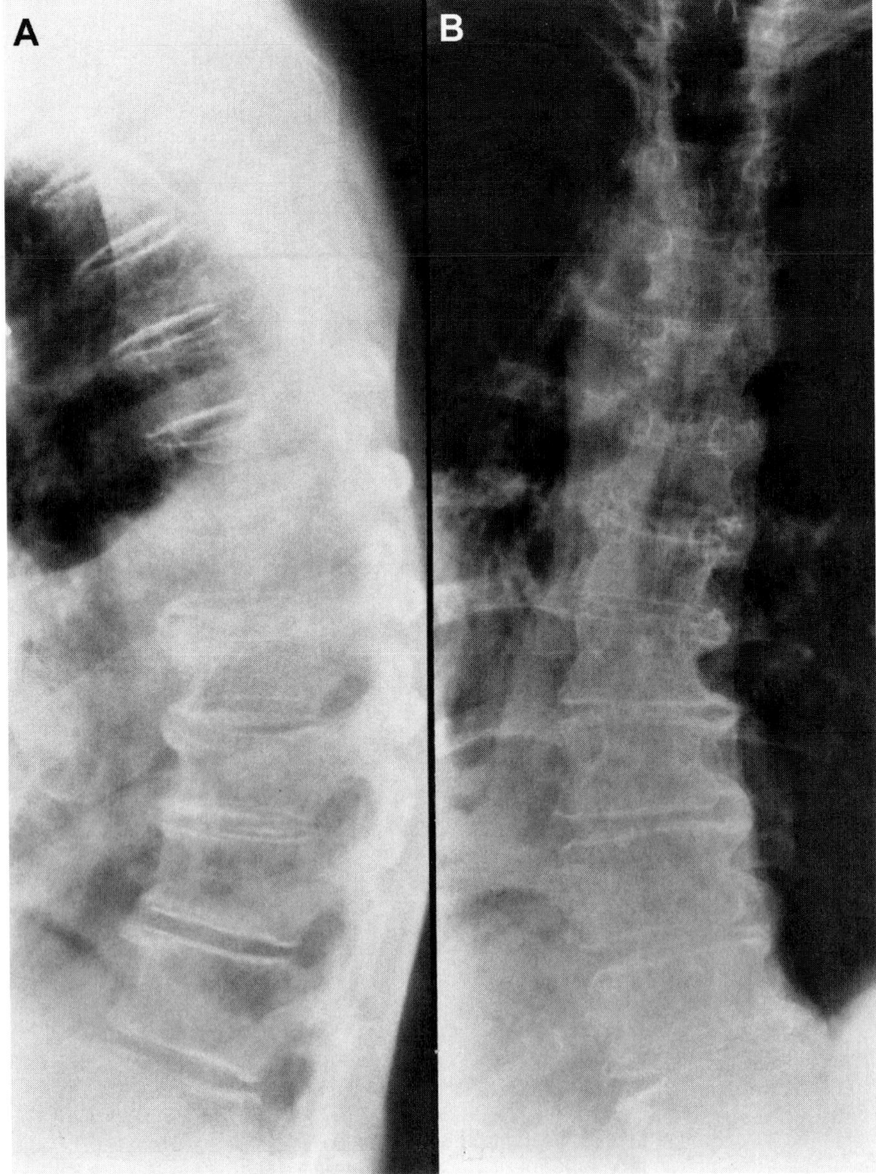

Figure 1–32. Patient with carcinoma of the breast with a history of back pain and osteolytic metastases. **(A,B)** Plain roentgenograms of the thoracic spine in the lateral and anterior posterior projections were normal. A bone scan was also normal. **(C)** Sagittal multiplanar-gradient echo T_2-weighted image reveals multiple hyperintense foci (arrows) indicating osteolytic metastases. **(D,E)** Sagittal T_1-weighted images of thoracic and lumbar spine reveal multiple hypointense foci (arrows) affecting almost all of the visualized vertebral bodies. (*continued*)

With respect to the MRI characteristics of radiation necrosis, most lesions consist of an enhancing mass (Figs. 1–37 to 1–42) with a central area of necrosis. The lesions are single or multiple. The enhancing characteristics of radiation necrosis commonly seen are a ring lesion with a central "soap bubble"–like interior (Fig. 1–38E), solid lesions (Fig. 1–40), or a "Swiss cheese"–like interior (Fig. 1–41A,B). Contrast enhancement of these lesions is secondary to radiation-induced endothelial damage,

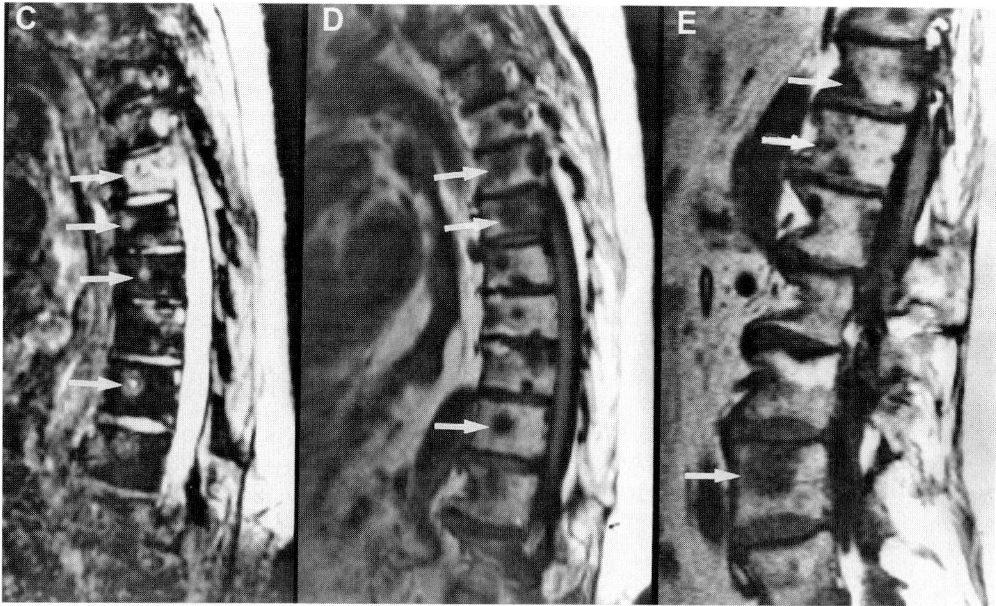

Figure 1–32. (*Continued*)

which leads to the breakdown of the BBB. The use of platinum-based chemotherapy drugs such as cisplatin and carboplatin combined with radiation therapy (RT) may contribute to the development of radiation-induced necrosis (Kumar et al., 2000).

In addition to the most common form of radiation necrosis, which consists of a single lesion arising at the site of the original primary tumor (Fig. 1–37), other less common patterns may be observed, such as *(1)* multiple lesions (Fig. 1–41); *(2)* lesions occurring within the ipsilateral hemisphere distant from the site of primary tumor (Fig. 1–38A–E); *(3)* lesions in the contralateral hemisphere (Fig. 1–39); and *(4)* lesions arising remotely from a primary site, for example in the cerebellum (Fig. 1–40), brain stem (Fig. 1–37), and subependymal lesions. Periventricular white matter is especially vulnerable to radiation necrosis. This neuroanatomic region has a relatively poor blood supply from long medullary arteries that lack collateral vessels, creating a susceptibility to ischemic effects produced by postradiation vasculopathy (Moody et al., 1990; Nelson et al., 1991). The corpus callosum is also vulnerable to radiation necrosis.

The incidence of radiation necrosis after conventional therapy ranges from 5% to 24%, with higher rates at autopsy (Burger et al., 1979; Marks et al., 1981). Kumar et al. (2000) have reported results from a cohort of 148 adult patients who underwent surgical resection of malignant brain (glial) tumors. The patients were subsequently entered into a research protocol that consisted of accelerated RT with carboplatin followed by chemotherapy (procarbazine, lomustine, vincristine). Pure radiation necrosis developed in 20 patients (13.5%). Sixteen patients (10.8%) manifested a mixture predominantly of radiation necrosis with limited recurrent and/or residual tumor (less than 20% of resected tissue). These findings were demonstrated by histopathologic examination at surgery or autopsy in 22 of the 56 patients with anaplastic gliomas (VA Levin, unpublished information, 2001) and in 14 of the 92 patients with glioblastomas under protocols DM 88–133 (Levin et al., 1995). The necrosis of the brain was attributed to the combined effects of RT and chemotherapy.

Radiation-induced necrosis is a dynamic pathophysiologic process with several possible clinical outcomes. Although continued necrotic growth with attendant cytologic edema and mass effect is commonly seen, lethal progression is not inevitable. Some lesions will stabilize, whereas others will regress (Fig. 1–42). In some cases, surgery may be required to reduce mass effect and, despite advances in special imaging techniques, to establish an accurate histologic diagnosis. Finally, even after gross total surgical resection, radiation necrosis recurrence will be observed in some cases. The MRI spectrum of RT-induced injury to the brain includes, in addition to necrosis, radiation-induced vasculopathy, white matter demyelination (Fig. 1–43), radiation-induced cranial neuropathy, mineralizing microangiopathy (Fig. 1–44), and radiation-induced neoplasms. The role of single-photon emission tomography and PET in distinguishing recurrent brain tumor from radiation necrosis is discussed in more detail in Chapter 2.

ADVANCED MAGNETIC RESONANCE IMAGING TECHNIQUES IN NEUROIMAGING

From the mid-1980s through the mid-1990s, proton density-weighted (PDW), T_1-weighted (T1W) with and without contrast agent enhancement, and T_2-weighted (T2W) acquisitions provided the standard set of MR images with which intracranial lesions were evaluated. In the mid-1990s, fluid attenuated inversion recovery (FLAIR) and magnetization transfer contrast sequences were added to, or used in place of, one or more of the standard set of PDW, T1W, and T2W images.

The FLAIR images have significantly improved visualization of neoplasm versus edema, cortical strokes, and periventricular multiple sclerosis plaques, for example, where magnetization transfer contrast images have been reported to improve the conspicuity of small metastases. These two additional sequences are not, however, radical departures from the standard imaging sequences used since the mid-1980s. Instead, they have essentially been made robust and rapid enough for routine clinical applications.

In the late 1990s significant improvements were made in the magnetic gradient field subsystems of commercial scanners. The maximum gradient field amplitudes (Tesla/meter, T/m) increased by a factor of 2 to 4, and the time required to switch the gradient fields on and off (the rise time, in seconds) decreased by nearly equal factors. This results in gradient field slew rates (T/m/sec) that increased by factors of 4 to 16. Coupled with improvements in the data acquisition sampling rates, these gradient subsystem changes resulted in scan times as rapid as 30 to 50 msec/image. Such acquisition rates have opened up entirely new neuroimaging options that result in images that depict not only anatomy but function. This section discusses some of these new options in neuroimaging, each of which depends on high-speed image acquisition techniques. In addition, advances in

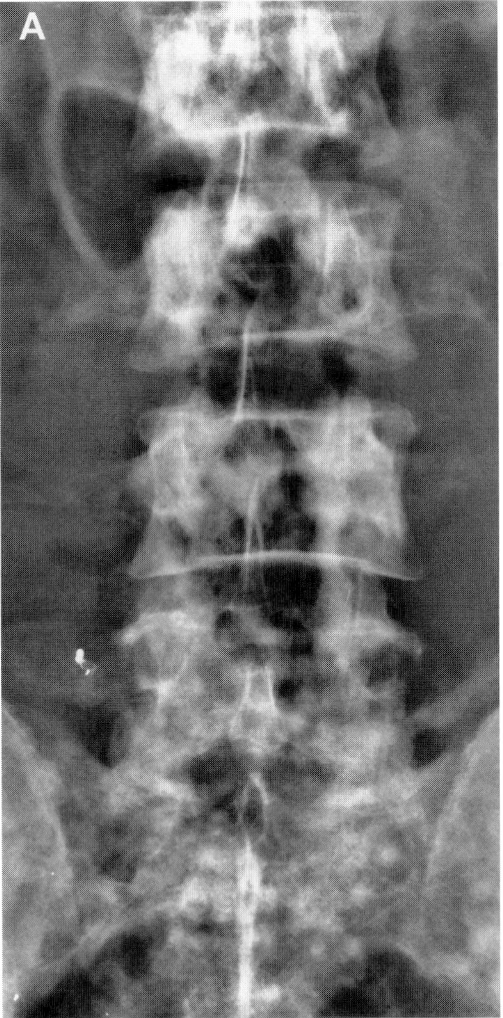

Figure 1–33. Patient with prostatic cancer and multiple osteoblastic metastases within the lumbar spine. **(A)** Antero-posterior projection of lumbar spine reveals multiple large and small nodules of increased density within the lumbar spine and sacrum, which look like cotton balls. **(B)** Sagittal T_1-weighted image of the lumbar spine shows multiple hypointense foci (arrows) affecting all lumbar vertebral bodies and the sacrum. **(C)** Sagittal T_2-weighted image reveals that all lesions remain hypointense, indicating that the lesions are osteoblastic metastases. *(continued)*

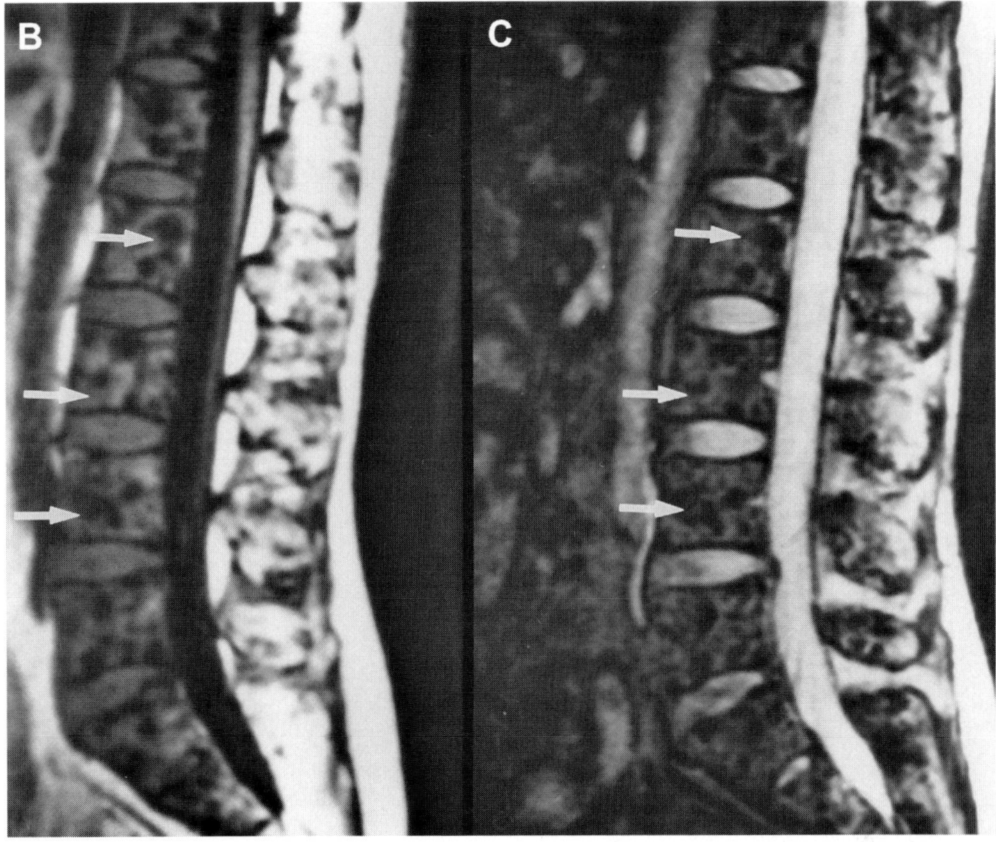

Figure 1–33. (*Continued*)

spectroscopic data acquisition and processing capabilities, which may have important applications in the management of tumor patients, are briefly reviewed.

Perfusion Imaging Pulse Sequences

It is commonly accepted that tumors cannot grow beyond a few millimeters in diameter without altering the local vascular environment. Furthermore, tumors with highly permeable and plentiful blood vessels appear to be more likely to metastasize and, in general, are associated with a poorer prognosis. Treatment-related changes, on the other hand, are variably associated with increases in vascular density and permeability. Therefore, the ability to assess vascular volume, flow, and permeability may be highly valuable in the noninvasive characterization of intracranial lesions and may provide a means of more reliably determining tumor progression versus treatment-related changes that are often difficult or impossible to distinguish even with the wide range of image contrasts provided by standard MRI techniques. Techniques available to noninvasively monitor tissue vascularity should prove highly useful for assessing the efficacy of antiangiogenic agents currently in clinical trials.

Two MR-based techniques have been developed for mapping regional cerebral blood flow (rCBF) and regional cerebral blood volume (rCBV). The first technique, often referred to as *dynamic susceptibility contrast* (DSC) mapping, takes advantage of the transient susceptibility change that occurs as a bolus of paramagnetic contrast agent passes through the microvascular vessels (Sanders and Orrison, 1995; Ostergaard et al., 1996a,b; Sorensen and Rosen, 1996; Sorensen et al., 1997). These transient susceptibility changes are manifested as short-lived, localized, inhomogeneities in the local magnetic field. Such changes cause enhanced dephasing of the local nuclear spins by decreasing the "apparent" T_2 relax-

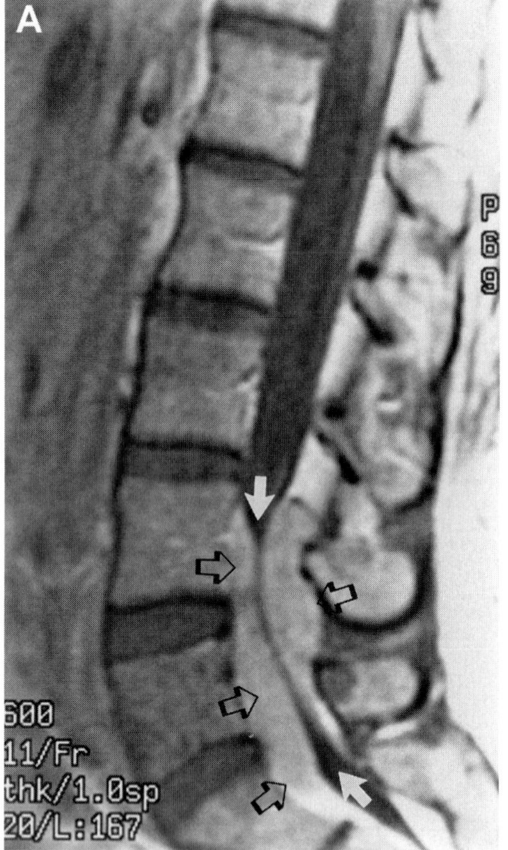

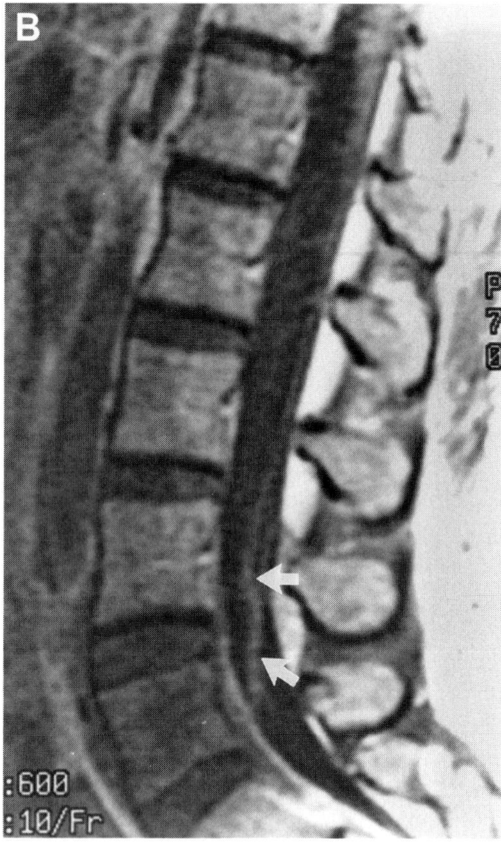

Figure 1–34. Hodgkin's disease of the lumbar spinal canal with epidural mass. **(A,B)** Post-contrast sagittal T_1-weighted images. **(A)** There is extensive ventral and dorsal epidural tumor (open arrows) squeezing the lumbar subarachnoid space and nerve roots (white arrows). **(B)** Post-radiation therapy follow-up MRI scan reveals near-complete disappearance of the epidural tumor with expansion of the lumbar subarachnoid space, which shows an excellent response to therapy. Some residual thickening of the nerve roots (arrows) is noted.

ation time (T_2*). This dephasing results in a transient decrease in signal intensity on T2W or T2*W images as the bolus passes (Fig. 1–45). The higher the rCBV, the greater the magnitude of the transient signal loss. Assuming that the contrast agent remains in the vasculature, that is, there is no BBB break down, such images can be used to construct maps of rCBV (Fig. 1–46). If, however, the BBB is fenestrated and contrast agent "leaks" from the vascular to the interstitial space, the DSC mapping technique can underestimate the rCBV measures due to loss of compartmentalization of the contrast agent and local decreases in the T_1 relaxation times (Sorensen and Rosen, 1996).

This can be particularly problematic with the current class of commonly utilized paramagnetic contrast agents that are FDA approved for clinical use. All three of these agents, gadolinium dimeglumine, gadodiamide, and gadoteridol, have relatively small molecular weights (on the order of 600 daltons) and readily extravasate in cases of BBB fenestration. Several higher molecular weight (greater than 25,000 dalton) contrast agents are currently in phase I and phase II clinical trials and promise to greatly expand the use of DSC mapping of vascular volume and flow in both neuroimaging applications and body imaging applications, where the absence of a BBB exacerbates the contrast leakage problem. An advantage of the DSC technique, however, is the favorable signal-to-noise ratio of the resulting rCBV maps, particularly if double-dose bolus injections are utilized. If the mean transit time (MTT) of the contrast agent can be de-

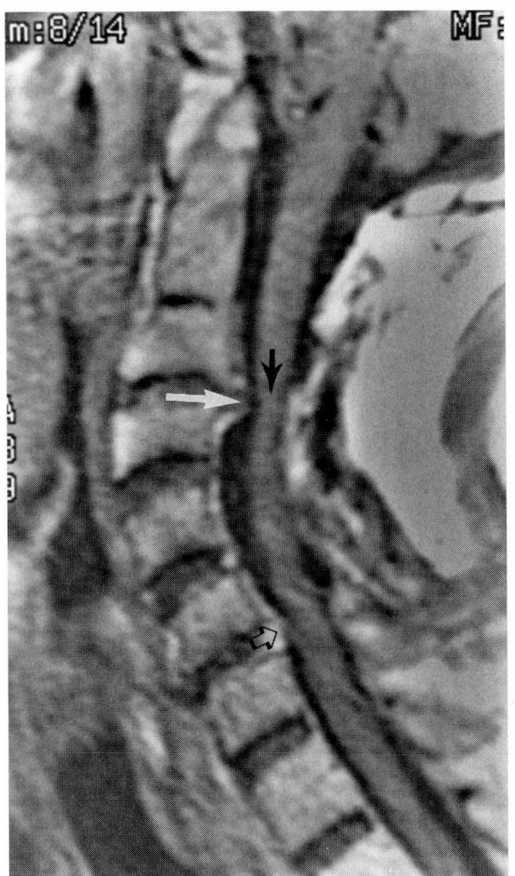

Figure 1–35. Patient with melanoma who presented with acute radiating pain to the arm. Sagittal T_1-weighted image of the cervical spine reveals a herniated disc at the C4–C5 level (white arrow) with cervical cord compression (black arrow). A smaller herniated disc is also seen at the C6–C7 level (open arrow).

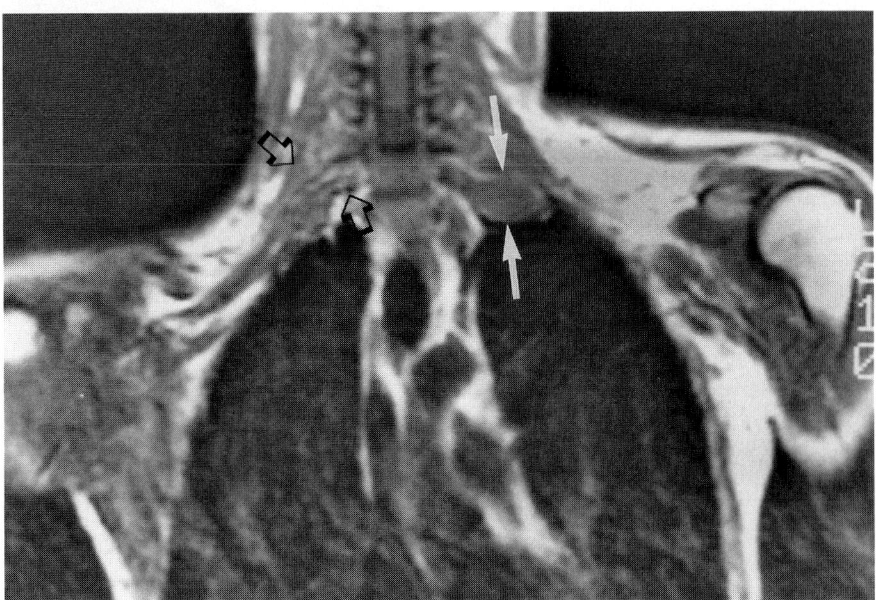

Figure 1–36. Dumbbell-shaped neurofibroma involving the right brachial plexus. There is a large neurofibroma originating from the left brachial plexus (white arrows) compared with the normal brachial plexus on the right (open arrows).

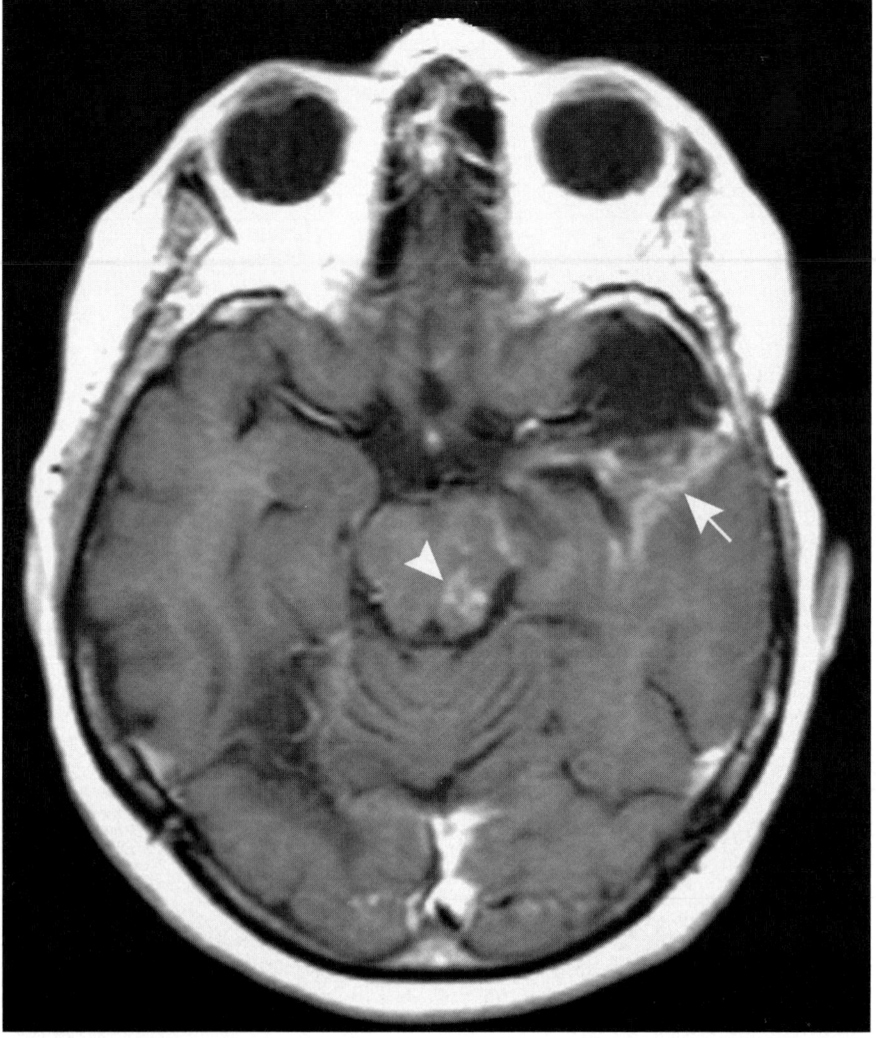

Figure 1–37. Post-contrast axial T_1-weighted MR image. Irregular enhancing lesions (arrow) posterior to the surgical cavity within the left temporal lobe and in the midbrain (arrowhead) were proved to be radiation necrosis at autopsy. The patient was status postsurgery with accelerated radiation therapy and chemotherapy for an anaplastic astrocytoma.

termined (e.g., from the signal intensity change in an intracranial artery) then the rCBV can be converted to rCBF using the central volume theorem, rCBF = rCBV/MTT.

The second MR technique used for assessing cerebral microvascular changes requires no exogenous contrast agent. This technique, known as *arterial spin tagging* (AST), relies on time-of-flight signal loss in an imaging section that occurs from inversion of flowing spins in a section a few centimeters away (Detre et al., 1992; Edelman et al., 1994; Alsop and Detre, 1996). The inverted spins from the "tagged" section yield decreased signal intensity when imaged in the section of interest. Knowing the location of the tagging section, the T_1 relaxation times in the section of interest, and the blood–tissue partition coefficient (approximately constant with a value of ~0.9), rCBF can be computed in the section of interest. The totally noninvasive nature of the AST rCBF measures makes this approach more advantageous than the DSC approach described above. The signal-to-noise ratio of the DSC technique is significantly higher, however, and obtaining good-quality AST measures of rCBF from multiple sections is more difficult due to mag-

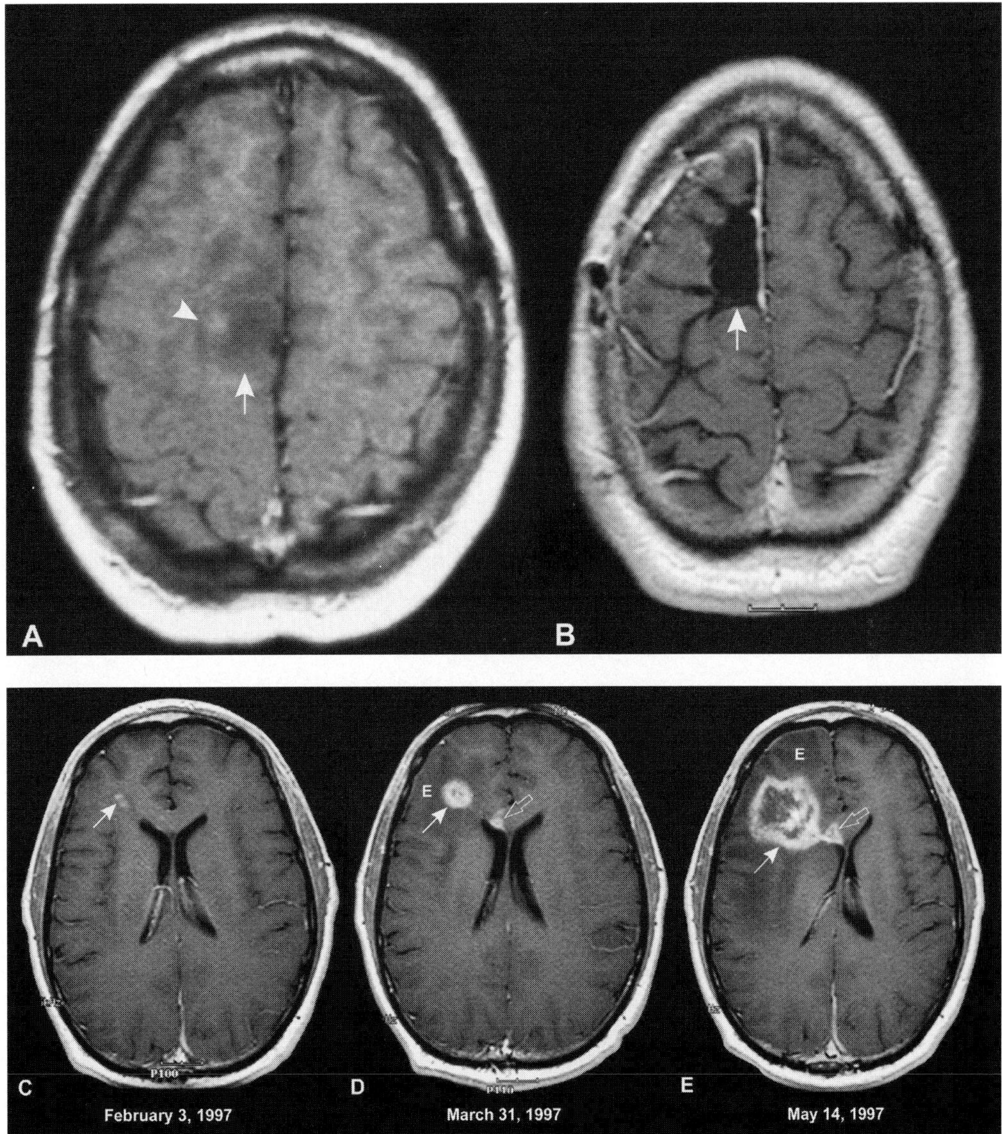

Figure 1–38. Post-contrast MR images (A–E). A nonenhancing tumor (arrow) with an enhancing nodule (arrowhead) occupying the right frontal lobe high-convexity region was noted in a 29-year-old male **(A).** The tumor was resected (resection cavity is shown in **B,** arrow). The tumor was an oligodendroglioma, and the patient was treated with radiation therapy (RT) and chemotherapy. The patient developed a small enhancing lesion in the right frontal lobe 8 months after completion of RT (arrow in **C**) that progressively increased in size in follow-up studies (arrows in **D** and **E**). There is also a progressive increase in the degree of edema (E) and mass effect on the right lateral ventricle. Surgical excision of the mass at this point revealed extensive radiation necrosis. Radiation necrosis affecting the corpus callosum is also shown (open arrows in D and E). Note that the radiation necrosis within the right frontal lobe (C–E) occurred remotely from the primary tumor (A).

netization transfer effects. Because of the lower signal-to-noise ratio, obtaining AST acquisitions is currently more time consuming than obtaining DSC acquisitions. More recent ultra-high-field systems, with static magnetic fields at or greater than 3 Tesla, however, may provide adequate AST signal-to-noise ratios in scan times that begin to rival those required for current DSC techniques.

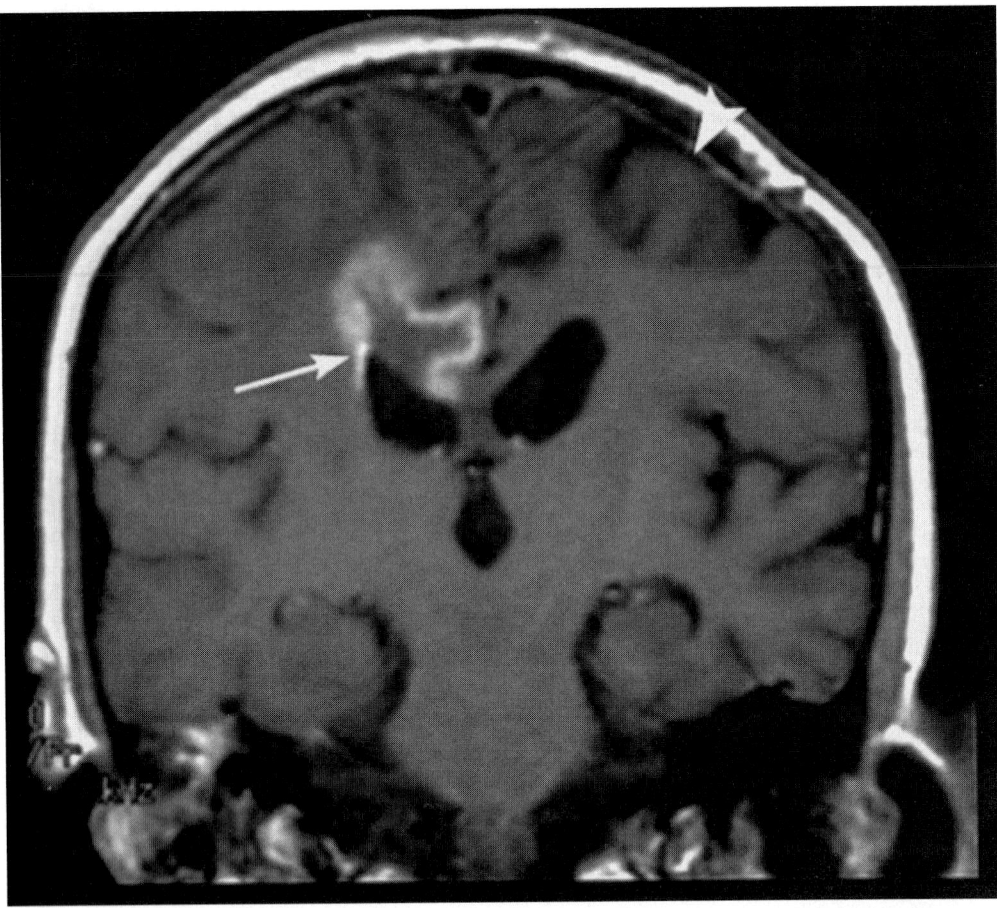

Figure 1–39. Post-contrast coronal T_1-weighted MRI of the brain. Biopsy-proven radiation necrosis affected the contralateral hemisphere (arrow) and involved the corpus callosum (C). The patient was status post-resection of glioblastoma in the left frontal lobe (arrowhead points to craniotomy site) followed by radiation and chemotherapy.

It should be noted that both the DSC and AST techniques for mapping rCBV and/or rCBF require very rapid imaging capabilities. Typically, this is best achieved using systems capable of single-shot, spin-echo, echo-planar imaging (EPI) techniques, which allow image acquisition rates as high as 50 msec/image.

Dynamic Contrast Magnetic Resonance Imaging Techniques

The use of static pre- and post-contrast agent-enhanced MR scans has been routine in neuroimaging since the mid-1980s. However, the kinetics of contrast agent uptake are infrequently used. The rapid acquisition of T1W images before, during, and after the infusion of a bolus of paramagnetic contrast agent, however, allows the rates of contrast agent uptake and washout between a lesion and the vasculature to be assessed. In theory, simple two-compartment pharmacokinetic modeling of the contrast agent kinetics can be used to *(1)* map the fractional plasma volume (vascular volume), *(2)* determine endothelial transfer coefficient (permeability–surface area product) when contrast leakage is not flow rate limited, *(3)* assess extraction-flow product when leakage is great enough to be flow limited (Tofts, 1997), and *(4)* obtain the contrast agent reflux rate. Such noninvasive measures of vascular endothelial parameters might be highly useful in determining the penetration of novel chemotherapeutic agents, assessing the efficacy of novel antiangiogenic agents, and more specif-

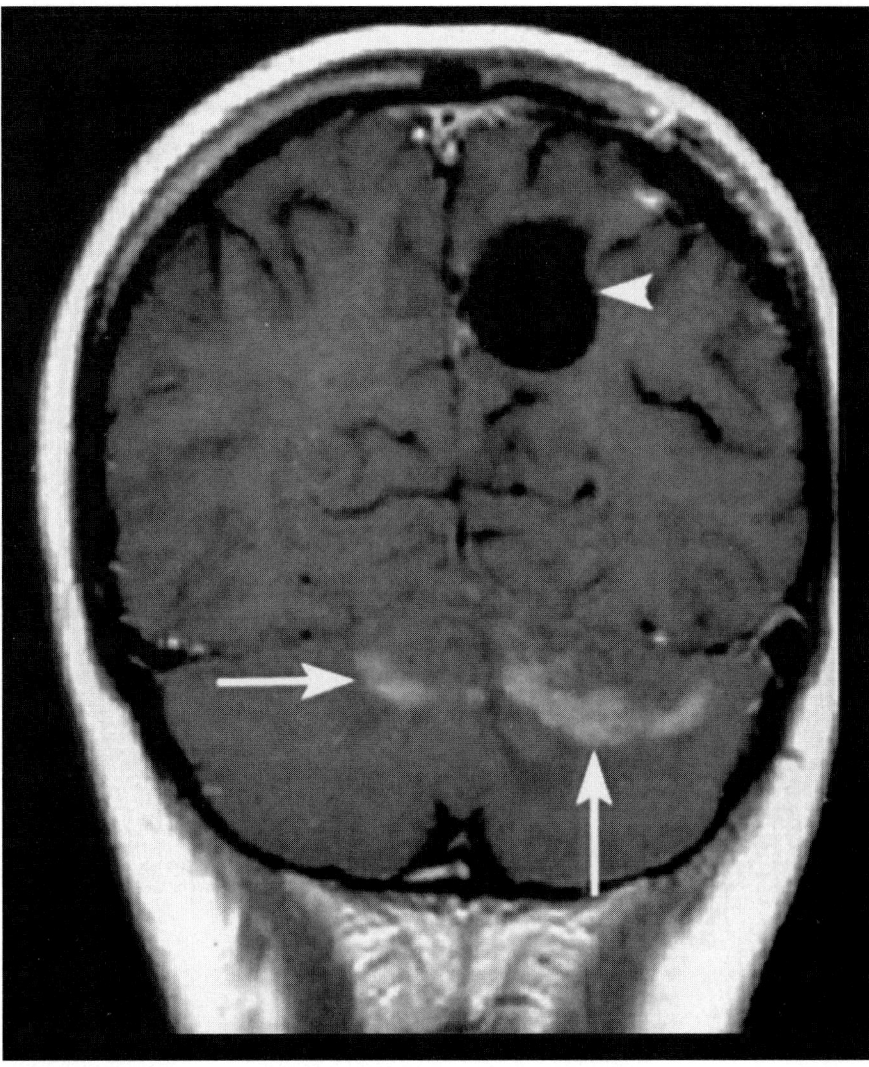

Figure 1–40. Post-contrast coronal T_1-weighted MRI of the brain shows radiation necrosis of the cerebellar hemispheres (arrows) that developed after resection of a parietal lobe glioblastoma and accelerated radiation therapy with chemotherapy to the brain (arrowhead points to the surgical cavity).

ically characterizing lesions in a noninvasive manner (e.g., differentiating between tumor progression and treatment-related changes).

Qualitative or semiquantitative applications of dynamic contrast agent–enhanced MRI to neuroimaging of patients with intracranial neoplasms have been previously reported. The utility of such scans in differentiating treatment-related changes from primary brain tumors, metastases, and meningiomas has been previously described (Hazle et al., 1997), and significant correlations between outcome measures and dynamic contrast MRI measures in anaplastic astrocytoma and glioblastoma multiforme patients have been reported by Wong et al. (1998). In addition to these studies based on empirical modeling of the dynamic data, several pharmacokinetic studies have been reported in which the endothelial transfer coefficient, contrast reflux rate, and fractional plasma volume have been determined (Larsson et al., 1990; Tofts and Kermode, 1991; Tofts, 1997; Parker and Tofts, 1999). When such calculations are performed on a pixel-by-pixel basis, the rapidly acquired source images can

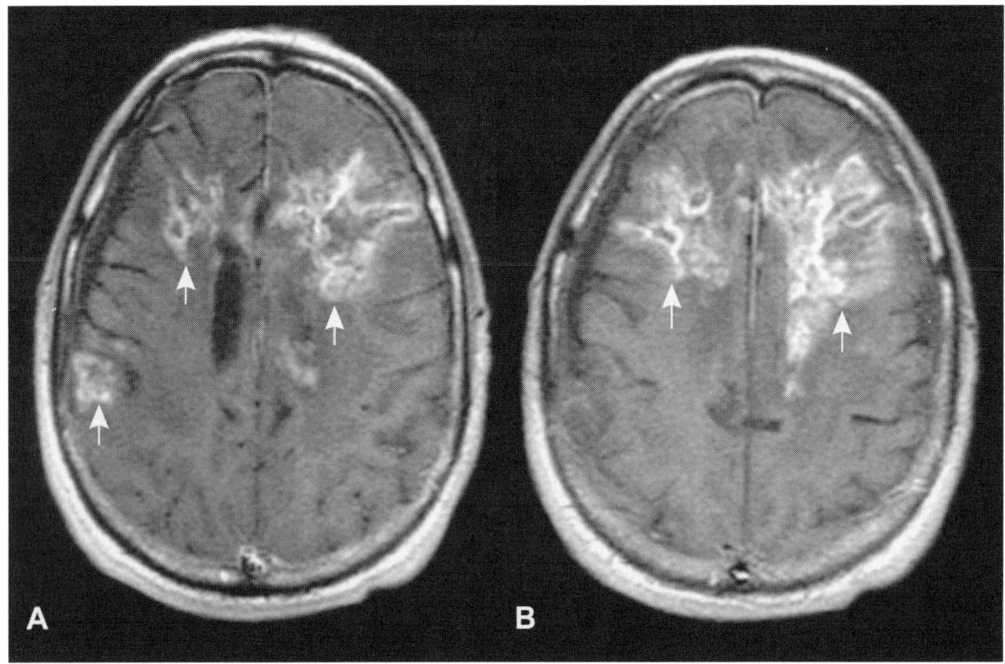

Figure 1–41. Post-contrast coronal T_1-weighted MR images **(A,B)** of the brain show extensive heterogeneous enhancing lesions involving both frontal lobes (arrows) with "Swiss cheese"–like interior, produced by radiation necrosis. Despite the large sized lesions, there is no mass effect secondary to involution of the brain. The patient was status postsurgery with accelerated radiation therapy and chemotherapy for a right frontal lobe anaplastic astrocytoma.

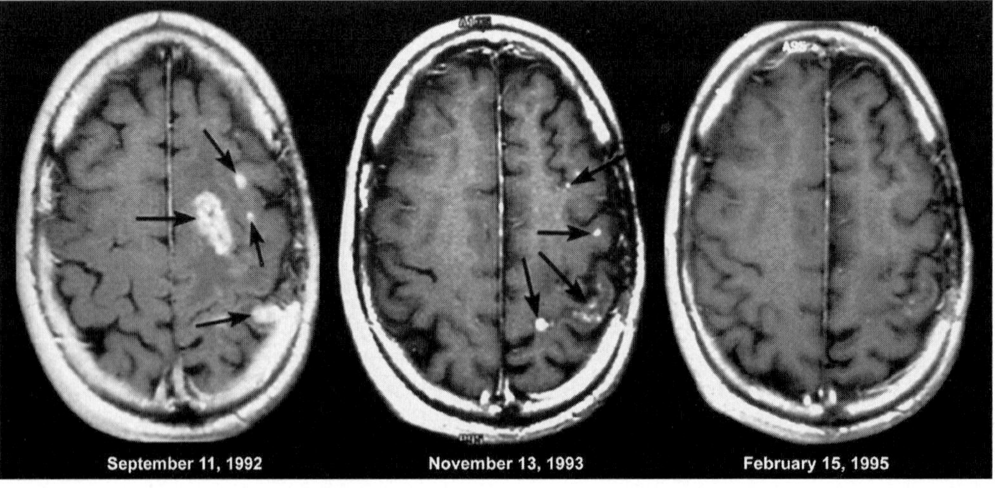

Figure 1–42. Post-contrast axial T_1-weighted MR images of the brain show spontaneous regression of radiation-induced enhancing lesions (arrows) within lesions in the left frontoparietal lobe. The patient is status postsurgery with accelerated radiation therapy and chemotherapy for a nonenhancing anaplastic astrocytoma involving the parietal lobe.

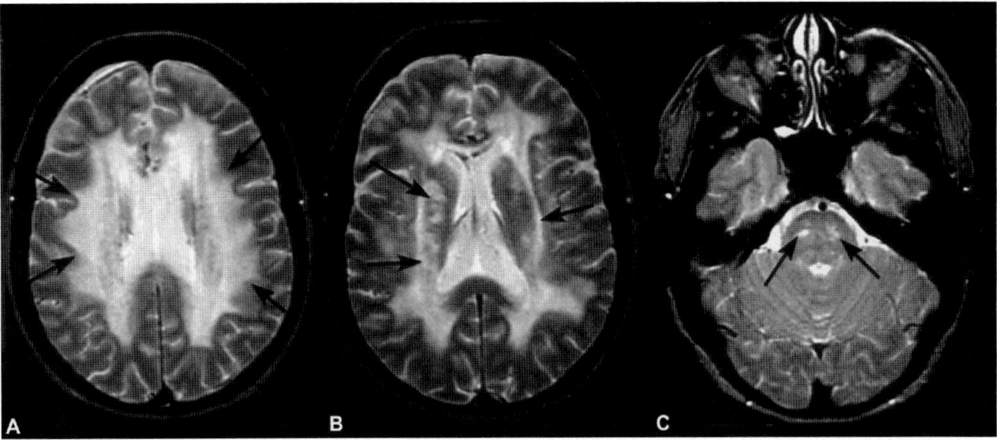

Figure 1–43. Axial T_2-weighted images **(A–C)** of the brain demonstrate radiation- and chemotherapy-induced periventricular leukoencephalopathy affecting the white matter (arrows in A) and two tracts (arrows in B and C).

be used to generate maps of each of the above parameters (Parker et al., 1997). Such *parametric maps* allow for improved assessment of lesion heterogeneity, thereby avoiding the potential for "sampling error," which is commonly a point of concern in histopathologic analyses of tissue samples. Examples of parametric maps of fractional plasma volume and endothelial transfer coefficient in a patient with pathologically proven anaplastic astrocytoma are shown in Color Figure 1–47.

As with perfusion imaging techniques, dynamic contrast agent–enhanced scans require rapid image acquisition rates, particularly to obtain fractional plasma volume measures. Furthermore, if accurate measures of permeability–surface area product are desired, contrast agents with larger molecular weights than those currently available may be required for lesions associated with significant BBB breakdown. Otherwise, as mentioned above, contrast agent extravasation may be flow limited, leading to possible erroneous permeability–surface area measurements. As an example, extracranial lesion studies in animals have previously demonstrated improved correlations between permeability–surface area product and fractional plasma volume with histopathologic results when using higher molecular weight agents (~90,000 daltons) compared with FDA-approved low molecular weight agents (~600 daltons) (Daldrup et al., 1998).

Diffusion Imaging Techniques

If appropriate gradient pulses are applied within the echo time of a spin-echo EPI sequence, the resulting image contrast can be made to depend strongly on the rate of diffusion, or Brownian motion, of the nuclear spins of interest. The larger the area under the applied diffusion-sensitizing gradients, the greater the influence of diffusion on the image contrast. This area is directly related to the often-quoted "*b*-factor" value. More specifically, the degree of attenuation of the signal from a given tissue in diffusion-weighted images is proportional to e^{-bD}, where b is the *b*-factor value and D is the diffusion coefficient. Thus, for a given *b*-factor, larger diffusion coefficient levels are associated with larger degrees of signal attenuation. Similarly, for a given diffusion coefficient level, the degree of signal attenuation increases with increasing values of b. Therefore, in *diffusion-weighted images,* regions where diffusion is more restricted are hyperintense relative to regions of unrestricted diffusion.

In general, to obtain the degree of diffusion sensitization necessary for acceptable image contrast, the *b*-factor values must be rather large (e.g., 1000 sec/mm^2). Therefore, the areas of the diffusion-sensitizing gradient pulses are large, and the minimum echo time is relatively long, resulting in T2W source image contrast. Because the images are T2W, substances with long T_2 values may not be as hy-

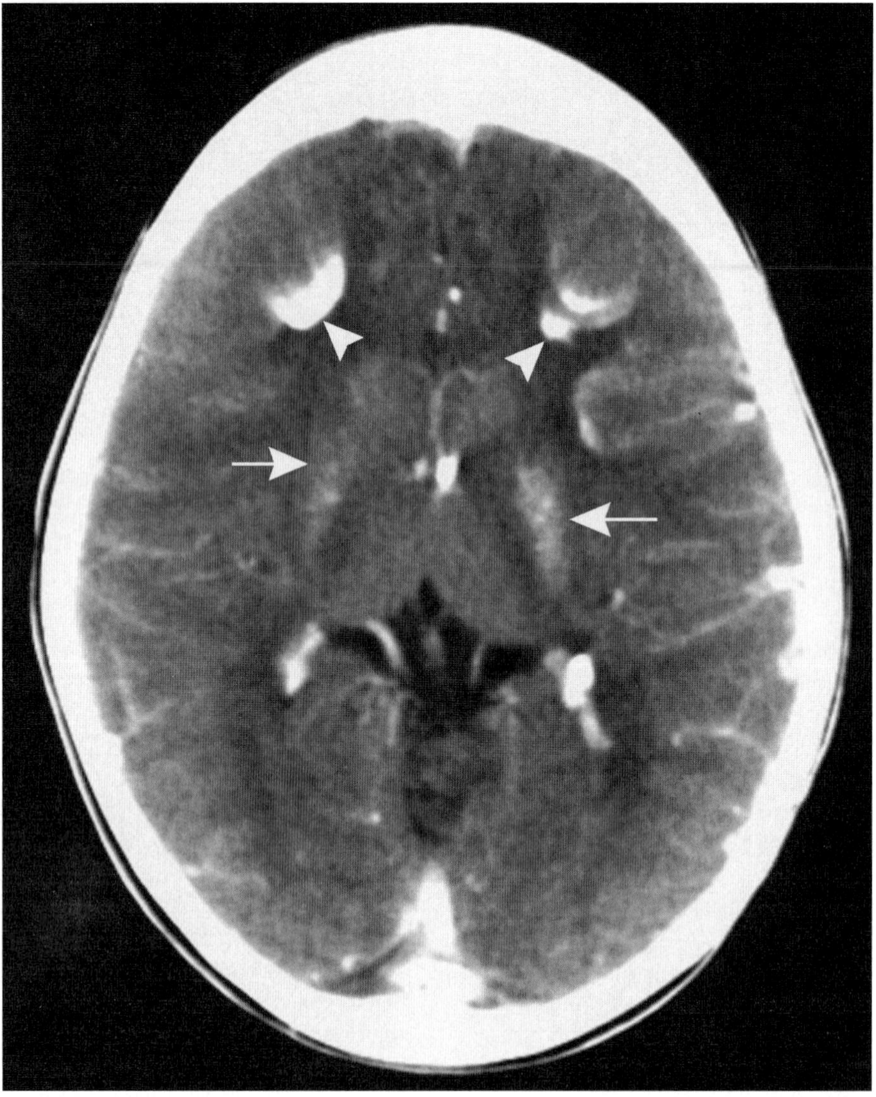

Figure 1–44. Radiation-induced mineralizing microangiopathy in a 13-year-old girl who underwent resection of an astrocytoma of the vermis followed by 45 Gy to the posterior fossa and 30 Gy to the whole brain. The patient developed multifocal calcifications 3 years after treatment. Non-contrast axial CT scan of the brain at that time revealed dense calcifications involving the basal ganglion (arrows) and subcortical white matter (arrowheads).

pointense as expected based solely on the rate of diffusion, resulting in "T_2 shine-through" of such substances in the diffusion-weighted images. To remove such confounding shine-through effects, image contrast may be based on the "apparent diffusion coefficient" (or ADC) (Le Bihan et al., 1992; Le Bihan and Turner, 1993; Sanders and Orrison, 1995). The ADC images are computed from a set of diffusion-weighted images obtained with multiple (~2 to 5), *b*-factor values. Of note is the fact that the contrast on *ADC*-weighted images is the inverse of the contrast obtained on diffusion-weighted images; regions where diffusion is restricted are hypointense, and regions where diffusion is unrestricted are hyperintense.

Of importance also is the fact that diffusion in some tissues is anisotropic (Moseley et al., 1990). For ex-

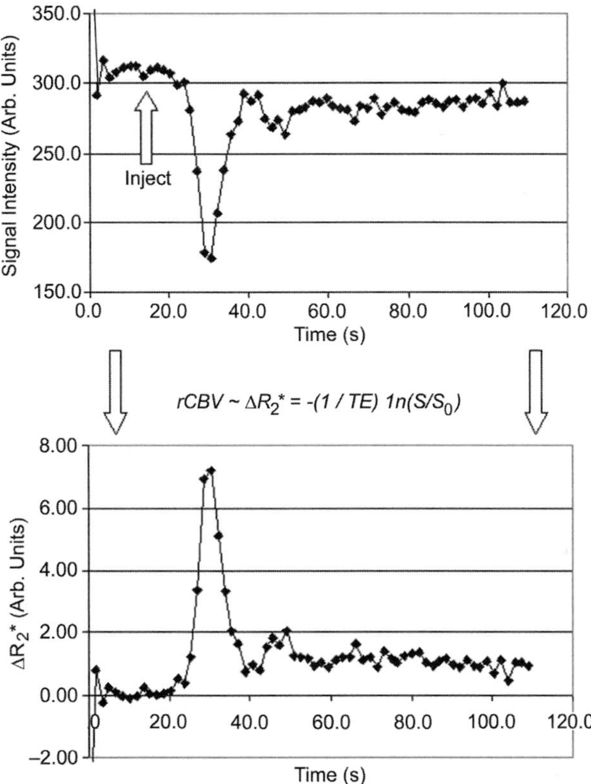

Figure 1–45. Dynamic susceptibility contrast (DSC) regional cerebral blood volume (rCBV) mapping. **(Top)** A typical signal intensity versus time curve from a region of interest in the parietal cortex. Note the dramatic signal loss in the cortex during the bolus transit and the recovery to baseline following the first pass. **(Bottom)** The change in signal intensity can be converted to a change in apparent T_2 relaxation rate ($\Delta R2^*$). Because rCBV $\propto$ [Gd] $\propto$ $\Delta R2^*$, the regional cerebral blood volume can then be determined (see Ostergaard et al., 1996b, for complete details.)

ample, diffusion along white matter tracts is much less restricted than diffusion across the tracts (Fig. 1–48). Therefore, if diffusion-sensitizing gradient pulses are applied only in one direction, it is difficult to know if signal variations in the image plane are due to true differences in diffusion rates or to white matter diffusion anisotropy. To remove this confound, diffusion-sensitizing gradients are typically applied in each of the three orthogonal directions, and the results are averaged together to yield the average or "trace" diffusion-weighted image in which the anisotropic diffusion rate information is suppressed (Fig. 1–48). On the other hand, the fact that white matter tract diffusion is anisotropic does allow the use of diffusion tensor imaging techniques for noninvasively mapping the white matter tracts (Fig. 1–49) (Pierpaoli et al., 1996; Pajevic and Pierpaoli, 1999; Virta et al., 1999).

Thus far, the primary clinical application of diffusion imaging has been the detection of acute stroke (van Gelderen et al., 1994; Sorensen and Rosen, 1996; Beauchamp et al., 1998). On diffusion-weighted images, areas of restricted extracellular water diffusion, secondary to increased cellular volume, appear hyperintense in acute ischemic injury. These signal changes have been shown to occur well before detectable changes occur on T2W or FLAIR images and have been useful in the detection and staging of ischemic injury. Coupled with perfusion imaging techniques, diffusion imaging techniques might permit assessment of the ischemic penumbra and assist in treatment decisions using current and novel stroke

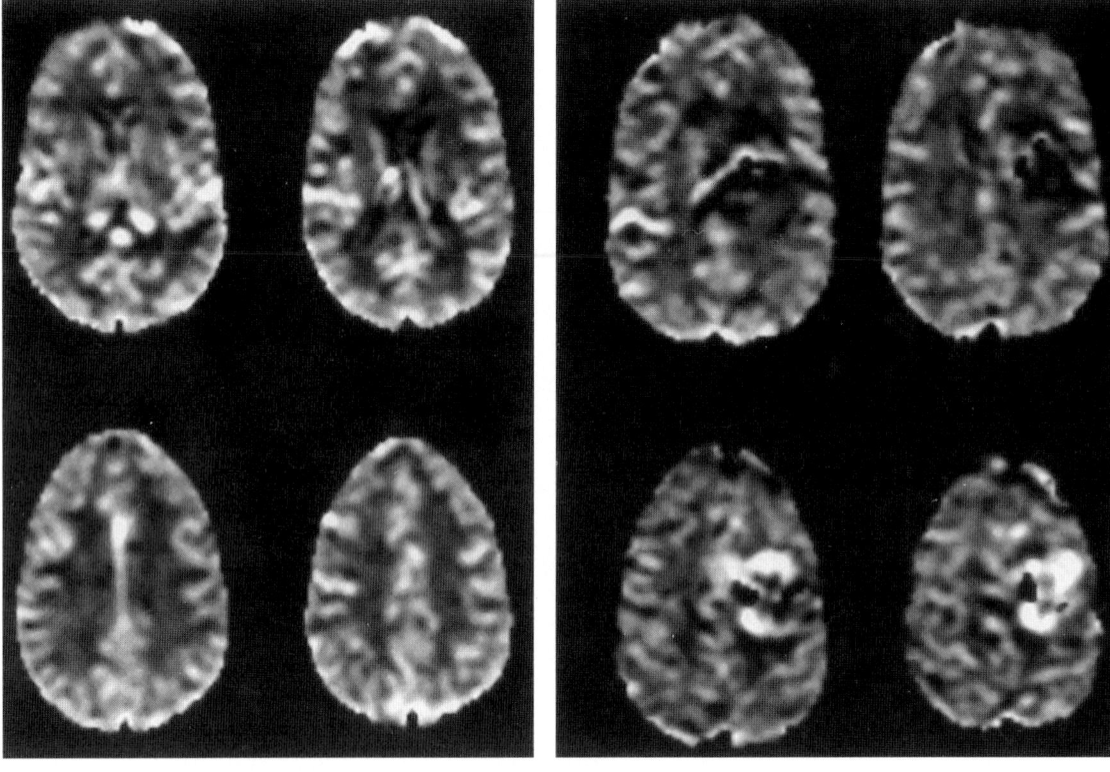

Figure 1–46. Dynamic susceptibility contrast (DSC) regional cerebral blood volume (rCBV) maps showing normal perfusion contrast **(left)** and increased rCBV **(right)** in a patient with pathologically proven anaplastic astrocytoma (right).

therapies (Beauchamp et al., 1998). Furthermore, quantitative diffusion imaging, by providing a means of noninvasively assessing the degree of cellularity (Chenevert et al., 1997), may prove useful in improved characterization of intracranial lesions.

As with perfusion imaging techniques, diffusion imaging requires very high-speed imaging capabilities. In fact, of all of the current advanced neuroimaging techniques, diffusion imaging is the most demanding of the MR scanner hardware. The large gradient field pulses push the limit of even state-of-the-art scanners and typically require relatively long echo times, potentially increasing the T_2 shine-through problem. Furthermore, the large amplitude of rapidly switched gradient field pulses requires good eddy current compensation performance to prevent unacceptable levels of artifact. (Eddy currents induced in the surrounding metallic components in the magnet give rise to transient magnetic fields that oppose the applied gradient fields and limit the speed with which the images can be acquired without substantial artifacts.) Typically, single-shot, spin-echo EPI sequences are used for diffusion imaging to capture the small-scale motion represented by the diffusion process in a background of larger scale motions due to involuntary and voluntary patient motion and motion due to CSF pulsation.

Functional Imaging of Neuronal Task Activation

Before recent developments in MRI, the only image modality that was capable of imaging areas of neuronal function was PET. Other techniques for mapping areas of activation (e.g., electroencephalography [EEG] and magnetoencephalography [MEG]), were not image based, and spatial localization of the activated areas was coarse, at best. In 1991 and 1992, two new functional MRI (fMRI) techniques for indirectly mapping areas of neuronal activation in response to a visual stimulus were reported (Belliveau et al., 1991; Kwong et al., 1992). The underlying phys-

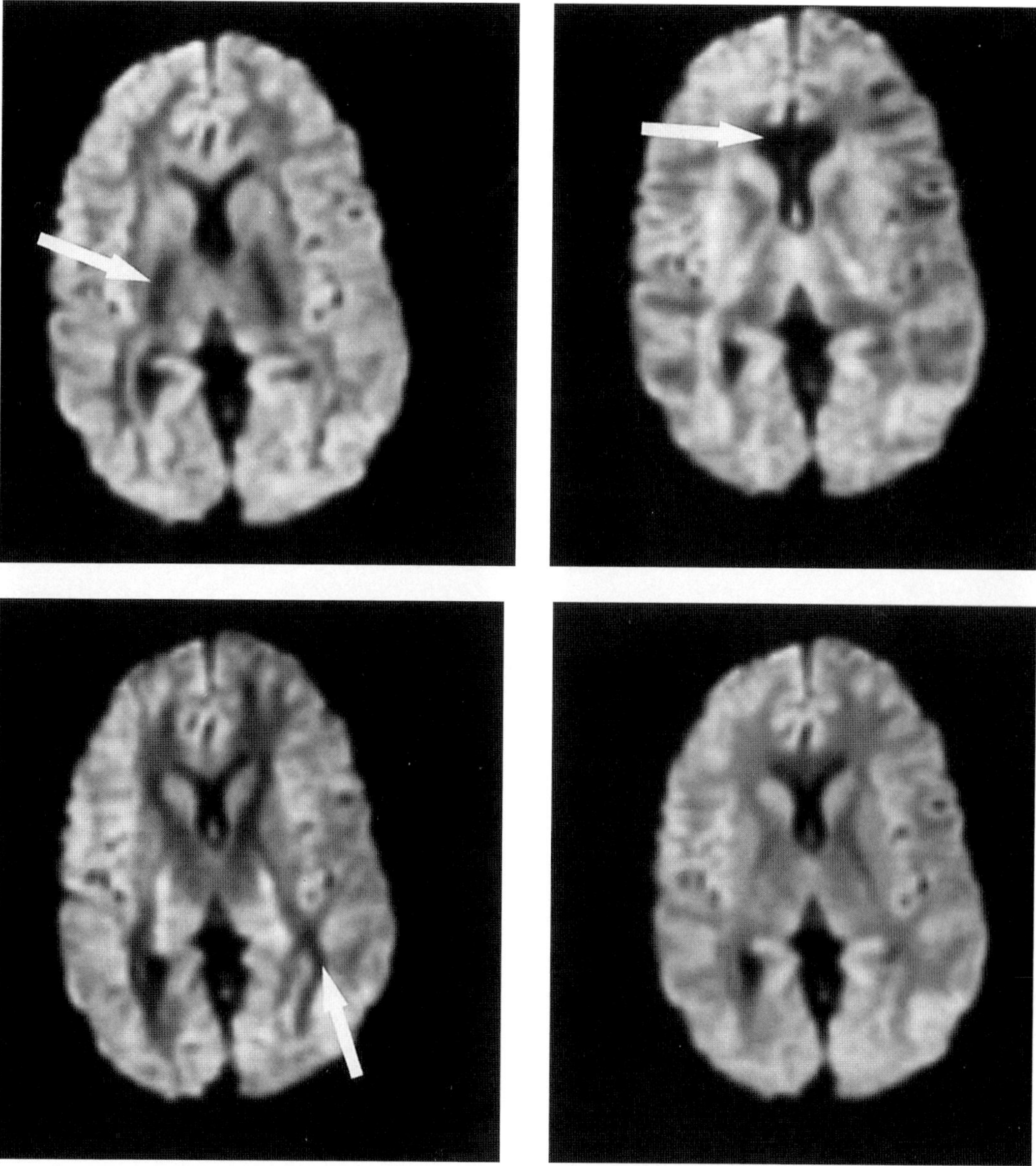

Figure 1–48. Diffusion-weighted MR images with diffusion-sensitizing gradients applied in the superoinferior **(top left)**, right–left **(top right)**, and anteroposterior **(bottom left)** directions. Note the dramatic differences in image appearance due to the anisotropic nature of water diffusion within the white matter tracts (arrows). Signal intensity is hypointense in directions of less restricted diffusion (along the tracts). The trace image **(lower right)** does not exhibit such anisotropic effects.

iologic principle of both techniques is that the neuronal activation that occurs in response to a stimulus, such as a visual task, results in local vasodilatation and a concomitant local increase in rCBV and rCBF. The first fMRI technique used to map this increase was the bolus contrast agent–enhanced DSC perfusion imaging acquisition discussed previously. First, a resting rCBV map was acquired. Then, during a given functional task, a second bolus of contrast agent was administered and a second rCBV map was obtained. The difference in the two images provided a map of areas of the brain that exhibited increased

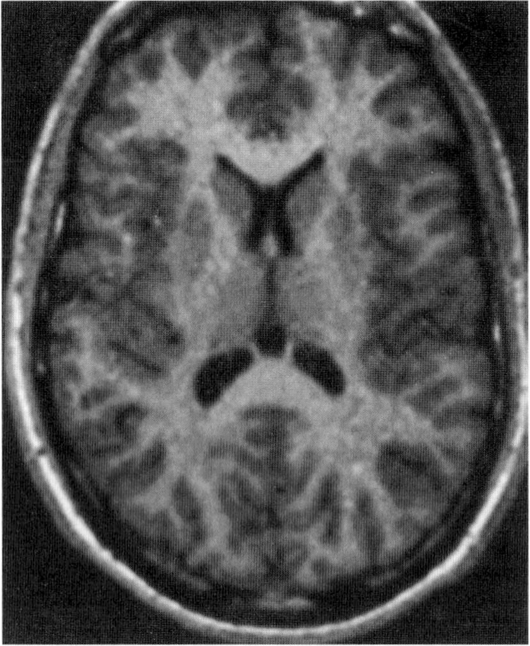

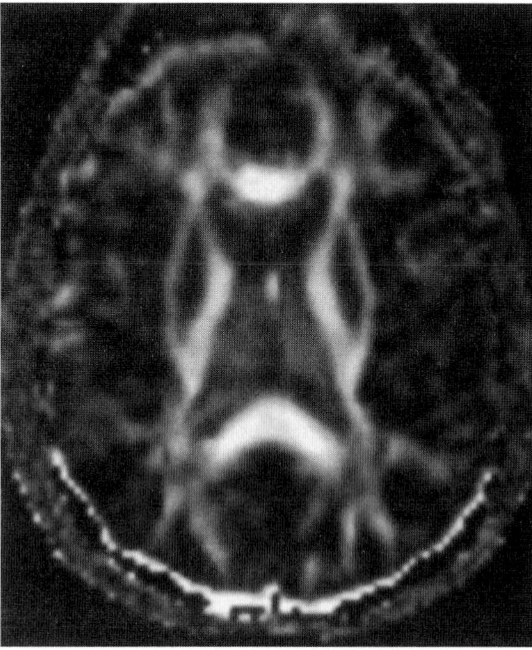

Figure 1–49. Diffusion tensor imaging to depict white matter tracts. **(Left)** T1W image. **(Right)** MR "tractogram."

rCBV during the task. The advantage of the DSC fMRI technique is that the signal intensity change between rest and activation is approximately 30% at 1.5 Tesla. The disadvantage of this technique is that it requires two contrast agent infusions per set of functional images and limits the number of tasks that can be evaluated in a single imaging session as well as how soon sessions can be repeated.

The second fMRI technique is based on *b*lood *o*xygen *l*evel *d*ependent (BOLD) contrast and is currently the most commonly used approach for imaging areas of neuronal activation. In this technique, no exogenous contrast agent is administered. Instead, advantage is made of the fact that deoxyhemoglobin is a paramagnetic substance and oxyhemoglobin is a diamagnetic substance. As noted with the DSC perfusion imaging technique, paramagnetic substances cause increased dephasing of the MR signal on T2W or T2*W images due to susceptibility effects. On the other hand, diamagnetic substances have minimal effect on signal dephasing. Therefore, a given amount of deoxyhemoglobin (paramagnetic) results in more signal loss relative to the same amount of oxyhemoglobin (diamagnetic). In regions of neuronal activation, local increases in rCBV and rCBF result in local increases in the oxyhemoglobin concentration, and, as shown by previous PET studies (Fox and Raichle, 1986), the rate of oxygen extraction is significantly less than the rate of oxyhemoglobin delivery. Therefore, in areas of activation, there is a net increase in the oxyhemoglobin/deoxyhemoglobin ratio and a concomitant increase in signal intensity on T2W and T2*W images.

The key advantages of this technique are that it is totally noninvasive and the resolution of the resulting activation maps is on the order of 1.5 to 2.0 mm, significantly better than those obtained using PET. However, the change in signal intensity at 1.5 Tesla is only about 1% to 3%, requiring excellent stability of the MR scanner and well-designed test paradigms and signal processing strategies. (The BOLD signal increases supralinearly with field strength, and much of the recent interest in 3 and 4 Tesla scanners stems primarily from the improved BOLD signal response relative to 1.5 Tesla scanners.)

Since the publication of the first fMRI studies of neuronal function in 1991, there have been many reports of BOLD fMRI studies for widely varying applications, including studies of visual stimulation, auditory stimulation, memory, language, sensorimotor stimulation, psychiatric disorders, and pain (e.g., Sanders and Orrison, 1995; Sorensen and Rosen,

1996; Buckner and Koutstaal, 1998; Tootell et al., 1998; Turner et al., 1998; and references therein). Examples of fMRI mapping for presurgical planning purposes are given in Color Figure 1–50.

In Vivo Spectroscopic Techniques

One of the earliest practical applications of the nuclear magnetic resonance phenomenon was the determination of chemical structure based on MR spectral data. It is not surprising, therefore, that investigators began developing and attempting to apply in vivo MR spectroscopy (MRS) techniques to whole-body scanners as soon as they were commercially available (in the mid-1980s). Clinical MRS applications have, however, lagged significantly behind rapidly advancing imaging capabilities. Nevertheless, the promise of being able to obtain biochemical information in a completely noninvasive manner continues to drive the transition of in vivo MRS from a research tool to a clinical application. Furthermore, many of the advances in scanner hardware that have allowed imaging techniques to evolve from a means of obtaining purely anatomic information to a means of obtaining physiologic information have also greatly improved MRS capabilities on state-of-the-art scanners.

It is well beyond the scope of this section to provide detailed descriptions of the acquisition, processing, and clinical applications of in vivo MRS. Instead, each of these topics is briefly reviewed and references are made to the rather extensive literature available on these subjects.

There are three basic requirements for performing an in vivo MRS examination on a clinical imaging system. First, an appropriate non-zero spin nucleus must be selected, and the system must be capable of transmitting and receiving signals at the frequency appropriate for the chosen nucleus of interest. Although it is theoretically possible to obtain MRS data from a range of different nuclei in the human body, natural abundance and relative MR sensitivity considerations generally limit clinical applications to ^{1}H and ^{31}P studies. The second basic requirement is a means of accurately localizing the region from which the MRS data are obtained. Numerous localization schemes have been proposed, but the most commonly used techniques in clinical applications are the single voxel (SV) technique and the spectroscopic imaging (SI) technique (Fig. 1–51). In the SV technique, spectral data are acquired from a single volume of interest (VOI) at a time. (An SV ^{1}H spectrum from a patient with glioblastoma multiforme is shown in Fig. 1–52.) On the other hand, SI techniques acquire spectral data from a number of VOIs simultaneously.

Both techniques have advantages and disadvantages. For example, one key criterion for obtaining good quality spectral data is that the magnetic field in the VOI is highly uniform. The magnetic field homogeneity can typically be better optimized on a small volume of tissue, like the VOI in an SV acquisition, than the larger volume typically examined using SI techniques. The SI technique, however, allows for obtaining spectra from multiple VOIs that are individually much smaller than an SV VOI, thereby permitting assessment of the heterogeneity of a given lesion and surrounding tissue. Furthermore, low-resolution "metabolite maps" can be computed from the SI data, allowing visualization of the spatial distribution of various compounds (Color Figs. 1–53 and 1–54). An additional requirement of the chosen acquisition technique, at least for ^{1}H MRS acquisitions, is the ability to suppress the signal from water, as the concentrations of the compounds of interest are typically 5000 to 10,000 times less than the concentration of water.

The third basic requirement for clinical MRS examinations is a means of analyzing the spectral data. Spectral data can be analyzed in three primary ways. The first is visual inspection of the spectral peaks—clearly the simplest, but most highly subjective, method to implement. The second commonly used method is to form ratios of spectral peak heights, or areas, with respect to a chosen reference peak. With ^{1}H brain spectra, for example, the most common reference peak is the creatine/phosphocreatine resonance, which varies minimally with spatial position within the brain. This approach is more quantitative and less subjective than the visual inspection method. In disease processes, however, changes in spectral peak ratios may reflect concentration changes in the compound of interest, in the reference compound, or in both.

The third method for analyzing spectral data is to obtain absolute metabolite concentrations from the associated spectral peak areas. Although obviously the most objective technique, this method of analysis is notoriously difficult. To convert from peak areas to absolute concentration requires a reference peak from a compound with known concentration. This

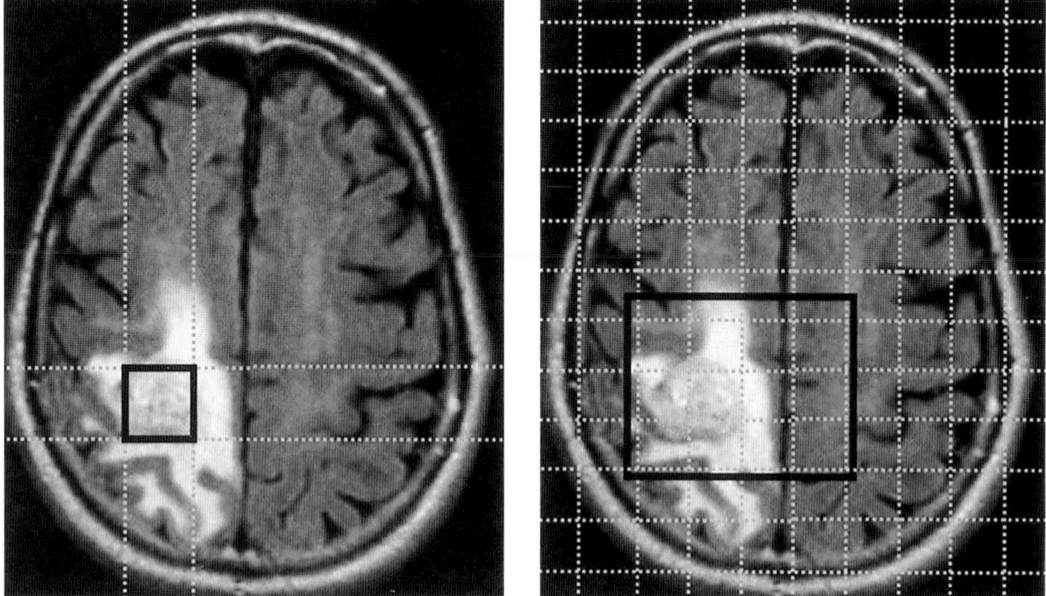

Figure 1–51. Proton MRS localization techniques. **(Left)** Single voxel (SV) technique used to acquire spectral data from one volume of at a time. The intersection of three planes, defined by the through-plane slice and two orthogonal "slices" (dotted lines), defines the VOI (black square). **(Right)** Spectroscopic imaging (SI) technique used to obtain spectral data from multiple VOIs in a single acquisition. Typically, a large volume is initially defined as in the SV technique (black rectangle). Phase-encoding techniques are then used to obtain individual spectra from multiple VOIs within the large volume of interest.

reference compound may be either an internal—most commonly water—or an external standard from which a spectrum is obtained just before or just after in vivo MRS data acquisition. The internal standard approach may be problematic in disease states where the internal reference compound concentration changes, whereas in the external standard approach it can be difficult to position and obtain a spectrum from the reference standard under the same conditions that occurred during in vivo MRS acquisition. Given the lack of objectivity of the visual inspection technique and the inherent difficulties of the

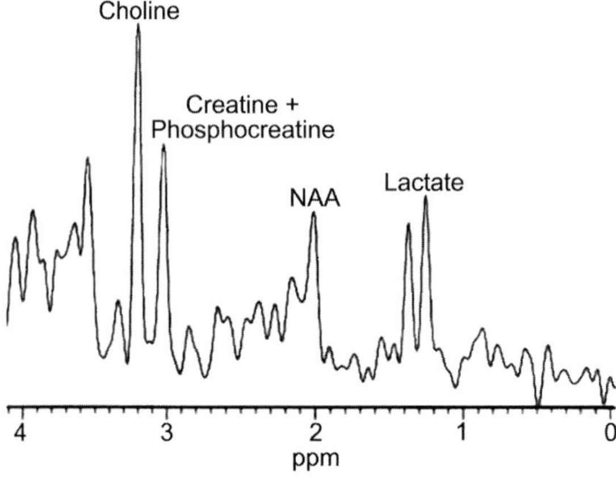

Figure 1–52. SV spectrum (echo time = 30 ms, repetition time = 2000 ms) from a glioblastoma multiforme showing greatly decreased levels of *N*-acetylaspartate, elevated lactate, and elevated choline.

absolute concentration technique, many investigators have settled on spectral peak ratios as the method of choice for routine analysis of spectral data. Because the T_1 and T_2 relaxation times of the various compounds of interest vary, however, it should be noted that the spectral peak heights, areas, and ratios depend strongly on echo time (TE) and, to a lesser degree, on repetition time (TR). Therefore, when comparing spectral data to literature values or between examinations, it is most important to take the TE and TR values into account. Several review articles and texts describe the wide range of clinical applications of in vivo MRS (Cady, 1990; Negendank, 1992; Barker et al., 1993; Howe et al., 1993; Ross and Michaelis, 1994, 1996; Vion-Dury et al., 1994; Cox, 1996; Falini et al., 1996; Danielsen and Ross, 1999; Jackson, 1999; Nelson et al., 1999).

Although many research investigations using both ^1H and ^{31}P MRS, as well as other less abundant nuclei, have been reported, undoubtedly the most common clinical application is ^1H MRS of the brain. In a normal human brain spectrum, the most prominent spectral peak is due to *N*-acetylaspartate (NAA). Although the exact biochemical role of NAA has yet to be fully elucidated, it is present in abundance only in viable neurons (Birken and Oldendorf, 1989). Reductions in the normal levels of NAA are sensitive indicators of neuronal degradation, but are nonspecific. The next most prominent spectral peaks in the normal brain spectrum are due to creatine/phosphocreatine and choline-containing compounds. Less prominent peaks due to *myo*-inositol and, for short TE spectra, glutamate/glutamine, are also visible. Lactate peaks are typically below detection limits in normal brain tissue, but may be visible in disease states, including ischemic injury and some neoplasms. Spectral peaks from lipids, abundant in the myelin, are not seen in normal brain due to the rigid structure of the lipids within the myelin. In some disease states, however, lipid peaks and peaks from macromolecular breakdown products may be present in spectra acquired with short echo times. (The effective T_2 relaxation times of these breakdown products are relatively short, resulting in the absence of peaks in spectra such as are acquired with long echo times.) In neoplastic lesions, the most common findings are elevated levels of choline-containing compounds, decreased levels of creatine/phosphocreatine, and decreased levels of NAA. Lactate peaks may, or may not, be present. Therefore, using the spectral peak ratio method of analysis, the most common finding in neoplastic lesions is elevated choline/creatine and choline/NAA ratios relative to normal brain tissue levels. Treatment-related changes, such as radiation necrosis, do not typically demonstrate such highly elevated choline/creatine ratios and are often associated with the presence of peaks due to lipids and other macromolecular breakdown products (in short TE spectra).

Outside of the brain, the most common clinical oncologic application of in vivo MRS has been in the prostate, where the level of citrate in ^1H spectra has been used to differentiate between benign prostate hyperplasia and neoplasm (Hahn et al., 1997; Heerschap et al., 1997; Liney et al., 1999).

Summary of Advanced MRI Techniques

In the last 5 years, significant improvements in MR scanner technology have allowed for new neuroimaging techniques, which have changed MRI from a means of acquiring images with exquisite anatomic detail and soft tissue contrast to a means of acquiring images of tissue function. Whereas many of these functional imaging techniques are currently in a transitional stage from basic research to clinical practice, several are poised to make a significant impact on clinical patient management and outcome. Newer imaging techniques, including more specific contrast agents and novel image contrast mechanisms, will undoubtedly continue to propel the expanding use of MRI in neuroimaging applications. In addition, significant improvements in automated SV and SI in vivo MRS data acquisition and processing techniques have allowed for "routine" acquisition of biochemical information that can be used, for example, to aid in the often difficult differentiation between tumor progression and treatment-related changes.

REFERENCES

Alsop DC, Detre JA. 1996. Reduced transit-time sensitivity in noninvasive magnetic resonance imaging of human cerebral blood flow. J Cereb Blood Flow Metab 16:1236–1249.

Ball WS, Jr, Prenger EC, Ballard ET. 1992. Neurotoxicity of radio/chemotherapy in children: pathologic and MR correlation. Am J Neuroradiol 13:761–776.

Barker PB, Glickson JD, Bryan RN. 1993. In vivo magnetic resonance spectroscopy of human brain tumors. Top Magn Reson Imaging 5:32–45.

Beauchamp NJ, Jr, Ulug AM, Passe TJ, van Zijl PC. 1998. MR diffusion imaging in stroke: review and controversies. RadioGraphics 18:1269–1283.

Belliveau JW, Kennedy DN, Jr, McKinstry RC, et al. 1991. Functional mapping of the human visual cortex by magnetic resonance imaging. Science 254:716–719.

Birken DL, Oldendorf WH. 1989. *N*-acetyl-L-aspartic acid: a literature review of a compound prominent in ^{1}H-NMR spectroscopic studies of brain. Neurosci Biobehav Rev 13:23–31.

Blood CH, Zetter BR. 1990. Tumor interactions with vasculature angiogenesis and tumor metastasis. Biochim Biophys Acta 1032:89–118.

Buckner RL, Koutstaal W. 1998. Functional neuroimaging studies of encoding, priming, and explicit memory retrieval. Proc Natl Acad Sci USA 95:891–898.

Burger PC, Boyko OB. 1991. The pathology of central nervous system radiation injury. In: Gutin PH, Leibel SA, Sheline GE (eds), Radiation Injury to the Nervous System. New York: Raven Press, p 191.

Burger PC, Mahley MS, Jr, Dudka L, Vogel FS. 1979. The morphologic effects of radiation administered therapeutically for intracranial gliomas: a postmortem study of 25 cases. Cancer 44:1256–1272.

Cady EB. 1990. Clinical Magnetic Resonance Spectroscopy. New York: Plenum Press, 278 pp.

Castel JC, Caille JM. 1989. Imaging of irradiated brain tumours. Value of magnetic resonance imaging. J Neuroradiol 16:81–132.

Chenevert TL, McKeever PE, Ross BD. 1997. Monitoring early response of experimental brain tumors to therapy using diffusion magnetic resonance imaging. Clin Cancer Res 3:1457–1466.

Choucair AK, Levin VA, Gutin PH, et al. 1986. Development of multiple lesions during radiation therapy and chemotherapy in patients with gliomas. J Neurosurg 65:654–658.

Cowley AR. 1983. Influence of fiber tracts on the CT appearance of cerebral edema: anatomic pathologic correlation. AJNR (Am J Neuroradiol) 4:915–925.

Cox IJ. 1996. Development and applications of in vivo clinical magnetic resonance spectroscopy. Prog Biophys Mol Biol 65:45–81.

Daldrup H, Shames DM, Wendland M, et al. 1998. Correlation of dynamic contrast-enhanced MR imaging with histologic tumor grade: comparison of macromolecular and small-molecular contrast media. AJR (Am J Roentgenol) 171: 941–949.

Danielsen ER, Ross BD. 1999. Clinical cases. In: Danielsen ER, Ross B (eds), Magnetic Resonance Spectroscopy Diagnosis of Neurological Diseases. New York: Marcel Dekker, pp 53–302.

Davis PC, Hudgins PA, Peterman SB, Hoffman JC, Jr. 1991. Diagnosis of cerebral metastases: double dose delayed CT vs contrast-enhanced MR imaging. AJNR (Am J Neuroradiol) 12:293–300.

Detre JA, Leigh JS, Williams DS, Koretsky AP. 1992. Perfusion imaging. Magn Reson Med 23:37–45.

Doyle WK, Budinger TF, Valk PE, Levin VA, Gutin PH. 1987. Differentiation of cerebral radiation necrosis from tumor recurrence by [18F]FDG and 82Rb positron emission tomography. J Comput Assist Tomogr 11(4):563–570.

Ebner F, Ranner G, Slavc I et al. 1989. MR findings in methotrexate induced CNS abnormalities. AJR (Am J Roentgenol) 153:1283–1288.

Edelman RR, Siewert B, Darby DG, et al. 1994. Qualitative mapping of cerebral blood flow and functional localization with echo-planar MR imaging and signal targeting with alternating radio frequency. Radiology 192:513–520.

Elster AD, Chen MY. 1992. Can nonenhancing white matter lesions in cancer patients be disregarded? AJNR (Am J Neuroradiol) 13:1309–1318.

Falini A, Calabrese G, Origgi D, et al. 1996. Proton magnetic resonance spectroscopy and intracranial tumours: clinical perspectives. J Neurol 243:706–714.

Fike JR, Sheline GE, Cann CE, David RL. 1984. Radiation necrosis. Prog Exp Tumor Res 28:136–151.

Fox PT, Raichle ME. 1986. Focal physiological uncoupling of cerebral blood flow and oxidative metabolism during somatosensory stimulation in human subjects. Proc Natl Acad Sci USA 83:1140–1144.

Frank JA, Girton M, Dwyer AJ, et al. 1987. Ocular and cerebral metastases in the VX2 rabbit tumor model: contrast-enhanced MR imaging. Radiology 164:527–530.

Hahn P, Smith IC, Leboldus L, Littman C, Somorjai RL, Bezabeh T. 1997. The classification of benign and malignant human prostate tissue by multivariate analysis of ^{1}H magnetic resonance spectra. Cancer Res 57:3398–3401.

Hazle JD, Jackson EF, Schomer DF, Leeds NE. 1997. Dynamic imaging of intracranial lesions using fast spin-echo imaging: differentiation of brain tumors and treatment effects. J Magn Reson Imaging 7:1084–1093.

Heerschap A, Jager GJ, van der Graaf M, et al. 1997. In vivo proton MR spectroscopy reveals altered metabolite content in malignant prostate tissue. Anticancer Res 17:1455–1460.

Heier LA, Zimmerman RD. 1992. Commentary: can nonenhancing white matter lesions be disregarded? Am J Neuroradiol 13:1316.

Hoffman WF, Levin VA, Wilson CB. 1979. Evaluation of malignant glioma patients during the postirradiation period. J Neurosurg 50:624–628.

Howe FA, Maxwell RJ, Saunders DE, Brown MM, Griffiths JR. 1993. Proton spectroscopy in vivo. Magn Reson Q 9:31–59.

Jackson EF. 1999. Magnetic resonance spectroscopy: physical principles and applications. In: Kim EE, Jackson EF (eds), Molecular Imaging in Oncology: PET, MRI, and MRS. Berlin: Springer, pp 47–70.

Kumar AJ, Leeds NE, Fuller GN, et al. 2000. Malignant gliomas: MR imaging spectrum of radiation therapy- and chemotherapy-induced necrosis of the brain after treatment. Radiology 217:377–384.

Kwong KK, Belliveau JW, Chesler DA, et al. 1992. Dynamic magnetic resonance imaging of human brain activity during primary sensory stimulation. Proc Natl Acad Sci USA 89:5675–5679.

Kyritsis AP, Levin VA, Yung WK, Leeds NE. 1993. Imaging patterns of multifocal gliomas. Eur J Radiol 16:163–170.

Larsson HB, Stubgaard M, Frederiksen JL, Jensen M, Henriksen O, Paulson OB. 1990. Quantitation of blood–brain barrier defect by magnetic resonance imaging and gadolinium-DTPA in patients with multiple sclerosis and brain tumors. Magn Reson Med 16:117–131.

Le Bihan D, Turner R. 1993. Diffusion and perfusion nuclear magnetic resonance imaging. In: Potchen EJ, Haacke EM,

Siebert JE, Gottschalk A (eds), Magnetic Resonance Angiography. Concepts and Applications. St Louis: Mosby Year Book, pp 323–342.

Le Bihan D, Turner R, Dovek P, Patronas N. 1992. Diffusion MR imaging: clinical applications. AJR (Am J Roentgenol) 159:591–599.

Levin VA, Maor MH, Thall PF, et al. 1995. Phase II study of accelerated fractionation radiation therapy with carboplatin followed by vincristine chemotherapy for the treatment of glioblastoma multiforme. Int J Radiat Oncol Biol Phys 33:357–364.

Liney GP, Turnbull LW, Knowles AJ. 1999. In vivo magnetic resonance spectroscopy and dynamic contrast enhanced imaging of the prostate gland. NMR Biomed 12:39–44.

Marks JE, Baglan RJ, Prassad SC, Blank WF. 1981. Cerebral radionecrosis: incidence and risk in relation to dose, time, fractionation and volume. Int J Radiat Oncol Biol Phys 7:243–252.

Moody DM, Bell MA, Challa VR. 1990. Features of the cerebral vascular pattern that predict vulnerability to perfusion or oxygenation deficiency: an anatomic study. AJNR (Am J Neuroradiol) 11:431–439.

Moseley ME, Cohen Y, Kucharczyk J. 1990. Diffusion-weighted MR imaging of anisotropic water diffusion in cat central nervous system. Radiology 176:439–445.

Negendank W. 1992. Studies of human tumors by MRS: a review. NMR Biomed 5:303–324.

Nelson MD, Jr, Gonzalez-Gomez I, Gilles FH. 1991. Dyke award. The search for human telencephallic ventriculofugal arteries. AJNR (Am J Neuroradiol) 12:215–222.

Nelson SJ, Vigneron DB, Dillon WP. 1999. Serial evaluation of patients with brain tumors using volume MRI and 3D ^{1}H MRSI. NMR Biomed 12:123–138.

Ostergaard L, Sorensen AG, Kwong KK, Wiesskoff RM, Gyldensted C, Rosen BR. 1996a. High resolution measurement of cerebral blood flow using intravascular tracer bolus passages. Part II: Experimental comparison and preliminary results. Magn Reson Med 36:726–736.

Ostergaard L, Weisskoff RM, Chesler DA, Gyldensted C, Rosen BR. 1996b. High resolution measurement of cerebral blood flow using intravascular tracer bolus passages. Part I: Mathematical approach and statistical analysis. Magn Reson Med 36:715–725.

Pajevic S, Pierpaoli C. 1999. Color schemes to represent the orientation of anisotropic tissues from diffusion tensor data: application to white matter fiber tract mapping in the human brain. Magn Reson Med 42:526–540.

Parker GJ, Suckling J, Tanner SF, et al. 1997. Probing tumor microvascularity by measurement, analysis and display of contrast agent uptake kinetics. J Magn Reson Imaging 7:564–574.

Parker GJ, Tofts PS. 1999. Pharmacokinetic analysis of neoplasms using contrast-enhanced dynamic magnetic resonance imaging. Top Magn Reson Imaging 10:130–142.

Pierpaoli C, Jezzard P, Basser PJ, Barnett A, Di Chiro G. 1996. Diffusion tensor MR imaging of the human brain. Radiology 201:637–648.

Ross B, Michaelis T. 1994. Clinical applications of magnetic resonance spectroscopy. Magn Reson Q 10:191–247.

Ross B, Michaelis T. 1996. MR spectroscopy of the brain: neurospectroscopy. In: Edelman RR, Hessselink JR, Zlatkin M (eds), Clinical Magnetic Resonance Imaging. Philadelphia: WB Saunders, pp 928–981.

Sanders JA, Orrison WW, Jr. 1995. Functional magnetic resonance imaging. In: Orrison WW, Jr, Lewine JD, Sanders JA, Hartshorne MF (eds), Functional Brain Imaging. St Louis: Mosby Year Book, pp 239–326.

Schorner W, Laniado M, Niendorf HP, Schubert C, Felix R. 1986. Time-dependent changes in image contrast in brain tumors after gadolinium-DTPA. AJNR (Am J Neuroradiol) 7:1013–1020.

Sorensen AG, Rosen BR. 1996. Functional MRI of the brain. In: Atlas SW (ed), Magnetic Resonance Imaging of the Brain and Spine. New York: Raven Press, pp 1501–1545.

Sorensen AG, Tievsky AL, Ostergaard L, Weisskoff RM, Rosen BR. 1997. Contrast agents in functional MR imaging. J Magn Reson Imaging 7:47–55.

Sze G, Milano E, Johnson C, Heier L. 1990. Detection of brain metastases: comparison of contrast-enhanced MR with unenhanced MR and enhanced CT. AJNR (Am J Neuroradiol) 11:785–791.

Sze G, Soletsky S, Bronen R, Krol G. 1989. MR imaging of the cranial meninges with emphasis on contrast enhancement and meningeal carcinomatosis. AJR (Am J Roentgenol) 153:1039–1049.

Tofts PS. 1997. Modeling tracer kinetics in dynamic Gd-DTPA MR imaging. J Magn Reson Imaging 7:91–101.

Tofts PS, Kermode AG. 1991. Measurement of the blood–brain barrier permeability and leakage space using dynamic MR imaging. 1. Fundamental concepts. Magn Reson Med 17:357–367.

Tootell RB, Hadjikhani NK, Vanduffel W, et al. 1998. Functional analysis of primary visual cortex (V1) in humans. Proc Natl Acad Sci USA 95:811–817.

Turner R, Howseman A, Rees GE, Josephus O, Friston K. 1998. Functional magnetic resonance imaging of the human brain: data acquisition and analysis. Exp Brain Res 123:5–12.

Valk PE, Dillon WP. 1991. Radiation injury of the brain. AJNR (Am J Neuroradiol) 12:45–62.

van Gelderen P, de Vleeschouwer MH, DesPres D, Pekar J, van Zijl PC, Moonen CT. 1994. Water diffusion and acute stroke. Magn Reson Med 31:154–163.

Virta A, Barnett A, Pierpaoli C. 1999. Visualizing and characterizing white matter fiber structure and architecture in the human pyramidal tract using diffusion tensor MRI. Magn Reson Imaging 17:1121–1133.

Vion-Dury J, Meyerhoff DJ, Cozzone PJ, et al. 1994. What might be the impact on neurology of the analysis of brain metabolism by in vivo magnetic resonance spectroscopy? J Neurol 241:354–371.

Wong ET, Jackson EF, Hess KR, et al. 1998. Correlation between dynamic MRI and outcome in patients with malignant glioma. Neurology 50:777–781.

Yuh WT, Engelken JD, Muhonen MG, Mayr NA, Fisher DJ, Ernhardt JC. 1992. Experience with high-dose gadolinium MR imaging in the evaluation of brain metastases. AJNR (Am J Neuroradiol) 13:335–345.

2

Nuclear Medicine in Neuro-Oncology

FRANKLIN C. WONG AND E. EDMUND KIM

The usefulness of radionuclides in medicine has been well established through in vitro studies, diagnostic imaging, and the treatment of malignant and nonmalignant disease. The myriad permutations and developments in the use of radionuclides in medicine are directly reflected in the extensive medical literature on this subject. The specialty of nuclear medicine has involved translating this large body of data in a meaningful and efficacious way into clinical practice and research. This chapter examines the clinical application of nuclear medicine in neuro-oncology, particularly incorporating the results of in vitro and in vivo studies and diagnostic imaging into therapeutic schemes to improve patient care.

TRANSLATION BETWEEN IN VITRO AND IN VIVO STUDIES

Because of the high specific activities (i.e., radioactivities or disintegration per second per mass) of available radionuclides, their sensitivity of detection is also very high. For instance, ^{99m}Technetium (^{99m}Tc) is available at 1000 Ci/g, a level of radioactivity that translates into 3.7×10^{13} disintegrations per second per gram, or 3.7×10^{14} counts per second per mole. With a 10% counting efficiency, only approximately 0.3 pm of material is thus required to achieve a statistically significant count of 10,000 for 100 seconds of counting and detection. Radiopharmaceuticals commonly used in medical practice are in the subnanomolar concentration range. In general, the biologic effects from chemicals used at this low concentration are physiologically negligible. Because of this, only radioactivity units (e.g., Curie [Ci], mCi, or μCi), are used in nuclear medicine. These units represent the only measurable quantities that remain after initial quality control procedures are performed. This superior ability to detect subnanomolar ranges of molecular change confers advantages for nuclear medicine that surpass conventional radiology, including computed tomography (CT) and magnetic resonance imaging (MRI). CT and MRI can only deal with water and proton alterations at molar and millimolar levels. In contrast, radionuclide labels cause little perturbation in the chemical structure of host molecules. As a result, they provide true measures of in vivo physiology and pathology in terms of minute changes of biochemicals. This is especially true for ^{11}Carbon (^{11}C)- and ^{15}Oxygen (^{15}O)-labeled biochemicals that have nearly identical behavior compared with similar, unlabeled biochemicals.

The high sensitivity and low level of chemical perturbation from radionuclides enables accurate translation of results between in vitro, in vivo, and in situ studies. For instance, ^{64}Copper (^{64}Cu)-labeled Cu-pyruvaldehyde-bis(N4-methylthiosemicarbazone) (Cu-PTSM) was used to label C6 glioma cells in rats and to trace their biologic routes following intravenous injection. A micro positron emission tomography (PET) instrument capable of 2 mm resolution was used to monitor in vivo distribution of glioma cells for as long as 24 hours (Adonai et al., 2000). Although concordance between findings from in vitro and in vivo studies is often the rule, discordance was illustrated by a comparative study of peripheral benzodiazepine receptors in human brain tumors. 1-(2-Chlorophenyl)-*N*-methyl-*N*-(1-methylpropyl)-3-isoquinoline carboxamide (PK11195) in vitro binding to gliomas demonstrated more than a 20-fold elevated receptor density on the tumor cells (Price et al., 1990). Ex vivo autoradiography confirmed only an approximately sixfold elevated receptor density when the tissue was sectioned in thin layers and exposed to the ligand (Pappata et al., 1991). Human ^{11}C PK11195 PET images revealed a mere twofold increase in signal detected in tumor compared with that in surrounding brain tissue (Starosta-Rubinstein et al., 1990). The explanation for this loss of signal/noise ratio may be the multiple factors involved in biodistribution of any drug: transport, diffusion, endogenous competition, ligand binding, internalization of receptor, and imperfect detection of the signal in the living organism. Loss of signal between in vitro and in vivo studies is not unique to the brain or brain tumors and has been observed in other tumors and structures in the body.

Exaggeration of signals from in vitro experiments is occasionally encountered during in vivo studies. In the case of human meningioma detection by ^{111}Indium (^{111}In)-labeled octreotide (a somatostatin receptor ligand), very intense signal is usually the rule. However, in vitro receptor binding studies did not detect somatostatin receptors in about one-half of the meningioma surgical specimens assayed (Krenning et al., 1995). However, florid expression of somatostatin receptors occurred in the endothelium of the blood vessels surrounding the tumors. Such discordance between in vitro and in vivo studies is encountered in all medical disciplines. The use of radionuclides is often the first and only feasible approach that can be taken to verify concordance or to discover discordance. These observations, in turn, help direct rational planning of appropriate diagnostic and therapeutic strategies.

CONVENTIONAL SCINTIGRAPHY

Single-Photon Emission Computed Tomography, Brain Perfusion, and Cerebrospinal Fluid Circulation

The application of conventional scintigraphy to study cerebral structural integrity has largely been replaced by CT and MRI, which provide superior spatial resolution at the submillimeter level. The current resolution for PET and single-photon emission computed tomography (SPECT) is in the 5 to 10 mm range. PET and SPECT are important tools for evaluating physiologic functions and pathologies in neuro-oncology because of their ability to detect molecular changes near the submicromolar range. The practical lower limit of CT, MRI, or functional MRI is, however, at a millimolar level. Furthermore, the diagnostic imaging industry has provided clinicians with only a handful of CT and MRI contrast agents, and gram quantities are required for their use in humans. In contrast, hundreds of radionuclides have been synthesized that can be applied to study tumors, making the technology even more attractive.

Traditional SPECT techniques involve producing multiple planar images in quick succession followed with their reprojection according to algorithms similar to those used in CT and MRI. This approach has helped to delineate small structures deep within the body and head. It is limited clinically because no algorithm is available that allows absolute quantification of results. Nevertheless, this approach has provided invaluable qualitative and semiquantitative clinical information for tracer distribution in different parts of the body, including the brain. For patients without brain tumors, SPECT using ^{99m}Tc hetamethylpropyl-eneamine oxide (HMPAO) has been extensively applied to study the integrity of cerebral perfusion under pathologic conditions. One study has even correlated reversible perfusion defects with neuropsychological deficits in oncology patients receiving interferon (Meyers et al., 1994).

Figure 2–1 illustrates the use of ^{67}Gallium (^{67}Ga) to detect CNS lymphoma. ^{67}Ga empirically accumulates in many tumors with a high signal-to-background ratio. Although its uptake may be related to the transferin receptors that exist on lymphoma cells, the exact mechanism of localization remains unclear.

Early reports provide data for the use of ^{201}Thallium (^{201}Tl) SPECT, with its high uptake by tumor, to confirm recurrent glioma. In contrast, uptake in normal brain tissue or in necrotic tissue is quite low (Black et al., 1989). In this technique, typically, as much as 4 mCi of ^{201}Tl chloride is injected intravenously, followed shortly by acquisition of SPECT images. The advantage of ^{201}Tl-SPECT is that because normal brain tissue has little tracer uptake, malignant tissue with its high uptake appears with a high contrast ratio and can thus be defined. Uptake is usually

A
13.7+C
Jun 17
02:31:59
Mag =
FL:
ROT:
B
17
18
21
22
Coronal

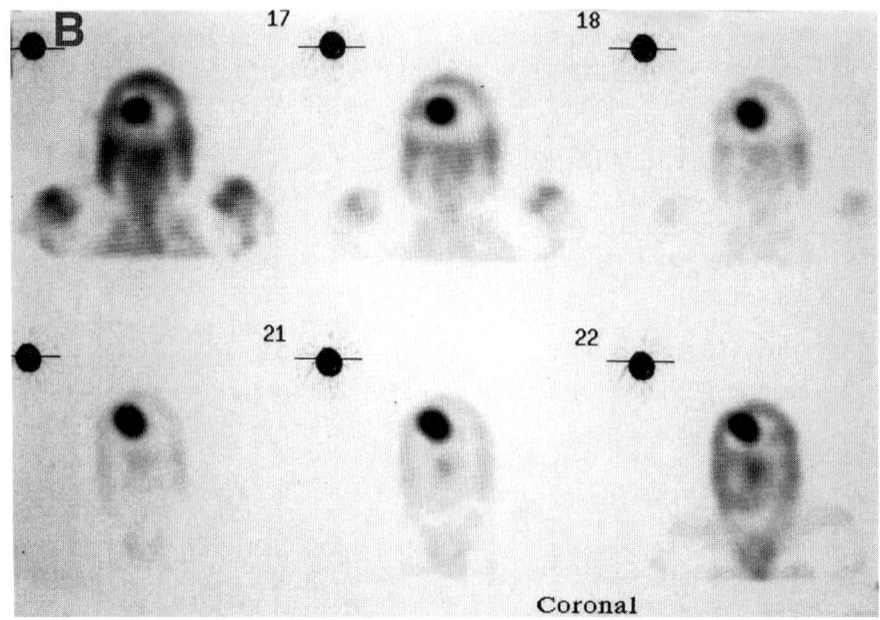

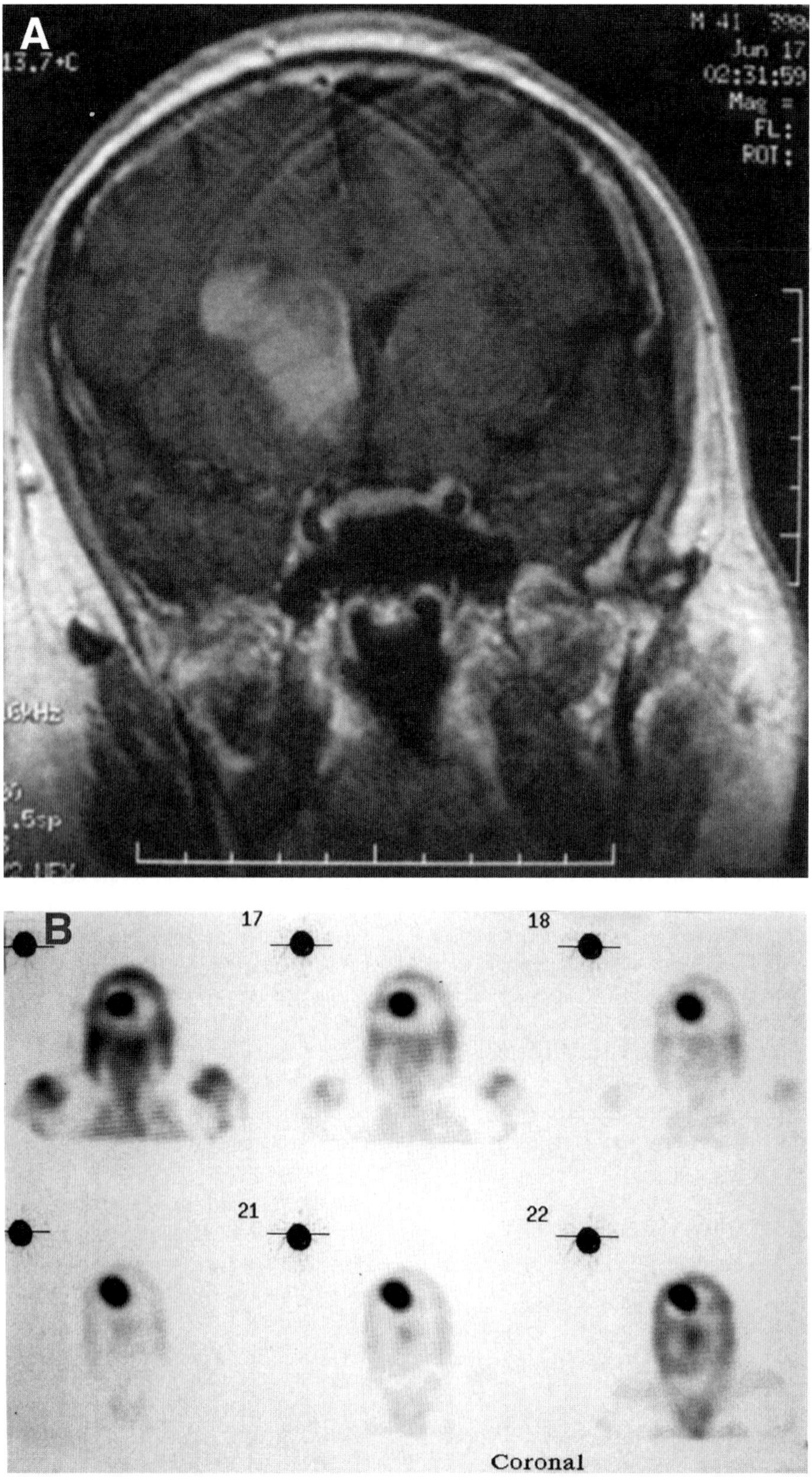

measured against either contralateral normal brain structures or the contralateral scalp, which has a relatively stable uptake (Holman et al., 1991). Earlier studies established lesion-to-scalp ratios above 3.5 for malignant tissue and ratios of 1.5 or below as being in the nonmalignant tumor range. This classification has defined ratios between 1.5 and 3.5 as undecided or nonspecific. Earlier investigators have attempted to use the perfusion index of tumor-to-cerebellum ratios to further distinguish lesions in this nonspecific range (Carvalho et al., 1992). The combined ^{201}Tl-SPECT and ^{99m}Tc-HMPAO SPECT approach is, however, technically demanding and time-consuming. Subsequent studies and our experience in patient care have failed to find this combined SPECT approach to be clinically feasible. Instead, our approach has been to adopt a maximum tumor-to-scalp ratio greater than 2.5 as a conclusive cut-off point for the diagnosis of recurrent tumor. For the range between 1.5 and 2.5, collaborative evidence, including conformation of lesion and temporal changes from measurements of varied intensities, are required to accurately interpret ^{201}Tl-SPECT data. Figure 2–2 shows a patient with recurrent anaplastic astrocytoma who had a high lesion-to-scalp ratio of 3.0.

^{99m}Tc-labeled sestamibi (MIBI) is an FDA-approved agent used to detect breast cancer. Although the exact mechanism of tumor uptake has not been established, it is energy dependent and requires mitochondrial integrity. The use of MIBI in detecting brain tumors in adults and children has been reported (O'Tuama et al., 1993). Its advantages include a higher allowable injected radiation dosage (to 40 mCi). However, because MIBI accumulates in the choroid plexus in a manner that cannot be suppressed by other drugs, false-positive or false-negative findings might ensue, particularly if the clinician chooses to ignore uptake in ventricular or periventricular areas where the choroid plexus resides. Nevertheless, recent reports in nuclear medicine have indicated that MIBI may provide better clinical confirmation of tumor recurrence than ^{201}Tl (Yamamoto et al., 2000). In a manner analogous to the study of the myocardium, temporal changes of ^{201}Tl uptake in tumors have been delineated with early results (15 to 30 minutes) compared with results from later (3 hour) phases. In other types of tumors, such analysis has yielded interesting correlations with the presence of recurrent tumor, although brain tumors have not been specifically addressed.

Other SPECT agents have been developed to measure altered metabolic pathways in brain tumors. For instance, ^{123}I-iodomethyltyrosine (IMT) has been extensively studied in Europe and Asia. The critical step in tumor IMT uptake is via a neutral amino acid transporter. Indeed, the level of IMT uptake in human brain tumor has been found to directly correlate with patient survival (Weber et al., 2000). Radioiodine analogues (^{123}I, ^{131}I, and ^{124}I) of iododeoxyuridine (IrdU) have also been applied to tomographic studies of brain tumor to nondestructively assay their elevated nucleotide production (Tjuvajev et al., 1994). Their correlations with tumor presence and grade were found to be independent of glucose metabolism.

In addition to tomographic imaging, dynamic or sequential images measured over different durations provide invaluable physiologic and pathologic information for neuro-oncologists. Determination of brain death is a task occasionally encountered in neuro-oncology. Although brain death as the sole determinant of death is somewhat controversial in the United States, realization of brain death per se can be difficult because administration of multiple medications and electroencephalographic variances can sometimes confound its determination. Scintigraphic dynamic and static imaging using either ^{99m}Tc-DTPA, ^{99m}Tc-neurolite (ECD), or ^{99m}Tc-ceretec (HMPAO) remain the most reliable methods to assess cerebral perfusion as an ancillary test for the determination of brain death. Typically, the imaging study itself is performed under stringent quality control. The absence of blood flow (radioactivity) in the parenchyma of the entire brain can be used as one of the ancillary criteria for brain death.

Dynamic and static scintigraphic images are helpful for evaluating cerebrospinal fluid (CSF) flow in neuro-oncologic patients, especially those with leptomeningeal metastasis who require intrathecal ther-

Figure 2–1. A patient with a history of central nervous system lymphoma presented with an enhancing lesion in the right basal ganglia extending to the periventricular area on MRI **(A).** The 48 hour delayed ^{67}Ga-SPECT (7 mCi, IV) showed intense uptake corresponding to the same location while the rest of the brain did not demonstrate significant uptake **(B).** Only small amounts of tracer are seen in the scalp, nasopharnx, and shoulders.

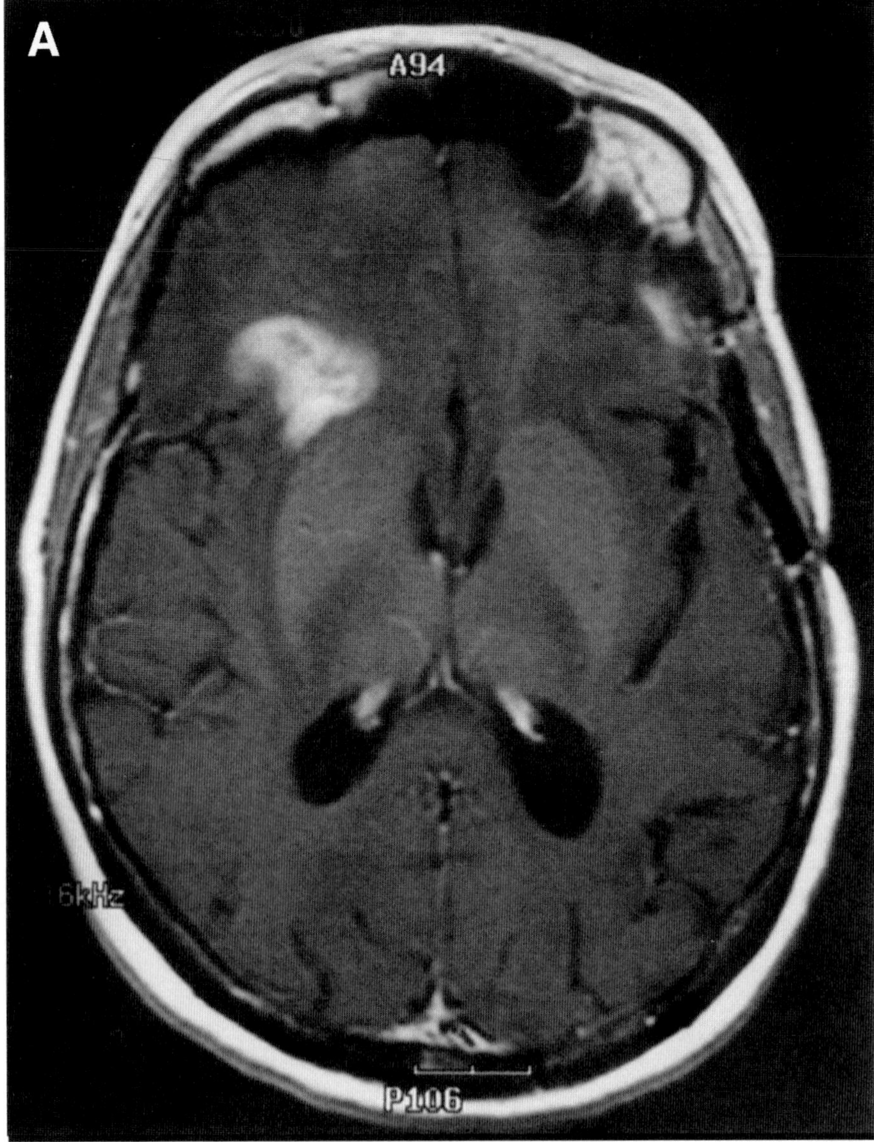

Figure 2–2. A patient with a history of treated anaplastic astrocytoma presented with a new enhancing MRI lesion **(A)** in the right posterior frontal lobe. The 30 minute delayed ^{201}Tl-SPECT (4 mCi, IV) in coronal, sagittal, and transverse projections **(B)** revealed an intense uptake in the lesion with a lesion-to-scalp ratio of 3.0, which is consistent with recurrent tumor. There is minimal tracer activity in the rest of the brain and physiologic tracer activity in the nasopharynx and scalp. The anterior planar image (lower right, B) of the head did not show enough signal-to-background activity to reveal the tumor. *(continued)*

apy. Our group has developed an algorithm to semi-quantitatively measure CSF flow from four serial whole-body images over 24 hours. Considering the entire CSF space as a single compartment, the effective half-life (Te) of ^{111}In-DTPA has been determined to be 12 to 20 hours (Wong et al., 1998a) with a mono-exponential decline. Cerebrospinal fluid flow rates can be altered by a CSF leak or by turning on the valve of a ventriculoperitoneal (VP) shunt (Wong et al., 1999); both result in a significantly shortened Te (3

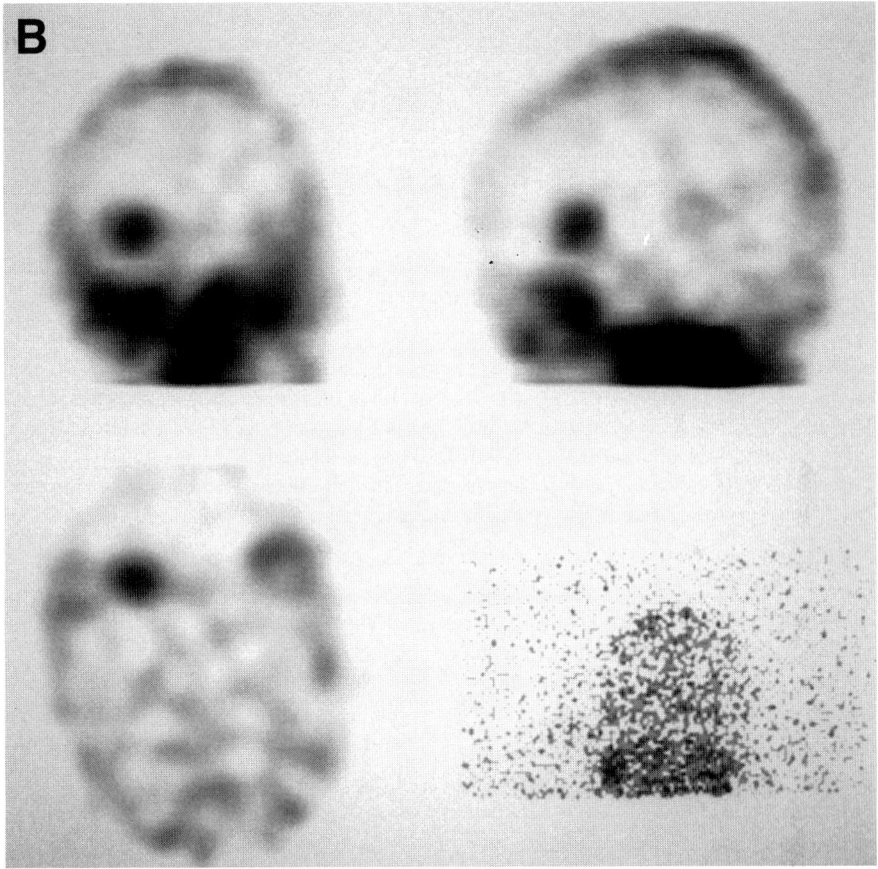

Figure 2–2. (*Continued*)

to 10 hours; Wong et al., 2000a). On the other hand, obstructive symptoms lengthen Te to over 20 hours (Wong et al., 1998b). Figure 2–3 illustrates that opening a closed VP shunt valve decreased Te from 40 hours to 7 hours in a patient with obstructive symptoms. The therapeutic implication of Te is that, owing to its monoexponential decline, total intrathecal tracer exposure (measured by the area under the curve [AUC]) is directly proportional to the tracer Te (Loevinger et al., 1988). For instance, methotrexate is a small, ionized molecule whose intrathecal pharmacokinetics are similar to those of ^{111}In-DTPA by simultaneous CSF sampling (Mason et al., 1998). Therefore, determining the Te of ^{111}In-DTPA will also provide an estimation of the effects of exposure to methotrexate or to similar drugs that are predominantly cleared from the CSF by bulk flow. This parallelism is not limited by whether the patient has a VP shunt or whether the VP valve is in the on or off position as long as the predominant route of clearance of the drug is via bulk CSF flow. In fact, Te measurement may be applied to guide the adjustment of intrathecal dosages of methotrexate or similar drugs in pathologic situations where the Te of ^{111}In-DTPA markedly deviates from the normal range.

The different techniques available in conventional scintigraphy continue to provide invaluable temporal and spatial information about brain tumor physiology and pathology.

APPLICATION OF POSITRON EMISSION TOMOGRAPHY IN NEURO-ONCOLOGY

The development of PET preceded that of MRI but was limited by medical practice policy, including the

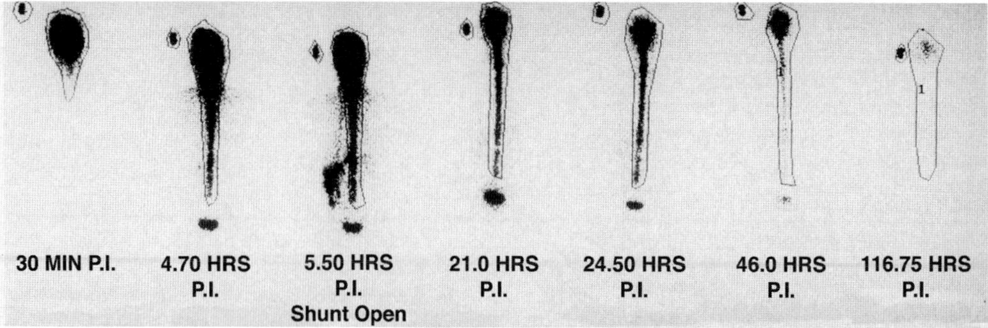

Figure 2–3. Whole-body images of a patient suffering from leptomeningeal metastasis from breast cancer. As part of an evaluation of the patency of CSF, she was injected with 0.5 mCi ^{111}In-DTPA via an Ommayo reservoir, which was connected with a ventriculoperitoneal shunt via an on–off valve. The dotted line encircling each image indicates where the level of radioactivity was measured for the one-compartment model. The valve was in the closed position for the first 5 hours. Initial effective half-life was 40 hours. Upon opening the valve, radioactivity is seen along the shunt and in the abdomen. The effective half-life after opening the valve was 7 hours, indicating communication between the CSF and extrathecal space P.I., postinjection.

lack of insurance reimbursement. With PET, after initial electronic gating for coincidence, tomographic images are obtained using reconstruction algorithms (and iterative methods) similar to those used in CT and MRI. Successful application of PET depends on effective utilization of the scanner, careful choice of PET radiopharmaceuticals, and the relevant interpretation of physiologic and pathologic findings. Currently, there are only a handful of available PET scanner models (GE, Seimens, Philips, and Imagtron). These models basically evolved from similar designs, and their performance depends on a combination of hardware that is used to collect high temporal and spatial resolution and software that is used to present the collected images in a meaningful fashion.

The latest generation of a PET multiple-slice scanner with the highest resolution available was developed at the M. D. Anderson Cancer Center. Called the MDAPET, it has a resolution down to 2.8 mm in plane and 2.9 mm axial (Uribe et al., 1999; Wong et al., 1996). This scanner was designed to use an innovative quadrant-sharing scheme to deploy detectors (Wong et al., 1993). Initial brain phantom studies show details similar to those derived from a low-end MRI. The development of other high-resolution PET scanners with similar detector schemes is being undertaken by several vendors in the industry. Furthermore, the development of combined CT-PET instruments is close to the marketing stage with the enticement of contemporaneous acquisition and registration of anatomic images (by CT) and metabolic images (by PET).

The study of human brain tumors using PET began in the 1970s. Gross pathology at the vascular level, such as perfusion abnormalities, was reported using ^{15}O-water PET (Ito et al., 1982). Breakdown of blood–brain barriers were reported with ^{68}Ga-PET (Yamamoto et al., 1977). Differential vascular responses between vessels in tumor versus brain were demonstrated via adenosine pharmacologic stimulation using ^{15}O-water PET (Baba et al., 1990). Vascular responses to physiologic stimulation have been assessed in patients with brain tumors for the purpose of identifying motor and sensory representation in brain parenchyma, data that have been used as a clinical tool for presurgical planning (Nariai et al., 1997). Since the 1970s, the regional perfusion of tumors has been investigated at cellular and subcellular levels, with particular attention being paid to oxygen consumption and glucose utilization. Although other specific PET tracers have been synthesized to study in situ cancer metabolism of sugar, lipid, amino acid, and nucleotides, ^{18}Fluorine (^{18}F)-fluoro-2-deoxy-D-glucose (FDG) remains the most commonly used tracer. It has gained federal approval for reimbursement in the clinical evaluation of lymphoma, melanoma, lung, esophageal, and colorectal tumors.

Tumor grading and staging are important tasks for the clinical oncologist. In the 1980s, increased ^{18}F-FDG uptake in gliomas was correlated with tumor grades (Di Chiro et al., 1982; Di Chiro, 1987). Because of its uptake by the normal cerebrum, ^{18}F-FDG is still the main tracer used to study the brains of patients with and without tumors. Despite the popular use of FDG in PET, the mechanism of action of FDG is not fully understood. Putative mechanisms include increased hexose kinase activity (Weber, 1977), increased uptake by surrounding macrophages (Kubota et al., 1994), and increased levels of glucose transporters in tumors (Fulham et al., 1994).

Tomographic images are typically acquired between 40 and 60 minutes after intravenous injection of 5 to 10 mCi of FDG followed by the acquisition and evaluation of qualitative images. Semiquantitative evaluation may involve measuring the standard uptake value (SUV), which is the measured radioactivity calibrated for injected dose and body weight. The SUV approach is applicable to all tracers and is more effective than visual inspection of the images alone. Exact quantification requires multiple image sessions over short durations along with arterial catheterization to obtain the arterial input function for deconvolution of the measured pharmacokinetic and pharmacodynamic parameters. Application of this approach is illustrated by a study of ^{11}C-*N*-methyspiperone (NMSP) used to compare the quantification of dopamine receptors on pituitary adenomas with postmortem in vitro binding data (Yung et al., 1993). However, the marginal gain achieved in clinical benefit from this type of vigorous maneuvering has not been established and at the moment is perhaps best suited to a research setting.

The clinical utility of PET resides in extrapolation of its results to treatment planning. Most PET studies of brain tumors are of primary brain tumors (i.e., gliomas) with the findings directing subsequent treatment plans, such as continuing chemotherapy, further surgery, or observation. The usefulness of FDG-PET in the routine clinical evaluation of brain tumors other than gliomas, however, is not known. Meningiomas and metastases have only been scantily investigated vis-à-vis PET because treatment is directed by surgery for meningiomas and directed by treatment of the primary tumor for metastases. The use of PET is also limited in both meningiomas and metastases because of their variable uptake of FDG, which ranges from hypermetabolism to hypometabolism. With gliomas, a group of brain tumors of varying grade, there is an apparent trend of a higher uptake by higher grade tumors. Few studies, however, have delineated specific FDG uptake by specific glioma histology.

FDG-PET remains useful for differentiating recurrent tumor and post-treatment necrosis. In contradistinction, MRI of post-treatment patients often reveals persistent contrast enhancement. This is due to alterations in the architecture of normal brain parenchyma caused by the tumor or by the treatment for the tumor. Thus, grossly abnormal CT and MRI signals, including contrast enhancement, remain whether there is or is not recurrent tumor. In PET, necrotic tissues often have low FDG uptake, whereas tumors have a markedly elevated uptake. Immediately after radiation treatment, FDG uptake by brain and tumor may increase slightly, return to baseline, but then become subnormal after a few weeks (Valk et al., 1988). Surgery and administration of systemic steroids produced no significant changes in FDG uptake in the few days that followed in this study. Determining the location of a metabolic lesion (e.g., in gray matter versus in white matter) may help to distinguish recurrent tumor from post-treatment necrosis because there is a preferential and variable physiologic uptake of FDG by the gray matter. Some might argue that the PET findings are not necessary because a patient with primary glioma is expected to have multiple foci of tumor and infiltrating tumor fronts that spread throughout the entire brain, including in post-treatment necrotic tissues. A recent trend in this area has been to assess the temporal change of ^{18}F-FDG uptake in tumors. One study took measurements using a 3 hour window after injection. Uptake in the tumor rose in contrast to a pattern of steady or decreasing uptake in inflammation (Zhuang et al., 2000). Preliminary studies have indicated that rising FDG uptake over time correlates with the presence of tumor. Whether this finding is relevant to brain tumors is unknown.

Although the use of ^{11}C-methionine PET has been restricted mainly to research centers, it is a promising alternative to ^{18}F-FDG PET. Because there is minimal background activity in the brain, the lesions are well enhanced. The technology is, however, limited by a very short synthesis time due to the short half-life of ^{11}C-methionine (20 minutes). Occasionally, post-treatment necrosis also exhibits high uptake of the tracer. In one series of 29 patients, ^{11}C-methionine PET was reported to have better sensitivity (90%

versus 80%) than ^{18}F-FDG PET, although their specificities were comparable (70%) (Haynie et al., 1993; Wong, 1993). The search for tumor-specific markers in PET continues, with increasing emphasis on tumor-specific molecules such as essential amino acids (e.g., L-^{11}C-methionine) (O'Tuama et al., 1988), nucleotides such as ^{124}I-IUDR (Carnochan and Brooks, 1999), dopamine D2 receptors (Yung et al., 1993), and peripheral benzodiazepine receptors. A recent emphasis has been the development of ^{18}F-labeled compounds for tumor imaging. Tumor-related hypoxia may be studied using ^{18}F-labeled imidazole analogues (Yang et al., 1995). ^{18}Fluoro-ethyl-L-tyrosine (FET) is a new PET agent used for detection of tyrosine transporters on human brain tumors, producing results that compare favorably with those from ^{11}C-methionine (Derlon, 1989). ^{18}F-(3′-deoxy-fluorothymidine), or FLT, is a tracer that is retained in the cell after phosphorylation by thymidine kinase in a manner analogous to the relationship between FDG and hexose kinase. Tumor uptake of FLT is markedly elevated against background activities on PET (Dohman et al., 2000). ^{18}F-labeled PET tracers have the obvious advantage of a longer physical half-life, which allows regional distribution shortly after synthesis from the cyclotron to imaging facilities in the vicinity up to 100 miles away. Confirmation of the usefulness of these tracers awaits large-scale human studies of various tumor types to determine specificity.

Although the application of PET in the routine care of neuro-oncology patients is still under development, advances in PET technology have been furthered through the development of PET instrumentation with high spatial and temporal resolutions, along with novel specific PET metabolic tracers percolating down from the laboratory to the clinical arena. Recent efforts to co-register anatomic images with metabolic images permits exact determination of the location of metabolic lesions. With established co-registration algorithms (Woods et al., 1993), MRI and PET images are fused, pixel to pixel, so that the metabolic lesion is clearly identified on the anatomic image, as seen in Color Figure 2–4. Research in this area has been bolstered by an infusion of federal research money for clinical studies, ushering in a new era in PET technology for use in oncology. These developments, along with supported research, are creating vast opportunities for improved patient care, as well as state-of-the-art clinical and basic research in neuro-oncology.

RADIONUCLIDE THERAPY IN NEURO-ONCOLOGY

External beam radiation therapy with various schemes to achieve high target to nontarget delivery remains in the mainstream of radiotherapy. The use of radionuclides in therapy nevertheless may prove advantageous in selected types of cancer. Beta-emitters (in contrast to gamma-emitters) with their short millimeter ranges and high radiation absorbed dose deposited in a small volume are theoretically useful in cancer treatment. However, except for thyroid cancers and their cerebral metastases, systemic administration does not deliver enough radioactivity to brain tumor sites (usually $<0.1\%$ of injected dose/gram) to be effective and simultaneously subjects the rest of the body to excessive toxicity.

Interestingly, for systemic applications outside of the central nervous system, two beta-emitters have been shown to be effective and have received FDA approval for the palliation of painful osseous metastasis. ^{89}Strontium (^{89}Sr) chloride (Metastron) (Nair, 1999) and ^{153}Samarium-EDTMP (^{153}Sm-EDTMP) (Quadramet) (Resche et al., 1997) have physical half-lives of 50 days and 2 days, respectively. They bind to osteoblastic centers in osseous metastases and serve as a localized irradiation source against metastatic tumors. As many as 80% of patients receive sustained relief of pain from osseous metastasis for several months or longer. Empirically, the onset of pain relief is faster (in 2 to 3 days) with ^{153}Sm-EDTMP than with ^{89}Sr (2 to 3 weeks). The faster onset of action of ^{153}Sm-EDTMP is probably related to its quick deposit of one-half of its radiation within a shorter duration.

There are few similar examples of effective radiopharmaceuticals to treat brain tumors. The approach is usually locoregional (Akabani et al., 2000a). Brachytherapy using ^{125}I seeds has been reported with mixed results that showed a benefit primarily in smaller glioblastoma tumors (Mehta and Sneed, 1997). Injection of ^{32}P-colloid is another approach with limited success in cystic glioma, and it also has been limited by producing systemic toxicity (reviewed by Harbert, 1996b). Direct injection of a small amount (0.5 mCi) of ^{201}Tl into experimental intracerebral gliomas in rats resulted in eradication of the tumors by Auger electrons (Sjoholm et al., 1995), but no human studies have been reported. More recently, intracavitary brachytherapy using inflatable double-lumen balloons filled with ^{125}I-iodo-hydroxybenzene sulfonate (Iotrex) in amounts as high as 532 mCi and as long as 16 hours of exposure has had few incremental adverse effects (deGuzman et al., 2000). A phase I study of intralesional continuous infusion into a glioma mass of ^{131}I-labeled chimeric antibodies against DNA/histone complexes has also been reported and demonstrates quadruple tracer retention through multiple-catheter injection (Spicer et al., 2000).

An Italian study of intralesional injection of monoclonal antibodies (BC4) against tenascin into patients with glioblastoma multiforme reported improved survival with ^{90}Y-labled BC4 and ^{131}I-labeled BC4. The overall median survival rates for ^{90}Y-BC4 in this study were 17 and 32 months for bulky disease and small remnant disease, respectively, and 14 months and 24 months, respectively, for ^{131}I-BC4 (Riva et al., 2000). The study population was composed of patients who had multiple previous failed therapy regimens, including radioimmunotherapy. Studies in more stratified patient populations are necessary to confirm the significance of results obtained thus far.

Alpha-emitters may provide a higher radiation absorbed dose to a more confined volume. This occurs because a high level of energy is emitted from the massive particle and delivered at a close range that is less than 0.1 mm in diameter. In theory, one particle is sufficient to destroy a cell. Such a high potential for destruction can also engender nonspecific toxicity because essentially all tissues in the immediate vicinity are subject to destruction along with tumor tissue. The clinical use of alpha-emitters will require specific knowledge of dosimetry at organ, tissue, cellular, and subcellular levels (microdosimetry). Despite these potential barriers, the clinical applications of alpha-emitters will increase because of their greater availability following the Cold War. In fact, the use of postsurgical intracavitary injection of up to 10 mCi of ^{213}Bi-81C6 antibodies in human glioma has been reported to cause low systemic toxicity in a phase I human study (Akabani et al., 2000b). Dosimetric estimates have also been derived (McLendon et al., 1999), confirming a high absorption of radiation in tumor contrasted with low levels of radiation absorption by the rest of the body.

Locoregional use of gold radiocolloid for intrathecal treatment of leptomeningeal metastasis has had partial success, limited by hematotoxicity, myelopathy, and radiculopathy, the last being due to sequestration of colloid in the thecal sac (Harbert, 1996a). Several groups reported the use of intrathecal ^{131}I-labeled monoclonal and polyclonal antibodies to treat leptomeningeal metastasis (Bigner et al., 1995). Using a ^{131}I dosage as high as 140 mCi with 60 mg proteins, scientists reported promising results, with hematotoxicity as the dose-limiting factor. However, what contribution antigen–antibody binding makes to the effectiveness of this treatment has not been established. In fact, this hypothesis may be in doubt because of the multiple biologic barriers that antibodies must overcome to reach and remain bound to the limited supply of antigens. The radiation dosimetry in CSF from this class of radiopharmaceuticals is only marginally better than that from ^{131}I-sodium iodide (Wong et al., 2000b) or ^{131}I-labeled human serum albumin (Johnston et al., 1972; Stabin and Evans, 1999), both of which have no tumor binding affinity.

The disadvantages of monoclonal antibodies (MoAbs) include their limited availability, the presence of foreign protein in the CSF, and the prolonged retention of ^{131}I that directly correlates with hematotoxicity (Wahl et al., 1998). One recent study employed ^{90}Y-labeled biotin in postsurgical cavities, with and without pre-targeting with biotinylated anti-tenascin MoAbs to treat glioblastoma patients. The preliminary results have demonstrated slight improvement in outcome with MoAb (one more patient in partial remission) but no difference in survival (Bartolomei et al., 2000). In fact, our laboratories are studying whether intrathecal application of beta-emitting radiopharmaceuticals with no tumor affinity is sufficient for treating leptomeningeal metastasis. Earlier simulations have demonstrated a promising radiation dose delivery to tumors in the CSF, with little effects on the brain and spinal cord (Wong et al., 2000c). A phase I human study is underway at M. D. Anderson Cancer Center. It is hoped that the results from this trial will show that locoregional application of nonspecific beta-emitters in the CSF may provide sufficient radiation to treat tumor cells in the CSF and surrounding leptomeninges.

With the availability of more radionuclides, a better understanding of radiation biology, and establishment of more precise dosimetric measurements, the use of alpha- and beta-emitters in neuro-oncology therapy may prove to be desirable alternatives after conventional therapeutic avenues have been exhausted.

CONCLUSION

Both nuclear medicine and neuro-oncology have shared in the benefits derived from the explosive growth of medical knowledge during the last few decades. Along with a constant flux of theoretical and empirical changes in medicine, the role of nuclear medicine in neuro-oncology has continued to evolve. Its initial role in evaluation of anatomic integrity has been transformed into a confirmatory role of physiologic and pathologic anomalies in brain tumors in which anatomic alterations have already been established. An increased understanding of how radionuclides interact with tissues has also enabled beta-emitters, and possibly alpha-emitters, to be used in cancer therapy. Whereas one of the current trends in medicine is to provide more specific diagnostic insights and therapeutic strategies aimed at the molecular level, nuclear medicine techniques have become invaluable in the practice of oncology and neuro-oncology. Nuclear medicine applications will play increasingly important roles in the future of clinical medicine because of the advantages of picomolar sensitivity and low chemical perturbation, along with the development of new instruments for monitoring and new molecular markers that can be used as probes on the organ level as well as on a subnucleotide level.

REFERENCES

Adonai N, Nguyen K, Walsh J, et al. 2000. Ex vivo Cu-PTSM labeling of cells as a method to image in vivo cell trafficking with PET. J Nucl Med 41:256P.

Akabani G, Cokgor I, Coleman RE, et al. 2000a. Dosimetry and dose–response relationships in newly diagnosed patients with malignant gliomas treated with iodine-131–labeled anti-tenascin monoclonal antibody 81C6 therapy. Int J Radiat Oncol Biol Phys 46:947–958.

Akabani G, McLendon RE, Bigner DD, Zalutsky MR. 2000b. Microdosimetry of alpha-particle–emitting At-211–labelled monoclonal antibody (MAb) using histological images of malignant brain tumors. J Nucl Med 41:84P.

Baba T, Fukui M, Takeshita I, Ichiya Y, Kuwabara Y, Hasuo K. 1990. Selective enhancement of intratumoral blood flow in malignant gliomas using intra-arterial adenosine triphosphate. J Neurosurg 72:907–911.

Bartolomei M, Grana G, Farrari M, Cremonesi M, Chinol M, Paganelli G. 2000. Pretargeting ^{90}Y-biotin radiotherapy in glioblastoma patients. Eur J Nucl Med 27:A941.

Bigner DD, Brown M, Coleman E, et al. 1995. Phase I studies of treatment of malignant gliomas and neoplastic meningitis with ^{131}I-radiolabeled monoclonal antibodies anti-tenascin 81C6 and anti-chondroitin proteoglycan sulfate me1-14 F (ab) 2—a preliminary report. Neuro-Oncol 24:109–122.

Black KL, Hawkins RA, Kim KT, Becker DP, Lerner C, Marciano D. 1989. Use of thallium-201 SPECT to quantitate malignancy grade of gliomas. J Neurosurg 71:342–346.

Carnochan P, Brooks R. 1999. Radiolabelled 5′-iodo-2′-deoxyuridine: a promising alternative to [18F]-2-fluoro-2-deoxy-D-glucose for PET studies of early response to anticancer treatment. Nucl Med Biol 26:667–672.

Carvalho PA, Schwartz RB, Alexander E 3d, et al. 1992. Detection of recurrent gliomas with quantitative thallium-201/technetium-99m HMPAO single-photon emission computerized tomography. J Neurosurg 74:565–570.

deGuzman AF, Karvelis SKC, Shaw EG, et al. 2000. Brachytherapy of re-resected malignant glioma cavity margins using an inflatable balloon catheter and liquid 125I source: a phase I study. J Nucl Med 41:274P (abstract).

Derlon JM, Bourdet C, Bustany P, et al. [11C]L-methionine uptake in gliomas. Neurosurgery 25:720–728.

Di Chiro G. 1987. Positron emission tomography using (18F) fluorodeoxyglucose in brain tumors. A powerful diagnostic and prognostic tool. Invest Radiol 22:360–371.

Di Chiro G, DeLaPaz RL, Brooks RA, et al. 1982. Glucose utilization of cerebral gliomas measured by [18F]fluorodeoxyglucose and PET. Neurology 32:1323–1329.

Dohman BM, Dittmann H, Wei R, et al. 2000. ^{18}F FLT Vs ^{18}F FDG for tumor PET: first results of a comparative study. J Nucl Med 41:274P.

Fulham MJ, Melisi JW, Nishimiya J, et al. 1994. Neuroimaging of juvenile pilocytic astrocytomas: an enigma. Radiology 189:221–225.

Harbert J. 1996a. Intrathecal radiocolloids in meningeal leukemia. In: Harbert JC, Eckelman WC, Neumann RD (eds), Nuclear Medicine: Diagnosis and Therapy. New York: Thieme Medical Publishers, pp 1157–1162.

Harbert JC. 1996b. Radionuclide therapy of cystic brain tumors in meningeal leukemia. In: Harbert JC, Eckelman WC, Neumann RD (eds), Nuclear Medicine: Diagnosis and Therapy. New York: Thieme Medical Publishers, pp 1083–1092.

Haynie TP, Wong FC, Kim EE, et al. 1993. Comparison of C-11 methionine and F-18 FDG for tumor imaging with positron emission tomography (PET). Eur J Nucl Med 20:829.

Holman BL, Zimmerman RE, Johnson KA, et al. 1991. Computer-assisted superimposition of magnetic resonance and high-resolution technetium-99m–HMPAO and thallium-201 SPECT images of the brain. J Nucl Med 32:1478–1484.

Ito M, Lammertsma AA, Wise RJ, et al. 1982. Measurement of regional cerebral blood flow and oxygen utilisation in patients with cerebral tumours using ^{15}O and positron emission tomography: analytical techniques and preliminary results. Neuroradiology 23:63–74.

Johnston RE, Staab E, Brill AB, Allen JH. 1972. Radiation dosimetry associated with the intrathecal administration of ^{131}I human serum albumin. Br J Radiol 45:444–451.

Krenning EP, Kwekkeboom DJ, Panwels S, Kvols LK, Reubi JC. 1995. Somatostatin receptor scintigraphy. In: Freeman LM (ed), Nuclear Medicine Annual, New York: Raven Press, pp 1–50.

Kubota R, Kubota K, Yamada S, Tada M, Ido T, Tamahashi N. 1994. Active and passive mechanisms of [F-18] fluorodeoxyglucose uptake by proliferating and prenecrotic cancer cells in vivo: a microautoradiographic study. J Nucl Med 35:1067–1075.

Loevinger R, Budinger TF, Watson EE. 1988. Chapter 1. Introduction, MIRD Primer for Absorbed Dose Calculations. New York: Society of Nuclear Medicine, pp 1–20.

Mason WP, Yeh SDJ, DeAngelis LM. 1998. 111Indium-diethylenetriamine pentaacetic acid cerebrospinal fluid flow studies predict distribution of intrathecally administered chemotherapy and outcome in patients with leptomeningeal metastases. Neurology 50:438–444.

McLendon RE, Archer GE, Larsen RH, Akabani G, Bigner DD, Zalutsky MR. 1999. Radiotoxicity of systemically administered 211at-labeled human/mouse chimeric monoclonal antibody: a long-term survival study with histologic analysis. Int J Radiat Oncol Biol Phys 45:491–499.

Mehta MP, Sneed PK. 1997. Insterstitial radiation therapy for brain tumors. In: Nag S (ed), Principles and Practice of Brachytherapy. Armonk, NY: Futurea, pp 247–267.

Meyers CA, Valentine AD, Wong FC, et al. 1994. Reversible neurotoxicity of interleukin-2 and tumor necrosis factor: correlation of SPECT with neuropsychological testing. J Neuropsychiatry Clin Neurosci 6:285–288.

Nair N. 1999. Relative efficacy of 32P and 89Sr in palliation in skeletal metastases. J Nucl Med 40:256–261.

Nariai T, Senda M, Ishii K, et al. 1997. Three-dimensional imaging of cortical structure, function and glioma for tumor resection. J Nucl Med 38:1563–1568.

O'Tuama LA, Guilarte TR, Douglass KH, et al. 1988. Assessment of [11C]-L-methionine transport into the human brian. J Cereb Blood Flow Metab 8:341–345.

O'Tuama LA, Treves ST, Larar JN, et al. 1993. Tallium-201 versus technetium-99m-MIBI SPECT in evaluation of childhood brain tumors: a within-subject comparison. J Nucl Med 34:1045–1051.

Pappata S, Cornu P, Samson Y, et al. 1991. PET study of carbon-11–PK-11195 binding to peripheral type benzodiazepine sites in glioblastoma: a case report. J Nucl Med 32:1608–1610.

Price GW, Ahier RG, Hume SP. 1990. In vivo binding to peripheral benzodiazepine binding sites in lesioned rat brain: comparison between [^{3}H]PK11195 and [^{18}F]PK14105 as markers for neuronal damage. J Neurochem 55:175–185.

Resche I, Chatal JF, Pecking A, et al. 1997. A dose-controlled study of 153Sm-ethylenediaminetetramethylenephosphonate (EDTMP) in the treatment of patients with painful bone metastases. Eur J Cancer 33:1583–1591.

Riva P, Franceschi G, Frattarelli M, et al. 2000. Intralesional radioimmunotherapy of glioblastoma. Comparison of the results obtained with I-131 and Y-90–labelled antitenascin monoclonal Antibodies. J Nucl Med 41:A272P.

Sjoholm H, Ljunggren K, Adeli R, et al. 1995. Necrosis of malignant gliomas after intratumoral injection of 201Tl in vivo in the rat. Anticancer Drugs 6:109–114.

Spicer KM, Patel S, Gordon L, Van Tassel P, Bloodworth G. 2000. Intracerebral distribution of I-131-chTNT 1/B: Comparison of Drug vs. tumor volume with single/dual catheter infusions. J Nucl Med 41:272P (abstract).

Stabin MG, Evans JF. 1999. The Radiation Dosimetry of Intrathecally Administrated Radionuclides. Sixth International Radiopharmaceutical Dosimetry Symposium, Oak Ridge Associated Universities 99-0164, pp 500–512.

Starosta-Rubinstein S, Ciliax BJ, Penney JB, McKeever P, Young AB. 1990. Imaging of a glioma using peripheral benzodiazepine receptor ligands. Proc Natl Acad Sci USA 84: 891–895.

Tjuvajev JG, Macapinlac HA, Daghighian F, et al. 1994. Imaging of brain tumor proliferative activity with iodine-131-iododeoxyuridine. J Nucl Med 35:1407–1417.

Uribe J, Baghaei H, Li H, et al. 1999. Basic imaging performance charactieristics of a variable field of view PET camera using quandrant sharing detector design. IEEE T Nucl Sci 46:491–497.

Valk PE, Budinger TF, Levin VA, Silver P, Gutin PH, Doyle WK. 1988. PET of malignant cerebral tumors after interstitial brachytherapy. Demonstration of metabolic activity and correlation with clinical outcome. J Neurosurg 69:830–838.

Wahl RL, Kroll S, Zasadny KR. 1998. Patient-specific whole-body dosimetry: principles and a simplified method for clinical implementation. J Nucl Med 39:14S–20S.

Weber G. 1977. Enzymology of cancer cells (first of two parts). N Engl J Med 296:486–492.

Weber W, Grosu A, Dick S, et al. 2000. Prognostic value of residual I-123-alpha-methyl-L-tyrosine (IMT) uptake after resection of primary brain tumors. J Nucl Med 41:A69P.

Wong FC, Jaeckle KA, Kim EE, et al. 1998a. Whole-body ommayogram in the evaluation of CSF flow in patients with leptomeningeal carcinomatosis (LC). Eur J Nucl Med 25(8):A1075.

Wong FC, Jaeckle KA, Kim EE, McCullough S, Macey D, Podoloff DA. 1998b. Delayed clearance of in-111 DTPA from cerebral spinal fluid (CFS) correlates with signs of obstruction in patients with leptomeningeal carcinomatosis (LC). Neurology 50:A382.

Wong FC, Jaeckle KA, Kim EE, Podoloff DA. 1999. Whole-body scintigraphic estimation of clearance of In-111 DTPA in the CSF of patients with VP shunt. Neurology 52:A198.

Wong FC, Kim EE, Jaeckle KA, et al. 2000a. CSF Leakage is associated with shortened effective tracer half-life (TE) during a whole-body cisternogram. Eur J Nucl Med 27:A1117.

Wong FC, Sparks R, Kim EE, et al. 2000b. Dosimetric considerations for intrathecal beta-emitters for ablative therapy (IBEAT) against leptomeningeal metastasis (LM) using beta-emitting radiopharmaceuticals. Neurology 54:A37.

Wong FC, Sparks R, Kim EE, Podoloff DA. 2000c. Simulated dosimetry of intraventrically-injected beta-emitters for ablative therapy against leptomeningeal metastasis in patients with or without CSF stasis. J Nucl Med 41:A237P.

Wong FCL, Kim EE, Korkmaz M, et al. 1993. Semi-quantitative PET assessment of recurrent brain tumors using C11-methionine and F-18 FDG. J Nucl Med 34:A206.

Wong WH. 1993. A positron camera detector design with cross-coupled scintillators and quadrant sharing photomultipliers. IEEE T Nucl Sci 40:962–966.

Wong WH, Uribe J, Lu W, et al. 1996. Design of a variable field prototype pet camera. IEEE Trans Nucl Sci 43:1915–1920 (abstract).

Woods RP, Mazziotta JC, Cherry SR. 1993. MRI-PET registration with automated algorithm. J Comput Assist Tomogr 17:536–546.

Yamamoto Y, Nishiyama Y, Takahashi K, et al. 2000. Clinical role of 99mTc and 201Tl SPECT in differentiation between recurrent brain tumors and post-treatment necrosis. J Nucl Med 41:A69P.

Yamamoto YL, Thompson CJ, Meyer E, Robertson JS, Feindel W. 1977. Dynamic positron emission tomography for study of cerebral hemodynamics in a cross section of the head using positron-emitting 68 Ga-EDTA and 77 Kr. J Comput Assist Tomogr 1:43–56.

Yang DJ, Wallace S, Cherif A, et al. 1995. Development of F-18–labeled fluoroerythronitroimidazole as a PET agent for imaging tumor hypoxia. Radiology 194:795–800.

Yung BCK, Wand GS, Blevins L, et al. 1993. In vivo assessment of dopamine receptor density in pituitary macroadenoma and correlation with in vitro assay. J Nucl Med 34:133P.

Zhuang HM, Lee JH, Lambright E, et al. 2000. Experimental evidence in support of dual-time point FDG-PET imaging for differentiating malignancy from inflammation. J Nucl Med 41:114P.

Part II

Primary Central Nervous System Tumors

3

Primary Cerebral Tumors

MITCHEL S. BERGER, STEVEN A. LEIBEL, JANET M. BRUNER, JONATHAN L. FINLAY, AND VICTOR A. LEVIN

The intracranial supratentorial compartment is the most common site for central nervous system (CNS) tumors. Understanding tumors that arise within the supratentorial brain is, therefore, of the utmost importance. This chapter provides the reader with a reasonably thorough understanding of *(1)* the symptoms and signs of tumors that arise within the various supratentorial locations; *(2)* the various approaches to surgical intervention, from biopsy to cortical mapping, for tumors in eloquent sites of the brain; *(3)* the pathologic classification and grading schemes used around the world for the various supratentorial tumors; *(4)* conventional as well as other radiation approaches such as brachytherapy, radiosurgery, three-dimensional conformal radiotherapy, and proton beam treatment for the tumors; and *(5)* the progress and limitations of chemotherapy used with radiation and as independent therapy. In addition, some major and subtle differences between children and adult patients with primary brain tumors are noted. Therapeutic approaches to tumors in infants are not covered in this chapter as they are rare and too specialized for this text.

SYMPTOMS AND SIGNS

Neurologic symptoms and physical signs reflect the location of tumor rather than tumor histology. Symptoms are at two levels: general symptoms, associated with increased intracranial pressure; and focal symptoms, related to tumor location.

General symptoms are headache, gastrointestinal upset such as nausea and vomiting, personality changes, and slowing of psychomotor function. Because the brain parenchyma does not have pain-sensitive structures, headache has been attributed to local swelling and distortion of pain-sensitive nerve endings associated with blood vessels, primarily in the meninges. Many tumors grow without headache as a prominent symptom, but others rapidly lead to headache either because of the tumor's proximity to pain-sensitive fibers or due to its rapid growth and the achievement of a critical volume that causes compression and displacement of brain. Under the latter circumstances, the onset and disappearance of headache correlate with changes in intracranial pressure. Headaches can vary in severity and quality; frequently they occur in the early morning hours or upon first awakening. Sometimes patients complain of an uncomfortable feeling in the head rather than headache.

Gastrointestinal symptoms such as loss of appetite, queasiness, nausea, and occasionally vomiting can occur in all patients but are most common in children and in patients harboring infratentorial rather than supratentorial tumors. Changes in personality, mood, mental capacity, and concentration can be noted early or can be the only abnormalities observed. In general, patients with brain tumors tend to sleep longer at night and nap during the day. These symptoms are not unique to individuals with brain tumors and can easily be confused with depression, neurasthenia, and other psychological problems.

Focal symptoms can be episodic (seizures) or progressive. Seizures are important harbingers of brain tumors; although only 10% of patients presenting with seizures are diagnosed with a brain tumor, the association increases with increasing patient age. Seizures are a presenting symptom in approximately 20% of patients with supratentorial brain tumors. Rapidly growing, infiltrative malignant gliomas are likely to produce complex partial motor or sensory seizures, although generalized grand mal seizures are also common. In patients with slowly growing astrocytomas, gangliogliomas, and oligodendrogliomas, generalized seizures may antedate the clinical diagnosis by months to years. The etiology of seizures associated with these tumors is unclear, although experimental evidence implicates a depletion of gamma aminobutyric acid (GABA) and somatostatin-immunoreactive neurons in the adjacent, nontumor-infiltrated epileptogenic brain (Haglund et al., 1992). Focal seizures that occur in patients older than 40 years of age are indicative of a brain tumor until proven otherwise.

The distribution of infiltrative parenchymal tumors in the brain has a direct relationship to the mass of the affected lobe or region. The most frequently involved locations in the cerebrum are, in descending order of frequency, frontal, parietal, temporal, and occipital lobes. Clinical patterns of tumor growth in the various brain locations are less stereotypic than those observed after strokes; nonetheless, understanding the nature of the various syndromes that present will help clinicians to better understand the effect of tumor growth in the CNS.

Frontal lobe tumors can be asymptomatic or can produce mild slowing of contralateral hand movements, contralateral spastic hemiplegia, marked elevation in mood or loss of initiative, and dysphasia (if the involved lobe is the dominant lobe). Bifrontal disease is, unfortunately, all too common and can cause bilateral hemiparesis, spastic bulbar palsy, severe impairment of intellect, lability of mood, and dementia.

Temporal lobe tumors can be clinically silent or can produce impairment of recent memory, homonymous quadrantanopsia, auditory hallucinations, and even aggressive behavior. Involvement of the nondominant temporal lobe can lead to minor perceptual problems and spatial disorientation. Dominant temporal lobe involvement can lead to dysnomia, impaired perception of verbal commands, and even full-blown, fluent Wernicke-like aphasia. Bilateral disease involving both temporal lobes is rare compared with the common occurrence of bilateral disease in frontal lobe tumors that readily cross through the corpus callosum. However, in some cases, use of opposed lateral field radiation portals can lead to bilateral temporal lobe damage that can be devastating for the patient as it produces impairment of recent memory and can lead to dementia.

Parietal lobe tumors affect sensory and perceptual functions more than motor functions, although mild hemiparesis is sometimes seen with extensive parietal lobe tumors. Abnormalities may range from mild, and observable only by formal testing, to severe sensory loss leading to hemianesthesia and/or other hemisensory abnormalities. In addition to homonymous hemianopsia or visual inattention, involvement of the nondominant parietal lobe can lead to perceptual abnormalities, anosognosia, and an apraxia for dressing oneself; dominant parietal lobe tumors lead to alexia, dysgraphia, and other types of apraxia.

Occipital lobe tumors can produce contralateral homonymous hemianopsia or visual aberrations that take the form of imperception of color, object size, or object location. Bilateral occipital damage rarely occurs as a result of tumor invasion, but it can be produced in herniation syndromes and can lead to cortical blindness.

Thalamic and basal ganglia tumors can reach 3 to 4 cm in diameter before the patient experiences symptoms, which can be nonspecific headaches resulting from hydrocephalus and increased intracranial pressure secondary to trapping of the lateral horn of one of the ventricles. Patients can also present with contralateral sensory abnormalities detected only by testing for sensory extinction or, rarely, with a severe neuropathic pain syndrome. Some patients complain of intermittent paresthesias on the contralateral side; these are at times so episodic that anticonvulsant drugs are prescribed. Contralateral intention tremor and hemiballistic-like movement disorders are uncommon.

GENERAL SURGICAL METHODS AND TECHNIQUES

Biopsy Techniques

A simple and readily available method that can be used to obtain a biopsy specimen is with computer tomography (CT) or magnetic resonance imaging (MRI) guidance. After a localizing CT or MRI scan is done, a small twist drill opening is made in the skull and a biopsy needle is placed into it and imaged to ensure correct placement; a tumor sample is then taken and a repeat scan performed to make sure no hemorrhage has occurred. A comparison of the freehand method with one using a stereotactic apparatus, found no significant difference in morbidity and mortality between the two procedures (Wen et al., 1993).

An alternative biopsy approach involves the use of ultrasonography via a burr hole (Berger, 1986; Enzmann et al., 1984; Tsutsumi et al., 1989). This has been performed very accurately on lesions greater than 7 to 10 mm and provides immediate feedback after the procedure to ensure that a hemorrhage has not occurred. In a study comparing this method to CT-guided stereotactic techniques, the diagnostic yield rate was found to be comparable for CT-guided and ultrasound-guided approaches (94% versus 91%) (Di Lorenzo et al., 1991). Both methods resulted in a similar number of complications. The ultrasound biopsy method, however, had a shorter operative time and was significantly less costly.

With the advent of CT-coupled stereotactic frames in the late 1970s and early 1980s, surgeons had the capability of obtaining tissue specimens with millimeter accuracy. The components of the most commonly used apparatus, the Brown-Roberts-Wells frame, included a base ring that was fixed to the skull and a localizing ring with nine graphite rods to allow lesions to be referenced in three dimensions (Heilbrun et al., 1983). An arc guidance system fit into the base ring allows any two points in three-dimensional space to be traversed (e.g., entry and target points). This represented a tremendous step forward in neurosurgical instrumentation and precision. Experience has shown that tumor biopsy accuracy has been greatest when directed to the tumor center and the immediately surrounding contrast-enhancing tissue. The diagnostic accuracy for grade and type of lesion may be enhanced by including cytologic squash preparations with the histology (Cappabianca et al., 1991).

Comparing histologic findings from lesions that were biopsied and subsequently resected, the discrepancy rate was greatest with astrocytic tumors in terms of their grade (Chandrasoma et al., 1989). This is clearly a problem when small samples are obtained, especially when differentiating between low-grade gliomas and reactive gliosis (Taratuto et al., 1991). Notwithstanding that, the stereotactic biopsy technique is the most accurate method for obtaining tissue, regardless of the type of frame used, and this method is the standard against which all other methods of obtaining small tissue samples should be compared.

Stereotactic-Guided Volumetric Resections

Kelly and colleagues (1982, 1983) developed an innovative technique that coupled imaging with computer-assisted stereotactic resection of tumors. Reconstructed tumor sections based on CT and MRI results are displayed to the surgeon on a video terminal during surgery, allowing for precise, stereotactic laser vaporization of any intracranial target. It became apparent early in their experience that this approach was more beneficial for patients with circumscribed lesions (i.e., metastasis, pilocytic astrocytoma, and so forth) than for those with more infiltrative glial tumors (Kelly et al., 1986). The morbidity associated with this procedure is acceptable; however, the outcome for malignant glial tumors was disappointing. Survival data were not significantly different compared with those from conventional radical resections (Kelly, 1988).

The limitations of all surgical approaches have more to do with the infiltrative nature of gliomas than with surgical technique. Stereotactic biopsy samples from brain adjacent to the contrast-enhanced and hypodense areas in high- and low-grade gliomas demonstrated isolated tumor cells well beyond the bulk of the image-defined tumor mass (Kelly et al., 1987; Kelly, 1993). Extending the resection into these areas without consideration for functional white matter tracts will result in unacceptable morbidity, emphasizing the need to consider in the overall treatment plan the infiltrated brain adjacent to the main tumor nidus.

Frameless Navigational Resection Devices

The next generation of image-based computerized localization for tumor resection will not use frames attached to the skull for three-dimensional reference of an intracranial target. The primary components of any contemporary navigational system are registering the surgical target with respect to surrounding structures and physical space, interacting with a localization device, integrating real-time data, and interfacing with a computer. Contemporary frameless navigation systems include ultrasonic digitizer systems, magnetic field digitizers, multijointed encoder arms, infrared flash systems, and robotic systems (Zakhary et al., 1999). The majority of these newer systems use a localizing arm that initializes and calibrates fiducial markers that are attached to the patient's head during the preoperative scan and at the time of surgery. Changes in the position of the localizing arm are updated using acoustic transit times between the sound sources and the fiducial markers (Roberts et al., 1986; Barnett et al., 1993); other systems use mechanical sensors (Watanabe et al., 1987) or light emitters.

Regardless of the system employed, surgeons will ultimately use this technology to preoperatively plan incisions and bone flaps as well as to guide the initial phases of the resection. Shifting of the brain contents will necessarily limit the utility of these methods when intra-axial tumors are resected because localization is based on findings from the preoperative scan. This will not, however, be a factor during complex skull base surgery.

Intraoperative Imaging Techniques

Unlike frameless and frame-based systems that are limited by their reliance on preoperative imaging, both intraoperative CT and MR scanning provide intraoperative updates of data sets for navigational systems. Intraoperative re-registration of target anatomy eliminates the problem of brain shift that may be caused by resection or brain retractors and allows the surgeon to more precisely achieve resection control and to modify the preplanned surgical approach, if necessary. Use of intraoperative MR requires MR-compatible instruments (i.e., titanium or ceramic) to minimize artifact. Surgical instruments can be tracked with the use of light-emitting diode sensors to provide image guidance during movements and interactive feedback on corresponding images (Black et al., 1997; Tronnier et al., 1997; Steinmeier et al., 1998).

Intraoperative Localization of Tumor and Margins

For neurosurgeons, gross visualization for consistency and color has been the sine qua non used to distinguish normal brain from tumor at the time of surgery. Low-grade glial tumors differ from their malignant counterparts in both texture (firmer than normal brain) and color (slightly paler than white matter). Most malignant gliomas have a very soft and often necrotic grayish appearance; characteristic thrombosed veins are almost always seen with glioblastoma. These tumors are usually highly vascular with vascularization corresponding to the contrast-enhancing rim on the imaging studies.

Following the opening of the dura, the cortex is inspected for expanded gyri and red "arterialized" veins, which are pathognomonic for malignant gliomas secondary to reduced oxygen extraction with increased blood flow (Fig. 3–1). Before the resection begins, it is helpful to use ultrasound localization to determine the overall tumor size, depth, and underlying cystic structures. Tumor volumes, as seen on both CT and MRI scans, closely correspond to high- and low-grade gliomas that have been previously unresected and untreated (LeRoux et al., 1989, 1993). Once these are operated on and radiated, gliosis accumulates and increases the echogenic background, which tends to overestimate the true size of the tumor.

Intraoperative verification of tumor and of the transition zone between the tumor and the adjacent tumor-infiltrated brain is best achieved with serial frozen sections or smear preparations (Reyes et al., 1991). This is often a very time-consuming process and is complicated by the need to distinguish reactive astrocytes from infiltrating tumor cells. Alternative ways to intraoperatively document the extent of tumor removal involve imaging with dedicated CT and MRI, laser activation of hematoporphyrin (Perria et al., 1988), fluorescent dyes (Poon et al., 1992), intravenous (IV) indocyanine green (Hansen et al., 1993), and IV fluorescein with ultraviolet photoactivation (Moore, 1947).

Functional Mapping-Guided Tumor Resection

As radical resective surgery becomes more commonplace in modern neurosurgical practice and teaching, the risks of functional morbidity will certainly be the rate-limiting factor for most surgeons. Over the past several years, functional mapping of cortical and subcortical regions using both intraoperative and extraoperative techniques has become an indispensable adjunct to avoid morbidity while performing wide, radical tumor resections in eloquent brain areas. For example, in the dominant cerebral

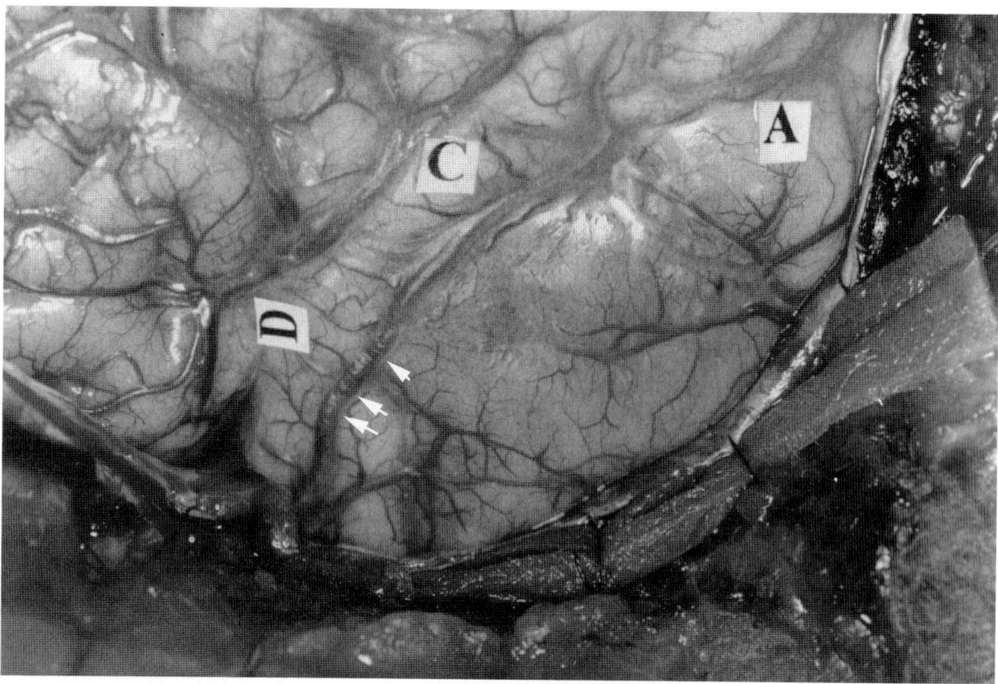

Figure 3–1. Intraoperative photograph demonstrating swollen gyri infiltrated with a glioblastoma multiforme. Tumor margins are depicted as A, D, and C. A large, arterialized vein is seen draining the tumor.

hemisphere, language testing for reading, speech, and naming must be done before tumors that involve the posterior frontal, anterior parietal, and temporal lobes are resected. Preoperative deficits in these language functions could be due either to swelling or to tumor infiltration into essential language sites; a preoperative trial of high-dose dexamethasone will usually distinguish between the two causes. The motor cortex is located within 3 to 5 cm behind the coronal suture superiorly and a similar distance posterior to the outer border of the sphenoid wing. The region is flanked posteriorly by the primary somatosensory cortex and near the vertex by the supplementary motor area anteriorly. The presence of any tumor on either side of the motor cortex should dictate that stimulation mapping be done to identify the cortical motor neurons and also their descending motor tracts in the subcortical white matter. These include the corona radiata, internal capsule, cerebral peduncles, and the corticospinal pathways to the brain stem and spinal cord. Tumors involving the insula, thalamus, and basal ganglia often abut the descending motor tracts, which may be readily stimulated.

Because seizures associated with low-grade gliomas are often medically refractory, neurosurgical approaches have been adapted from epilepsy surgery to provide better seizure control. Intraoperative mapping of seizure foci using electrocorticography will readily identify epileptogenic areas and, combined with the functional brain map, will allow for removal of these regions without associated deficits.

Not all patients will be good candidates for functional mapping resections. Preoperative planning begins with a thorough neurologic assessment to decide whether the patient is a candidate for mapping. If a dense hemiparesis is present despite administration of steroids, it is unlikely that intraoperative stimulation will elicit motor responses. In that setting, somatosensory evoked responses may be used to identify the central sulcus by documenting a phase reversal potential across this sulcus (Woolsey et al., 1979). Because the motor cortex in young children is often unexcitable by direct stimulation mapping, evoked potentials should also be available for this particular patient population (Goldring and Gregorie, 1984). Language function is assessed by having the

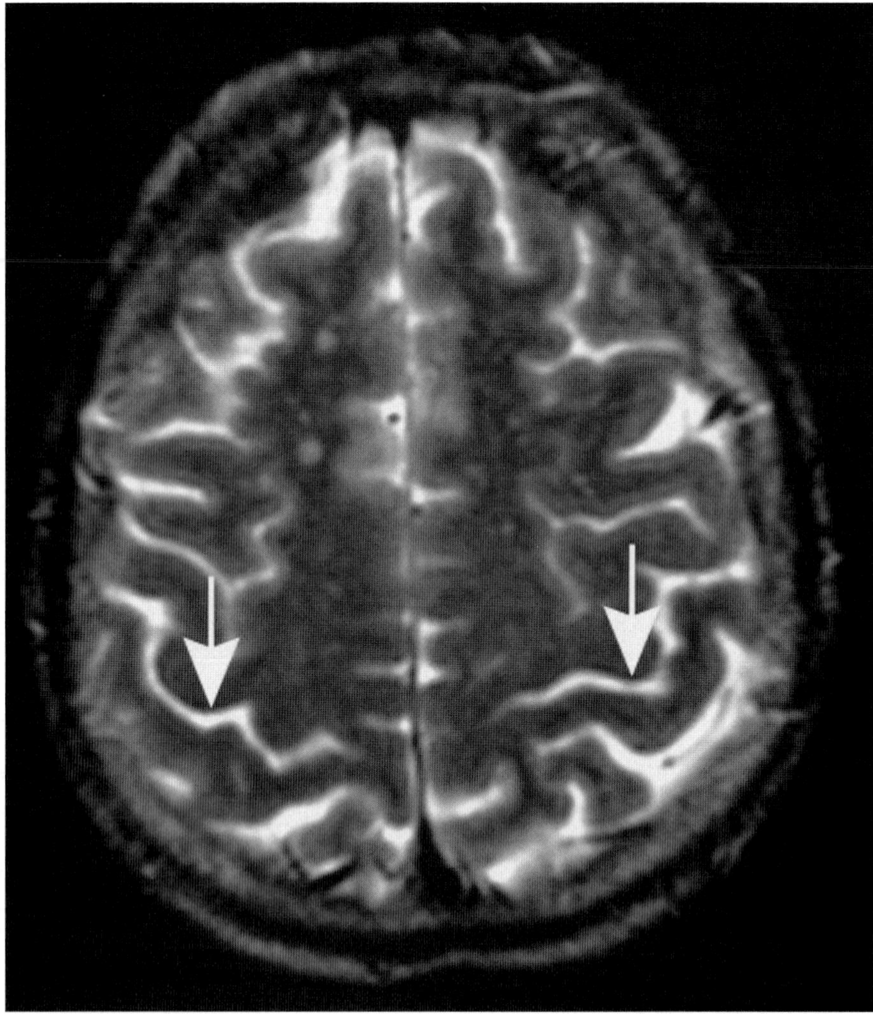

Figure 3–2. T_2-weighted axial image with arrows pointing to the precentral sulcus immediately anterior to the motor cortex.

patient count to 10 and stick out his or her tongue, which verifies that Broca's area and the inferior face motor cortex are intact. The patient is then shown a series of picture slides with common objects to name. A baseline naming error rate greater than 25% will prevent functional mapping from providing reliable information.

The MRI scan is used to identify the motor cortex by localizing two mirror image lines on both sides of the midline that represent the central sulcus (Berger, 1990; Berger et al., 1990b). This is best seen on the high T_2-weighted axial images (Fig. 3–2). Sagittal and far-sagittal scans may be used to identify the marginal sulcus and an imaginary line drawn from the back of the insular triangle, respectively, which mark the combined sensorimotor (i.e., Rolandic) cortex.

With the patient awake and the cortex exposed, the sensory and motor cortex is easily stimulated using currents as low as 2 mA and usually not greater than 6 mA. The current is produced with a constant current generator, which elicits a train of biphasic square wave pulses (frequency, 60 Hz; duration per phase, 1.25 msec) via a bipolar electrode. Patients who are asleep will require higher currents (i.e., 6 to 16 mA maximum). Using multichannel electromyographic recordings in addition to visual observation of motor activity results in greater sensitivity, allowing the use of lower stimulation levels and facilitating detection

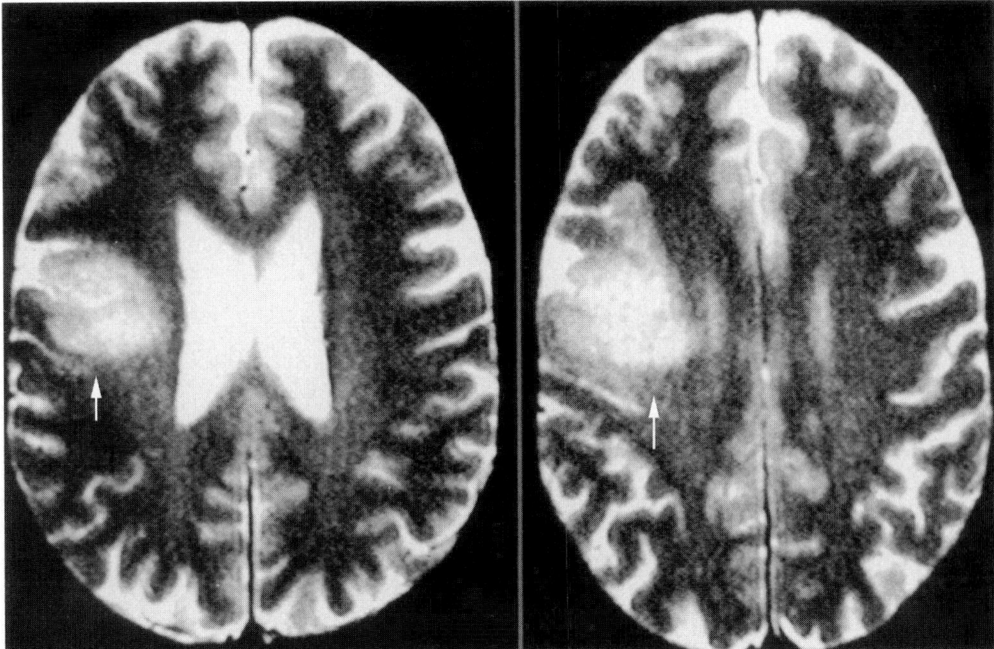

Figure 3–3. T_2-weighted axial image demonstrating a hyperintense glioma infiltrating the face motor cortex.

of stimulation-induced seizure activity (Yingling et al., 1999). A current greater than 16 mA has never been necessary to evoke sensory or motor responses. At this point, cold Ringer's lactate solution should be immediately available for irrigation of the stimulated cortex if a focal motor seizure develops. The best management of intraoperative stimulation-induced focal motor seizures is rapid cortical irrigation at the stimulation site with ice-cold Ringer's solution, which will abruptly stop the seizure activity originating from the irritated cortex without using short-acting barbiturates (Sartorius and Berger, 1998). The current should be elevated in 1 and 2 mA increments for awake and asleep patients, respectively. When operating near the vertex, the leg motor cortex will be hidden along the falx. Thus, a strip electrode should be inserted between the midline cortex and the falx to evoke stimulation-induced responses of the leg and foot. The same or a slightly higher current may be used to stimulate subcortical motor tracts without concern for current spread, which remains limited to within 2 to 4 mm of the bipolar electrode contacts.

Figure 3–3 demonstrates the utility of mapping the cortex and the underlying white matter in a patient with an infiltrative astrocytic glioma involving the face motor cortex in the nondominant hemisphere. The cortex was mapped to evoke orofacial movements in addition to finger and wrist flexion and extension (Fig. 3–4). The face motor cortex was resected in its entirety, and the tumor was removed until subcortical stimulation demonstrated hand movements (Figs. 3–5 and 3–6). The patient had a left-sided facial droop, which cleared in 3 weeks, and brief hand weakness, which lasted a few days.

Following localization of Broca's area based on stimulation-induced counting arrest, naming is tested as a language measure that best predicts postoperative deficits (Penfield and Roberts, 1959). Before testing it is essential to determine the optimal stimulation current based on recording after discharge potentials from the cortex following bipolar stimulation. This is done to ensure that subclinical seizure activity is not the cause of speech dysfunction during the mapping. The current to be used will vary between 2 and 8 mA and should be adjusted to 1 mA below the current that causes after-discharge potentials. A wide surface area is tested after sterile numbered tickets are placed on the cortex for documentation purposes. Approximately 15 to 25 sites are tested, with each site being stimulated at least three times. Errors in naming take the form of hesitation or complete anomia. Hesitation in naming is not con-

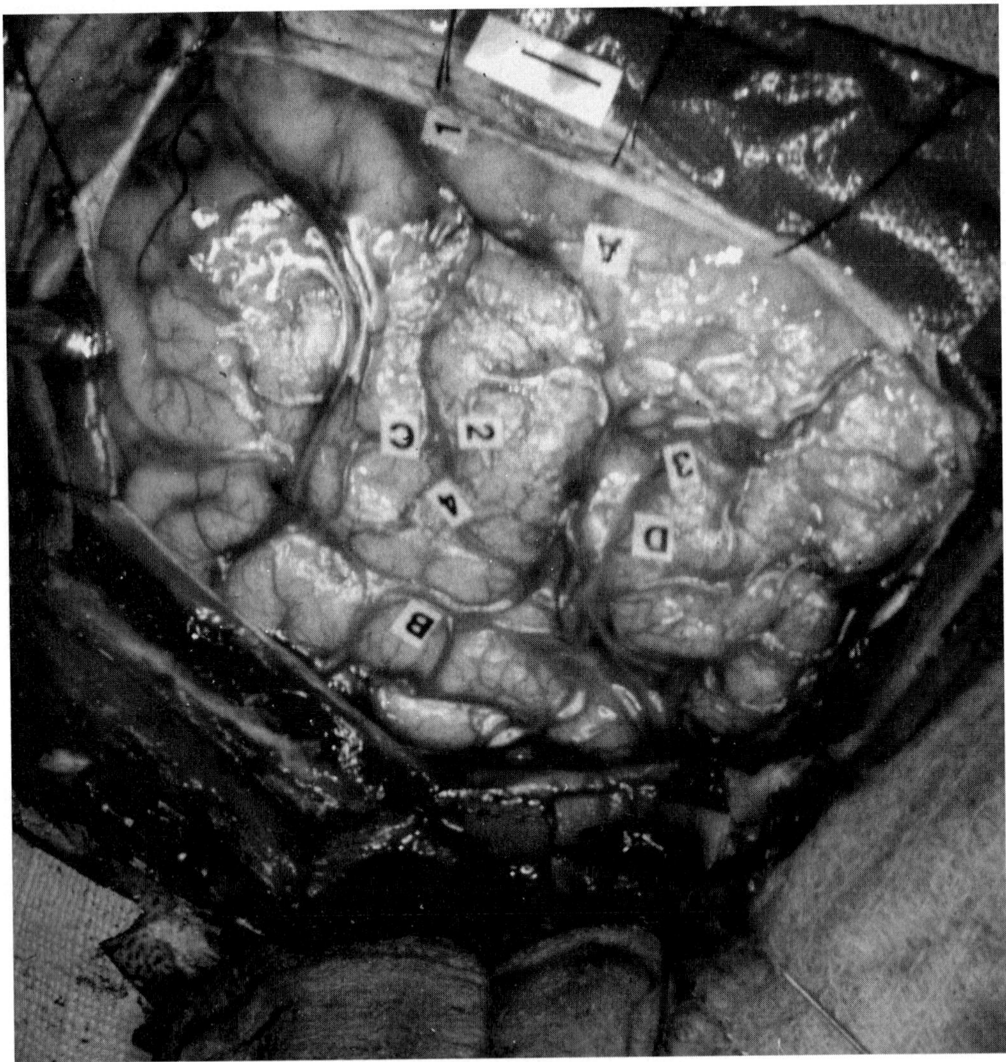

Figure 3–4. Intraoperative photograph following stimulation mapping of the face (2, 3, 4) and hand (1) motor cortex. Tumor margins are A–D.

sidered critical, whereas difficulty with naming is a critical function and denotes an essential language site.

In a series of 117 patients who had language testing when undergoing operation on the left, dominant hemisphere, essential language sites were randomly identified throughout that hemisphere, with the heaviest concentration of sites located around the perisylvian cortex (Ojemann et al., 1989). At least 67% had more than one essential language site, and in 16% of the population tested no temporoparietal language sites could be found. A companion study to this evaluation of temporal lobe language in patients with gliomas in the same region showed a number of findings that again emphasized that language localization cannot be determined anatomically but must rely on stimulation mapping (Haglund et al., 1993). In that study, we failed to identify a language function in the inferior temporal gyrus, whereas the superior temporal gyrus was nearly twice as likely as the middle temporal gyrus to have stimulation-induced language errors. Contrary to accepted neurosurgical teaching,

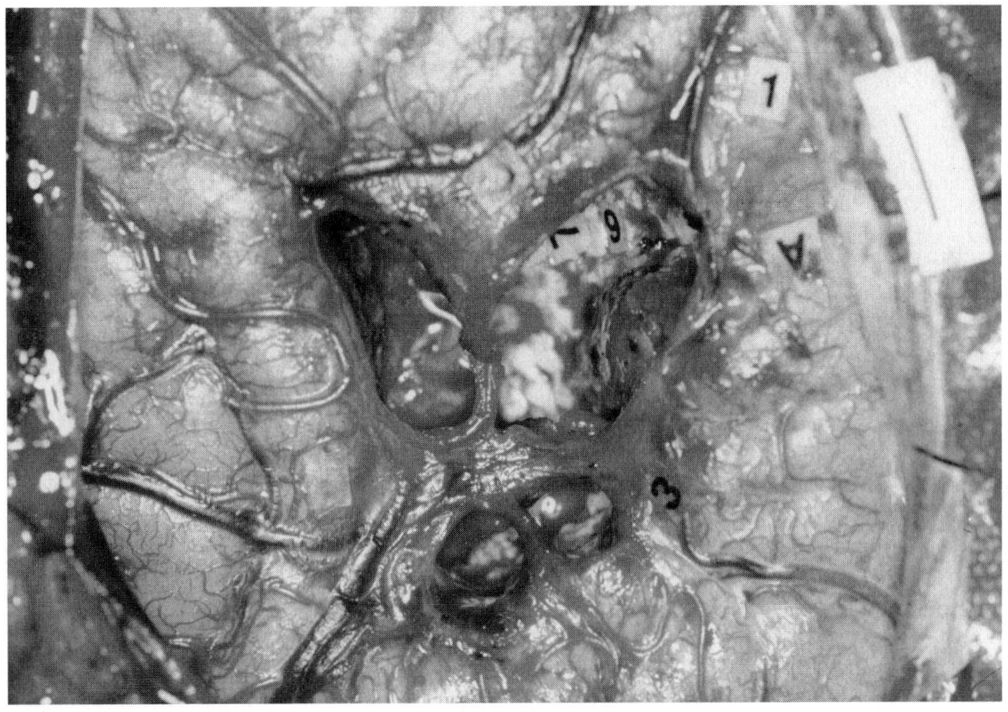

Figure 3–5. Subcortical hand motor fibers (6, 7) are seen following resection of the overlying cortex. A indicates a tumor margin.

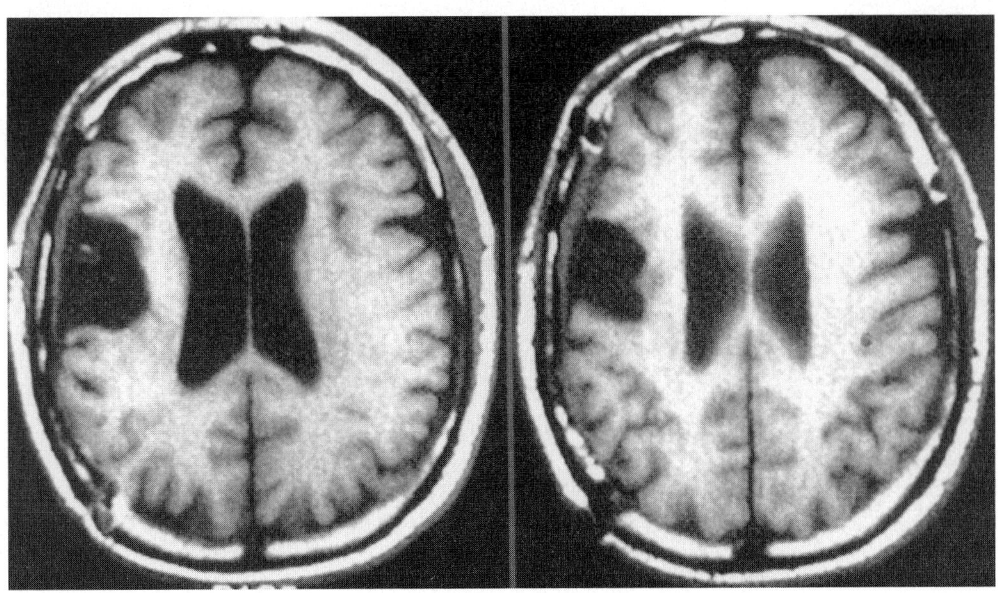

Figure 3–6. Postoperative T_1-weighted axial image showing the resection cavity.

essential naming sites were found in the anterior temporal lobe (i.e., first 3 cm) in nearly 15% of patients with temporal lobe gliomas. It was also learned from this study that resecting the tumor within 7 mm of an essential language site results in a permanent naming deficit 40% of the time. However, if the resection is further than 1 cm from the essential naming cortex, no permanent deficits will result. Knowing this, we are now able to avoid permanent morbidity while removing tumors from the dominant cerebral hemisphere when language is mapped before resection.

An example of the utility of speech mapping during tumor resection is shown in Figure 3–7. In this case, the patient had a brief history of seizure activity accompanied by postictal confusion and naming errors, which resolved after each seizure. A MRI scan revealed a non–contrast-enhancing tumor in the posterior parietal lobe on the left side. Intraoperative speech mapping demonstrated repetitive errors in naming at three essential sites between 1 and 3 cm in front of the tumor nidus (Fig. 3–8). The lesion was resected completely using intraoperative ultrasound guidance, and the resection cavity did not come closer than 1 cm to the nearest essential language site (Figs. 3–9 and 3–10). Postoperatively, the patient had a severe dysnomia, which cleared within 4 to 6 weeks following surgery, and his neurologic functions returned to baseline.

PATHOLOGY OF DIFFUSE INFILTRATIVE GLIOMAS

The most common tumors of the cranial–spinal axis are those that infiltrate or displace the brain parenchyma of the intracranial supratentorial compartment. Of these tumors, histologically, the most common belong to the glioma family of tumors.

General Features

The astrocytic gliomas, the most common class of supratentorial glial neoplasms, are derived from and have an appearance simulating normal astrocytes. Astrocytes occur most commonly in the white matter, but are also found in the cerebral cortex. Astrocytomas are diffusely infiltrating neoplasms of the cerebral hemispheres, and there is evidence that their prognosis and survival depend on the tumor's histologic grade (Burger et al., 1985; Fulling and Nelson,

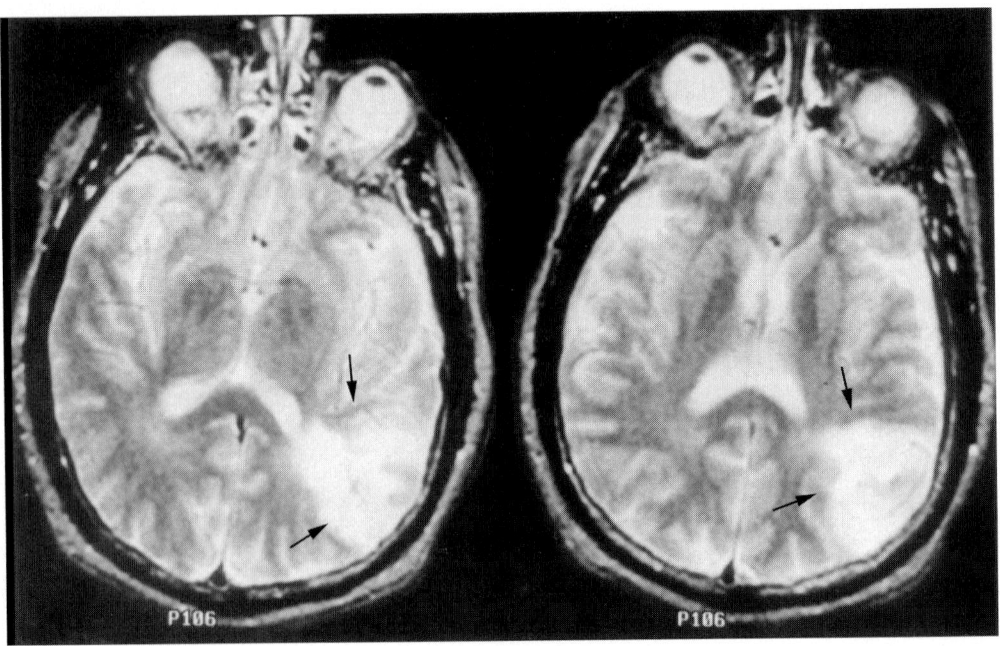

Figure 3–7. T_2-weighted axial image showing a hyperintense glioma involving the angular and supramarginal gyri of the dominant hemisphere.

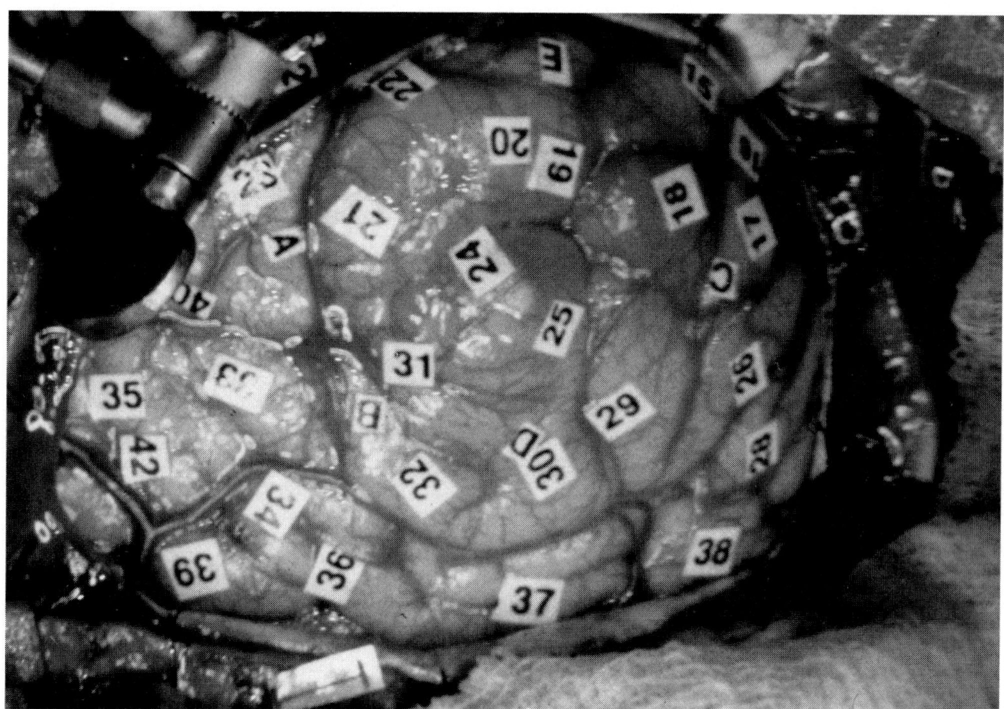

Figure 3–8. Intraoperative photograph of the tumor and adjacent brain following awake stimulation mapping of the cortex. Repetitive errors in naming were documented in numbers 33, 34, and 35. Numbers 24 and 25 overlie the center of the tumor.

1984; Kim et al., 1991). All grades of diffuse infiltrative cerebral astrocytoma should be considered malignant, even if only by virtue of their location within the enclosed bony skull, because almost none of these tumors is cured by surgical excision alone.

Astrocytes are supporting glial cells and generally have small round nuclei with inconspicuous micronucleoli. Under normal circumstances in routinely stained histologic sections, astrocytes do not have visible cytoplasm, but ultrastructural studies reveal short cytoplasmic processes containing intermediate filaments. These filaments are known, through immunohistochemical studies, to be composed of glial fibrillary acidic protein, a specific type of astrocytic protein (Fig. 3–11). Tumors can be confirmed as astrocytomas by specific immunostaining of tumor cells for glial fibrillary acidic protein. Astrocytes can react to brain injury by increasing the amount of their cytoplasm and the complement of filaments filling it. Their cytoplasmic processes become elongated and thickened, their cell bodies become enlarged, and their cytoplasm is then visible in routine sections. These enlarged, reactive astrocytes are called *gemistocytes.*

Astrocytic neoplasms exhibit a stereotypic range of features that become more prominent with increasing grades of anaplastic malignancy. In general, the features we use to grade tumor malignancy are those that permit us to diagnose the tumors. These features include degree of cellularity, nuclear and cytoplasmic pleomorphism of individual cells, mitotic activity, vascular changes such as small vessel proliferation or vascular mural cell proliferation, and tumor necrosis. None of these features in isolation is specifically diagnostic of malignancy, but the combined spectrum is used for both diagnosis and tumor grading. Other histologic features that suggest a diagnosis of tumor and tend to suggest increasing malignancy, but are not statistically significant in studies of histologic grading, include tumor invasion of the cerebral cortex, microcystic areas (indirectly correlated with grade), presence of tumor gemistocytes, and pial or subpial invasion by tumor cells.

Most astrocytomas are derived from fibrillary astrocytes of white matter and arise in the subcortical white matter. Low-grade astrocytomas show an increased cellularity over normal white matter, and the cell nuclei are slightly enlarged. No mitotic activity is

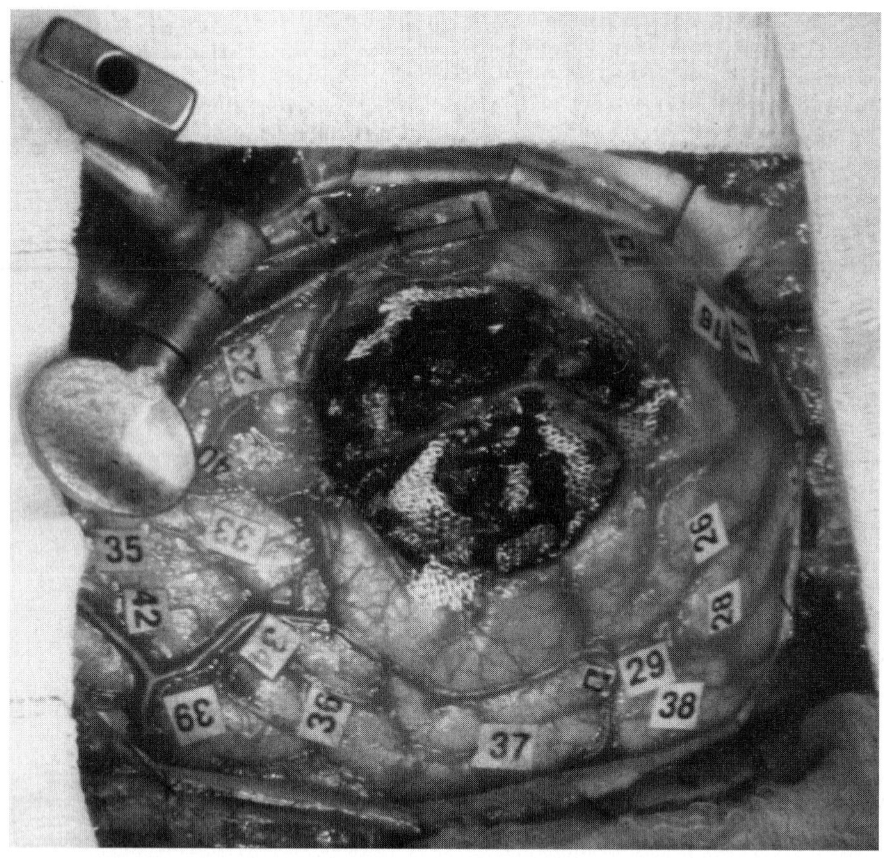

Figure 3–9. Post-resection photograph with essential language sites preserved.

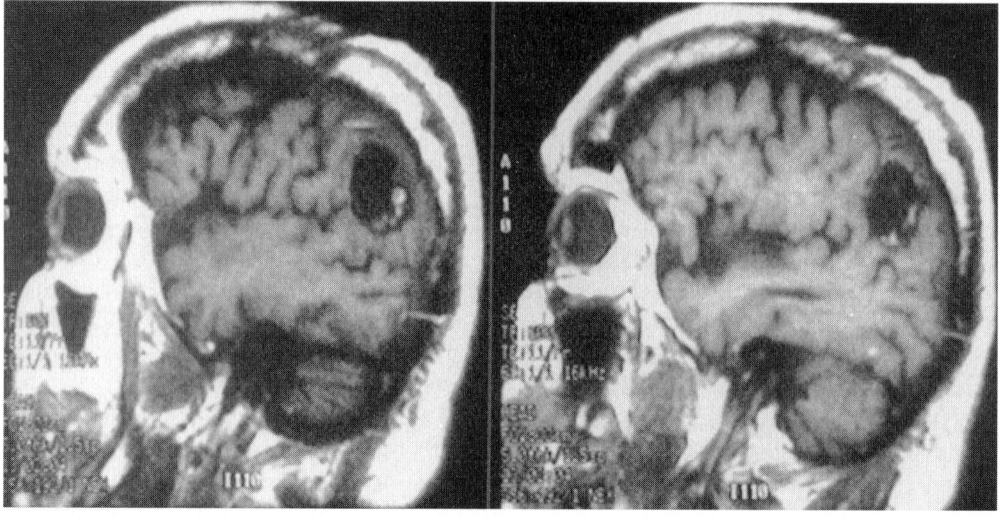

Figure 3–10. Postoperative T_1-weighted sagittal images of the resection cavity.

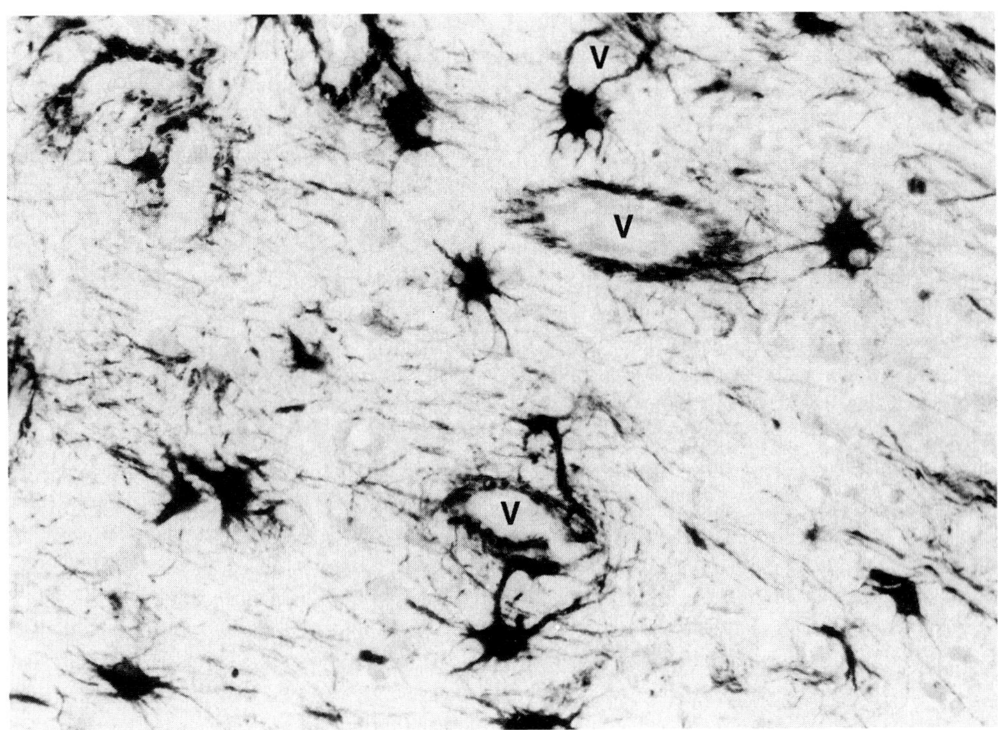

Figure 3–11. Reactive supporting astrocytes. Supporting reactive astrocytes have voluminous cytoplasm filled with dark-staining immunoreactive filaments of glial fibrillary acidic protein. They send foot processes to surround blood vessels (V) and form part of the blood–brain barrier. Immunoperoxidase for glial fibrillary acidic protein with aminoethylcarbazole-hematoxylin. Original magnification, ×200.

seen, vessels are not abnormal, and necrosis is not identified. Small nucleoli may become more prominent, but the nuclei themselves are regular in outline without much pleomorphism. Microcysts may be a distinctive feature and may contain proteinaceous fluid. Astrocytomas derived from the protoplasmic astrocytes of the cerebral cortex are relatively filament-poor and arise within the cortex itself. These tumor cells have short, delicate processes and poor immunoreactivity for glial fibrillary acidic protein.

As cellularity and pleomorphism, either nuclear or cytoplasmic, increase, the tumor becomes more anaplastic. Anaplastic astrocytomas may have moderate degrees of all these features. In addition, mitotic activity is present. Anaplastic astrocytomas are more likely to show cortical invasion or subpial accumulation of neoplastic cells. Any astrocytoma with gemistocytic change involving greater than about 20% of the cells should be graded as an anaplastic astrocytoma (Krouwer et al., 1991), although designation as a gemistocytic astrocytoma requires that approximately 60% of the tumor cells be gemistocytes.

The distinguishing histologic features of glioblastoma, the highest malignant grade of astrocytoma, are the presence of vascular mural cell proliferation or coagulative tumor necrosis (Burger and Green, 1987; Kleihues and Cavenee, 2000). Necrosis may be accompanied by pseudopalisading of neoplastic cells around it, but evidence of palisading is not required by most neuropathologists to make the diagnosis of glioblastoma (Burger et al., 1985).

In addition to specific histologic features of malignancy grades, astrocytomas may have a widely variable histology from one microscopic field to another within the same tumor, a feature known as *heterogeneity*. Tumor heterogeneity is thought to arise from a predominance of various transformed clones of astrocytes in different regions of the tumor during its growth. As the name *multiforme* suggests, glioblastomas are especially noted for their variable histology.

Approaches to Grading Gliomas

Whereas for most tumors it is recognized that higher grades of malignancy are associated with a poorer patient prognosis, the grading criteria for gliomas in most grading schemes are subjective. Within a single grade, the prognosis for tumors in individual patients may be difficult to predict on the basis of grade alone (i.e., astrocytomas with similar histologic features may behave in widely disparate clinical fashions). Any scheme of histologic grading has two main goals: the tumor grade must predict behavior, and the grading criteria must be sufficiently objective and defined to minimize variation among observers and to maximize reproducibility (Fulling and Nelson, 1984). Numerous grading systems have been used for astrocytomas, most of them utilizing three or four grades of malignancy (Burger et al., 1985, 1991; Fulling and Nelson, 1984; Svien et al., 1949; Kernohan et al., 1949; Ringertz, 1950; Nelson et al., 1983; Burger and Green, 1987; Daumas-Duport et al., 1988b; Kleihues and Cavenee, 2000). Histologic criteria used to define these grades vary somewhat for different schemes (Table 3–1). Increasingly, more malignant tumors show a continuum of histologic features that permits their classification into grades.

The first systems for grading gliomas were presented at about the same time (Svien et al., 1949; Kernohan et al., 1949; Ringertz, 1950). Svien and Kernohan each used a four-grade system (designated as grades 1 through 4) that was patterned after the histologic grading system for epithelial neoplasms used at the Mayo Clinic. Ringertz's system had three grades of astrocytoma malignancy: astrocytoma, intermediate-type astrocytoma, and glioblastoma multiforme. Necrosis was used to divide the intermediate-type astrocytoma from the glioblastoma. Although the three systems defined histologic grade according to the presence of cellular anaplasia, the systems of Svien and Kernohan determined tumor grade according to the proportion of normal tissue remaining mixed with the invading tumor and on the type of invading edge of tumor into normal tissue. Because of the infiltrative growth pattern of gliomas, this feature is notoriously difficult to distinguish, especially in well-differentiated tumors. Also, it has subsequently been considered that the presence of even a single highly malignant focus of glioblastoma in an otherwise lower-grade astrocytoma portends a grave prognosis. Data from the original publications (Svien et al., 1949; Kernohan et al., 1949) showed no clinical distinction between grades II and III astrocytomas, whereas there was a clear survival difference among the three groups of patients in Ringertz's study. Thus, the three-tiered grading schemes were popularized.

Three-tiered grading systems have been shown to be closely correlated with the clinical prognosis for astrocytomas and are widely used today in diagnostic neuropathology. These grading systems include those of Ringertz, with its modifications (Ringertz, 1950; Fulling and Nelson, 1984; Nelson et al., 1983; Burger et al., 1985; Burger and Green, 1987), and a scheme widely called the *St. Anne-Mayo system* (Daumas-Duport et al., 1988b). The St. Anne-Mayo scheme designates four histologic features to be used in grading and nominally has four grades of astrocytoma. Their grade 1 tumor, however, is exceedingly rare (<0.25% in one series), and the other three grades produce three distinct survival curves; thus, this scheme should also be considered as a three-tiered scale (Kim et al., 1991).

Histologic features used to grade astrocytomas include increasing cellularity; microcysts (which suggest an improved prognosis); nuclear and cellular

Table 3–1. Comparison of Astrocytoma Grading Systems

Modified Ringertz	*St. Anne-Mayo, 1988*	*WHO 2000*
Astrocytoma (low grade)	Astrocytoma, grades 1 and 2	Diffuse astrocytoma (II)
	Astrocytoma, grade 3	Anaplastic astrocytoma (III)
Anaplastic astrocytoma		
	Astrocytoma, grade 4	Glioblastoma multiforme (IV)
Glioblastoma multiforme		

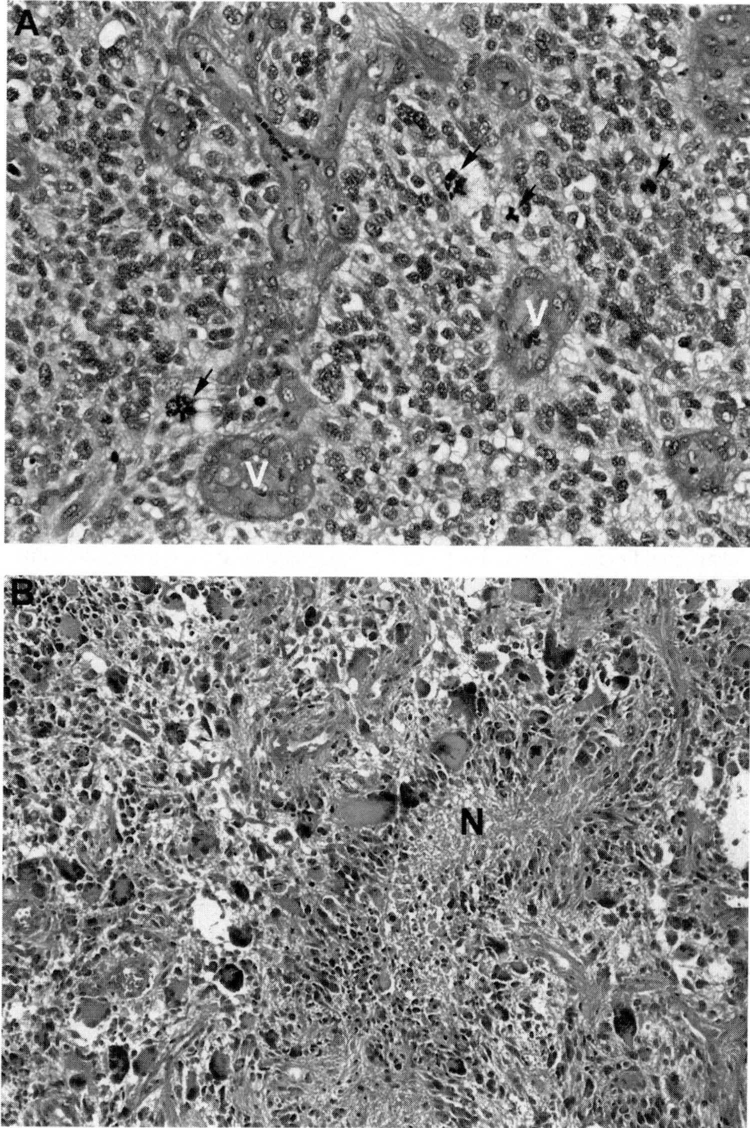

Figure 3–12. Histologic features used to grade astrocytoma malignancy. **(A)** High cellularity, microvascular proliferation (V), and frequent mitotic figures (arrows) are features of an anaplastic astrocytoma. Original magnification, ×200. **(B)** Focus of coagulation necrosis (N) with peripheral pseudopalisading of neoplastic cells that also show marked nuclear and cytoplasmic pleomorphism. These are features of a glioblastoma multiforme. Original magnification, ×100. Both are hematoxylin and eosin stained.

pleomorphism; vascular mural cell proliferation; mitotic activity; and coagulative tumor necrosis (Fig. 3–12). The St. Anne-Mayo system rates cellular pleomorphism, mitotic activity, vascular endothelial proliferation, and necrosis within a standardized and objective numeric scale. When present, each feature receives one scoring point, and the grades are based solely on the total numeric score. Concordance among individual pathologists who use the St. Anne-Mayo system is reported to be as high as 94% (Kim et al., 1991). That single study examined 251 astrocytoma cases and suggested, because of survival data, that the presence of necrosis should cause a tumor to immediately be classified as grade 4, even using their system. In this discussion, the terms *low-grade astrocytoma, anaplastic astrocytoma,* and *glioblas-*

toma are used. In most cases it can be assumed that the glioblastoma is primarily derived from astrocytes, even though its morphology may be so bizarre as to obscure such recognition, and sometimes it follows an earlier diagnosis of oligodendroglioma.

The most recent World Health Organization (WHO) classification also incorporates grading of nervous system neoplasms (Kleihues and Cavenee, 2000). The WHO criteria and general grading for astrocytomas are analogous to the St. Anne-Mayo system, but the terms used are *diffuse astrocytoma* (low grade), *anaplastic astrocytoma,* and *glioblastoma.* They are considered as WHO grades II, III, or IV, respectively (Daumas-Duport et al., 1988b; Kleihues and Cavenee, 2000).

Previous grading schemes for oligodendrogliomas are not as well correlated with patient survival as are those for astrocytomas (Smith et al., 1983; Burger et al., 1987; Shaw et al., 1992; Mork et al., 1985; Kros et al., 1988, 1990). Well-differentiated oligodendrogliomas are considered as WHO grade II neoplasms, whereas anaplastic oligodendrogliomas are WHO grade III (Kleihues and Cavenee, 2000). Grading oligodendrogliomas using WHO criteria has been shown to be clinically significant (Dehghani et al., 1998). Only these two grades of malignancy are accepted by the WHO. Many features used to grade oligodendrogliomas are similar to those for astrocytomas: cellularity, pleomorphism, mitotic activity, vascular changes, and necrosis (Smith et al., 1983; Burger et al., 1987). Sometimes lower grade oligodendrogliomas may have microcysts as well (Mork et al., 1986). Oligodendrogliomas of all histologic grades tend to infiltrate the cortex readily to form clusters of neoplastic cells in the subpial region and around neurons and blood vessels.

Grading systems for the other types of gliomas are much less well defined. For ependymomas, most authors have found little correlation between postoperative survival and tumor grade (Schiffer et al., 1991; Fokes and Earle, 1969; Ross and Rubinstein, 1989; Chiu et al., 1992).

Specific Tumor Characteristics

Low-Grade Astrocytoma

Diffuse low-grade astrocytomas are WHO grade II (Kleihues and Cavenee, 2000). Even though low-grade astrocytomas might be considered slow-growing tumors, most neuropathologists and neurosurgeons do not consider them benign because of their invasive quality and their location within the confines of the bony calvarium. These astrocytomas are rarely cured because they cannot be completely excised and because their ability to expand without damage to the host is limited by the skull. Thus, patients may die from recurrent astrocytomas, sometimes even lower grade ones, because of associated increased intracranial pressure or invasion of vital CNS structures.

Diffuse fibrillary astrocytomas are the most common morphologic subtype and usually arise in the white matter, which is the location of their normal cellular counterparts. The lobar distribution of these tumors is similar to that of the amount of white matter present in each brain lobe, with a higher incidence in the frontal regions (Burger et al., 1991). Grossly, these tumors are slightly discolored yellow or gray and have indistinct margins with the surrounding brain. The usually discrete border between cerebral white matter and gray matter may be blurred by the tumor. The tumor consistency is variably reported as firm, almost rubbery, or soft and gelatinous. This character may depend on the degree of fibrillarity of the individual cells within the neoplasm.

Histologically, low-grade astrocytomas show increased cellularity compared with normal brain tissue and have mild or moderate nuclear pleomorphism. The increase in cellularity may be only slight, producing a challenge for the diagnostic pathologist, and may simulate the slightly increased cellularity of reactive astrocytosis, a repair process. However, reactive astrocytic cells show generally more abundant and luxuriant cytoplasmic processes than do neoplastic astrocytes, with a more even cellular distribution and smaller, darker nuclei. The nuclei of astrocytoma cells are enlarged and show more prominent chromatin granules. Microcysts may be a useful feature for making a differential diagnosis with gliosis because this feature is rare in gliosis but common in low-grade astrocytomas. Astrocytoma cytoplasmic processes may be evident in routine sections but can be better visualized after immunohistochemical staining for glial fibrillary acidic protein. Other features of anaplasia, such as mitotic activity, vascular proliferative changes, and necrosis, are absent. Microcalcifications can be present in as many as 15% of astrocytomas. Although these tumors are diffusely invasive into the surrounding brain, their invasion is largely limited to white matter. Invasion of the cerebral cortex with perineuronal satellitosis and subpial accumulation suggests a more aggressive astrocytoma or an oligodendroglioma.

Astrocytomas, especially low-grade examples, may occur as mixed tumors with neuronal or other glial components. Mixtures with oligodendroglioma are especially common, but other elements should be present in significant proportions to justify a diagnosis of mixed glioma.

Anaplastic Astrocytoma

The gross appearance of anaplastic astrocytomas is similar to that of the lower grade tumors, except that the anaplastic astrocytomas have a softer consistency because they usually lack extreme fibrillarity. Diffuse infiltration remains a feature, without evidence of necrosis in the tumor, although the relatively greater difference with surrounding normal brain tissue may falsely suggest a more discrete lesion.

The histologic features of anaplastic astrocytomas are similar to those of low-grade astrocytomas but these features are more abundant and exaggerated. These tumors are WHO grade III (Kleihues and Cavenee, 2000). Cellularity is more increased, as are nuclear and cellular pleomorphism. These features may be extreme, with back-to-back cells and bizarre, hyperchromatic nuclei. Cytoplasm may be scanty, with nuclear lobation and enlargement indicating anaplasia. Alternatively, the abundant eosinophilic cytoplasm of gemistocytes may be prominent, with relatively small and uniform nuclei. Gemistocytic astrocytic foci generally occur in tumors with other more usual fibrillary areas. The presence of more than 20% of gemistocytes in a glial neoplasm is a poor prognostic sign (Krouwer et al., 1991); thus, gemistocytic astrocytomas should be considered anaplastic. Mitotic activity is easily recognized in most anaplastic astrocytomas but inexplicably may be absent in the gemistocytic areas. Despite this seeming anomaly, gemistocytic cells commonly transform to more highly anaplastic small cells.

The range of anaplasia in this grade is broad, with some examples showing low cellularity and pleomorphism with a few mitotic figures and others being highly cellular and pleomorphic with frequent mitoses, lacking only the necrosis required for a histologic diagnosis of glioblastoma. For this reason, it is useful to have a more objective indicator of behavior, and some markers of cell proliferation have been used in an attempt to predict prognosis more accurately. The most used markers in this area have been antibodies to bromodeoxyuridine (BrdU) and Ki-67. The cellular incorporation of BrdU is a specific marker of the DNA synthesis phase of the cell cycle, whereas the Ki-67 antibody labels an antigen that is present in all phases of the cell cycle except G0. Both antibodies can be identified by immunohistochemical staining in paraffin-embedded tissue sections. In longer use, the BrdU labeling index was found to correlate with tumor grade and prognosis in all grades of astrocytoma and oligodendroglioma (Hoshino et al., 1993; Prados et al., 1998b; Lamborn et al., 1999), but not within the glioblastoma multiforme histology (Ritter et al., 1994). The BrdU labeling index appears to be an age-independent predictor of survival only in low-grade and anaplastic astrocytomas (Ito et al., 1994).

Because BrdU must be introduced into the tumor by injection into the patient before surgery, the MIB-1 antibody to the Ki-67 antigen is far more popular today. The MIB-1 antibody can be used in paraffin tissue sections and appears reliable for labeling index prognostications (Key et al., 1993; Davis et al., 1995) in a manner similar to BrdU. Some studies suggest that astrocytomas with MIB-1 labeling indices of >5% or >7.5% are associated with shorter survival times and an anaplastic histologic grade (Jaros et al., 1992; Montine et al., 1994).

Glioblastoma

Glioblastoma, also known as glioblastoma multiforme, is the glioma with the highest grade of malignancy, WHO grade IV (Kleihues and Cavenee, 2000). It represents 15% to 23% of intracranial tumors and about 50% to 60% of astrocytomas. Most examples are generally considered to arise from astrocytes because glial fibrillary acidic protein can be identified in the cell cytoplasm. Some examples, however, apparently arise from other glial lineages, such as oligodendrocytes. Glioblastoma is the most frequently occurring astrocytoma. Autopsy and serial biopsy studies have shown that some astrocytomas progress through the grades of malignancy with transformation from low-grade to anaplastic astrocytoma to glioblastoma (Muller et al., 1977). But, because some examples of glioblastoma appear to arise rapidly in otherwise normal patients and are recognized when they are small, it is thought that this variety of glioblastoma can also arise directly from malignant transformation of astrocyte precursor cells without passing through the lower grades of malignancy (Kleihues and Ohgaki, 1997, 1999).

Tumor necrosis is the characteristic gross feature that distinguishes glioblastoma from anaplastic astrocytoma (Fulling and Nelson, 1984; Nelson et al., 1983; Burger et al., 1985; Burger and Green, 1987). Another microscopic feature that is distinctive and diagnostic is the presence of proliferative vascular changes within the tumor. These changes may occur in the endothelial cells (vascular endothelial hyperplasia or proliferation) or in the cells of the vessel wall itself (vascular mural cell proliferation). Both types of change are sometimes considered together as microvascular proliferation. Glioblastomas may show evidence of older or more recent hemorrhage, and their cellularity is usually extremely high. The individual cells may be small, with a high nuclear/cytoplasmic ratio, or very large and bizarre, with abundant eosinophilic cytoplasm. With cell proliferation labeling studies, the small cells are the more proliferative ones, and these small cell glioblastomas have a more aggressive course, with even shorter patient survival times than those of highly pleomorphic or better differentiated astrocytes (Burger and Green, 1987). Some glioblastomas may be so highly cellular that the population of small anaplastic cells simulates primitive neuroectodermal tumors such as the medulloblastoma. These same small cells may appear to condense in rows around areas of tumor necrosis, forming the characteristic pseudopalisades. They also have a propensity to infiltrate the brain extensively, spreading even to distant locations and giving the appearance of a multifocal glioma. Although some examples are truly multifocal (i.e., arising in multiple simultaneous primary sites), many of these multifocal tumors show a histologic connection when the whole brain is examined at autopsy.

The histologic morphology of glioblastoma can be highly variable, conferring the name *multiforme.* Some tumors are largely spindled and simulate a fibrosarcoma. Others show cytoplasmic lipidization or epithelioid structures that imitate squamous or glandular patterns with positive keratin immunoreactivity (Rosenblum et al., 1991; Gherardi et al., 1986; Galloway and Roessmann, 1986). A myxoid or chondroid type of appearance has also been seen (Kepes et al., 1984). The astrocytic origin of these diverse morphologic cell types can be confirmed by a positive glial fibrillary acidic protein immunostain.

The regional distribution of glioblastomas is similar to that of other astrocytomas, although these neoplasms occur relatively frequently in the brain stem and spinal cord in younger patients. If the tumors gain access to the ventricular system or the subarachnoid space, these pathways become avenues for wide dissemination.

Gliosarcoma

Gliosarcoma is a variant of glioblastoma in which a distinct component of sarcoma is admixed with the glioma. The frequency of gliosarcoma in glioblastoma is reported to be from 2% to 8% (Morantz et al., 1976; Meis et al., 1991). In some cases, this change is recognized at recurrence of an anaplastic astrocytoma or glioblastoma and may also be seen de novo. The sarcoma element may be of any histologic type, with fibrosarcoma being the usual one. Other types include malignant fibrous histiocytoma, osteosarcoma, rhabdomyosarcoma, and chondrosarcoma. Currently, the sarcomatous element is thought to be derived from a mesenchymal cell associated with the vascular adventitia. Differentiation into endothelium, smooth muscle, or pericytes can occur (Miller et al., 1991; Haddad et al., 1991). The prognosis of gliosarcoma is similar to that of glioblastoma.

Oligodendroglial Tumors

Oligodendrogliomas, like astrocytomas, mimic the histology of their presumed cell of origin. They also arise primarily in the white matter but tend to infiltrate the cerebral cortex more than do astrocytomas of a similar grade of malignancy. Like astrocytomas, grading schemes of histologic malignancy have been used for oligodendrogliomas, but these correlate less well with prognosis than those used for astrocytomas. Many of the histologic features used to grade oligodendrogliomas are similar to those used for astrocytomas: cellularity, pleomorphism, mitotic activity, vascular changes, and necrosis. Lower grade oligodendrogliomas may have microcysts. Oligodendrogliomas of all histologic grades tend to infiltrate the cortex readily and to form clusters of neoplastic cells in the subpial region, around neurons, and around blood vessels. In general, the cells of oligodendrogliomas have round, regular nuclei and dis-

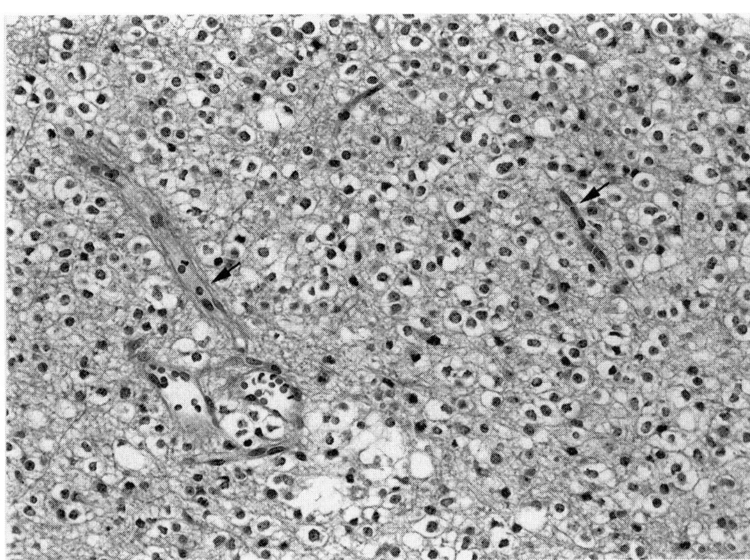

Figure 3–13. Low-grade oligodendroglioma. Proliferation of cells with round nuclei and cleared cytoplasm ("fried egg" cells). The oligodendroglioma cells are more numerous than would be seen in normal brain tissue, but neuropil is present between the neoplastic cells. Small, thin-walled capillaries (arrows) are also a feature. Hematoxylin and eosin. Original magnification, ×200.

tinct cytoplasmic borders with clearing of the cytoplasm (Fig. 3–13). Their cytologic appearance has been compared to "fried eggs." The neoplastic cells do not have fibrillary cytoplasmic processes. Another fairly distinctive and diagnostically helpful feature is the vascular pattern of oligodendrogliomas, referred to as "chicken wire" vessels. The blood vessels divide the tumor into discrete lobules. For this reason and because of the not uncommonly seen discrete margin between oligodendrogliomas and adjacent white matter, some are mistaken for metastatic carcinomas. Variants of the usual clear cells are recognized. Some oligodendrogliomas can have cells with a small rim of eosinophilic cytoplasm. These cells are distinctive and are called *mini-gemistocytes.* Despite the cytoplasm, there are few or no cell processes, and these mini-gemistocytes are believed to be true oligodendrocytes rather than astrocytes (Herpers and Budka, 1984).

As might be expected, this rim of eosinophilic cytoplasm may contain intermediate filaments ultrastructurally (Kros et al., 1992), and it shows positive immunoreactivity for glial fibrillary acidic protein. In addition, most oligodendrocytes show positive nuclear and cytoplasmic reactivity for S-100 protein, a characteristic that can help in distinguishing them from other clear cell tumors in the brain and that can be useful if these tumors are nonimmunoreactive (as might be expected) for glial fibrillary acidic protein. With increasing anaplasia, oligodendrogliomas can become highly cellular and pleomorphic, approaching an appearance of glioblastoma multiforme with the presence of necrosis. Although it is correct to classify these as anaplastic oligodendrogliomas, some would use the term *glioblastoma* once necrosis is identified in any high-grade glial neoplasm. One justification for separating anaplastic oligodendrogliomas from astrocytic glioblastomas is the slightly better prognosis of the former, even in this highest grade of malignancy (Ludwig et al., 1986; Dehghani et al., 1998). Some authors have reported that an MIB-1 labeling index of >3% to 5% predicts a worse prognosis in oligodendrogliomas (Heegard et al., 1995; Kros et al., 1996; Coons et al., 1997; Cairncross et al., 1998; Dehghani et al., 1998).

Oligoastrocytomas

Many, if not most, oligodendrogliomas occur with a regional or intimate cellular mixture of astrocytoma. For the diagnosis of mixed glioma, the proportion of each should be substantial, but authors have differing opinions with respect to exact numbers; usually a mixture with a range from 10% to 25% of the minor element is used to diagnose a mixed glioma. Oligoastrocytomas and anaplastic oligoastrocytomas correspond to WHO grade II or grade III, respectively (Kleihues and Cavenee, 2000). Histologic features of anaplasia may be present in either component and will affect the prognosis adversely. Such features include marked cellular pleomorphism, high cellularity, and a high mitotic rate. Microvascular proliferation and necrosis may also be seen. Prognosis and response to therapy have not been shown to depend on the proportion of the oligodendroglial versus the astrocytic component of the tumor (Shaw et al., 1994).

Supratentorial Ependymomas

Ependymomas are tumors that arise from the ependymal cells of the ventricles. Although more common in the posterior fossa of children, they are also well-recognized supratentorial gliomas. In contrast to the posterior fossa examples, supratentorial ependymomas often arise with no direct connection to the cerebral ventricles (Burger et al., 1991; Bigner et al., 1998). They have a distinctive, almost epithelial, appearance and are commonly calcified. One diagnostic feature is the presence of true ependymal rosettes, but these are rare. A feature that serves to suggest the diagnosis is the alternating appearance of zones with fairly uniform round nuclei alternating with eosinophilic anuclear zones. These anuclear zones occur most commonly around blood vessels and represent ependymal cell cytoplasmic processes. True ependymal rosettes may be impossible to find without resorting to ultrastructural studies.

Ependymomas may have some immunoreactivity to glial fibrillary acidic protein and may also react with antikeratin antibodies. Other ultrastructural features that attest to these tumors' histologic origin are a columnar cell shape, a definite polar orientation with respect to blood vessels, basal lamina near the vessel, and abundant microvilli on the cell surface distant from the vessel. True cilia may be recognized but may be difficult to find. Many supratentorial ependymomas have regions with clear cells, simulating a mixture of oligodendroglial cells. However, these clear cells are thought to be a variant of ependymal cells. Ependymomas are classified with WHO grade II tumors. Anaplastic ependymomas are WHO grade III (Kleihues and Cavenee, 2000). Ominous features that suggest a higher grade include very high cellularity and frequent mitoses. Vascular mural cell proliferation and necrosis do not seem to be predictive of poor prognosis in ependymomas.

PATHOLOGY OF NONINFILTRATIVE GLIOMAS

The following sections of this chapter discuss the very low-grade, noninfiltrating gliomas and other low-grade infiltrating gliomas whose prognosis, while quite good for brain tumor patients, is less favorable than that of patients with noninfiltrating gliomas. Most low-grade glioma patients are children, adolescents, or young adults; therefore, special consideration with respect to surgery, perioperative care, radiotherapy, and chemotherapy is discussed.

In addition to the diffuse supratentorial astrocytomas that are histologically graded according to the above scheme, special variants of astrocytoma exist that do not conform to these grades and that occur in specific clinical situations. These include the juvenile pilocytic astrocytoma, which is the most common tumor in this group; the pleomorphic xanthoastrocytoma; the desmoplastic astrocytoma; and the subependymal giant cell astrocytoma of tuberous sclerosis. Other more uncommon variants of mixed neuronal–glial and mature neuronal tumors include the desmoplastic infantile ganglioglioma, the dysembryoplastic neuroepithelial tumor, the central neurocytoma, and the ganglioglioma.

Characteristics of Specific Tumors

Juvenile Pilocytic Astrocytoma

The most common locations of supratentorial juvenile pilocytic astrocytomas, considered as WHO grade I, are the cerebral hemispheres followed by, in order of decreasing frequency, optic pathways, hypothalamus, and thalamus (Clark et al., 1985; Sutton, 1987). Juvenile pilocytic astrocytomas of the cerebral hemispheres are usually cystic, with a tumor nidus presenting as a mural nodule (Palma and Guidetti, 1985; Tomita et al., 1986). On occasion, the tumor is arranged in a plaque-like fashion at the perimeter of the cyst, which is brightly enhanced on CT following the administration of IV contrast agents (Maiuri, 1988). It should be noted, however, that not all cystic hemispheric lesions, with or without the appearance of a mural nodule, are astrocytic in nature. The clinical differential diagnosis of these tumors includes ependymoma, hemangioblastoma, neuroblastoma, meningioma, and primitive neuroectodermal tumor.

The vast majority of patients with juvenile pilocytic astrocytomas develop symptoms in the first three decades of life, in particular between the ages of 10 and 25 years (Clark et al., 1985; Garcia and Fulling, 1985; Schisano et al., 1963). The duration of symptoms before surgery is usually 3 to 5 years. The most common symptoms of cerebral hemisphere tumors are related to mass effect and location and include headaches, nausea and vomiting, weakness, visual disturbances, and seizures. Tumors of the hypothalamus and thalamus can cause precocious puberty, "diencephalic syndrome" (Scott and Mickle, 1987), and hemiparesis, respectively. Children less than 1 to 2 years of age may also present with macrocephaly. This finding of an enlarged head in an infant or newborn who also is failing to thrive indicates a tumor in the hypothalamic area until proven otherwise (Wisoff et al., 1990). Obstructive hydrocephalus results from a tumor, usually of a pilocytic phenotype, occurring in the posterior optic pathway, optic–hypothalamic region, or the anterior thalamus (Nishio et al., 1993). Anatomically, the tumor occludes the anterior third ventricle, blocking either the aqueduct of Sylvius or the foramen of Monro. Anteriorly located optic pathway tumors are rarely associated with hydrocephalus.

Astrocytomas of the third ventricle region, optic apparatus, and cerebellum in children have a similar histologic appearance and biologic behavior. Their singular common feature is the presence of elongated, spindled astrocytes, the so-called pilocytes or "hair-like" cells (Burger et al., 1991). These cells have spindle-shaped nuclei and long, thin, eosinophilic cytoplasmic processes that extend from the cells in a bipolar array. Another usual histologic feature is the presence of Rosenthal fibers within the tumor or at its periphery and the interface with surrounding brain. These distinctive eosinophilic beaded structures are derived from astrocytic processes. Ultrastructurally, the eosinophilic material is electron dense, and residual intermediate filaments can be distinguished at its periphery. Immunocytochemically, studies for glial fibrillary acidic protein usually show peripheral positive reactivity in Rosenthal fibers, with a largely negative reaction in the center.

In addition to this common feature, tumors of the separate locations have some distinctive features. The parenchymal pilocytic astrocytomas are commonly described as cystic with a mural nodule. This nodule has a fleshy, dark red appearance grossly and is distinguished histologically by its biphasic nature. It appears as an irregular alternating pattern of pilocytic areas and looser microcystic areas (Fig. 3–14). The microcysts contain eosinophilic, acellular, proteinaceous material. The cells in the looser areas are more stellate, with multiple short cell processes and round nuclei. The pilocytic areas are commonly located around blood vessels. The numerous blood vessels can show thickening and hyalinization of their walls, with endothelial cell hypertrophy or proliferation, simulating the vascular mural cell proliferation seen in malignant astrocytomas of the cerebral hemispheres. However, in the pilocytic astrocytomas of children, these vascular changes do not portend an ominous prognosis. Other areas of these tumors may show cells with clear cytoplasm, resembling oligodendroglioma. Individual nuclei of the pilocytes can be enlarged, hyperchromatic, and pleomorphic, but these nuclear features again are not associated with a worse behavior. It is thought that this nuclear pleomorphism represents a degenerative change. The pilocytic astrocytomas with the biphasic pattern have been termed *juvenile* pilocytic astrocytomas to distinguish them from the diffuse astrocytomas having a pilocytic growth pattern that occurs in the cerebral hemispheres of adults or in the brain stem. These diffuse pilocytic astrocytomas are typically graded according to the usual criteria for malignant astrocytomas and behave as such.

Pilocytic astrocytomas of the optic apparatus and third ventricle region are less commonly biphasic than are the hemispheric parenchymal examples, but have the distinctive pilocytes and lack mitotic activity (Fig. 3–14). These tumors distort the usual organizational pattern of the optic nerves and chiasm, expanding and then obliterating the septate structure. There is an increase in glial cellularity but little pleomorphism. An exuberant growth of connective tissue is also a common feature, and the tumors can grow into the leptomeninges of the optic structures. Rosenthal fibers are a common finding. Metastatic spread in the cerebrospinal fluid has been described, even in the absence of increased histologic anaplasia (Obana et al., 1991).

Pilocytic astrocytomas show strong cytoplasmic glial fibrillary acidic protein immunoreactivity in the pilocytic cells with diffuse reactivity in the stellate

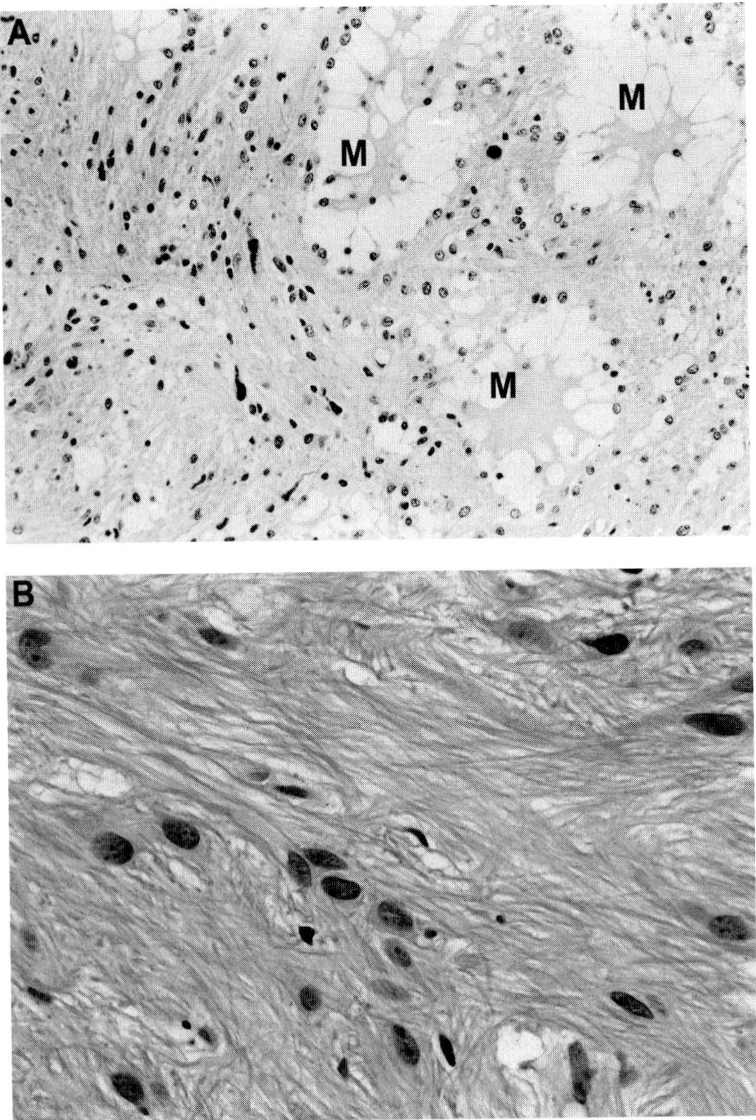

Figure 3–14. Low-grade pilocytic astrocytoma. **(A)** The "juvenile" type shows a biphasic solid and microcystic (M) growth pattern. Hematoxylin and eosin. Original magnification, ×200. **(B)** The diffuse type of pilocytic astrocytoma shows elongated "hair-like" cells without the microcystic component. No mitotic activity is present. Hematoxylin and eosin. Original magnification, ×300.

cells. Vascular structures fail to stain with glial fibrillary acidic protein, but can be delineated with a Masson trichrome, reticulin, or Factor VIII immunostain. These three methods label the perivascular collagen, connective tissue fibers, or endothelial cells, respectively.

Tuberous Sclerosis (Bourneville's Disease)

Tuberous sclerosis is a phakomatosis associated with supratentorial noninfiltrative gliomas. Children and young adults afflicted with this syndrome are typically cognitively retarded and have seizures that are often refractory to medical care and dermatologic manifestations of facial adenoma sebaceum. Cortical hamartomas are the rule and are associated with periventricular calcified nodules (Pinto-Lord et al., 1986). These latter lesions are typically located near the foramen of Monro and histologically are subependymal giant cell astrocytomas (McLaurin and Towbin, 1986), a lesion that has not been documented in patients without tuberous sclerosis (Shepherd et al., 1991). If the subependymal nodule grows, it will block the foramen of Monro and cause obstructive hydrocephalus. Often this is a very indolent process with a gradual onset of symptoms.

Subependymal Giant Cell Astrocytoma

The subependymal giant cell astrocytoma is a tumor of uncertain histogenesis that is usually included with astrocytomas. It is classified as WHO grade I (Kleihues and Cavenee, 2000). The degree of histologic pleomorphism of the cells may suggest a diagnosis of glioblastoma multiforme, but mitotic activity and necrosis are lacking. The subependymal giant cell astrocytoma generally occurs in the setting of tuberous sclerosis and is located, as its name suggests, in the subependymal region, two features that may be helpful in suggesting the correct diagnosis. However, sporadic examples in patients without a history of tuberous sclerosis do occur (Boesel et al., 1979). The tumor cells are large and bizarre, and the tumor is highly cellular. Abundant eosinophilic cytoplasm is a usual feature. The nuclei are very enlarged and have prominent nucleoli, even suggesting a neuronal origin (Nakamura and Becker, 1983). Ultrastructurally, intermediate filaments are numerous, as are long, thickened cytoplasmic processes. Immunohistochemical studies, however, failed to reveal a defined histogenesis for this neoplasm, as tumor cells may mark poorly for both glial and neuronal antigens or may mark for both. This tumor is usually considered benign and is curable by surgical excision alone (Shepherd et al., 1991).

Pleomorphic Xanthoastrocytoma

Another tumor found to involve the cerebral hemispheres in children and young adults is the pleomorphic xanthoastrocytoma. This lesion is almost always superficial in location and often abuts a leptomeningeal surface (Kepes et al., 1979). The temporal lobe is most commonly involved, followed in frequency by the parietal lobe. In our experience, seizures are the most common form of presentation, and the duration of symptoms may extend up to several years before the surgical diagnosis. Although usually described as a benign and indolent lesion and classified as WHO grade II, the clinical course and outcome of this tumor are controversial because of the difficulty in arriving at a histologic diagnosis due to its pleomorphic and giant cell appearance. Nonetheless, cases have been reported with a rapidly progressive tumor growth resulting in death (Weldon-Linne et al., 1983). Xanthoastrocytomas, like other gliomas, have been found in patients with neurofibromatosis (Ozek et al., 1993).

The pleomorphic xanthoastrocytoma is a distinctive astrocytoma variant known for its extreme histologic pleomorphism in the absence of significant mitotic activity and necrosis (Kepes et al., 1979; Kepes, 1993). The importance of recognizing this variant is that it should not be mistaken for glioblastoma multiforme. This superficially located tumor of early adulthood is usually considered benign and is surgically curable. The individual tumor cells, in addition to showing marked pleomorphism tending even toward the bizarre, have a high content of lipid, revealed in frozen sections by staining for neutral fat with oil red O. The astrocytic nature of these foamy, lipidized cells is revealed by positive cytoplasmic immunoreactivity for glial fibrillary acidic protein (Grant and Gallagher, 1986). The finding of mitotic activity or necrosis or the occurrence of this neoplasm in patients beyond the third decade of life should raise caution about the diagnosis and prognosis. These examples may be classified as WHO grade III (Giannini et al., 1999). Some examples have been shown to transform to glioblastoma or to behave in a malignant fashion (Weldon-Linne et al., 1983).

Desmoplastic Cerebral Astrocytoma

The desmoplastic infantile astrocytoma is another distinctive variant that occurs in a stereotypical clinical situation. It corresponds to WHO grade I (Kleihues and Cavenee, 2000). This tumor is generally one of infancy and childhood (VandenBerg, 1993; Louis et al., 1992; de Chadarevian et al., 1990). A few examples in adults have been described. The singular histologic feature is the extreme spindling of astrocytes within an extensive collagen matrix. The tumor may be superficially located in the hemisphere, and it has been postulated that the collagen arises from growth of the tumor into the pia with collagen proliferation from that source. These tumors may even resemble a sarcoma, but immunohistochemical studies positive for glial fibrillary acidic protein again reveal their astrocytic nature. The prognosis for these tumors is considered favorable with complete excision, but they occur very infrequently.

A tumor having similar histology but also exhibiting primitive small cells and neuronal differentiation occurs in very young children, generally under 2 years of age (VandenBerg et al., 1987; VandenBerg, 1993). These are the desmoplastic infantile gangliogliomas, which are discussed below.

Mixed Neuronal–Glial Tumors

Mixed neuronal–glial tumors include a broad histologic spectrum, ranging from the typical ganglioglioma, with its complement of atypical but well-differentiated neuronal elements, to the more complex examples of desmoplastic infantile ganglioglioma and dysembryoplastic neuroepithelial tumor.

Dysembryoplastic Neuroepithelial Tumor. The dysembryoplastic neuroepithelial tumor is found exclusively in patients who undergo cortical resections for intractable epilepsy (Daumas-Duport et al., 1988a). This tumor is described as showing multiple intracortical nodules of glial proliferative elements combined with a dysplastic cerebral cortex and a columnar orientation of a "specific glioneuronal element" composed of oligodendroglia, neurons, and capillaries (Daumas-Duport, 1993). The astrocytic component is generally pilocytic and forms nodules that may be microcystic. Mitotic activity is not seen, and necrosis is not a feature of this tumor. These are considered WHO grade I (Kleihues and Cavenee, 2000). The tumor's intracortical location and nodular architecture, with associated cortical dysplasia, distinguish it from the typical ganglioglioma. After resection for epilepsy treatment, recurrence or progression of dysembryoplastic neuroepithelial tumor has not been demonstrated.

Dysembryoplastic neuroepithelial tumors have a predilection for the temporal lobe in young patients who have difficult-to-control seizure activity. These tumors are well circumscribed grossly and on diagnostic imaging studies (Koeller and Dillon, 1992). They are typically very indolent lesions with a long natural history (Daumas-Duport, 1993).

Ganglioglioma. Gangliogliomas usually have a long duration of symptoms, sometimes up to 15 to 20 years, before definitive clinical diagnosis (Kalyan-Raman and Oliverio, 1987; Silver et al., 1991). Gangliogliomas have a predilection for the temporal and frontal lobes and almost always are associated with seizures (i.e., complex partial epilepsy, with or without secondary generalization). Often patients with these tumors present with medically refractory epilepsy that requires intraoperative electrocorticography (see below) to improve seizure control (Pilcher et al., 1993).

The ganglioglioma is a biphasic tumor that has a mature but atypical neuronal component mixed with a neoplastic glial component. Gangliomas may be WHO grade I or II (Kleihues and Cavenee, 2000). The tumor's histologic appearance is quite characteristic, with a prominent vascular septa dividing it into a lobular pattern. Mature lymphocytes can be a feature of the vascular component. The glial component is usually astrocytic and low grade, with rare or absent mitotic figures (Haddad et al., 1992). The glial morphology may suggest a pilocytic astrocytoma. Intermixed with the astrocytic component is a population of atypical neurons, which are manifested in their size and shape, arrangement, and neurohistology. Multinucleated forms may be seen. Because large, gemistocytic astrocytes may simulate atypical neurons with their abundant eosinophilic cytoplasm, special immunohistochemical markers of neuronal differentiation, such as synaptophysin or neurofilament protein, may be required to confirm the diagnosis (Miller et al., 1993).

Desmoplastic Infantile Ganglioglioma. The desmoplastic infantile ganglioglioma is a distinctive and rare tumor that occurs in infants, generally within the first 2 years of life (VandenBerg, 1993). These tumors are very similar to the superficial cerebral astrocytoma with dural attachment described by Taratuto et al. (1984) and tend to be located in the frontal and parietal regions. These tumors may be large, with a prominent cystic or multicystic appearance, and generally have a superficial hemispheric location. They have a predominant desmoplastic character, resulting in a firm gross consistency, and often have a large amount of proteinaceous fluid. Despite this, they infiltrate into brain. The desmoplasia consists of admixed fibrous collagen and glial elements. The astrocytic component may be moderately pleomorphic but is identified by its positive cytoplasmic immunoreactivity for glial fibrillary acidic protein. The neuronal elements range from mature neurons to primitive small cells and can be recognized by immunohistochemical stains for synaptophysin or neurofilament protein. The neuronal elements are usually seen in the less desmoplastic areas of the tumor and may be of variable amounts. Mitoses and necrosis are more likely to be found in association with the small cell component. Despite their cellular heterogeneity and primitive small cell component, these tumors are associated with a prolonged survival provided that the tumor is maximally resected. They are WHO grade I (Kleihues and Cavenee, 2000).

Central Neurocytoma

Neurocytomas are neoplasms of small mature neurons that may arise within the ventricles (intraventricular or central neurocytoma) or in the brain parenchyma (cerebral neurocytoma) (Burger et al., 1991; Hassoun et al., 1993; Hessler et al., 1992). The classic central neurocytoma is a supratentorial, often calcified, mass within the lateral ventricle. It may arise from the septum pellucidum (Kim et al., 1992).

Histologically, this neoplasm is characterized by a diffuse proliferation of small, clear cells with round nuclei and finely punctate chromatin. Fibrillary zones may be interspersed and may help to distinguish this tumor from oligodendroglioma. The tumor is not anaplastic, mitotic figures are rare, and necrosis is unusual. It corresponds to WHO grade II. The diagnostic feature is evidence of neuronal differentiation, either immunohistochemically or ultrastructurally (Hessler et al., 1992). Tumor cells are positive for the neuronal markers synaptophysin and neurofilament and negative for glial fibrillary acidic protein. Electron microscopy reveals dense-cored granules within the cell bodies (Hassoun et al., 1993). These diagnostic studies can distinguish neurocytomas from ependymomas and oligodendrogliomas. With complete removal, neurocytomas seem to behave in a benign fashion and generally do not recur (Kim et al., 1992).

OUTCOME VARIABLES

Several patient and tumor characteristics influence outcome in those with astrocytomas. The most important prognostic variables are patient age at diagnosis, functional status, completeness of resection, and tumor histology. Young age (Leibel et al., 1975; Marsa et al., 1975; Laws et al., 1985; Piepmeier, 1987; Medbery et al., 1988; Shaw et al., 1989; North et al., 1990; Whitton and Bloom, 1990), absence of postoperative performance deficits, alteration of consciousness and personality change (Laws et al., 1985; Piepmeier, 1987; Medbery et al., 1988; Shaw et al., 1989; North et al., 1990), and more extensive surgery (Leibel et al., 1975; Laws et al., 1985; Shaw et al., 1989; Soffietti et al., 1989; North et al., 1990) are associated with an improved outcome. Patients with mixed oligoastrocytomas have a better prognosis than do those with pure astrocytomas (Shaw et al., 1991). Oligodendrogliomas, however, have a significantly better long-term survival than mixed oligoastrocytomas and astrocytomas (Shaw et al., 1997). While sometimes included with grade II astrocytomas, in general, survival of patients with gemistocytic astrocytoma is similar to those with anaplastic astrocytomas.

SURGICAL TREATMENT AND ITS IMPACT

The belief that most gliomas are infiltrative into adjacent brain has been strengthened in recent years by studies based on diagnostic imaging and neuroimage-guided stereotactic biopsies of these tumors and their surrounding periphery. This, along with technical advances in neurosurgical instrumentation allowing for precise tissue sampling using image-coupled reference frames, has had a significant effect on the role of surgery in managing the patient with a glioma.

In a study correlating results of CT scans with results of postmortem examination for extent of disease in patients with glioblastoma, Burger and colleagues (1988) found tumor beyond the contrast-enhancing rim at autopsy in most cases that had shown hypodense regions on the scan. However, there was a delay of several weeks between the imaging study and death; also the cause of death was the actual tumor in fewer than 50% of cases. Furthermore, the authors stated that the "methodology to identify neoplastic cells (in adjacent brain) has significant limitations."

Daumas-Duport et al. (1987) optimized tissue fixation methods to be able to define in greater detail cells that appeared to be neoplastic and had been obtained stereotactically from peripheral glioma zones. In addition, this group implanted corresponding specimens into nude mice, and the implants formed tumors composed of astrocytes. There was no attempt made to correlate the regions from where these isolated tumor cells were taken and patterns of recurrence in patients on the basis of follow-up imaging studies. Making a qualitative interpretation of neoplastic versus reactive astrocytes suffers from the lack of specific tumor cell markers. Extending beyond the CT era, biopsy material obtained from hyperintense, T_2-weighted signal regions seen on MR imaging studies also verified isolated tumor cells outside the contrast-enhancing rim in high-grade glial tumors (Kelly, 1993).

Despite the knowledge base surgeons have acquired about the histologic limits of infiltrative gliomas, clinical studies have supported a localized pattern of tumor recurrence. Reports by Liang et al. (1991) and Hochberg and Pruitt (1980) documented recurrent disease within 2 cm of the contrast-enhancing rim in 85% to 90% of their patients. These two studies were done 10 years apart, and even with improvements in imaging, the conclusions were the same. Similarly, in another study Gaspar et al. (1992) found tumor recurrence in all cases within 4 cm of the contrast margin and not beyond this imaging line of demarcation.

Low-Grade Infiltrative Gliomas

Controversy continues to exist with regard to extent of tumor removal and outcome in patients with supratentorial low-grade glial tumors, which, in most circumstances, involve the cerebral hemispheres. Several points regarding the prognostic effect of tumor removal remain unclear, and management strategies are almost always based on class III evidence (i.e., evidence provided by expert opinions, nonrandomized historic controls, or case reports) (Bampoe and Bernstein, 1999; Eddy, 1990). A review by the Guidelines and Outlines Committee of the American Association of Neurological Surgeons (1998), based on data published between 1966 to 1994 on low-grade gliomas showed that the only available standard for adults with suspected or known supratentorial nonoptic pathway low-grade glioma is to obtain tissue diagnosis before active treatment. Several critical issues (e.g., the need for biopsy before observation and the effects of observation, resection, and radiotherapy on outcome) remained unclear. There were no standards or guidelines that could be supported by class I evidence (randomized controlled clinical trial) or class II evidence (case–control or cohort studies). Therefore, all current management strategies were considered as practice options based on class III evidence.

It is generally believed that the survival rate is higher for patients with gross total tumor resections compared with those with biopsy only. Unfortunately, no prospective randomized study has ever been done to evaluate the relationship between amount of tumor removed and subsequent influence on recurrence patterns and survival. Most studies are retrospective. Reports have been based on the surgeon's impression at the time of surgery, appearance of the postoperative CT or MRI images, or measurement of perpendicular tumor diameters as seen on contrast-enhanced neuroimages. In addition, several studies include pediatric patients and evaluate survival characteristics for a combination of adult and pediatric patients, without taking into account that age is the strongest prognostic indicator within a histologic subgroup. This approach results in longer survival times and better overall outcomes for series incorporating younger patients.

Another common methodologic problem arises when various histologies with different natural histories are combined and evaluated together without manipulating the data to separate individual histologic subtypes. In several studies, pilocytic or gemistocytic astrocytomas are included in the study population. These heterogeneous populations make the data harder to interpret, and conflicting results are often obtained in studies evaluating the efficiency of a particular treatment option. Currently, there are only a few hemispheric low-grade glioma series with more than 75 patients that exclude the pediatric age group as well as gemistocytic and pilocytic histologies. All of these studies with relatively homogeneous patient populations show a statistically significant advantage in terms of survival for low-grade glioma patients who receive the most extensive resections (Leighton et al., 1997; Philippon et al., 1993; Rajan et al., 1993; Soffietti et al., 1989; van Veelen et al., 1998). None of these studies, however, offers class I evidence (randomized controlled clinical trial).

Of additional importance in interpreting surgical results is the fact that a large number of low-grade gliomas recur with a more malignant tumor grade (Afra et al., 1978; Laws et al., 1985; North et al., 1990; Piepmeier et al., 1987).

We previously analyzed our database, using a computerized image analysis technique (Duong et al., 1992) that yields a quantitative, volumetric determination of preoperative and postoperative tumor volumes, including percent of resection, to ascertain whether these parameters influence recurrence patterns. By measurement we found a mean preoperative tumor volume of 26.6 cc (based on T_2-weighted MR signal) and found no tumor recurrence (mean follow-up, 42 months) when the preoperative volume was <10 cc (Berger et al., 1994). The likelihood of recurrence was greater and the time to tumor progression shorter when the volume increased (e.g., 41% recurrence rate at a median 30 months for patients with tumors >30 cc). Other studies have found radical resection to favorably influence outcome for patients who have a low-grade glioma. Data on the amount of resection were based on the operative report or on the qualitative assessment of the postoperative scans, without an attempt to use volumetric analysis (Guthrie and Laws, 1990; Laws et al., 1985; North et al., 1990). These data are similar to those reported by the Japanese Brain Tumor Registry during the past 25 years (1992), which include 5 year survival rates of 48% for biopsy and subtotal resections of 50% or less versus a 70% survival for those with greater than 90% resections (Brain Tumor Registry of Japan, 1992).

These data also parallel studies that evaluated postoperative tumor volume and survival time for high-grade gliomas (Levin et al., 1980b). Using volumetric measurements (based on tumor measurements in 3 intersecting directions), it was found that when the postoperative tumor volume was >10 cc the chance of recurrence was 46% (median time to tumor progression, 30 months) compared with a tumor volume of <10 cc, which had a chance of recurrence of 15% (median, 50 months); there were no recurrences following complete resection at a mean follow-up time of 54 months.

The timing of surgical intervention following a diagnosis based on imaging studies is also controversial, with some studies recommending immediate intervention (Laws et al., 1985; Morantz, 1987; Weingart et al., 1991) and others advocating a less urgent approach (Cairncross and Laperriere, 1989; Recht et al., 1992). One study that quantified the tumor area as being less than or greater than 25 cc found a significant difference in survival when patients with smaller tumors were operated on earlier (Shibamoto et al., 1993). Another retrospective review of patients whose surgery was deferred until disease progressed demonstrated that in nearly 50% of the cases malignancy was documented at the time of the biopsy even though the lesions had a classic low-grade appearance on the initial imaging studies (Recht et al., 1992). Although controversy will continue about biopsy versus radical resection as well as about the timing of surgery, such data as are presented in this section show a trend toward an increasing risk of early and malignant recurrence when a conservative approach is taken once the presumptive diagnosis of low-grade glioma is made.

Very few data exist on what role extensive surgery plays in determining the outcomes of patients with oligodendroglioma. Survival was positively influenced by total tumor resection in some studies (Chin et al., 1980; Shaw et al., 1992; Varma et al., 1983; Mork et al., 1985; Celli et al., 1994; Schiffer et al., 1997). This contrasts with studies by Sun and colleagues (1988) and others (Kros et al., 1994; Daumas-Duport et al., 1997) in which survival was not affected by the extent of resection. In one analysis, radiotherapy did not affect outcome following total tumor removal, implying that, unlike other infiltrative low-grade gliomas, oligodendroglioma may be more amenable to a complete tumor resection because of its somewhat circumscribed nature associated with macroscopically distinct margins (Lindegaard et al., 1987). As with all low-grade gliomas, the surgical strategy should favor radical tumor removal when at all feasible.

Finally, because low-grade tumors tend to have an indolent growth pattern, they are often associated with seizure activity that is infrequently not refractory to medical care. This is especially true for oligodendrogliomas, gangliogliomas, and astrocytic gliomas (Arseni and Petrovici, 1971; Hirsch et al., 1989; Pilcher et al., 1993). A controversial surgical issue involves the role of intraoperative electrocorticography during tumor resection used to minimize postoperative seizures. For most patients with intermittent seizures that are well controlled with antiepileptic drugs, removing the tumor alone without seizure mapping is sufficient and results in good control of tumor-associated epilepsy (Cascino et al., 1990; Cascino, 1990; Franceschetti et al., 1990; Goldring et al., 1986; Hirsch et al., 1989). In some low-grade glioma patients who have intractable seizures, tumor removal by itself often will not diminish seizure activity (Awad et al., 1991; Cascino et al., 1990; Spencer et al., 1984; Zentner et al., 1997). Our approach has been to use electrocorticography during the tumor resection to identify separate seizure foci adjacent to the tumor nidus (Berger et al., 1993). Of our adult patients,

88% became seizure free with (47%) or without (41%) antiepileptic drugs. Even the few patients who had persistent seizure activity while taking medication benefited from surgery and had fewer seizures that were often less intense. Each child and adolescent in our series was seizure free and not taking medication except for two children who continued therapy with antiepileptic drugs because they had a few seizures following surgery. These data are also supported by other investigators who use electrocorticography to control postoperative seizures in this particular patient population (Awad et al., 1991; Drake et al., 1987; Gonzalez and Elvidge, 1962; Rasmussen, 1975; Ribaric et al., 1991).

Juvenile Pilocytic Astrocytomas and Other Noninfiltrative Gliomas

The goal of surgical intervention in patients with cerebral hemispheric juvenile pilocytic astrocytomas is to evacuate the cyst contents and remove all contrast-enhanced tissue documented on the preoperative CT or MRI studies. This includes the mural nodule and any or all parts of the cyst that are contrast enhanced. Failure to remove the lesion while simply draining the cyst will uniformly result in re-accumulation of the cyst contents. Several studies have documented that the cyst wall is gliotic without neoplastic cells when it does not enhance with contrast administration (Maiuri, 1988; Tomita et al., 1986). If the cyst wall enhances, it must be completely resected to avoid tumor recurrence (Morota et al., 1990). The mural nodule is quite discrete and has a reddish-brown appearance. It is friable and moderately bloody. At the end of the resection, the adjacent, noninfiltrated white matter should be clearly visible. As expected, there is a distinct microscopic margin between the tumor and the contiguous white matter (Garcia and Fulling, 1985). Because the cyst is often in continuity with the ependymal surface of the ventricular system, we do not recommend, as do some authors, that the cyst be fenestrated into the ventricle (Palma et al., 1983; Mercuri et al., 1981). Following removal of the tumor, the cyst will not recur. In addition, debris from the resection cavity may seep into the ventricle and cause a communicating hydrocephalus.

With solid juvenile pilocytic astrocytomas it is somewhat more difficult to achieve a gross total resection, especially when the tumor is deep or attached to subcortical functional tracts. Solid tumors should be aggressively resected, however, unless excessive or unacceptable morbidity would result. The long-term results without radiotherapy or chemotherapy are excellent following a complete resection. Nevertheless, as a precautionary measure we advocate careful and routine follow up every 6 to 12 months for the first several years after surgery. The 10 year survival rate for a completely resected pilocytic hemispheric astrocytoma, verified with postoperative imaging studies, should approach 100% (Wallner et al., 1988a; Shaw et al., 1989). This favorable outcome also pertains to adult patients with this diagnosis (Garcia and Fulling, 1985). Although incompletely resected tumors may have a protracted course, recurrence is likely over a period of several years, necessitating routine follow up (Palma and Guidetti, 1985).

Thalamic juvenile pilocytic astrocytomas tend to be well circumscribed and may be associated with a cyst (Wald et al., 1982). Anterior thalamic tumors are best resected via a parasagittal incision in front of the premotor cortex, thus entering the ventricle anteriorly. These lesions displace the internal capsule laterally, whereas posterior thalamic masses push the posterior limb of the internal capsule forward. Therefore, the best approach in the latter circumstance is through the posterior ventricle (i.e., the atrium). It is critical to localize the capsular motor fibers using subcortical stimulation methods to avoid morbidity while maximizing the extent of resection (Berger et al., 1990). An alternative surgical approach is to volumetrically resect the pilocytic tumor using computer-assisted stereotactic methods (Lyons and Kelly, 1992). This technology is very accurate and effective, but is expensive and is not available to most neurosurgeons.

Because subependymal giant cell astrocytomas are always located within the anterior horn of the lateral ventricle, the preferred approach to them depends on the ventricular size. Ventricular dilatation is the rule for symptomatic patients because of the relationship between the tumor and the foramen of Monro. Therefore, in most circumstances a frontal transventricular approach is performed to gain the necessary exposure, taking advantage of the large ventricles. However, some surgeons still recommend a transcallosal exposure because there is less brain retraction and less potential risk of postoperative epilepsy, although this latter point is debatable (McLaurin and Towbin, 1986). Regardless of approach, virtually all surgeons agree that these lesions should only be removed when symptoms of ventricular obstruction exist.

The supratentorial ependymoma and pleomorphic xanthoastrocytoma appear grossly as an encapsulated mass distinct from the adjacent brain. However, the latter lesion tends to have more of a contiguous relationship with the leptomeninges (Kepes et al., 1989), making its resection more difficult, especially when the tumor occurs within the sylvian fissure. With both lesions, a superficial (i.e., pial-based) attachment should alert the surgeon that these tumors are circumscribed and amenable to complete resection. One review of the literature, however, revealed that even with complete resection of a pleomorphic xanthoastrocytoma, there is a 30% chance of recurrence (Macaulay et al., 1993); thus, routine surveillance with postoperative imaging studies is mandatory.

While there is universal agreement among surgeons that cerebral hemispheric gangliogliomas should be completely resected (Silver et al., 1991; Otsubo et al., 1992), controversy exists regarding the extent of resection as it pertains to optimal tumor control. If the literature is reviewed with respect to seizure control and extent of surgical resection, it appears that a complete tumor resection results in a 50% seizure-free condition, a rate not greatly dissimilar to that with incomplete tumor removal (Haddad et al., 1992). However, when intraoperative electrocorticography is used to map epileptogenic foci so as to include them as part of the operative procedure, the likelihood that patients with a gross total tumor resection would achieve complete seizure control was 92% (Pilcher et al., 1993). This outcome is significantly better than that for removing only the tumor. Even when the tumor was removed and the epileptic focus incompletely resected, a 95% reduction in postoperative seizures was demonstrated. Therefore, intraoperative electrocorticography is indispensable for patients who have intractable epilepsy associated with gangliogliomas or other similar, yet less frequently occurring, lesions (e.g., desmoplastic infantile gangliogliomas and dysembryoplastic neuroepithelial tumors). For the latter two noninfiltrative, circumscribed tumor types, the goal of surgery is complete resection, which positively influences outcome for control of recurrence and seizures (VandenBerg, 1993; Daumas-Duport, 1993).

High-Grade Gliomas

Unlike for low-grade gliomas, surgeons have been much more willing to use cytoreductive surgery for bulky malignant gliomas to alleviate mass effect associated with symptoms and signs of increased intracranial pressure. Moreover, areas of necrosis are more amenable to surgical aspiration than is firm white matter infiltrated with a low-grade glial tumor. However, the idea that the extent of resection sufficiently influences survival of patients with malignant gliomas is still not universally accepted; thus, treatment recommendations will vary among surgeons. For example, in a retrospective study that analyzed outcome after a limited (i.e., stereotactic) biopsy, the median survival times for patients with glioblastoma and anaplastic astrocytoma were each less than 30 weeks; if deep midline tumors were excluded, the median survivals improved to 47 and 129 weeks, respectively. In this study, the few patients who received cytoreductive surgery exhibited no statistical difference in outcome when biopsy was compared with a more aggressive surgery, although in the latter situation no information was provided about the extent of resection (Coffey et al., 1988). Kelly (1990) demonstrated a survival advantage for those patients with glioblastoma who underwent complete stereotactically guided resection (48 weeks) over those patients who had a biopsy or a standard craniotomy and resection (30 and 38 weeks, respectively). Comparing results from these two studies suggests that biopsy is not a substitute for a good tumor resection.

A number of radiographic studies have shown an inverse relationship between postsurgical tumor volume and survival (Levin et al., 1980b; Wood et al., 1988). Volumetric analysis of 107 operations on patients with hemispheric glioblastoma multiforme showed that patients who underwent a total tumor resection with no residual disease had a significantly longer time to tumor progression and survival (Keles et al., 1999). In this study, as volume of residual tumor increased, a shorter time to progression and a longer survival were observed. Most cooperative prospective multimodality trials show a survival advantage for subtotal and gross total resection compared with biopsy.

In addition to the concept that an aggressive resection, as opposed to limited tumor removal, will positively influence outcome (Chang et al., 1983; Levin et al., 1980b; Walker et al., 1978; Dinapoli et al., 1993), quality of life also becomes a critical issue, which is influenced by surgery. It has been recognized for quite some time that removal of a very small tumor or biopsy specimen may result in excessive morbidity from swelling or hemorrhage (Fadul et al., 1988). Studies (Ammirati et al., 1987; Ciric et al., 1987; Keles et al., 1999) have demonstrated that patients usually improve neurologically or remain the same with aggressive tumor removal. This has also been our experience, and, combined with neurophysiologic cortical and subcortical mapping methods, the likelihood of creating a permanent deficit with current surgical techniques should be less than 3% to 5%.

The role of radical resection for children with malignant supratentorial gliomas has not been as rigorously examined as for adults. In the few studies that address this issue without any reference to how extent of resection was determined, it appears that children who received a radical resection rather than a biopsy survived longer (Allen et al., 1986; Artico et al., 1993). In a study evaluating extent of resection on survival conducted by the Childrens Cancer Group (CCG-945), the 5 year progression-free survival (PFS) rates for anaplastic astrocytoma were 44% following gross total resection and 22% for less radically resected tumors; for glioblastoma the 5 year PFS rates were 26% for gross total resection and only 4% for children with less radical resections (Wisoff et al., 1998).

Gliosarcoma continues to be a difficult problem for the surgeon because of its highly invasive nature. Often, the lesion may appear somewhat circumscribed (Maiuri et al., 1990), but it is extremely vascular and frequently invades the overlying dura (Morantz et al., 1976). Too few studies have been done to determine whether the extent of surgery influences survival for this tumor type, although the data will likely be similar to those for glioblastoma.

Gliomatosis cerebri is mentioned in this section, although it is an unusual finding. These very extensive, diffusely infiltrating gliomas usually present with symptoms and signs of increased intracranial pressure. A biopsy is mandatory and will suffice along with the MRI sequences (Spagnoli et al., 1987). There is no indication for extensive resection, and a stereotactic procedure should be directed at any contrast-enhancing tissue when present. Because of the intracranial hypertension associated with a large tumor mass, a biopsy may result in rapid neurologic deterioration (Ross et al., 1991); therefore, the patient should be observed in the intensive care unit overnight following biopsy.

In summary, radical tumor resections performed under the proper conditions will usually preserve or improve a patient's functional status and augment survival for a longer period of time than when more limited tumor resections are performed (Mornex et al., 1993; Chandler et al., 1993; Kornblith et al., 1993; Kaplan, 1993). This applies not only to glioblastoma but to other anaplastic (including gemistocytic), astrocytic, and oligodendroglial tumors (Krouwer et al., 1991; Winger et al., 1989; Prados et al., 1992a). However, in the anaplastic subtypes, the advantage of surgery must be considered to be strongly influenced by age at diagnosis because that is a known key prognostic variable for malignant gliomas (Curran et al., 1992a; Winger et al., 1989) in terms of tumor biology and in biasing the surgeon to be more aggressive.

Ependymomas

Few reports are available that describe the rationale for surgical resection of supratentorial ependymomas. Similar to other tumors that arise within the ventricle and extend into the cerebral hemispheres, surgical excision is designed to relieve mass effect and unblock the ventricular system. By itself, total tumor removal for ependymomas and mixed ependymoma astrocytomas will often result in long-term survival without the need for radiation (Palma et al., 1993). However, this is not the case with the malignant variant of this lesion, which requires focal radiation and sometimes chemotherapy to achieve similar results. Unfortunately, most studies that comment on survival in relation to extent of tumor removal do so without separating supratentorial from fourth ventricular tumors. Nonetheless, there is a distinct survival advantage for a radical tumor resection in the majority of series (Kovalic et al., 1993; Vanuytsel et al., 1992; Undjian and Marinov, 1990; Papadopoulos et al., 1990).

In a series from Boston that combined tumors in both supratentorial and fourth ventricular locations, it is important to note a discrepancy between the operative report and the postoperative imaging study (i.e., overestimation in 33% of the cases) (Healey et al., 1991). This discrepancy will certainly change as MRI replaces CT scans in the postoperative analyses of future studies. In the Boston study, the survivals at 10 years after surgery were 75% for those patients without radiographic evidence of residual tumor and 0% for patients with residual disease. Two other series, incorporating multivariate analyses, reported significantly longer PFS and overall survival rates for patients who underwent gross total resections (Rousseau et al., 1993; Pollack et al., 1995).

In the Italian Pediatric Neuro-oncology Group study, which included 92 patients, radical surgery was the only prognostic factor found in multivariate analysis to have a statistically significant effect in predicting both PFS and overall survival (Perilongo et al., 1997). Recently, in a multi-institutional study, including patients from 11 United States pediatric oncology centers, less than gross total resection was a significant adverse risk factor for event-free and overall survival (Horn et al., 1999).

Two studies dispute these findings, however. The authors claim that, in their collective experience, radical surgery is not prognostically important (Goldwein et al., 1990; Rawlings et al., 1988). Only in the Goldwein et al. (1990) study were postoperative imaging scans obtained. Notwithstanding these two studies, current neurosurgical management of ependymomas, regardless of histology, involves achieving a radical resection of the lesion without removing more than 5 to 10 mm of adjacent white matter. The prevailing consensus is that greater extent of resection seems to improve outcome and can be maximized by careful preoperative planning, a meticulous but aggressive surgical strategy, and excellent postoperative care (Smyth et al., 2000).

RATIONALE FOR REOPERATION

With heightened interest in treating patients who have failed first-line therapy, the role of reoperation must be critically evaluated in terms of the benefits versus risks. Clearly, for those patients who have mass effect, cytoreductive surgery is an important therapeutic modality that can be carried out if the patient is to have a good quality of life during the retreatment phase. Historically, a few important retrospective studies have analyzed patients who had malignant gliomas; these studies defined important clinical parameters that predicted a good outcome (survival advantage and an improved quality of life) following reoperation. Prognostically significant factors included duration of time from initial resection to tumor progression, age, and Karnofsky performance status (KPS) (Wilson, 1975; Young et al., 1981; Salcman et al., 1982). Overall, patients with glioblastoma and anaplastic astrocytoma may expect median survivals of 36 weeks and 88 weeks, respectively, following reoperation and subsequent chemotherapy (Harsh et al., 1987). Somewhat better figures have been reported by Berger et al. (1992) when the interval of time between initial surgery and reoperation is long, the KPS is 70 or greater, and the age of the patient at the time of reoperation is less than 60 years. They found for glioblastoma a mean survival time of approximately 70 weeks when the Karnofsky score before reoperation was 70 or better; for a small group of patients with anaplastic astrocytoma, the mean survival time after reoperation was 135 weeks. The interval between initial surgery and diagnosis to reoperation was predictive: patients with disease progression within 6 months of the initial operation had a mean survival of 40 weeks after reoperation versus 150 weeks if the tumor did not recur until 1 year following the original surgery. From these studies we conclude that patients who benefit most from reoperation with a malignant glioma are younger than 60 years old, have a good functional status, and have a prolonged period of disease stability following the initial operation.

RADIOTHERAPY AND CHEMOTHERAPY TREATMENT

Approaches for Low-Grade Infiltrating Gliomas

Radiotherapy

Until recently, there have been no randomized trials to clarify many of the issues surrounding the treatment of low-grade astrocytomas; thus, therapeutic decisions generally have been based on information obtained from retrospective reports. Some series do not separate patients with pilocytic astrocytomas from those with nonpilocytic tumors, although this distinction is important in the therapeutic decision-mak-

Table 3–2. Supratentorial Astrocytoma: 5 and 10 Year Survival Rates

Author	*No. of Cases*	*Treatment*	*Survival Rate (%)*	
			5 Year	*10 Year*
Levy and Elvidge (1956)	42	S	26	NA
	45	S + RT	36	NA
Bouchard (1980)	105	S + RT	49	NA
Leibel et al. (1975)	35	S	23	15
	49	S + RT	35	24
Marsa et al. (1975)	40	S + RT	40	20
Fazekas (1977)	18	S	22	NA
	36	S + RT	50	18
Laws et al. (1984)	461	S, S + RT	36	20
	167	S	34	NA
	74	S + RT	49	NA
Garcia et al. (1985)	23	S	21	10
	57	S + RT	50	25
Medbery et al. (1988)	50	S + RT	45	32
		≥50 Gy	55	45
		<50 Gy	22	13
Shaw et al. (1989)	19	S	32	11
	35	S + RT ≥53 Gy	68	39
	67	S + RT <53 Gy	47	21
Whitton and Bloom (1990)	60	S + RT	36	26
North et al. (1990)	77	S, S + RT	55	43
	52	45–59 Gy	66	NA
McCormack et al. (1992)	53	S + RT	64	48
Shibamoto et al. (1993)	71	S + RT	54 (age >30)	33
Philippon et al. (1993)	179	S	65	NA
		S + RT	55	NA
Eyre et al. (1993)	54	S + RT	50	30
Karim et al. (1996)	391	S + RT (45 Gy)	58	NA
		S + RT (59.4 Gy)	59	NA
Leighton et al. (1997)	167	S, S + RT	72	50
Shaw et al. (1998)	203	S + RT (50.4 Gy)	73	NA
		S + RT (64.8 Gy)	68 ($p = 0.57$)	NA
Karim et al. (1998)	311	S + immediate RT	63 (PFS 44%)*	NA
		S + delayed RT	66 (PFS 37%)	NA

S, surgery alone; S + RT, surgery and postoperative irradiation; N, data not available; PFS, 5 year progression-free survival.

*Difference significant, $p = 0.02$.

ing process. Representative survival rates for supratentorial astrocytomas treated with surgery or surgery and radiation therapy are summarized in Table 3–2. The outcomes of patients diagnosed and treated in the era of modern neuroimaging are notably better than those reported in older studies when the conditions for making a diagnosis were less sophisticated (Philippon et al., 1993).

Median survival times in recent series range from 7.2 to 12.9 years, raising concerns over the value today of the older literature in making treatment decisions. The improved outcome appears to be related to the earlier diagnosis of neurologically intact patients who exhibited only seizures at the time of diagnosis (Piepmeier, 1987; Cairncross and Laperriere, 1989; McCormack et al., 1992; Philippon et al.,

1993). As mentioned, survival is significantly affected by the age of the patient at diagnosis, presence of seizures at presentation, KPS, as well as whether the lesion enhances with IV contrast administration. Using a recursive partition analysis, Bauman et al. (1999a) were able to distinguish four distinct prognostic subgroups of adult, supratentorial, low-grade glioma (including oligodendroglioma) patients: group 1 (<70, age >40 years), median survival time 1 year; group II (≥70, age >40 years, the tumor enhances on CT/MRI), median survival time 3.8 years; group III (<70, age 18 to 40 years or ≥70, age >40, the tumor does not enhance), median survival time 7.2 years; and group IV (≥70, age 18 to 40 years), median survival time 10.7 years.

Using a BrdU labeling index, Hoshino et al. (1988) found that 10% (3/29) of patients with tumors exhibiting a labeling index <1% died within a 3.5 year follow-up period, whereas 50% (9/18) of patients with a labeling index >1% died within the same time interval. This concept has been corroborated in subsequent studies as well (Ito et al., 1994; Lamborn et al., 1999). These data emphasize that low-grade astrocytomas may vary considerably in their biologic behavior even though they have similar histologic appearances. Repeat biopsy specimens and autopsy studies indicate that over time at least 50% of astrocytomas transform into more anaplastic lesions (Laws et al., 1985; Muller et al., 1977; Rubinstein, 1972; Soffietti et al., 1989). Thus, whereas astrocytomas are generally considered to be benign, slow-growing tumors, in some cases they may be highly lethal.

Opinions differ regarding the need for postoperative irradiation when a complete surgical resection has been performed. The 5 year recurrence-free survival rates for patients with supratentorial astrocytomas or mixed oligoastrocytomas who undergo total or radical subtotal tumor resection range from 52% to 95% (Fazekas, 1977; Garcia et al., 1985; Hirsch et al., 1989; Leibel et al., 1975; Medbery et al., 1988; Shaw et al., 1989). The variations in outcome reflect prognostic differences related to age, the inclusion of patients with radical subtotal resections, and the reliance on retrospective evaluations of operative reports to determine the completeness of resection in the era before the availability of CT and MRI studies. Because recurrences are infrequent in children whose astrocytomas have been completely resected, postoperative irradiation is generally not recommended (Hirsh et al., 1989; Nishio et al., 1989; Mercuri et al., 1981). In contrast, the outcomes in adult patients after total or radical subtotal resection have been found in some series to be similar to those of patients undergoing less extensive surgery (Fazekas, 1977; Garcia et al., 1985; Shaw et al., 1989). Thus, some authors have recommended postoperative irradiation after complete resection in adults (Garcia et al., 1985; Shaw et al., 1989, 1991), whereas others suggest that radiation therapy be withheld until there is evidence of tumor recurrence (Leibel et al., 1975; Morantz, 1987; Soffietti et al., 1989; Wara, 1985).

Postoperative irradiation appears to prolong the survival of patients with incompletely excised supratentorial astrocytomas (Fazekas, 1977; Garcia et al., 1985; Leibel et al., 1975; Levy and Elvidge, 1956; Shaw et al., 1989). On average, the 5 and 10 year survival rates for patients who receive radiation therapy are 52% and 26%, respectively, compared with 26% and 12% for patients who do not (Table 3–2). Leibel et al. (1975) reported the outcomes of 108 patients of all ages with incompletely resected lesions. Of those, 71 patients received postoperative irradiation and 37 did not. Only 6% of tumors were pilocytic, whereas 78% arose in the cerebral hemispheres. The age distribution and performance status of the patients in the two groups were similar. The 5 year recurrence-free survival rate after incomplete resection alone was 19%, whereas it was 46% after incomplete resection and irradiation. For adult patients, the 5 year survival rate was 10% after surgery alone, compared with 32% when radiation therapy was added. The survival of patients undergoing incomplete resection and postoperative irradiation was superior to that of patients treated by surgery alone at all follow-up time intervals from 3 to 20 years. All patients not receiving radiation therapy had died by 20 years, whereas 23% of those who did remained alive and free of disease.

In their series of adult patients with cerebral astrocytomas, Garcia et al. (1985) reported an actuarial 5 year survival rate of 21% after resection alone compared with 50% after resection and postoperative irradiation ($p = 0.02$). Shaw et al. (1989) found that patients receiving high-dose postoperative irradiation had a significantly longer survival than those receiving low-dose irradiation or surgery alone. The 5 year survival rate was 68% for patients receiving a dose of at least 53 Gy, 47% for those receiving less than 53 Gy, and 32% for those receiving none ($p = 0.04$).

Older patients appear to benefit most from postoperative irradiation (Garcia et al., 1985; Laws et al., 1985; Shaw et al., 1989). Shaw et al. (1989) found that patients 35 years of age or older who received postoperative irradiation had 5 and 10 year survival rates of 67% and 45%, respectively, compared with 37% and 5% for patients treated with low-dose irradiation or surgery alone ($p = 0.008$). For patients 34 years of age or less, the 5 year survival rate was 70% with high-dose irradiation compared with 53% with low-dose irradiation or surgery alone ($p = 0.69$).

The fact that low-grade astrocytomas are diagnosed earlier in their natural history has raised questions regarding whether radiotherapy should be administered immediately after surgery or be delayed until recurrence or progression has been demonstrated. It is generally agreed that patients with intractable seizures or those with large, progressive, symptomatic, unresectable or incompletely resected tumors should undergo immediate radiotherapy. However, radiotherapy is commonly deferred in patients with medically controlled seizures who present with asymptomatic, indolent tumors (MacDonald, 1994). Proponents of this approach argue that it is unclear whether early irradiation provides an outcome advantage over delayed irradiation or whether such treatment delays or prevents tumor dedifferentiation (Cairncross and Laperriere, 1989; Whitten and Bloom, 1990).

This issue was clarified in a clinical trial conducted by the European Organization for Research and Treatment of Cancer (EORTC) and British Medical Research Council Brain Tumour Working Party (MRC). Patients with low-grade astrocytomas (65%), oligodendrogliomas (25%), or mixed tumors (10%) were randomized to receive immediate postoperative irradiation to a dose of 54 Gy or no further treatment until there was evidence of disease progression. Among those in the deferred treatment arm, 65% of patients received subsequent radiotherapy, 19% underwent surgery and/or chemotherapy, and the remainder received only supportive care. A preliminary analysis of the study demonstrated that immediate irradiation significantly improved the 5 year PFS (44% versus 37%, $p = 0.02$). However, there was no improvement in overall 5 year survival (63% versus 66%) (Karim et al., 1998). The outcomes of patients with astrocytomas strongly correlate with the proliferative potential of the tumor as measured by an antibody to BrdU incorporation into tumor cells (Hoshino et al., 1988) and the MIB-1 antibody to the Ki-67 protein (Shibuya et al., 1993). The development of such immunohistochemical and molecular markers to better predict the prognosis for an individual patient may provide an opportunity for earlier intervention and improvement in outcome for the prognostically more unfavorable subsets of patients.

Limited radiation fields are used in the treatment of low-grade astrocytomas. Recurrences are nearly always found at the original primary tumor site (Medbery et al., 1988; Shaw et al., 1989), and there is no difference in the survival distributions or patterns of failure between patients receiving partial and those receiving whole-brain irradiation (Medbery et al., 1988; North et al., 1990; Shaw et al., 1989). Fields should encompass the T_2-weighted MRI abnormality, which tends to be larger than the CT-defined lesion, with a margin of 1 to 2 cm (Kun, 1992; Shaw et al., 1991; Karlsson et al., 1992). Complex three-dimensional treatment plans are used whenever appropriate to limit the high-dose volume and to minimize the risk of long-term radiation sequelae (Ellenberg et al., 1987).

The optimal dose of radiation for astrocytomas is not well defined. The standard dose for adult patients is 54 Gy, administered in daily fractions of 1.8 to 2.0 Gy. This dose level is relatively conservative so as to decrease the risk of excessive treatment-related morbidity (Bloom, 1982). At this dose level about 75% of patients will improve neurologically, and the maximum radiographic improvement occurs within a median of 2.8 months (Bauman et al., 1999b). Two randomized trials have shown that higher dose levels do not improve patient outcome (at least at 5 years). In a trial conducted by the EORTC, patients were randomized to receive 45 Gy in 25 fractions or 59.4 Gy in 33 fractions. No difference in survival was observed between the two dose levels. The 5 year survival rates were 58% for 45 Gy and 59% for 59.4 Gy. The PFS rates were also similar (47% versus 50%, respectively) (Karim et al., 1996).

Similarly, a combined North Central Cancer Treatment Group (NCCTG), Radiation Therapy Oncology Group (RTOG), and Eastern Cooperative Oncology Group (ECOG) trial randomized adult patients with supratentorial astrocytomas to receive 50.4 Gy in 28 fractions or 64.8 Gy in 36 fractions. As in the EORTC study, the 5 year survival rates were similar for the two dose levels studied: 73% for 50.4 Gy and 68%

for 64.8 Gy (Shaw et al., 1998). An increase in functional sequelae (Kiebert et al., 1998) and radiation necrosis (Shaw et al., 1998) was observed in patients treated in the high-dose arms of these studies. These data support the use of lower radiation levels for low-grade gliomas.

The 4 year overall survival of children with cerebral hemispheric astrocytomas is 90% (Gajjar et al., 1997). Radiation therapy is likely to lead to unacceptable sequelae in children younger than 3 to 5 years of age. Therefore, in this age group, radiation therapy is postponed for as long as possible provided that no significant neurologic deficits or changes indicative of rapid tumor progression are present. Periodic imaging studies are performed to monitor the disease status. The radiation dose is reduced to 50 Gy for children under 5 years of age. Management decisions are also frequently individualized in older children with incompletely resected astrocytomas who, compared with adults, have a generally better prognosis, a less pronounced survival improvement with postoperative irradiation, and a greater risk of late radiation sequelae (Hirsch et al., 1989; Mercuri et al., 1981; Nishio et al., 1989; Yule et al., 2001).

Chemotherapy

Low-grade astrocytomas account for 40% to 50% of brain tumors in childhood. The use of chemotherapy in the management of children and adults with low-grade astrocytomas is currently evolving. It is unclear how great an effect chemotherapy will have on patients with low-grade astrocytomas as these tumors have a history of being relatively indolent, and uncertainty remains as to the timing of radiation therapy as well as chemotherapy. Because of concern about the toxic effects of radiation in young children, several studies have focused on the use of chemotherapy in an attempt to delay the need for radiation therapy in young children with low-grade astrocytomas in general (Pons et al., 1992; Packer et al., 1993) and optic/chiasmatic/hypothalamic astrocytomas in particular (Packer et al., 1988). These studies have each used a weekly "back-bone" therapy of IV vincristine, with the addition of actinomycin-D, or etoposide, or carboplatin. Results have demonstrated that *(1)* objective radiographic responses can be observed in patients with either recurrent or newly diagnosed low-grade astrocytomas; *(2)* prolonged disease stabilization, often for several years, can be achieved even in the absence of objective radiographic responses; and *(3)* radiation therapy can be delayed for up to several years with the use of such therapeutic strategies, either alone or combined with judicious surgical debulking.

The actual effect of chemotherapy on overall survival and on quality of survival will take many years to establish. At least for children with low-grade astrocytomas, it is hoped that to address this question the Pediatric Oncology Group and the Childrens Cancer Group (of North America) will conduct randomized trials of observation versus chemotherapy in children less than 5 years of age who have newly diagnosed low-grade astrocytomas. To date, prospective trials of chemotherapy for astrocytoma in adults have been impossible to conduct because of the small numbers of patients with low-grade astrocytoma available for study.

With increasing patient age, histologically low-grade astrocytomas assume a biologic malignancy that leads many clinicians to treat those who present with these tumors after age 45 years more aggressively than younger patients with higher dose radiation (60 Gy instead of 54 Gy) and to add chemotherapy. Other clinicians adhere to the histologic criteria of malignancy and withhold chemotherapy until tumor recurrence. Even more controversial is the use of chemotherapy for those patients under the age of 45 years. In a Southwest Oncology Group trial, patients with incompletely excised low-grade gliomas were randomized to receive radiation therapy alone (n = 19; median age 36 years) or radiation therapy and CCNU (n = 35; median age 39 years). The median survival time of the 54 evaluable patients was 4.4 years with no difference between the two treatment arms (Eyre et al., 1993).

Based on the observation of Piepmeier (1987) that patients with contrast-enhancing low-grade astrocytomas have shorter survival times than those with non–contrast-enhancing low-grade astrocytomas (3.9 versus 7.8 years), Levin et al. (1995) treated a subset of the CT-based contrast-enhanced low-grade glioma group with aggressive chemoradiation and adjuvant chemotherapy. Twenty-two consecutive patients received BrdU during radiation therapy followed by combination chemotherapy with procarbazine, lomustine, and vincristine (PCV) for 1 year after irradiation (Levin et al., 1995). Seventy percent of patients survived nearly 7 years. As a result of this study, during the last 10 years, Levin et al. have treated most histologically low-grade infiltrating astrocytomas in adults younger than 45 years with three courses of lomustine and procarbazine followed by limited-field radiation. Controversy surrounds this practice.

One of the problems with adjuvant chemotherapy programs for patients with low-grade astrocytoma is that it is difficult to conduct randomized trials because of the relative rarity of the tumor in the general population, the bias of clinicians with respect to its management, and the length of time required to conduct trials. When low-grade astrocytomas recur, approximately 50% do so with the original low-grade histology, whereas the rest recur as a more aggressive anaplastic astrocytoma or glioblastoma multiforme (Afra et al., 1978; Laws et al., 1984; Muller et al., 1977; Rubinstein, 1972; Soffietti et al., 1989). When the recurrence is either a low- or mid-grade astrocytoma, chemotherapy is frequently beneficial, although cure at that point is not a likely outcome. The drugs and schedules cited in the section on anaplastic gliomas and in Tables 3–3 and 3–4 should be referred to for chemotherapeutic approaches for the patient with recurrent low-grade astrocytoma.

Juvenile Pilocytic Astrocytomas

Radiotherapy

Because the long-term survival of patients with supratentorial juvenile pilocytic astrocytomas approaches 100% when a complete or near-complete (>90%, equivalent to 1 log of cells) surgical resection has been performed, postoperative irradiation is not in-

Table 3–3. Single-Agent Chemotherapy for Recurrent and Progressive Supratentorial Glioblastoma Multiforme and Anaplastic Astrocytomas

Treatment	*GBM, % R + SD*	*GBM, MTP (Weeks)*	*AA, % R + SD*	*AA, MTP (Weeks)*
Carmustine (Levin, 1985; Wilson et al., 1976)	29	22	64	22
PCNU (Levin et al., 1984)	33	8	69	28
Procarbazine (Rodriquez et al., 1989)	27	30	28	49
Diaziquone, 5 day bolus (Schold et al., 1984; Decker et al., 1985)			24	24
Diaziquone, 5 day bolus (EORTC Brain Tumor Cooperative Group, 1985)	41	18*	44	18*
Melphalan, oral (Chamberlain et al., 1988)	0	NA	7	NA
Cisplatin (Bertolone et al., 1989)†	73	8	83	12
Cisplatin (Sexauer et al., 1985)†	0	NA	7	NA
Carboplatin (Yung et al., 1991a)	40	20	57	21
Eflornithine (Levin et al., 1992)	21	NA	44	48
Betaseron (Yung et al., 1991b)	51	18	50	16
Cis-retinoic acid (Yung et al., 1993)	58	43	48	25
Trans-retinoic acid (Kaba et al., 1997)	26	16	71	18
Ifosfamide/mesna (Elliott et al., 1991)	0	NA	0	NA
Temozolomide (Yung et al., 1999, 2000)	46	20	58	41
Tamoxifen (Chamberlain and Kormanik, 1999)			63	78
Irinotecan (Friedman et al., 1999)	71	NA	70	NA

GMB, glioblastoma multiforme; AA, anaplastic astrocytoma; % R + SD, percent of all treated patients who responded or had stable disease; MTP, median time to tumor progression; EORTC, European Oncology Radiation and Treatment Committee; NA, not available; PCNU, 1-(2-chloroethyl)-3-(2,6-dioxo-1-piperidyl)-1-nitrosourea.

*Report combined GBM and AA groups because histologies were not separated or there were too few patients in each group to separate activity by histology.

†Childhood tumor data.

Table 3–4. Combination Chemotherapy for Recurrent and Progressive Supratentorial Glioblastoma Multiforme and Anaplastic Astrocytomas

Treatment	*GBM, % R + SD*	*GBM MTP (Weeks)*	*AA % R + SD*	*AA, MTP (Weeks)*
Procarbazine, lomustine, vincristine (Gutin et al., 1975; Levin et al., 1980a)	45	15	65	27
Carmustine, 5-fluorouracil, hydroxyurea, 6-mercaptopurine (Levin et al., 1986a)	55	23	71	46
Elfornithine, carmustine (Prados et al., 1989)	30	8	57	76
Eflornithine, methyl bisguanylhydrazone (Levin et al., 1987)			72	49
6-Thioguanine, procarbazine, dibromodulcitol, lomustine, 5-fluorouracil, hydroxyurea (Levin et al., 1993)	61	40	92	65
Diaziquone, carmustine (Schold et al., 1987; Yung et al., 1989)	0–28	9	80	37
Diaziquone, procarbazine (Schold et al., 1987)	31	25	53	42
Cyclophosphamide, vincristine (Longee et al., 1990)	60	15	78	35
Carboplatin, 5-fluorouracil, procarbazine (Flowers et al., 1993)	32	20	57	36
Carboplatin, etoposide (Jeremic et al., 1992)	50	43	75	38
Mechlorethamine, vincristine, procarbazine (Coyle et al., 1990)	38	43	100	54
Etoposide, cisplatin (Buckner et al., 1990)	39	NA	15	NA
6-Thioguanine, procarbazine, CCNU, hydroxyurea (Kyritsis et al., 1996)	33	21	77	38
Nitrogen mustard, vincristine, procarbazine (Galanis et al., 1998)	4	11	18	16–19
Carboplatin, *cis*-retinoic acid (Kunschner et al., 1999)	52	30		

GBM, glioblastoma multiforme; AA, anaplastic astrocytoma; % R + SD, percent of all treated patients who responded or had stable disease; MTP, median time to tumor progression; NA, not available.

dicated (Garcia et al., 1985; Hirsch et al., 1989; Mercuri et al., 1981; Shaw et al., 1989; Wallner et al., 1988a). The efficacy of radiation therapy for incompletely resected pilocytic astrocytomas is not well established (Shaw et al., 1989; Wallner et al., 1988a). Shaw et al. (1989) found that patients who underwent subtotal resection or biopsy and postoperative irradiation survived longer than those who did not, although the number of patients treated with surgery alone was small. The 5 year survival rate for patients who did not receive radiation therapy was 50% compared with 85% for those who received postoperative irradiation ($p = 0.08$). Therefore, after subtotal resection the recommendation may be either immediate irradiation or close follow up, deferring treatment until there is clinical or radiographic evidence of disease progression.

Chemotherapy

Chemotherapy in the treatment of juvenile pilocytic tumors is generally limited to recurrent disease in patients previously treated with surgery and irradiation. Frequently, chemotherapy is initiated after reoperation. The dearth and diversity of these tumors has led to anecdotal experience but no prospective studies. The most commonly used therapies have been with cell-cycle phase nonspecific drugs such as alkylating agents. In our experience, nitrosourea-based drug combinations have been capable of long-term palliation. Therapies such as procarbazine, lomustine (CCNU), and vincristine (Rodriguez et al., 1990; Petronio et al., 1991) and a combination of 6-thioguanine, dibromodulcitol, lomustine, procarbazine, and vincristine (Petronio et al., 1991; Chamberlain and Levin, 1989) have been quite active. Based on the low level of activity of cisplatin and etoposide in infiltrative low-grade astrocytomas, these are not the first choice for the treatment of recurrent noninfiltrating gliomas.

Malignant Astrocytomas

Radiation Therapy

The importance of radiation therapy for malignant gliomas was demonstrated in prospective clinical studies conducted by the Brain Tumor Cooperative Group (BTCG) (formerly the Brain Tumor Study Group) (Walker et al., 1978, 1980) and the Scandinavian Glioblastoma Study Group (Kristiansen et al., 1981). Patients who received postoperative irradiation had a longer survival time than those treated with either supportive care or chemotherapy alone.

The practice of prescribing a radiation dose of 60 Gy in conventional fractionation schemes is based on data from clinical studies and on limitations imposed by the radiation tolerance of normal brain tissue (Leibel and Sheline, 1991). A randomized trial conducted by the Radiation Therapy Oncology Group (RTOG) and the Eastern Cooperative Oncology Group (ECOG) compared 60 Gy whole-brain irradiation with 60 Gy delivered to the whole brain plus an additional 10 Gy delivered to the tumor volume. No survival improvement was noted with the 70 Gy regimen (Chang et al., 1983; Nelson et al., 1988). Thus, it is customary to treat anaplastic astrocytomas and glioblastoma multiforme to 60 Gy given in single daily fractions of 1.8 to 2.0 Gy for 5 days per week (Leibel and Sheline, 1987).

With conventional radiation radiotherapeutic techniques the median survival time for patients with glioblastoma multiforme is 9 to 10 months, whereas the 3 year survival rate is only 2% to 6% (Leibel et al., 1975, 1994; MRC Working Group, 2001). Less firm is the median survival time for patients with anaplastic astrocytoma treated with irradiation only. Estimates of median survivals of 13 to 19 months have been reported (Leibel et al., 1975; MRC Working Group Party, 2001). In a mixed group of high-grade glioma patients treated between 1974 and 1989 with radiation therapy and variable types and amounts of chemotherapy on RTOG protocols, a recursive partition analysis based on age, histology, mental status, duration of symptoms, neurologic functional status, extent of surgery, and radiation dose identified six prognostic classes of malignant glioma patients with median survival times ranging from 4.6 to 58.6 months (Curran et al., 1993) (Table 3–5).

The amount of tissue to include within the treatment volume has been a subject of considerable discussion. Studies that compared cerebral angiography and pneumoencephalography interpretations of tumor extent with autopsy findings demonstrated that malignant gliomas were usually more extensive than had been determined clinically (Concannon et al., 1960; Kramer, 1969; Salazar et al., 1976). Although patients included in these series had very advanced tumors and often died soon after diagnosis, the conclusion that treatment failure could be due to inadequate tumor coverage led to a recommendation that the whole brain be irradiated (Kramer, 1969; Salazar and Rubin, 1976).

Other studies comparing CT and MRI scans with pathologic findings and patterns of failure after radiation therapy support treating malignant gliomas with limited-field rather than with whole-brain irradiation. These investigations have shown that *(1)* malignant gliomas are localized, and microscopic invasion of the peritumoral brain tissue is limited at the time of initial diagnosis (Burger et al., 1983); *(2)* only 1.1% to 7.3% of patients with glioblastoma and 4.4% of all patients with astrocytomas present with multifocal lesions (Choucair et al., 1986; Kyritsis et al., 1992); *(3)* after initial treatment, most tumors recur at or within 1 to 2 cm of their original location (Hochberg and Pruitt, 1980; Wallner et al., 1989; Gaspar et al., 1992); *(4)* following resection of recurrent tumors, second tumor recurrences develop at the original primary tumor location (Massey and Wallner, 1990); and *(5)* cognitive impairment and frank dementia occurred all too frequently in patients treated with whole-brain radiation fields. On the other hand, in biopsy (Kelly et al., 1987) and autopsy (Burger et al., 1988) studies, isolated tumor cells have been found to infiltrate into edematous brain tissue surrounding the primary lesion. These observations have suggested that radiation fields should extend to the periphery of CT-defined peritumoral hypodense regions or should encompass tissues that have a prolonged T_2-weighted MRI signal. However, analyses of recurrence patterns after conventional irradiation have not demonstrated a propensity for tumors to recur within edematous areas at a distance from the primary tumor site (Wallner et al., 1989). It is possible that all the observed

Table 3–5. Outcomes of Patients with Malignant Astrocytic Gliomas According to Prognostic Class Based on a Recursive Partition Analysis of the RTOG Database of 1578 Patients Treated Between 1974 and 1989

Class	*Characteristics*	*Median Survival (Months)*	*2 Year Survival (%)*
I	AAF, age <50 years, normal mental status	58.6	76
II	AAF, age ≥50 years, KPS 70–100, time from first symptom to diagnosis >3 months	37.4	68
	AAF, age <50 years, abnormal mental status		
III	*or*	17.9	35
	GBM, age <50 years, KPS 90–100		
	GBM, age <50 years, KPS <90		
	or		
IV	AAF, age ≥50 years, time from first symptom to diagnosis ≤3 months	11.1	15
	or		
	GBM, KPS 70–100, ≥partial resection, "work" neurologic functional status		
	GBM, age ≥50 years, KPS 70–100, ≥partial resection, "home" or "hospital" neurologic functional status		
	or		
V	GBM, age ≥50 years, KPS 70–100, biopsy only, received >54.4 Gy	8.9	6
	or		
	GBM, age ≥50 years, KPS <70, normal mental status		
	GBM, age ≥50 years, KPS 70–100, biopsy only, received ≤54.4 Gy		
VI	*or*	4.6	4
	GBM, age ≥50 years, KPS <70, abnormal mental status		

AAF, astrocytoma with atypical or anaplastic features; GBM, glioblastoma multiforme; KPS, Karnofsky performance status.

Data from Curran et al. (1993).

isolated tumor cells were not tumorigenic because a critical mass of tumor cells was not present.

As there is no apparent survival advantage to irradiating the whole brain compared with irradiating more limited fields (Leibel and Sheline, 1990; Levin et al., 1995) and because many patients who survive for prolonged periods after whole-brain irradiation and chemotherapy develop significant treatment-related sequelae (Shapiro, 1986), partial brain field irradiation is accepted as a standard approach in the treatment of malignant gliomas. The fields are designed to encompass the perimeter of the contrast-enhancing tumor with a 2.5 to 3.0 cm margin of tissue based on preoperative diagnostic imaging studies. If the tumor and associated edema are limited, the surrounding edema may initially be included in the treatment volume (Leibel et al., 1991b). However, if the tumor is extensive and accompanied by a large volume of peritumoral edema, coverage of the entire hypodense region would require treatment of a large volume of brain tissue for what will probably be minimal or no therapeutic gain (Wallner, 1991). Radiation portals should, when possible, be designed with three-dimensional conformal techniques to spare, to the extent possible, the surrounding normal tissues.

The response of malignant gliomas to standard radiation therapy techniques is limited by their striking inherent radioresistance and the radiosensitivity of the surrounding normal brain tissue. Accordingly, a considerable amount of research has been directed at improving the efficacy of radiotherapy. In addition to incorporating chemical radiation-response modifiers and pursuing more effective chemotherapy programs (see below), areas of investigation have included the use of altered fractionation schemes, dose escalation with interstitial brachytherapy, radiosurgery, and three-dimensional conformal radiotherapy and the application of heavy particle irradiation.

Hyperfractionated irradiation differs from conventionally fractionated irradiation in that with the former, two or more treatments are given daily with fraction sizes smaller than the usual dose fractions. The goal of this approach is to deliver a higher total radiation dose in the same overall time (6 to 6.5 weeks) as a conventional treatment schedule. Compared with rapidly proliferating glioma cells, normal neural tissues exhibit a slow rate or absence of cell division and have a greater capacity to repair sublethal radiation damage. The size of the radiation dose per fraction has a predominant effect on the incidence of late toxic effects in neural tissue (Leibel and Sheline, 1991). Therefore, the tolerance of these tissues to radiation should be improved by reducing the size of the fractional dose (Nelson et al., 1986). Because rapidly proliferating tumor cells are less affected by the reduction in fraction size, tumor control probability should improve with hyperfractionation, whereas late toxic effects should be equivalent to those observed with conventional fractionation schedules. The 6 to 8 hour interval between dose fractions allows the normal tissues to repair sublethal radiation damage. On the other hand, rapidly proliferating tumor cells progress into more radiosensitive phases of the cell cycle during the interval between fractions. Target cells for late sequelae proliferate slowly; thus, for these tissues little cell cycle reassortment or "self-sensitization" occurs during irradiation (Withers, 1985).

A randomized phase II dose-escalation study conducted by the RTOG found that patients receiving 72 Gy in 1.2 Gy fractions twice daily had a longer median survival time (14.2 months) and a higher 18 month survival rate (44%) than patients who received 81.6 Gy (11.7 months and 28%, respectively). The inferior outcome in the 81.6 Gy arm of the study was attributed in part to excess neurotoxicity. On the basis of findings from a randomized phase II dose-escalation study (Werner-Wasik et al., 1996), the RTOG carried out a randomized trial comparing the hyperfractionated irradiation to 72 Gy with conventional fractionated irradiation to 60 Gy with carmustine (BCNU) given in both study arms. Hyperfractionation did not lead to an improved outcome. The median survival times for patients with glioblastoma multiforme in the two treatment arms were similar—10.2 months with the hyperfractionated regimen and 11.2 months with conventional fractionation ($p = 0.44$). Similarly, for patients with anaplastic astrocytoma the median survival times were 43.5 months with hyperfractionation and 49.5 months with conventional fractionation ($p = 0.81$) (Scott et al., 1998).

Another fractionation option, accelerated fractionation, attempts to improve radiation-induced tumor cell kill in rapidly proliferating tumors by reducing the length of time needed to complete the course of treatment (Fowler, 1990). Conventional size dose fractions (1.6 to 2.0 Gy) are given two or three times daily. This treatment schedule may also improve the therapeutic ratio by reducing tumor cell repopulation during treatment, thereby increasing the probability of tumor control for a given dose level (Withers, 1985). Several trials using accelerated regimens have been conducted, but none has shown a survival benefit over conventional irradiation for these regimens (Simpson and Platts, 1976; Keim et al., 1987; Shenouda et al., 1991; Prados et al., 2001). These studies, however, indicate that the overall treatment time can be shortened, which may be especially appropriate for patients with relatively short survival expectancies (Simpson and Platts, 1976).

Because most gliomas are localized to a single area of the brain (Choucair et al., 1986; Hochberg and Pruitt, 1980; Kyritsis et al., 1992), they should be controllable if sufficiently high radiation doses can be delivered without damaging the surrounding normal brain tissue. Therefore, as a second strategy for improving the outcome of malignant gliomas, interstitial brachytherapy, radiosurgery, and three-dimensional proton beam and photon radiation therapy are being used as an adjunct to conventional irradiation to augment the dose to the primary tumor.

Interstitial brachytherapy has been extensively studied as an approach for increasing the tumor dose. Unlike conventional radiation therapy, the intratumoral placement of encapsulated radioactive sources results in maximal doses to the tumor while the surrounding normal tissues receive considerably lower radiation doses (Leibel et al., 1989a,b). 125-Iodine and 192-Iridium sources have most frequently been used in clinical practice, and stereotactic techniques have been devised for the placement of afterloading catheters, which are removed after the prescribed dose has been given.

Well-circumscribed, peripheral supratentorial tumors measuring up to 5 cm are best suited to receive implantation. Patients with multifocal tumors or lesions with poorly defined borders, as well as those with corpus callosum involvement and subependymal spread, and tumors of the cerebellum, midbrain, and brain stem are not considered for this technique. To be eligible for radiation implantation, the patient should have good neurologic function and a KPS of at least 70. Based on these criteria, approximately 33% of patients with newly diagnosed malignant gliomas are candidates for brachytherapy (Florell et al., 1992).

The limiting aftereffect associated with interstitial brachytherapy is focal peritumoral radiation injury to the brain. The clinical and radiographic changes caused by implanted radioactive sources may be indistinguishable from signs of tumor progression. Brachytherapy-induced neurologic deterioration and steroid dependency may be effectively reversed by resection of the necrotic tissue, a step necessary in approximately 40% of implanted patients (Leibel et al., 1991a).

Initially, interstitial implantation was used for retreating previously irradiated patients who had recurrent malignant gliomas. When improvements in survival and quality of life were demonstrated (Gutin et al., 1987; Leibel et al., 1989a), this treatment was integrated into the primary management of patients with newly diagnosed malignant gliomas. As shown in Table 3–6, early phase II studies demonstrated survival improvements in patients with glioblastoma multiforme who received a combination of external beam irradiation and interstitial brachytherapy to total doses of 110 to 120 Gy compared with patients treated with conventional radiation therapy (alone or with chemotherapy) but who otherwise satisfied the criteria for implantation (Florell et al., 1992; Gutin et al., 1991; Loeffler et al., 1990; Prados et al., 1992b; Scharfen et al., 1992). Such comparisons, however, are subject to considerable patient selection bias (Florell et al., 1992).

The brachytherapy approach was studied in three randomized trials. The BTCG compared interstitial implantation (60 Gy at 10 Gy per day) preceding external irradiation (60.2 Gy at 1.72 Gy per fraction) and BCNU with external irradiation and BCNU alone. Implanted patients experienced a significant improvement in median survival (16 versus 13 months) and 18 month survival (47% versus 32%) compared with those who did not receive brachytherapy (Green at al., 1994). However, in another trial, Laperriere et al. (1998) found no difference in outcome of patients randomized to receive external beam irradiation alone to 50 Gy or external beam irradiation and a ^{125}I implant delivering a minimum tumor dose of 60 Gy. The median survival time of patients receiving external beam irradiation and brachytherapy was 13.8 months compared with 13.2 months for those treated with external beam irradiation alone (p = 0.49).

A randomized trial testing the addition of interstitial microwave hyperthermia to the brachytherapy boost after external irradiation in newly diagnosed patients with glioblastoma multiforme was conducted at the University of California, San Francisco. Time to progression and survival (median survival 85 versus 76 weeks; 2 year survival 31% versus 15%) were significantly longer in patients receiving hyperthermia than in those treated with external beam irradiation and brachytherapy alone ($p = 0.045$ and $p = 0.02$, respectively) (Sneed et al., 1998).

Table 3–6. Effect of ^{125}I Implantation on Survival of Patients with Glioblastoma Multiforme

				Median Survival		
Study	*No. of Cases*	*Treatment*	*Dose (Gy)*	*Months*	*1 Year (%)*	*2 Years (%)*
Florell et al. (1992)	68	Ext RT	60	14	55	12
Loeffler et al. (1990)	40	Ext RT	60	10	40	12
Loeffler et al. (1990)	35	Ext + ^{125}I	110	NR	87	57
Scharfen et al. (1992)	106	Ext + ^{125}I	110–120	22	86	29

Ext RT, external beam irradiation; Ext + ^{125}I, external beam irradiation plus ^{125}I implantation; NR, not reached.

Stereotactic radiosurgery has also been used to increase the tumor dose. Radiosurgery is a method of focused, closed-skull external beam irradiation that uses an imaging-compatible stereotactic device for precise target localization. The relationship between the stereotactic coordinate system and the radiation source allows accurate delivery of radiation to the target volume (Larson et al., 1992). Radiosurgery may be delivered using multiple cobalt beams (as in the "gamma knife"), modified linear accelerators, or charged particle beams. The radiation beams intersect at one (sometimes two or more) point(s) within the skull after entering through numerous points or arcs distributed over the surface of the skull (Larson et al., 1990). This technique was designed to deliver a high radiation dose to an intracranial target in a single session without delivering significant radiation to adjacent normal tissues. To maintain a steep dose gradient at the edges of the field, the target volume must be small. Furthermore, because the dose that can be safely administered in a single fraction is limited by the volume irradiated, the application of radiosurgery in effective single doses is restricted to lesions measuring approximately 4 cm or less in diameter (Wilson et al., 1992).

Stereotactic radiosurgery techniques have been used to treat a variety of benign intracranial processes, most frequently small arteriovenous malformations as well as benign tumors such as pituitary adenomas, acoustic neurinomas, and meningiomas. The role of radiosurgery as a boost after conventional radiation therapy for malignant gliomas is currently an area of active research (Loeffler et al., 1992). Shrieve et al. (1999) used radiosurgery as a boost after standard external beam irradiation (59.4 Gy) in 78 patients with newly diagnosed glioblastoma multiforme. Patients with discrete, geometrically spherical lesions measuring 4 cm or less in diameter and a KPS of 70 or higher were selected for radiosurgery. The median tumor volume at the time of radiosurgery was 9.3 cm^3, and the median minimum tumor dose was 12 Gy. The median survival time was 19.9 months, and the 1 and 2 year survival rates were 88.5% and 35.9%, respectively. Similar to brachytherapy, 50% of the patients required reoperation to resect necrotic tissue or recurrent tumor. Based on tumor size and geometry and functional status criteria (Loeffler et al., 1992), only 9% of patients are eligible for this procedure (Curran et al., 1992b). The median survival time for radiosurgery-eligible glioblastoma multiforme patients was 12.5 months compared with 10.5 months for ineligible patients ($p = 0.07$). A comparison of these data with those reported by Shrieve et al. (1999) suggests that for glioblastoma multiforme a survival advantage of approximately 7 months is conferred when radiosurgery is actually given. The benefit of radiosurgery diminishes when broader selection criteria are used (Mehta et al., 1994), whereas a better outcome is associated with lower pathologic grade, younger age, higher KPS, smaller tumor volume, and unifocal tumors. (Larson et al., 1996) Although radiosurgery is biologically at the opposite end of the fractionation spectrum from brachytherapy, the therapeutic ratios of these two modalities appear to be similar (Larson et al., 1993). Stereotactic radiosurgery offers several advantages over brachytherapy. Radiosurgery is noninvasive, thus avoiding the risks of hemorrhage, infection, and tumor seeding. Furthermore, prolonged hospitalization is not required. Thus, for the most part, radiosurgery has replaced brachytherapy for selected patients to augment the tumor dose.

Radiosurgery may also be used to re-treat patients with small, previously irradiated tumors. In one series, the median survival time of 86 patients with recurrent glioblastoma multiforme was 10 months from the time of radiosurgery, similar to the published experience with brachytherapy at recurrence (Shrieve et al., 1995).

Three-dimensional conformal photon radiation therapy is another method of treatment planning and delivery designed to enhance the conformation of the radiation dose to the target volume while maximally restricting the dose delivered to normal tissue outside the treatment volume. When applied to cerebral tumors, conformal treatment planning techniques have permitted a 30% to 50% reduction in the volume of normal brain tissue irradiated at high doses (Thornton et al., 1991, 1992). This new approach to treatment planning may not only decrease the risk of normal tissue injury but may allow higher than traditional radiation doses to be safely administered to patients with malignant gliomas. In an ongoing study at the University of Michigan, doses as high as 90 Gy have been administered using three-dimensional techniques (Lee et al., 1999; AS Lichter, personal communication, 2000).

Protons and helium ion beams, which feature sharp lateral beam edges and have a finite range in tissue, may also be used to deliver higher radiation doses to limited tumor volumes while keeping the dose to neighboring critical structures at a safe level.

The depth of radiation penetration can be tailored to the tumor target by varying the energy of the beam or by interposition of bolus material in the beam path. Proton beam arrangements designed with three-dimensional treatment planning systems are being used as boost therapy for glioblastoma multiforme (approximately 60 cc in volume) after conventional radiation therapy (Suit and Urie, 1992). Fitzek et al. (1999) treated 23 patients with glioblastoma multiforme using combined photon and proton beams to administer a tumor dose of 90 cobalt gray equivalent (CGE) with an accelerated fractionation approach. The median survival time was 20 months (a 5 to 11 month improvement compared with patients with comparable risk factors treated with conventional radiotherapy). The 2 and 3 year actuarial survival rates were 34% and 18%, respectively. Tumor regrowth, demonstrated by histologic tissue examination, occurred most commonly in regions that received dose levels of 70 CGE or less, whereas tumor was found in the 90 CGE dose volume in only one case.

Chemotherapy with Irradiation

For patients with malignant astrocytomas, chemotherapy has been given before, during, and after radiotherapy to improve survival. In the past, the most common forms of chemotherapy have been cytotoxic drugs. The earliest question asked was whether the use of chemotherapy added to the survival benefit already achieved by surgery and radiotherapy. Historically, the nitrosoureas (carmustine and lomustine) have been the most frequently studied agents (Chang et al., 1983; Walker et al., 1978, 1980). A meta-analysis of the results of eight randomized trials reported between 1976 and 1985 showed that the addition of a nitrosourea agent to radiation therapy provided a significant, albeit limited, benefit over radiation therapy. The 1 year survival rate was increased by only 9% ($p = 0.002$) and the 2 year survival rate by only 3.5% ($p = 0.046$) (Stenning et al., 1987). Patients younger than 60 years of age ($p < 0.01$) appear to benefit most from carmustine, whereas carmustine is less beneficial for older patients (Chang et al., 1983; Nelson et al., 1988). Based on these studies, the combination of conventional irradiation and carmustine became the standard treatment regimen for malignant gliomas (Deutsch et al., 1989).

In an effort to improve on these data, a number of chemotherapy combinations were evaluated in clinical trials. The most widely used combination of procarbazine, lomustine, and vincristine (PCV) was reported by Levin and colleagues (1990, 1995) in trials where PCV was given after surgery and radiation therapy. Tables 3–7 and 3–8 summarize some of the adjuvant chemotherapy trials conducted and published through 1999.

Table 3–7. Comparison of Survivals of Patients with Anaplastic Glioma

Treatment	*No.*	*50% Survival (Weeks)*	*25% Survival (Weeks)*
WBRT, HU, carmustine	37	82	157
WBRT, HU, PCV (Levin et al., 1990)	36	157	NA (>317)
WBRT, mPCV (Jeremic et al., 1992)	31	148	NA
LFRT, PCNU versus	50	74	204
LFRT, carmustine (Dinapoli et al., 1993)	46	88	208
BrdU, LFRT, PCV (Levin et al., 1995)	138	208	NA
LFRT, 6TG, carmustine (Prados et al., 1998b)	110	>284	NA
WB/LFRT, carmustine	257	168	NA
WB/LFRT, PCV (RTOG retrospective study reported by Prados et al.,1999a)	175	>168	NA
LFRT, PCV versus	92	?	NA
LFRT, BrdU, PCV (Prados et al., 1999b)	97	?	NA

WBRT, whole-brain radiotherapy; LFRT, limited-field radiation therapy; HU, hydroxyurea; PCV, procarbazine, lomustine, vincristine; mPCV, dose-modified PCV; BrdU, bromodeoxyuridine; 6TG, 6-thioguanine; NA, not available.

Table 3–8. Comparison of Survival Among Studies that Evaluated Glioblastoma Patients as a Distinct Histology

Treatment	*No.*	*50% Survival (Weeks)*	*25% Survival (Weeks)*
WBRT, HU, carmustine (Levin et al., 1990)	29	57	71
WBRT, HU, PCV (Levin et al., 1990)	31	50	94
WBRT, mPCV (Jeremic et al., 1992)		62	69
LFRT, PCNU versus	118	42	62
LFRT, carmustine (Dinapoli et al., 1993)	120	41	73
5FU, lomustine, LFRT, MISO, HU, PCB, VCR, BCNU, 5 FU (Levin et al., 1986b)	64	50	NA
BrdU, LFRT, PCV (Phillips, et al., 1991)	160	62	104
CARBO, AFLFRT, PCV (Levin et al, 1995)	74	55	91
LFRT and PCV versus	134	60	82
LFRT and PCV, DFMO (Levin et al., 2000b)	138	58	78
BrdU, AFLRT, PCV (Groves et al., 1999)	70	57	79
AFLRT versus	231	40	
LFRT versus		37	
AFLRT and DFMO during RT versus		42	
LFRT and DFMO during RT (Prados et al., 2001)		34	
LFRT versus	226	39	57
LFRT and PCV (MRC Working Group Party, 2001)	223	40	61

WBRT, whole-brain radiotherapy; LFRT, limited-field radiation therapy; HU, hydroxyurea; PCV, procarbazine, lomustine, vincristine; mPCV, dose-modified PCV; MISO, misonidazole; BrdU, bromodeoxyuridine; CARBO, carboplatin; DFMO, difluoromethylornithine (eflornithine); AFLRT, accelerated fractionated radiation therapy; VCR, vincristine; NA, not available.

The two variables having the most impact on chemotherapy studies are age at diagnosis and tumor histology. As an approximation, survival appears to be inversely correlated to age and grade of malignancy: young patients survive longer than the elderly, and patients with low-grade gliomas live longer than those with high-grade gliomas. In a randomized trial conducted by the Childrens Cancer Group, children receiving radiation therapy and the combination of lomustine (CCNU), vincristine, and prednisone had a 5 year event-free survival rate of 46% compared with 17% for children who received radiation therapy alone ($p = 0.026$). When patients who underwent at least a partial resection were separated by pathology groups, chemotherapy was found to be beneficial to children with glioblastoma multiforme (5 year event-free survival, $p = 0.011$; 5 year survival, $p = 0.044$) but not to those with anaplastic astrocytomas. This is comparable to our experience with adults with glioblastoma for whom 5 year survival is closer to 5%.

There is no doubt that patients with anaplastic gliomas respond better to chemotherapy than those with glioblastoma (Levin et al., 2001). In addition, there are data that show that adjuvant (after surgery and radiotherapy) combination chemotherapy of procarbazine, CCNU, and vincristine (PCV) or 6-thioguanine and BCNU leads to longer survival for patients with anaplastic astrocytoma and other anaplastic gliomas (see Tables 3–7 and 3–8) than does monotherapy with adjuvant nitrosourea or procarbazine. The median survival in three studies ranges between 3 and 5 years (Levin et al., 1990, 1995; Prados et al., 1998a).

In addition to pursuing more effective chemotherapy programs, investigational research efforts are directed at improving the therapeutic efficacy of external irradiation. One strategy has focused on techniques designed to selectively enhance tumor cell killing using methods to overcome tumor cell hypoxia, halogenated pyrimidine analogue radiation sensitizers, and modified radiation time–dose fractionation schedules such as hyperfractionation and accelerated fractionation.

Hypoxia protects cells against the effects of radiation. Hypoxic but viable cells may be found in regions of coagulation necrosis that are present in glioblastoma multiforme (Nelson et al., 1986). Even when only 2% to 3% of such resistant cells are present, the radiation dose required to completely eradicate a tumor may double (Dische, 1991). Various methods to modify the effects of hypoxia have been studied, including irradiation under hyperbaric oxygen conditions (Chang, 1977) and combining radiation therapy with electron-affinic hypoxic cell radiation sensitizers such as misonidazole (Bleehen, 1990). To date, neither of these approaches has resulted in an improvement in outcome over that produced by conventional radiation therapy alone. Treatment with high-linear energy transfer radiations (i.e., neutrons and heavy ions) that are less dependent on oxygen tension than conventional (low-linear energy transfer) photon irradiation has also not improved survival rates (Castro et al., 1982; Laramore et al., 1988).

The halogenated pyrimidine analogues are radiation sensitizers that are incorporated into rapidly dividing cells undergoing DNA synthesis because of their similarity to the DNA precursor thymidine. When the analogue is substituted for thymidine in the DNA chain, the cell becomes more susceptible to radiation injury (Djordjevic and Szybalski, 1960). These analogues appear to enhance the effects of a given dose of radiation by a factor of 1.5 to 2 (Mitchell et al., 1983). Tumors located in the brain are ideally suited for halogenated pyrimidine analogue radiosensitization because the clonogenic cells undergo division more rapidly and, therefore, incorporate more drug into DNA than do the surrounding normal neural tissues. Two analogues, BrdU and iododeoxyuridine, have been evaluated in patients with malignant gliomas. The initial impression from these studies was that BrdU with radiation therapy produced survival improvement for patients who had anaplastic astrocytomas (Levin et al., 1995) but not for those with glioblastoma multiforme (Goffman et al., 1992; Phillips et al., 1991; Groves et al., 1999).

Unfortunately, recent publications bring this conclusion into question. First, a retrospective analysis of RTOG and Northern California Oncology Group (NCOG) databases since 1974 suggested that there might be a subset of relatively younger glioblastoma patients who were most likely to benefit from BrdU therapy during irradiation. The data from that study were, however, inconclusive (Prados et al., 1998b). Disappointing was the recent closure of a multigroup open-label randomized phase III trial in newly diagnosed patients with anaplastic glioma comparing radiotherapy plus adjuvant PCV chemotherapy with or without BrdU given as a 96 hour infusion each week of radiotherapy. The study was closed early because a conditional power analysis indicated that even with an additional 12 months of accrual and follow up the probability of detecting a difference between the two arms was less than 0.01% (Prados et al., 1999b). The final report of this study will be available in 2002.

Chemotherapy of Malignant Astrocytomas of Childhood

Although the major effect of chemotherapy on the outcomes of adult patients with malignant astrocytomas has, to date, been limited to anaplastic gliomas, therapeutic trials during the last 15 years in children with these tumors have demonstrated some benefit, even for those with glioblastoma multiforme. This finding suggests that high-grade astrocytomas have a somewhat different biology in adults and children.

In 1976, the Childrens Cancer Group embarked on a randomized trial in children newly diagnosed with high-grade astrocytomas in which involved-field irradiation alone was compared with involved-field irradiation plus adjuvant chemotherapy (vincristine, CCNU, and prednisone) for a duration of approximately 1 year. Although the number of fully evaluable patients accrued to this randomized study was small ($n = 58$), an advantage for adjuvant chemotherapy was observed for patients with glioblastoma multiforme: those receiving radiation alone died of progressive disease, whereas 49% of patients receiving the adjuvant chemotherapy remained free of tumor progression beyond 5 years. Because of the small numbers of patients enrolled in the study, no advantage for chemotherapy could be statistically confirmed in patients with anaplastic astrocytoma despite a 20% 5 year PFS rate for children with radiation alone versus 45% for children with radiation plus chemotherapy. The most powerful factor predictive of outcome, in addition to the use of chemotherapy, was extent of resection (Sposto et al., 1989).

Based on results from the above study, in 1985 the Childrens Cancer Group embarked on a second randomized therapeutic trial in which the regimen of CCNU and PCV from the earlier study served as the "standard therapy" arm and was compared with the "eight drugs in one day" regimen, a chemotherapeutic regimen that actually incorporated seven drugs (vincristine, CCNU, procarbazine, hydroxyurea, cisplatin, cytosine arabinoside, and either cyclophosphamide or dacarbazine) in addition to methylprednisolone for antiedema and antiemetic effects. In 1991, when the study closed, 185 children had been entered and randomized to a treatment group, and an additional 40 children younger than 3 years of age were nonrandomly assigned to receive the experimental treatment in addition to radiation. Results showed no benefit for the more intensive experimental therapy compared with control arm therapy; nevertheless, the study reaffirmed the benefit of adjuvant chemotherapy for childhood high-grade astrocytomas. Again, the prognostic impact of extent of resection is observed in this study, with virtually all patients who underwent a biopsy or a partial resection having died of disease progression (Finlay et al., 1995).

Of children younger than 3 years treated with the "8-in-1" chemotherapy regimen with the intent of delaying or avoiding irradiation, 35% were alive without disease progression beyond 3 years after diagnosis, a finding similar to that for older children. This more favorable outcome in young children may reflect an idiosyncratic biologic behavior of these tumors to certain cytotoxic chemotherapy agents in very young children. Certainly the time to disease progression is much shorter for younger children (less than 6 months) than for older ones. Young children also display a more dramatic radiographic response to chemotherapy than older children, indicating the promising potential of chemotherapeutic strategies without irradiation for the treatment of younger children with high-grade astrocytomas. These children have traditionally fared poorly with any therapy and are particularly vulnerable to the devastating consequences of cranial irradiation (Geyer et al., 1995).

Results of phase II trials evaluating new agents or older drugs used in new, more dose-intensive strategies have been most encouraging for the medulloblastoma/primitive neuroectodermal family of tumors but far less so for children or adults with high-grade astrocytomas. In trials a decade ago, ifosfamide and etoposide in combination produced a 6% response rate (with no complete responses) among 16 patients with recurrent high-grade astrocytomas (Miser et al., 1991). Ifosfamide alone demonstrated no activity in eight patients with recurrent astrocytoma (Chastagner et al., 1993). Partial and minor response rates varying from 0% to 38% have been reported in children with recurrent high-grade astrocytomas treated with carboplatin (Allen et al., 1987) or cisplatin (Bertolone et al., 1989). The original experience with the "8-in-1" regimen showed overall response rates of 22% to 44% in 27 patients with recurrent high-grade astrocytoma treated in three studies. In the Childrens Cancer Group protocol 945 discussed above, however, the partial response rate was less than 10% in 80 children (Finlay et al., 1994). Clearly, these chemotherapeutic agents, alone or in combination and at conventional or dose-intensive strategies, have a minimal ability to produce significant tumor shrinkage in high-grade astrocytomas in children.

An approach initiated in the mid-1980s for children with recurrent brain tumors was the use of myeloablative doses of chemotherapy followed by bone marrow rescue with the patient's own previously cryopreserved marrow. One initial regimen utilized thiotepa plus etoposide (Finlay et al., 1990); this regimen demonstrated a 20% 2 year disease PFS rate among patients with recurrent high-grade astrocytomas. Among patients so treated following radical surgical resection and who had no gross evidence of residual disease or had achieved a complete response to the myeloablative chemotherapy, approximately 33% were alive beyond 2 years post-diagnosis. Because of these early results, the regimens were subsequently intensified for patients with recurrent tumor, and high-dose carboplatin was added (Finlay, 1992b). Additionally, children with newly diagnosed anaplastic astrocytoma or glioblastoma multiforme were treated with high-dose chemotherapy (thiotepa, etoposide, and carmustine) followed by marrow rescue and subsequent involved-field irradiation; this was the basis for a Childrens Cancer Group multicenter trial in North America for such children and young adults between the ages of 3 and 25 years (CCG-9921; Groves et al., 1999).

Chemotherapy for Malignant Astrocytomas in Adults

Chemotherapy for glioblastoma multiforme is, for the most part, a frustrating experience for both the physician and the patient. During the last 25 years, chemotherapy has provided small gains measured in added months rather than years of life. Most agents found to be active in phase II clinical trials produce short-duration responses of 3 to 9 months in patients with progressive or recurrent glioblastoma. Response rates vary from 0% to 70%, depending on the criteria used to define response. For anaplastic astrocytomas, the gains have been much greater: Response rates of 25% to 90% have been reported, with median times to progression of 6 to 15 months depending on the drugs and drug combinations used.

Because the most important measure of the activity of a chemotherapuetic drug or regimen is time to treatment failure (when the tumor grows), what is needed to assess the value of therapy are precise, reliable criteria to define and determine tumor progression. Even though clinical considerations are important in good patient management, clinical stability or deterioration alone is insufficient to guide treatment.

Over the years, a variety of methods have been used to assess response. These have included electroencephalography, radionuclide brain scans, CT scans, and, most recently, MRI. Of these, MRI is the most informative method, providing precise anatomic localization as well as information on tumor growth, associated edema and mass effect, hydrocephalus, brain atrophy, radiation damage, leptomeningeal spread of tumor, and intracranial (or tumoral) bleeding.

Tables 3–3 and 3–4, respectively, summarize single-agent and combination phase II chemotherapy trial results for many, but not all, published trials. It is our belief that an effective treatment must be durable in at least a subset of patients. Response alone is insufficient as a measure of benefit unless it can be maintained. For single agents, a "good" therapy for glioblastoma multiforme should produce a median time to tumor progression of 20 to 30 weeks in 30% to 40% of patients. For anaplastic astrocytomas, a "good" median time to progression is 30 to 50 weeks in 40% to 60% of patients.

Two recent publications have addressed response covariates and study approaches that address the issue of durability of treatment benefit. In the first, the authors analyzed eight consecutive phase II trials that included 225 glioblastoma and 150 anaplastic astrocytoma patients (Wong et al., 1999). The data are summarized in Table 3–9. Based on their data, the investigators propose that phase II studies could utilize PFS at 6 months for glioblastoma as an outcome measure and be quite comfortable with a new therapy that substantially exceeded the 15% observed in their study. On the other hand, for anaplastic astrocytoma patients the PFS at 6 months was 31%, and this group of patients responds longer to chemotherapy than glioblastoma patients. This suggests that PFS at 9 months or 1 year would be a better study endpoint for anaplastic astrocytoma. This approach is addressed in a recent paper by Hess et al. (1999).

Excluding studies utilizing radiosurgical approaches, the best published results today for the treatment of glioblastoma by surgery, radiation, and chemotherapy have included chemotherapy during radiation therapy to potentiate radiation followed by the PCV combination after radiation. Table 3–8 summarizes current data. There certainly have been no giant steps made in the success of any one therapy. This is important to keep in mind because many of the approaches being proposed today have public appeal because they utilize twenty-first century technology: gene therapy, radiosurgery, the gamma knife, bone marrow transplantation, osmotic opening of the blood–brain barrier to improve drug access to the brain and tumor, and toxin immunoconjugates. Perhaps in the future one or more of these approaches will have a place in the therapy for malignant gliomas,

Table 3–9. Outcome Analysis of Phase II Studies for Recurrent Malignant Gliomas

Variable	*No.*	*CR and PR*	*CR, PR, MR, and SD*	*PFS 6 Months*	*PFS 1 Year*	*OS 1 Year*
Anaplastic astrocytoma	150	14%	48%	31%	20%	47%
Glioblastoma multiforme	225	6%	33%	15%	8%	21%

CR, complete response; PR, partial response; MR, minor response; SD, stable disease; PFS, progression-free survival; OS, overall survival.

Data from Wong et al. (1999).

but currently their benefits are inconsistent and for the most part problematic. One must be wary of referring patients for costly and marginally effective treatments without sound scientific principles underlying the proposed treatment plan.

Another concern is that current treatments add little to the survival or quality of life of older patients (Grant et al., 1995), particularly those older than 60 years. All clinical trials to date have found precipitous declines in survival after 60 to 65 years of age. This is not to say that surgery should not be carried out aggressively in these patients, but rather to inject caution about expectations from radiation and chemotherapy. Cytotoxic chemotherapy especially is not likely to improve survival for older patients.

For anaplastic gliomas, the story is quite different. Although advanced age is an important variable that negatively influences survival, chemotherapy can increase survival substantially. Treatment advances are in part due to *(1)* drugs such as the nitrosoureas (CCNU, carmustine), procarbazine, carboplatin, temozolomide, and *cis*-retinoic acid; and *(2)* some drug combination schedules. Table 3–7 summarizes some of the gains made in adjuvant chemotherapy for anaplastic gliomas. Survival gains have increased from 1.5 to 5 years during the last decade. It is likely that temozolomide (Temodar), an alkylating agent approved by the U.S. Federal Drug Administration in August 1999, will create new opportunities for drug combination therapy against malignant gliomas as well as medulloblastomas. In appears to be well tolerated with less morbidity than many of the drugs currently used to treat brain tumors.

The future will likely be characterized by slow increases in the length of patient survival unless there is a research breakthrough that will provide a new chemotherapeutic approach. Tumor-specific and selective therapies at the genetic and chemical levels will be required for any truly meaningful progress in lengthening survival times. Achieving this task will require major research commitments and a good deal of luck.

Oligodendrogliomas and Oligoastrocytomas

Radiation Therapy

The infrequent occurrence of oligodendrogliomas as well as their variable and often long prediagnosis and post-treatment natural history make it difficult to evaluate the effect of radiation therapy on these tumors (Sheline, 1983). Representative survival data for oligodendrogliomas are summarized in Table 3–10. Ten year survival rates vary, ranging from 8% to 59%. In contemporary series, median survival times of as long as 16 years have been reported (Olson et al., 2000).

The role of postoperative irradiation for patients with oligodendrogliomas is controversial, and conclusions regarding its value are contradictory. Some authors recommend immediate postoperative irradiation for patients with incompletely resected lesions (Chin et al., 1980; Griffin et al., 1992; Lindegaard et al., 1987; Wallner et al., 1988b), whereas others have been unable to show that postoperative irradiation is of benefit (Bullard et al., 1987; Sun et al., 1988). It has also been suggested that radiation therapy be deferred until there is evidence of tumor progression or recurrence (Reedy et al., 1983; Olson et al., 2000) or that only patients with anaplastic tumors or mixed oligoastrocytomas should receive radiation treatment.

Caution should be exercised when drawing firm conclusions from retrospective studies. For example, most retrospective studies comparing surgery alone with surgery plus radiation therapy do not contain analyses to ensure that the distribution of patients in the two treatment groups are comparable with respect to prognostic variables such as age (Bullard et al., 1987), completeness of resection (Mork et al., 1985; Whitton and Bloom, 1990), neurologic signs and symptoms (Bullard et al., 1987; Griffin et al., 1992), and histopathologic features (Bullard et al., 1987; Griffin et al., 1992; Mork et al., 1986). Furthermore, treatment selection factors are either not stated or are unknown (Lindegaard et al., 1987), and changes in the quality of surgery, radiation therapy, and patient management over the long time intervals spanned by the studies are not taken into consideration. In addition, carefully performed pathologic studies suggest that certain histologic and cytologic features have a significant effect on prognosis (Mork et al., 1986; Ludwig et al., 1986), making it important that pathologic material be independently reviewed.

Taken together, the data shown in Table 3–10 suggest that there may be a benefit to radiation therapy for oligodendrogliomas during the first 5 years after treatment, but this effect appears to diminish over time. Gannett et al. (1994) found a significant improvement in survival with postoperative irradiation.

Table 3–10. 5 Year and 10 Year Survival Rates for Patients with Oligodendroglioma

Study	*No. of Cases*	*Treatment*	*Survival Rate (%)*	
			5 Year	*10 Year*
Marsa et al. (1975)	14	S + RT	74	36
Chin et al. (1980)	11	S	82	—
	24	S + RT	100	—
Reedy et al. (1983)	21	S	67	46*
	27	S + RT	63	51*
Lindegaard et al. (1987)	62	S	27	12
	108	S + RT	36	8
Bullard et al. (1987)	34	S	48†	17†
	37	S + RT	60	15†
Wallner et al. (1988b)	11	S	55†	18
	14	S + RT l 45 Gy	78†	56
Sun et al. (1988)	16	S	31	16
	30	S + RT	57	43
Shaw et al. (1991)	8	S	25	25
	26	S + RT <50 Gy	39	20
	29	S + RT >50 Gy	62	31
Griffin et al. (1992)	14	S	45	13
	27	S + RT	78	43

S, surgery alone; S + RT, surgery and postoperative irradiation; —, data not available.

*Percent survival at 8 years.

†Data estimated from graphs.

Patients treated with surgery alone had 5 and 10 year survival rates of 51% and 36%, respectively, compared with 83% and 46%, respectively, for patients who received radiation therapy ($p = 0.032$). Lindegaard et al. (1987) reported that radiation therapy prolonged the median survival time of patients with incompletely resected tumor (37 months with radiotherapy versus 26 months for surgery alone; $p = 0.0089$) but did not influence the overall cure rate. The studies by Wallner et al. (1988b) and Shaw et al. (1992) suggested a survival advantage for patients with incompletely resected tumors who received at least 45 to 50 Gy. However, the advantage of irradiation versus nonirradiation did not reach statistical significance. On the other hand, Bullard et al. (1987) found no improvement in the time to clinical deterioration, time to tumor recurrence, or median survival time with the addition of radiation therapy, although the percentage of patients surviving with radiation therapy was consistently higher than those surviving without radiation therapy during the first 5 years after treatment. A meta-analysis on reports from the current literature concluded that postoperative irradiation conferred a 14% improvement in 5 year survival ($p \leq 0.01$) (Shimizu et al., 1993). The data presented in these studies suggest that more effective therapies are needed to improve the long-term outcomes of patients with oligodendrogliomas.

As for low-grade astrocytomas, it is also difficult to take a categorical position regarding the role of radiation therapy in the treatment of oligodendrogliomas. Patients with completely resected low-grade oligodendrogliomas as well as those with small, asymptomatic (except for seizures controlled with anticonvulsant medication), incompletely resected lesions can be observed, deferring radiotherapy until the time of recurrence. Large, symptomatic, unresectable or incompletely resected tumors should receive postoperative irradiation (Macdonald, 1994). Proliferation markers such as the MIB-1 labeling index may help to distinguish patients who require aggressive treatment from those who can merely undergo observation (Schiffer et al., 1997).

Radiation therapy is given using fields that encompass the tumor volume with a 2 to 2.5 cm margin. A dose of 54 Gy in daily 1.8 Gy fractions is given

Table 3–11. Effects of Histologic Classification Schemas on Median Survival Time for Patients with Oligodendrogliomas

	Histologic Type	
Series	*Low Grade** *(Months)*	*High Grade†* *(Months)*
Smith et al. (1983)	94	17
Kros et al. (1988)	113	15
Shaw et al. (1992)	117	47
Mean (±SD)	108 (±12)	26 (±18)

Mean, mean of reported median survival duration; SD, standard deviation.

*Smith type A and St. Anne-Mayo low grade.

†Smith type D and St. Anne-Mayo high grade.

to adults, and that dose is reduced to 50.4 Gy for children (Karlsson et al., 1992). The dose is increased to 59.4 Gy with a reduced field for patients with anaplastic oligodendrogliomas (Bauman and Cairncross, 2001). Complex three-dimensional techniques should be used for treatment planning and delivery when appropriate. PCV chemotherapy (see next section) may be useful in reducing the size of large tumors before radiotherapy is begun (Streffer et al., 2000).

Chemotherapy for Oligodendrogliomas

As previously discussed, oligodendroglial tumors can be categorized by histologic features that correlate with survival. Table 3–11 summarizes survivals for low-grade and high-grade oligodendrogliomas using the "A to D" and the St. Anne-Mayo grading schemes. From the reports cited it can be concluded that patients with low-grade tumors survive 108 months (9 years) compared with 26 months (2.2 years) for those with high-grade tumors. In general, the patients reported (Smith et al., 1983; Shaw et al., 1989, 1992) were treated with surgery and irradiation; few were formally treated with chemotherapy. It is clear from Table 3–12, given the sensitivity of oligodendrogliomas to chemotherapy, that the survival of anaplastic oligodendroglioma patients treated with adjuvant chemotherapy (or chemotherapy at tumor progression) will easily exceed the median 2.2 years.

Table 3–12 summarizes adjuvant chemotherapy (pre-radiation and/or post-radiation) with two different dose schedules of procarbazine, CCNU, and vincristine (PCV and slightly higher dose mPCV). The response and stable disease rates are nearly 100%, and the number of patients without progression at 2 years range from 50% to 85%. PCV combinations have been used widely in the treatment of recurrent oligodendroglioma and oligoastrocytoma tumors with complete response rates of 12% to 33%, partial response rates of 40% to 50%, and stable disease rates of 19% to 31% (Cairncross et al., 1994; Soffietti et al., 1998; van den Bent et al., 1998). Taken together, the three studies yield PFS values of 31 months for complete response, 16 months for partial response, and 14 months for stable disease.

There is little doubt that other chemotherapy approaches that utilize combinations of cytotoxic agents such as carboplatin and temozolomide would be expected to be active against oligodendrogliomas. As a

Table 3–12. Initial treatment of Oligodendrogliomas, Anaplastic Oligodendrogliomas, and Oligoastrocytomas

Series	*Treatment*	*No.*	*% R + SD*	*% 2 Year TTP*
Anaplastic oligodendroglioma				
Glass et al. (1992)	mPCV + RT	5	100	50*
Kyritsis et al. (1993)	PCV + RT	8	100	62
Oligoastrocytoma				
Glass et al. (1992)	mPCV + RT	14	92	85†
Kyritsis et al. (1993)	PCV + RT	12	100	75

PCV, procarbazine, lomustine, and vincristine; mPCV, different PCV schedule; RT, radiation therapy; TTP, time to tumor progression, % R + SD, percent of all patients who respond or have stable disease.

*Three pre-radiation PCV courses.

†Three no radiation at evaluation; 10 pre-radiation PCV; 2 year survival projected because no patient has been evaluated long enough.

conservative approach, while we wait for newer drugs and better approaches to chemotherapy for oligodendrogliomas, it is reasonable to advocate using a combination of procarbazine, CCNU, and vincristine or simply the combination of CCNU and procarbazine for patients with recurrent tumors and to anticipate that adjuvant chemotherapy with surgery and radiation may also turn out to be efficacious.

Chemotherapy for Mixed Oligoastrocytomas

Although most high-grade astrocytic tumors in adults and children are either glioblastoma multiforme or anaplastic astrocytoma, a few patients have mixed malignant gliomas. These are usually anaplastic astrocytoma with oligodendroglioma or, less commonly, anaplastic astrocytoma and ependymoma. Only limited information on chemotherapy for children with these tumors is available. In the Childrens Cancer Group protocol 945, 14 patients were considered to have mixed gliomas, with PFS and overall survival at 5 years of 64% and 71%, respectively.

Adjuvant chemotherapy trials for adults with mixed oligoastrocytomas are also listed in Table 3–12. As with oligodendrogliomas, response to therapy in these tumors is high, with more of these patients than those with anaplastic oligodendroglioma having no tumor progression at 2 years (80% versus 56%). Most patients received the PCV combination. Based on these data, it seems most appropriate to treat children as well as adults with a PCV combination until a better therapy comes along. As part of the initial treatment, we normally advocate that a nitrosourea-based chemotherapy regimen such as PCV be used after limited-field irradiation.

Ependymoma

Radiation Therapy

Most supratentorial ependymomas cannot be completely excised because of their location and growth characteristics (Marks and Adler, 1982; Kricheff et al., 1964). Historically, 0% to 15% of patients with supratentorial tumors treated with surgery survived 5 years (Ringertz and Reymond, 1949; Mork and Loken, 1977). More recently, with improved surgical techniques, survival gains have been realized. Palma et al. (1993) reported on 20 patients between the ages of 1 and 20 years. Of the 18 who survived surgery, 12 (67%) were alive and disease free at a mean follow-up of 12 years (range 5.2 to 21 years); there were nine ependymoma, one anaplastic ependymoma, and two subependymoma patients in this surviving group.

Radiation therapy significantly improves tumor control and survival and is an accepted part of the standard treatment for ependymomas. As shown in Table 3–13, 5 year survival rates for patients who re-

Table 3–13. 5 Year Survival Rates for Patients Receiving Radiation Therapy for Supratentorial Ependymomas

Studies	*Cases*	*Treatment*	*5 Year Survival (%)*
Ringertz and Reymond (1949)	13	S	15
Mork and Loken (1977)	14	S	0
		S + RT	
Phillips et al. (1964)	12	S + RT	80
		S + RT >45 Gy	
Kim and Fayos (1977)	11	S + RT	46
Bouchard (1980)	17	S + RT	65
Marks and Adler (1982)	20	S + RT	35
Pierre-Kahn et al. (1983)	15	S + RT	51
Salazar et al. (1983)	20	S + RT	35
Read (1984)	19	S + RT	40 (adults) 17 (children)
Goldwein et al. (1990)	18	S + RT	35
Vanuytsel et al. (1992)	40	S + RT	48

S, surgery alone; S + RT, surgery and postoperative radiation therapy.

ceived radiation therapy range from 30% to 80%. The correlation between survival and histopathologic grade is controversial, although we found it to be an important predictor of tumor behavior and outcome (Leibel and Sheline, 1987).

Supratentorial tumors generally have a poorer prognosis than their infratentorial counterparts, probably because a greater proportion of them are high grade (Chin et al., 1982) and because there is a tendency for larger volumes of residual disease to be present after surgical resection at this location (Marks and Adler, 1982). Unlike other brain tumors, young children with ependymomas tend to have a poorer outcome than older children or adults (Garrett and Simpson, 1983; Goldwein et al., 1990; Shaw et al., 1987). This may reflect the practice of reducing the dose of radiation for very young children (Goldwein et al., 1990, 1991; Marks and Adler, 1982).

The amount of normal CNS tissue that should be included in the treatment volume is a major area of controversy. Differences in opinion are based on the potential for ependymomas to spread into the ventricular system and to disseminate into the spinal subarachnoid space. In some reports, the inclusion of ependymoblastomas, which are known for their propensity to disseminate throughout the CNS, tends to overestimate the risk of seeding of the spinal subarachnoid space (Goldwein et al., 1991; Ross and Rubinstein, 1989). Autopsy and clinical studies show that patients who develop intracranial and intraventricular spread also have recurrent or persistent disease at the primary tumor site (Marks and Adler, 1982; Salazar et al., 1983; Wallner et al., 1986). Spinal seeding is uncommon in supratentorial ependymomas, occurring in only 1.6% of cases in a literature review by Vanuytsel and Brada (1991). In that review, no patient with high-grade supratentorial lesions developed spinal subarachnoid seeding, whereas the incidence of seeding in low-grade supratentorial lesions was 2.7%. Relapse of the primary tumor had the greatest effect on the subsequent development of spinal seeding, regardless of tumor grade or site. Spinal dissemination occurred in 3.3% of patients with locally controlled tumors, whereas 9.5% with uncontrolled primary lesions developed seeding ($p < 0.05$). The frequency of seeding was not affected by whether prophylactic spinal irradiation was given.

The treatment volumes recommended for low-grade supratentorial ependymomas vary from generous local fields (Goldwein et al., 1990; Leibel and Sheline, 1987; Pierre-Kahn et al., 1983; Shaw et al., 1987; Wallner et al., 1986; Vanuytsel et al., 1992) to fields encompassing the whole brain (Salazar et al., 1983). However, the survival and local tumor control rates achieved by partial brain irradiation (Goldwein et al., 1990; Vanuytsel et al., 1992; Wallner et al., 1986) are comparable with those obtained with whole-brain irradiation (Salazar et al., 1983). As nearly all recurrences are limited to the original primary tumor site, whole-brain irradiation would not be expected to improve the chance of cure. Patients are treated using a generous target volume, based on operative and radiographic findings, to a dose of at least 54 Gy. Pretreatment myelography, spinal MRI, and CSF evaluation are not performed unless there is evidence of ventricular involvement or signs of subarachnoid metastases.

In the past most authors recommended inclusion of the entire craniospinal axis in the treatment of anaplastic supratentorial ependymomas (Salazar et al., 1983; Wallner et al., 1986; Vanuytsel et al., 1992), although some recommended whole-brain irradiation with an additional boost for high-grade supratentorial lesions located away from the CSF pathways (Pierre-Kahn et al., 1983; Goldwein et al., 1990) if there was no evidence of leptomeningeal spread. However, despite the apparent superiority of craniospinal radiation therapy noted in some series (Salazar et al., 1983), the findings that *(1)* local recurrence is the primary pattern of failure (Goldwein et al., 1991; Salazar et al., 1983; Marks and Adler, 1982; Shaw et al., 1987; Vanuytsel et al., 1992; Merchant et al., 1997; McLaughlin et al., 1998; Schild et al., 1998), *(2)* spinal seeding is uncommon in the absence of local recurrence (Leibel and Sheline, 1987; Marks and Adler, 1982; Vanuytsel and Brada, 1991; Schild et al., 1998), *(3)* the patterns of failure are similar in patients with high-grade tumors treated with local fields or with craniospinal axis irradiation (Goldwein et al., 1991a; Vanuytsel et al., 1992; McLaughlin, 1998), and *(4)* prophylactic treatment may not prevent spinal metastases have led many investigators to question whether the routine use of craniospinal or whole-brain irradiation leads to improved survival (Goldwein et al., 1991; Vanuytsel and Brada, 1991; Vanuytsel et al., 1992).

Merchant et al. (1997) reviewed the outcomes of 28 pediatric patients with anaplastic ependymoma treated either with or without craniospinal irradiation. The actuarial 5 and 10 year survival rates were

56% and 38%, respectively. A benefit from craniospinal irradiation could not be demonstrated. All 19 patients who failed radiotherapy relapsed at the primary site, and one of these also developed subarachnoid dissemination. On the basis of these and other data, craniospinal irradiation is generally not recommended for patients with supratentorial anaplastic (high-grade) ependymomas unless evidence of leptomeningeal spread is pathologically or radiographically documented (Vanuytsel and Brada, 1991; Goldwein et al., 1991; Goldwein and Lefkowitz, 1991; Merchant et al., 1997; McLaughlin, 1998). Although dose levels of 54 Gy have typically been used to treat anaplastic ependymomas, the administration of 59.4 Gy with conformal techniques would appear to be warranted.

Because the inability to eradicate the primary tumor remains the single most important factor leading to treatment failure (Vanuytsel et al., 1992), more aggressive local therapies to improve local tumor control, in both low- and high-grade ependymomas, are being explored. These include the use of boosts with stereotactic radiotherapy or conformal radiotherapy techniques as well as hyperfractionated radiation schedules (McLaughlin, 1998; Schuller et al., 1999).

Chemotherapy

Supratentorial ependymomas are uncommon tumors, probably representing fewer than 30% of all ependymomas. While firm data on age incidence for these supratentorial tumors are unavailable, in our experience these tumors are most often seen in the first two decades of life. Also, there may be a higher proportion of anaplastic (or malignant) ependymomas than of the more common cellular (or low-grade) ependymomas. In most series, supratentorial ependymomas occur nearly as frequently as infratentorial ependymomas. When supratentorial ependymomas recur, they almost always do so at the primary tumor site, regardless of pathology.

The value of chemotherapy for ependymomas in general and for supratentorial ependymomas in particular remains unclear (Puccetti and Finlay, 1992). No distinction has been made in phase II chemotherapy trials between supratentorial and infratentorial ependymomas. Table 3–14 summarizes therapies for ependymomas in both locations. Single agents vary in the quality of responses and the durability of responses that they produce. Those yielding good responses and longer duration of response activity are carmustine (Levin et al., 1993), dibromodulcitol (Levin et al., 1984), and diaziquone (Ettinger et al., 1990). Cisplatin and carboplatin appear less effective; more recent trials with ifosfamide have shown similar activity.

Unfortunately, no studies to date have demonstrated a survival advantage with single-agent chemotherapy plus irradiation compared with irradiation alone in children or adults with newly diagnosed ependymomas (Goldwein and Lefkowitz, 1991). Levin and colleagues (2000a) reported on 17 patients with malignant ependymoma treated with a combination of 6-thioguanine, procarbazine, dibromodulcitol, CCNU, and vincristine (TPDCV) chemotherapy and craniospinal radiation. With the combined chemotherapy–radiotherapy protocol, 65% of patients failed, with a median time to progression of 141 weeks and a median survival of 42 months, and there

Table 3–14. Chemotherapy for Recurrent Ependymoma and Anaplastic Ependymoma Regardless of Location

Series	*Drug*	*No.*	*% R + SD*	*50% TTP (Months)*	*25% TTP (Months)*
Levin et al. (1984)	Dibromodulcitol	12	75	16	20
Levin et al. (1987)	Carmustine	14	78	13	24
Bertolone et al. (1989)	Cisplatin	8	75	3.8	4.3
Goldwein et al. (1990)	Various*	37 trials/16 patients	22	9	10
Gaynon et al. (1990)	Carboplatin	14	28	14	NA
Ettinger et al. (1990)	Diaziquone	12	42	10	16
Prados et al. (1991)	TPDCV	11	82	21.6	NA

% R + SD, percent of patients who responded or had stable disease; TTP, time to tumor progression; TPDCV, 6-thioguanine, procarbazine, dibromodulcitol, lomustine, and vincristine (MD Prados and VA Levin, personal communication); NA, not attained yet.

*Various combinations of vincristine, cisplatin, lomustine, procarbazine, etoposide, and ifosfamide combinations.

were 8 patients alive at a median of 9 years after study entry.

Therapy for ependymomas relies first on surgery, second on radiation, and third on chemotherapy. In most cases, failure of the first two approaches forces consideration of chemotherapy. Although we advocate no specific chemotherapy at this time, we believe that platinum-based therapies are not particularly active and should be avoided. Unfortunately, few adjuvant chemotherapy studies of the treatment of anaplastic ependymoma are ongoing at this time.

PRIMITIVE NEUROECTODERMAL TUMORS

Pathology

The term *primitive neuroectodermal tumor* (PNET) was originally used to describe small cell, predominantly undifferentiated, tumors occurring in the cerebral hemispheres of young patients (Hart and Earle, 1973). Some tumors showed minor components of glial or neuronal differentiation. The common histologic feature of all of these tumors is, however, some component of immature, small embryonal-like cells. Most have frequent mitotic activity and zones of necrosis. Subsequently, the term *cerebral neuroblastoma* has been used for those morphologically similar tumors that show evidence of primitive or more advanced neuronal differentiation. The features of neuronal differentiation include the presence of Homer-Wright fibrillary rosettes and large neuron-like cells with more abundant eosinophilic cytoplasm, large round nuclei, and prominent nucleoli. Cerebral neuroblastomas also tend to have an abundant component of connective tissue and a desmoplastic appearance. Small cell, undifferentiated tumors that show astrocytic differentiation or both neuronal and astrocytic differentiation may be called PNET with glial or with divergent differentiation.

Most pathologists accept positive immunoreactivity for glial fibrillary acidic protein (GFAP) in neoplastic cells as evidence of astrocytic differentiation. Positive immunoreactivity for synaptophysin or for neurofilament protein confirms neuronal or neuroblastic components. Examples with definite epithelial ependymal rosettes are designated ependymoblastomas, or PNET with ependymal differentiation. Tumors arising in the pineal region are pineoblastomas.

Clinical Features

Primitive neuroectodermal tumors occur most commonly in the first two decades of life, although they are increasingly recognized in adults into the sixth decade. Following the initial description of primary cerebral neuroblastoma by Horten and Rubinstein (1976), a distinction in clinical behavior and outcome between that entity and supratentorial PNET (Hart and Earle, 1973) has been emphasized by some authors but not by others. Both types of tumors demonstrate similar clinical and diagnostic features, although the in vivo appearance of each may be somewhat different. Either lesion may be cystic, grayish-granular, sharply demarcated, and hemispheric in location (Kosnik et al., 1978). In addition to being cystic, the cerebral neuroblastoma may also have a mural tumor nodule that is not seen in PNET. The latter lesion often shows gross areas of necrosis, which are not typical of the cerebral neuroblastoma.

Staging for extent of tumor is similar to that for infratentorial medulloblastoma, although the yield of positive studies at initial diagnosis is lower. Patients must undergo imaging of the entire neuraxis by brain and spine MRI, as well as a diagnostic lumbar puncture within 2 to 3 weeks following surgery for cytologic evaluation of CSF for malignant cells.

Surgery

The goal of surgery is complete tumor resection whenever feasible. Because of the tumor's hemispheric location, it may be necessary to utilize physiologic mapping to achieve that goal, as previously described. There are sparse data on how extent of resection affects outcome. Although several reports of long-term survival appear to coincide with radical resection of either tumor type (Duffner et al., 1981; Halperin et al., 1993; Gaffney et al., 1985), this is not always the case (Tomita et al., 1988). The patients who benefit most from total resection have cystic cerebral neuroblastomas (Berger et al., 1983).

Although PNET may occur in the first three decades of life (unlike neuroblastomas, which always affect younger children), both lesions must be distinguished from the adult central neurocytoma, which is an intraventricular, neuronally derived tumor originating from the septum pellucidum (Hassoun et al., 1993). Central neurocytomas are histologically distinct from the neuroblastic and neuroectodermal tumors described above. Complete resection of the central neurocytoma is usually curative without further adjuvant therapy (Kim et al., 1992).

Radiation Therapy

The general consensus is that patients with PNET should receive postoperative radiation therapy (Humphrey et al., 1981). Although radiation therapy appears to increase survival time (Duffner et al., 1981; Jenkin, 1981), the outcome is usually poor, and most patients develop local or regional recurrences. Because of their propensity to spread throughout the subarachnoid space (Kosnik et al., 1978; Parker et al., 1975; Knapp et al., 1981; Ashwal et al., 1984; Humphrey et al., 1981), PNET are treated with craniospinal axis irradiation (Jenkin, 1981; Gaffney et al., 1985). The primary tumor is given 54 to 55 Gy, and the remainder of the axis receives 36 Gy. The dose should be reduced for very young children (Gaffney et al., 1985).

Chemotherapy is usually a part of the treatment program. Although primitive neuroectodermal tumors are included in pediatric cooperative group protocols designed for high-risk medulloblastoma patients, they are less radiocurable than medulloblastomas (Gaffney et al., 1985; Humphrey et al., 1981). In some series 1 year survival rates are as low as 10% (Kosnik et al., 1978), whereas others report 5 year survival rates of 20% to 47% (Gaffney et al., 1985; Humphrey et al., 1981; Paulino and Melian, 1999). The disparity in survival figures reflects the heterogeneity of malignancies that are classified under the term *primitive neuroectodermal tumors* (Rubinstein, 1985). For example, in a series of 14 patients reported by Gaffney et al. (1985), the 3 year survival rate was 29%. None of the patients with tumors containing more than 90% undifferentiated elements were alive at 3 years, whereas 60% of those with less primitive tumors survived 3 years.

An important question is raised by the relative infrequency of neuraxis dissemination at diagnosis of supratentorial nonpineal region PNET compared with infratentorial medulloblastoma. Because the outcome for patients with residual tumor in the absence of metastases remains so poor even in the face of full-dose craniospinal irradiation, one might argue that for such patients restricting irradiation to involved fields might permit greater tolerance of dose intensification of chemotherapy with improved outcome. It is important to remember that almost 40% of the body's bone marrow resides in the spinal vertebrae and that, following craniospinal irradiation at the standard dose of 36 Gy, the patient's ability to tolerate even modest doses of chemotherapy is significantly impaired. For patients with pineoblastomas, who are known to experience a very high rate of neuraxis dissemination at diagnosis and relapse, restricting the irradiation field (especially in older children and adults) is probably inappropriate; however, in patients with other supratentorial PNET this may be appropriate within the conduct of a formal clinical trial. One other approach to permit intensification of chemotherapy is to deliver such treatment in a therapeutic window before the delivery of craniospinal irradiation.

Cerebral neuroblastomas are biologically distinct from other PNET. They tend to be less malignant, have a better outcome, and are less likely to disseminate throughout the craniospinal axis (Cohen and Duffner, 1984). This tumor may present as a cystic lesion with a peripheral nodule or as a solid mass, and the tumor's morphologic appearance is related to prognosis. Berger et al. (1983) reported the outcomes of 11 patients with cerebral neuroblastoma. Six patients presented with cystic tumors, and five had solid lesions. Gross total resection was achieved in only two patients, both with cystic tumors. All patients received postoperative irradiation. Seven of the 11 patients, all treated with local irradiation to an average of 52 Gy, remained alive with no evidence of tumor progression. None of the six patients with cystic tumors developed recurrent disease, whereas four of the five patients with solid tumors had a relapse at the primary site within 8 to 31 months after treatment. The only patient with a solid lesion who did not have a tumor recurrence received adjuvant chemotherapy. Although subarachnoid dissemination is found in autopsied cases (Horten and Rubinstein, 1976), this pattern of spread does not represent a significant clinical problem. Thus, localized cerebral neuroblastomas are treated with limited-field irradiation to 54 Gy. The craniospinal axis is included only if there is evidence of tumor dissemination beyond the site of origin by imaging studies or CSF cytology.

Chemotherapy

Although the mainstay of therapy for PNET is surgery and irradiation, young patient age, incomplete resection, and recurrent tumor require the addition of chemotherapy. Several single-institution reports on supratentorial PNET have indicated a poor prognosis following surgical resection alone or combined with postoperative irradiation; this reflects a high incidence of primary site recurrence as well as neuraxis dissemination throughout the leptomeninges, even in the face of prophylactic craniospinal irradiation. This is particularly true of pineoblastomas, which have a high rate of neuraxis dissemination at both initial presentation and subsequent recurrence. Patient age at onset of these tumors may also have a powerful prognostic importance; most studies indicate that very young children fare worse than older patients, with higher rates of dissemination at diagnosis and recurrence and a shorter time to recurrence. Chemotherapy alone is now generally employed for children younger than 3 years with supratentorial PNET.

The site of origin of PNET has been documented as an important prognostic indicator in a large phase III trial conducted by the Childrens Cancer Group in North America (the CCG-921 study). In that study, both posterior fossa and supratentorial PNET were randomized to one of two chemotherapy-containing regimens; all patients underwent maximal surgical resection of the primary site tumor and were given postoperative craniospinal irradiation with a boost to the primary tumor site. Chemotherapy with CCNU, vincristine, and prednisone was compared with the 8-in-1 regimen of CCNU, vincristine, cisplatin, hydroxyurea, cytosine arabinoside, cyclophosphamide, and methylprednisolone. The most recently published reports from this study (Jakacki et al., 1995; Cohen et al., 1995; Zeltzer et al., 1999) demonstrate some surprising differences between patients with pineal region PNET, other nonpineal region PNET, and infratentorial PNET or medulloblastoma. For patients with pineal PNET, the 3 year PFS was 61% ± 13%, whereas the corresponding 3 year PFS for patients with nonpineal supratentorial PNET was only 33% ± 9%, a statistically significant difference. Considering both extent of resection and tumor stage, patients with supratentorial PNET have a poorer PFS and overall survival rate than do patients with infratentorial PNET.

In the above cooperative group study, the infratentorial PNET were primarily medulloblastoma, whereas the supratentorial PNET carried other diagnostic labels; no differentiation was made between cerebral neuroblastomas and other supratentorial PNET. Interestingly, greater than 40% of infratentorial tumors showed evidence of neuraxis dissemination at diagnosis (either positive CSF cytology and/or radiographic evidence of intracranial or spinal leptomeningeal dissemination on head CT scan or myelogram), whereas only 21% of patients with supratentorial PNET showed such dissemination. The outcome for patients with supratentorial PNET was significantly affected by neuraxis dissemination; patients without neuraxis dissemination had a 3 year PFS of 56%, whereas all patients with evidence of neuraxis dissemination at diagnosis ultimately relapsed.

An additional effect of volume of residual tumor was observed in patients with nonpineal PNET treated in the CCG-921 study; those with residual tumor volume less than 1.5 cm^2 on postoperative scans had a 4 year survival of 40% ± 22% compared with 13% ± 8% for those with greater residual tumor volume. Because of small patient numbers, however, this difference did not attain statistical significance (Albright et al., 1995). The even smaller patient numbers with pineal PNET obviated any valid comparisons, but suggest that patients with bulky residual disease relapsed at a higher rate and earlier following diagnosis (Jakacki et al., 1995). Subsequent pediatric cooperative group trials attempted to improve upon the poor results for patients with supratentorial PNET with either significant residual tumor postoperatively and/or neuraxis dissemination. The studies employed intensification of chemotherapy with agents known to be efficacious against PNET (e.g., alkylating agents such as cyclophosphamide or ifosfamide at high doses, and cisplatin or carboplatin). Again, however, evidence of benefit over conventional chemotherapy is lacking.

Because the occurrence of supratentorial PNET is not uncommon within the first 3 years of life, and because children with these tumors are particularly vulnerable to the deleterious effects of whole-brain irradiation on the developing brain, chemotherapy is now routinely used instead of irradiation either to avoid entirely or to at least delay the need for or restrict the volume and dose of radiation to the brain. In the Childrens Cancer Group CCG-921 study, children younger than 18 months with medulloblastoma/PNET were nonrandomly assigned to receive the 8-in-1 chemotherapy regimen with the intent of delaying irradiation until the completion of at least 1 year of chemotherapy. In a publication reporting the

CCG-921 study, all children younger than 18 months of age at diagnosis of pineoblastoma died following tumor recurrence at a median of just 4 months from diagnosis (Jakacki et al., 1995).

The outcome for young children with nonpineal region supratentorial PNET is less clear. All nine children aged 19 to 36 months treated with reduced-dose irradiation to the spine (23.4 Gy) and the primary site (45 Gy) as well as with chemotherapy relapsed and died (Albright et al., 1995). However, those children younger than 18 months of age treated with 8-in-1 chemotherapy without irradiation achieved a 55% ± 16% 3 year PFS, comparable with the survival rate of children older than 36 months of age treated with full-dose irradiation and the same chemotherapy regimen (Geyer et al., 1994). This unusually favorable outcome in a small number of patients (n = 11) contrasts with other reports indicating equally poor outcomes for infants with pineal and nonpineal supratentorial PNET treated with chemotherapy alone (Duffner et al., 1993).

To avoid irradiation for children younger than 6 years of age with supratentorial PNET and for children younger than 3 years of age with PNET in any location, the "Head Start I" chemotherapy regimen was developed (Mason et al., 1998). This regimen uses five cycles of intensive induction chemotherapy (cisplatin, vincristine, high-dose cyclophosphamide, and etoposide) followed by a single cycle of myeloablative chemotherapy (thiotepa, etoposide, and carboplatin) with autologous hemopoietic stem cell rescue. The most recent update (Golomb et al., 1999) indicates a 4 year PFS of almost 50% for patients with supratentorial PNET, with avoidance of irradiation for more than 80% of patients. The more recent protocol, "Head Start II," being conducted in a multinational setting, employs the same regimen as Head Start I but with intensification in induction using high-dose methotrexate for patients with neuraxis dissemination at diagnosis and increasing the age of eligibility for patients with supratentorial tumors to 10 years.

For recurrences of supratentorial PNET, the subsequent course of management must be tailored to the individual patient, depending on the extent of disease at recurrence, prior exposure to irradiation and/or chemotherapy, the patient's general condition, and specific organ function at time of recurrence. For those with localized recurrence, radical surgical resection should be considered as a first step. In the presence of leptomeningeal dissemination, surgical debulking of mass lesions is more problematic, although at times it can contribute toward an improved level of palliation.

Postoperative chemotherapy approaches for patients with tumor recurrence range from the use of new investigational agents to myeloablative chemotherapy regimens with autologous hemopoietic stem cell rescue if the patient can be brought to a state of minimal residual tumor either through surgical resection of localized tumor or through reinduction chemotherapy. This intensive approach is particularly warranted for young children who have not received irradiation before recurrence and for the small proportion of patients for whom myeloablative chemotherapy with autologous stem cell rescue followed by irradiation may afford cure of disease (Guruangan et al., 1998).

CHOROID PLEXUS PAPILLOMAS AND CARCINOMAS

Pathology

Benign or malignant proliferations of choroid plexus epithelium are termed *papillomas* or *carcinomas,* respectively. Both are rare, occurring most often in the first decade of life (Matson and Crofton, 1960; Bigner et al., 1998). Congenital examples have been described (Tomita and Naidich, 1987). The papilloma is usually cured surgically (McGirr et al., 1988). These tumors may arise at any choroid plexus site, but the lateral and third ventricles are more common sites in children, whereas the fourth ventricle is more common in adults (Burger et al., 1991; Bigner et al., 1998). Symptoms are usually referable to hydrocephalus, a sequela either of ventricular outflow obstruction by the mass or of active oversecretion of CSF by the proliferating choroid plexus epithelium, or both (Boyd and Steinbok, 1987; Eisenberg et al., 1974).

The diagnosis of choroid plexus papilloma hinges on the presence of an unusually large mass of choroid plexus tissue and some cellular crowding and pseudostratification (Burger et al., 1991) with almost no mitotic activity. The histologic features are remarkably similar to those of normal choroid plexus epithelium. Foci of bone, cartilage, or oncocytic change may be seen (Bonnin et al., 1987). Even histologically benign lesions have been reported to seed the subarachnoid space, but they do not invade the cerebral parenchyma (Bigner et al., 1998).

Choroid plexus carcinomas are highly anaplastic, malignant, and invasive neoplasms (Lewis, 1967; Packer et al., 1992; Paulus and Janisch, 1990). They appear as poorly differentiated carcinomas, with ultrastructural features of adenocarcinomas, such as cilia, microvilli, and well-formed cytoplasmic junctions (Burger et al., 1991; Bigner et al., 1998). The differential diagnoses are intraventricular ependymoma and metastatic carcinoma. The distinction from ependymoma can usually be made by identifying the neoplastic stroma as either glial (ependymoma) or mesenchymal (choroid plexus neoplasm). Immunostaining for glial fibrillary acidic protein is usually strongly and diffusely positive in an ependymoma but focal in a choroid plexus tumor (Coffin et al., 1986; Mannoji and Becker, 1988; Miettenen et al., 1986; Bigner et al., 1998). In contrast, cytokeratins are present in choroid plexus tumors as carcinoembryonic antigen may be present in carcinomas, whereas both agents are focal or absent in ependymomas (Coffin et al., 1986; McComb and Burger, 1983).

The role of transthyretin (prealbumin) immunostaining in making a diagnosis is still controversial (Herbert et al., 1990; Paulus and Janisch, 1990). Although this substance is produced in normal choroid plexus and immunoreactivity is seen in most papillomas, the extent and intensity of reactivity decrease with increasing anaplasia (Matsushima et al., 1988). The presence of transthyretin immunoreactivity is, however, not entirely specific for choroid plexus epithelium as other systemic (metastatic) neoplasms may also react (Albrecht et al., 1991).

In adults, the rarity of choroid plexus neoplasms mandates that metastatic carcinoma be the preferred diagnosis unless it is absolutely and rigorously eliminated (Gottschalk et al., 1993; Bigner et al., 1998).

Surgery

Choroid plexus tumors present a difficult challenge to the surgeon because of their large size and enormous blood volume. These lesions are often found in the lateral and third ventricles during childhood and in the fourth ventricle in adults. The goals of surgery include gross total resection and management of the massive ventriculomegaly that often results. In the past, the mortality from surgery approached 20% to 30% as a result of excessive bleeding (Hawkins, 1980), and neurologic morbidity was unacceptably high.

The approach to the lesion depends on the position it occupies in the ventricle. Lateral ventricular tumors are best approached through the posterior temporal lobe, inferior to the middle gyrus (dominant hemisphere), and via the middle to superior gyrus in the nondominant hemisphere (Spallone et al., 1990). Tumors situated in the third ventricle may be approached by a transcortical (superior frontal gyrus) incision or through the transcallosal route (Schijman et al., 1990). The tumor must be mobilized to find the arterial pedicle from the anterior choroidal artery in the case of a lateral ventricular lesion entering into its inferomedial surface (Raimondi and Gutierrez, 1975). However, this approach is not always possible due to the massive size of the tumor. In this setting, the tumor must be removed piecemeal with bipolar coagulation (Tomita and Naidich, 1987) as opposed to an en bloc delivery, which is the ideal surgical approach. In neonates and infants, the blood volume may range between 250 and 500 ml, thus requiring massive transfusions to replete the rapid bleeding that often occurs with piecemeal removal.

Tumor in the third ventricle will protrude through the foramen of Monro (Fig. 3–15) and derives its vascular pedicle from the roof of the third ventricle. It may be necessary to split both fornices or to maneuver under the lateral ventricle choroid plexus to enter the mid to posterior third ventricle. Venous drainage also becomes a problem because of massive distention due to increased tumor blood volume and the fragility of the draining veins in a young child. Once the tumor is removed, a drain should be left in place for 2 to 3 days to remove all bloody CSF and tumor debris. In most circumstances, a larger subdural effusion will develop, although some surgeons claim that this can be obviated by sealing the cortical opening with fibrin glue (Boyd and Steinbok, 1987). The treatment of choice for this problem if it is symptomatic or does not resolve within 3 to 6 months is to place a subdural–peritoneal shunt.

The etiology of the hydrocephalus is thought to be secondary to overproduction of CSF (Eisenberg et al., 1974), although the altered flow of CSF along with its elevated protein concentration may also be implicated (Rekate et al., 1985). Usually, removal of the tumor

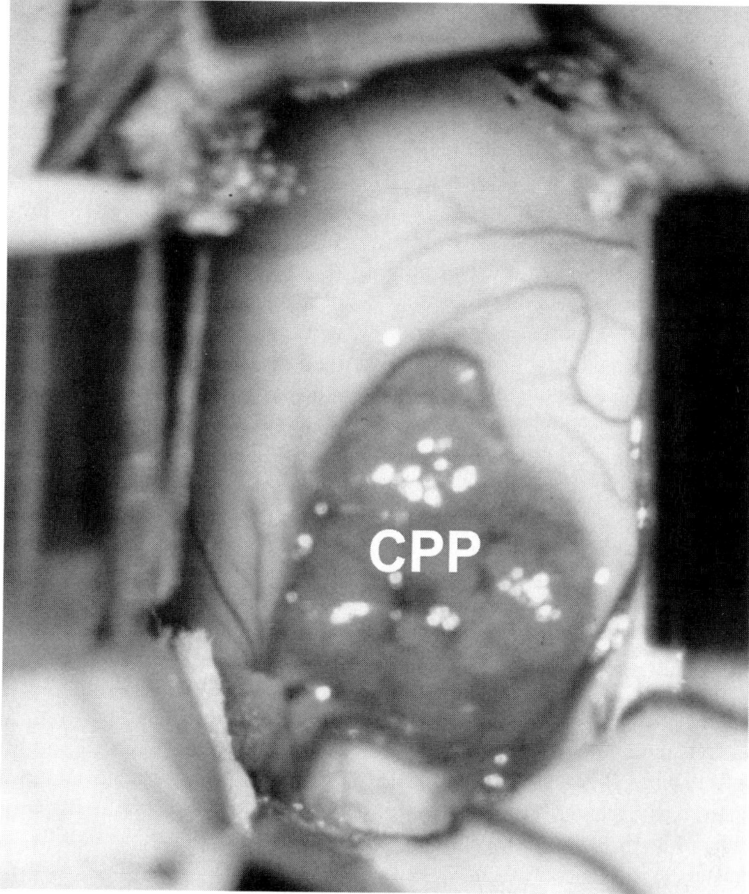

Figure 3–15. Choroid plexus papilloma (CPP) protruding through the foramen of Monro.

will reduce the hydrocephalus and the need for permanent ventriculoperitoneal shunting, which is required in 20% or more of cases (Hawkins, 1980).

Choroid plexus carcinomas should likewise be completely resected if possible, as this has been more effective in determining long-term outcome than has adjuvant therapy (Ellenbogen et al., 1989; St. Clair et al., 1991).

Radiation

Because choroid plexus papillomas are often cured by total surgical excision (McEvoy et al., 2000), not much information exists about their response to irradiation (Cohen and Duffner, 1984). The studies that are available do not provide sufficient detail or data to allow an assessment of the value of radiation therapy for these lesions. Pathology specimens from patients who received low-dose preoperative irradiation (approximately 30 Gy) demonstrated a significant reduction in tumor size, obliteration of the tumor capillary bed, and necrosis, although at this dose level there was little change observed in neoplastic choroidal cells (Carrea and Polak, 1977). Naguib et al. (1981) reported a case of an inoperable cerebellopontine angle choroid plexus papilloma that extensively involved the adjacent mastoid bone. This patient received 49.5 Gy in 32 treatment fractions over a period of 33 days. Within 16 months after completion of radiation therapy, the mass was markedly reduced in size. Such anecdotal reports suggest that it is reasonable to offer local irradiation to patients with inoperable or recurrent choroid plexus papillomas (Cohen and Duffner, 1984).

Radiation therapy may be beneficial for patients with choroid plexus carcinomas (Ausman et al.,

1984; Carpenter et al., 1982; Chow et al., 1999). Subarachnoid tumor seeding has been identified in as many as 44% of cases (Ausman et al., 1984). Therefore consideration should be given to irradiating the entire craniospinal axis; however, data to support this approach are not available. Chow et al. (1999) recommend that patients with completely excised, localized choroid plexus carcinomas be treated with either adjunctive chemotherapy or limited-field irradiation provided that their spinal MRI and CSF cytology studies are negative. Because of potential intellectual and endocrinologic sequelae, radiotherapy is used sparingly for infants and young children. However, radiotherapy appears to be helpful to those also receiving chemotherapy who develop progressive disease. Both chemotherapy and craniospinal axis irradiation may be indicated for patients with incompletely excised tumors and for those with evidence of leptomeningeal spread (Chow et al., 1999).

Chemotherapy

The role of chemotherapy in the management of choroid plexus tumors remains ill defined. Several phase II trials of chemotherapeutic agents in recurrent pediatric brain tumors have included occasional patients with choroid plexus carcinomas, and objective radiographic responses to such agents have been observed. A small number of reports have focused on the efficacy of chemotherapy for choroid plexus carcinomas and have demonstrated objective radiographic responses to *(1)* a combination of cisplatin and etoposide, *(2)* myeloablative doses of thiotepa and etoposide, *(3)* the 8-in-1 regimen (J Finlay, personal communications, 1993), and *(4)* cyclophosphamide-based therapies with or without intraventricular chemotherapy (VA Levin personal communications, 1993; Souweidane et al., 1999).

Even though chemotherapy has produced objective responses in patients with choroid plexus carcinoma, it does not follow that such drugs have a clear role in improving the outcome for newly diagnosed tumors in children. It seems clear that the single most powerful prognostic factor of a favorable outcome for children with choroid plexus tumors is extent of surgical resection; children who undergo a successful gross total resection of tumor at diagnosis have an excellent survival; it is unclear whether such children require any additional therapy, either irradiation or chemotherapy. Volumetric reduction with preoperative chemotherapy may improve the ability to perform a complete resection (Souweidane et al., 1999). However, the outcomes for patients with incompletely resected or metastatic choroid plexus carcinoma is poor, even with the addition of radiation therapy and/or conventional chemotherapy. Given that the carcinomas have shown sensitivity to chemotherapy, it is appropriate to advocate intensive chemotherapy regimens for children with newly diagnosed, incompletely resected, and/or metastatic choroid plexus carcinoma, with avoidance of irradiation, as most of these children will be younger than 6 years of age and at greatest risk for tumor recurrence and profound developmental and psychosocial dysfunction if subjected to cranial irradiation. In light of the importance of radical surgical resection, any child with localized but incompletely resected primary choroid plexus papilloma or carcinoma should be considered for reoperation to achieve gross total resection.

REFERENCES

Afra D, Muller W, Benoist G, Schroder R. 1978. Supratentorial recurrences of gliomas. Results of reoperations on astrocytomas and oligodendrogliomas. Acta Neurochir (Wien) 43:217–227.

Albrecht S, Rouah E, Becker LE, Bruner J. 1991. Transthyretin immunoreactivity in choroid plexus neoplasms and brain metastases. Mod Pathol 4:610–614.

Albright AL, Wisoff JH, Zeltzer PM, et al. 1995. Prognostic factors in children with supratentorial (nonpineal) primitive neuroectodermal tumors. A neurosurgical perspective from the Childrens Cancer Group. Pediatr Neurosurg 22:1–7.

Allen JC, Bloom J, Ertel I, et al. 1986. Brain tumors in children: current cooperative and institutional chemotherapy trials in newly diagnosed and recurrent disease. Semin Oncol 13:110–122.

Allen JC, Walker R, Luks E, Jennings M, Barfoot S, Tan C. 1987. Carboplatin and recurrent childhood brain tumors. J Clin Oncol 5:459–463.

Ammirati M, Vick N, Liao Y, Ciric I, Mikhael M. 1987. Effect of extent of surgical resection on survival and quality of life in patients with supratentorial glioblastomas and anaplastic astrocytomas. Neurosurgery 21:201–206.

Arseni C, Petrovici IN. 1971. Epilepsy in temporal lobe tumors. Eur Neurol 5:201–214.

Artico M, Cervoni L, Celli P, Salvati M, Palma L. 1993. Supratentorial glioblastoma in children: a series of 27 surgically treated cases. Childs Nerv Syst 9:7–9.

Ashwal S, Hinshaw DB, Bedros A. 1984. CNS primitive neuroectodermal tumors of childhood. Med Pediatr Oncol 12:180–188.

Ausman JI, Schrontz C, Chason J, Knighton RS, Pak H, Patel S. 1984. Aggressive choroid plexus papilloma. Surg Neurol 22:472–476.

Awad IA, Rosenfeld J, Ahl J, Hahn JF, Luders H. 1991. Intractable epilepsy and structural lesions of the brain: mapping, resection strategies and seizure outcome. Epilepsia 32:179–186.

Bampoe J, Bernstein M. 1999. The role of surgery in low grade gliomas. J Neurooncol 42:259–269.

Barnett GH, Kormos DW, Steiner CP, Weisenberger J. 1993. Use of a frameless, armless stereotactic wand for brain tumor localization with two-dimensional and three-dimensional neuroimaging. Neurosurgery 33:674–678.

Bauman GS, Cairncross JG. 2001. Multidisciplinary management of adult anaplastic oligodendrogliomas and anaplastic mixed oligo-astrocytomas. Semin Radiat Oncol 11:170–180.

Bauman G, Lote K, Larson D, et al. 1999a. Pretreatment factors predict overall survival for patients with low-grade glioma: a recursive partitioning analysis. Int J Radiat Oncol Biol Phys 45:923–929.

Bauman G, Pahapill P, Macdonald D, Fisher B, Leighton C, Cairncross G. 1999b. Low grade glioma: a measuring radiographic response to radiotherapy. Can J Neurol Sci 26:18–22.

Berger MS. 1986. Ultrasound-guided stereotaxic biopsy using a new apparatus. J Neurosurg 65:550–554.

Berger MS, Cohen W, Ojemann GA. 1990b. Correlation of motor cortex brain mapping data with magnetic resonance imaging. J Neurosurg 72:383–387.

Berger MS, Deliganis AV, Dobbins J, Keles GE. 1994. The effect of extent of resection on recurrence in patients with low grade cerebral hemisphere gliomas. Cancer 74:1784–1791.

Berger MS, Edwards MS, Wara WM, Levin VA, Wilson CB. 1983. Primary cerebral neuroblastoma. Long-term follow-up review and therapeutic guidelines. J Neurosurg 59:418–423.

Berger MS, Ghatan S, Haglund MM, Dobbins J, Ojemann GA. 1993. Low-grade gliomas associated with intractable epilepsy: seizure outcome utilizing electrocorticography during tumor resection. J Neurosurg 79:62–69.

Berger MS, Ojemann GA, Lettich E. 1990a. Neurophysiological monitoring during astrocytoma surgery. Neurosurg Clin Am 1:65–80.

Berger MS, Tucker A, Spence A, Winn HR. 1992. Reoperation for glioma. Clin Neurosurg 39:172–186.

Bertolone SJ, Baum ES, Krivit W, Hammond GD. 1989. A phase II study of cisplatin therapy in recurrent childhood brain tumors. A report from the Childrens Cancer Study Group. J Neurooncol 7:5–11.

Bigner DD, McLendon R, Bruner JM. 1998. Russell and Rubinstein's Pathology of Tumors of the Nervous System, 6th ed. London: Edward Arnold, 757 pp.

Black PM, Moriarty T, Alexander E 3d, et al. 1997. Development and implementation of intraoperative magnetic resonance imaging and its neurosurgical applications. Neurosurgery 41:831–845.

Bleehen NM. 1990. Studies of high grade cerebral gliomas. Int J Radiat Oncol Biol Phys 18:811–813.

Bloom HJ. 1982. Intracranial tumors: response and resistance to therapeutic endeavors, 1970–1980. Int J Radiat Oncol Biol Phys 8:1083–1113.

Boesel CP, Paulson GW, Kosnik EJ, Earle KM. 1979. Brain hamartomas and tumors associated with tuberous sclerosis. Neurosurgery 4:410–417.

Bonnin JM, Colon LE, Morawetz RB. 1987. Focal glial differentiation and oncocytic transformation in choroid plexus papilloma. Acta Neuropathol (Berl) 72:277–280.

Bouchard J. 1980. Central nervous system. In: Fletcher GH (ed), Textbook of Radiotherapy, 3rd ed. Philadelphia: Lea & Febiger, p 444.

Boyd MC, Steinbok P. 1987. Choroid plexus tumors: problems in diagnosis and management. J Neurosurg 66:800–805.

Brain Tumor Registry of Japan. 1992. Neurol Medico-Chir 32:385–547.

Buckner JC, Brown LD, Cascino TL, et al. 1990. Phase II evaluation of infusional etoposide and cisplatin in patients with recurrent astrocytoma. J Neurooncol 9:249–254.

Bullard DE, Rawlings CE 3d, Phillips B, et al. 1987. Oligodendroglioma. An analysis of the value of radiation therapy. Cancer 60:2179–2188.

Burger PC, Dubois PJ, Schold SC, et al. 1983. Computerized tomographic and pathologic studies of the untreated, quiescent, and recurrent glioblastoma multiforme. J Neurosurg 58:159–169.

Burger PC, Green SB. 1987. Patient age, histologic features, and length of survival in patients with glioblastoma multiforme. Cancer 59:1617–1625.

Burger PC, Heinz ER, Shibata T, Kleihues P. 1988. Topographic anatomy and CT correlations in the untreated glioblastoma multiforme. J Neurosurg 68:698–704.

Burger PC, Rawlings CE, Cox EB, McLendon RF, Schold SC, Bullard DE. 1987. Clinicopathologic correlations in the oligodendroglioma. Cancer 59:1345–1352.

Burger PC, Scheithauer BW, Vogel FS. 1991. Surgical Pathology of the Nervous System and Its Coverings, 3rd ed. New York: Churchill Livingstone, 737 pp.

Burger PC, Vogel FS, Green SB, Strike TA. 1985. Glioblastoma multiforme and anaplastic astrocytoma. Pathologic criteria and prognostic implications. Cancer 56:1106–1111.

Cairncross JG, Laperriere NJ. 1989. Low-grade glioma. To treat or not to treat? Arch Neurol 46:1238–1239.

Cairncross G, Macdonald D, Ludwin S, et al. 1994. Chemotherapy for anaplastic oligodendroglioma. National Cancer Institute of Canada Clinical Trials Group. J Clin Oncol 12:2013–21.

Cairncross JG, Ueki K, Zlatescu MC, et al. 1998. Specific genetic predictors of chemotherapeutic response and survival in patients with anaplastic oligodendrogliomas. J Natl Cancer Inst 90:1473–1479.

Cappabianca P, Spaziante R, Caputi F, et al. 1991. Accuracy of the analysis of multiple small fragments of glial tumors obtained by stereotactic biopsy. Acta Cytol 35:505–511.

Carpenter DB, Michelsen WJ, Hays AP. 1982. Carcinoma of the choroid plexus. Case report. J Neurosurg 56:722–727.

Carrea R, Polak M. 1977. Preoperative radiotherapy in the management of posterior fossa choroid plexus papillomas. Childs Brain 3:12–24.

Cascino GD. 1990. Epilepsy and brain tumors: implications for treatment. Epilepsia 31:S37–S44.

Cascino GD, Kelly PJ, Hirschorn KA, Marsh WR, Sharbrough FW. 1990. Stereotactic resection of intra-axial cerebral lesions in partial epilepsy. Mayo Clin Proc 65:1053–1060.

Castro JR, Saunders WM, Tobias CA, et al. 1982. Treatment of cancer with heavy charged particles. Int J Radiat Oncol Biol Phys 8:2191–2198.

Celli P, Nofrone I, Palma L, Cantore G, Fortuna A. 1994. Cerebral oligodendroglioma: prognostic factors and life history. Neurosurgery 35:1018–1035.

Chamberlain MC, Kormanik PA. 1999. Salvage chemotherapy with tamoxifen for recurrent anaplastic astrocytomas. Arch Neurol 56:703–708.

Chamberlain MC, Levin VA. 1989. Chemotherapeutic treatment of the diencephalic syndrome. A case report. Cancer 63:1681–1684.

Chamberlain MC, Prados MD, Silver P, Levin VA. 1988. A phase I/II study of 24 hour intravenous AZQ in recurrent primary brain tumors. J Neurooncol 6:319–323.

Chandler KL, Prados MD, Malec M, Wilson CB. 1993. Long-term survival in patients with glioblastoma multiforme. Neurosurgery 32:716–720.

Chandrasoma PT, Smith MM, Apuzzo ML. 1989. Stereotactic biopsy in the diagnosis of brain masses: comparison of results of biopsy and resected surgical specimen. Neurosurgery 24:160–165.

Chang CH. 1977. Hyperbaric oxygen and radiation therapy in the management of glioblastoma. Natl Cancer Inst Monogr 46:163–169.

Chang CH, Horton J, Schoenfeld D, et al. 1983. Comparison of postoperative radiotherapy and combined postoperative radiotherapy and chemotherapy in the multidisciplinary management of malignant gliomas. A joint Radiation Therapy Oncology Group and Eastern Cooperative Oncology Group study. Cancer 52:997–1007.

Chastagner P, Sommelet-Olive D, Kalifa C, et al. 1993. Phase II study of ifosfamide in childhood brain tumors: a report by the French Society of Pediatric Oncology (SFOP). Med Pediatr Oncol 21:49–53.

Chin HW, Hazel JJ, Kim TH, Webster JH. 1980. Oligodendrogliomas. I. A clinical study of cerebral oligodendrogliomas. Cancer 45:1458–1466.

Chin HW, Maruyama Y, Markesbery W, Young AB. 1982. Intracranial ependymoma. Results of radiotherapy at the University of Kentucky. Cancer 49:2276–2280.

Chiu JK, Woo SY, Ater J, et al. 1992. Intracranial ependymoma in children: analysis of prognostic factors. J Neurooncol 13:283–290.

Choucair AK, Levin VA, Gutin PH, et al. 1986. Development of multiple lesions during radiation therapy and chemotherapy in patients with gliomas. J Neurosurg 65:654–658.

Chow E, Reardon DA, Shah AB, et al. 1999 Pediatric choroid plexus neoplasms. Int J Radiat Oncol Biol Phys 44:249–254.

Ciric I, Ammirati M, Vick N, Mikhael M. 1987. Supratentorial gliomas: surgical considerations and immediate postoperative results. Gross total resection versus partial resection. Neurosurgery 21:21–26.

Clark GB, Henry JM, McKeever PE. 1985. Cerebral pilocytic astrocytoma. Cancer 56:1128–1133.

Coffey RJ, Lunsford LD, Taylor FH. 1988. Survival after stereotactic biopsy of malignant gliomas. Neurosurgery 22:465–473.

Coffin CM, Wick MR, Braun JT, Dehner LP. 1986. Choroid plexus neoplasms. Clinicopathologic and immunohistochemical studies. Am J Surg Pathol 10:394–404.

Cohen BH, Zeltzer PM, Boyett JM, et al. 1995. Prognostic factors and treatment results for supratentorial primitive neuroectodermal tumors in children using radiation and chemotherapy: a Childrens Cancer Group randomized trial. J Clin Oncol 13:1687–1696.

Cohen ME, Duffner PK. 1984. Miscellaneous: primitive neuroectodermal tumors, oligodendrogliomas, choroid plexus papillomas. In: Cohen ME, Duffner PK (eds) Brain Tumors in Children: Principles of Diagnosis and Treatment. New York: Raven Press, p 273.

Concannon JP, Kramer S, Berry R. 1960. The extent of intracranial gliomas at autopsy and its relationship to techniques used in radiation therapy of brain tumors. Am J Roentgen 84:99–107.

Coons SW, Johnson PC, Pearl DK. 1997. The prognostic significance of Ki-67 labeling indices for oligodendrogliomas. Neurosurgery 41:878–884.

Coyle T, Baptista J, Winfield J, et al. 1990. Mechlorethamine, vincristine, and procarbazine chemotherapy for recurrent high-grade glioma in adults: a phase II study. J Clin Oncol 8:2014–2018.

Curran WJ, Scott CB, Horton J, et al. 1992a. Does extent of surgery influence outcome for astrocytoma with atypical or anaplastic foci (AAF)? A report from three Radiation Therapy Oncology Group (RTOG) trials. J Neurooncol 12:219–227.

Curran WJ, Scott CB, Horton J, et al. 1993. Recursive partitioning analysis of prognostic factors in three Radiation Therapy Oncology Group malignant glioma trials. J Natl Cancer Inst 85:704–710.

Curran WJ, Scott CB, Nelson JS, et al. 1992b. Survival comparison of radiosurgery eligible and ineligible malignant glioma patients treated with hyperfractionated radiation therapy (RT) and BCNU: a report of Radiation Therapy Oncology Group (RTOG) 83-02. Int J Radiat Oncol Biol Phys 24(suppl 1):A29.

Daumas-Duport C. 1993. Dysembryoplastic neuroepithelial tumours. Brain Pathol 3:283–295.

Daumas-Duport C, Scheithauer BW, Chodkeiwicz JP, Laws ER, Vedrenne C. 1988a. Dysembryoplastic neuroepithelial tumor: a surgically curable tumor of young patients with intractable partial seizures. Report of thirty-nine cases. Neurosurgery 23:545–556.

Daumas-Duport C, Scheithauer BW, Kelly PJ. 1987. A histologic and cytologic method for the spatial definition of gliomas. Mayo Clin Proc 62:435–449.

Daumas-Duport C, Scheithauer BW, O'Fallon J, Kelly P. 1988b. Grading of astrocytomas. A simple and reproducible method. Cancer 62:2152–2165.

Daumas-Duport C, Tucker ML, Kolles H, et al. 1997. Oligodendrogliomas. Part II: a new grading system based on morphological and imaging criteria. J Neurooncol 34:61–78.

Davis RL, Onda K, Shubuya M, Lamborn K, Hoshino T. 1995. Proliferation markers in gliomas: a comparison of BUDR, KI-67, and MIB-1. J Neurooncol 24:9–12.

de Chadarevian JP, Pattisapu JV, Faerber EN. 1990. Desmoplastic cerebral astrocytoma of infancy. Light microscopy, immunocytochemistry, and ultrastructure. Cancer 66:173–179.

Decker DA, Al Sarraf M, Kresge C, Austin D, Wilner HI. 1985. Phase II study of aziridinylbenzoquinone (AZQ: NSC-

182986) in the treatment of malignant gliomas recurrent after radiation. Preliminary report. J Neurooncol 3:19–21.

Dehghani F, Schachenmayr W, Laun A, Krof HW. 1998. Prognostic implication of histopathological, immunohistochemical and clinical features of oligodendrogliomas: a study of 89 cases. Acta Neuropathol (Berl) 95:493–504.

Deutsch M, Green SB, Strike TA, et al. 1989. Results of a randomized trial comparing BCNU plus radiotherapy, streptozotocin plus radiotherapy, BCNU plus hyperfrationated radiotherapy, and BCNU following misonidazole plus radiotherapy in the postoperative treatment of malignant glioma. Int J Radiat Oncol Biol Phys 16:1389–1396.

Di Lorenzo N, Esposito V, Lunardi P, Delfini R, Fortuna A, Cantore G. 1991. A comparison of computerized tomography-guided stereotactic and ultrasound-guided techniques for brain biopsy. J Neurosurg 75:763–765.

Dinapoli RP, Brown LD, Arusell RM, et al. 1993. Phase III comparative evaluation of PCNU and carmustine combined with radiation therapy for high-grade glioma. J Clin Oncol 11:1316–1321.

Dische S. 1991. A review of hypoxic cell radiosensitization. Int J Radiat Oncol Biol Phys 20:147–152.

Djordjevic B, Szybalski W. 1960. Genetics of human cell lines. III. Incorporation of 5-bromo and 5-iododeoxyuridine into the deoxyribonucleic acid of human cells and its effect on radiation sensitivity. J Exp Med 112:509–531.

Drake J, Hoffman HJ, Kobayashi J, Hwang P, Becker LE. 1987. Surgical management of children with temporal lobe epilepsy and mass lesions. Neurosurgery 21:792–797.

Duffner PK, Cohen ME, Heffner RR, Freeman AI. 1981. Primitive neuroectodermal tumors of childhood. An approach to therapy. J Neurosurg 55:376–381.

Duffner PK, Horowitz ME, Krischer JP, et al. 1993. Postoperative chemotherapy and delayed radiation in children less than three years of age with malignant brain tumors. N Engl J Med 328:1725–1731.

Duong DH, Rostomily RC, Haynor DR, Keles GE, Berger MS. 1992. Measurement of tumor resection volumes from computerized images. Technical note. J Neurosurg 77:151–154.

Eddy DM. 1990. Designing a practice policy. Standards, guidelines, and options. JAMA 263:3077–3084.

Eisenberg HM, McComb JG, Lorenzo AV. 1974. Cerebrospinal fluid overproduction and hydrocephalus associated with choroid plexus papilloma. J Neurosurg 40:381–385.

Ellenberg L, McComb JG, Siegel SE, Stowe S. 1987. Factors affecting intellectual outcome in pediatric brain tumor patients. Neurosurgery 21:638–644.

Ellenbogen RG, Winston KR, Kupsky WJ. 1989. Tumors of the choroid plexus in children. Neurosurgery 25:327–335.

Elliott TE, Buckner JC, Cascino TL, Levitt R, O'Fallon JR, Scheithauer BW. 1991. Phase II study of ifosfamide with mesna in adult patients with recurrent diffuse astrocytoma. J Neurooncol 10:27–30.

Enzmann DR, Irvin KM, Marshall WH, Silverberg GD, Britt RH, Hanbery JW. 1984. Intraoperative sonography through a burr hole: guide for brain biopsy. AJNR Am J Neuroradiol 5:243–246.

EORTC Brain Tumour Cooperative Group. 1985. Effect of AZQ (1,4-cyclohexadiene-1,4-diacarbamic acid-2,5-bis(1-aziridinyl)-3,6-dioxodiethylester) in recurring supratentorial malignant brain gliomas—a phase II study. Eur J Cancer Clin Oncol 21:143–146.

Ettinger LJ, Ru N, Krailo M, Ruccione KS, Krivit W, Hammond GD. 1990. A phase II study of diaziquone in children with recurrent or progressive primary brain tumors: a report from the Childrens Cancer Study Group. J Neurooncol 9:69–76.

Eyre HJ, Crowley JJ, Townsend JJ, et al. 1993. A randomized trial of radiotherapy versus radiotherapy plus CCNU for incompletely resected low-grade gliomas: a Southwest Oncology Group study. J Neurosurg 78:909–914.

Fadul C, Wood J, Thaler H, Galicich J, Patterson RH, Posner JB. 1988. Morbidity and mortality of craniotomy for excision of supratentorial gliomas. Neurology 38:1374–1379.

Fazekas JT. 1977. Treatment of grades I and II brain astrocytomas. The role of radiotherapy. Int J Radiat Oncol Biol Phys 2:661–666.

Finlay JL. 1992b. High-dose chemotherapy followed by bone marrow "rescue" for recurrent brain tumors. In: Packer RJ, Bleyer WA, Pochedly C (eds), Pediatric Neuro-oncology: New Trends in Clinical Research. New York: Harwood Academic Publishers, pp 278–297.

Finlay JL, August C, Packer R, et al. 1990. High-dose multiagent chemotherapy followed by bone marrow "rescue" for malignant astrocytomas of childhood and adolescence. J Neurooncol 9:239–248.

Finlay JL, Boyett JM, Yates AJ, et al. 1995. Randomized phase III trial in childhood high-grade astrocytoma comparing vincristine, lomustine, and prednisone with the eight-drugs-in-1-day regimen. Childrens Cancer Group. J Clin Oncol 13: 112–123.

Finlay JL, Geyer JR, Turski PA, et al. 1994. Pre-irradiation chemotherapy in children with high-grade astrocytoma: tumor response to two cycles of the "8-drug-in-1-day" regimen. A Childrens Cancer Group study CCG-945. J Neurooncol 21:255–265.

Fitzek MM, Thornton AF, Rabinov JD, et al. 1999. Accelerated fractionation proton/photon irradiation to 90 cobalt gray equivalent for glioblastoma multiforme: results of a phase II prospective trial. J Neurosurg 91:251–260.

Florell RC, Macdonald DR, Irish WD, et al. 1992. Selection bias, survival, and brachytherapy for glioma. J Neurosurg 76:179–183.

Flowers A, Gleason MJ, Levin VA, et al. 1993. Combination chemotherapy with carboplatin, 5-fluorouracil (5FU) and procarbazine (PCB) for recurrent malignant gliomas. Proc Am Soc Clin Oncol 12:180.

Fokes EC, Earle KM. 1969. Ependymomas: clinical and pathological aspects. J Neurosurg 30:585–594.

Fowler JF. 1990. How worthwhile are short schedules in radiotherapy? A series of exploratory calculations. Radiother Oncol 18:165–181.

Franceschetti S, Binelli S, Casazza M, et al. 1990. Influence of surgery and antiepileptic drugs on seizures symptomatic of cerebral tumours. Acta Neurochir (Wien) 103:47–51.

Friedman HS, Petros WP, Friedman AH, et al. 1999. Irinotecan therapy in adults with recurrent or progressive malignant glioma. J Clin Oncol 17:1516–1525.

Fulling KH, Nelson JS. 1984. Cerebral astrocytic neoplasms in the adult: contribution of histologic examination to the assessment of prognosis. Semin Diagn Pathol 1:152–163.

Gaffney CC, Sloane JP, Bradley NJ, Bloom HJ. 1985. Primitive neuroectodermal tumors of the cerebrum. Pathology and treatment. J Neurooncol 3:23–33.

Gajjar A, Sanford RA, Heideman R, et al. 1997. Low-grade astrocytoma: a decade of experience at St. Jude Children's Research Hospital. J Clin Oncol 15:2792–2799.

Galanis E, Buckner JC, Burch PA, et al. 1998. Phase II trial of nitrogen mustard, vincristine, and procarbazine in patients with recurrent glioma: North Central Cancer Treatment Group results. J Clin Oncol 16:2953–2958.

Galloway PG, Roessmann U. 1986. Anaplastic astrocytoma mimicking metastatic carcinoma. Am J Surg Pathol 10:728–732.

Gannett DE, Wisbeck WM, Silbergeld DL, Berger MS. 1994. The role of postoperative irradiation in the treatment of oligodendroglioma. Int J Radiat Oncol Biol Phys 30:567–573.

Garcia DM, Fulling KH. 1985. Juvenile pilocytic astrocytoma of the cerebrum in adults. A distinctive neoplasm with favorable prognosis. J Neurosurg 63:382–386.

Garcia DM, Fulling KH, Marks JE. 1985. The value of radiation therapy in addition to surgery for astrocytomas of the adult cerebrum. Cancer 55:919–927.

Garrett PG, Simpson WJ. 1983. Ependymomas: results of radiation treatment. Int J Radiat Oncol Biol Phys 9:1121–1124.

Gaspar LE, Fisher BJ, Macdonald DR, et al. 1992. Supratentorial malignant glioma: patterns of recurrence and implications for external beam local treatment. Int J Radiat Oncol Biol Phys 24:55–57.

Gaynon PS, Ettinger LJ, Baum ES, Siegel SE, Krailo MD, Hammond GD. 1990. Carboplatin in childhood brain tumors. A Children's Cancer Study Group phase II trial. Cancer 66:2465–2469.

Geyer JR, Finlay JL, Boyett JM, et al. 1995. Survival of infants with malignant astrocytomas: a report from the Childrens Cancer Group. Cancer 75:1045–1050.

Geyer JR, Zeltzer PM, Boyett JM, et al. 1994. Survival of infants with primitive neuroectodermal tumors or malignant ependymomas of the CNS treated with eight drugs in 1 day: a report from the Childrens Cancer Group. J Clin Oncol 12:1607–1615.

Gherardi R, Baudrimont M, Nguyen JP, et al. 1986. Monstrocellular heavily lipidized malignant glioma. Acta Neuropathol (Berl) 69:28–32.

Giannini C, Scheithauer BW, Burger PC, et al. 1999. Pleomorphic xanthoastrocytoma: what do we really know about it? Cancer 85:2033–2045.

Glass J, Hochberg FH, Gruber ML, Louis DN, Smith D, Rattner B. 1992. The treatment of oligodendrogliomas and mixed oligodendroglioma-astrocytomas with PCV chemotherapy. J Neurosurg 76:741–745.

Goffman TE, Dachowski LJ, Bobo H, et al. 1992. Long-term follow-up on National Cancer Institute phase I/II study of glioblastoma multiforme treated with iododeoxyuridine and hyperfractionated irradiation. J Clin Oncol 10:264–268.

Goldring S, Gregorie EM. 1984. Surgical management of epilepsy using epidural recordings to localize the seizure focus. Review of 100 cases. J Neurosurg 60:457–466.

Goldring S, Rich KM, Picker S. 1986. Experience with gliomas in patients presenting with a chronic seizure disorder. Clin Neurosurg 33:15–42.

Goldwein JW, Corn BW, Finlay JL, Packer RJ, Rorke LB, Schut L. 1991. Is craniospinal irradiation required to cure children with malignant (anaplastic) intracranial ependymomas? Cancer 67:2766–2771.

Goldwein JW, Leahy JM, Packer RJ, et al. 1990. Intracranial ependymomas in children. Int J Radiat Oncol Biol Phys 19:1497–1502.

Goldwein JW, Lefkowitz I. 1991. Advances in ependymomas: radiation and chemotherapy. In: Packer RJ, Bleyer WA, Pochedly C (eds), Pediatric Neuro-oncology: New Trends in Clinical Research. New York: Harwood Academic Publishers, pp 242–253.

Golomb L, Gardner S, Sapp M, et al. 1999. Chemotherapy only for young children with newly-diagnosed malignant brain tumors: an update on the "Head Start" protocol. Med Pediatr Oncol 33:201.

Gonzalez D, Elvidge AR. 1962. On the occurrence of epilepsy caused by astrocytoma of the cerebral hemispheres. J Neurosurg 19:470–482.

Gottschalk J, Jautzke G, Paulus W, Goebel S, Cervos-Navarro J. 1993. The use of immunomorphology to differentiate choroid plexus tumors from metastatic carcinomas. Cancer 72:1343–1349.

Grant JW, Gallagher PJ. 1986. Pleomorphic xanthoastrocytoma: Immunohistochemical methods for differentiation from fibrous histiocytomas with similar morphology. Am J Sug Pathol 10:336–341.

Grant R, Liang BC, Page MA, Crane DL, Greenberg HS, Junck L. 1995. Age influences chemotherapy response in astrocytomas. Neurology 45:929–933.

Green SB, Shapiro WR, Burger PC, et al. 1994. A randomized trial of interstitial radiotherapy (RT) for newly diagnosed malignant glioma: Brain Tumor Cooperative Group (BTCG) trial 8701. Proc Am Soc Clin Oncol 13:174.

Griffin BR, Silbergeld DL, Berger MS, Wisbeck W, Gannett DE. 1992. Oligodendrogliomas: postoperative radiotherapy increases survival. Int J Radiat Oncol Biol Phys 24(suppl 1):142.

Grovas AC, Boyett JM, Lindsley K, Rosenblum M, Yates AJ, Finlay JL. 1999. Regimen related toxicity of myeloablative chemotherapy with BCNU, thiotepa and etoposide followed by autologous stem cell rescue for children. Med Pediatr Oncol 33:83–87.

Groves MD, Maor MH, Meyers C, et al. 1999. Kyritsis AP, Jaeckle KA, Yung WKA, Sawaya RE, Hess K, Bruner JM, Peterson P, Levin VA. A phase II trial of high-dose bromodeoxyuridine with accelerated fractionation radiotherapy followed by procarbazine, lomustine, and vincristine for glioblastoma multiforme. Int J Radiat Oncol Biol Phys. 45:127–135.

Guidelines and Outcomes Committee of the AANS. 1998. Practice parameters in adults with suspected or known supratentorial nonoptic pathway low-grade glioma. Neurosurg Focus 4, Article 10.

Guruangan S, Dunkel IJ, Goldman S, et al. 1998. Myeloablative chemotherapy with autologous bone marrow rescue in young children with recurrent malignant brain tumors. J Clin Oncol 16:2486–2493.

Guthrie BL, Laws ER. 1990. Supratentorial low-grade gliomas. Neurosurg Clin North Am 1:37–48.

Gutin PH, Leibel SA, Wara WM, et al. 1987. Recurrent malignant gliomas: survival following interstitial brachytherapy with high-activity iodine-125 sources. J Neurosurg 67:864–873.

Gutin PH, Prados MD, Phillips TL, et al. 1991. External irradiation followed by an interstitial high activity iodine-125 implant "boost" in the initial treatment of malignant gliomas: NCOG study 6G-82-2. Int J Radiat Oncol Biol Phys 21:601–606.

Gutin PH, Wilson CB, Kumar AR, et al. 1975. Phase II study of procarbazine, CCNU, and vincristine combination chemotherapy in the treatment of malignant brain tumors. Cancer 35:1398–1404.

Haddad SF, Moore SA, Menezes AH, VanGilder JC. 1992. Ganglioglioma: 13 years of experience. Neurosurgery 31:171–178.

Haddad SF, Moore SA, Schelper RL, Goeken J. 1991. Smooth muscle cells can comprise the sarcomatous component of gliosarcomas. J Neuropathol Exp Neurol 50:291A.

Haglund MM, Berger MS, Kunkel DD, Franck JE, Ghatan S, Ojemann GA. 1992. Changes in gamma-aminobutyric acid and somatostatin in epileptic cortex associated with low-grade gliomas. J Neurosurg 77:209–216.

Haglund MM, Berger MS, Shamseldin M, Lettich E, Ojemann GA. 1993. Cortical localization of temporal lobe language sites in patients with gliomas. Neurosurgery 34:567–576.

Halperin EC, Friedman HS, Schold SC, et al. 1993. Surgery, hyperfractionated craniospinal irradiation, and adjuvant chemotherapy in the management of supratentorial embryonal neuroepithelial neoplasms in children. Surg Neurol 40:278–283.

Hansen DA, Spence AM, Carski T, Berger MS. 1993. Indocyanine green (ICG) staining and demarcation of tumor margins in a rat glioma model. Surg Neurol 40:451–456.

Harsh GR, Levin VA, Gutin PH, Seager M, Silver P, Wilson CB. 1987. Reoperation for recurrent glioblastoma and anaplastic astrocytoma. Neurosurgery 21:615–621.

Hart MN, Earle KM. 1973. Primitive neuroectodermal tumors of the brain in children. Cancer 32:890–897.

Hassoun J, Soylemezoglu F, Gambarelli D, Figarella-Branger D, von Ammon K, Kleihues P. 1993. Central neurocytoma: a synopsis of clinical and histological features. Brain Pathol 3:297–306.

Hawkins JC 3d. 1980. Treatment of choroid plexus papillomas in children: a brief analysis of twenty years' experience. Neurosurgery 6:380–384.

Healey EA, Barnes PD, Kupsky WJ, et al. 1991. The prognostic significance of postoperative residual tumor in ependymoma. Neurosurgery 28:666–672.

Heegard S, Sommer HM, Broholm H, Broendstrup O. 1995. Proliferating cell nuclear antigen and Ki-67 immunohistochemistry of oligodendrogliomas with special reference to prognosis. Cancer 76:1809–1813.

Heilbrun MP, Roberts TS, Apuzzo ML, Wells TH, Sabshin JK. 1983. Preliminary experience with Brown-Roberts-Wells (BRW) computerized tomography stereotaxic guidance system. J Neurosurg 59:217–222.

Herbert J, Cavallaro T, Dwork AJ. 1990. A marker for primary choroid plexus neoplasms. Am J Pathol 136:1317–1325.

Herpers MJ, Budka H. 1984. Glial fibrillary acidic protein (GFAP) in oligodendroglial tumors: gliofibrillary oligodendroglioma and transitional oligoastrocytoma as subtypes of oligodendroglioma. Acta Neuropathol (Berl) 64:265–272.

Hess KR, Wong ET, Jaeckle KA, et al. 1999. Response and progression in recurrent malignant glioma. Neuro-Oncology 1:282–288.

Hessler RB, Lopes MB, Frankfurter A, Reidy J, VandenBerg SR. 1992. Cytoskeletal immunohistochemistry of central neurocytomas. Am J Surg Pathol 16:1031–1038.

Hirsch JF, Sainte Rose C, Pierre-Khan A, Pfister A, Hoppe-Hirsch E. 1989. Benign astrocytic and oligodendrocytic tumors of the cerebral hemispheres in children. J Neurosurg 70:568–572.

Hochberg FH, Pruitt A. 1980. Assumptions in the radiotherapy of glioblastoma. Neurology 30:907–911.

Horn B, Heideman R, Geyer R, et al. 1999. A multi-institutional retrospective study of intracranial ependymoma in children: identification of risk factors. J Pediatr Hematol Oncol 21:203–211.

Horten BC, Rubinstein LJ. 1976. Primary cerebral neuroblastoma. A clinicopathological study of 35 cases. Brain 99:735–756.

Hoshino T, Ahn D, Prados MD, Lamborn K, Wilson CB. 1993. Prognostic significance of the proliferative potential of intracranial gliomas measured by bromodeoxyuridine labeling. Int J Cancer 53:550–555.

Hoshino T, Rodriguez LA, Cho KG, et al. 1988. Prognostic implications of the proliferative potential of low-grade astrocytomas. J Neurosurg 69:839–842.

Humphrey GB, Dehner LP, Kaplan RJ, et al. 1981. Overview on the management of primitive neuroectodermal tumors. In: Humphrey GB, Dehner LP (eds), Pediatric Oncology I. The Hague: M Nijhoff, p 289.

Ito S, Chandler KL, Prados MD, Lamborn K, Wynne J, Malec MK, Wilson CB, Davis RL, Hoshino T. 1994. Proliferative potential and prognostic evaluation of low-grade astrocytomas. J Neurooncol 19:1–9.

Jakacki RI, Zeltzer PM, Boyett JM, et al. 1995. Survival and prognostic factors following radiation and/or chemotherapy for primitive neuroectodermal tumors of the pineal region in infants and children: a report of the Childrens Cancer Group. J Clin Oncol 13:1377–1383.

Jaros E, Perry RH, Adam L, et al. 1992. Prognostic implications of p53 protein, epidermal growth factor receptor, and Ki-67 labeling in brain tumours. Br J Cancer 66:373–385.

Jenkin D. 1981. Primitive neuroectodermal tumor. In: Humphrey GB, Dehner LP (eds), Pediatric Oncology I. The Hague: M Nijhoff, p 243.

Jeremic B, Grujicic D, Jevremovic S, et al. 1992. Carboplatin and etoposide chemotherapy regimen for recurrent malignant glioma: a phase II study. J Clin Oncol 10:1074–1077.

Kaba SE, Kyritsis AP, Conrad C, et al. 1997. The treatment of recurrent cerebral gliomas with all-*trans*-retinoic acid (tretinoin). J Neurooncol 34:145–151.

Kalyan-Raman UP, Olivero WC. 1987. Ganglioglioma: a correlative clinicopathological and radiological study of ten surgically treated cases with follow-up. Neurosurgery 20:428–433.

Kaplan RS. 1993. Supratentorial malignant gliomas: risk patterns and therapy. J Natl Cancer Inst 85:690–691.

Karim AB, Cornu P, Bleehan N, et al. 1998. Immediate postoperative radiotherapy in low grade glioma improves progression free survival but not overall survival: preliminary results of an EORTC/MRC randomized phase III trial. Proc Am Soc Clin Oncol 17:400A.

Karim AB, Maat B, Hatlevoll R, et al. 1996. A randomized trial on dose–response in radiation therapy of low-grade cerebral glioma: European Organization for Research and Treatment of Cancer (EORTC) Study 22844. Int J Radiat Oncol Biol Phys 36:549–556.

Karlsson UL, Leibel SA, Wallner K, et al. 1992. Brain. In: Perez CA, Brady LW (eds), Principles and Practice of Radiation Oncology, 2nd ed. Philadelphia: JB Lippincott, p 515.

Keim H, Potthoff PC, Schmidt K, Schiebusch M, Neiss A, Trott KR. 1987. Survival and quality of life after continuous accelerated radiotherapy of glioblastomas. Radiother Oncol 9:21–26.

Keles GE, Anderson B, Berger MS. 1999. The effect of extent of resection on time to tumor progression and survival in patients with glioblastoma multiforme of the cerebral hemisphere. Surg Neurol 52:371–379.

Kelly PJ. 1988. Volumetric stereotactic surgical resection of intra-axial brain mass lesions. Mayo Clin Proc 63:1186–1198.

Kelly PJ. 1990. Image-directed tumor resection. In: Rosenblum ML (ed), Neurosurgery Clinics of North America. The Role of Surgery in Brain Tumor Management, vol 1. Philadelphia: WB Saunders, pp 81–95.

Kelly PJ. 1993. Computed tomography and histologic limits in glial neoplasms: tumor types and selection for volumetric resection. Surg Neurol 39:458–465.

Kelly PJ, Alker GJ, Goerss S. 1982. Computer-assisted stereotactic microsurgery for the treatment of intracranial neoplasms. Neurosurgery 10:324–331.

Kelly PJ, Daumas-Duport C, Kispert DB, Kall BA, Scheithauer BW, Illig JJ. 1987. Imaging-based stereotaxic serial biopsies in untreated intracranial glial neoplasms. J Neurosurg 66:865–874.

Kelly PJ, Kall B, Goerss S, Alker GJ. 1983. Precision resection of intra-axial CNS lesions by CT-based stereotactic craniotomy and computer monitored CO_2 laser. Acta Neurochir (Wein) 68:1–9.

Kelly PJ, Kall BA, Goerss S, Earnest F. 1986. Computer-assisted stereotaxic laser resection of intra-axial brain neoplasms. J Neurosurg 64:427–439.

Kepes JJ. 1993. Pleomorphic xanthoastrocytoma. The birth of a diagnosis and concept. Brain Pathol 3:269–274.

Kepes JJ, Rubinstein LJ, Ansbacher L, Schreiber DJ. 1989. Histopathological features of recurrent pleomorphic xanthoastrocytomas: further corroboration of the glial nature of this neoplasm. A study of 3 cases. Acta Neuropathol (Berl) 78:585–593.

Kepes JJ, Rubinstein LJ, Chiang H. 1984. The role of astrocytes in the formation of cartilage in gliomas. An immunohistochemical study of four cases. Am J Pathol 117:471–483.

Kepes JJ, Rubinstein LJ, Eng LF. 1979. Pleomorphic xanthoastrocytoma: a distinctive meningocerebral glioma of young subjects with relatively favorable prognosis. A study of 12 cases. Cancer 44:1839–1852.

Kernohan JW, Mabon RF, Svien HJ, Adson AW. 1949. A simplified classification of the gliomas. Proc Staff Meet Mayo Clin 24:71–75.

Key G, Becker MH, Baron B, et al. 1993. New Ki-67–equivalent murine monoclonal antibodies (MIB 1–3) generated against bacterially expressed parts of the Ki-67 cDNA containing three 62 base pair repetitive elements encoding for the Ki-67 epitope. Lab Invest 68:629–636.

Kiebert GM, Curran D, Aaronson NK, et al. 1998. Quality of life after radiation therapy of cerebral low-grade gliomas of the adult: results of a randomised phase III trial on dose response (EORTC trial 22844). EORTC Radiotherapy Co-operative Group. Eur J Cancer 34:1902–1909.

Kim DG, Chi JG, Park SH, et al. 1992. Intraventricular neurocytoma: clinicopathological analysis of seven cases. J Neurosurg 76:759–765.

Kim YH, Fayos JV. 1977. Intracranial ependymomas. Radiology 124:805–808.

Kim TS, Halliday AL, Hedley-Whyte ET, Convery K. 1991. Correlates of survival and the Daumas-Duport grading system for astrocytomas. J Neurosurg 74:27–37.

Kleihues P, Cavenee WK. 2000. Pathology and Genetics of Tumors of the Nervous System. Lyon: IARC Press.

Kleihues P, Ohgaki H. 1997. Genetics of glioma progression and the definition of primary and secondary glioblastoma. Brain Pathol 7:1131–1136.

Kleihues P, Ohgaki H. 1999. Primary and secondary glioblastoma: from concept to clinical diagnosis. Neuro-Oncology 1:44–51.

Knapp J, Francini D, Van Eys J, Cangir A. 1981. Primitive neuroectodermal tumors of brain in childhood: literature review and the M. D. Anderson experience. In: Humphrey GB, Dehner LP (eds), Pediatric Oncology I. The Hague: M Nijhoff, p 215.

Koeller KK, Dillon WP. 1992. Dysembryoplastic neuroepithelial tumors: MR appearance. AJNR Am J Neuroradiol 13:1319–1325.

Kornblith PK, Welch WC, Bradley MK. 1993. The future of therapy for glioblastoma. Surg Neurol 39:538–543.

Kosnik EJ, Boesel CP, Bay J, Sayers MP. 1978. Primitive neuroectodermal tumors of the central nervous system in children. J Neurosurg 48:741–746.

Kovalic JJ, Flaris N, Grigsby PW, Pirkowski M, Simpson JR, Roth KA. 1993. Intracranial ependymoma long term outcome, patterns of failure. J Neurooncol 15:125–131.

Kramer S. 1969. Tumor extent as a determining factor in radiotherapy of glioblastomas. Acta Radiol Ther Phys Biol 8:111–117.

Kricheff II, Becker M, Schneck SA, Taveras JM. 1964. Intracranial ependymomas. A study of survival in 65 cases treated by surgery and irradiation. Am J Roentgenol 91:167–175.

Kristiansen K, Hagen S, Kollevold T, et al. 1981. Combined modality therapy of operated astrocytomas grade III and IV. Confirmation of the value of postoperative irradiation and lack of potentiation of bleomycin on survival time: a prospective multicenter trial of the Scandinavian Glioblastoma Study Group. Cancer 47:649–652.

Kros JM, de Jong AA, van der Kwast TH. 1992. Ultrastructural characterization of transitional cells in oligodendrogliomas. J Neuropathol Exp Neurol 51:186–193.

Kros JM, Hop WC, Godschalk JJ, Krishnadath KK. 1996. Prognostic value of the proliferation-related antigen Ki-67 in oligodendrogliomas. Cancer 78:1107–1113.

Kros JM, Pieterman H, van Eden CG, Avezaat CJ. 1994. Oligodendroglioma: the Rotterdam-Dijkzigt experience. Neurosurgery 34:959–966.

Kros JM, Troost D, Van Eden CG, van der Werf AJ, Uylings HB. 1988. Oligodendroglioma. A comparison of two grading systems. Cancer 61:2251–2259.

Kros JM, Van Eden CG, Stefanko SZ, Waayer-Van Batenburg M, van der Kwast TH. 1990. Prognostic implications of glial fibrillary acidic protein containing cell types in oligodendrogliomas. Cancer 66:1204–1212.

Krouwer HG, Davis RL, Silver P, Prados M. 1991. Gemistocytic astrocytomas: a reappraisal. J Neurosurg 74:399–406.

Kun LE. 1992. Brain tumors in children. In: Perez CA, Brady LW (eds), Principles and Practice of Radiation Oncology, 2nd ed. Philadelphia: JB Lippincott, p 417.

Kunschner LJ, Yung WK, Levin VA, Jaeckle KA. 1999. Carboplatin and 13-*cis*-retinoic acid for recurrent glioblastoma multiforme. Neuro-Oncology 1:320.

Kyritsis AP, Yung WK, Bruner J, Gleason MJ, Levin VA. 1993. The treatment of anaplastic oligodendrogliomas and mixed gliomas. Neurosurgery 32:365–371.

Kyritsis AP, Yung WK, Jaeckle KA, et al. 1996. Combination of 6-thioguanine, procarbazine, lomustine, and hydroxyurea for patients with recurrent malignant gliomas. Neurosurgery 39:921–926.

Kyritsis AP, Yung WK, Leeds NE, Bruner J, Gleason MJ, Levin VA. 1992. Multifocal cerebral gliomas associated with secondary malignancies [letter]. Lancet 339:1229–1230.

Lamborn KR, Prados MD, Kaplan SB, Davis RL. 1999. Final report on the University of California San Francisco experience with bromodeoxyuridine labeling index as a prognostic factor for the survival of glioma patients. Cancer 85:925–935.

Laperriere NJ, Leung PM, McKenzie S, et al. 1998. Randomized study of brachytherapy in the initial management of patients with malignant astrocytoma. Int J Radiat Oncol Biol Phys 41:1005–1011.

Laramore GE, Diener-West M, Griffin TW, et al. 1988. Randomized neutron dose searching study for malignant gliomas of the brain: results of an RTOG study. Radiation Therapy Oncology Group. Int J Radiat Oncol Biol Phys 14:1093–1102.

Larson DA, Flickinger JC, Loeffler JS. 1993. The radiobiology of radiosurgery. Int J Radiat Oncol Biol Phys 25:557–561.

Larson DA, Gutin PH, Leibel SA, Phillips TL, Sneed PK, Wara WM. 1990. Stereotaxic irradiation of brain tumors. Cancer 65:792–799.

Larson DA, Gutin PH, McDermott M, et al. 1996. Gamma knife for glioma: selection factors and survival. Int J Radiat Oncol Biol Phys 36:1045–1053.

Larson DA, Wasserman TH, Dryzmala DE, Simpson JR. 1992. Stereotactic External-beam irradiation. In: Perez CA, Brady LW (eds), Principles and Practice of Radiation Oncology, 2d ed. Philadelphia: JB Lippincott, p 530.

Laws ER, Taylor WF, Bergstralh EJ, Okazaki H, Clifton MB. 1985. The neurosurgical management of low-grade astrocytoma. Clin Neurosurg 33:575–588.

Laws ER, Taylor WF, Clifton MB, Okazaki H. 1984. Neurosurgical management of low-grade astrocytoma of the cerebral hemispheres. J Neurosurg 61:665–673.

Lee SW, Fraass BA, Marsh LH, et al. 1999. Patterns of failure following high-dose 3-D conformal radiotherapy for high-grade astrocytomas: a quantitative dosimetric study. Int J Radiat Oncol Biol Phys 43:79–88.

Leibel SA. 1990. Teleradiotherapy: methods and expectations. In Apuzzo MLJ (ed), Malignant Cerebral Glioma. Park Ridge, IL: American Association of Neurological Surgeons, p 159.

Leibel SA, Gutin, PH, Davis RL. 1991a. Factors affecting radiation injury after interstitial brachytherapy for brain tumors. In: Gutin PH, Leibel SA, Sheline GE (eds), Radiation Injury to the Nervous System. New York: Raven Press, p 257.

Leibel SA, Gutin PH, Sneed PK, et al. 1989a. Interstitial irradiation for the treatment of primary and metastatic brain tumors. Principles Practice Oncol Updates 3:1–11.

Leibel SA, Gutin PH, Wara WM, et al. 1989b. Survival and quality of life after interstitial implantation of removable high-activity iodine-125 sources for the treatment of patients with recurrent malignant gliomas. Int J Radiat Oncol Biol Phys 17:1129–1139.

Leibel SA, Scott CB, Loeffler JS. 1994. Contemporary approaches to the treatment of malignant gliomas with radiation therapy. Semin Oncol 21:198–219.

Leibel SA, Scott CB, Pajak TF. 1991b. The management of malignant gliomas with radiation therapy: therapeutic results and research strategies. Semin Radiat Oncol 1:32–49.

Leibel SA, Sheline GE. 1987. Radiation therapy for neoplasms of the brain. J Neurosurg 66:1–22.

Leibel SA, Sheline GE. 1990. Radiotherapy in the treatment of cerebral astrocytomas. In: Thomas DGT (ed), Neuro-oncology: Primary Malignant Brain Tumours. Baltimore: Johns Hopkins University Press, p 193.

Leibel SA, Sheline GE. 1991. Tolerance of the brain and spinal cord to conventional irradiation. In: Gutin PH, Leibel SA, Sheline GE (eds), Radiation Injury to the Nervous System. New York: Raven Press, p 239.

Leibel SA, Sheline GE, Wara WM, Boldrey EB, Nielsen SL. 1975. The role of radiation therapy in the treatment of astrocytomas. Cancer 35:1551–1557.

Leighton C, Fisher B, Bauman G, et al. 1997. Supratentorial low-grade glioma in adults: an analysis of prognostic factors and timing of radiation. J Clin Oncol 15:1294–1301.

LeRoux PD, Berger MS, Ojemann GA, Wang K, Mack LA. 1989. Correlation of intraoperative ultrasound tumor volumes and margins with preoperative computed tomography scans. An intraoperative method to enhance tumor resection. J Neurosurg 71:691–698.

LeRoux PD, Winter TC, Berger MS, Mack LA, Wang K, Elliott P. 1994. A comparison between preoperative magnetic resonance scans and intraoperative ultrasound tumor volumes and margins. J Clin Ultrasound 22:29–36.

Levin VA. 1985. Chemotherapy of primary brain tumors. In: Vick NA, Bigner DD (eds), Neuro-Oncology, Neurologic Clinics of North America, 3d ed. Philadelphia: WB Saunders, p 855.

Levin VA, Prados MD, Yung WK, Gleason MJ, Ictech S, Malec M. 1992. Treatment of recurrent gliomas with eflornithine. J Natl Cancer Inst 84:1432–1437.

Levin VA, Chamberlain MC, Prados MD, et al. 1987. Phase I–II study of eflornithine and mitoguazone combined in the treatment of recurrent primary brain tumors. Cancer Treat Rep 71:459–464.

Levin VA, Edwards MS, Wright DC, et al. 1980a. Modified procarbazine, CCNU, and vincristine (PCV 3) combination chemotherapy in the treatment of malignant brain tumors. Cancer Treat Rep 64:237–244.

Levin VA, Hoffman WF, Heilbron DC, Norman D. 1980b. Prognostic significance of the pretreatment CT scan on time to progression for patients with malignant gliomas. J Neurosurg 52:642–647.

Levin VA, Lamborn K, Wara W, et al. 2000a. Phase II study of 6-thioguanine, procarbazine, dibromodulcitol, lomustine, and vincristine chemotherapy with radiotherapy for treating malignant gliomas in children. Neuro-Oncology 2:22–28.

Levin VA, Leibel SA, Gutin PH. 2001. Neoplasms of the central nervous system. In: DeVita VT Jr, Hellman S, Rosenberg SA (eds), Cancer: Principles and Practice of Oncology, 6th ed. Philadelphia: Lippincott-Raven, pp 2022–2082.

Levin VA, Phuphanich S, Liu HC, et al. 1986a. Phase II study of combined carmustine, 5-fluorouracil, hydroxyurea, and 6-mercaptopurine (BFHM) for the treatment of malignant gliomas. Cancer Treat Rep 70:1271–1274.

Levin VA, Prados MR, Wara WM, et al. 1995. Radiation therapy with bromodeoxyuridine chemotherapy followed by procarbazine, lomustine, and vincristine for the treatment of anaplastic gliomas. Int J Radiat Oncol Biol Phys 32:75–83.

Levin VA, Resser K, McGrath L, Vestnys P, Nutik S, Wilson CB. 1984. PCNU treatment for recurrent malignant gliomas. Cancer Treat Rep 68: 969–973.

Levin VA, Silver P, Hannigan J, et al. 1990. Superiority of post-radiotherapy adjuvant chemotherapy with CCNU, procarbazine, and vincristine (PCV) over BCNU for anaplastic gliomas: NCOG 6G61 final report. Int J Radiat Oncol Biol Phys 18:321–324.

Levin VA, Thall PF, Maor MH, et al. 1995. Phase II study of accelerated fractionation radiation therapy with carboplatin followed by PCV chemotherapy for the treatment of glioblastoma multiforme. Int J Radiat Oncol Biol Phys 33:357–364.

Levin VA, Uhm JH, Jaeckle KA, et al. 2000b. Phase III randomized study of post-radiotherapy chemotherapy with alpha-difluoromethylornithine-procarbazine, N-(2-chloroethyl)-N′-cyclohexyl-N-nitrosurea, vincristine (DFMO-PCV) versus PCV for glioblastoma multiforme. Clin Cancer Res 6:3878–3884.

Levin VA, Wara WM, Davis RL, et al. 1986b. Northern California Oncology Group protocol 6G91: response to treatment with radiation therapy and seven-drug chemotherapy in patients with glioblastoma multiforme. Cancer Treat Rep 70:739–744.

Levy LF, Elvidge AR. 1956. Astrocytoma of the brain and spinal cord—a review of 176 cases, 1940–1949. J Neurosurg 13:413–443.

Lewis P. 1967. Carcinoma of the choroid plexus. Brain 90:177–186.

Liang BC, Thornton AF, Sandler HM, Greenberger HS. 1991. Malignant astrocytomas: focal tumor recurrence after focal external beam radiation therapy. J Neurosurg 75:559–563.

Lindegaard KF, Mork SJ, Eide GE, et al. 1987. Statistical analysis of clinicopathological features, radiotherapy, and survival in 170 cases of oligodendroglioma. J Neurosurg 67:224–230.

Loeffler JS, Alexander E 3d, Shea WM, et al. 1992. Radiosurgery as part of the initial management of patients with malignant gliomas. J Clin Oncol 10:1379–1385.

Loeffler JS, Alexander E 3d, Wen PY, et al. 1990. Results of stereotactic brachytherapy used in the initial management of patients with glioblastoma. J Natl Cancer Inst 82:1918–1921.

Longee DC, Friedman HS, Albright RE, et al. 1990. Treatment of patients with recurrent gliomas with cyclophosphamide and vincristine. J Neurosurg 72:583–588.

Louis DN, von Deimling A, Dickersin GR, Dooling EC, Seizinger BR. 1992. Desmoplastic cerebral astrocytomas of infancy: a histopathological, immunohistochemical, ultrastructural, and molecular genetic study. Hum Pathol 23:1402–1409.

Ludwig CL, Smith MT, Godfrey AD, Armbrustmacher VW. 1986. A clinicopathological study of 323 patients with oligodendrogliomas. Ann Neurol 19:15–21.

Lyons MK, Kelly PJ. 1992. Computer-assisted stereotactic biopsy and volumetric resection of thalamic pilocytic astrocytomas. Report of 23 cases. Stereotact Funct Neurosurg 59:100–104.

Macaulay RJ, Jay V, Hoffman HJ, Becker LE. 1993. Increased mitotic activity as a negative prognostic indicator in pleomorphic xanthoastrocytoma. Case report. J Neurosurg 79:761–768.

MacDonald DR. 1994. Low-grade gliomas, mixed gliomas, and oligodendrogliomas. Semin Oncol 21:236–248.

Maiuri F. 1988. Cysts with mural tumor nodules in the cerebral hemispheres. Neurosurgery 22:703–706.

Maiuri F, Stella L, Benvenuti D, Giamundo A, Pettinato G. 1990. Cerebral gliosarcomas: correlation of computed tomographic findings, surgical aspect, pathological features, and prognosis. Neurosurgery 26:261–267.

Mannoji H, Becker LE. 1988. Ependymal and choroid plexus tumors. Cytokeratin and GFAP expression. Cancer 61:1377–1385.

Marks JE, Adler SJ. 1982. A comparative study of ependymomas by site of origin. Int J Radiat Oncol Biol Phys 8:37–43.

Marsa GW, Goffinet DR, Rubinstein LJ, Bagshaw MA. 1975. Megavoltage irradiation in the treatment of gliomas of the brain and spinal cord. Cancer 36:1681–1689.

Mason WP, Grovas A, Halpern S, et al. 1998. Intensive chemotherapy and bone marrow rescue for young children with newly diagnosed malignant brain tumors. J Clin Oncol 16:210–221.

Massey V, Wallner KE. 1990. Patterns of second recurrence of malignant astrocytomas. Int J Radiat Oncol Biol Phys 18:395–398.

Matson DD, Crofton FDL. 1960. Papilloma of the choroid plexus in childhood. J Neurosurg 17:1002–1027.

Matsushima T, Inoue T, Takeshita I, Fukui M, Iwaki T, Kitamoto T. 1988. Choroid plexus papillomas: an immunohistochemical study with particular reference to the coexpression of prealbumin. Neurosurgery 23:384–389.

McComb R, Burger PC. 1983. Choroid plexus carcinoma. Report of a case with immunohistochemical and ultrastructural observations. Cancer 51:470–475.

McCormack BM, Miller DC, Budzilovich GN, Voorhees GJ, Ransohoff J. 1992. Treatment and survival of low-grade astrocytoma in adults—1977–1988. Neurosurgery 31:636–642.

McEvoy AW, Harding BN, Phipps KP, et al. 2000. Management of choroid plexus tumours in children: 20 years experience at a single neurosurgical centre. Pediatr Neurosurg 32:192–199.

McGirr SJ, Ebersold MJ, Scheithauer BW, Quast LM, Shaw EG. 1988. Choroid plexus papillomas: long-term follow-up results in a surgically treated series. J Neurosurg 69:843–849.

McLaughlin MP, Marcus RB, Buatti JM, et al. 1998. Ependymoma: results, prognostic factors and treatment recommendations. Int J Radiat Oncol Biol Phys 40:845–850.

McLaurin RL, Towbin RB. 1986. Tuberous sclerosis: diagnostic and surgical considerations. Pediatr Neurosci 12:43–48.

Medbery CA 3d, Straus KL, Steinberg SM, Cotelingam JD, Fisher WS. 1988. Low-grade astrocytomas: treatment results and prognostic variables. Int J Radiat Oncol Biol Phys 15:837–841.

Mehta MP, Masciopinto J, et al. 1994. Stereotactic radiosurgery for glioblastoma multiforme: report of a prospective study evaluating prognostic factors and analyzing long-term survival advantage. Int J Radiat Oncol Biol Phys 30:541–549.

Meis JM, Martz KL, Nelson JS. 1991. Mixed glioblastoma multiforme and sarcoma. A clinicopathologic study of 26 Radiation Therapy Oncology Group cases. Cancer 67:2342–2349.

Merchant TE, Haida T, Wang MH, Finlay JL, Leibel SA. 1997. Anaplastic ependymoma: treatment of pediatric patients with or without craniospinal radiation therapy. J Neurosurg 86:943–949.

Mercuri S, Russo A, Palma L. 1981. Hemispheric supratentorial astrocytomas in children. Long-term results in 29 cases. J Neurosurg 55:170–173.

Miettinen M, Clark R, Virtanen I. 1986. Intermediate filament proteins in choroid plexus and ependyma and their tumors. Am J Pathol 123:231–240.

Miller DC, Lang FF, Epstein FJ. 1993. Central nervous system gangliogliomas. Part 1: pathology. J Neurosurg 79:859–866.

Miller LL, Ostrow PT, Chau R. 1991. Characterization of gliosarcomas by image analysis of superimposed serial sections. J Neuropathol Exp Neurol 50:365A.

Miser J, Krailo M, Smithson W Belasco J, Ortega J, Hammond GD. 1989. Treatment of children with recurrent brain tumors with ifosphamide, etoposide and mesna. Results of a phase II Childrens Cancer Study Group trial. Proc Am Soc Clin Oncol 8:A328.

Mitchell JB, Kinsella TJ, Russo A, et al. 1983. Radiosensitization of hematopoietic precursor cells (CFUc) in glioblastoma patients receiving intermittent intravenous infusions of bromodeoxyuridine (BUdR). Int J Radiat Oncol Biol Phys 9:457–463.

Montine TJ, Vandersteenhoven JJ, Aguzzi A, et al. 1994. Prognostic significance of Ki-67 proliferation index in supratentorial fibrillary astrocytic neoplasms. Neurosurgery 34:674–678.

Moore GE. 1947. Fluorescein as an agent in the differentiation of normal and malignant tissues. Science 106:130–131.

Morantz RA. 1987. Radiation therapy in the treatment of cerebral astrocytoma. Neurosurgery 20:975–982.

Morantz RA, Feigin R, Ransohoff J 3d. 1976. Clinical and pathological study of 24 cases of gliosarcoma. J Neurosurg 45:398–408.

Mork SJ, Halvorsen TB, Lindegaard KF, Eide GE. 1986. Oligodendroglioma. Histologic evaluation and prognosis. J Neuropathol Exp Neurol 45:65–78.

Mork SJ, Lindegaard KF, Halvorsen TB, et al. 1985. Oligodendroglioma: incidence and biological behavior in a defined population. J Neurosurg 63:881–889.

Mork SJ, Loken AC. 1977. Ependymoma: a follow-up study of 101 cases. Cancer 40:907–915.

Mornex F, Nayel H, Taillandier L. 1993. Radiation therapy for malignant astrocytomas in adults. Radiother Oncol 27:181–192.

Morota N, Sakamoto K, Kobayashi N, Hashimoto K. 1990. Recurrent low-grade glioma in children with special reference to computed tomography findings and pathological changes. Childs Nerv Syst 6:155–160.

MRC Working Group Party. 2001. Randomized trial of procarbazine, lomustine, and vincristine in the adjuvant treatment of high-grade astrocytoma: a Medical Research Council trial. J Clin Oncol 19:509–518.

Muller W, Afra D, Schroder R. 1977. Supratentorial recurrences of gliomas. Morphological studies in relation to time intervals with astrocytomas. Acta Neurochir (Wien) 37:75–91.

Naguib MG, Chou SN, Mastri A. 1981. Radiation therapy of a choroid plexus papilloma of the cerebellopontine angle wtih bone involvenment. J Neurosurg 52:245–247.

Nakamura Y, Becker LE. 1983. Subependymal giant cell tumor: astrocytic or neuronal? Acta Neuropathol (Berl) 60:271–277.

Nelson DF, Diener-West M, Horton J, Chang CH, Schoenfeld D, Nelson JS. 1988. Combined modality approach to treatment of malignant gliomas—re-evaluation of RTOG 7401/ECOG 1374 with long-term follow-up. A joint study of the Radiation Therapy Oncology Group and the Eastern Cooperative Oncology Group. NCI Monogr 6:279–284.

Nelson DF, Urtasun RC, Saunders WM, Gutin PH, Sheline GE. 1986. Recent and current investigations of radiation therapy of malignant gliomas. Semin Oncol 13:46–55.

Nelson JS, Tsukada Y, Schoenfeld D, Fulling K, Lamarche J, Peress N. 1983. Necrosis as a prognostic criterion in malignant supratentorial, astrocytic gliomas. Cancer 52:550–554.

Nishio S, Takeshita I, Fujii K, Fukui M. 1989. Supratentorial astrocytic tumours of childhood: a clinicopathological study of 41 cases. Acta Neurochir (Wien) 101:3–8.

Nishio S, Takeshita I, Fujiwara S, Fukui M. 1993. Optico-hypothalamic glioma: an analysis of 16 cases. Childs Nerv Syst 9:334–338.

North CA, North RB, Epstein JA, Piantadosi S, Wharam MD. 1990. Low-grade cerebral astrocytomas. Survival and quality of life after radiation therapy. Cancer 66:6–14.

Obana WG, Cogen PH, Davis RL, Edwards MS. 1991. Metastatic juvenile pilocytic astrocytoma. Case report. J Neurosurg 75:972–975.

Ojemann G, Ojemann J, Lettich E, Berger M. 1989. Cortical language localization in left, dominant hemisphere. An electrical stimulation mapping investigation in 117 patients. J Neurosurg 17:316–326.

Olson JD, Riedel E, DeAngelis LM. 2000. Long-term outcome of low-grade oligodendroglioma and mixed glioma. Neurology 54:1442–1448.

Otsubo H, Hoffman HJ, Humphries RP, et al. 1992. Detection and management of gangliogliomas in children. Surg Neurol 38:371–378.

Ozek MM, Sav A, Pamir MN, Ozer AF, Ozek E, Erzen C. 1993. Pleomorphic xanthoastrocytoma associated with von Recklinghausen neurofibromatosis. Childs Nerv Syst 9:39–42.

Packer RJ, Lange B, Ater J, et al. 1993. Carboplatin and vincristine for progressive, recurrent and newly diagnosed low-grade gliomas of childhood. J Clin Oncol 11:850–856.

Packer RJ, Perilongo G, Johnson D, et al. 1992. Choroid plexus carcinoma of childhood. Cancer 69:580–585.

Packer RJ, Sutton L, Bilaniuk L, et al. 1988. Treatment of chiasmatic/hypothalamic gliomas of childhood with chemotherapy: an update. Ann Neurol 23:79–85.

Palma L, Celli P, Cantore G. 1993. Supratentorial ependymomas of the first two decades of life. Long-term follow-up of 20 cases (including two subependymomas). Neurosurgery 32:169–175.

Palma L, Guidetti B. 1985. Cystic pilocytic astrocytomas of the cerebral hemispheres. Surgical experience with 51 cases and long-term results. J Neurosurg 62:811–815.

Palma L, Russo A, Mercuri S. 1983. Cystic cerebral astrocytomas in infancy and childhood: long-term results. Childs Brain 10:79–91.

Papadopoulos DP, Giri S, Evans RG. 1990. Prognostic factors and management of intracranial ependymomas. Anticancer Res 10:689–692.

Parker JC, Mortara, RH, McCloskey JJ. 1975. Biological behavior of the primitive neuroectodermal tumors: significant supratentorial childhood gliomas. Surg Neurol 4:383–388.

Paulino AC, Melian E. 1999. Medulloblastoma and supratentorial primitive neuroectodermal tumors: an institutional experience. Cancer 86:142–148.

Paulus W, Janisch W. 1990. Clinicopathologic correlations in epithelial choroid plexus neoplasms: a study of 52 cases. Acta Neuropathol (Berl) 80:635–641.

Penfield W, Roberts L. 1959. Speech and Brain Mechanisms. Princeton, NJ: Princeton University Press, 286 pp.

Perilongo G, Massimino M, Sotti G, et al. 1997. Analyses of prognostic factors in a retrospective review of 92 children with ependymoma: Italian Pediatric Neuro-oncology Group. Med Pediatr Oncol 29:79–85.

Perria C, Carai M, Falzoi A, et al. 1988. Photodynamic therapy of malignant brain tumors: clinical results of, difficulties with, questions about, and future prospects for the neurosurgical applications. Neurosurgery 23:557–563.

Petronio J, Edwards MS, Prados M, et al. 1991. Management of chiasmal and hypothalamic gliomas of infancy and childhood with chemotherapy. J Neurosurg 74:701–708.

Philippon JH, Clemenceau SH, Fauchon FH, Foncin JF. 1993. Supratentorial low-grade astrocytomas in adults. Neurosurgery 32:554–559.

Phillips TL, Levin VA, Ahn DK, et al. 1991. Evaluation of bromodeoxyuridine in glioblastoma multiforme: a Northern Cancer Center Group Phase II study. Int J Radiat Oncol Biol Phys 21:709–714.

Phillips TL, Sheline GE, Boldrey E. 1964. Therapeutic considerations in tumors affecting the central nervous system: ependymomas. Radiology 83:98–105.

Piepmeier JM. 1987. Observations on the current treatment of low-grade astrocytic tumors of the cerebral hemisheres. J Neurosurg 67:177–181.

Pierre-Kahn A, Hirsch JF, Roux FX, Renier D, Sainte-Rose C. 1983. Intracranial ependymomas in childhood. Survival and functional results of 47 cases. Childs Brain 10:145–156.

Pilcher WH, Silbergeld DL, Berger MS, Ojemann GA. 1993. Intraoperative electrocorticography during tumor resection: impact on seizure outcome in patients with gangliogliomas. J Neurosurg 78:891–902.

Pinto-Lord MC, Abroms IF, Smith TW. 1986. Hyperdense cerebral lesion in childhood tuberous sclerosis: computed tomographic demonstration and neuropathologic analysis. Pediatr Neurol 2:245–248.

Pollack IF, Gerszten PC, Martinez AJ, et al. 1995. Intracranial ependymomas of childhood: long-term outcome and prognostic factors. Neurosurgery 37:655–667.

Pons M, Finlay JL, Walker RW, Puccetti D, Packer RJ, McElwain M. 1992. Chemotherapy with vincristine (VCR) and etoposide (VP-16) in children with low-grade astrocytoma. J Neurooncol 14:151–158.

Poon WS, Schomacker KT, Deutsch TF, Martuza RL. 1992. Laser-induced fluorescence: experimental intraoperative delineation of tumor resection margins. J Neurosurg 76: 679–686.

Prados MD, Gutin PH, Phillips TL, et al. 1992a. Highly anaplastic astrocytoma: a review of 357 patients treated between 1977 and 1989. Int J Radiat Oncol Biol Phys 23:3–8.

Prados MD, Gutin PH, Phillips TL, et al. 1992b. Interstitial brachytherapy for newly diagnosed patients with malignant gliomas: the UCSF experience. Int J Radiat Oncol Biol Phys 24:593–597.

Prados MD, Larson DA, Lamborn K, et al. 1998a. Radiation therapy and hydroxyurea followed by the combination of 6-thioguanine and BCNU for the treatment of primary malignant brain tumors. Int J Radiat Oncol Biol Phys 40:57–63.

Prados M, Rodriguez L, Chamberlain M, Silver P, Levin V. 1989. Treatment of recurrent gliomas with 1,3-bis(2-chloroethyl)-1-nitrosourea and alpha-difluoromethylornithine. Neurosurgery 24:806–809.

Prados MD, Scott C, Curran WJ, Nelson DF, Leibel S, Kramer S. 1999a. Procarbazine, lomustine, and vincristine (PCV) chemotherapy for anaplastic astrocytoma: a retrospective review of Radiation Therapy Oncology Group protocols comparing survival with carmustine or PCV adjuvant chemotherapy. J Clin Oncol 17:3389–3395.

Prados MD, Scott CB, Rotman M, et al. 1998b. Influence of bromodeoxyuridine radiosensitization on malignant glioma patient survival: a retrospective comparison of survival data from the Northern California Oncology Group (NCOG) and Radiation Therapy Oncology Group trials (RTOG) for glioblastoma multiforme and anaplastic astrocytoma. Int J Radiat Oncol Biol Phys 40:653–659.

Prados MD, Scott C, Sandler H, Buckner JC, et al. 1999b. A phase 3 randomized study of radiotherapy plus procarbazine, CCNU, and vincristine (PCV) with or without BUdR for the treatment of anaplastic astrocytoma: a preliminary report of RTOG 9404. Int J Radiat Oncol Biol Phys 45:1109–1115.

Prados MD, Wara WM, Sneed PK, et al. 2001. Phase III trial of accelerated hyperfractionation with or without difluromethylornithine (DFMO) versus standard fractionated radiotherapy with or without DFMO for newly diagnosed patients with glioblastoma multiforme. Int J Radiat Oncol Biol Phys 49:71–77.

Puccetti D, Finlay JL. 1992. Current treatment of intracranial ependymomas in children. Crit Rev Neurosurg 2:93–107.

Raimondi AJ, Gutierrez FA. 1975. Diagnosis and surgical treatment of choroid plexus papillomas. Childs Brain 1:81–115.

Rajan B, Pickuth D, Ashley S, et al. 1993. The management of histologically unverified presumed cerebral gliomas with radiotherapy. Int J Radiat Oncol Biol Phys 28:405–413.

Rasmussen TB. 1975. Surgery of epilepsy associated with brain tumors. Adv Neurol 8:227–239.

Rawlings CE III, Giangaspero F, Burger PC, et al. 1988. Ependymomas: a clinicopathologic study. Surg Neurol 29:271–281.

Read G. 1984. The treatment of ependymoma of the brain and spinal canal by radiotherapy: a report of 79 cases. Clin Radiol 35:163–166.

Recht LD, Lew R, Smith TW. 1992. Suspected low-grade glioma: is deferring treatment safe? Ann Neurol 31:431–436.

Reedy DP, Bay JW, Hahn JF. 1983. Role of radiation therapy in the treatment of cerebral oligodendroglioma: an analysis of 57 cases and a literature review. Neurosurgery 13:499–503.

Rekate HL, Erwood S, Brodkey JA, et al. 1985. Etiology of ventriculomegaly in choroid plexus papilloma. Pediatr Neurosci 12:196–201.

Reyes MG, Homsi MF, McDonald LW, Glick RP. 1991. Imprints, smears and frozen sections of brain tumors. Neurosurgery 29:575–579.

Ribaric I, Nagulic M, Djurovic B. 1991. Surgical treatment of epilepsy: our experiences with 34 children. Childs Nerv Syst 7:402–404.

Ringertz N. 1950. "Grading" of gliomas. Acta Pathol Microbiol Scand 27:51–64.

Ringertz N, Reymond A. 1949. Ependymomas and choroid plexus papillomas. J Neuropathol Exp Neurol 8:355–380.

Ritter AM, Sawaya R, Hess KR, Levin VA, Bruner JM. 1994. Prognostic significance of bromodeoxyuridine labeling in primary and recurrent glioblastoma multiforme. Neurosurgery 35:192–198.

Roberts DW, Strohbehn JW, Hatch JF, Murray W, Kettenberger H. 1986. A frameless stereotaxic integration of computerized tomographic imaging and the operating microscope. J Neurosurg 65:545–549.

Rodriguez LA, Edwards MS, Levin VA. 1990. Management of hypothalamic gliomas in children: an analysis of 33 cases. Neurosurgery 26:242–247.

Rodriguez LA, Prados M, Silver P, Levin VA. 1989. Re-evaluation of procarbazine for the treatment of recurrent malignant CNS tumors. Cancer, 64:2420–2423.

Rosenblum MK, Erlandson RA, Budzilovich GN. 1991. The lipid-rich epitheliod glioblastoma. Am J Surg Pathol 15:925–934.

Ross GW, Rubinstein LJ. 1989. Lack of histopathological correlation of malignant ependymomas with postoperative survival. J Neurosurg 70:31–36.

Ross IB, Robitaille Y, Villemure JG, Tampieri D. 1991. Diagnosis and management of gliomatosis cerebri: recent trends. Surg Neurol 36:431–440.

Rousseau P, Habrand JL, Sarrazin D, et al. 1993. Treatment of intracranial ependymomas of children: review of a 15-year experience. Int J Radiat Oncol Biol Phys 28:381–386.

Rubinstein LJ. 1972. Tumors of the Central Nervous System. Atlas of Tumor Pathology, Series 2, Fascicle 6. Washington, DC: Armed Forces Institute of Pathology, p 1.

Rubinstein LJ. 1985. Embryonal central neuroepithelial tumors and their differentiating potential. A cytogenetic view of a complex neuro-oncological problem. J Neurosurg 62:795–805.

Salazar OM, Castro-Vita H, VanHoutte P, Rubin P, Aygun C. 1983. Improved survival in cases of intracranial ependymoma after radiation therapy. Late report and recommendations. J Neurosurg 59:652–659.

Salazar OM, Rubin P. 1976. The spread of glioblastoma multiforme as a determining factor in the radiation treatment volume. Int J Radiat Oncol Biol Phys 1:627–637.

Salazar OM, Rubin P, McDonald JV, Feldstein ML. 1976. Patterns of failure in intracranial astrocytomas after irradiation: Analysis of dose and field factors. Am J Roentgenol 126:279–292.

Salcman M, Kaplan RS, Durken TB, Abdo H, Montgomery E. 1982. Effect of age and reoperation on survival in the combined modality treatment of malignant astrocytoma. Neurosurgery 10:454–463.

Sartorius CJ, Berger MS. 1988. Rapid termination of intraoperative stimulation-evoked seizures with application of cold Ringer's lactate to the cortex. Technical note. J Neurosurg 88:349–351.

Scharfen CO, Sneed PK, Wara WM, et al. 1992. High activity iodine-125 interstitial implant for gliomas. Int J Radiat Oncol Biol Phys 24:583–591.

Schiffer D, Chio A, Cravioto H, et al. 1991. Ependymoma: Internal correlations among pathologic signs: the anaplastic variant. Neurosurgery 29:206–210.

Schiffer D, Dutto A, Cavalla P, et al. 1997. Bosone I, Chio A, Villani R, Bellotti C (eds), Prognostic Factors in Oligodendroglioma. Can J Neurol Sci 24:313–319.

Schijman E, Monges J, Raimondi AJ, Tomita T. 1990. Choroid plexus papillomas of the III ventricle in childhood. The diagnosis and surgical management. Childs Nerv Syst 6:331–334.

Schild SE, Nisi K, Scheithauer BW, et al. 1998. The results of radiotherapy for ependymomas: the Mayo Clinic experience. Int J Radiat Oncol Biol Phys 42:953–958.

Schisano G, Tovi D, Nordenstam H. 1963. Spongioblastoma polare of the cerebral hemisphere. J Neurosurg 20:241–251.

Schold SC, Friedman HS, Bjornsson TD, Falletta JM. 1984. Treatment of patients with recurrent primary brain tumors with AZQ. Neurology 34:615–619.

Schold SC, Mahaley MS, Vick NA, et al. 1987. Phase II diaziquone-based chemotherapy trials in patients with anaplastic supratentorial astrocytic neoplasms. J Clin Oncol 5:464–471.

Schuller P, Schafer U, Micke O, Willich N. 1999. Radiotherapy for intracranial and spinal ependymomas. A retrospective analysis. Strahlenther Onkol 175:105–111.

Scott CB, Curran W, Yung WK, et al. 1998. Long term results of RTOG 9006: randomized trial of hyperfractionated radiotherapy (RT) to 72 Gy & carmustine vs standard RT & carmustine for malignant glioma patients with emphasis on anaplastic astrocytoma patients. Proc Am Soc Clin Oncol 17:40A.

Scott EW, Mickle JP. 1987. Pediatric diencephalic gliomas—a review of 18 cases. Pediatr Neurosci 13:225–232.

Sexauer CL, Khan A, Burger PC, et al. 1985. Cisplatin in recurrent pediatric brain tumors. A POG phase II study. A Pediatric Oncology Group Study. Cancer 56:1497–1501.

Shapiro WR. 1986. Therapy of adult malignant brain tumors: what have the clinical trials taught us? Semin Oncol 13:38–45.

Shaw E, Arusell R, Scheithauer B, et al. 1998. A prospective randomized trial of low- versus high-dose radiation therapy in adults with supratentorial low-grade glioma: initial report of a NCCG-RTOG-ECOG study. Proc Am Soc Clin Oncol 17:401A.

Shaw EG, Daumas-Duport C, Scheithauer BW, et al. 1989. Radiation therapy in the management of low-grade supratentorial astrocytomas. J Neurosurg 70:853–861.

Shaw EG, Evans RG, Scheithauer BW, Istrup DM, Earle JD. 1987. Postoperative radiotherapy of intracranial ependymoma in pediatric and adult patients. Int J Radiat Oncol Biol Phys 13:1457–1462.

Shaw EG, Scheithauer BW, O'Fallon JR. 1991. Management of supratentorial low-grade gliomas. Oncology (Huntingt) 7:94–111.

Shaw EG, Scheithauer BW, O'Fallon JR. 1997. Supratentorial gliomas: a comparative study by grade and histologic type. J Neurooncol 31:273–278.

Shaw EG, Scheithauer BW, O'Fallon JR, Davis DH. 1994. Mixed oligoastrocytomas: a survival and prognostic factor analysis. Neurosurgery 34:577–582.

Shaw EG, Scheithauer BW, O'Fallon JR Tazelaar HD, Davis DH. 1992. Oligodendrogliomas. The Mayo Clinic experience. J Neurosurg 76:428–434.

Sheline GE. 1983. Radiotherapy of adult primary cerebral neoplasms. In: Walker MD (ed), Oncology of the Nervous System. Boston: M Nijhoff, p 223.

Shenouda G, Souhami J, Freeman C, Hazel J, Lehnert S, Joseph L. 1991. Accelerated fractionation for high-grade cerebral astrocytomas. Preliminary treatment results. Cancer 67:2247–2252.

Shepherd CW, Scheithauer BW, Gomez MR, Altermatt HJ, Katzmann JA. 1991. Subependymal giant cell astrocytoma: a clincial, pathological, and flow cytometric study. Neurosurgery 28:864–868.

Shibamoto Y, Kitakabu Y, Takahashi M, et al. 1993. Supratentorial low-grade astrocytoma. Correlation of computed tomography findings with effect of radiotherapy and prognostic variables. Cancer 72:190–195.

Shibuya M, Ito S, Miwa T, Davis RL, Wilson CB, Hoshino T. 1993. Proliferative potential of brain tumors. Analyses with Ki-67 and anti-DNA polymerase alpha monoclonal antibodies, bromodeoxyuridine labeling, and nuclear organizer region counts. Cancer 71:199–206.

Shimizu KT, Tran LM, Mark RJ, Selch MT. 1993. Management of oligodendrogliomas. Radiology 186:569–572.

Shrieve DC, Alexander E 3d, Black PM, et al. 1999. Treatment of patients with primary glioblastoma multiforme with standard postoperative radiotherapy and radiosurgical boost: prognostic factors and long-term outcome. J Neurosurg 90:72–77.

Shrieve DC, Alexander E, Wen PY, et al. 1995. Comparison of stereotactic radiosurgery and brachytherapy in the treatment of recurrent glioblastoma multiforme. Neurosurgery 36:275–282.

Silver JM, Rawlings CE 3d, Rossitch E Zeidman SM, Friedman AH. 1991. Ganglioglioma: a clinical study with long-term follow-up. Surg Neurol 35:261–266.

Simpson WJ, Platts ME. 1976. Fractionation study in the treatment of glioblastoma multiforme. Int J Radiat Oncol Biol Phys 1:639–644.

Smith MT, Ludwig CL, Godfrey AD, Armbrustmacher VW. 1983. Grading of oligodendrogliomas. Cancer 52:2107–2114.

Smyth MD, Horn BN, Russo C, Berger MS. 2000. Intracranial ependymomas of childhood: current management strategies. Pediatr Neurosurg 33:138–150.

Sneed PK, Stauffer PR, McDermott MW, et al. 1998. Survival benefit of hyperthermia in a prospective randomized trial of brachytherapy boost +/− hyperthermia for glioblastoma multiforme. Int J Radiat Oncol Biol Phys 40:287–295.

Soffietti R, Chio A, Giordana MT, Vasario E, Schiffer D. 1989. Prognostic factors in well-differentiated cerebral astrocytomas in the adult. Neurosurgery 24:686–692.

Soffietti R, Ruda R, Bradac GB, Schiffer D. 1998. PCV chemotherapy for recurrent oligodendrogliomas and oligoastrocytomas. Neurosurgery 43:1066–1073.

Souweidane MM, Johnson JH, Lis E. 1999. Volumetric reduction of a choroid plexus carcinoma using preoperative chemotherapy. J Neurooncol 43:167–171.

Spagnoli MV, Grossman RI, Packer RJ, et al. 1987. Magnetic resonance imaging determination of gliomatosis cerebri. Neuroradiology 29:15–18.

Spallone A, Pastore FS, Guiffre R, Giudetti B. 1990. Choroid plexus papillomas in infancy and childhood. Childs Nerv Syst 6:71–74.

Spencer DD, Spencer SS, Mattson RH, Williamson PD. 1984. Intracerebral masses in patients with intractable partial epilepsy. Neurology 34:432–436.

Sposto R, Ertel IJ, Jenkin RD, et al. 1989. The effectiveness of chemotherapy for treatment of high-grade astrocytoma in children; results of a randomized trial. A report from the Childrens Cancer Study Group. J Neurooncol 7:165–177.

St Clair SK, Humphreys RP, Pillay PK, Hoffman HJ, Blaser SI, Becker LE. 1991. Current management of choroid plexus carcinoma in children. Pediatr Neurosurg 17:225–233.

Steinmeier R, Fahlbusch O, Ganslandt O, et al. 1998. Intraoperative magnetic resonance imaging with the magnetom open scanner: concepts, neurosurgical indications, and procedures: a preliminary report. Neurosurgery 43:739–748.

Stenning SP, Freedman LS, Bleehen NM. 1987. An overview of published results from randomized studies of nitrosoureas in primary high grade malignant glioma [letter to editor]. Br J Cancer 56:89–90.

Streffer J, Schabet M, Bamberg M, et al. 2000. A role for preirradiation PCV chemotherapy for oligodendroglial brain tumors. J Neurol 247:297–302.

Suit H, Urie M. 1992. Proton beams in radiation therapy. J Natl Cancer Inst 84:155–164.

Sun ZM, Genka S, Shitara N, Akanuma A, Takakura K. 1988. Factors possibly influencing the prognosis of oligodendroglioma. Neurosurgery 22:886–891.

Sutton LN. 1987. Current management of low-grade astrocytomas of childhood. Pediatr Neurosci 13:98–107.

Svien HJ, Mabon RF, Kernohan JW, Adson AW. 1949. Astrocytomas. Proc Staff Meet Mayo Clinic 24:54–63.

Taratuto AL, Monges J, Lylyk P, Leiguarda R. 1984. Superficial cerebral astrocytoma attached to dura. Report of six cases in infants. Cancer 54:2505–2512.

Taratuto AL, Sevlever G, Piccardo P. 1991. Clues and pitfalls in stereotactic biopsy of the central nervous system. Arch Pathol Lab Med 115:596–602.

Thornton AF, Hegarty TJ, Ten Haken RK, et al. 1991. Three-dimensional treatment planning of astrocytomas: a dosimetric study of cerebral irradiation. Int J Radiat Oncol Biol Phys 20:1309–1315.

Thornton AF, Sandler HM, Ten Haken RK, et al. 1992. The clinical utility of magnetic resonance imaging in 3-dimensional treatment planning of brain neoplasms. Int J Radiat Oncol Biol Phys 24:767–775.

Tomita T, McLone DG, Naidich TP. 1986. Mural tumors with cysts in the cerebral hemispheres of children. Neurosurgery 19:998–1005.

Tomita T, McLone DG, Yasue M. 1988. Cerebral primitive neuroectodermal tumors in childhood. J Neurooncol 6:233–243.

Tomita T, Naidich TP. 1987. Successful resection of choroid plexus papillomas diagnosed at birth: Report of two cases. Neurosurgery 20:774–779.

Tronnier VM, Wirtz CR, Knauth M, et al. 1997. Intraoperative diagnostic and interventional magnetic resonance imaging in neurosurgery. Neurosurgery 40:891–902.

Tsutsumi Y, Andoh Y, Sakaguchi J. 1989. A new ultrasound-guided brain biopsy technique through a burr hole. Technical note. Acta Neurochir (Wien) 96:72–75.

Undjian S, Marinov M. 1990. Intracranial ependymomas in children. Childs Nerv Syst 6:131–134.

van den Bent MJ, Kros JM, Heimans JJ, et al. 1998. Response rate and prognostic factors of recurrent oligodendroglioma treated with procarbazine, CCNU, and vincristine chemotherapy. Dutch Neuro-oncology Group. Neurology 51:1140–1145.

VandenBerg SR. 1993. Desmoplastic infantile ganglioglioma and desmoplastic cerebral astrocytoma of infancy. Brain Pathol 3:275–281.

VandenBerg SR, May EE, Rubinstein LJ, et al. 1987. Desmoplastic supratentorial neuroepithelial tumors of infancy with divergent differentiation potential ("desmoplastic infantile gangliogliomas"). Report on 11 cases of a distinctive embryonal tumor with favorable prognosis. J Neurosurg 66:58–71.

Vanuytsel LJ, Bessell EM, Ashley SE, Bloom HJ, Brada M. 1992. Intracranial ependymoma: long-term results of a policy of surgery and radiotherapy. Int J Radiat Oncol Biol Phys 23:313–319.

Vanuytsel L, Brada M. 1991. The role of prophylactic spinal irradiation in localized intracranial ependymoma. Int J Radiat Oncol Biol Phys 21:825–830.

van Veelen ML, Avezaat CJ, Kros JM, van Putten W, Vecht C. 1998. Supratentorial low grade astrocytoma: prognostic factors, dedifferentiation, and the isuue of early versus late surgery. J Neurol Neurosurg Psychiatry 64:581–587.

Varma RR, Crumrine PK, Bergman I, et al. 1983. Childhood oligdendrogliomas presenting with seizures and low-density lesions on computed tomography. Neurology 33:806–808.

Wald SL, Fogelson H, McLaurin RL. 1982. Cystic thalamic gliomas. Childs Brain 9:381–393.

Walker MD, Alexander E, Hunt WE, et al. 1978. Evaluation of BCNU and/or radiotherapy in the treatment of anaplastic gliomas. A cooperative clinical trial. J Neurosurg 49:333–343.

Walker MD, Green SB, Byar DP, et al. 1980. Randomized comparisons of radiotherapy and nitrosoureas for the treatment of malignant glioma after surgery. N Engl J Med 303:1323–1329.

Wallner KE. 1991. Radiation treatment planning for malignant astrocytomas. Semin Radiat Oncol 1:17–22.

Wallner KE, Galicich JH, Krol G, Arbit E, Malkin MG. 1989. Patterns of failure following treatment for glioblastoma multiforme and anaplastic astrocytoma. Int J Radiat Oncol Biol Phys 16:1405–1409.

Wallner KE, Gonzales MF, Edwards MS, Wara WM, Sheline GE. 1988a. Treatment results of juvenile pilocytic astrocytoma. J Neurosurg 69:171–176.

Wallner KE, Gonzales M, Sheline GE. 1988b. Treatment of oligodendrogliomas with or without postoperative irradiation. J Neurosurg 68:684–688.

Wallner KE, Wara WM, Sheline GE, Davis RL. 1986. Intracranial ependymomas: results of treatment with partial or whole brain irradiation without spinal irradiation. Int J Radiat Oncol Biol Phys 12:1937–1941.

Wara WM. 1985. Radiation therapy for brain tumors. Cancer 55:2291–2295.

Watanabe E, Watanabe T, Manaka S, Mayanagi Y, Takakura K. 1987. Three-dimensional digitizer (neuronavigator): new equipment for computed tomography-guided stereotaxic surgery. Surg Neurol 27:543–547.

Weingart J, Olivi A, Brem H. 1991. Supratentorial low-grade astrocytomas in adults. Neurosurg Q 1:141–159.

Weldon-Linne CM, Victor TA, Groothius DR, Vick NA. 1983. Pleomorphic xanthoastrocytoma. Ultrastructural and immunohistochemical study of a case with a rapidly fatal outcome following surgery. Cancer 52:2055–2063.

Wen DY, Hall WA, Miller DA, Seljeskog EL, Maxwell RE. 1993. Targeted brain biopsy: a comparison of freehand computed tomography-guided and stereotactic techniques. Neurosurgery 32:407–413.

Werner-Wasik M, Scott CB, Nelson DF, et al. 1996. Final report of a phase I/II trial of hyperfractionated and accelerated hyperfractionated radiation therapy and carmustine for adults with supratentorial malignant gliomas. Radiation Therapy Oncology Group Study 83-02. Cancer 77:1535–1543.

Whitton AC, Bloom HJ. 1990. Low grade glioma of the cerebral hemispheres in adults: a retrospective analysis of 88 cases. Int J Radiat Oncol Biol Phys 18:783–786.

Wilson CB. 1975. Reoperation for primary tumors. Semin Oncol 2:19–20.

Wilson CB, Gutin PH, Boldrey EB, Drafts D, Levin VA, Enot KJ. 1976. Single-agent chemotherapy of brain tumors. A five-year review. Arch Neurol 33:739–744.

Wilson CB, Larson DA, Gutin PH. 1992. Radiosurgery: a new application? J Clin Oncol 10:1373–1374.

Winger MJ, Macdonald DR, Cairncross JG. 1989. Supratentorial anaplastic gliomas in adults. The prognostic importance of extent of resection and prior low-grade glioma. J Neurosurg 71:487–493.

Winger MJ, Macdonald DR, Schold SC, Cairncross JG. 1989. Selection bias in clinical trials of anaplastic glioma. Ann Neurol 26:531–534.

Wisoff JH, Abbott R, Epstein F. 1990. Surgical management of exophytic chiasmatic-hypothalamic tumors of childhood. J Neurosurg 73:661–667.

Wisoff JH, Boyett JM, Berger MS, et al. 1998. Current neurosurgical management and the impact of the extent of resection in the treatment of malignant gliomas of childhood: a report of the Children's Cancer Group trial no. CCG-945. J Neurosurg 89:52–59.

Withers HR. 1985. Biologic basis for altered fractionation schemes. Cancer 55:2086–2095.

Wong ET, Hess KR, Gleason MJ, et al. 1999. Outcomes and prognostic factors in recurrent glioma patients enrolled onto phase II clinical trials. J Clin Oncol 17:2572–2578.

Wood JR, Green SB, Shapiro WR. 1988. The prognostic importance of tumor size in malignant gliomas: a computed tomographic scan study by the Brain Tumor Cooperative Group. J Clin Oncol 6:338–343.

Woolsey CN, Erickson TC, Gilson WE. 1979. Localization in somatic sensory and motor areas of human cerebral cortex as determined by direct recording of evoked potentials and electrical stimulation. J Neurosurg 51:476–506.

Yingling CD, Ojemann S, Dodson B, Harrington MJ, Berger MS. 1999. Identification of motor pathways during tumor surgery facilitated by multichannel electromyographic recording. J Neurosurg 91:922–927.

Young B, Oldfield EH, Markesbery WR, et al. 1981. Reoperation for glioblastoma. J Neurosurg 55:917–921.

Yule SM, Hide TA, Cranney M, Simpson E, Barrett A. 2001. Low grade astrocytomas in the West of Scotland 1987–96: treatment, outcome and cognitive functioning. Arch Dis Child 84:61–64.

Yung WK, Albright RE, Olson J, et al. 2000. A phase II study of temozolomide vs. procarbazine in patients with glioblastoma multiforme at first relapse. Br J Cancer 83:588–593.

Yung WK, Harris MI, Bruner JM, Feun LG. 1989. Intravenous BCNU and AZQ in patients with recurrent malignant gliomas. J Neurooncol 7:237–240.

Yung WK, Mechtler L, Gleason MJ. 1991a. Intravenous carboplatin for recurrent malignant gliomas: a phase II study. J Clin Oncol 9:860–864.

Yung WK, Prados MD, Levin VA, et al. 1991b. Intravenous recombinant interferon-beta in patients with recurrent malignant gliomas: a phase I/II study. J Clin Oncol 9:1945–1949.

Yung WK, Prados MD, Yaya-Tur R, et al. 1999. Multicenter phase II trial of temozolomide in patients with anaplastic astrocytoma or anaplastic oligoastrocytoma at first relapse. Temodal Brain Tumor Group. J Clin Oncol 17: 2762–2771.

Yung WK, Simaga M, Levin VA. 1993. 13-cis-retinoic acid: a new and potentially effective agent for recurrent malignant astrocytomas. Proc Ann Meet Am Soc Clin Oncol 12: A497.

Zakhary R, Keles GE, Berger MS. 1999. Intraoperative imaging techniques in the treatment of brain tumors. Curr Opin Oncol 11:152–156.

Zeltzer PM, Boyett JM, Finlay JL, et al. 1999. Metastasis stage, adjuvant treatment, and residual tumor are prognostic factors for medulloblastoma in children: conclusions from the Children's Cancer Group 921 randomized phase III study. J Clin Oncol 17: 832–845.

Zentner J, Hufnagel A, Wolf HK, et al. 1997. Surgical treatment of neoplasms associated with medically intractable epilepsy. Neurosurgery 41:378–387.

4

Primary Spinal Cord Tumors

ERIC MARMOR AND ZIYA L. GOKASLAN

The first successful resection of a spinal cord tumor was performed by Victor Horsley in 1887 (Stein and McCormick, 1996). The diagnosis and treatment of intramedullary spinal cord tumors was first described in detail by Elsberg in 1925 (Stein and McCormick, 1996), and Greenwood reported the first large modern series in 1967. Since then, numerous radiographic, microsurgical, and electrophysiologic advances have enabled the clinician to better manage patients with these challenging tumors. Today a skilled and knowledgeable surgeon is able to cure many patients harboring such tumors. Despite these improvements, much remains to be learned about the optimal management of patients with spinal cord tumors.

EPIDEMIOLOGY

Very few reliable epidemiologic data on primary intraspinal tumors are found in the literature, with most series consisting of authors' personal experiences, which are often biased by referral patterns. The few existing population-based studies indicate that the annual incidence of these tumors ranges from 0.5 to 1.4 per 100,000 (Helseth and Mork, 1989; Sasanelli et al., 1983). The majority of the tumors included in these series consist of meningiomas and schwannomas, which are not discussed in this chapter. Classifications of spinal tumors are frequently made on the basis of their anatomic location, as depicted in Table 4–1. Approximately 25% of intraspinal tumors in adults and the majority of these tumors in children are intramedullary. Of the true intramedullary spinal cord tumors, the vast majority are gliomas, with ependymomas occurring most frequently in the adult population and astrocytomas accounting for about 60% of pediatric intramedullary tumors (Nadkarni and Rekate, 1999; Cristante and Herrmann, 1994; O'Sullivan et al., 1994; Epstein et al., 1992; Cooper, 1989). Most spinal gliomas are low grade, with glioblastomas representing only 7.5% of all intramedullary gliomas (Ciappetta et al., 1991; Cohen et al., 1989; Helseth and Mork, 1989).

Hemangioblastomas, which occur sporadically or are associated with von Hippel-Lindau syndrome, are the third most common intramedullary tumor type to occur in adults and represent only approximately 4% of intramedullary tumors (Hoff et al., 1993; Trost et al., 1993; Solomon and Stein, 1988). In contrast to the gliomas, which occur with approximately equal incidence in both sexes, hemangioblastomas occur more frequently in males (Cristante and Herrmann, 1999; Cooper, 1996; Murota and Symon, 1989). Even less frequently encountered tumors in this location include gangliogliomas, primitive neuroectodermal tumors, lipomas (usually associated with congenital defects), ganglioneurocytomas, and neurocytomas (Constantini and Epstein, 1996; Tatter et al., 1994). Myxopapillary ependymomas, histologic variants of ependymomas, are most commonly found in the filum terminale. These tumors infrequently invade the thecal sac, are usually well circumscribed, and are often completely resectable. All of these factors account

Table 4–1 Classification of Spinal Tumors by Location

Location	*Tumor*
EXTRADURAL	Metastatic (carcinoma, lymphoma, melanoma, sarcoma), chordoma, epidermoid, teratoma, dermoid, lipoma
INTRADURAL	
Extramedullary	Nerve sheath tumors (schwannoma), epidermoid, teratoma, dermoid, lipoma, neurenteric cyst
Intramedullary	Astrocytoma, ependymoma, hemangioblastoma

for the generally favorable outcome that patients harboring these rare tumors can expect (Freeman and Cahill, 1996).

RADIOLOGY

Magnetic resonance imaging (MRI) is the radiographic method of choice in the diagnosis of primary spinal cord tumors. All MRI studies done on suspected intramedullary tumors should include T_1- and T_2-weighted images as well as images taken after the administration of a contrast agent. Computed tomography (CT) with myelography, which was the diagnostic tool of choice for intramedullary tumors in the 1970s and 1980s, continues to be used when MRI is not available. Although CT with myelography can reliably identify the presence of spinal cord pathology, it is an invasive test and does not define the spinal cord anatomy as well as MRI. In addition, in the presence of a complete spinal block, it may be necessary to perform a C1–C2 puncture to define the rostral extent of the tumor.

More recently, emphasis has been placed on making a pathologic diagnosis from MRI characteristics, with particular attention paid toward differentiating astrocytomas from ependymomas. Despite the improving quality of MRI and our increasing experience with this diagnostic modality, the only way to ascertain a definitive diagnosis is by obtaining a surgical specimen of the tumor. Furthermore, the surgical resectability of these tumors is not reliably predicted by their MRI characteristics.

In general, intramedullary ependymomas appear isointense on T_1-weighted images. All have a hyperintense signal on T_2-weighted images and are enhanced after administration of a contrast agent (Fine et al., 1995). The enhancement borders are sharply defined, and the tumor is characteristically found to be centrally located in an expanded spinal cord (Epstein et al., 1993) (Fig. 4–1). Hemosiderin is often found at the periphery of cervical ependymomas (Fine et al., 1995).

Astrocytomas similarly show diffuse cord enlargement on T_1-weighted images, with increased signal on T_2-weighted images (Epstein et al., 1993); however, contrast enhancement in astrocytomas is often heterogeneous and the borders are often irregular (Epstein et al., 1993; Dillon et al., 1989). Furthermore, astrocytomas are less frequently associated with a syrinx than are ependymomas or hemangioblastomas (Samii and Klekamp, 1994). Regardless of the pathology, the more rostral the tumor, the more likely it is to be associated with a syrinx (Samii and Klekamp, 1994).

Hemangioblastomas are isointense or slightly hyperintense on T_1-weighted images. Classically, they are known to contain an intensely enhancing tumor nodule surrounded by edema and are associated with a cyst or a syrinx (Xu et al., 1994; Hoff et al., 1993). Spinal angiography in hemangioblastomas will often demonstrate the compact tumor nodule, feeding arteries, and main draining vein and is useful for diagnosing these tumors as it most clearly defines the regional vascular anatomy (Spetzger et al., 1996). Spinal angiography can also be used therapeutically for preoperative embolization (Tampieri et al., 1993), but is not indicated if MRI characteristics are suggestive of an astrocytoma or ependymoma.

CLINICAL PRESENTATION

The clinical presentation for primary spinal cord tumors usually involves an indolent course. The most common presenting symptoms include pain along the spinal axis, sensory disturbances, motor weakness, and gait disturbance. Bowel and bladder as well as

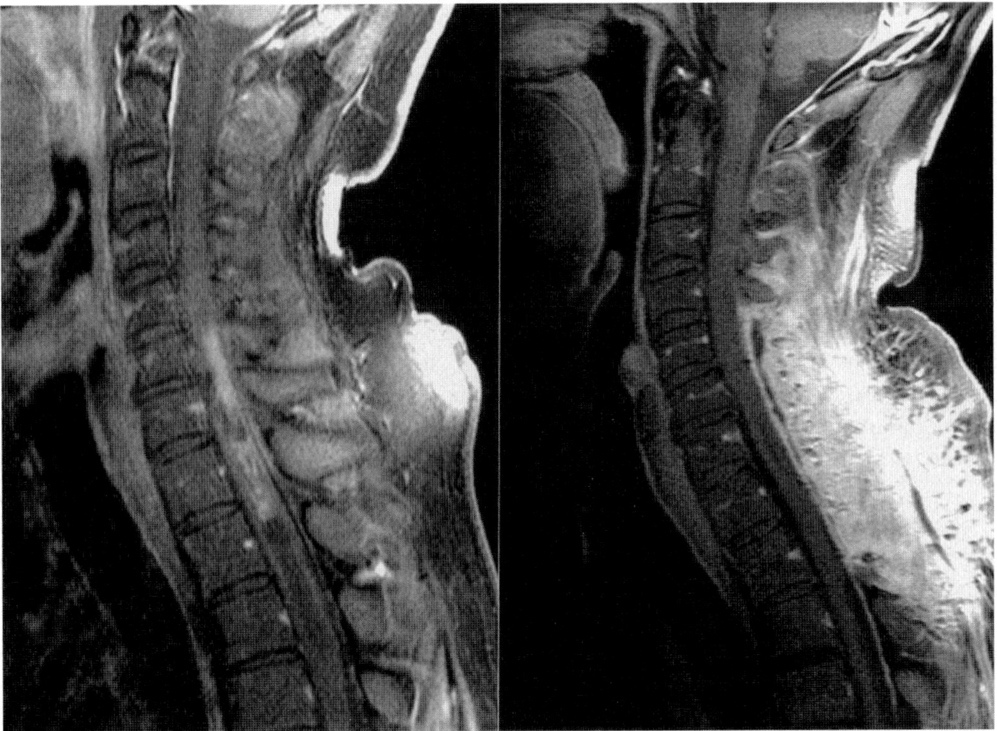

Figure 4–1. Pre- and postoperative T_1-weighted images of a patient with cervicothoracic region ependymoma, after contrast injection. Preoperative study (left) demonstrates a relatively well-circumscribed enhancing intramedullary lesion associated with syrinx and spinal cord enlargement. Postoperative MRI (right) shows complete excision of intramedullary tumor and almost complete resolution of syrinx.

sexual dysfunction are considerably less frequent but well-described symptoms found on presentation (Lee et al., 1998). Radicular pain occurs in approximately 10% of patients and is usually limited to one or two cervical, thoracic, or lumbar dermatomes (Constantini and Epstein, 1996).

On examination, variable motor deficits, sensory disturbances, reflex changes, and long tract findings may be detected (Lee et al., 1998). In the pediatric population, these tumors may additionally present with torticollis and progressive kyphoscoliosis (Constantini et al., 1996; Rossitch et al., 1990).

The duration of symptoms before presentation for astrocytomas and ependymomas varies depending on the series. Cooper (1989), in a review of 51 patients, reported means of 7.7 and 6.4 years of symptoms before surgery for astrocytomas and ependymomas, respectively. Others report a shorter range of several months to several years for both of these tumor types (Jyothirmayi et al., 1997; Minehan et al., 1995; Waldron et al., 1993). In contrast, malignant gliomas have a much shorter prodrome of only several weeks to several months before presentation (Cristante and Herrmann, 1994). In addition, patients with these malignant tumors may present with headaches, and of these patients ultimately 50% to 60% will develop concurrent hydrocephalus (Ciappetta et al., 1991; Cohen et al., 1989). Even patients with a more benign pathology can develop hydrocephalus, albeit at a significantly lower frequency. The pathophysiology of the development of hydrocephalus in these patients is thought to be related either to markedly increased protein concentration in the cerebrospinal fluid or to dissemination of tumor in the subarachnoid space, as seen with malignant gliomas (Rifkinson-Mann et al., 1990).

As stated previously, the only definitive way to make a pathologic diagnosis is to evaluate tissue from the tumor. However, by combining the patient's clinical presentation with imaging information, it is frequently possible to predict whether a particular intramedullary tumor is benign. In general, when a patient presents with a mild neurologic deficit and significant cord enlargement is seen on MRI, the tumor's histology will be benign. If, however, the patient presents with a severe neurologic deficit with only modest cord enlargement, then the tumor is likely to be malignant.

Hemangioblastomas have presenting features similar to other intramedullary tumors and are symptomatic for a mean of approximately 2 years before presentation (Cristante and Herrmann, 1999). In addition, these tumors have been reported to present acutely, mimicking a typical intracranial subarachnoid hemorrhage, or with acute onset of paraplegia secondary to hemorrhage into the tumor (Yu et al., 1994; Cerejo et al., 1990).

SURGERY

General Considerations

Surgery for primary spinal cord tumors is one of the most technically challenging procedures performed by neurosurgeons. These tumors are rare, and, as a result, no practice guidelines have been established for their optimal treatment. It is the authors' opinion, however, that surgery is indicated for virtually all patients who are found to have radiographic evidence of an intramedullary tumor, with the exception of the rare patient who is medically unable to tolerate an operation. Patients who do not have neurologic deficit may be followed very closely but should undergo surgery at the earliest hint of neurologic dysfunction or of radiographic evidence of tumor enlargement. Even patients who have a complete neurologic deficit below the spinal level of the tumor should undergo surgery to establish a diagnosis and prevent the onset of neurologic deficits at a higher spinal level, particularly if the tumor extends above T4.

The goals of surgery are to establish a diagnosis and to resect the maximal amount of tumor possible without causing any deterioration in the patient's neurologic condition. These goals can be attained by always establishing adequate exposure and meticulously minimizing manipulation of the spinal cord. Intraoperative ultrasonography should be used before the dura is opened to ensure that sufficient bone has been removed to permit safe resection of the tumor. Ultrasonography is also useful in planning the placement of the myelotomy and confirming that there is no residual tumor once the resection has been completed (Epstein et al., 1991). Available instruments that facilitate the resection of these tumors include the Cavitron ultrasonic aspirator (CUSA) and the laser.

Ependymomas have a distinct surgical plane between the tumor and the spinal cord, and thus a total resection is often feasible, although internal debulking is frequently required to prevent excessive retraction of the spinal cord (Hoshimaru et al., 1999; Epstein et al., 1993) (Fig. 4–2). Hemangioblastomas also display a clear interface between the tumor and normal tissue; however, the surgeon is advised to refrain from internally debulking these vascular tumors (Cristante and Herrmann, 1999; Murota and Symon, 1989).

Conversely, astrocytomas normally do not have a distinct plane of demarcation between the tumor and spinal cord and must be debulked internally, with the surgeon using his or her discretion as to when to stop the resection (Fig. 4–3). If a frozen section is sent for diagnosis intraoperatively, particular care must be used, as tanycytic ependymomas can easily be mistaken for astrocytomas. Detailed descriptions of the resection of these tumors are beyond the scope of this chapter and are well described elsewhere (Cooper, 1996; Stein and McCormick, 1996).

The role of intraoperative somatosensory evoked potential (SSEP) monitoring during resection of intramedullary tumors is unclear, and no statistically valid evidence exists to support use of this technique (Cooper, 1996). Nevertheless, most surgeons performing this operation use SSEP monitoring. Problems with SSEP monitoring for intramedullary tumors include the frequently abnormal responses seen before the resection is started. In addition, the delay inherent in this monitoring system will often indicate that injury has occurred only after it has become irreversible. Furthermore the system monitors sensory pathways and does not reflect the integrity of the motor pathways.

Motor evoked potential (MEP) monitoring is a newer technique that directly measures the integrity of motor pathways and is being used at an increasing number of medical centers. Preliminary studies indicate that this technique provides good functional outcome prognosis in adults, but it has not yet been determined whether it improves surgical outcome

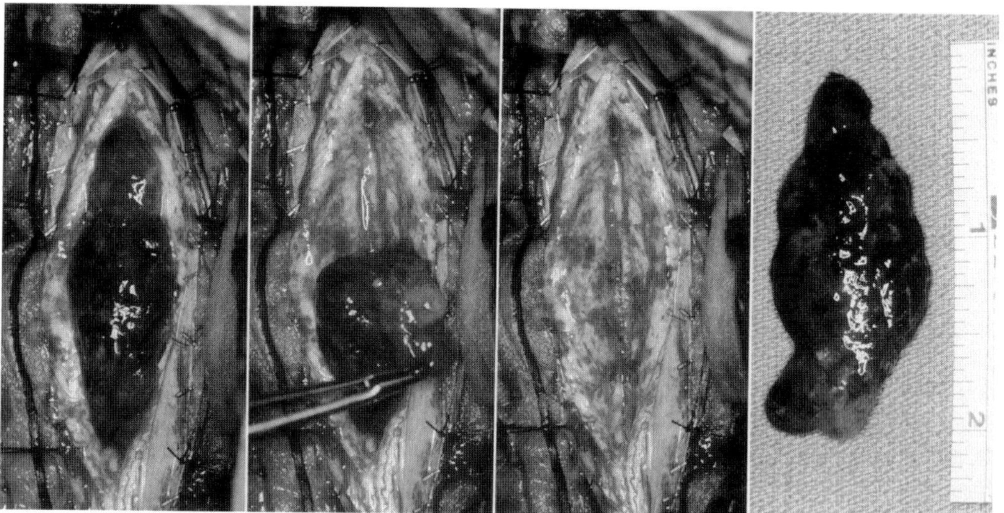

Figure 4–2. Serial intraoperative photographs (from left to right) of the patient in Figure 4–1 show the characteristic features of an ependymoma. After a dorsal midline myelotomy, a typical well-circumscribed, beefy-red-appearing mass is observed. After tedious dissection using the operating microscope, the tumor is gradually being lifted off the normal spinal cord. The tumor specimen, which has been removed in toto, measures almost 2 inches in length.

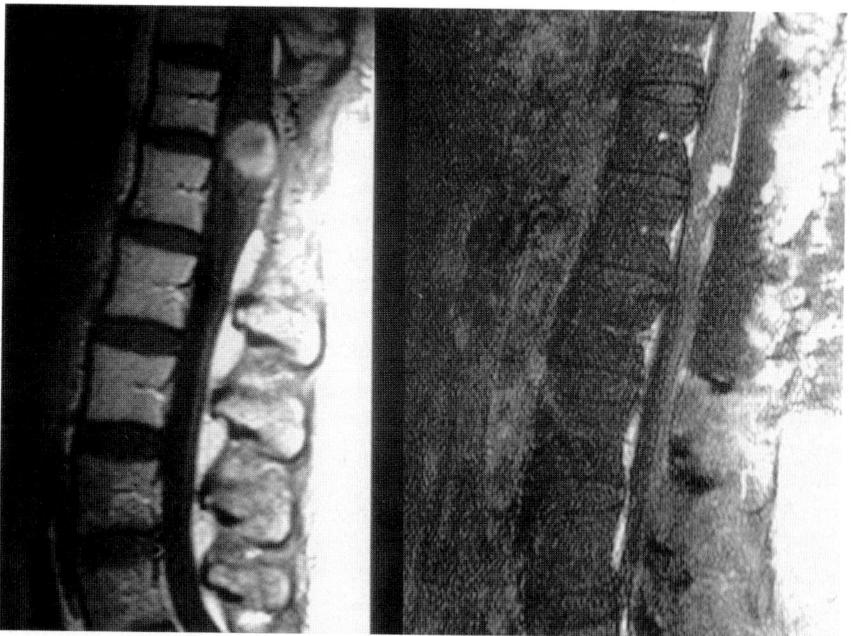

Figure 4–3. Pre- and postoperative MR images (after gadolinium injection) of a patient with anaplastic astrocytoma of the conus region. Despite the relatively well-circumscribed radiographic appearance of the tumor on preoperative MR images (left), intraoperative explorations revealed infiltration of the conus with no distinct surgical plane. Thus, as seen on the postoperative MR image (right), residual tumor infiltrating the spinal cord was not removed to avoid causing any neurologic deficit.

(Morota et al., 1997). This monitoring technique is less useful in pediatric patients because of the nature of their immature nervous systems (Morota et al., 1997).

Surgical Complications

The postoperative course of patients with intramedullary tumors is frequently characterized by a transient deterioration in neurologic condition, lasting from a few days to months before recovery occurs (Samii and Klekamp, 1994). Some investigators do not report any motor deterioration in the immediate postoperative period in patients with benign gliomas, even after aggressive resection (Epstein et al., 1992). Patients with severe preoperative disability are more likely to deteriorate as a result of surgery (Constantini and Epstein, 1996). Patients who have a syrinx associated with their tumor tend to recover more rapidly (Samii and Klekamp, 1994).

Loss of proprioception is a common complication that can be very debilitating, even in the presence of preserved motor function. The development or progression of kyphoscoliosis can occur postoperatively, especially in the pediatric population, and may necessitate a second operation for fusion and instrumentation. Cerebrospinal fluid leaks and concomitant meningitis may also occur despite meticulous surgical technique, particularly if the region has been irradiated previously.

RADIATION THERAPY

In general, when radiotherapy is employed, approximately 50 Gy are administered to the involved site (with rostral/caudal margins of at least 3 cm) in 16 to 20 fractions over a 4 to 5 week period (Shirato et al., 1995). There has not yet been any prospective, randomized study demonstrating the efficacy of radiation therapy in treating primary spinal cord tumors. However, until a more definitive study is done, generalizations can be drawn from the many retrospective series that exist.

In the treatment of benign ependymomas, prior studies show that postoperative radiotherapy is not indicated if a gross total resection of the tumor has been achieved (Ohata et al., 1999; Lee et al., 1998; McLaughlin et al., 1998; Shirato et al., 1995; Clover et al., 1993; Epstein et al., 1993; Waldron et al., 1993; Wen et al., 1991; Whitaker et al., 1991; McCormick et al., 1990). The same studies recommend radiotherapy when there is residual tumor. Some also recommend postoperative radiotherapy if the tumor has been removed in a piecemeal fashion (McLaughlin et al., 1998; Wen et al., 1991), whereas others vehemently disagree (Epstein et al., 1993). Despite the recommendations above, it must be emphasized that no definitive study has demonstrated a benefit of radiation exceeding that of clinical follow-up and reoperation for residual tumor (Lee et al., 1998).

Most reported series recommend postoperative radiotherapy in the treatment of low-grade astrocytomas, regardless of the degree of surgical resection (McLaughlin et al., 1998; Jyothirmayi et al., 1997; Minehan et al., 1995; Shirato et al., 1995; Huddart et al., 1993; Cooper, 1989). Others suggest that close observation without radiotherapy is a better alternative, with either reoperation or radiotherapy should the tumor recur (Innocenzi et al., 1997; Brotchi et al., 1992; Epstein et al., 1992). All malignant gliomas of the spinal cord are treated with postoperative radiotherapy, although there is no clinical evidence for the efficacy of this treatment.

There is no evidence to support the use of either pre- or postoperative radiotherapy in the treatment of hemangioblastomas (Murota and Symon, 1989). The hazards of administrating radiotherapy in the pediatric population have been well described (Duffner et al., 1993). As a result, postoperative radiation treatment should not routinely be used in this cohort of patients with primary spinal cord tumors except for the treatment of malignant tumors or in the setting of recurrence (Goh et al., 1997; Przybylski et al., 1997; Constantini et al., 1996).

CHEMOTHERAPY

The adjuvant role of chemotherapy in the treatment of malignant primary spinal cord tumors is even less well defined than that of radiation therapy. Several small retrospective series that have examined the optimal management of these lesions recommend chemotherapy, although it is unclear whether this therapeutic modality changes the uniformly poor outcome associated with these tumors (Ciappetta et al., 1991; Cohen et al., 1989). More recently, limited trials using experimental chemotherapeutic regimens in pediatric populations have shown some limited success (Allen et al., 1998; Lowis et al., 1998; Doireau et al., 1999). The exact role that chemotherapy has in the treatment of intramedullary tumors thus remains uncertain, and no clear guidelines for its use can be established at the present time.

OUTCOME

Of patients with astrocytomas of the spinal cord, 50% to 73% survive 5 years and 23% to 54% survive for 10 years (reviewed by Abdel-Wahab et al., 1999). The histologic type and grade of the tumor are the most important features in predicting prognosis (Abdel-Wahab et al., 1999; McLaughlin et al., 1998; Innocenzi et al., 1997; Jyothirmayi et al., 1997; Huddart et al., 1993). Among the low-grade astrocytomas, patients with pilocytic tumors had significantly improved survival rates (81% at 5 years) compared with those with fibrillary tumors (15% at 5 years) (Minehan et al., 1995). Prognostically significant clinical features were the length of history of the disease and the patient's pre- and postoperative neurologic status, with both a longer disease history and good neurologic status predicting a favorable outcome (Innocenzi et al., 1997; Cristante and Herrmann, 1994; Samii and Klekamp, 1994). Some series report an association between female gender and a favorable prognosis (Abdel-Wahab et al., 1999; Huddart et al., 1993). The extent of surgical resection in patients with low-grade astrocytomas was found by most to not have a significant impact on survival (Abdel-Wahab et al., 1999; Jyothirmayi et al., 1997; Minehan et al., 1995; Huddart et al., 1993; Sandler et al., 1992; Cooper, 1989). However, in a retrospective review of intramedullary astrocytomas, Epstein et al. (1992) suggest that radical resection of these tumors does improve patient outcome, although no control group was provided. Biopsy of these lesions carries the same risk as more aggressive resection. Furthermore, there is no correlation between increased postoperative radiation doses and improved survival (Jyothirmayi et al., 1997; Minehan et al., 1995; Wen et al., 1991).

All patients with malignant astrocytomas have a very poor prognosis, with overall median postoperative survival times in the range of 6 months to 1 year (Innocenzi et al., 1997; Cohen et al., 1989). Furthermore, surgery on these patients does not halt the decline in their neurologic function (Epstein et al., 1992). Neither a greater extent of surgical resection nor the administration of radiotherapy or chemotherapy have been shown to improve outcome (Epstein et al., 1992; Ciappetta et al., 1991; Cohen et al., 1989).

The overall 10 year survival for patients with intramedullary ependymomas ranges from about 50% to 95% and is better than that observed for astrocytomas (Abdel-Wahab et al., 1999; Waldron et al., 1993). The most important factors in determining long-term outcome for patients with ependymomas include whether total surgical resection is attained, the preoperative neurologic status of the patient, and the histologic grade of the tumor (Hoshimaru et al., 1999; Whitaker et al., 1991; Cooper, 1989). Several groups report 100% long-term survival in patients undergoing radical resection of ependymomas without postoperative radiotherapy (Epstein et al., 1993; McCormick et al., 1990). Patients with incomplete resection of primary spinal ependymomas have an approximately 62% 10 year survival rate when treated with postoperative radiation (Whitaker et al., 1991). The survival rates of ependymoma patients who undergo subtotal resection or biopsy and do not receive radiotherapy are not known.

The incidence of intramedullary hemangioblastomas is very low, and as a result outcome analysis for these tumors is lacking. One study examining recurrence rates of hemangioblastomas that had been surgically treated found that recurrence was correlated with younger age, association with von Hippel-Lindau syndrome, and the presence of multicentric tumors of the nervous system at the time of presentation (de la Monte and Horowitz, 1989). Investigations of neurologic outcome after surgical resection of these tumors report long-term clinical improvement in 40% to 72% of patients (Cristante and Herrmann, 1999; Murota and Symon, 1989).

Outcome in the pediatric population appears to be similar to that in adults, and patients with ependymomas have the longest recurrence-free survival (Goh et al., 1997; Przybylski et al., 1997). As in adults, the histologic grade of the tumor and the patient's preoperative neurologic condition are the most frequently identified prognostic indicators (Nadkarni and Rekate, 1999; Bouffet et al., 1998). Children with malignant gliomas generally have poor survival; however, a small minority of these children with anaplastic astrocytomas survive longer than 10 years (Merchant et al., 1999).

CONCLUSION

The management of patients with primary spinal cord tumors remains a formidable challenge to the clinician. These tumors are very rare, and the presenting symptoms will often initially mimic more common benign pathologies. Even after the diagnosis has been made, the ideal treatment of these tumors remains somewhat controversial. Overall, the tumors are best treated with aggressive surgical resection early in the course of the disease and performed by a surgeon experienced with all aspects of their management.

The exact role of postoperative adjunctive therapy is controversial, but certainly there is no role for radiotherapy after total resection of an ependymoma. There remains much room for improvement in treating patients with malignant primary spinal cord tumors, and clearly new therapies will have to be found to deal with these devastating tumors.

REFERENCES

Abdel-Wahab M, Corn B, Wolfson A, et al. 1999. Prognostic factors and survival in patients with spinal cord gliomas after radiation therapy. Am J Clin Oncol 22:344–351.

Allen JC, Aviner S, Yates AJ, et al. 1998. Treatment of high-grade spinal cord astrocytoma of childhood with "8-in-1" chemotherapy and radiotherapy: a pilot study of CCG-945. Children's Cancer Group. J Neurosurg 88:215–220.

Bouffet E, Pierre-Kahn A, Marchal JC, et al. 1998. Prognostic factors in pediatric spinal cord astrocytomas. Cancer 83:2391–2399.

Brotchi J, Noterman J, Baleriaux D. 1992. Surgery of intramedullary spinal cord tumours. Acta Neurochir (Wien) 116:176–178.

Cerejo A, Vaz R, Feyo PB, Cruz C. 1990. Spinal cord hemangioblastoma with subarachnoid hemorrhage. Neurosurgery 27:991–993.

Ciappetta P, Salvati M, Capoccia G, Artico M, Raco A, Fortuna A. 1991. Spinal glioblastomas: report of seven cases and review of the literature. Neurosurgery 28:302–306.

Clover LL, Hazuka MB, Kinzie JJ. 1993. Spinal cord ependymomas treated with surgery and radiation therapy. Am J Clin Oncol 16:350–353.

Cohen AR, Wisoff JH, Allen JC, Epstein F. 1989. Malignant astrocytomas of the spinal cord. J Neurosurg 70:50–54.

Constantini S, Epstein FJ. 1996. Primary spinal cord tumors. In: Levin VA (ed), Cancer in the Nervous System. New York: Churchill Livingstone, pp 127–128.

Constantini S, Houten J, Miller DC, et al. 1996. Intramedullary spinal cord tumors in children under the age of 3 years. J Neurosurg 85:1036–1043.

Cooper PR. 1989. Outcome after operative treatment of intramedullary spinal cord tumors in adults: intermediate and long-term results in 51 patients. Neurosurgery 25:855–859.

Cooper PR. 1996. Management of intramedullary spinal cord tumors. In: Tindall GT, Cooper PR, Barrow DL (eds), The Practice of Neurosurgery. Baltimore: Williams & Wilkins, pp 1335–1346.

Cristante L, Herrmann HD. 1994. Surgical management of intramedullary spinal cord tumors: functional outcome and sources of morbidity. Neurosurgery 35:69–76.

Cristante L, Herrmann HD. 1999. Surgical management of intramedullary hemangioblastoma of the spinal cord. Acta Neurochir (Wien) 141:333–340.

de la Monte SM, Horowitz SA. 1989. Hemangioblastomas: clinical and histopathological factors correlated with recurrence. Neurosurgery 25:695–698.

Dillon WP, Norman D, Newton TH, Bolla K, Mark A. 1989. Intradural spinal cord lesions: Gd-DTPA-enhanced MR imaging. Radiology 170:229–237.

Doireau V, Grill J, et al. 1999. Chemotherapy for unresectable and recurrent intramedullary glial tumours in children. Brain Tumours Subcommittee of the French Society of Paediatric Oncology (SFOP). Br J Cancer 81:835–840.

Duffner PK, Horowitz ME, Krischer JP, et al. 1993. Postoperative chemotherapy and delayed radiation in children less than three years of age with malignant brain tumors. N Engl J Med 328:1725–1731.

Epstein FJ, Farmer JP, Freed D. 1992. Adult intramedullary astrocytomas of the spinal cord. J Neurosurg 77:355–359.

Epstein FJ, Farmer JP, Freed D. 1993. Adult intramedullary spinal cord ependymomas: the result of surgery in 38 patients. J Neurosurg 79:204–209.

Epstein FJ, Farmer JP, Schneider SJ. 1991. Intraoperative ultrasonography: an important surgical adjunct for intramedullary tumors. J Neurosurg 74:729–733.

Fine MJ, Kricheff II, Freed D, Epstein FJ. 1995. Spinal cord ependymomas: MR imaging features. Radiology 197:655–658.

Freeman TB, Cahill DW. 1996. Management of intradural extramedullary tumors. In: Tindall GT, Cooper PR, Barrow DL (eds), The Practice of Neurosurgery. Baltimore: Williams & Wilkins, pp 1323–1334.

Goh KY, Velasquez L, Epstein FJ. 1997. Pediatric intramedullary spinal cord tumors: is surgery alone enough? Pediatr Neurosurg 27:34–39.

Greenwood J Jr. 1967. Surgical removal of intramedullary tumors. J Neurosurg 26:276–282.

Helseth A, Mork SJ. 1989. Primary intraspinal neoplasms in Norway, 1955 to 1986. A population based survey of 467 patients. J Neurosurg 71:842–845.

Hoff DJ, Tampieri D, Just N. 1993. Imaging of spinal cord hemangioblastomas. Can Assoc Radiol J 44:377–383.

Hoshimaru M, Koyama T, Hashimoto N, Kikuchi H. 1999. Results of microsurgical treatment for intramedullary spinal cord ependymomas: analysis of 36 cases. Neurosurgery 44:264–269.

Huddart R, Traish D, Ashley S, Moore A, Brada M. 1993. Management of spinal astrocytoma with conservative surgery and radiotherapy. Br J Neurosurg 7:473–481.

Innocenzi G, Salvati M, Cervoni L, Delfini R, Cantore G. 1997. Prognostic factors in intramedullary astrocytomas. Clin Neurol Neurosurg 99:1–5.

Jyothirmayi R, Madhavan J, Nair MK, Rajan B. 1997. Conservative surgery and radiotherapy in the treatment of spinal cord astrocytoma. J Neurooncol 33:205–211.

Lee TT, Gromelski EB, Green BA. 1998. Surgical treatment of spinal ependymoma and post-operative radiotherapy. Acta Neurochir (Wien) 140:309–313.

Lowis SP, Pizer BL, Coakham H, Nelson RJ, Bouffet E. 1998. Chemotherapy for spinal cord astrocytoma: can natural history be modified? Childs Nerv Syst 14:317–321.

McCormick PC, Torres R, Post KD, Stein BM. 1990. Intramedullary ependymoma of the spinal cord. J Neurosurg 72:523–532.

McLaughlin MP, Buatti JM, Marcus RB Jr, Maria BL, Mickle PJ, Kedar A. 1998. Outcome after radiotherapy of primary spinal cord glial tumors. Radiat Oncol Invest 6:276–280.

Merchant TE, Nguyen D, Thompson SJ, Reardon DA, Kun LE, Sanford RA. 1999. High-grade pediatric spinal cord tumors. Pediatr Neurosurg 30:1–5.

Minehan KJ, Shaw EG, Scheithauer BW, Davis DL, Onofrio BM. 1995. Spinal cord astrocytoma: pathological and treatment considerations. J Neurosurg 83:590–595.

Morota N, Deletis V, Constantini S, Kofler M, Cohen H, Epstein FJ. 1997. The role of motor evoked potentials during surgery for intramedullary spinal cord tumors. Neurosurgery 41:1327–1336.

Murota T, Symon L. 1989. Surgical management of hemangioblastoma of the spinal cord: a report of 18 cases. Neurosurgery 25:699–708.

Nadkarni TD, Rekate HL. 1999. Pediatric intramedullary spinal cord tumors. Childs Nerv Syst 15:17–28.

Ohata K, Takami T, Gotou T, El-Bahy K. 1999. Surgical outcome of intramedullary spinal cord ependymoma. Acta Neurochir (Wien) 141:341–347.

O'Sullivan C, Jenkin RD, Doherty MA, Hoffman HJ, Greenberg ML. 1994. Spinal cord tumors in children: long-term results of combined surgical and radiation treatment. J Neurosurg 81:507–512.

Przybylski GJ, Albright AL, Martinez AJ. 1997. Spinal cord astrocytomas: long-term results comparing treatments in children. Childs Nerv Syst13:375–382.

Rifkinson-Mann S, Wisoff JH, Epstein F. 1990. The association of hydrocephalus with intramedullary spinal cord tumors: a series of 25 patients. Neurosurgery 27:749–754.

Rossitch E Jr, Zeidman SM, Burger PC, et al. 1990. Clinical and pathological analysis of spinal cord astrocytomas in children. Neurosurgery 27:193–196.

Samii M, Klekamp J. 1994. Surgical results of 100 intramedullary tumors in relation to accompanying syringomyelia. Neurosurgery 35:865–873.

Sandler HM, Papadopoulos SM, Thornton AF Jr, Ross DA. 1992. Spinal cord astrocytomas: results of therapy. Neurosurgery 30:490–493.

Sasanelli F, Beghi E, Kurland LT. 1983. Primary intraspinal neoplasms in Rochester, Minnesota, 1935–1981. Neuroepidemiology 2:156–163.

Shirato H, Kamada T, Hida K, et al. 1995. The role of radiotherapy in the management of spinal cord glioma. Int J Radiat Oncol Biol Phys 33:323–328.

Solomon RA, Stein BM. 1988. Unusual spinal enlargement related to intramedullary hemangioblastoma. J Neurosurg 68:550–553.

Spetzger U, Bertalanffy H, Huffmann B, Mayfrank L, Reul J, Gilsbach JM. 1996. Hemangioblastomas of the spinal cord and the brainstem: diagnostic and therapeutic features. Neurosurg Rev 19:147–51

Stein B, McCormick PC. 1996. Spinal intradural tumors. In: Wilkins RH, Rengachary SS (eds), Neurosurgery. New York: McGraw Hill, pp 1769–1781.

Tampieri D, Leblanc R, TerBrugge K. 1993. Preoperative embolization of brain and spinal hemangioblastomas. Neurosurgery 33:502–505.

Tatter SB, Borges LF, Louis DN. 1994. Central neurocytomas of the cervical spinal cord. Report of two cases. J Neurosurg 81:288–293.

Trost HA, Seifert V, Stolke D. 1993. Advances in diagnosis and treatment of spinal hemangioblastomas. Neurosurg Rev 16:205–209.

Waldron JN, Laperriere NJ, Jaakkimainen L, et al. 1993. Spinal cord ependymomas: a retrospective analysis of 59 cases. Int J Radiat Oncol Biol Phys 27:223–229.

Wen BC, Hussey DH, Hitchon PW. 1991. The role of radiation therapy in the management of ependymomas of the spinal cord. Int J Radiat Oncol Biol Phys 20:781–786.

Whitaker SJ, Bessell EM, Ashley SE, Bloom HJ, Bell BA, Brada M. 1991. Postoperative radiotherapy in the management of spinal cord ependymoma. J Neurosurg 74:720–728.

Xu QW, Bao WM, Mao RL, Yang GY. 1994. Magnetic resonance imaging and microsurgical treatment of intramedullary hemangioblastoma of the spinal cord. Neurosurgery 35:671–676.

Yu JS, Short MP, Schumacher J, Chapman PH, Harsh GR 4th. 1994. Intramedullary hemorrhage in spinal cord hemangioblastoma. Report of two cases. J Neurosurg 81:937–940.

5

Optic Nerve, Chiasmal, and Hypothalamic Tumors

JOANN ATER, NANCY J. TARBELL, AND EDWARD LAWS, JR.

Gliomas are the most common tumors in the optic nerve, chiasmal, and hypothalamic regions of the central nervous system (CNS). As such, they are the focus of this chapter. For completeness, the less common tumors of these regions—meningiomas and craniopharyngiomas—are also covered. Germ cell tumors can also occur in this region but are discussed in Chapter 7.

GLIOMAS

Gliomas that affect the optic nerves, chiasm, and hypothalamus represent a unique type of tumor with a variable clinical course. Histologically, most other midline astrocytomas of childhood are of the pilocytic subtype. These gliomas are among the neoplasms of the nervous system whose tumor type and prognosis are age related. Except for infants, the prognosis for patients with these tumors is inversely related to age at onset, with older individuals having a poorer prognosis. In infancy, tumors affecting the optic pathways can be malignant in their course, although the reasons for this are not known. Gliomas of the optic nerves and chiasm are strongly associated with neurofibromatosis type 1. Several large series report obvious signs of neurofibromatosis in as many as 54% of affected children (Alvord and Lofton, 1988; Hoyt and Baghdassarian, 1969; Listernick et al., 1988; Packer et al., 1983; Manera et al., 1994). Gliomas affecting the hypothalamus and anterior third ventricle are also strongly associated with neurofibromatosis and may be found in tuberous sclerosis, another hereditary condition.

The pathology of optic pathway gliomas runs the gamut from very benign astrocytomas, considered by some to be hamartomas, to tumors that are glioblastoma multiforme. The typical histologic picture of a glioma of the optic nerve is one of dense arachnoid proliferation around an infiltrating pilocytic glioma, with thin hair-like tumor cells intermixed among the fibers of the optic nerve itself. The low-grade gliomas that tend to affect the optic chiasm, anterior third ventricle, and hypothalamus frequently are characterized as juvenile pilocytic astrocytomas, having few mitoses, no malignant features, or degenerative changes such as Rosenthal fibers. Despite their relatively "benign" histology, these tumors can progress and cause considerable morbidity in young children. Occasionally, anterior third ventricle tumors are discovered in conjunction with tuberous sclerosis; these tumors are generally noninfiltrating, relatively benign subependymal giant cell astrocytoma (see Chapter 3). Overall, approximately 4% to 5% of optic pathway tumors are frankly malignant, and those usually have many of the characteristics typical of glioblastoma multiforme. The tumors with malignant histology occur most commonly in adolescents and older individuals.

In addition to patient age, anatomic distinctions are extremely important in the evolution and prognosis of these tumors. Optic nerve gliomas can be conveniently grouped into two major categories: the anterior optic nerve glioma, which primarily affects the optic nerve or nerves; and the posterior optic nerve glioma, usually centered in the optic chiasm. Obviously, tumors in both categories affect the visual system, but the two types differ in pace and progression. Anterior optic nerve gliomas, which usually occur in childhood, are ordinarily quite benign and progress very slowly. Some of these tumors do not progress at all or progress over many years. Posterior optic nerve gliomas, which occur in very young children or older individuals, tend to form larger masses and present with more symptoms. These tumors may become large enough to affect the physiology of the hypothalamus and/or obstruct the anterior third ventricle, producing hydrocephalus. In infants who present with optic nerve or chiasmal gliomas, the spectrum ranges from indolent tumors to aggressive tumors that can spread throughout the optic pathway from the globe back to the occipital cortex.

Tumors arising primarily in the hypothalamus or anterior third ventricle are less common and less often associated with neurofibromatosis. Hamartomatous lesions also occur in the hypothalamus and in the interpeduncular fossa. More typical juvenile astrocytomas can occur in this region, along with standard anaplastic astrocytomas and other malignant forms.

Clinical Presentation

Optic gliomas occur primarily in children, with more than 71% diagnosed in patients younger than 10 years of age and 90% diagnosed during the first two decades of life (Dutton, 1991). The tumors can range from mild fusiform enlargement of the optic nerve or nerves within the orbit to very large, globular exophytic masses that extend from the chiasm and are virtually indistinguishable from a primary hypothalamic tumor.

In one series, more than 60% of optic pathway tumors involved the optic chiasm (Tenny et al., 1982). The signs and symptoms in children with optic pathway tumors who presented to The University of Texas M. D. Anderson Cancer Center between 1975 and 1993 are listed in Table 5–1 (Manera et al., 1994). The clinical picture of a patient with a lesion affecting the optic nerves, chiasm, or hypothalamus is usually one of progressive visual loss. In unilateral optic nerve tumors, this begins as a unilateral loss of optic nerve function; in other tumors, mixed variants of optic nerve and chiasmal patterns of visual loss can occur, with an asymmetric bitemporal hemianopsia being the most common finding in a chiasmal glioma.

In addition, behavioral changes, possibly related to elevated intracranial pressure or hypothalamic involvement, are prominent. Irritability, depression, social withdrawal, somnolence, and aggressive behavior have been reported. Because of the frequent involvement of the suprasellar-hypothalamic region, children with optic nerve tumors of these areas can also present with endocrine abnormalities. Although endocrine manifestations can occur with any of the suprasellar lesions, such presentations are particularly common in lesions that arise in the hypothalamus or floor of the third ventricle. The hypothalamic dysfunction produced by these lesions can range from varying forms and degrees of hypopituitarism to endocrine-active syndromes produced by tumors that secrete hypothalamic-releasing factors. Tumors that affect the physiology of the appropriate nuclei in the hypothalamus or of the pituitary stalk can result in diabetes insipidus. Finally, hypothalamic hamartomas that present in the interpeduncular fossa are also associated with precocious puberty. In a report of 33 children with optic chiasmatic-hypothalamic tumors, 5 (14%) of 33 presented with symptoms of endocrine dysfunction and 14 (56%) of 25 demonstrated endocrine abnormalities on laboratory evaluation. Growth hormone deficiency was the most common abnormality, followed by precocious puberty, delayed puberty, and diabetes insipidus. In addition, 7 (21%) of 33 patients failed to thrive and had the diencephalic syndrome (Rodriguez et al., 1990), which is characterized by severe emaciation and an inability to gain weight even when caloric intake is adequate (Russell, 1951).

Evaluations of endocrine function in children with diencephalic syndrome usually reveal normal thyroid function and elevated levels of cortisol and growth hormone. Usually the child is young at the time of diagnosis and frequently has been subjected to extensive failure-to-thrive evaluations before the diagnosis is made. Because the only neurologic findings on examination may be decreased visual acuity, visual field cuts, optic atrophy, or nystagmus, which are difficult to evaluate in a child younger than 3 years, these signs may be overlooked in a less than thorough examination.

The association of optic nerve gliomas with neurofibromatosis is well known. Optic nerve gliomas ac-

Table 5–1. Optic Pathway/Hypothalamic Tumors Referred to the Pediatric Brain Tumor Clinic at The University of Texas M. D. Anderson Cancer Center, 1980 to 1993*

	No.	%
Demographics		
Total	60	100
Neurofibromatosis (NF)	31	54
Male	34	57
Female	26	43
Symptoms at diagnosis		
Decreased visual acuity or blindness	28	47
Visual field deficit	12	20
Nausea/vomiting	17	46
Headache	19	32
Failure to thrive and diencephalic syndrome	6	10
Behavioral problems (irritability, social withdrawal, somnolence, aggressive behavior)	12	20
No symptoms with NF	12	7
Endocrine complaints	4	7
Radiographic findings		
Multilobular suprasellar-optic chiasmal masses	35	58
Optic nerve and chiasmal swelling	17	32
Isolated optic nerve	6	10
Hydrocephalus	23	38

*Median age at diagnosis was 5.2 (range, 0.75 to 14.3) years.

count for only 4% to 8% of all brain tumors in childhood (Pollock, 1994), but as many as 70% of the optic nerve glioma cases are found in individuals with neurofibromatosis type 1 (Stern et al., 1979). In a prospective study of children referred to a neurofibromatosis clinic who had no specific ocular complaints, 15% were found to have optic nerve gliomas, 30% unilateral, 30% bilateral, and 40% involving the optic chiasm (Listernick et al., 1989). In addition, all children who had plexiform neurofibromas of the eyelid and glaucoma were found through comprehensive neuroimaging to have optic nerve gliomas. Whether the natural history of these tumors in children with neurofibromatosis is the same or different from the rest of the population remains controversial.

Prognosis and Natural History

The natural history of optic pathway tumors has been debated for nearly a century, with some early investigators (Hoyt and Baghdassarian, 1969) believing that these tumors are not neoplasms, but rather are hamartomas that do not grow continuously. From the literature, however, it is clear that the clinical course of optic pathway tumors can be quite variable, ranging from rare reports of spontaneous tumor regression (Brzowski et al., 1992), to tumors that remain stable for life, as suggested by Hoyt and Baghdassarian (1969), to aggressive tumors that over time carry considerable risk of visual loss and death (Alvord and Lofton, 1988). Several factors have now been identified that at diagnosis predict favorable and poor outcomes (Kanamori et al., 1985). Table 5–2 summarizes these factors.

Most investigators have divided optic pathway tumors into two groups: anterior optic nerve gliomas with isolated optic nerve enlargement and posterior optic nerve gliomas with optic chiasmal involvement. Ten to 20 year survival rates are excellent (approximately 90%) for patients with optic nerve tumors (Weiss et al., 1987) and more variable (40%

Table 5–2. Classification of Optic Glioma by Factors Influencing Prognosis

	FAVORABLE PROGNOSIS
Age at onset	Early childhood to adolescence
Clinical features	Visual loss with laterality
	Slowly progressive or arrested course
	Incidental finding in child with neurofibromatosis
	No symptoms of endocrine dysfunction or hydrocephalus
	Does not have diencephalic syndrome
Radiographic features	Intrinsic optic nerve and/or chiasmal location
	POOR PROGNOSIS
Age at onset	Infancy to early childhood and adulthood
Clinical feature	Hypothalamic symptoms and/or signs of increased intracranial pressure
	Severely affected vision in both eyes
Radiographic features	Large exophytic chiasmal tumor with posterior extension
	Extension into third ventricle
	Hydrocephalus

Adapted from Kanamori et al. (1985) and Alvord and Lofton (1988).

to 90%) for those with optic chiasmal tumors (Packer et al., 1983; Pierce et al., 1990; Horwich and Bloom, 1985; Tao et al., 1997). Upon careful examination, it can be observed that chiasmal involvement that is not extensive and not associated with a large exophytic mass may also carry an excellent prognosis. The characteristics of tumors with the worst prognosis include early onset in infancy, hypothalamic symptoms, signs of hydrocephalus, presence of diencephalic syndrome, third ventricular involvement, and large chiasmal tumors extending posteriorly. It is most difficult to determine the best treatment for young children with these characteristics because aggressive treatment with surgery and irradiation do not necessarily lead to the best survival rates or the best quality of life (Jannoun and Bloom, 1990).

In evaluating the effects of the tumor itself and the treatment of optic chiasmal gliomas, the series from San Francisco (Hoyt and Baghdassarian, 1969; Imes and Hoyt, 1986) is useful because of its long-term follow-up period and its evaluation of the actual causes of death. In the original 1969 report, 8 of 28 patients were dead, and at follow up 15 years later 8 more had died, leaving only 12 (46%) of 28 surviving at a median follow up of 20 years. Nine of the 16 deaths occurred in patients with neurofibromatosis; only two of these patients had died of their chiasmal tumors. The remaining died of other malignant gliomas of the brain, neurofibrosarcomas of peripheral nerves, or complications of management of cervical neurofibromas. Of the seven who died without neurofibromatosis, five died as a result of tumor and three died of unrelated medical illnesses. Of those patients treated with radiation, 4 of 14 patients died because of their tumor, whereas only 5 of 14 who did not receive radiation died, 1 from tumor and 4 from other causes.

On the basis of these data, no benefit from radiotherapy (RT) could be demonstrated. In addition, the risk of death from tumor was greatest in the early follow-up period. However, most other investigators have concluded that RT does improve survival and does prolong the interval before disease progression (Alvord and Lofton, 1988; Pierce et al., 1990; Horwich and Bloom, 1985; Tao et al., 1997). For example, in a series of 26 children with chiasmal gliomas treated with RT at the Joint Center for Radiation Therapy, 60% had objective tumor shrinkage that occurred gradually over a period of 5 years. Vision either improved or stabilized in 72.7% of the children. The 15 year overall survival rate was 85.1% and freedom from progression was 82.1%, with median follow up of 108 months (Tao et al., 1997).

Management of Optic Gliomas

The literature abounds with inconsistencies, controversy, and disparate conclusions about the prognosis, natural history, and management of optic pathway gliomas. Although only 4% to 8% of childhood brain tumors originate from the optic tract, the potential morbidity of these tumors and their treatment in the face of good survival rates has resulted in extensive literature about the best forms of treatment to optimize cure rates and minimize morbidity. However, because of the relative infrequency of occurrence of these tumors and their heterogeneous behavior related to patient age and tumor location and size, most series have not reported numbers adequate to allow definitive conclusions about this relatively rare subgroup of gliomas, and randomized trials could not be conducted with them. Furthermore, as Sutton et al. (1995) aptly stated, "It is unlikely that any single modality (surgery, RT, or chemotherapy) will be the optimum treatment for all children with hypothalamic/chiasmatic astrocytoma. The challenge for the future is to determine the most appropriate treatment for each patient, based on rate of tumor progression, age, radiographic demonstration of extension of tumor, prior therapy, and visual/endocrine status." It is therefore extremely difficult to arrive at any "standard recommended treatment" for these tumors. Recognizing that controversies exist, we have adapted the following guidelines for the evaluation, treatment, and follow up of children with optic pathway gliomas.

Diagnosis

The evaluation of patients with optic pathway gliomas involves a thorough family history, an accurate assessment of visual status, evaluation for signs and symptoms of increased intracranial pressure, and delineation of the patient's endocrine status, looking for both hypopituitarism and endocrine-active syndromes. Physical examination should be directed toward these points, noting the presence of papilledema or optic atrophy, deficiencies in visual acuity or visual fields, and the general intellectual and neurologic state of the patient. Careful attention should be paid to growth and development parameters and to the presence of any lesions suggestive of neurofibromatosis or tuberous sclerosis. For asymptomatic children with neurofibromatosis with no previous diagnosis of optic glioma, routine screening with imaging or visual evoked potentials is not warranted, and tests should be determined by findings on clinical examination (Gutmann et al., 1997).

Diagnostic evaluation consists of appropriate laboratory testing, including measurement of pertinent pituitary hormones, a formal visual examination and measurement of acuity and visual fields, and imaging diagnosis, which currently rests on magnetic resonance imaging (MRI) with gadolinium enhancement for the most accurate delineation of the lesions involved.

In children with neurofibromatosis and optic nerve enlargement, characteristic findings on MRI or computed tomography (CT) scans are adequate to allow diagnosis. Unless there is a history of acute visual loss or neurologic changes, these such patients can be evaluated and followed up for objective evidence of progression. The baseline and follow-up evaluations should include complete physical and neurologic examination, careful ophthalmologic examination, including visual fields and MRI, or CT scan evaluations. The MRI scan is superior to the CT scan for detecting change, relationship of tumor to the optic chiasm, and tumor extension into adjacent brain. Visual evoked potentials can be useful if the baseline value is normal and can be very sensitive in detecting disease progression. Once vision is impaired, however, we have not found the visual evoked potentials to be very useful, especially when visual field defects are present. Unfortunately, for young, uncooperative children the visual evoked potential studies were not as useful as we had hoped. For very young children, the most useful evaluation of vision appears to be that performed by a child neurologist or pediatric ophthalmologist.

At diagnosis, it is often unclear from the patient's history how rapidly visual change is occurring; therefore, for the first 6 months to 1 year, we perform radiographic and physical examinations every 3 months. If no change is observed, evaluation intervals can be safely decreased to yearly. For children without neurofibromatosis, these guidelines can also be followed in cases of isolated optic nerve enlargement. When tumor progression is identified, options for further treatment include surgery, radiation, and chemotherapy. The pros and cons of these approaches are discussed separately.

Surgery

When a suprasellar mass is present at diagnosis, surgical resection or biopsy is usually recommended.

The extent of resection depends on the extent and location of the tumor. A biopsy is necessary to confirm the diagnosis in patients who present with a suprasellar-hypothalamic mass. Frequently, the origin of the tumor cannot be determined by radiography, and craniopharyngiomas may be indistinguishable from suprasellar germinomas. Because management of these two entities differs somewhat, a definitive diagnosis is needed.

In addition, careful surgical removal from the chiasm of the portion of the tumor that is exophytic can sometimes improve vision by relieving external pressure on the adjacent optic nerve (Oakes, 1990). Sometimes surgical debulking can also relieve hydrocephalus. These goals must, however, be balanced against the risks of increased visual loss and increased postoperative hypothalamic dysfunction, which can result in a disturbed sleep–wake cycle, distorted appetite and thirst, hyperactivity, memory dysfunction, and panhypopituitarism.

The indication for surgery varies with the type and location of the tumors affecting the optic pathways. For the typical unilateral optic nerve glioma located within the orbit, the indication for surgery is progressive visual loss and progressive proptosis. Surgery is generally the treatment of choice when there is loss of vision in an eye without extension of tumor into the chiasm. Surgical excision of the lesion when it has not reached the optic chiasm can be curative, but the eye remains blind. Current surgical techniques allow for preservation of the globe and a good cosmetic result. Patients known to have optic nerve gliomas with little proptosis and preserved functional vision can be evaluated with periodic imaging studies and visual assessments. If there is any evidence of the tumor extending toward the optic chiasm, treatment should be planned early. When surgery is indicated, the operation involves a frontal craniotomy and unroofing of the orbit, sectioning of the optic nerve at its junction with the globe, and removal of the optic nerve, including its intracanalicular segment up to its junction with the optic chiasm. Results are excellent provided that the tumor is totally excised and the remaining optic nerve is free of disease.

Astrocytomas that involve the optic chiasm cannot be resected without causing significant visual impairment. Unfortunately, the characteristics of this type of tumor, as shown by neuroimaging scans, are still not specific enough to allow a histologic diagnosis without biopsy. In these cases, the goal is to perform a safe but effective biopsy of the lesion without producing additional visual impairment. This is ordinarily accomplished with a frontotemporal type of craniotomy using microsurgical techniques for the tumor biopsy. Some tumors in this region are large enough so that the exophytic component extending from the chiasm produces obstructive hydrocephalus; in such cases, a tumor debulking that preserves the portion involving the optic chiasm can be accomplished to relieve the ventricular obstruction. This procedure can be performed accurately and safely using careful microsurgical techniques. There are reports of very satisfactory results of removal of some hypothalamic hamartomas using similar techniques, with reversal of some of the endocrine deficits, particularly precocious puberty.

Despite the risks, several neurosurgical groups have advocated radical resection as primary treatment for children with hypothalamic gliomas. Wisoff et al. (1990) reported a series of 16 children with chiasmatic-hypothalamic tumors treated with radical resection, with 11 of 16 "alive and well" 4 months to 4.5 years after surgery, most without other therapy. Infants were most likely to progress after surgery and require other therapy. It is evident that significant surgical judgment and skill are necessary to deal with these difficult lesions, as the dysfunction produced by overzealous resections can have serious, life-threatening consequences, such as memory loss, inappropriate thirst, and severe diabetes insipidus, which can ultimately result in an individual's requiring constant care. In addition, of 11 children with diencephalic syndrome after surgical intervention in an M. D. Anderson Cancer Center series (Manera et al., 1994), 9 (82%) eventually became obese and suffered multiple endocrine deficits. The progression to morbid obesity and endocrine deficits can also occur after RT and during the natural course of tumor progression, but the manifestation is usually not acute.

When the tumor is infiltrative, extensive, and difficult to remove in bulk, hydrocephalus may be treated with a shunting procedure. Depending on the circumstances, one can consider either a ventriculoperitoneal or a ventriculocisternal (Torkildsen) type of shunt procedure.

In summary, we recommend a conservative surgical approach primarily for diagnosis. Once the diagnosis is made, children who exhibit favorable characteristics are followed up until signs of tumor progression occur. For those who show unfavorable characteristics (Table 5–2), either RT or chemotherapy is recommended for most, depending on the age of the individual. For patients who have extensive tumors invading the hypothalamus, extending to the third ventricular region, with massive infiltration along the optic tracts, or with clear-cut evidence of rapidly progressive disease at the time of diagnosis, a delay in treatment is not recommended. However, in those few cases of tumors where surgical decompression and improvement of vision have occurred, especially in young children, very close follow up without intervention until objective signs of progression occur is also an acceptable alternative.

Radiation

Most modern reports utilizing megavoltage RT document an advantage for patients who have progressive chiasmal gliomas (Pierce et al., 1990; Horwich and Bloom, 1985; Wong et al., 1987; Tao et al., 1997). Radiation therapy is generally the treatment of choice for symptomatic chiasmatic/hypothalamic gliomas in older children. Many recent series report excellent survival after RT—generally 90% at 10 years (Pierce et al., 1990; Horwich and Bloom, 1985; Tao et al., 1997). However, deaths can occur from disease progression many years after treatment, and, thus, long-term follow up is critical in the management of this disease.

Outcome in terms of vision is an important measure of treatment success for chiasmal/hypothalamic gliomas. Following RT, vision is improved in approximately one-third of patients, with most patients experiencing visual stabilization (Pierce et al., 1990; Tao et al., 1997). This success in maintaining or improving vision is possible only if treatment is initiated before severe visual damage has occurred. Therefore, documented visual deterioration is a major indication for the prompt initiation of therapy.

The overall survival rate for patients with optic system gliomas is excellent. However, conventional RT has been associated with significant morbidity. Most radiation fields cover not only the tumor bed (tumor volume) but also tissues thought to be at risk for microscopic disease to allow for uncertainty in tumor definition and for inconsistencies in the daily treatment set-up (target volume). The tolerance of the normal brain parenchyma and its vascular and supporting structures becomes, therefore, the limiting parameter of external-beam therapy, and the risks of acute and long-term sequelae are major dose-limiting factors. Permanent radiation injury can include pituitary-hypothalamic dysfunction as well as memory and intellectual deficits. Young children are at greater risk than adults (Glauser and Packer, 1991; Ellenberg et al., 1987; Ater et al., 1999). After irradiation, 72% of children treated at the Joint Center for Radiation Therapy developed new onset of hypopituitarism, most commonly growth hormone deficiency in 59%, with panhypopituitarism in 21% (Tao et al., 1997).

With conventional fractionation schedules (1.8 Gy/day), total doses of 50 to 54 Gy are considered standard for the treatment of optic gliomas. Late effects appear in a predictable manner in terms of radiation dose, volume, and fractionation. Fractionation exploits the differences in response to irradiation between normal brain and tumor tissue; normal tissues tolerate multiple small doses of irradiation much better than they tolerate a single, large fraction.

Until recently, greater precision in the delivery of conventional RT was limited by an incomplete diagnostic definition of tumor volumes, unsophisticated treatment planning systems, and imprecise immobilization devices. Computed tomography and MRI now provide much improved delineation of CNS neoplasms, and three-dimensional treatment planning systems are currently available. These technological advances allow for accurate focal administration of a dose to the target area and have thus promoted the widespread use of radiosurgery techniques.

Stereotactic Radiosurgery

Stereotactic radiosurgery is a highly accurate and precise technique that utilizes stereotactically directed convergent beams of ionizing radiation to treat a small and distinct volume of tissue with a single radiation dose. The multiple-beam approach of radiosurgery results in sharp dose fall-off beyond the target, thus sparing adjacent normal tissue. The technique must, however, be reserved for select small lesions because it ablates both normal and abnormal tissue within the treatment volume. Some investigators have advocated using stereotactic radiosurgery to reduce the treatment volumes of discrete, well-circumscribed lesions, although certain parameters, including the size and location of the target volume, are associated with complications from radiosurgery (Marks and Spencer, 1991; Loeffler and Alexander, 1993; Tishler et al., 1993). Certain intracranial lesions cannot be treated safely or effectively with radiosurgery once the target volume becomes relatively large or is located near brain stem, retina, and the optic pathways. For example, the maximum radiation tolerance of the optic nerve appears to be between 8 and 10 Gy; if more than 1 cm of the eighth nerve is treated with radiosurgery, hearing loss is predictable even with doses as low as 15 Gy (Tishler et al., 1993). Kjellberg and others have published isoeffect data predicting the incidence rates of brain necrosis using a proton facility (Kjellberg et al., 1983; Flickinger, 1989). These isoeffect curves demonstrate the relationship between tumor necrosis, radiation dose, and field size and demonstrate the limitations of using large single fractions for intracranial lesions that involve critical structures such as the optic system. Therefore, although stereotactic radiosurgery is precise in the administration of large single fractions, complications associated with larger volumes (greater than 3 cm) and with certain locations (brain stem, visual pathways) limit the use of this procedure in the primary management of pediatric tumors, particularly in the management of patients with optic pathway tumors.

Stereotactic Radiotherapy

Fractionation of the daily dose of radiation combined with the precision of radiosurgical techniques may be the optimal way to treat relatively small, symptomatic optic tumors that do not show extensive involvement along the optic tracts. Stereotactic RT is defined as the use of stereotactic radiosurgery hardware and software (stereotactic head frame and support system, small-field collimators, and three-dimensional planing) combined with radiation routine fractionation (1.8 Gy/day) or some form of altered fractionation such as hypofractionation (a few large fractions of 4.0 to 8.0 Gy). Basic requirements necessary to administer stereotactic RT include specially designed software and reproducible repeat head fixation and localization systems.

Dose-optimization treatment using stereotactic RT or other conformal techniques has now become routine for lesions that are well controlled by conventional RT. These RT techniques may become the treatment of choice for many diseases such as incompletely resected craniopharyngioma, pituitary adenoma, and small optic pathway tumors. The radiation dose to nearby nontarget volume structures vital for memory (mesial temporal lobe), for endocrine function (hypothalamic-pituitary axis), and for normal structural development (skull, mandible, and soft tissues of the scalp) is markedly reduced with these techniques. This technique of dose optimization is particularly important in the pediatric population. For many pediatric intracranial tumors, focal RT techniques will largely replace conventional RT in order to reduce the long-term side effects of therapy (Dunbar et al., 1994; Loeffler et al., 1999).

In general, the use of stereotactic techniques as definitive treatment should be restricted to lesions that *(1)* are distinct on imaging scans, *(2)* are of relatively small volume, and *(3)* are noninvasive or noninfiltrating. Although stereotactic techniques do not replace large-field RT in the treatment of widely infiltrating or seeding tumors, it is clear that conventional RT is no longer "acceptable" for a large subgroup of patients who have more focal intracranial tumors.

Chemotherapy for Optic Chiasmal Tumors

The use of chemotherapy for low-grade astrocytomas in children, especially optic chiasmal-hypothalamic tumors, has been investigated at several medical centers. In 1977, Packer and the group at Children's Hospital of Philadelphia started to treat patients younger than 6 years of age newly diagnosed with intracranial visual pathway gliomas with combination chemotherapy. Their justification for this approach was that the beneficial effects of radiation on vision could not be confirmed in their patient population as only 1 of 21 children demonstrated visual improvement after RT (Packer et al., 1983). In addition, these investigators found that progressive neurologic deterioration and visual loss did occur in patients who received radiation late in the course of their disease, usually 5 to 10 years after diagnosis.

Between 1977 and 1988, 32 children younger than 6 years of age were treated with vincristine and actinomycin D chemotherapy as initial therapy after diagnosis. At last report, 10 (31%) remained free of progressive disease and had not required additional therapy (Janss et al., 1995). For those whose disease progressed, the median time was 27 months after the initiation of treatment. Ten year overall survival for the entire group was 85% because of the success of salvage treatment.

Various chemotherapeutic agents, including lomustine; vincristine; a combination of procarbazine, lomustine, and vincristine; and cisplatin-containing combinations, have been somewhat effective in patients with recurrent low-grade gliomas (Edwards et al., 1980) and have been utilized for optic chiasmal tumors. In an M. D. Anderson Cancer Center trial of nitrogen mustard, vincristine, procarbazine, and prednisone (MOPP) given to children younger than 3 years of age with low-grade astrocytomas; six children either had hypothalamic or brain stem lesions. With a median follow up of more than 7 years, all patients survived with stable disease. However, five of six eventually received RT for tumor progression at a median of 1 year after diagnosis (Ater et al., 1988).

Combination chemotherapy with 6-thioguanine, procarbazine, dibromodulcitol, lomustine, and vincristine has been substituted effectively for RT for children with chiasmal and hypothalamic astrocytomas. Investigators at the University of California at San Francisco (Petronio et al., 1991) initially reported results for 19 infants and children (median age, 3.2 years) with chiasmal and hypothalamic gliomas who received chemotherapy, 12 at diagnosis and 7 at the time of tumor progression. Most received 6-thioguanine, procarbazine, dibromodulcitol, lomustine, and vincristine chemotherapy, and two received other combinations. Of the 18 patients with evaluable disease initially managed with chemotherapy, tumors in 15 (83%) either responded to therapy or stabilized. With a median follow-up period of 18 months, all are surviving; disease progressed in only 4 of 15 and was successfully treated with radiation. Vision initially improved or stabilized in 16 (88%) patients. This series was updated in 1997 and now includes a group of 42 children with a mean age of 5 years. The median time to progression was 132 weeks, with a 5 year survival rate of 78% (95% CI, 60% to 87%) (Prados et al., 1997).

In low-grade hypothalamic and chiasmal gliomas, the criteria used to evaluate the usefulness of the chemotherapy are different from those in the usual phase II studies that assess tumor response. For low-grade astrocytomas, prolonged stable disease has been considered a "response" by some investigators. Friedman and the Pediatric Oncology Group (1992) studied the response of pediatric brain tumors to carboplatin. Based on results from 13 children with clearly progressive, low-grade astrocytomas of the optic pathway, third ventricle, thalamus and suprasellar region, and temporal region, in which 73% achieved stable disease and one had a partial response, Friedman's group determined that carboplatin is active against low-grade astrocytomas. The duration of stable disease in this subgroup of patients ranged from 3 months to greater than 68 months (median, >40 months).

A multi-institutional group studied the combination of weekly low-dose carboplatin plus vincristine given for low-grade gliomas (Packer et al., 1993, 1997). At the most recent report, 78 children with newly diagnosed progressive low-grade gliomas with a median age of 3.1 years were treated with this regimen. Fifty-eight were chiasmatic-hypothalamic in location, and the remainder occurred in other locations. Forty-five (56%) children had objective tumor response. Tumor response did not correlate with length of disease control. The only significant factor predictive of outcome was age, with a 2-year progression-free survival rate for children younger than 5 years at start of treatment of 81% compared with 58% in older children ($p < 0.01$) (Packer et al., 1997).

Partly because of variability in prognostic factors such as age, the most effective regimen cannot be gleaned from these single-arm studies. Therefore, a national randomized trial in the Children's Cancer Group (CCG) is currently underway testing the efficacy of chemotherapy for progressive low-grade gliomas in children younger than 10 years old, comparing the carboplatin-vincristine regimen to the CCNU-based regimen reported by Prados et al. (1997). Neuropsychological and endocrine outcome of children treated with chemotherapy will also be evaluated in this trial.

Long-term Follow-up and Complications of Therapy

The use of chemotherapy for hypothalamic-chiasmal gliomas is gaining support not only because of the previously mentioned risks of extensive surgery but also because of the consequences of conventional RT. For young patients, there is a risk of increased endocrine deficits and intellectual impairment following RT delivered to the hypothalamic region (Moore et al., 1992; Ater et al., 1997, 1999; Tao et al., 1997). Serial IQ scores before radiation showed no decline, but among those receiving radiation, IQ scores fell a median of 12 points from baseline (Janss et al., 1995). Also, several reports (Rajakulasingam et al., 1979; Mitchell et al., 1991) have recognized the risk of radiation-induced moyamoya vascular change in the suprasellar region, which can result in vasospasm, transient ischemic-type episodes, seizures, and strokes. The actual incidence of moyamoya is not known, but it may be higher than suspected because the symptoms may also be attributed to progressive disease. The risk of moyamoya appears to be related to the patient's age at radiation, and the condition has been seen generally in children receiving radiation before 3 years of age or in association with neurofibromatosis type 1 (Poussaint et al., 1995).

When patients experience new symptoms that suggest progressive disease, especially many years after treatment, MRI or CT scans can provide essential information, but definitively distinguishing progressive disease from another cause can remain difficult. At times the MRI scan can be diagnostic, revealing hemorrhage, stroke, or tumor growth. However, in a report by Epstein et al. (1992), three children with chiasmatic-hypothalamic gliomas who had symptoms of tumor progression 9.5, 11.5, and 2 years after RT were found to have misleading radiographic findings. Neuroradiographic studies including angiography showed large mass lesions. These were presumed to be tumor recurrences and chemotherapy was initiated. However, on autopsy of two and biopsy of the third, the bulk of the mass was found to consist of numerous vessels of variable size. The authors proposed that these lesions probably represented "incorporation of the rich vasculature in the chiasmal region into the tumor, which underwent degeneration secondary to radiation therapy" (Epstein et al., 1992). Further prospective evaluation of the vascular phenomenon associated with these tumors and their treatment is needed.

MENINGIOMAS

Clinical Presentation

Meningiomas can occur anywhere within the cranium and are related to the arachnoid cap cells of the pacchionian granulations, where spinal fluid is absorbed into the venous sinuses. Meningiomas arise from these structures and are attached to the dura. They occur most commonly in females, and several different subtypes of meningioma can specifically affect the visual apparatus and the hypothalamus. Arising peripherally, meningiomas may grow out of the optic nerve sheath itself. These tumors tend to involve the dura of the optic nerve and ultimately strangulate the nerve; they may also occlude the blood supply to the ophthalmic artery. Direct surgery on these tumors usually results in devascularization of the optic nerve and blindness. The indications for surgery are progressive visual loss and proptosis, similar to the scenario with optic nerve gliomas but with a less favorable prognosis, as meningiomas can extend readily from the intraorbital segment of the optic nerve sheath through the optic canal to involve the intracranial dura.

Meningiomas may also arise from the dura around the optic foramen in which case these lesions may strangulate the optic nerve and affect the ophthalmic artery. Both optic nerve sheath meningiomas and meningiomas of the optic foramen can be bilateral. This is most commonly seen in optic foramen meningiomas where tumor cells may bridge from one optic foramen to the other or may arise as two separate, nearly symmetric, lesions around the optic foramen. More common are meningiomas that arise from the dura of the planum sphenoidale or the tuberculum sellae. The former cause optic nerve-type visual loss, compressing the optic nerves from above and pushing them inferiorly. The latter tend to be suprasellar tumors and may affect either the optic nerves or the optic chiasm or both. Some meningiomas arise from the dura of the diaphragma sellae and also act like suprasellar tumors, producing chiasmal-type visual loss and sometimes compressing the pituitary stalk, causing distortions of pituitary-hypothalamic function. Tumors arising from the dura of the inner third of the sphenoid wing commonly involve both the cavernous sinus (and the nerves within it) and the optic nerve on the same side. Patients afflicted with these tumors may present with double vision, ptosis, pupillary abnormalities, and optic nerve-type visual loss.

Management

Diagnosis

As with gliomas affecting the optic nerves and chiasm, patients with meningiomas in similar regions need careful documentation of their visual function and visual fields. Basic laboratory tests that include hormonal evaluations are important. The diagnostic imaging method of choice is an MRI scan with gadolinium contrast, which clearly shows the meningioma and frequently its areas of origin from the dura. Such scans accurately reveal the effects of the tumor on the surrounding anatomy and help guide the surgeon in devising a safe and effective approach.

Surgery

Indications for surgery of meningiomas generally are those of progressive enlargement of the tumor along with the progressive visual and neurologic signs that may accompany such growth. A number of meningiomas reach a certain size and stop growing, so an argument can be made for careful follow up in some cases.

Basic surgical principles include the planning of a craniotomy that provides excellent exposure of the lesion with the ability to protect and preserve normal neurologic structures. Adjuncts such as intraoperative corticosteroids and mannitol to shrink the brain temporarily are most helpful, and the surgery is carried out with precise microsurgical techniques. Occasionally, a laser or ultrasonic surgical aspirator allows the surgeon to manage difficult tumors that may have a very firm consistency.

Because the vast majority of meningiomas are benign, surgery may not be indicated for patients whose vision is preserved without it when curative surgery could produce blindness or other forms of neurologic deficit. In such instances, RT has been beneficial in a reasonable number of patients.

Radiation Therapy

The largest use of radiation for menigiomas has been with conventional RT (Goldsmith et al., 1994). Postoperative RT is indicated for malignant menigiomas, subtotally resected tumors, tumors with atypical histologies, or multiply recurrent meningiomas. Focused radiosurgery also has its role in the management of small meningiomas, and many promising results have been reported (Hakim et al., 1998).

CRANIOPHARYNGIOMA

Clinical Presentation

Craniopharyngiomas are developmental lesions thought to arise from squamous remnants of Rathke's pouch. Although these tumors tend to appear as tumors of childhood, they can actually occur at any age; there are three basic types of clinical presentation that are age related. In childhood, craniopharyngiomas tend to be large, cystic suprasellar lesions that present as failure of growth and development, which are related to the tumor's effects on the hypothalamus. Craniopharyngiomas may also present with progressive visual loss of the chiasmal type along with obstructive hydrocephalus in large lesions that affect the third ventricle. In young adulthood, craniopharyngiomas tend to present in a fashion similar to pituitary adenomas. In women, the amenorrhea-galactorrhea syndrome is a common presentation and may or may not be associated with progressive chiasmal-type visual loss. Men may develop hypopituitarism and impotence along with visual symptoms. In the elderly, these tumors usually present with mental function changes, but may also produce increased intracranial pressure and visual loss.

Management

Diagnosis

Medical evaluation for craniopharyngiomas should include a careful history and physical examination, paying particular attention in children to their growth and development, including secondary sexual characteristics, and to sexual function in older patients. Careful evaluation of the visual system, including visual acuity and visual field determinations, should be carried out. Laboratory evaluation should include a careful review of pituitary hormone status. Because craniopharyngiomas frequently arise from the pituitary stalk, some patients, particularly children, present with diabetes insipidus; appropriate laboratory tests should be ordered if this is one of the features of clinical presentation.

Patients with increased intracranial pressure usually have headaches and may have papilledema. The imaging procedure used for diagnosis is an MRI scan with gadolinium contrast. This modality usually is fairly diagnostic for craniopharyngioma. Because many of these lesions are calcified, a CT scan or even a plain skull X-ray may show the presence and position of calcified portions of the tumor. For the evaluation of postoperative residual disease, CT and MRI scans are often complementary, with CT demonstrating residual calcification (not easily seen on MRI) and MRI most often demonstrating possible residual cystic or solid craniopharnygioma.

Surgery

The surgical principles utilized in the management of craniopharyngioma are a subject of some controversy. It is clear that a proportion of these lesions, particularly cystic lesions in children, can be totally excised. Ordinarily this is accomplished using a craniotomy for those lesions that are suprasellar. The craniotomy procedure utilized to attack a craniopharyngioma can be tailored to the position and extent of the lesion. Subfrontal, frontotemporal (pterional), and a variety of skull base approaches can be utilized to approach and effectively remove these lesions. A scrupulous microsurgical technique is essential and can provide good results in both extent of tumor removal and preservation or restoration of vision. If a craniopharyngioma is associated with significant enlargement of the sella, then the tumor may have had its origin below the diaphragma sella and may be amenable to total removal using the transsphenoidal approach. For these lesions, the size of the sella, whether the tumor is primarily cystic or primarily solid, and whether calcifications are present can be important factors in determining the extent of debulking. Many suprasellar craniopharyngiomas, particularly in older patients, are intimately associated with the floor of the third ventricle, the hypothalamus, and the optic chiasm. In such cases, attempts at total removal can produce significant neurologic damage; thus the surgeon must use good judgment in attempting complete tumor removal. Often, it is better to remove the bulk of the tumor and to treat the small remnants adherent to vital structures with postoperative irradiation.

Radiotherapy

Conventional RT has been effective for craniopharyngiomas (Hetelekidis et al., 1993). For the reasons stated previously, however, conventional RT is not recommended for the immature brain (generally, children 3 years of age or younger). Stereotactic techniques include radiosurgery, stereotactic RT, and direct colloid instillation into cystic craniopharyngiomas. Radiosurgery has been utilized for adjunctive management of craniopharyngiomas. However, because the chiasm is often in close proximity, the same constraints as discussed earlier apply for craniopharyngiomas (Tarbell et al., 1994).

Radiosurgery should only be considered when there is a very small area (less than 2 cm) of residual/recurrent tumor that is away from the optic chiasm. Direct instillation of colloidal radioisotopes into the cysts of primarily cystic tumors appears effective when appropriately applied. This technique has been widely used in Europe with limited experience in the United States. Stereotactic radiation or conformal radiation treatments using conventional fractionation may be the safest mode of treatment for patients with a solid component of residual disease.

REFERENCES

Alvord EC Jr, Lofton S. 1988. Gliomas of the optic nerve or chiasm: outcome by patients' age, tumor site, and treatment. J Neurosurg 68:85–98.

Ater JL, Moore BD, Slopis J, Copeland D. 1999. Neuropsychological effects of focal cranial radiation therapy on children treated for brain tumors. ASCO Proc 18:149A.

Ater JL, van Eys J, Woo SY, et al. 1997. MOPP chemotherapy without irradiation as primary postsurgical therapy for brain tumors in infants and young children. J Neurooncol 32:243–252.

Ater JL, Woo SY, van Eys J. 1988. Update on MOPP chemotherapy as primary therapy for infant brain tumors. Pediatr Neurosci 14:153.

Brzowski AE, Bazan C 3d, Mumma JV, Ryan SG. 1992. Spontaneous regression of optic glioma in a patient with neurofibromatosis. Neurology 42:679–681.

Dunbar SF, Tarbell NJ, Kooy HM, et al. 1994. Stereotactic radiotherapy for pediatric and adult brain tumors: preliminary report. Int J Radiat Oncol Biol Phys 30:531–539.

Dutton JJ. 1991. Optic nerve gliomas and meningiomas. Neurol Clin 9:163–177.

Edwards MS, Levin VA, Wilson CB. 1980. Brain tumor chemotherapy: an evaluation of agents in current use for phase II and III trials. Cancer Treat Rep 64:1179–1205.

Ellenberg L, McComb JG, Siegel SE, Stowe S. 1987. Factors affecting intellectual outcome in pediatric brain tumor patients. Neurosurgery 21:638–644.

Epstein MA, Packer RJ, Rorke LB, et al. 1992. Vascular malformation with radiation vasculopathy after treatment of chiasmatic/hypothalamic glioma. Cancer 70:887–893.

Flickinger JC. 1989. An integrated logistic formula for prediction of complications from radiosurgery. Int J Radiat Oncol Biol Phys 17:879–885.

Friedman HS, Krischer JP, Burger P, et al. 1992. Treatment of children with progressive of recurrent brain tumors with carboplatin or iproplatin: a Pediatric Oncology Group Randomized phase II study. J Clin Oncol 10:249–256.

Glauser TA, Packer RJ. 1991. Cognitive deficits in long-term survivors of childhood brain tumors. Childs Nerv Syst 7:2–12.

Goldsmith BJ, Wara WM, Wilson CB, Larson DA. 1994. Postoperative irradiation for subtotally resected meningiomas: a retrospective analysis of 140 patients treated from 1987 to 1990. J Neurosurg 80:195–201.

Gutmann DH, Aylsworth A, Carey JC, et al. 1997. The diagnostic evaluation and multidisciplinary management of neurofibromatosis 1 and neurofibromatosis 2. JAMA 278:51–57.

Hakim R, Alexander E 3rd, Loeffler JS, et al. 1998. Results of linear accelerator-based radiosurgery for intracranial meningiomas. Neurosurgery 42:446–453.

Hetelekidis S, Barnes PD, Tao ML, et al. 1993. 20-year experience in childhood craniopharyngioma. Int J Radiat Oncol Biol Phys 27:189–195.

Horwich A, Bloom HJ. 1985. Optic gliomas: radiation therapy and prognosis. Int J Radiat Oncol Biol Phys. 11:1067–1079.

Hoyt WF, Baghdassarian SA. 1969. Optic glioma of childhood. Natural history and rationale for conservative management. Br J Ophthalmol 53:793–798.

Imes RK, Hoyt WF. 1986. Childhood chiasmal gliomas: update on the fate of patients in the 1969 San Francisco study. Br J Ophthalmol 70:179–182.

Jannoun L, Bloom HJ. 1990. Long-term psychological effects in children treated for intracranial tumors. Int J Radiat Oncol Biol Phys 18:747–753.

Janss AJ, Grundy R, Cnaan A, et al. 1995. Optic pathway and hypothalamic/chiasmatic gliomas in children younger than 5 years with a 6-year follow-up. Cancer 75:1051–1059.

Kanamori M, Shibuya M, Yoshida J, Takayasu M, Kageyama N. 1985. Long-term follow-up of patients with optic glioma. Childs Nerv Syst 1:272–278.

Kjellberg RN, Hanamura T, Davis KR, Lyons SL, Adams RD. 1983. Bragg-peak proton-beam therapy for arteriovenous malformations of the brain. N Engl J Med 309:269–274.

Listernick R , Charrow J, Greenwald MJ, Esterly NB. 1989. Optic gliomas in children with neurofibromatosis type 1. J Pediatr 114:788–792.

Loeffler JS, Alexander E III. 1993. Radiosurgery for the treatment of intracranial metastases. In: Alexander E III, Loeffler JS, Lunsford LD (eds), Stereotactic Radiosurgery. New York: McGraw-Hill, pp 197–206.

Loeffler JS, Kooy HM, Terbell NJ. 1999. The emergence of conformal radiotherapy: special implications for pediatric neuro-oncology. Int J Radiat Oncol Biol Phys 44:237–238.

Manera RB, Ater JL, Leeds N, et al. 1994. Treatment outcome and neurological, neuroendocrine and neurobehavioral profile of children with supratentorial midline brain tumors. Pediatr Neurosurg 21:265.

Marks LB, Spencer DP. 1991. The influence of volume on the tolerance of the brain to radiosurgery. J Neurosurg 75:177–180.

Mitchell WG, Fishman LS, Miller JH, et al. 1991. Stroke as a late sequela of cranial irradiation for childhood brain tumors. J Child Neurol 6:128–133.

Moore BD 3rd, Ater JL, Copeland DR. 1992. Improved neuropsychological outcome in children with brain tumors diagnosed during infancy and treated without cranial irradiation. J Child Neurol 7:81–290.

Oakes WJ. 1990. Recent experience with the resection of pilocytic astrocytomas of the hypothalamus. In: AE Marlin (ed), Concepts in Pediatric Neurosurgery, vol 10. Basel: Karger, pp 108–117.

Packer RJ, Ater J, Allen J, et al. 1997. Carboplatin and vincristine chemotherapy for children with newly diagnosed progressive low-grade gliomas. J Neurosurg 86:747–754.

Packer RJ, Lange B, Ater J, et al. 1993. Carboplatin and vincristine for recurrent and newly diagnosed low-grade gliomas of childhood. J Clin Oncol 11:850–856.

Packer RJ, Savino PJ, Bilaniuk LT, et al. 1983. Chiasmatic gliomas of childhood. A reappraisal of natural history and effectiveness of cranial irradiation. Childs Brain 10:393–403.

Petronio J, Edwards MS, Prados M, et al. 1991. Management of chiasmal and hypothalamic gliomas of infancy and childhood with chemotherapy. J Neurosurg 74:701–708.

Pierce SM, Barnes PD, Loeffler JS, McGinn C, Tarbell NJ. 1990. Definitive radiation therapy in the management of symptomatic patients with optic glioma. Cancer 65:45–52.

Pollock IF. 1994. Brain tumors in children. N Engl J Med 331:1500–1507.

Poussaint TY, Siffert J, Barnes PD, et al. 1995. Hemorraghic vasculopathy after the treatment of central nervous system neoplasia in childhood: diagnosis and follow-up. Am J Neuroradiol 16:693–699.

Prados MD, Edwards MS, Rabbitt J, Lamborn K, Davis RL, Levin VA. 1997. Treatment of pediatric low-grade gliomas with a nitrosourea-based multiagent chemotherapy regimen. J Neurooncol 32:235–241.

Rajakulasingam K, Cerullo LJ, Raimondi AJ. 1979. Childhood moyamoya syndrome. Postradiation pathogenesis. Childs Brain 5:467–475.

Rodriguez LA, Edwards MS, Levin VA. 1990. Management of hypothalamic gliomas in children: an analysis of 33 cases. Neurosurgery 26:242–246.

Russell A. 1951. A diencephalic syndrome of emaciation in infancy and childhood. Arch Dis Child 26:274–275.

Stern J, DiGiacinto GV, Housespian EM. 1979. Neurofibromatosis and optic glioma: clinical and morphological correlations. Neurosurgery 4:524–528.

Sutton LN, Molloy PT, Sernyak H, et al. 1995. Long-term outcome of hypothalamic/chiasmatic astrocytomas in children treated with conservative surgery. J Neurosurg 83:583–589.

Tao ML, Barnes PD, Billett AL, et al. 1997. Childhood optic chiasm gliomas: radiographic response following radiotherapy and long-term clinical outcome. Int J Radiat Oncol Biol Phys 39:579–587.

Tarbell NJ, Barnes P, Scott RM, et al. 1994. Advances in radiation therapy for craniopharyngiomas. Pediatr Neurosurg 21(suppl 1):101–107.

Tenny RT, Laws ER Jr, Younge BR, Rush JA. 1982. The neurosurgical management of optic glioma. Results in 104 patients. J Neurosurg 57:452–458.

Tishler RB, Loeffler JS, Lunsford LD, et al. 1993. Tolerance of cranial nerves of the cavernous sinus to radiosurgery. Int J Radiat Oncol Biol Phys 27:215–221.

Weiss L, Sagerman RH, King GA, Chung CT, Dubowy RL. 1987. Controversy in the management of optic nerve glioma. Cancer 59:1000–1004.

Wisoff JH, Abbott R, Epstein F. 1990. Surgical management of exophytic chiasmatic-hypothalamic tumors of childhood. J Neurosurg 73:661–667.

Wong JY, Uhl V, Wara WM, Sheline GE. 1987. Optic gliomas. A reanalysis of the University of California, San Francisco experience. Cancer, 60:1847–1855.

6

Tumors of the Brain Stem, Cerebellum, and Fourth Ventricle

ROGER J. PACKER, HENRY S. FRIEDMAN,
LARRY E. KUN, AND GREGORY N. FULLER

The posterior fossa is a small region of brain cradled on all sides by bone and limited above by the tentorium. The brain stem, cerebellum, and fourth ventricle occupy this region of brain. Expansion of a mass in this infratentorial area occurs at the expense of the normal structures in the region and may result in brain stem or cerebellar dysfunction, often associated with blockage of the fourth ventricle and hydrocephalus. Although many different tumor types may arise in the posterior fossa and affect the brain stem, cerebellum, and fourth ventricle, the majority are either medulloblastomas, cerebellar astrocytomas (rarely, higher grade cerebellar glial tumors), brain stem gliomas, or ependymomas. Other tumor types, which may arise less frequently, include choroid plexus papillomas, germ cell tumors, and dermoid lesions. Because tumors do not respect discrete compartmental landmarks, those that arise in the thalamus or suprasellar region can extend inferiorly into the posterior fossa. Similarly, lesions that arise from the spinal cord can extend up into the medullary area and cause symptoms of brain stem dysfunction.

Fewer than 5% of all adult tumors originate in the posterior fossa, whereas approximately 50% of primary central nervous system (CNS) tumors occurring in patients younger than 15 years of age arise in the fourth ventricular region. For unclear reasons, lower grade lesions in children are more frequently found in the posterior fossa than those in adults. Ependymomas, which are more frequent in a supratentorial region in adulthood, are more frequently found in the posterior fossa in childhood.

With the modern neuroimaging techniques, which have replaced previously used tests such as pneumoencephalography and angiography, these tumors can now be diagnosed at earlier stages of disease. Computed tomography (CT) delineates the presence of tumor in greater than 95% of patients with posterior fossa tumors, but, due to bone artifact obfuscation, this technique has limited applicability. For lesions that arise deep within the posterior fossa, especially those at the cervicomedullary junction, and for lesions that infiltrate the brain stem, magnetic resonance imaging (MRI) has become the procedure of choice. The beauty of MRI is that it allows scanning in all planes without reformatting, which makes it easier to anatomically define a lesion in the brain stem or deep in the cerebellum. The extent of the infiltrating component of posterior fossa tumors, especially those that infiltrate the brain stem, are visualized considerably better with MRI than with CT.

The clinical presentation associated with posterior fossa tumors is essentially similar in adults and children. In general, the briefer the history, the more likely the tumor is to be growing rapidly and arising in the axial midline of the posterior fossa, obstructing cerebrospinal fluid (CSF) flow. Late in the course of illness, symptoms usually include increased intracranial pressure, focal neurologic deficits secondary to compromise of brain stem or cerebellar tissue, and meningeal irritation, whereas early in the course of illness nonspecific complaints of vague, intermittent headache, fatigue, and personality change may predominate. The clinical triad of increased intracranial pressure—headache, vomiting, and blurred or double vision—is the hallmark of an infratentorial tumor. Although a classic headache of increased intracranial pressure is common late in the disease, early on the headache may be far less specific. Similarly, vomiting, which occurs in the morning and is associated with relief of head pain, is a footprint of posterior fossa tumors that have obstructed the fourth ventricle. Less frequently, vomiting may occur secondary to tumors that invade or compress the floor of the fourth ventricle, especially in the medullary area. The vomiting pattern from such lesions is usually more constant during the day and is associated with persistent nausea, anorexia, and significant weight loss.

Cerebellar deficits occur in most patients with posterior fossa tumors. In midline lesions, compromise of the anterior and posterior lobes of the cerebellum causes truncal and gait ataxia manifested by unsteadiness when sitting and a staggering gait. Limb ataxia occurs more frequently in lesions that involve the lateral cerebellar hemispheres, most commonly cerebellar astrocytomas. However, brain stem lesions that infiltrate the cerebellar peduncles will frequently cause cerebellar symptomatology.

Other focal neurologic deficits may occur in patients with posterior symptoms. Ocular motor deficits are relatively frequent and tend to be of localizing value, except for a sixth nerve palsy, which may be present secondary to diffuse increased intracranial pressure. Epileptic seizures rarely occur in children or adults with subtentorial tumors except in patients with infiltrating masses that extend into the subcortical areas and in patients with lesions that have disseminated into the nervous system. Alterations in consciousness may occur, but tend to be a late finding. Acute hemorrhage into a posterior fossa tumor may result in acute coma.

Infants and young children with posterior fossa tumors are notoriously difficult to diagnose, although they may have increasing head circumference due to their open sutures and fontanelles.

SPECIFIC TUMORS

Medulloblastoma

Medulloblastomas are common tumors of childhood in the posterior fossa. They typically arise in the vermis but can arise in the cerebellar hemisphere (Fig. 6–1). Medulloblastomas are classic "small round blue cell" tumors in which neoplastic cells may exhibit various organizational patterns, including unstructured sheets, nests, and cords. Four named morphologic variants are recognized by the current WHO classification: classic medulloblastoma, desmoplastic medulloblastoma, medulloblastoma with extensive nodularity and advanced neuronal differentiation, and large cell medulloblastoma. In addition, there are two very rare related neoplasms: melanotic medulloblastoma and medullomyoblastoma (medulloblastoma with skeletal muscle differentiation). All medulloblastoma variants are malignant neoplasms in which mitotic figures are typically numerous and necrosis is often present. Rapid growth with secondary involvement of the fourth ventricle and seeding via CSF pathways is common.

The desmoplastic medulloblastoma, a histologic variant of the medulloblastoma, received its name from the abundance of connective tissue present, which can be seen particularly well with reticulin or Masson trichrome stains. The distinctive appearance of this tumor derives from the contrast of background with scattered circumscribed areas that lack a connective tissue stroma, so-called "pale islands" (Fig. 6–2). Such foci often exhibit glial or neuronal differentiation demonstrated by immunopositivity for glial fibrillary acidic protein or synaptophysin, respectively. The prognostic significance of the desmoplastic variant and glial/neuronal differentiation is not yet known.

In addition to medulloblastoma, another entity in the differential diagnosis of a malignant neoplasm arising in the cerebellum of a young child is atypical teratoid/rhabdoid tumor (ATRT). These neoplasms can resemble medulloblastoma, particularly the large cell medulloblastoma variant. In general ATRTs are more heterogeneous and pleomorphic than medulloblastomas and their immunophenotypic profile is distinctive: All are immunopositive for vimentin, the vast majority (95%) are positive for epithelial membrane antigen (EMA), and a large percentage (60% to 75%) show positivity for smooth muscle antigen.

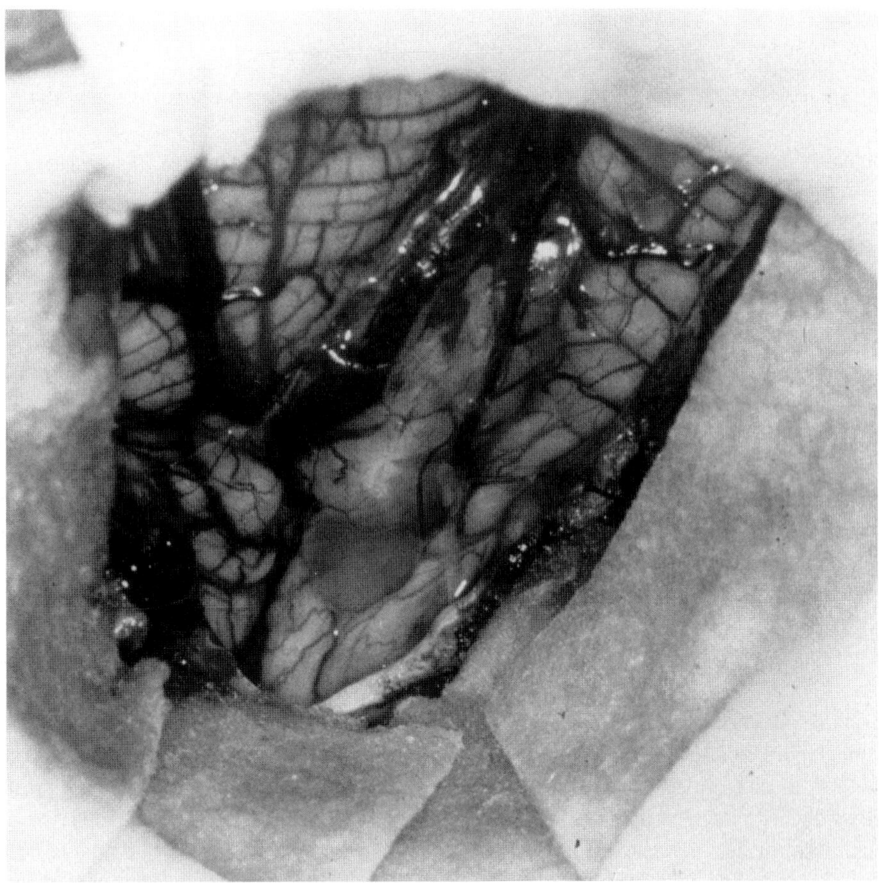

Figure 6–1. Medulloblastoma visible in vermis at time of surgery. Note herniation of cerebellar tonsils.

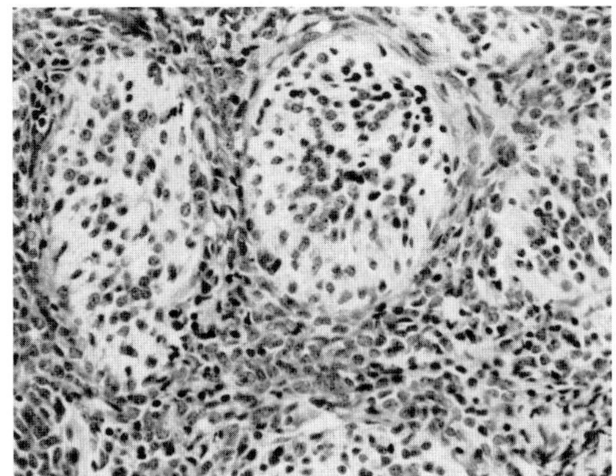

Figure 6–2. Desmoplastic medulloblastoma. Like all medulloblastomas, this variant is composed of small neoplastic cells with hyperchromatic nuclei and scant cytoplasm. In desmoplastic medulloblastomas, there is an abundant reticulin stroma throughout the tumor, except in scattered, roughly spherical, aggregates termed "pale islands," thus imparting a distinctive architectural pattern.

In addition to these markers, a wide range of other antigens may be expressed, including epithelial (keratins) and neural (GFAP, synaptophysin) markers (Kleihues and Cavenee, 2000). ATRTs are aggressive tumors with a tendency for widespread dissemination via cerebrospinal pathways.

Presentation

Patients with medulloblastoma typically present with vomiting, headache, and an ataxic gait (Cushing, 1930). Manifestations of obstruction of the fourth ventricular outlet include vomiting, headache, lethargy, and occasionally papilledema. Vomiting secondary to a medulloblastoma usually occurs when the child awakens in the morning and may precede resolution of complaints for the remainder of the day. Progressive awkwardness and clumsiness, with difficulty standing or walking alone, results from in-

Table 6–1. Staging of Patients with Medulloblastoma

	Average Risk	*Intermediate Risk*	*Poor Risk*
Age (years)	Older than 3 years of age	Older than 3 years of age; less than 3 years of age with increased TrkC	Younger than 3 years of age
Tumor resection	Total/near-total localized	? Partial	Biopsy and/or partial
Extent		? Disseminated with increased TrkC; ? brain stem involvement	Disseminated alone or with ? decreased TrkC

TrkC, type C tyrosine kinase neurotrophin receptor.

? Signifies possible but not conclusively proven to date.

volvement of cerebellar hemispheres. These findings may be more common in adults, as tumors in adults are somewhat more frequently lateral lesions arising in the cerebellopontine angle. Cranial nerve palsies, particularly of the sixth and seventh nerves, may also be seen. In some patients, medulloblastomas will hemorrhage and cause acute neurologic compromise, including coma.

Staging

Staging is one of the cornerstones of managing patients with medulloblastoma (Table 6–1). Approximately one-third of children with medulloblastoma will have disseminated disease at the time of diagnosis, and an even higher percentage of children younger than 2 years of age will manifest such dissemination. The rate of dissemination in adult patients is poorly characterized, but probably occurs in 10% to 20% of patients at diagnosis. As would be expected, disseminated disease carries a poorer prognosis than localized disease (Zeltzer et al., 1999).

Patients with medulloblastoma are staged with either pre- or postoperative MRI of the entire neuraxis, and CSF cytology is generally performed following surgery. Some patients have free-floating tumor cells present after surgery that disappear spontaneously. Positive CSF cytology on studies performed 2 to 3 weeks after surgery has been related with a poorer outcome. Lumbar CSF cytology is more sensitive for detecting free-floating tumor cells than ventricular fluid analysis (Gajjar et al., 1999).

Although, in the past, bone scans and bone marrow examinations were utilized to determine the extent of dissemination, their yield is quite low, and such investigations are now usually limited to those patients at highest risk, including children younger than 3 years of age or those with disseminated disease in the leptomeninges.

Based on staging studies and on the extent of surgical resection, most patients with medulloblastoma can be stratified into two major risk groups. The first includes patients with localized disease at the time of diagnosis and extensive (total or near-total) resections. Such patients are thought to have average-risk disease and constitute approximately 60% to 70% of patients (possibly more in adults) and have a 60% to 65% chance of 5 year progression-free survival (PFS) after treatment with craniospinal and local radiotherapy. Patients with disseminated disease or partially resected tumor have "poor-risk" disease. Patients with "poor-risk" disease have approximately a 40% likelihood of 5 year PFS after treatment with craniospinal and local radiotherapy. The presence of brain stem involvement at the time of diagnosis was initially thought to be of prognostic importance, but in more recent studies brain stem involvement at the time of diagnosis has not been shown to predict outcome (Zeltzer et al., 1999). Age is a powerful predictor of outcome, as younger patients (primarily those younger than 3 years of age at diagnosis) fare poorly. All these factors are affected by treatment, and in some studies the predictive significance of any one parameter or parameters may be abrogated by altering treatment (such as adding chemotherapy). More recently, determination of neurotrophin expression in medulloblastoma tissue has been found to be a strong predictive factor, as patients with higher expression of type C tyrosine kinase neurotrophin receptor (TrkC) have a better prognosis (Grotzer et al., 2000). The predictive interaction between extent of tumor at diagnosis, age, TrkC expression, and treatment is still being delineated.

Surgery

The aim of surgery for medulloblastoma is total removal. Because these tumors are malignant, adjunctive therapy is necessary for their management (Deutsch, 1988; Jenkin et al., 1990; Levin et al., 1988; Rutka et al., 1990). The best results are obtained when the tumor is totally or almost totally removed with no evidence of metastatic deposit (Tomita and McLone, 1986; Zeltzer et al., 1999). Approximately 30% to 50% of children with medulloblastoma will require permanent ventriculoperitoneal shunting after surgery, although some surgeons believe that this need is lessened when patients are diagnosed early and have smaller tumors. Some patients have a transient need for CSF diversion before or immediately after surgery, which can be accomplished by external ventricular drainage. Some surgeons prefer to place a catheter between the third ventricle and cisterna magna at the time of craniectomy and tumor removal (Hoffman et al., 1976) as ventriculoperitoneal shunting is not without complications in this patient population. In addition to the potential for CSF infections, young children may require shunt modification to keep pace with growth, and sometimes their hydrocephalus is associated with extremely low pressure, making incorporation of a valve in the shunting path problematic and shunt revisions a likelihood.

Radiotherapy

The principles of radiotherapy are similar for medulloblastoma, ependymoblastoma, and the putative undifferentiated primitive neuroectodermal tumor (PNET). These tumors classically spread through CSF pathways, suggesting that the role of craniospinal irradiation is to systematically encompass the entire subarachnoid space. Craniospinal irradiation is a technically demanding treatment requiring immobilization in the prone position for all patients except the very young. Therapy includes lateral craniocervical fields adjoined to posterior spinal fields to achieve homogeneous coverage of the neuraxis. Detailed attention to the subfrontal cribriform plate just above the eyes and the lower margin of the temporal fossa challenge the radiation oncologist in reproducibly ensuring appropriate treatment volume while avoiding direct irradiation of the eyes. In addition to craniospinal irradiation, a local posterior fossa boost is utilized to raise the dose to a higher level at the primary site.

The radiation dose for the posterior fossa is relatively well established in medulloblastoma based on the relative radiosensitivity of these tumors and the clinical observation in local posterior fossa disease that tumor control is optimal following doses of 54 to 55 Gy (Silverman and Simpson, 1982; Fertil and Malaise, 1985; Hughes et al., 1988; Jenkin et al., 1990).

Several recent studies confirming long-term survival in more than 50% of patients with medulloblastoma utilized craniospinal irradiation doses of 35 to 40 Gy to the neuraxis (Bloom et al., 1990; Jenkin et al., 1990; Halberg et al., 1991). The suggestion that a reduced neuraxis dose can provide equivalent disease control with potentially less late morbidity in selected "average-risk" populations (grossly resected, localized disease of limited extent) has been tested by two North American pediatric cooperative groups. A study conducted by the Pediatric Oncology Group and the Childrens Cancer Group demonstrated a higher rate of leptomeningeal disease control following 23.4 Gy craniospinal irradiation compared with the standard 36 Gy dose (Deutsch et al., 1996). However, further analysis revealed less of a difference in long-term disease control between patients treated with reduced-dose radiotherapy and those treated with conventional-dose craniospinal radiotherapy (Thomas et al., 1995).

The relative radiosensitivity of medulloblastoma and the exquisite relationship between dose per fraction and neurotoxicity suggest that hyperfractionated irradiation may be useful in treating this tumor (van der Kogel, 1991); but, to date, such trials have not demonstrated added efficacy (Allen et al., 1996; Kun et al., 1990; Prados et al., 1994; Prados et al., 1999).

Chemotherapy

Medulloblastoma is one of the more chemosensitive brain tumors of the pediatric population (Friedman and Oakes, 1987; Friedman et al., 1992). Nevertheless, results of three large randomized studies evaluating adjuvant chemotherapy have shown only modest benefits of this modality confined to patients with advanced disease (Evans et al., 1990; Tait et al., 1990; Krischer et al., 1991). Disappointment with these results must be tempered by recognition that all three studies included inadequately staged patients and incorporated chemotherapeutic agents now known to possess dubious anti-medulloblastoma activity.

Data from extensive preclinical studies with a panel of human medulloblastoma cell lines and transplantable xenografts in athymic mice as well as a series of phase II trials have confirmed the activity of cisplatin, cyclophosphamide, and melphalan against medulloblastoma (Friedman and Oakes, 1987; Friedman et al., 1988, 1989). Furthermore, current biochemical studies have revealed mechanisms underlying the limited activity of other agents used in the treatment of medulloblastoma. The minimal activity of nitrosoureas against medulloblastoma is due in large part to the high levels of O6-alkylguanine-DNA alkyltransferase (the protein that repairs methylating and chloroethylating agent-induced adducts) seen in this tumor (Schold et al., 1989; Mineura et al., 1993; Chen et al., 1992; He et al., 1992). The remarkable disease-free survival in children with poor-risk medulloblastoma treated with radiotherapy plus CCNU-cisplatin-vincristine (Packer et al., 1988, 1994b) presumably reflects the extraordinary activity of cisplatin. This study, albeit a single-arm trial with controversial criteria for high-risk assignment, considerably strengthens the belief that chemotherapy should play an important role in treating medulloblastoma in children. A randomized study performed by the German Oncology Group recently confirmed the "excellent" survival rate after treatment with radiotherapy and chemotherapy during and after radiation (Kortmann et al., 2000). To date, no chemotherapy trial has demonstrated a survival benefit for patients treated with pre-radiation chemotherapy (Zeltzer et al., 1999; Kuhl et al., 1998).

The apparent efficacy of chemotherapy in poor or high-risk disease has led some to postulate that combined chemotherapy and reduced-dose craniospinal irradiation may achieve effective disease control in selected average-risk medulloblastoma patients (Kun and Constine, 1991). A recent study completed by the Childrens Cancer Group demonstrated an 80% disease-free survival rate at 3 years after treatment with 23.4 Gy of craniospinal radiotherapy and post-radiotherapy chemotherapy with CCNU, vincristine, and cisplatinum (Packer et al., 1999). The current prospective, randomized Childrens Cancer Group and Pediatric Oncology Group trial is testing combined therapy with reduced-dose craniospinal irradiation (23.4 Gy) with one of two post-radiotherapy chemotherapy regimens for children with average-risk disease. The balance of survival and late treatment-related toxicities will be tested in the prospective clinical trial.

A prospective randomized trial in children with poor-risk disease, comparing CCNU and vincristine chemotherapy to pre-irradiation chemotherapy with the "8-drug-in-1-day" (8-in-1) regimen, has recently been completed. Patients who received the 8-in-1 regimen fared least well (Zeltzer et al., 1999). Other trials that have recently been completed utilizing even higher dose chemotherapy regimens have also not been beneficial (Kuhl et al., 1998). Concomitantly, among children with recurrent medulloblastoma, a subgroup of patients manifests long-term disease control after treatment with high-dose chemotherapy, especially thiotepa-based regimens (Finlay et al., 1996). These patients usually have localized disease at the time of relapse and/or tumors that can be totally resected after relapse.

These studies have resulted in a generation of trials utilizing chemotherapy at higher doses either during or after irradiation in children with poor-risk disease. Trials are ongoing with carboplatin during irradiation, and another trial is now being performed utilizing high-dose chemotherapy, a thiotepa-based regimen with peripheral stem cell rescue support.

Data from the experience with chemotherapy as the primary treatment for medulloblastoma, gathered from children younger than 3 years of age, have been disappointing. Treatment taking the Pediatric Oncology Group ("Baby POG") approach, with alternating cycles of cyclophosphamide, vincristine, and cisplatin VP-16, and studies utilizing a higher dose of treatment by the Childrens Cancer Group, have demonstrated that approximately 20% to 40% of patients, primarily those with localized disease at the time of diagnosis, can be treated with chemotherapy alone (Duffner et al., 1993; Geyer et al., 1994; Packer et al., 1998). For those patients with disseminated disease at the time of diagnosis, chemotherapy-alone regimens have resulted in much poorer disease control. Although many patients treated with chemotherapy will fail after completing treatment, leading to suggestions that radiation therapy be given after a finite period of chemotherapy, a subgroup will fail during chemotherapy, and a subgoup will fail during maintenance chemotherapy. The utility of maintenance chemotherapy for infants who have apparently responded to higher dose induction chemotherapy is questionable. Children with atypical teratoid tumors, who are usually younger than 3 years of age, fare poorly with any form of chemotherapy or radiotherapy (Rorke et al., 1996). More complex regimens utilizing high-dose chemotherapy have not yet been shown to be more effective than less-aggressive regimens (such as the MOPP regimen utilizing mechlorethamine, vincristine, prednisone and procarbazine) (Baram et al., 1987). Studies of high-dose chemotherapy in newly diagnosed patients with peripheral stem cell rescue are being completed. Future therapies are likely to be coupled with focal radiation therapy (Guruangan et al., 1998) or intrathecal chemotherapy to maximize disease control (Dupuis-Girod et al., 1996).

Adult Medulloblastoma

As is the case with children, an increase in 5 and 10 year survival rates has occurred in adults through improved neuroimaging techniques, safer surgery, more precise high-energy radiotherapy equipment, and better chemotherapies (Levin et al., 2001). Statistics gathered on patient survival during the past 40 years are limited by the use of retrospective data analyzed over decades and the different methods and parameters that were applied. Patients in earlier series not only were incompletely staged by today's standards, but, for the purposes of statistical analysis, this limitation is compounded by the myriad treatments that were used in different series. Taken together, these inconsistencies obfuscate the meaningfulness and predictive importance of factors such as extent of resection or tumor spread. Furthermore, treatment of medulloblastoma in adults has not been as well established in clinical trials as it has in children. Whereas this may reflect the increased frequency of occurrence of medulloblastoma in children, another factor is the impact that Childrens Cancer Group (CCG), Pediatric Oncology Group (POG), and International Society of Paediatric Oncology (SIOP) have had on medulloblastoma trials over the years. In addition, some of the chemotherapy approaches used for children, which involves administering multiple doses of vincristine and cisplatinum, may be difficult to complete in adults because of cumulative neurotoxicity. Analyzing data from adult medulloblastoma series dating from the 1960s, with these predominantly occurring from 1970 onward, 5 year survival rates range between 46% and 78%, with an average of approximately 60% (Kopelson et al., 1982; Hughes, 1984; Haie et al., 1985; Cornu et al., 1990; Hartsell et al. 1992; Hazuka et al., 1992; Carrie et al., 1993, 1994; Frost et al. 1995; Prados et al., 1995; Noel et al., 1997; Brandes et al., 1999; Giordana et al., 1999; Chan and Tarbell et al., 2000).

Cerebellar Pilocytic Astrocytomas

Cerebellar astrocytomas encroach on the fourth ventricle. Astrocytic neoplasms of the cerebellum span the full gamut from juvenile pilocytic astrocytomas to glioblastomas. Low-grade cerebellar tumors may occur in adults, but higher grade lesions are somewhat more frequent.

Early recognition of the pilocytic astrocytoma is important because it can be potentially cured through complete surgical excision. The histologic architecture of the pilocytic astrocytoma consists of clustered fascicles of elongated, bipolar neoplastic astrocytes (*pilocyte* literally means "hair cell") interspersed with less cellular, often microcystic, areas of stellate astrocytes (Fig. 6–3). It is also typical to find several markers of chronicity and degeneration, such as Rosenthal fibers, eosinophilic granular bodies ("protein droplets"), and nuclear atypia. The nuclear atypia together with the commonly encountered microvascular proliferation are not negative prognostic factors in pilocytic astrocytomas but may cause pilocytic astrocytomas to be erroneously overgraded as malignant astrocytomas (Fig. 6–4). Noninfiltrative, pilocytic, cerebellar astrocytomas occur primarily in children and constitute approximately 10% to 20% of all childhood primary CNS tumors and 30% to 40% of all posterior fossa tumors (Griffin et al., 1979; Matson, 1956). They occur most commonly during the latter portion of the first decade of life and have a second peak occurrence in the first half of the second decade. There is no clear sex predilection.

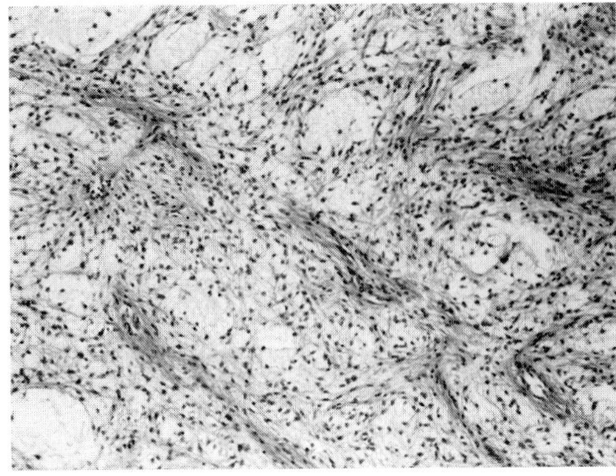

Figure 6–3. Pilocytic astrocytoma. Classic pilocytic astrocytoma architecture is biphasic, with compact areas of neoplastic pilocytes in juxtaposition to loose, microcystic stroma.

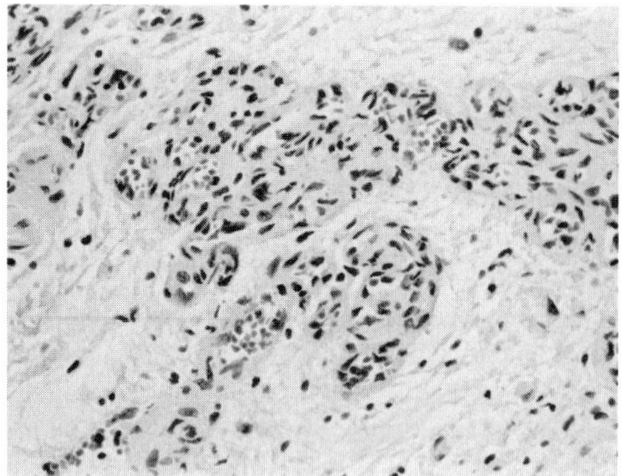

Figure 6–4. Pilocytic astrocytoma. Microvascular proliferation along with degenerative nuclear pleomorphism is commonly seen in pilocytic astrocytomas and constitutes a potential diagnostic pitfall for overgrading.

Fibrillary astrocytomas also occur in the cerebellum and, like their supratentorial counterparts, range from well differentiated to infrequent glioblastomas. It may be difficult to differentiate low-grade fibrillary astrocytomas from pilocytic astrocytomas with limited biopsy samples. Sometimes it is even difficult to distinguish infiltrating cerebellar astrocytomas from exophytic brain stem gliomas.

Presentation

Clinical signs and symptoms of cerebellar astrocytomas depend on the location of the tumor. For tumors that arise in the lateral portion of the cerebellum, unsteadiness and dysmetria predominate early in the course of illness (Griffin et al., 1979; Matson, 1956). Appendicular ataxia, unilateral to the site of the lesion, is then followed by truncal unsteadiness when the tumor or its cyst extends toward the midline. Later in the course of illness, cerebellar deficits are often overshadowed by signs of increased intracranial pressure, which is secondary to blockage of the fourth ventricle and hydrocephalus. The classic symptom of early morning headache, often relieved by nausea and vomiting, then occurs. When the tumor arises in the cerebellar vermis or other midline structures, truncal unsteadiness occurs early in the course of illness followed more rapidly by signs of increased intracranial pressure. In the first few years of life, irritability, anorexia, developmental delay, and, later, regression of intellectual and motor abilities may occur before the recognition of focal neurologic deficits.

At the time of diagnosis, common findings include papilledema, gait ataxia, unilateral or bilateral dysmetria, and cranial nerve abnormalities such as nystagmus or sixth nerve palsies. Head tilt may result from impaction of the cerebellar tonsils into the foramen magnum. Lower extremity hyperreflexia and spasticity may occur secondary to increased intracranial pressure, but are relatively infrequent signs. In infants and very young children, the "sunsetting sign" may be present, manifested by an impaired upgaze and a seemingly forced downward deviation of the eyes.

Surgery

From a surgical perspective, cerebellar tumors can be solid or cystic. Cystic tumors are of three types (Hoffman et al., 1990) (Figs. 6–5 and 6–6). The most common cystic tumor consists of a mural nodule with an associated cyst lined by a glial membrane. The false cystic tumors have a mural nodule with the wall of the cyst also lined by tumor. Another variation is a cyst wall lined by tumor without a mural nodule.

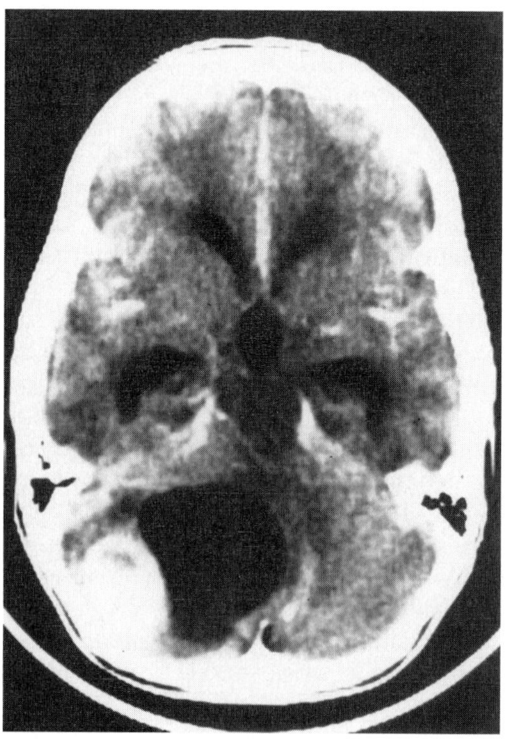

Figure 6–5. Axial enhanced CT scan of child with cystic cerebellar astrocytoma. Note the enhancement of nodule and not of cyst wall.

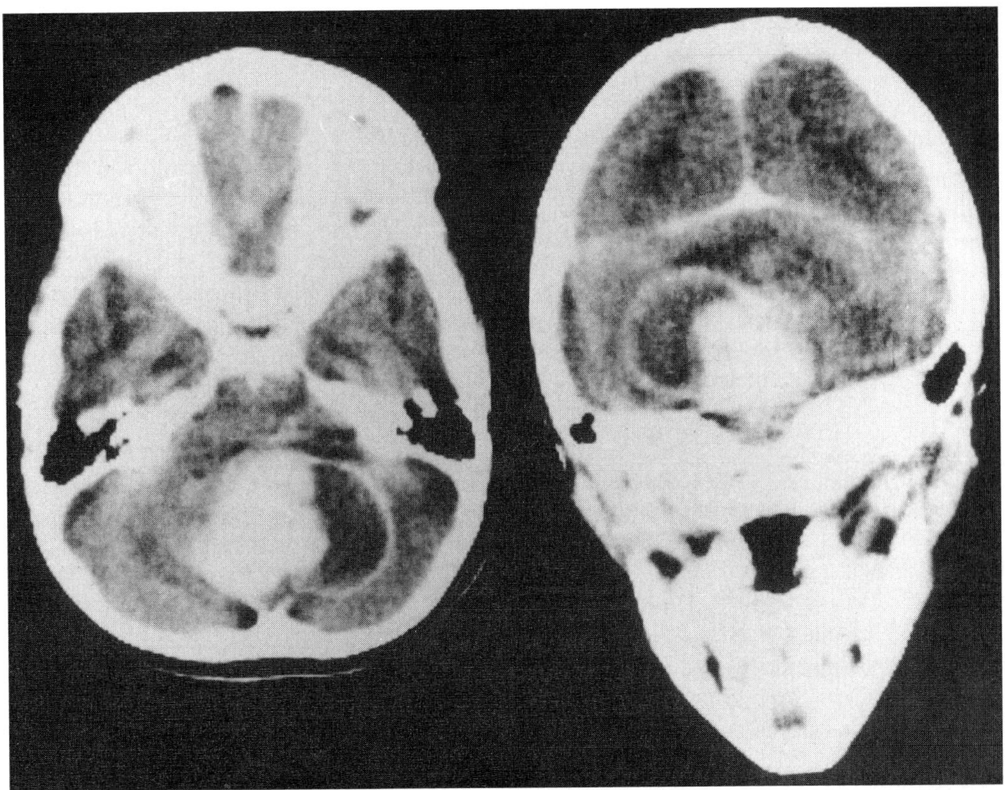

Figure 6–6. Axial and coronal enhanced CT scans of a child with false cystic cerebellar astrocytoma. Note enhancement of both mural nodule and cyst wall.

Radiologically, a distinction can be made between these types of cystic cerebellar astrocytoma because the cyst wall enhances if it is lined by tumor and does not enhance if it is a glial cyst.

Pilocytic cerebellar astrocytomas can normally be totally resected. Recurrences will occur when cystic infiltrative astrocytomas are mistaken for typical cystic pilocytic astrocytomas and part of the tumor cyst wall is left behind. After total resection the vast majority of children will require no further treatment, and 90% to 95% can be expected to be apparently cured. After subtotal resections, especially near-total resections of pilocytic tumors, some will not require further treatment for months or years. At the time of progression in these cases, reoperation and attempts at complete resection are probably indicated before other forms of treatment are initiated.

Radiotherapy

The efficacy of radiotherapy for incompletely resected pilocytic cerebellar astrocytomas is unproven (Leibel et al., 1975; Garcia et al., 1990). There is no evidence to support the use of radiotherapy for children with totally resected tumors (Geissinger, 1971; Gjerris and Klinken, 1978). Some reports suggest that radiotherapy prolongs the survival rate of patients who have only had a partial resection of tumor, although these are primarily retrospective reviews of patients collected over decades. Because the recurrences of pilocytic astrocytomas are infrequent and usually localized, it seems reasonable to withhold radiotherapy until there are signs of progression. Even at this point, the benefits of repeat resection versus radiotherapy remain uncertain (Leibel et al., 1975; Garcia et al., 1990).

Chemotherapy

Data showing the utility of chemotherapy for childhood pilocytic astrocytomas are even more scant (Edwards et al., 1980). There is no evidence that chemotherapy has a role as adjuvant treatment for children with totally resected tumors or for those children with partially resected tumors who then receive radiotherapy. There are scattered, mostly anecdotal, reports of the benefits of chemotherapy for patients with recurrent or progressive symptomatic tumors utilizing drugs such as carboplatin, vincristine, BCNU, and a combination such as TPDCV (6-thioguanine, procarbazine, dibromodulcitol, 1-[2-chloroethyl]-3-cyclohexyl-1-nitrosourea, and vincristine) (Prados et al., 1997; Petronio et al., 1991).

Diffuse, Infiltrating Cerebellar Astrocytomas

Presentation

Infiltrative gliomas of the cerebellum, which are more common in adults than in children (Hayostek et al., 1993), histologically range from low-grade astrocytomas to glioblastoma multiforme. As is the case for noninfiltrative gliomas, presentation depends on the location of the tumor in the cerebellum. In general, low-grade infiltrative astrocytomas tend to present more insidiously than pilocytic astrocytomas and cause greater midline cerebellar deficits early in the course of illness. Later, when the lesion obstructs the fourth ventricle, the more classic symptoms and signs of increased intracranial pressure, such as morning headaches and vomiting, become evident. Patients with higher grade lesions tend to present more explosively. This is especially true for patients with glioblastoma multiforme, as the symptoms and signs of increased intracranial pressure frequently overshadow cerebellar deficits.

At the time of diagnosis, most patients have unilateral or bilateral dysmetria, truncal unsteadiness, and papilledema. A sixth nerve palsy is a frequent finding, whereas other cranial nerve palsies occur less frequently. Other extraocular movement disorders, including ocular dysmetria, ocular flutter, and upbeat nystagmus, are common. Tumors that infiltrate the lower parts of the cerebellar vermis and compress the medullary regions may also cause downbeat nystagmus.

Surgery

Low-grade infiltrative astrocytomas and higher grade cerebellar gliomas tend to be refractory to total surgical resection. For "totally resected," low-grade infiltrative lesions, a period of observation before initiation of further therapy is likely indicated.

Radiotherapy

For those patients with subtotally resected low-grade infiltrative gliomas, there is little evidence that radiotherapy increases the rate of long-term disease control or survival (Leibel et al., 1975; Winston et al., 1977; Garcia et al., 1990). These tumors tend to recur locally, but leptomeningeal spread of these lesions at the time of disease relapse may occur, and patients should probably be staged by MRI of the spine for seeding at the time of local relapse.

Management of patients with higher grade cerebellar gliomas is more difficult. Although the majority of disease relapses occur at the primary tumor site, a significant percentage of patients (greater than 30% in some series) have evidence of leptomeningeal disease at presentation or at the time of progression (Packer et al., 1985). There is some evidence that craniospinal irradiation may be effective in controlling neuraxis disease (Salazar, 1981).

Chemotherapy

Similar to results in patients with high-grade cerebral malignancies, adjuvant chemotherapy may increase the chances of survival (Sposto et al., 1989; Chamberlain et al., 1990).

Brain Stem Gliomas

Brain stem gliomas may occur in any age group; however, approximately 75% of patients who develop such tumors will be younger than 20 years of age at diagnosis (Littman et al., 1980; Edwards et al., 1989; Albright et al., 1983). The peak incidence of these tumors is in the latter half of the first decade of life, and there is no sex predilection. It has been suggested that brain stem gliomas in adults tend to have a somewhat indolent course and are likely to be low grade and localized at the time of diagnosis (Edwards et al., 1989). Brain stem gliomas can generally be divided into three major subtypes: *(1)* diffuse intrinsic, *(2)* tectal, and *(3)* cervicomedullary. Occasionally, a true focal, often pilocytic, intrinsic brain stem glioma is seen (Table 6–2). The differential diagnosis of a brain stem mass is more difficult in adulthood, as metastatic and infectious lesions make up a higher proportion of lesions. Stereotactic biopsy of brain stem lesions has added importance for older patients in whom the vast majority of lesions are gliomas (Massager et al., 2000).

Table 6–2. Brain Stem Gliomas

Type	*Presentation*	*Treatment*	*Outcome*
Diffuse, intrinsic (usually pontine ± other regions)	Multiple cranial nerve deficits, long tract signs, sensory abnormalities	Surgery usually not indicated; local radiotherapy	10% or less 18 month PFS
Exophytic, cervicomedullary	Headache, vomiting, occasional ataxia and lower cranial nerve deficits	Gross total resection or partial resection plus local radiotherapy	80%–90% 5 year PFS
Focal, midbrain (usually tectal)	Headache, vomiting, hydrocephalus	Cerebrospinal fluid diversion; observation	67% stable for 5 years with other treatment
Focal, intrinsic (usually pontine)	Focal sixth and seventh cranial nerve palsies	Biopsy plus local radiotherapy	80%–90% 5 year PFS

PFS, progression-free survival.

Presentation

Brain stem gliomas tend to present insidiously; however, they will ultimately result in long tract signs, cranial neuropathies, and ataxia. Hydrocephalus and signs of increased intracranial pressure occur in fewer than one-third of patients at the time of diagnosis. In children, nonspecific signs such as headaches and behavioral changes may occur in as many as 50% of patients before diagnosis.

On examination, the sixth and seventh cranial nerves are most frequently involved; but depending on the location of the lesion within the brain stem, other cranial nerves may be impaired. If the brain stem glioma arises low in the medulla, it may cause slight cranial nerve deficits early in the course of illness (Albright et al., 1986). Symptoms of unsteadiness, vomiting, and nonspecific head pain tend to predominate. Later, dysphasia and speech difficulties are present. Less frequently, brain stem tumors may initially present as isolated cranial nerve palsies, including isolated sixth and seventh nerve palsies.

Since the advent of MRI, high midbrain tumors, especially those arising in the tectum, are being diagnosed more readily. Patients with these tumors tend to present with hydrocephalus and may or may not have signs of tectal dysfunction, such as upward gaze paresis, pupils that react better to accommodation than light, lid retraction, and convergence or retraction nystagmus ("Parinaud's syndrome"). Patients with this type of tectal presentation tend to have a long history of minor ocular symptoms and signs, behavioral changes, and, often, school difficulties before diagnosis.

Rarely, cortical symptoms are the presenting sign of brain stem gliomas. These symptoms, including behavioral changes and seizures, are probably due to subthalamic and/or subcortical tumor infiltration.

The median time to diagnosis of brain stem gliomas in older series was 4 to 6 months. With the advent and routine availability of better neuroimaging techniques, especially MRI, most patients are now diagnosed within 3 months of the onset of symptoms.

Various factors have been found to be of prognostic importance for children with diffuse, intrinsic brain stem gliomas (Albright et al., 1986). However, because overall outcome is so poor, the independent significance of a single factor has been questioned. In general, children and adults with longer clinical histories before diagnosis and those with more focal lesions, especially cervicomedullary and midbrain lesions, tend to fare best (Edwards et al., 1989; Albright et al., 1986; Barkovich et al., 1990–1991; Hoffman et al., 1980). The significance of histology, obtained by either open or stereotactic biopsy, remains unsettled. For patients with exophytic lesions, histology seems to impact outcome, and patients with benign histology tend to do better than those with anaplastic or malignant gliomas.

Surgery

In the appropriate clinical setting, diffusely infiltrating brain stem astrocytomas that present classic neuroimaging findings are often not biopsied. Studies of biopsied cases and postmortem specimens show a spectrum of differentiation ranging from low-grade infiltrative astrocytoma to glioblastoma; such findings, on biopsy, have not been prognostically important in diffuse tumors (Albright et al., 1993). Focal lesions and those arising in adulthood are more problematic, and stereotactic biopsy is often indicated. The diagnostic yield from such procedures is high, and morbidity is relatively low (Massager et al., 2000).

Modern neuroimaging has resulted in better categorization and understanding of brain stem gliomas, and at least some are amenable to surgical resection (Epstein and McLeary, 1986; Stroink et al., 1986). The diffuse intrinsic tumor is the most common brain stem glioma.

The dorsally exophytic brain stem tumors protrude posteriorly from the floor of the fourth ventricle, filling it (Hoffman et al., 1980). These tumors are typically low-grade astrocytomas and occasionally gangliogliomas. Patients present with hydrocephalus and rarely have cranial nerve signs. The bulk of the tumor can be removed, and, with such removal, additional therapy may not be necessary. However, surgery can cause significant morbidity, and it is unclear whether outcome is better for patients treated with radical surgery than with subtotal resection followed by local radiotherapy. In most series, 5 year survival rates after "gross-total" resection or partial resections followed by radiotherapy are in the 80% to 90% range (Epstein and McLeary, 1986).

Focal brain stem tumors occur in a segment of the brain stem, most commonly in the midbrain, especially in the tectum. These are usually solid, but they can be cystic. The majority are low-grade astrocytomas (Fig. 6–7). They are amenable to resection, but some tumors are so indolent that they can be observed without any specific treatment, other than cerebrospinal shunting, for weeks to months after detection. Approximately two-thirds of patients will have stable disease for 4 to 5 years after diagnosis and/or CSF diversion, without any other form of specific therapy (Pollack et al., 1994). Rarely, focal intrinsic pontine and medullary tumors may occur. They also may have an indolent course. Management options include observation, "total" surgical resection (with a risk of significant morbidity), or biopsy/partial resection followed by local radiotherapy.

Radiotherapy

Radiotherapy continues to be the primary treatment for the majority of adults and children with brain stem gliomas (Kim et al., 1980; Halperin et al., 1989). Most patients with diffuse intrinsic tumors will be treated with conventional or high-dose hyperfractionated radiotherapy and will experience clinical improvement; however, more than 90% of patients will succumb to their disease within 18 months of diagnosis. Hyperfractionated radiotherapy with total doses ranging between 68 and 78 Gy has been utilized for patients with brain stem gliomas (Edwards et al., 1989; Barkovich et al., 1990–1991; Packer et al., 1990). For children and adults with diffuse infiltrative lesions, there is yet no evidence that these higher doses of hyperfractionated radiotherapy result in better long-term tumor control (Edwards et al., 1989; Packer et al., 1990, 1994a). However, the majority of patients with high-grade infiltrative lesions will at least transiently respond to the higher doses of radiotherapy and show objective evidence of tumor shrinkage (Barkovich et al., 1990–1991; Packer et al., 1990). Higher doses of radiotherapy will, in a significant number of patients, cause transient neurologic worsening (Packer et al., 1990). Patients in these hyperfractionated radiotherapy series with localized lesions, especially midbrain masses, and those patients with exophytic lesions, which are histologically low grade, fare better than patients receiving hyperfractionated radiotherapy who have diffuse infiltrative masses (Edwards et al., 1989; Barkovich et al., 1990–1991; Mandell et al., 1999). More recent data suggest that patients with localized lesions or diffusely infiltrative pontine gliomas fare as well as with conventional fractionated doses of radiotherapy (180 cGy fractions) when given a total dose of 54 to 56 Gy.

Chemotherapy

Information concerning chemotherapy for patients with brain stem gliomas is largely based on data from patients treated at the time of recurrence (Rodriguez et al., 1988; Sexauer et al., 1985; Chastagner et al., 1997; Djerassi et al., 1977; Gaynon et al., 1990). Responses to a variety of drugs have been reported, including cisplatin, carboplatin, ifosfamide, CCNU (1-[2-cyclohexyl]-l-nitrosourea), and various drug combinations. Interferon-β has also been shown to be transiently effective in children with recurrent brain stem gliomas. To date, no adjuvant treatment trial, including one using interferon-β, has shown chemotherapy or other forms of adjuvant therapy to

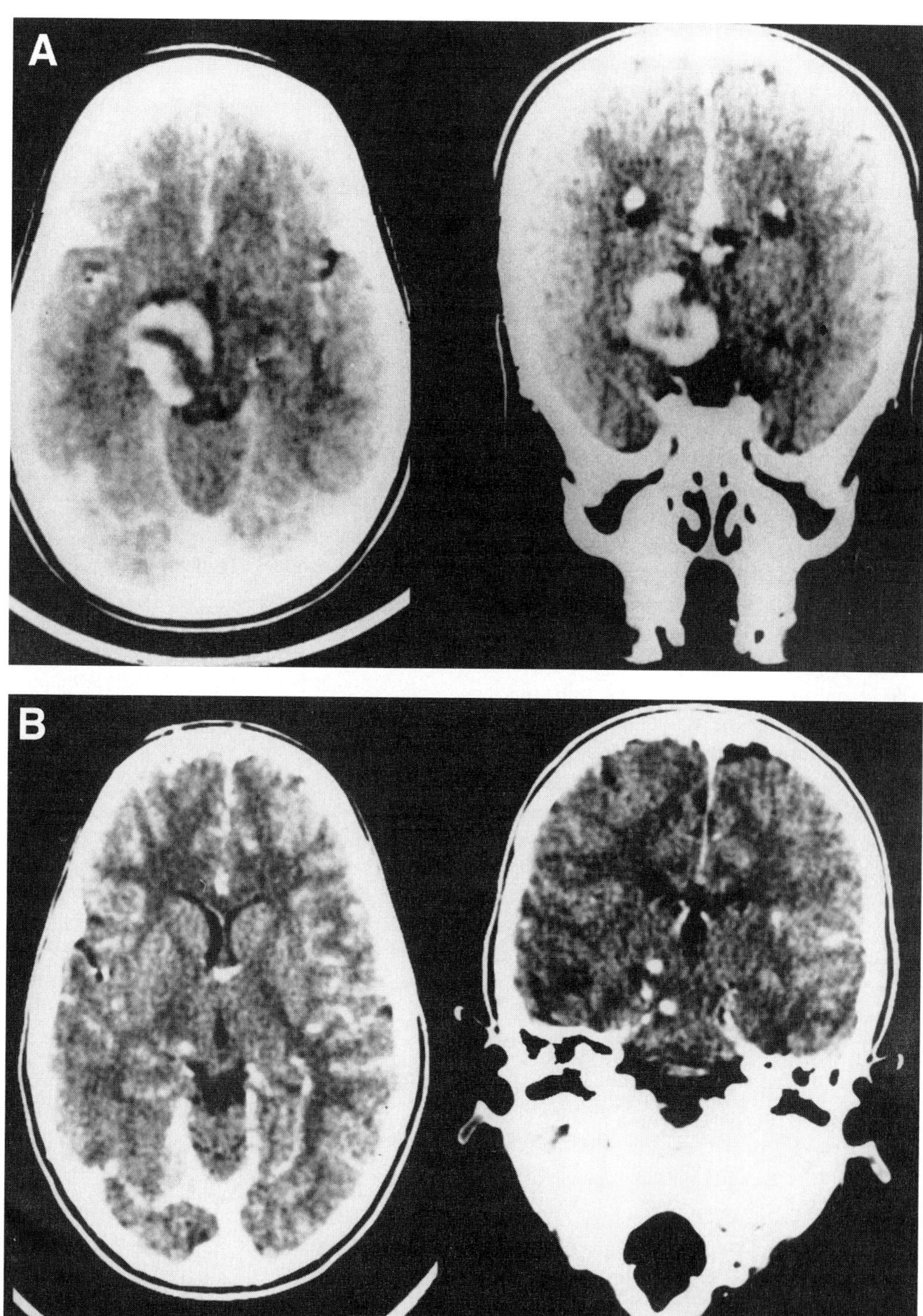

Figure 6–7. **(A)** Axial and coronal enhanced CT scans of 1-year-old child with focal low-grade midbrain astrocytoma before surgical resection. **(B)** Axial and coronal enhanced CT scan of same child 4 years after subtotal resection and a course of chemotherapy. The tumor shows a complete response.

be of substantial benefit to survival (Levin et al., 1984b). Exophytic, progressive low-grade tumors may respond to the combination of carboplatin and vincristine (Packer et al., 1997).

Ependymomas

Ependymomas occur in children and adults. In children, approximately two-thirds of ependymomas arise infratentorially and one-third arise supratentorially (Pierre-Kahn et al., 1983; Garret and Simpson, 1983; Wallner et al., 1986; Shaw et al., 1987). The opposite is true for adults. Ependymomas comprise between 10% and 20% of the posterior fossa tumors occurring in patients younger than 15 years of age. In children, ependymomas frequently fill the fourth ventricle and can penetrate the foramen of Luschka and even extend through the foramen of Magendie to the dorsal aspect of the spinal cord.

The two characteristic histologic features of ependymomas are anuclear perivascular collars of radiating cell processes ("perivascular pseudorosettes") and "true" rosettes of tumor cells, which possess a central lumen (Fig. 6–8). Perivascular pseudorosettes are seen more frequently than true rosettes. Immunohistochemically, the glial nature of these neoplasms is reflected in diffuse positivity for S-100 protein. Immunopositivity for glial fibrillary acidic protein is usually focally present, particularly around blood vessels in the cytoplasmic processes that compose the pseudorosettes. Ultrastructural examination often shows such markers of ependymal lineage as intercellular lumina filled with microvilli and cilia.

Presentation

Ependymomas vary in clinical presentation, and the initial symptoms are usually nonspecific and nonlocalizing (Djohrmann et al., 1976; Mork and Rubinstein, 1985; Pierre-Kahn et al., 1983; Garret and Simpson, 1983; Wallner et al., 1986; Shaw et al., 1987). The effects of increased intracranial pressure, including headaches, may occur early in the course of illness. Alternatively, ependymomas may mimic brain stem lesions and cause multiple cranial nerve palsies before the onset of signs of increased intracranial pressure. Tumors that arise in the cerebellopontine angle will cause unilateral sixth, seventh, and eighth nerve palsies and same-sided limb dysmetria early in illness. Ependymomas may also cause cerebellar deficits and be clinically indistinguishable from medulloblastomas. By and large, infratentorial ependymomas tend to cause symptoms and signs for 2 to 4 months before diagnosis. As these tumors have a tendency to infiltrate the upper portion of the cervical cord, they may also cause neck stiffness and head tilt.

Staging

Frequently, staging studies either before or after surgery are performed on patients with ependymomas, as some patients may have disseminated disease at di-

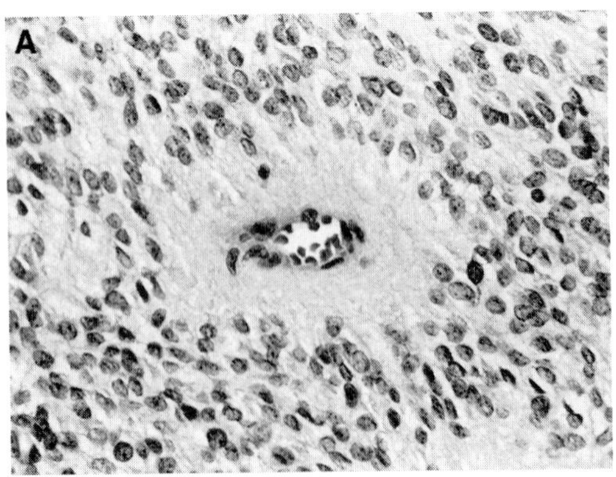

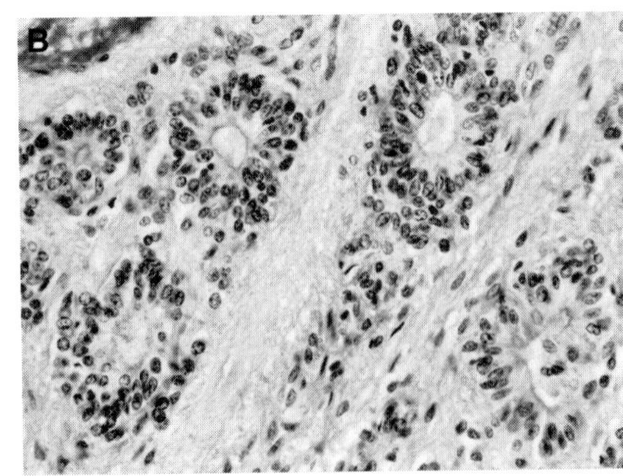

Figure 6–8. Ependymoma. The most characteristic features of most ependymomas are perivascular pseudorosettes **(A)**, which are encountered more frequently than are "true" rosettes **(B)**.

agnosis. Such dissemination is infrequent, occurring in fewer than 10% of patients. Despite this, postoperative (or in some cases preoperative) spinal MRI and CSF cytologic analyses are usually performed.

Surgery

The outcomes of patients who have ependymomas are for the most part proportional to the extent of surgical resection. Patients with totally resected tumors tend to have the best prognosis (Sutton et al., 1991). Approximately one-third of the ependymomas that occur in childhood appear histologically malignant with mitotic figures, pleomorphism, and necrosis. It is unclear if the prognosis for these patients differs from that of patients with less aggressive lesions. Some ependymomas are vascular and infiltrate into surrounding structures or extend into or arise in the cerebellopontine angle enveloping multiple cranial nerves; therefore, they do not lend themselves to total removal. About two-thirds of ependymomas in the posterior fossa have a histologically benign appearance; some of these tumors act aggressively (Pierre-Kahn et al., 1983; Jenkin et al., 1990; Nazar et al., 1990; Horn et al., 1999). If the ependymoma is free of the floor of the fourth ventricle and not intermixed with multiple cranial nerves, it can be totally removed; however, if the ependymoma invades the floor of the fourth ventricle or is wrapped around cranial nerves, it is frequently necessary to leave residual tumor. In such cases, hydrocephalus may continue, and it is therefore important to catheterize the aqueduct of Sylvius to maintain a patent CSF channel and avoid the need for a diversionary ventriculoperitoneal shunt (Jenkin et al., 1990).

Appropriate management for patients with totally resected ependymomas remains unsettled. Approximately 70% of children with totally resected tumors will be alive and free of tumor progression 5 years after surgery and adjuvant radiotherapy (Horn et al., 1999). There is no evidence that the addition of chemotherapy improves outcome. Some have suggested that no adjuvant treatment after total surgical resection is required, but this has not been documented in a prospective randomized study or even in a large retrospective series. The majority of those patients who have been treated with surgery alone have had supratentorial tumors.

Patients with subtotally resected tumors fare less well, with approximately 30% to 40% remaining free of disease 5 years after treatment with surgery, radiotherapy, and, for some, chemotherapy (Horn et al., 1999). Alternative treatment regimens are currently being evaluated for children with incompletely resected tumors.

Of note is the observation that occasionally residual tumor, following adjuvant therapy, will change in character, and sometimes a tumor that is nonresectable because of infiltration can become totally resectable following irradiation and/or chemotherapy.

Radiotherapy

Postoperative irradiation is a standard treatment for ependymomas. Long-term survival following surgery alone has been infrequent. Reports from the past 20 years indicate disease-free survival rates of 0% to 20% after surgical resection alone (Mork and Loken, 1977; Tomita et al., 1988a; Healey et al., 1991). These studies preceded the MRI era, making determinations of extent of resection and "total resection" less exact. Small series and case reports suggest a more favorable outcome after "total" resections alone, documented by MRI. Despite meaningfully higher disease control rates of 30% to 60% reported with postoperative irradiation, the pattern of failure for both differentiated ependymoma and anaplastic ependymoma remains overwhelmingly one of local recurrence (Goldwein et al., 1990b, 1991; Nazar et al., 1990; Rousseau et al., 1994).

There is continuing debate regarding the appropriate volume of radiotherapy to use in the treatment of ependymomas. The incidence of neuraxis dissemination is remarkably consistent in major series, reported at the 10% level. Tumor recurrence at the primary site usually precedes or occurs concurrently with tumor growth in the neuraxis; intracranial or CSF dissemination is rare as an initial post-treatment event (Kun, 1983; Bloom and Bessell, 1990; Goldwein et al., 1990a,b, 1991; Nazar et al., 1990; Vanuytsel and Brada, 1991; Rousseau et al., 1994). There does appear to be a higher frequency of subarachnoid seeding at diagnosis and at the time of initial failure in children younger than 3 years old (Tomita et al., 1988b; Duffner et al., 1993).

The relatively low rate of neuraxis involvement and the equivalent outcome in series comparing local versus full craniospinal irradiation argue strongly for restricting the radiation volume to the posterior fossa in children with ependymomas (Goldwein et al.,

1990b; Nazar et al., 1990; Shaw et al., 1987; Tomita et al., 1988b; Vanuytsel et al., 1992). The uncertain implication of high histologic grade (or anaplastic ependymoma) similarly favors the use of local fields (Rawlings et al., 1988; Goldwein et al., 1991; Rousseau et al., 1994). Only a prospective trial conducted to assess the local failure rate versus neuraxis failure rate following local posterior fossa irradiation will provide definitive information to clarify this aspect of radiotherapy. Even more localized irradiation, using conformal fields or fractionated stereotactic radiotherapy, have been recently utilized: The effects of such treatments are still under investigation.

Based on dose–response analyses for ependymomas, the typical radiation dose is between 50 and 55 Gy locally (Goldwein et al., 1990b; Vanuytsel et al., 1992; Rousseau et al., 1994). The high rate of local failure following incomplete resection has stimulated ongoing investigations of high-dose, hyperfractionated irradiation and precision-volume stereotactic radiosurgical "boosts" to residual disease sites.

Chemotherapy

The role of chemotherapy in the treatment of ependymomas is poorly defined, although a number of drug therapies have been tried. For patients with recurrent diseases, these therapies have been found to be primarily palliative unless preceded by or associated with "total" re-resections. A variety of different chemotherapeutic agents, including BCNU (1,3-bis-[2-chloroethyl]-1-nitrosourea), dibromodulcitol, cisplatin, ifosfamide, VP 16, and carboplatin, have been effective in the treatment of ependymomas at recurrence (Khan et al., 1982; Levin et al., 1984a, 2001; Miser et al., 1989; Robertson et al., 1998). Occasionally, patients can undergo prolonged remission after first recurrence and treatment with chemotherapy and reoperation. To date, however, there is no evidence that patients with infratentorial ependymomas benefit from adjuvant chemotherapy (Lefkowitz et al., 1989; Robertson et al., 1998). Children younger than 3 years of age, treated with alternating vincristine-cyclophosphamide and cisplatin-etoposide combinations following surgery, exhibited a 2 year PFS of 42%, permitting delayed radiotherapy (Duffner et al., 1993). However, it is unclear whether disease control was due to chemotherapy or was secondary to the degree of surgical resection. Clinical trials are now being conducted to evaluate the possible use of adjuvant chemotherapy, either before or after radiotherapy, for patients with subtotally resected infratentorial lesions.

OTHER TUMORS

Subependymomas

Subependymomas are rare tumors that may arise in the fourth ventricle. Initially, the majority of subependymomas were discovered in adults as an incidental finding at the time of autopsy, but with the advent of modern neuroimaging techniques, a higher percentage of patients are being diagnosed antemortem. These tumors exhibit a histologic cluster pattern, consisting of groups of benign-appearing, round to oval nuclei in a delicate fibrillary matrix (Fig. 6–9). Some tumors show prominent cystic change; and foci of calcification, hemorrhage, and other degenerative phenomena may be seen. All cases show immunopositivity for S-100 protein and glial fibrillary acidic protein. Ultrastructurally, ependymomal differentiation may be present. A subset of subependymomas exhibits foci of unequivocal ependymoma, which follow a more aggressive course similar to that of ependymomas.

Presentation

Whereas most subependymomas are asymptomatic, symptoms can occur when the tumor arises in the

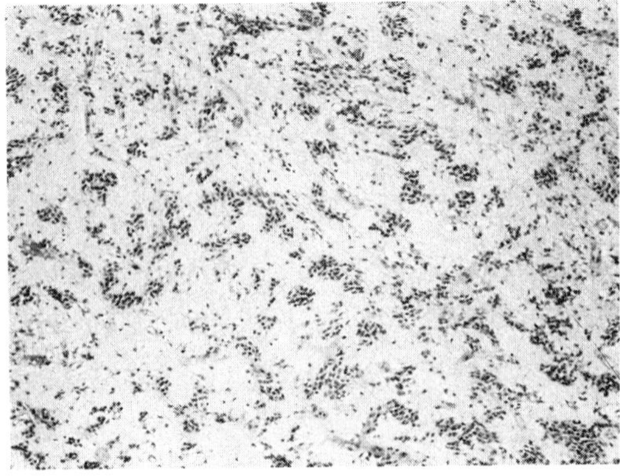

Figure 6–9. Subependymoma. The distinctive morphology of this low-grade neoplasm consists of clustered glial nuclei in a fibrillary stroma composed of cell processes.

fourth ventricle and produces obstructive hydrocephalus. The most common symptoms and signs are nystagmus, headaches, and vomiting; cranial nerve deficits and focal cerebellar signs are less frequent. Occasionally tumors can have elements of subependymomas intermixed with more prominent classic ependymal elements; while the intermixture of the two is common, the preponderance of the ependymal elements may alter the prognosis, which may approximate the fate of children with ependymomas.

Treatment

The treatment of choice for symptomatic tumors is surgical resection (Jooma et al., 1985). For patients with pure subependymomas, there is as yet little evidence that adjuvant radiotherapy or chemotherapy are beneficial. There is also little experience in the treatment of subependymomas with chemotherapy at the time of disease recurrence.

Choroid Plexus Papillomas

Normal choroid plexus consists of fibrovascular cores of connective tissue covered by modified ependymal cells ("choroid epithelium"). Choroid plexus papillomas closely mimic this architecture. These rare tumors arise from the choroid plexus of the fourth ventricle. They can be benign with no evidence of invasion and, thus, can be easily removed. Less histologic similarity to normal choroid plexus is found in the rarer choroid plexus carcinomas (Fig. 6–10), which can invade widely and metastasize.

Total surgical resection without additional therapy results in long-term disease control for children with choroid plexus papillomas and for some patients with carcinomas (Packer et al., 1992; Chow et al., 1999). The utility of adjuvant radiotherapy or chemotherapy for incompletely resected lesions, including carcinomas, has not been proved in a prospective clinical trial. Recently, however, Wolff and colleagues (1999) reported a retrospective analysis of 48 patients with choroid plexus carcinoma and total tumor resection, of whom one-half received postsurgical irradiation. They found a 5 year survival of 68% for the irradiated group compared with 16% for the nonirradiated group. Whereas the nonirradiated group was younger (median, 1.6 years) than those irradiated (median 3.9 years), they observed that older irradiated patients survived longer than younger patients. Subtotally resected or recurrent carcinomas may respond to radiotherapy or chemotherapy, but long-term disease control is usually poor (Packer et al., 1992; Duffner et al., 1993).

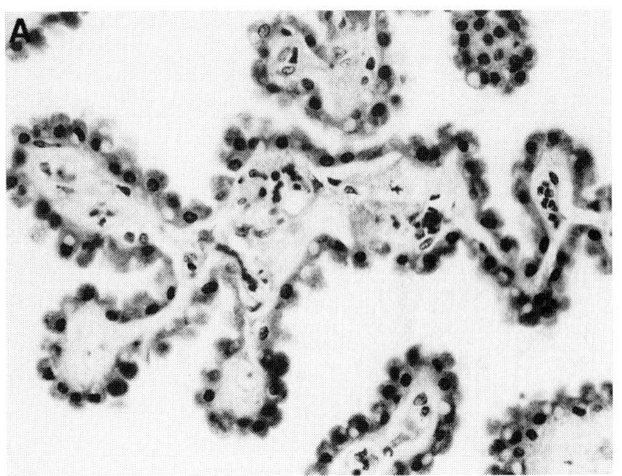

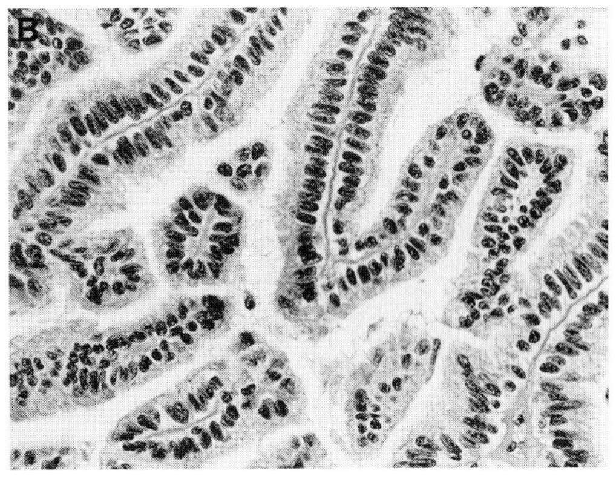

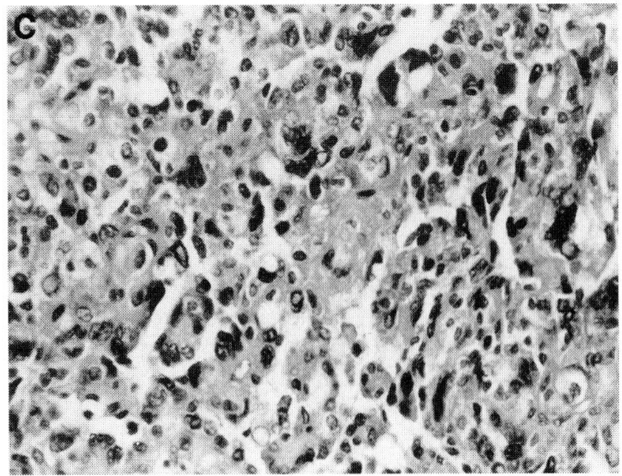

Figure 6–10. Choroid plexus papilloma. The architecture of normal choroid plexus **(A)** is closely mimicked by the choroid plexus papilloma **(B)** but significantly effaced in the rarer choroid plexus carcinoma **(C)**.

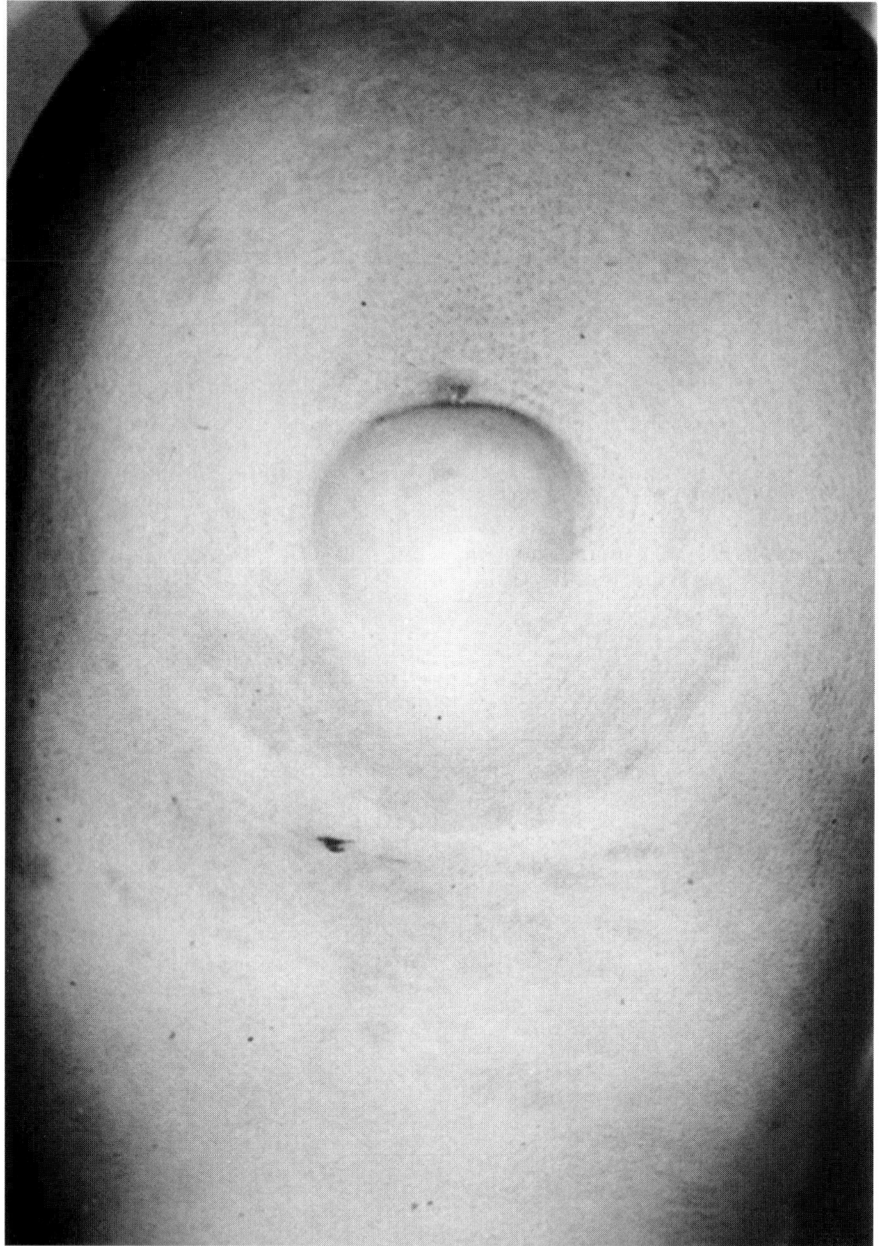

Figure 6–11. View of occiput of child with occipital dermal sinus and subcutaneous dermoid tumor, which extended through the calvarium and ended in a fourth ventricular dermoid tumor.

Dermoid Tumors

Dermoid tumors typically are midline tumors that in the posterior fossa occupy the vermis and encroach on the fourth ventricle (Fig. 6–11) and are usually associated with a dermal sinus, which typically runs in a caudal direction from a skin dimple near the inion. If a dimple is visualized in a child's occipital region, neuroimaging should be conducted to rule out an intracranial dermoid tumor. Dimples such as these are usually covered with hair and are frequently undetected until the child presents with a septic meningitis or until the tumor is precipitously enlarged due to abscess formation.

CONCLUSIONS

More than one-third of patients with fourth ventricular tumors, especially those with pilocytic cerebellar astrocytomas, will have a benign course, and their disease can be managed without adjuvant radiotherapy or chemotherapy. More than 50% of the malignant tumors of the fourth ventricle, especially medulloblastomas, are curable with modern techniques of radiotherapy and chemotherapy. Modern neuroimaging has led to earlier diagnosis and better understanding of the anatomy of such lesions by the neurosurgeon, and modern surgical tools have allowed the neurosurgeon to safely excise fourth ventricular tumors in a manner not possible in the past. Focal radiotherapy techniques are being studied for posterior fossa tumors. The role of chemotherapy is being better defined and, for medulloblastoma, is being expanded.

REFERENCES

Albright AL, Guthkelch AN, Packer RJ, Price RA, Rourke LB. 1986. Prognostic factors in pediatric brain-stem gliomas. J Neurosurg 65:751–755.

Albright AL, Packer RJ, Zimmerman R, Rorke LB, Byett J, Hammond GD. 1993. Magnetic resonance scans should replace biopsies for the diagnosis of diffuse brain stem gliomas: a report from the Children's Cancer Group. Neurosurgery 33:6:1026–1630.

Albright A, Price RA, Guthkelch AN. 1983. Brain stem gliomas of children. A clinicopathological study. Cancer 52:2313–2319

Allen JC, Donahue B, DaRosso R, Nirenberg A. 1996. Hyperfractionated craniospinal radiotherapy and adjuvant chemotherapy for children with newly diagnosed medulloblastoma and other primitive neuroectodermal tumors. Int J Radiat Oncol Biol Phys 36:1155–1161.

Baram TZ, van Eys J, Dowell RE, Cangir A, Pack B, Bruner JM. 1987. Survival and neurologic outcome of infants with medulloblastoma treated with surgery and MOPP chemotherapy. A preliminary report. Cancer 60:173–177.

Barkovich AJ, Krischer J, Kun LE, et al. 1990–1991. Brain stem gliomas: a classification system based on magnetic resonance imaging. Pediatr Neurosurg 16:73–83.

Bloom HJ, Glees J, Bell J, Ashley SE, Gorman C. 1990. The treatment and long-term prognosis of children with intracranial tumors: a study of 610 cases, 1950–1981. Int J Radiat Oncol Biol Phys 18:723–745.

Bloom HG, Bessell EM. 1990. Medulloblastoma in adults: a review of 47 patients treated between 1952 and 1981. Int J Radiat Oncol Biol Phys 18:763–777.

Brandes AA, Palmisano V, Monfardini S. 1999. Medulloblastoma in adults: clinical characteristics and treatment. Cancer Treat Rev 25:3–12.

Carrie C, Lasset C, Alapetite C. 1994. Multivariate analysis of prognostic factors in adult patients with medulloblastoma. Retrospective study of 156 patients. Cancer 74:2352–2360.

Carrie C, Lasset C, Blay JY, et al. 1993. Medulloblastoma in adults: survival and prognostic factors. Radiother Oncol 29:301–307.

Chamberlain MC, Silver P, Levin VA. 1990. Poorly differentiated gliomas of the cerebellum. A study of 18 patients. Cancer 65:337–340.

Chan AW, Tarbell NJ, Black PM, et al. 2000. Adult medulloblastoma: prognostic factors and patterns of relapse. Neurosurgery 47:623–631.

Chastagner P, Bracard S, Sommelet-Olive D, et al. 1997. Analysis of the treatment response and survival rate in two sequential series of 74 brain stem gliomas (BSG) treated in a single centre. Proc Annu Meet Am Soc Clin Oncol 16:A1419.

Chen JM, Zhang YP, Wang C, Sun Y, Fujimoto J, Ikenaga M. 1992. O6-methylguanine-DNA methyltransferase activity in human tumors. Carcinogenesis 13:1503–1507.

Chow E, Reardon DA, Shah AB, et al. 1999. Pediatric choroid plexus neoplasms. Int J Radiat Oncol Biol Phys 44:249–254.

Cornu P, Chatellier G, Fauchon F, et al. 1990. The prognosis of medulloblastoma in adults. Neurochirurgie 36:218–224.

Cushing H. 1930. Experiences with the cerebellar medulloblastoma. A critical review. Acta Phatol Microbiol Scand 7:1.

Deutsch M. 1988. Medulloblastoma: staging and treatment outcome. Int J Radiat Oncol Biol Phys 14:1103–1107.

Deutsch M, Thomas PR, Krischer J, et al. 1996. Results of a prospective randomized trial comparing standard dose neuraxis irradiation (3,600 cGy/20) with reduced neuraxis irradiation (2,340 cGy/13) in patients with low-stage medulloblastoma: a combined Children's Cancer Group-Pediatric Oncology Group Study. Pediatr Neurosurg 24:167–176.

Djerassi I, Kim JS, Shulman K. 1977. High-dose methotrexate-citrovorum factor rescue in the management of brain gliomas. Cancer Treat Rep 61:691–694.

Djohrmann GJ, Farwell JR, Flannery JT. 1976. Ependymomas and ependymoblastomas in children. J Neurosurg 45:273–283.

Duffner PK, Horowitz ME, Krischer JP, et al. 1993. Postoperative chemotherapy and delayed radiation in children less than three years of age with malignant brain tumors. N Engl J Med 328:1725–1731

Dupuis-Girod S, Hartmann O, Berhamou E, et al. 1996. Will high dose chemotherapy followed by autologous bone marrow transplantation supplant cranio-spinal irradiation in young children treated for medulloblastoma? J Neurooncol 27:87–98.

Edwards MS, Levin VA, Wilson CB. 1980. Chemotherapy of pediatric posterior fossa tumors. Childs Brain 7:252–260.

Edwards MS, Wara WM, Urtasun RC, et al. 1989. Hyperfractionated radiation therapy for brain-stem glioma: a phase I–II trial. J Neurosurg 70:691–700.

Epstein F, McCleary EL. 1986. Intrinsic brain-stem tumors of childhood: surgical indications. J Neurosurg 64:11–15.

Evans AE, Jenkin RD, Sposto R, et al. 1990. The treatment of medulloblastoma. Results of a prospective randomized trial of radiation therapy with and without CCNU, vincristine and prednisone. J Neurosurg 72:572–582.

Fertil B, Malaise EP. 1985. Intrinsic radiosensitivity of human cell lines is correlated with radioresponsiveness of human tumors: analysis of 101 published survival curves. Int J Radiat Oncol Biol Phys 11:1699–1707.

Finlay JL, Goldman S, Wong MC, et al. 1996. Pilot study of high-dose thiotepa and etoposide with autologous bone marrow rescue in children and young adults with recurrent CNS tumors. The Children's Cancer Group. J Clin Oncol 14:2495–2503.

Friedman HS, Colvin OM, Skapek SX, et al. 1988. Experimental chemotherapy of human medulloblastoma cell lines and transplantable xenografts with bifunctional alkylating agents. Cancer Res 48:4189–4195

Friedman HS, Dolan ME, Moschel RC, et al. 1992. Enhancement of nitrosourea activity in medulloblastoma and glioblastoma multiforme. J Natl Cancer Inst 84:1926–1931.

Friedman HS, Oakes WJ. 1987. The chemotherapy of posterior fossa tumors in childhood. J. Neurooncol 5:217–229.

Friedman HS, Schold SC Jr, Mahaley MS Jr, et al. 1989. Phase II treatment of medulloblastoma and pineoblastoma with melphalan: clinical therapy based on experimental models of human medulloblastoma. J Clin Oncol 7:904–911.

Frost PJ, Laperriere NJ, et al. 1995. Medulloblastoma in adults. Int J Radiat Oncol Biol Phys 32:851–957.

Gajjar A, Fouladi M, Walter AW, et al. 1999. Comparison of lumbar and shunt cerebrospinal fluid specimens for cytologic detection of leptomeningeal disease in pediatric patients with brain tumors. J Clin Oncol 17:1825–1828.

Garcia DM, Marks JE, Latifi HR, Klieforth AB. 1990. Childhood cerebellar astrocytomas: is there a role for postoperative irradiation? Int J Radiat Oncol Biol Phys 18:815–818.

Garrett PG, Simpson WJ. 1983. Ependymomas: results of radiation treatment. Int J Radiat Oncol Biol Phys 9:1121–1124.

Gaynon PS, Ettinger LJ, Baum ES, Siegel SE, Krailo MD, Hammond GD. 1990. Carboplatin in childhood brain tumors. A Children's Cancer Study Group phase II trial. Cancer 66:2465–2469.

Geissinger J. 1971. Astrocytomas of the cerebellum in children: long term study. Arch Neurol 24:125–135.

Geyer JR, Zeltzer PM, Boyett JM, et al. 1994. Survival of infants with primitive neuroectodermal tumors of malignant ependymomas of the CNS treated with eight-drugs-in-1-day: a report from the Childrens Cancer Group. J Clin Oncol 12:1607–1615.

Giordana MT, Schiffer P, Lanotte M, Girardi P, Chio A. 1999. Epidemiology of adult medulloblastoma. Int J Cancer 80:689–692.

Gjerris F, Klinken L. 1978. Long-term prognosis in children with benign cerebellar astrocytoma. J Neurosurg 49:179–184.

Goldwein JW, Corn BJ, Finlay JL, Packer RJ, Rorke LB, Schut L. 1991. Is craniospinal irradiation required to cure children with malignant (anaplastic) ependymomas? Cancer 67:2766–2771.

Goldwein JW, Glauser TA, Packer RJ, et al. 1990a. Recurrent intracranial ependymomas in children. Survival, patterns of failure, and prognostic factors. Cancer 66:557–563.

Goldwein JW, Leahy JM, Packer RJ, et al. 1990b. Intracranial ependymomas in children. Int J Radiat Oncol Biol Phys 19:1497–1502.

Griffin TW, Beaufait D, Blasko JC. 1979. Cystic cerebellar astrocytomas in childhood. Cancer 44:276–280.

Grotzer MA, Janss AJ, Fung K-M, et al. 2000. TrkC expression predicts good clinical outcome in primitive neuroectodermal brain tumors. J Clin Oncol 18:1027–1035.

Guruangan S, Dunkel IJ, Goldman S, et al. 1998. Myeloablative chemotherapy with autologous bone marrow rescue in young children with recurrent malignant brain tumors. J Clin Oncol 16:2486–2493.

Haie C, Schlienger M, Constans JP, Meder JF, Reynaud A, Ghenim C. 1985. Results of radiation treatment of medulloblastoma in adults. Int J Radiat Oncol Biol Phys 11:2051–2056.

Halberg FE, Wara WW, Fippin LF, et al. 1991. Low-dose craniospinal radiation therapy for medulloblastoma. Int J Radiat Oncol Biol Phys 20:651–654.

Halperin EC, Wehn SM, Scott JW, Djang W, Oakes WJ, Friedman HS. 1989. Selection of a management strategy for pediatric brainstem tumors. Med Pediatr Oncol 17:117–126.

Hartsell WF, Montag AG, Lydon J, Galinsky DL, Sarin P. 1992. Treatment of medulloblastoma in adults. Am J Clin Oncol 15:207–211.

Hayostek CJ, Shaw EG, Scheithauer B, et al. 1993. Astrocytomas of the cerebellum. Cancer 72:855–868.

Hazuka MB, DeBiose DA, Henderson RH, Kinzie JJ. 1992. Survival results in adult patients treated for medulloblastoma. Cancer 69:2143–2148.

He XM, Ostrowski LE, von Wronski MA, et al.1992. Expression of O6-methylguanine-DNA methyltransferase in six human medulloblastoma cell lines. Cancer Res 52:1144–1148.

Healey EA, Barnes PD, Kupsky WJ, et al. 1991. The prognostic significance of postoperative residual tumor in ependymoma. Neurosurgery 28:666–671.

Hoffman HJ, Becker L, Craven MA. 1980. A clinically and pathologically distinct group of benign brain stem gliomas. Neurosurgery 7:243–248.

Hoffman HJ, Berger MS, Becker LE. 1990. Cerebellar astrocytomas. In: Deutsch M (ed), Management of Childhood Brain Tumors. Boston: Kluwer Academic Publishers, 523 p.

Hoffman HJ, Hendrick EB, Humphreys RP. 1976. Metastasis via ventriculoperitoneal shunt in patients with medulloblastoma. J Neurosurg 44:562–566.

Horn B, Heideman R, Geyer R, et al. 1999. A multi-institutional retrospective study of intracranial ependymoma in children: identification of risk factors. J Pediatr Hematol Oncol 21:203–211.

Hughes EN, Shillito J, Sallan SE, Loeffler JS, Cassady JR, Tarbell NJ. 1988. Medulloblastoma at the Joint Center for Radiation Therapy between 1968 and 1984. The influence of radiation dose on the patterns of failure and survival. Cancer 61:1992–1998.

Hughes PG. 1984. Cerebellar medulloblastoma in adults. J Neurosurg 60:994–997.

Jenkin D, Goddard K, Armstrong D, et al. 1990. Posterior fossa medulloblastoma in childhood: treatment results and a proposal for a new staging system. Int J Radiat Oncol Biol Phys 19:265–274.

Jooma R, Torrens MJ, Bradshaw J, Brownell B. 1985. Subependymomas of the fourth ventricle. Surgical treatment in 12 cases. J Neurosurg 62:508–512.

Khan AB, D'Souza BJ, Wharam MD, et al. 1982. Cisplatin therapy in recurrent childhood brain tumors. Cancer Treat Rep 66:2013–2020.

Kim TH, Chin HW, Pollan S, Hazel JH, Webster JH. 1980. Radiotherapy of primary brain stem tumors. Int J Radiat Oncol Biol Phys 6:51–57.

Kleihues P, Cavenee W. 2000. Pathology and Genetics of Tumors of the Nervous System. Lyon: IARC Press.

Kortmann RD, Kuhl J, Timmermann B, et al. 2000. Postoperative neoadjuvant chemotherapy before radiotherapy as compared to immediate radiotherapy followed by maintenance chemotherapy in the treatment of medulloblastoma in childhood: results of the German prospective randomized trial HIT '91. Int J Radiat Oncol Biol Phys 46:269–279.

Kopelson G, Linggood RM, Kleinman GM. 1982. Medulloblastoma in adults: improved survival with supervoltage radiation therapy. Cancer 49:1334–1337.

Krischer JP, Ragab AH, Kun L, et al. 1991. Nitrogen mustard, vincristine, procarbazine, and prednisone as adjuvant chemotherapy in the treatment of medulloblastoma. A Pediatric Oncology Group study. J Neurosurg 74:905–909.

Kuhl J, Muller HL, Berthold F, et al. 1998. Preradiation chemotherapy of children and young adults with malignant brain tumors: results of the German pilot trial HIT '88/'89. Klin Padiatr 210:227–233.

Kun LE. 1983. Patterns of failure in tumors of the central nervous system. Cancer Treat Symp 2:285.

Kun LE, Constine LS. 1991. Medulloblastoma—caution regarding new treatment approaches. Int J Radiat Oncol Biol Phys 20:897–899.

Kun LE, Fontanesi J, Kovnar EH, et al. 1990. Hyperfractionated craniospinal irradiation: a phase I trial in children with malignant central nervous system tumors. Pediatr Neurosurg 16:112.

Lefkowitz I, Evans A, Sposto R, et al. 1989. Adjuvant chemotherapy of childhood posterior fossa (PF) ependymoma: craniospinal radiation with or without CCNU, vincristine (VCR) and prednisone (P). Proc Am Soc Clin Oncol 8:878.

Leibel SA, Sheline GE, Wara WM, Boldrey EB, Hielsen SL. 1975. The role of radiation therapy in the treatment of astrocytomas. Cancer 35:1551–1557.

Levin VA, Edwards MS, Gutin PH, et al. 1984a. Phase II evaluation of dibromodulcitol in the treatment of recurrent medulloblastoma, ependymoma, and malignant astrocytoma. J Neurosurg 61:1063–1068.

Levin VA, Edwards MS, Wara WM, Allen J, Ortega J, Vestnys P. 1984b. 5-Fluorouracil and 1-(2-chloroethyl)-cyclohexyl-l-nitrosourea (CCNU) followed by hydroxyurea, misonidazole, and irradiation for brain stem gliomas: a pilot study of the Brain Tumor Research Center and the Childrens Cancer Group. Neurosurg 14:679–681.

Levin VA, Leibel SA, Gutin PH. 2001. Neoplasms of the central nervous system. In: DeVita VT Jr, Hellman S Jr, Rosenberg SA (eds), Cancer: Principles and Practice of Oncology, 6th ed. Philadelphia: Lippincott-Raven.

Levin VA, Rodriguez LA, Edwards MS, et al. 1988. Treatment of medulloblastoma with procarbazine, hydroxyurea, and reduced radiation doses to whole brain and spine. J Neurosurg 68:383–387.

Littman P, Jarrett P, Bilaniuk LT, et al. 1980. Pediatric brain stem gliomas. Cancer 45:2787–2792.

Mandell LR, Kadota R, Freeman C. 1999. There is no role for hyperfractionated radiotherapy in the management of children with newly diagnosed diffuse intrinsic brainstem tumors: results of a Pediatric Oncology Group phase III trial comparing conventional vs. hyperfractionated radiotherapy. Int J Radiation Oncology Biol Phys 43:959–964.

Massager N, David P, Goldman S,, et al. 2000. Combined magnetic resonance imaging- and positron emission tomography-guided stereotactic biopsy in brainstem mass lesions: diagnostic yield in a series of 30 patients. J Neurosurg 93:951–957.

Matson D. 1956. Cerebellar astrocytoma in childhood. Pediatrics 18:150–155.

Mineura K, Izumi I, Watanabe K, et al. 1993. Influence of O6-methylguanine-DNA methyltransferase activity on chloroethylnitrosourea chemotherapy in brain tumors. Int J Cancer 55:76–81.

Miser J, Krailo M, Smithson W, et al. 1989. Treatment of children with recurrent brain tumors with ifosfamide (ifos), etoposide (VP-16), and mesna (M): results of a phase II trial. Proc Am Soc Clin Oncol 8:84.

Mork SJ, Loken AC. 1977. Ependymoma. A follow-up study of 101 cases. Cancer 40:907–915.

Mork SJ, Rubinstein LJ. 1985. Ependymoblastoma. A reappraisal of a rare embryonal tumor. Cancer 55:1536–1542.

Nazar GB, Hoffman HJ, Becker LE, Jenkin D, Humphreys RP, Hendrick EB. 1990. Infratentorial ependymomas in childhood: prognostic factors and treatment. J Neurosurg 72:408–417.

Noel G, J Merrer. 1997. Medulloblastoma in adults. Val-de-Grade hospital experience (1975–1994) and literature review. Cancer Radiother 1:60–67.

Packer RJ, Allen JC, Goldwein JL, et al. 1990. Hyperfractionated radiotherapy for children with brainstem gliomas: a pilot study utilizing 7,200 cGy. Ann Neurol 27:167–173.

Packer RJ, Ater J, Allen J, et al. 1997. Carboplatin and vincristine chemotherapy for children with newly diagnosed progressive low-grade gliomas. J Neurosurg 86:747–754.

Packer RJ, Boyett JM, Zimmerman RA, et al. 1994a. Outcome of children with brain stem gliomas after treatment with 7800 cGy of hyperfractionated radiotherapy: a Childrens Cancer Group phase I/II Trial. Cancer 74:1827–1834.

Packer RJ, Geyer R, Jennings M, et al. 1998. Disease control in infants and young children with medulloblastomas and ependymomas using chemotherapy alone: a Children's Cancer Group study. Ann Neurol 44:537.

Packer RJ, Goldwein J, Nicholson HS, et al. 1999. Treatment of children with medulloblastomas with reduced-dose craniospinal radiation therapy and adjuvant chemotherapy: a Children's Cancer Group study. J Clin Oncol 17:2127–2136.

Packer RJ, Perilongo G, Johnson D, et al. 1992. Choroid plexus carcinoma of childhood. Cancer 69:580–585.

Packer RJ, Seigel KR, Sutton LN, Litmann P, Bruce DA, Schutf L. 1985. Leptomeningeal dissemination of primary central nervous system tumors of childhood. Ann Neurol 18:217–221.

Packer RJ, Siegel KR, Sutton LN, et al. 1988. Efficacy of adjuvant chemotherapy for patients with poor-risk medulloblastoma: a preliminary report. Ann Neurol 24:503–508.

Packer RJ, Sutton LN, Elterman R, et al. 1994b. Outcome for children with medulloblastoma treated with radiation and cisplatin, CCNU, and vincristine chemotherapy. J Neurosurg 81:690–698.

Petronio J, Edwards MS, Prados M, et al. 1991. Management of chiasmal and hypothalamic gliomas of infancy and childhood with chemotherapy. J Neurosurg 74:701–708.

Pierre-Kahn A, Hirsch JF, Roux FX, Renier D, Sainte-Rose C. 1983. Intracranial ependymomas in childhood. Survival and results of 47 cases. Childs Brain 10:145–156.

Pollack IF, Pang D, Albright AL. 1994. The longterm outcome in children with late-onset aqueductal stenosis resulting from benign intrinsic tectal tumors. J Neurosurg 80:20–25.

Prados MD, Edwards MS, Chang SM, et al. 1999. Hyperfractionated craniospinal radiation therapy for primitive neuroectodermal tumors: results of a phase II study. Int J Radiat Oncol Biol Phys 43:279–285.

Prados MD, Edwards MS, Rabbitt J, Lamborn K, Davis RL, Levin VA. 1997. Treatment of pediatric low-grade gliomas with a nitrosourea-based multiagent chemotherapy regimen. J Neurooncol 32:235–241.

Prados MD, Wara WM, Edwards MS, Cogen PH. 1994. Hyperfractionated craniospinal radiation therapy for primitive neuroectodermal tumors: early results of a pilot study. Int J Radiat Oncol Biol Phys 28:431–438.

Prados MD, Warnick RE, et al. 1995. Medulloblastoma in adults. Int J Radiat Oncol Biol Phys 32:1145–1152.

Rawlings CE 3rd, Giangaspero F, Burger PC, Bullard DE. 1988. Ependymomas: a clinicopathologic study. Surg Neurol 29:271–281.

Robertson PL, Zeltzer PM, Boyett JM, et al. 1998. Survival and prognostic factors following radiation therapy and chemotherapy for ependymomas in children: a report of the Children's Cancer Group. J Neurosurg 88:695–703.

Rodriguez LA, Prados M, Fulton D, Edwards MS, Silver P, Levin V. 1988. Treatment of recurrent brain stem gliomas and other central nervous system tumors with 5-fluorouracil, CCNU, hydroxyurea, and 6-mercaptopurine. Neurosurgery 22:691–693.

Rorke LB, Packer RJ, Biegel JA. 1996. Central nervous system atypical teratoid/rhabdoid tumors of infancy and childhood: definition of an entity. J Neurosurg 85:56–65.

Rousseau P, Habrand JL, Sarrazin D, et al. 1994. Treatment of intracranial ependymomas of children: review of a 15-year experience. Int J Radiat Oncol Biol Phys 28:381–386.

Rutka JT, Hoffman HJ, Becker LE, et al. 1990. Medulloblastoma: the clinical problem, molecular genetics, and mitogenic factors. Dev Biol 1:407.

Salazar OM. 1981. Primary malignant cerebellar astrocytomas in children: a signal for postoperative craniospinal irradiation. Int J Radiat Oncol Biol Phys 7:1661–1665.

Schold SC Jr, Brent TP, von Hofe E, et al. 1989. O6-alkylguanine-DNA alkyltransferase and sensitivity to procarbazine in human brain tumor xenografts. J Neurosurg 70:573–577.

Sexauer CL, Khan A, Burger PC, et al. 1985. Cisplatin in recurrent pediatric brain tumors: a POG phase II study; a Pediatric Oncology Group Study. Cancer 56:1497–1501.

Shaw EG, Evans RG, Schelthauer BW, Ilstrup DM, Earle JD. 1987. Postoperative radiotherapy of intracranial ependymoma in pediatric and adult patients. Int J Radiat Oncol Biol Phys 13:1457–1462.

Silverman CL, Simpson JR. 1982. Cerebellar medulloblastoma: the importance of posterior fossa dose to survival and patterns of failure. Int J Radiat Oncol Biol Phys 8:1869–1876.

Sposto R, Ertel IJ, Jenkins RD, et al. 1989. The effectiveness of chemotherapy for treatment of high grade astrocytomas in children: result of a randomized trial. A report from the Childrens Cancer Study Group, J Neurooncol 7:165–177.

Stroink A, Hoffman HJ, Hendrick EB, Humphreys RP. 1986. Diagnosis and management of pediatric brain-stem gliomas. J Neurosurg 65:745–750.

Sutton LN, Goldwein J, Perilongo G, et al. 1991. Prognostic factors in childhood ependymomas. Pediatr Neurosurg 16:57–65.

Tait DM, Thornton-Jones H, Bloom HJG, Lemerle J, Morris-Jones P. 1990. Adjuvant chemotherapy for medulloblastoma: the first multi-centre control trial of the International Society of Paediatric Oncology (SIOP-I). Eur J Cancer 26:464–469.

Thomas PR, Deutsch M, Mulhern R, et al. 1995. Reduced dose vs standard dose neuraxis irradiation in low stage medulloblastoma: the POG and CCG study. Med Pediatr Oncol 24:277.

Tomita T, McLone DG. 1986. Medulloblastoma in childhood: results of radical resection and low-dose neuraxis radiation therapy. J Neurosurg 64:238–242.

Tomita T, McLone DG, Das L, Brand WN. 1988a. Benign ependymomas of the posterior fossa in childhood. Pediatr Neurosci 14:277–285.

Tomita T, McLone DG, Yasue M. 1988b. Cerebral primitive neuroectodermal tumors in childhood. J Neurooncol 6:233–243.

van der Kogel AJ. 1991. Central nervous system radiation injury in small animal models. In: Gutin PH, Leibel SA, Sheline GE (eds), Radiation Injury to the Nervous System. New York: Raven Press, pp 91–111.

Vanuytsel LJ, Bessell EM, Ashley SE, Bloom HJ, Brada M. 1992. Intracranial ependymoma: long-term results of a policy of surgery and radiotherapy. Int J Radiat Oncol Biol Phys 23:313–319.

Vanuytsel L, Brada M. 1991. The role of prophylactic spinal irradiation in localized intracranial ependymoma. Int J Radiat Oncol Biol Phys 21:825–830.

Wallner KE, Wara WM, Sheline GE, Davis RL. 1986. Intracranial ependymomas: results of treatment with partial or whole brain irradiation without spinal irradiation. Int J Radiat Oncol Biol Phys 12:1937–1941.

Winston K, Gilles F, Leviton A, Fulchiero A. 1977. Cerebellar gliomas in children. J Natl Cancer Inst 58:833–838.

Wolff JE, Sajedi M, Coppes MJ, et al. 1999. Radiation therapy and survival in choroid plexus carcinoma [letter]. Lancet 353:2126.

Zeltzer PM, Boyett JM, Finlay JL, et al. 1999. Metastasis stage, adjuvant treatment and residual tumor are prognostic factors for medulloblastoma in children: conclusions from the Children's Cancer Group 921 randomized phase III study. J Clin Oncol 17:832–845.

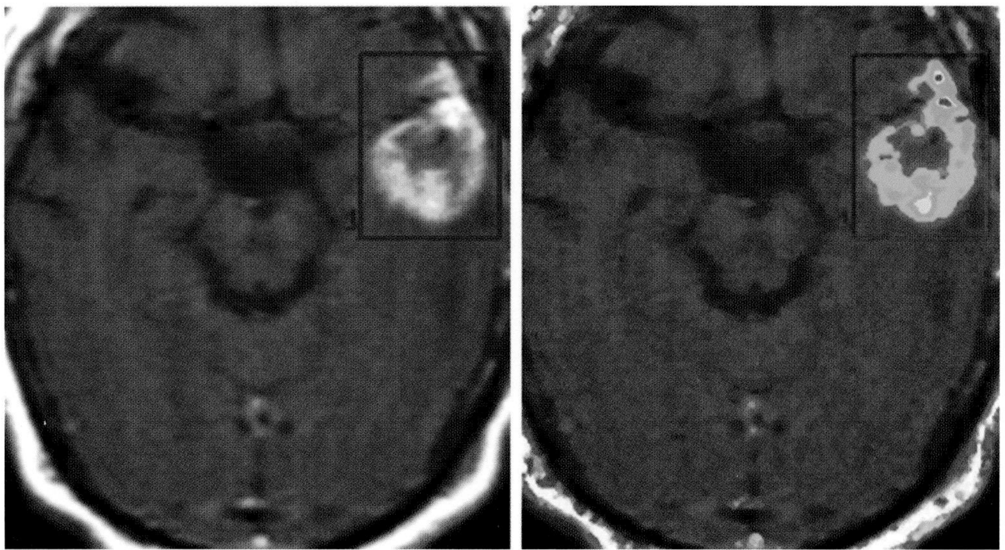

Color Figure 1–47. T1W post-contrast agent–enhanced image **(left)** and vascular endothelial transfer coefficient (permeability) parametric map **(right)** from a patient with pathologically proven anaplastic astrocytoma. In the parametric map, dark blue represents low permeability and red represents high permeability.

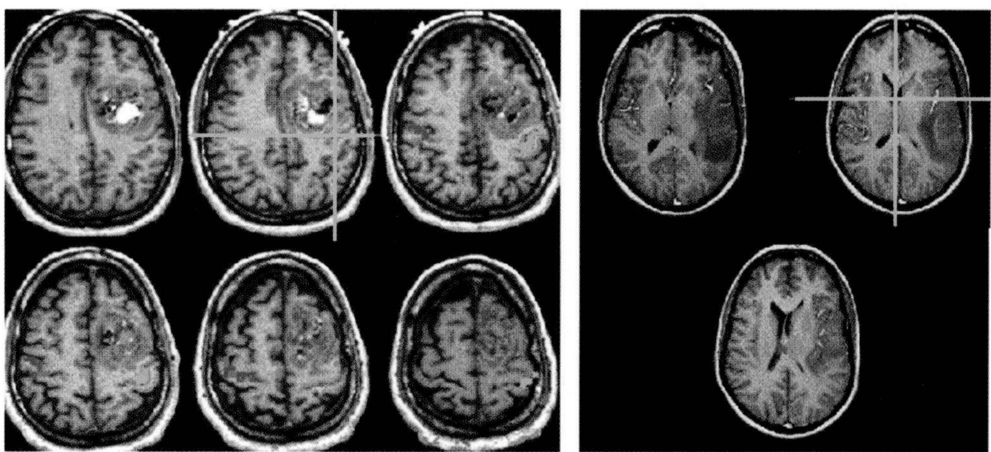

Color Figure 1–50. BOLD contrast fMRI maps for surgical planning. **(Left)** Bilateral upper extremity sensorimotor mapping (finger–thumb tapping task) in a patient with anaplastic astrocytoma (blue, left hand; orange, right hand). **(Right)** Expressive speech mapping (covert word generation task).

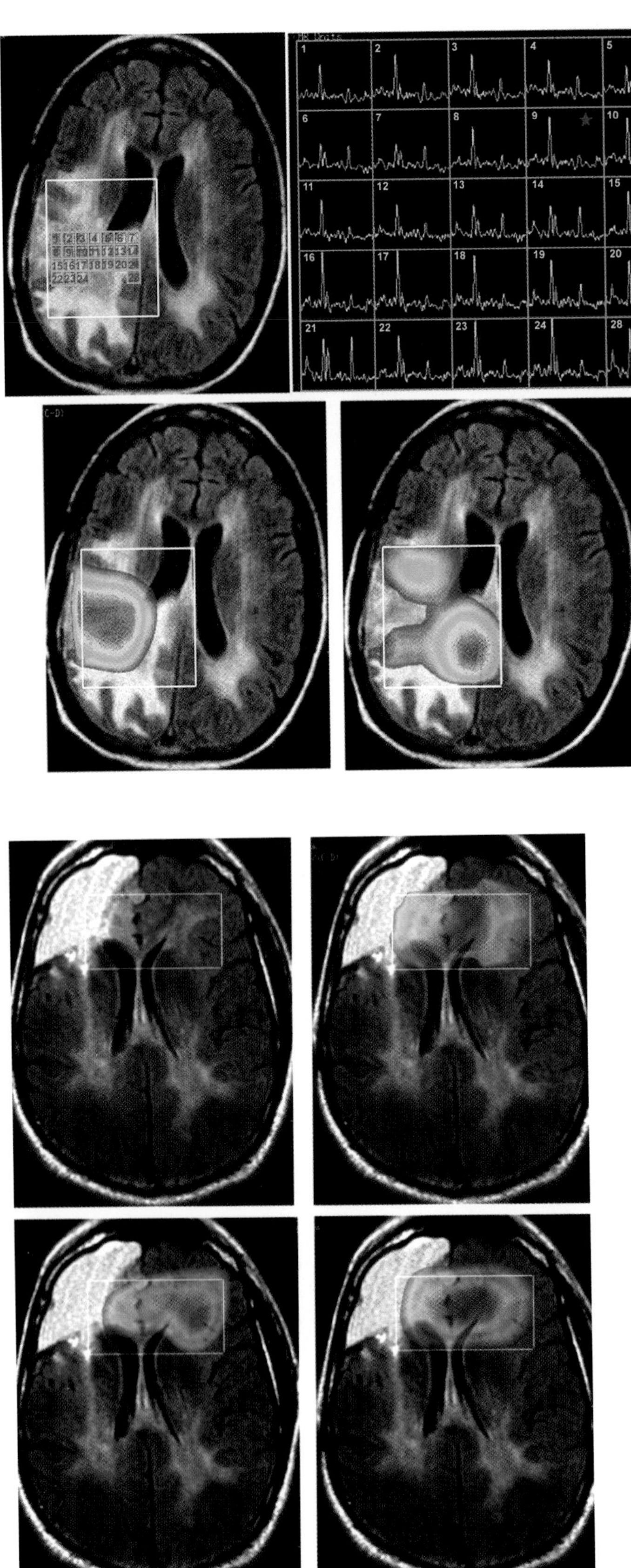

Color Figure 1–53. Spectroscopic imaging data from a patient with glioblastoma multiforme (echo time = 144 ms, repetition time = 1000 ms). **(Top left)** FLAIR image with selected volumes of interest (VOIs; blue squares) within the large excited volume (white rectangle). **(Top right)** Spectra from the numbered VOIs. Note the highly elevated choline levels in VOIs 9 and 10 (red stars) compared with the relatively normal spectrum from VOI 28 (lower left spectrum). **(Bottom left)** Computed choline-to-creatine "metabolite map" showing the areas of elevated choline/creatine ratio as red. **(Bottom right)** Computed *N*-acetylaspartate map.

Color Figure 1–54. (Top left) FLAIR image. **(Top right)** Computed choline/creatine ratio map showing elevated levels in red corresponding to transcallosal spread of the tumor into the contralateral hemisphere. **(Bottom left)** *N*-acetylaspartate map. **(Bottom right)** Choline map.

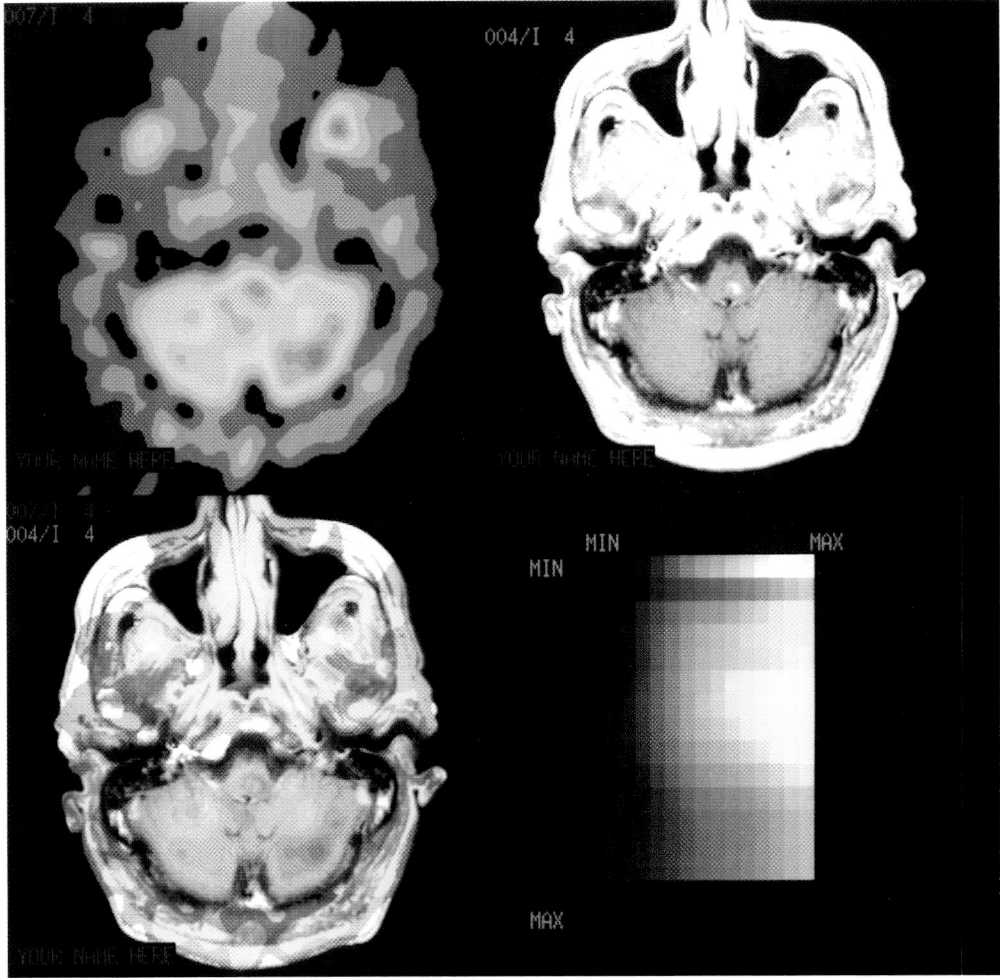

Color Figure 2–4. A patient with a history of central nervous system lymphoma in the periventricular area had responded favorably to previous treatment. He presented with an enhancing lesion in the brain stem on MRI. ^{18}F-FDG PET also showed a hypermetabolic lesion in the brain stem. The automatic image registration (AIR) algorithm (Woods et al., 1993) was used to localize the exact position of the metabolic lesion and found that it, indeed, corresponded with MRI enhancement.

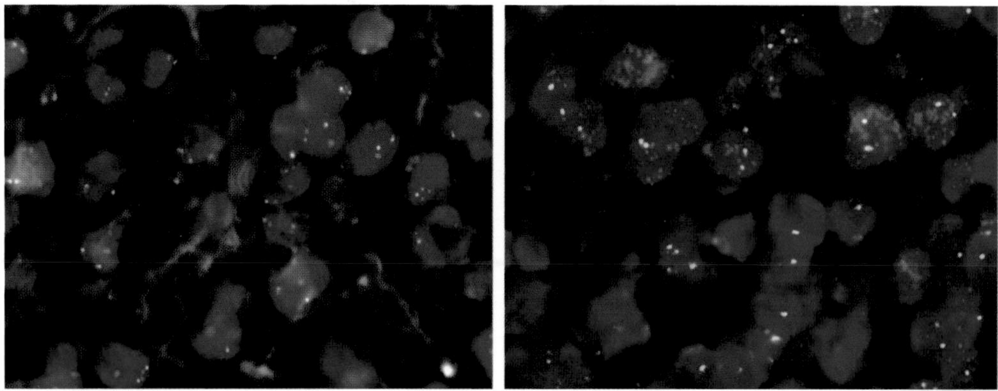

Color Figure 9–1. Epidermal growth factor receptor *(EGFR)* gene amplification detected in paraffin-embedded glioblastoma by FISH analysis.

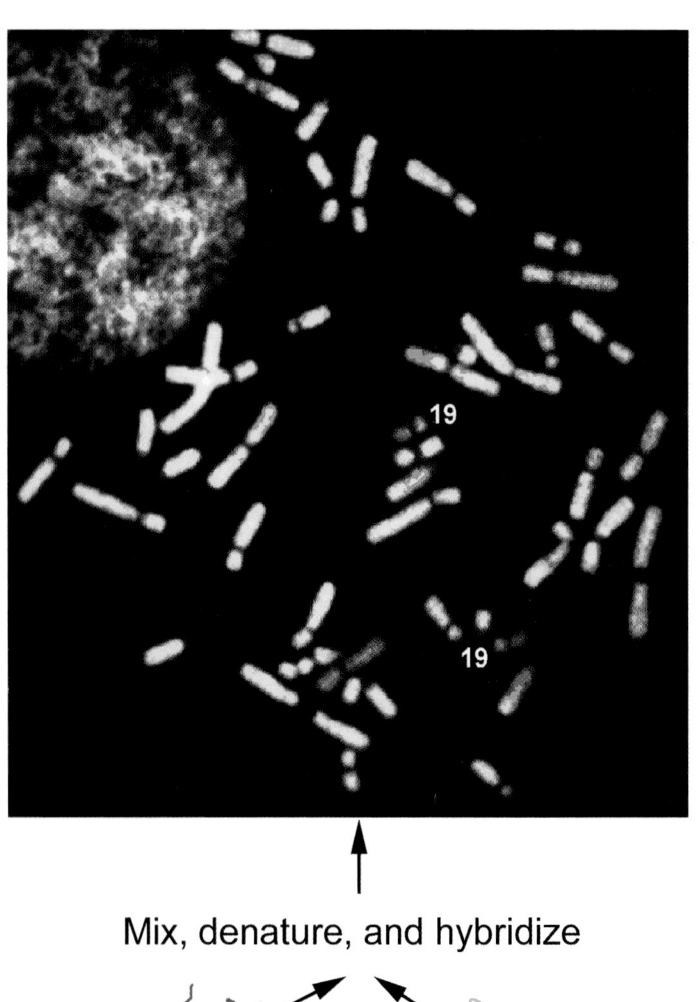

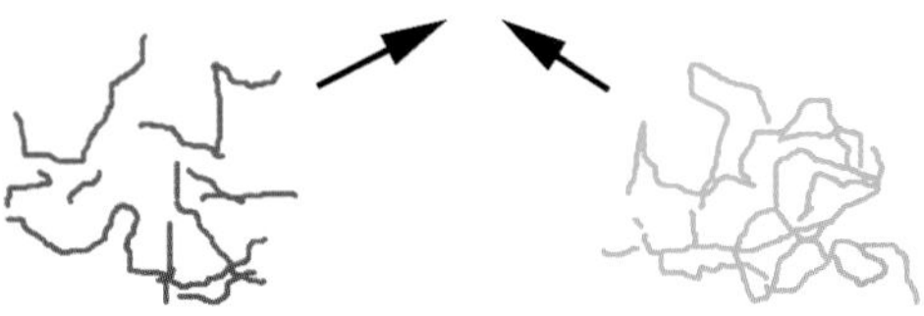

Color Figure 9–2. Comparative genomic hybridization (CGH). Total DNA from a patient's normal and tumor (oligodendroglioma) tissues were isolated and each labeled with a distinct fluorochrome (normal, red; tumor, green). The labeled DNAs were then mixed and hybridized to normal metaphase chromosomes (shown). Note the high level of red fluorescence from the long arm of chromosome 19 (19q), indicating a deletion of that region in the tumor DNA.

7

Pineal Region Tumors

JEFFREY C. ALLEN, JEFFREY BRUCE, LARRY E. KUN, AND LAUREN LANGFORD

Tumors of the pineal region can be divided into three categories (Rubinstein, 1970): *(1)* germ cell tumors, which range from surgically curable mature teratomas to the malignant germ cell tumors capable of metastasizing throughout the neuraxis; *(2)* pineal parenchymal tumors, such as the low-grade pineocytoma and the malignant pineoblastoma; and *(3)* other tumors such as intra-axial astrocytomas, ependymomas and mixed gliomas, and rare tumors of surrounding structures (meningioma, dermoid, epidermoid).

GERM CELL TUMORS

Background and Pathology

Germ cell tumors are relatively uncommon, constituting 3% to 5% of large institutional pediatric tumor series and 0.5% to 1% of adult brain tumor series (Hoffman et al., 1983). Table 7–1 summarizes the frequency of predominantly adult surgical pathology cases seen at the New York Neurologic Institute (Bruce and Stein, 1995). Germ cell tumor cases constituted 37% of their series of 160 cases. The origin of these non-neuroectodermal, primary brain tumors is unknown but may be related to an early period of ontogeny when the fetal germinal cells migrate widely throughout the body, including the central nervous system (CNS). Normally, germinal cells not residing in tissues destined to form sex organs become apoptotic and die; presumably some may occasionally survive and over many years transform into a neoplasm. The sites of origin of germ cell tumors in the CNS are unique, that is, extra-axial locations in proximity to the pineal gland and infundibulum. In unusual instances when germ cell tumors arise in the brain of infants or patients with Down's syndrome, other locations may predominate (Chik et al., 1999).

Germ cell tumors have several unique epidemiologic features such as the age at onset, sites of origin, and racial and sex predilections. The peak age at onset lies within the second and third decades of life, thereby including both the pediatric and adult populations. The primary sites of origin lie within midline extra-axial spaces such as the pineal region (45%), suprasellar region (35%), both regions (10%), and other locations (10%). Interestingly, the incidence of CNS germ cell tumors is extraordinarily high in the Japanese population, constituting 15% to 18% of primary CNS tumors in several large institutional series compared with 3% to 5% in North American reports (Jennings et al., 1985).

More than 95% of CNS germ cell tumors are biologically malignant, that is, capable of rapid growth, invasion, and metastasis. Histologically, approximately 65% of CNS germ cell tumors are pure germinomas, and most of the remaining ones are either pure nongerminomatous germ cell tumors (NGGCT) such as embryonal carcinoma, endodermal sinus or yolk sac tumor, choriocarcinoma, immature or malignant teratoma, or mixed malignant tumors. Mature teratomas that are slow growing and noninvasive are the least common variant (<5%). The pure germinomas are more commonly found in the pineal region, whereas NGGCT occur more frequently in the

Table 7–1. Summary of Pathology in 154 Patients Undergoing Surgery for Pineal Region Tumors at the New York Neurological Institute

Tumor Pathology	*No.*	*Sex (M/F)*	*Mean Age (Years)*
Germ cell	57 (37%)	51/6, 89% male	20.3
Germinoma	26		
Teratoma	9		
Lipoma	2		
Epidermoid	2		
Mixed malignant germ cell	14		
Immature teratoma	2		
Embryonal cell carcinoma	2		
Pineal cell	35 (23%)	19/16, 54% male	33.7
Pineocytoma	19		
Pineoblastoma	7		
Mixed pineal	9		
Glial cell	43 (28%)	21/22, 49% male	28.9
Astrocytoma	23		
Anaplastic astrocytoma	3		
Glioblastoma	4		
Ependymoma	10		
Oligodendroglioma	2		
Choroid plexus papilloma	1		
Miscellaneous	19 (12%)	11/8, 58% male	45.7
Pineal cyst	4		
Meningioma	9		
Other malignant	3		
Other benign	3		
Totals	154	102/52, 66% male	28.9

Data are from Bruce and Stein (1995).

suprasellar region (Edwards et al., 1988; Malogolowkin et al., 1990; Rueda-Pedraza et al., 1987). There exists a male predominance (3/1 [US] to 10/1 [Japanese]) in germ cell tumor series in the pineal location, but there is an equal sex distribution or female predominance for suprasellar primary tumors (Jennings et al., 1985).

Because the management and prognosis of patients with intracranial germ cell tumors is very dependent on histology, it is imperative to establish an unequivocal diagnosis prior to the administration of radiotherapy (RT) and/or chemotherapy. For example, germinomas are readily curable with RT alone or combinations of RT and chemotherapy; NGGCT are potentially curable with maximal surgical debulking and intensive chemotherapy and RT; and teratomas are curable with surgery alone (Jennings et al., 1985).

Primary intracranial germ cell neoplasms are histologically similar to gonadal germ cell tumors. Germinoma is histologically identical to the seminoma (testes) or dysgerminoma (ovary). Germinomas are typically composed of two cell types: large, uniform polyhedral cells with clear cytoplasm that resemble primordial germ cells; and smaller lymphoid cells. The large cells contain abundant intracytoplasmic glycogen. Their round nuclei contain one or more prominent nucleoli (Fig. 7–1). Although not neces-

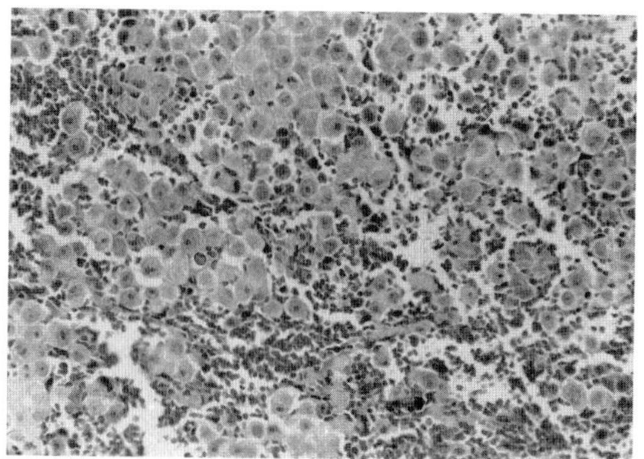

Figure 7–1. Germinomas contain large cells with clear cytoplasm and scattered lymphocytes. Hematoxylin and eosin, ×200.

sary for diagnosis, immunohistochemical studies can help in problem situations when only limited material is available. No single antigen, however, has been identified as "specific" for germinoma (Table 7–2). The lymphocytic component is immunopositive for antibodies to leukocyte common antigen, whereas the larger epithelioid cells may react to antibodies for placental alkaline phosphatase and cytokeratins (Felix and Becker, 1990). Some germinomas may also contain syncytiotrophoblastic cells, which are immunoreactive with antibodies to human β-chorionic gonadotropin.

From a treatment perspective, the malignant NGGCTs are the most challenging. Endodermal sinus tumor and choriocarcinoma resemble extra-embryonic tissues, and the embryonal carcinoma appears similar to fetal embryonal tissue. Endodermal sinus tumors (yolk sac tumor) consist of glomeruloid structures composed of a space lined by tumor cells with an invaginated vascular pedicle covered by a monolayer of the same cells. This tumor is considered to represent a neoplasm whose cells are partially differentiated into extra-embryonic structures that express yolk sac potential (Gonzalez-Crussi, 1979). Embryonal cell carcinoma is considered the most histogenetically primitive of the germ cell tumors, with features of anaplastic columnar to cuboidal cells arranged in sheets and cords (Bjornsson et al., 1985). This tumor shows a variable pattern of acinar, papillary tubular, or solid structures. A lymphocyte infiltrate may also be present but is not as abundant as in germinomas. Embryonal cell carcinoma may give rise to a multiplicity of tumor admixtures, with the most advanced form being teratoma. Choriocarcinomas are examples of differentiation along extraembryonic pathways and are composed solely of cytotrophoblastic and syncytiotrophoblastic cells without true villous formation. The primary immunohistochemical marker of this tumor is human β-chorionic gonadotropin, which is secreted by the syncytiotrophoblast; however, positive staining for human β-chorionic gonadotropin is not exclusively diagnostic of choriocarcinoma (Midgley and Pierce, 1962). Primary intracranial choriocarcinomas are rare (Bjornsson et al., 1986).

A relatively uncommon form of germ cell tumor is the pure teratoma, a tumor that is composed of mature tissues from all three germ cell layers (endoderm, mesoderm, and ectoderm). Pineal teratomas are complex mixtures of tissues that occur most frequently in males, in contrast to sacrococcygeal teratomas, which occur more often in females. Pineal teratomas are largely well differentiated or mature, but immature teratomas with malignant features do occur (Bjornsson et al., 1985). Any CNS teratoma,

Table 7–2. Tumor Marker Profile For Germ Cell Tumors

Tumor	*AFP*	*Cytokeratin*	*HCG*	*PLAP*
Germinoma			"+"	+
Choriocarcinoma		+	++	+/−
Embryonal carcinoma		+		+
Endodermal sinus tumors	++	+		+/−
Malignant teratoma	+/−	+		

+ = cases are positive; +/− = some cases are positive and some cases are negative; "+" = positive in special cases where syncytiotrophoblastic giant cells are seen; ++ = prominent immunohistochemistry appearance; AFP = α-Fetoprotein; HCG, β-chorionic gonadotropin; PLP, placental alkaline phosphatase.

however, can harbor foci of a malignant germ cell tumor; therefore, adequate sampling is of the utmost importance. If no other malignant elements are detectable, this variant can be managed with radical surgical resection alone. This strategy also pertains to other mature teratoid or embryonal tumors, such as dermoids and epidermoids.

Tumor Markers

The tumor markers α-fetoprotein (AFP), human β-chorionic gonadotropin (HCG), placental alkaline phosphatase, and lactic dehydrogenase isoenzymes are useful in the diagnosis and treatment monitoring of germ cell tumors. Elevations in levels of AFP alone in cerebrospinal fluid (CSF) and serum are found in pure endodermal sinus tumor. Elevated levels of both HCG and AFP are found in embryonal carcinoma, and high levels of HCG alone are found in choriocarcinoma. The serum and CSF levels in cells of AFP may be 10 to 100 times baseline. Serum HCG levels may be 100 times baseline, and there may be a CSF/serum gradient, especially when lumbar CSF is assayed. Modest elevations of HCG may be found in germinoma, usually in the presence of elevated placental alkaline phosphatase and/or lactic dehydrogenase isoenzymes (Allen, 1987). A serum or CSF HCG >50 IU/L and/or an AFP >25 ng/ml in the presence of a midline CNS tumor is supportive of a diagnosis of NGGCT (Calaminus et al., 1997).

Clinical Presentation

The clinical presentation of germ cell tumors varies with the site(s) of primary and/or metastatic disease. For suprasellar primary tumors, especially germinomas, the prodrome may be long, that is, from months to several years. Typically, a child may present with signs and symptoms of hypopituitarism (i.e., diabetes insipidus, growth failure, or secondary hypothyroidism) or precocious puberty. Initial neurodiagnostic studies may be noninformative. Children with acquired hypopituitarism are prime candidates to harbor germ cell tumors and should be followed expectantly with magnetic resonance imaging (MRI) scans at regular intervals. Visual field or acuity impairments and hydrocephalus occur late in the prodrome, when the tumor is large or disseminated. An MRI scan may disclose an extra-axial enhancing mass in the suprasellar and/or pineal region or intraventricular seeding in the third or lateral ventricles with hydrocephalus. A diagnostic surgical procedure is typically performed after a stress or therapeutic dose of corticosteroids is administered.

Patients with primary tumors arising in the pineal region tend to have a much shorter prodrome (i.e., weeks to several months). These patients usually present with signs and symptoms of raised intracranial pressure, such as headache, diplopia, and lethargy due to aqueductal obstruction. Tectal compression can cause Parinaud's syndrome (vertical gaze paresis, impaired pupillary light reflex, and convergence nystagmus). The MRI scan will reveal a pineal region-enhancing mass, which may protrude into the posterior region of the third ventricle with acute hydrocephalus (Fig. 7–2). Following high-dose corticosteroid therapy, the patient may need to be stabilized with ventriculostomy before definitive surgery.

General Management Considerations

The management of primary intracranial germ cell tumors is changing. Surgery is becoming an increasingly safer procedure for patients with suprasellar and pineal region tumors, and histologic documentation is a prerequisite for optimum therapy. The management of germ cell tumors is histology dependent and different protocols are emerging for patients with pure germinomas and nongerminoma germ cell tumors. During a prior era when surgical approaches to the pineal region were associated with considerable morbidity and mortality, the standard practice was to administer a therapeutic/diagnostic course of focal radiation therapy to 20 Gy. If the tumor underwent a major regression, a presumptive diagnosis of germinoma was made and the patient then received a full course (55 Gy) of focal and, in some institutions, craniospinal radiation. If the tumor did not respond to the 20 Gy dose, a diagnostic surgical procedure could be performed.

This approach is no longer favored for several reasons. Germinomas are not the most prevalent tumors in the pineal region in either pediatric or adult series, and the incidence of various tumor types is not readily predictable. For example, the incidence of germ cell tumors in the pineal region reported in two recent operative pediatric series from the Children's Hospital of Philadelphia (Packer et al., 1984) and the University of California, San Francisco (Edwards et al., 1988) were 32% and 61%, respectively. The in-

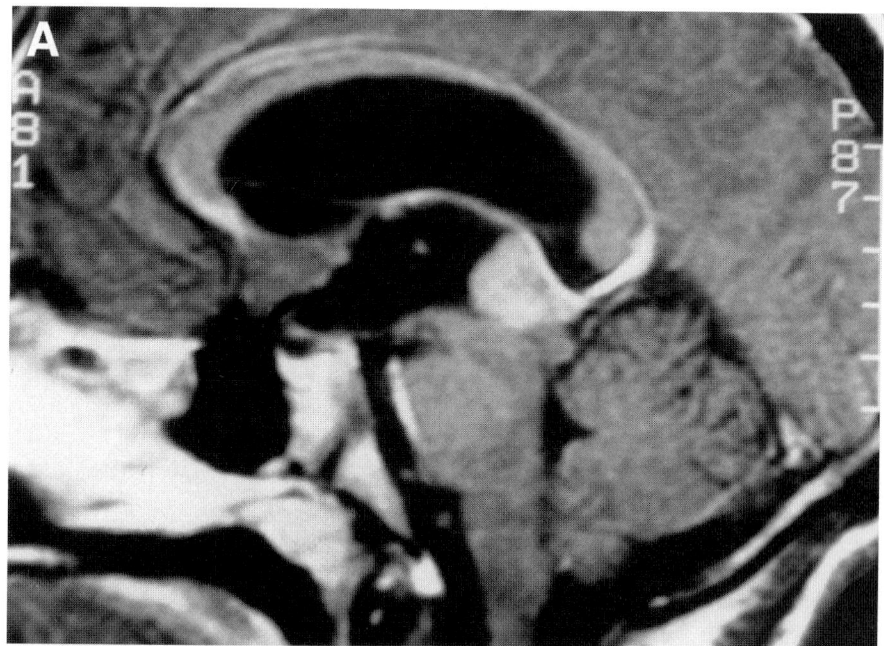

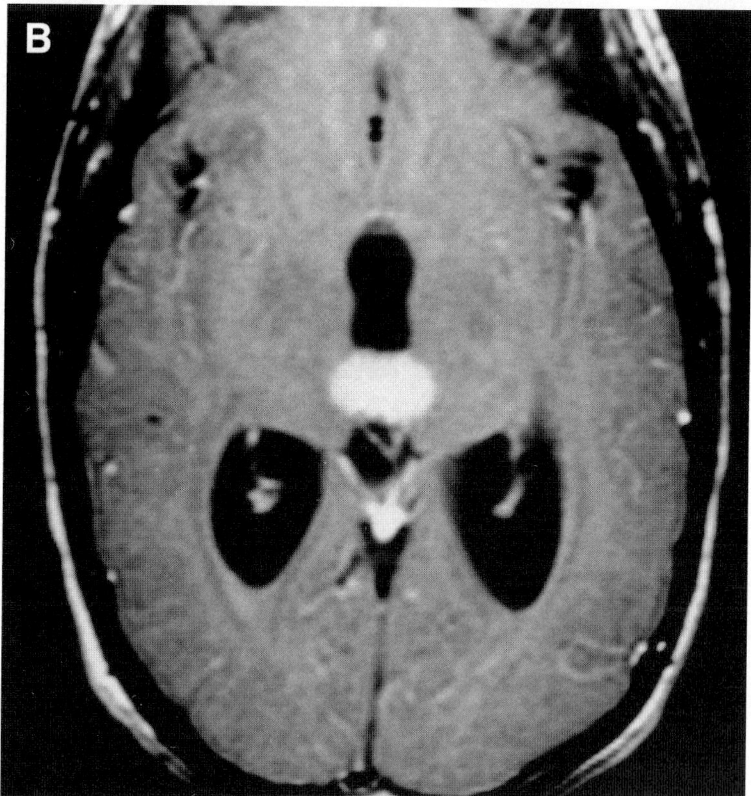

Figure 7–2. **(A)** Sagittal MRI scans with contrast of an 18-year-old man who presented with symptoms of increased intracranial pressure. The MRI shows a homogeneously enhancing pineal mass causing obstruction of the aqueduct of Sylvius. **(B)** Axial MRI of same patient. **(C)** Intraoperative photograph showing what turned out to be a germinoma. The superior colliculi are seen just inferior to the tumor. **(D)** Sagittal MRI 3 months after surgery and radiation therapy; no evidence of residual tumor is shown. (*continued*)

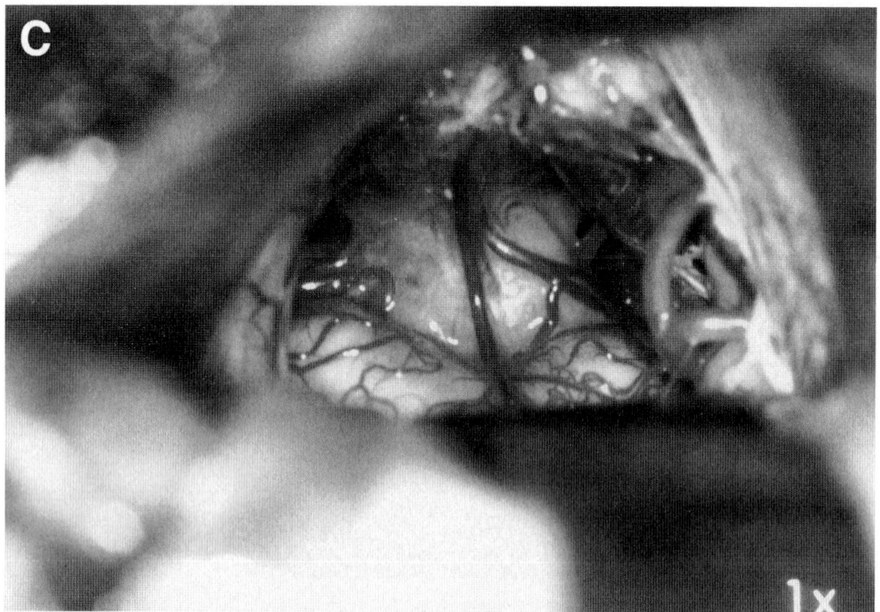

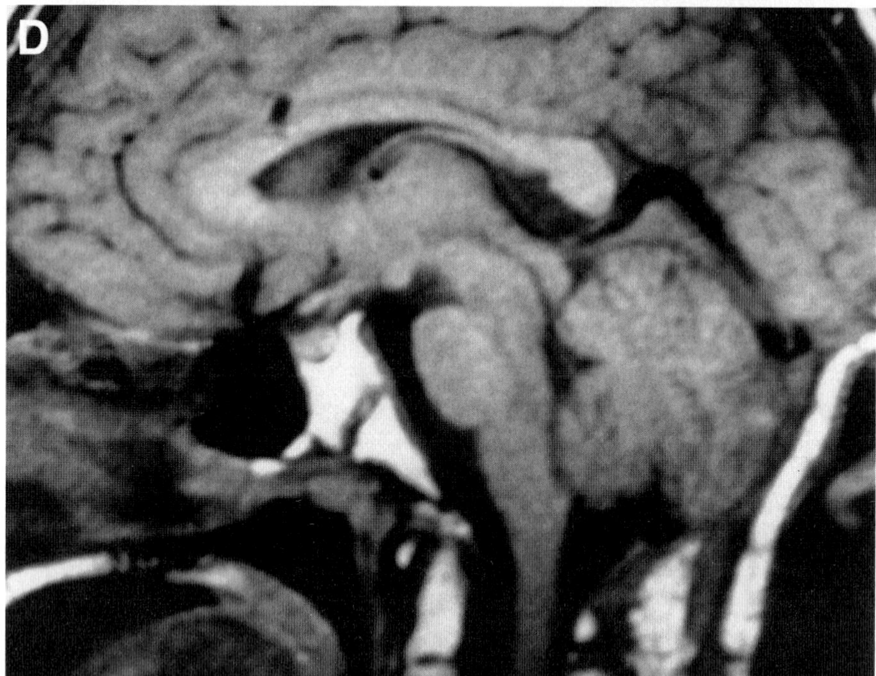

Figure 7–2. (*Continued*)

cidence in two adult series was 38% (Linggood and Chapman, 1992; Bruce and Stein, 1995). The incidence of pure germinoma in the two pediatric series was 20% (7/35) and 31% (11/36), respectively.

Other malignant tumors (pineoblastoma and malignant ependymoma) may respond to RT, but their management is quite different from that for germinoma. If a low-grade tumor such as an astrocytoma, pineocytoma, or teratoma exists, radical surgical resection alone rather than RT may be the treatment of choice. For certain tumors, such as ependymoma and malignant astrocytoma, focal RT is indicated; pineoblastomas and some germ cell tumors are generally treated with craniospinal RT. Most importantly, radiographic studies cannot reliably distinguish among these tumors. Surgery not only provides important diagnostic information, but radical resection of a malignant tumor may confer a therapeutic benefit. With modern neurosurgical techniques (operating microscope, image guidance, Cavitron, and so forth), the surgical morbidity is significantly reduced.

Figure 7–2 shows preoperative (Fig. 7–2A,B) and postoperative (Fig. 7–2D) MRI images of an 18-year-old male with a germinoma who presented with a 2 to 3 week history of progressive headache, nausea and vomiting, and diplopia whose examination revealed papilledema and Parinaud's syndrome. Figure 7–2A (saggital) and Figure 7–2B (axial) reveal a homogeneously enhancing pineal region mass extending into the posterior third ventricle. Aqueductal compression caused hydrocephalus. Figure 7–2C depicts the surgeon's view of the tumor through the operating microscope, and Figure 7–2D shows an MRI that confirms a radical resection.

Following surgery, the patient should be examined for possible CNS metastases. Central nervous system tumor dissemination may be present in 10% to 30% of patients with germ cell tumors at diagnosis (Allen, 1987; Hardenbergh et al., 1997). Complete staging includes lumbar Cerebrospinal fluid examination for malignant cells and tumor markers and MRI scans (head and spine) with gadolinium enhancement. CSF examination for malignant cells may not, however, be particularly helpful immediately after a surgical procedure; the accuracy of this examination increases over time and is more reliable 2 weeks or more after surgery. Like any CSF examination for malignant cytology, a negative result does not rule out leptomeningeal dissemination. As discussed earlier, germ cell tumor markers can be used in some cases to confirm the presence of a specific germ cell component. If detectable, these markers can also be used for tracking response to therapy or tumor recurrence. Table 7–2 indicates the expected tumor marker profile for each of the histologic tumor types.

Surgical Management

Objectives

Because a wide variety of histologic tumor subtypes can occur in the pineal region, establishing a definitive diagnosis is essential. Surgical biopsy is the only method for establishing a definitive diagnosis as features seen radiographically are not a reliable predictor of histology (Tien et al., 1990). Combined advances in surgical technique, neuroanesthesia, and postoperative management have decreased morbidity and mortality rates for pineal-region surgery to acceptable levels (Edwards et al., 1988; Neuwelt et al., 1979; Stein and Bruce, 1992). The specific tumor histology has important implications for determining prognosis, staging evaluation, choice of adjuvant treatment, and optimal strategies for long-term follow up. The one exception to the requirement for tissue diagnosis in a patient with a pineal-region tumor is the detection of elevated HCG or AFP in serum or CSF on the preoperative evaluation. The role of second-look surgery is more controversial. For patients with NGGCT who may be referred to a treatment center with subtotally resected disease, rather than attempting a radical resection before adjuvant therapy, the patient should first be treated with chemotherapy with or without RT. If the markers are still elevated or there is still residual disease on MRI, second-look surgery is indicated. Surgical resection may be curative. Residual tumor usually consists of benign germ cell elements that have been more resistant to therapy, with the malignant portions having been eradicated.

Control of Hydrocephalus

Nearly all patients with pineal-region tumors present with symptomatic hydrocephalus, which often requires urgent attention, either medically or surgically. This observation is useful in distinguishing neoplastic from benign conditions such as pineal cysts, which may be found incidentally in evaluating patients who have headache disorders. For patients who do not respond to high-dose corticosteroids, a ventriculostomy or shunt may be necessary. Preoperative control of hydrocephalus is desirable, as it allows a gradual decompression of the ventricles and intracranial pressure before surgical resection. Additionally, it facilitates CSF removal for tumor marker analysis and cytologic examination.

Several methods are available for controlling hydrocephalus, each with advantages and disadvantages. Placement of a permanent ventriculoperitoneal shunt alleviates the problem by diverting CSF from the cerebral ventricles to the peritoneal cavity, and it carries a low complication rate. However, shunt malfunction, infection, and, rarely, peritoneal seeding of malignant tumors are potential complications (Bruce and Stein, 1993). If the tumor can be removed, the patient may not need the shunt at all.

To avoid some of the drawbacks of shunts, an endoscopically guided third ventriculostomy is preferable (Goodman, 1993). By passing a small endoscope through a burr hole into the ventricles and floor of the third ventricle into the prepontine cistern, the surgeon may relieve obstructive hydrocephalus. This method avoids the risks of tumor seeding and shunt malfunction. The tumor may also be biopsied with this instrument. If a germinoma is diagnosed and the CSF markers are negative, then a craniotomy can be avoided as the patient has a medically curable disease. Major drawbacks of this method include the possibility that the ventriculostomy may close and a small risk of catastrophic hemorrhage during fenestration (Ferrer et al., 1997).

Patients who present with mild hydrocephalus and a tumor that appears resectable may be treated without any diversion of CSF. For these patients, a ventricular drain can be placed at the time of surgical resection. This drain is left in place for several days and removed when tolerated.

Optimum Methods of Obtaining Diagnostic Tissue

An open procedure, an endoscopic visually guided biopsy, and a stereotactic biopsy are the three methods available to secure tissue for diagnosis. An open procedure is nearly always preferred as it reduces the risk of sampling error. Ordinarily, a larger amount of tumor specimen will be available for histopathologic examination. This is critical not only because many pineal tumors are of mixed histology (Russell and Rubinstein, 1989; Stein and Bruce, 1992) but also because many of the histologic subtypes are rare and difficult even for experienced neuropathologists to interpret. An open operation with aggressive tumor resection is the preferred method of treatment for the one-third of pineal tumors that are benign (Stein and Bruce, 1992). Malignant tumors may also benefit from a thorough debulking to reduce the tumor burden before radiation therapy or chemotherapy (Stein and Bruce, 1992; Sano, 1976; Lapras and Patet, 1987). Surgical resection alone is sufficient treatment for some subgroups of slow-growing tumors such as pineocytomas, astrocytomas, ependymomas, and dermoids (Bruce and Stein, 1993).

Stereotactic biopsy guided by computed tomography (CT), which involves localizing a deep target lesion and passing a thin biopsy needle through it, is an alternative method for obtaining tissue (Dempsey et al., 1992). The biopsy needle secures a small core of tissue approximately 1×3 mm in size. Stereotactic biopsy can be performed relatively easily at a medical center where advanced stereotactic equipment is available. There are, however, considerable drawbacks to this procedure, the most significant being the potential for sampling error in a heterogeneous tumor or an erroneous diagnosis as only a small tissue sample is provided (Chandrasoma et al., 1989; Edwards et al., 1988). Because these are closed procedures performed by passing a probe through brain tissue, several anatomic features of pineal tumors make them undesirable for sampling by stereotactic biopsy for technical reasons. The risk of hemorrhage is heightened because of an adjacent deep venous system, the vascular nature of some malignant tumors, and their periventricular location, which allows minor bleeding to persist into the ventricle without tamponade by the surrounding tissue (Peragut et al., 1987). There have also been rare reports of implantation metastasis (Rosenfeld et al., 1990). The endoscopic biopsy procedure is attractive for patients who will undergo a third ventriculostomy and whose tumors protrude into the posterior third ventricle. The risks include limited biopsy material and hemorrhage.

Surgical Approaches to the Pineal Region

Three surgical approaches to the pineal region are used, each with advantages and disadvantages: infratentorial supracerebellar, suboccipital, and paramedian transcallosal (Bruce and Stein, 1993). The surgeon's degree of comfort and experience with the procedure play a major role in the approach chosen.

Surgical results depend more on the tumor's invasiveness and relationship with surrounding structures than on which approach is utilized. The deep location of these tumors makes surgery risky. An infratentorial approach is favored because it allows the most direct access to these midline tumors and, if a sitting position is used, allows gravity to work in the surgeon's favor when dissecting the tumor from the surrounding deep venous system. Supratentorial approaches are best suited for large tumors that have a significant lateral or supratentorial component.

Supratentorial approaches have the disadvantage of requiring brain retraction or sacrifice of bridging veins, which can lead to focal neurologic deficits.

Surgical Results

Most large surgical series reported by experienced neurosurgeons using microsurgical techniques report morbidity rates ranging from 0% to 12% and mortality rates ranging from 0% to 8% (Bruce and Stein, 1993). The largest series cited a mortality rate of 4% and a major morbidity rate of 3% (Stein and Bruce, 1992). Most series involving stereotactic biopsy demonstrated minimum mortality and morbidity; however, some errors in diagnosis occurred (Bruce and Stein, 1993). The most common operative-related complications involve extraocular movement dysfunction related to tectal trauma (Bruce and Stein, 1993). Altered mental status and ataxia can occur, but generally these deficits are temporary. Many of these problems are present preoperatively as a result of tumor compression and hydrocephalus and thus make it difficult to distinguish preoperative from postoperative morbidity. Ultimately, most complications are transient and improve with time. Shunt malfunction is another frequent complication (Bruce and Stein, 1993).

Multimodality Treatment Considerations

Much recent interest has been aroused concerning the application of adjuvant RT and/or chemotherapy following the diagnosis of a malignant germ cell tumor. Most clinical investigators use different treatment strategies for the management of germinomas and nongerminoma germ cell tumors such as endodermal sinus tumors, choriocarcinomas, embryonal carcinomas, and immature teratomas. Germinomas are readily curable with high-dose RT alone or with combinations of moderate-dose chemotherapy and RT, and the major concern is to minimize the late effects of therapy. NGGCTs are less responsive to therapy, and the goal is to improve survival by intensification of treatment.

Radiotherapy

Radiation has been the primary curative treatment for germinomas arising in the pineal and suprasellar regions. Durable disease control rates in excess of 65% to 90% are well documented in the literature (Linstadt et al., 1988; Legido et al., 1989; Dearnaley et al., 1990; Jenkin et al., 1990; Fuller et al., 1994). However, this survival rate is achieved at a high price as the late effects of RT on cognitive and neuroendocrine function may be significant. In addition, many medical centers also employ craniospinal RT (36 Gy) regardless of whether CNS metastases are present, and this therapy has additional late effects on spinal growth and cognition. Although responsive to irradiation, other malignant germ cell tumors such as endodermal sinus tumors, embryonal carcinomas, or choriocarcinomas in pure or mixed form are controlled in fewer than 10% to 25% of cases involving RT alone (Jennings et al., 1985; Dearnaley et al., 1990; Linggood and Chapman, 1992; Fuller et al., 1994).

The appropriate therapeutic radiation volume for pineal and suprasellar germinomas remains highly controversial. Recommendations vary from irradiation of limited local fields to coverage of the third ventricle, the entire ventricular system, the full cranium, or the entire neuraxis (craniospinal irradiation). The incidence of neuraxis dissemination is estimated at 10% to 20% in pineal germinomas and at 10% to 35% in suprasellar germinomas (Sung et al., 1978; Rich et al., 1985; Linstadt et al., 1988; Dearnaley et al., 1990; Jenkin et al., 1990; Fuller et al., 1994). A suggestion that biopsy predisposes to subarachnoid seeding, especially in lesions of the pineal region, is difficult to confirm, as benign tumor types may confuse outcome data among cases not undergoing biopsy (Linstadt et al., 1988; Dearnaley et al., 1990; Fuller et al., 1994). The excellent disease control and limited toxic effects following low-dose craniospinal irradiation in prepubertal patients favors administering craniospinal irradiation to 25 to 30 Gy followed by a local "boost" to the tumor site for a total of 50 Gy (Hardenbergh et al., 1997). Lower doses to the neuraxis may also be effective. A European pilot study (MAKEI 89) involving 49 germinoma patients reduced the craniospinal dose to 15 Gy while administering 45 Gy to the primary tumor. The 5 year progression-free survival in this series was 91% (Bamberg et al., 1999). A retrospective review of the Mayo Clinic experience involving 48 patients treated between 1935 and 1993 indicated that the spinal axis failure rate in patients who received partial brain volumes at 5 years from diagnosis was 49% compared with 0% for patients who received whole-brain or craniospinal treatment (Haddock et al., 1997).

Despite the obvious radiosensitivity of these tumors, dose–response data clearly indicate the necessity to deliver 50 Gy or more to the primary site. The "boost" encompasses the entire third ventricle for those with multiple midline germinomas, a relatively frequent adolescent presentation marked by two or more lesions around the midline structure (Rich et al., 1985; Dearnaley et al., 1990; Jenkin et al., 1990). There is little controversy that craniospinal irradiation is necessary in the few cases with neuraxis dissemination at diagnosis. Numerous recent series, however, question the necessity to treat beyond the local or third ventricular volume, as disease control rates in excess of 75% to 90% have been reported with more limited radiation volumes (Linstadt et al., 1988; Glanzmann and Seelentag, 1989; Dattoli and Newall, 1990; Fuller et al., 1994).

The majority opinion regarding treatment of both pineal and suprasellar germinomas appears to support wide local irradiation that includes the primary tumor with or without the adjacent third ventricle. This approach extrapolates to the 10% to 25% of adolescent males who present with multiple midline germinomas, which are believed to represent independent primary tumors or subependymal extension rather than subarachnoid seeding (Linstadt et al., 1988; Fuller et al., 1994). Some radiotherapists favor continued use of low-dose craniospinal irradiation for postpubertal patients based on a small but discernible benefit balanced against very limited added morbidity; for young children or patients who elect more limited treatment, wide local radiation fields can certainly be justified.

For the NGGCT types, an inferior survival rate with RT alone and the higher incidence of neuraxis recurrence supports the coordinated use of chemotherapy and craniospinal irradiation to near-tolerance levels (approximately 35 to 40 Gy) (Dearnaley et al., 1990; Allen, 1991; Fuller et al., 1994).

Chemotherapy

Chemotherapy is being utilized with increasing enthusiasm for both germinoma and nongerminoma germ cell tumors. For germinomas, attempts have been made to reduce or defer RT after a trial of neoadjuvant chemotherapy. In one study, following surgical confirmation of a pure germinoma and determination of the extent of CNS disease, two courses of high-dose cyclophosphamide were administered (Allen et al., 1987). A complete response (CR) or disappearance of all measurable disease was observed in 10 of 11 patients, and these 10 then received a 33% reduction in RT dose. The radiation volume (focal versus craniospinal) was determined by the extent of disease at diagnosis. Patients with localized disease at diagnosis who had a CR received involved-field RT only (30 Gy); those with disseminated disease received craniospinal therapy (24 Gy) plus a boost to the primary tumor. After a median of 5 years follow-up, only one patient developed a recurrence.

In an attempt to lower the risk of infertility after cyclophosphamide chemotherapy, the neoadjuvant chemotherapy has been changed to single-agent carboplatin. To date, the results of this trial show seven objective responses (six complete and one partial response) in eight patients with evaluative disease. The dose of RT was reduced in five patients who achieved a CR with carboplatin alone (Allen et al., 1994).

Pre-RT multidrug regimens have also been used with modifications of dose and volume of RT in attempts to lessen the late effects of RT. In a French study of 47 patients with germinoma, four courses of neoadjuvant chemotherapy (etoposide/carboplatin alternating with etoposide/ifosfamide) were administered before RT (40 Gy for localized disease). The 3-year, progression-free survival was 96% (Bouffet et al., 1999). Multidrug therapy with agents such as cisplatin and etoposide has also been used with encouraging results in a neoadjuvant setting with reduced-dose RT at the Mayo Clinic in a smaller pilot study of nine patients with germinoma (Buckner et al., 1999).

One study attempted to achieve long-term remission with chemotherapy alone. A multinational protocol developed at Memorial Sloan-Kettering Cancer Center administered six courses of carboplatin, etoposide, and bleomycin to 45 patients with germinoma and 26 with NGGCT. For those patients not experiencing a CR, two further courses of cyclophosphamide were administered. If a CR was achieved, RT was deferred. Although a CR was achieved in 78%, permitting a deferral of RT, 49% recurred after a median of 13 months of follow up. Most of these patients were salvaged with additional chemotherapy and high-dose RT (Balmaceda et al., 1996). These experiences support the continued use of multimodality therapy for newly diagnosed germinoma patients.

Based on these observations, multi-institutional and cooperative studies are underway to optimize pre-radiation chemotherapy and lower radiation doses and field sizes. Siffert and colleagues (2000) reported an ongoing study of patients with newly diagnosed germinoma who were treated with two courses of carboplatin and etoposide; if a CR was achieved they received reduced doses (typically 30.6 Gy) of radiation therapy and a reduced field if one site was involved. Patients who failed to achieve CR received two additional courses of cisplatin and cyclophosphamide before radiation therapy. This approach appears promising as 18 of 19 patients achieved a chemotherapy-induced CR with carboplatin and etoposide and reduced-dose radiation therapy.

Much progress has been made in the management of patients with NGGCT. A pilot multi-institutional study based at NYU Medical Center treated 18 NGGCT patients with a multimodality regimen employing chemotherapy (cisplatin/etoposide), RT, and then chemotherapy (bleomycin, vinblastine, carboplatin, and etoposide). The 4 year progression-free survival rate was 67% (Robertson et al., 1997). Another German/Italian pilot study treated 19 NGGCT patients with neoadjuvant chemotherapy (cisplatin/etoposide/ifosfamide) followed by RT. Preliminary results revealed an 81% progression-free survival rate at 12 months (Calaminus et al., 1997). Attempts to use single-modality therapy with either RT alone (Jennings et al., 1985) or chemotherapy alone (Balmaceda et al., 1996) produced an unacceptably high recurrence rate. Twelve of 13 patients in a French pilot study relapsed following 6 cycles of multiagent chemotherapy alone and deferral of RT (Baranzelli et al., 1998). Patients with NGGCT have a most favorable prognosis with combinations of chemotherapy, RT, and radical surgical resection either at diagnosis or for residual post-treatment disease.

Management of Recurrence

Because of the rarity of pineal tumors, standard regimens for their treatment at recurrence do not exist. Treatment decisions for recurrences should consider histologic diagnosis, previous response to treatment, and the time to recurrence. A second operation is useful for patients with slow-growing tumors of low malignancy. Chemotherapy, either conventional or high dose with stem cell support, can be useful for patients with recurrent malignant germ cell or pineal cell tumors, although their prognosis is poor. Radiosurgery (especially multiple-day fractions) is an attractive option for patients with localized tumor recurrences less than 3 cm in diameter. Fractionated conventional external-beam radiation is rarely a therapeutic option for recurrences, as it is generally given to its maximum allowable dose at initial tumor presentation. Patients with either germinomas or NGGCTs who have relapsed following chemotherapy alone can, however, be salvaged with multimodality therapy (Merchant et al., 1998; Baranzelli et al., 1998).

PINEOCYTOMA/PINEOBLASTOMA

Pathology

Neoplasms arising from pinealocytes or pineal parenchyma are rare. Traditionally these tumors have been categorized by grade as pineocytomas (low grade) and pineoblastomas (high grade) (Schild et al., 1993; Herrick and Rubinstein, 1979; D'Andrea et al., 1987). Pineocytomas occur in adolescence or adulthood. They are circumscribed, noninvasive, and slow growing. Histologically they resemble the normal pineal gland (Fig. 7–3).

Pineoblastomas are high-grade tumors resembling medulloblastomas in appearance and behavior. Morphologically they are composed of primitive, small cells that frequently form neuroblastic rosettes (Fig. 7–4). Pineoblastomas, in contrast to pineocytomas, have a propensity to seed the subarachnoid space.

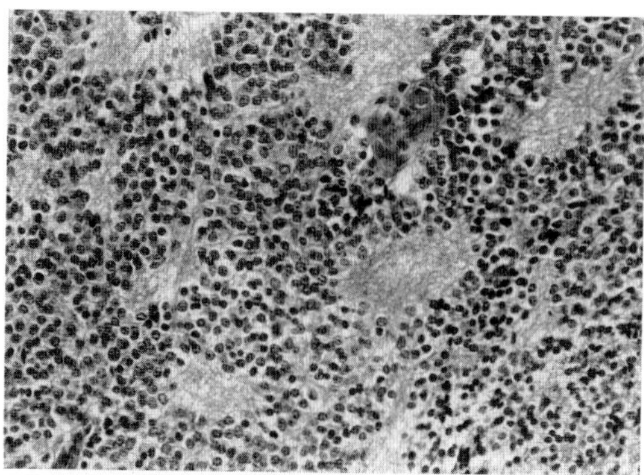

Figure 7–3. Pineocytomas have round nuclei and fibrillary cytoplasm compartmentalized into lobules. Hematoxylin and eosin, ×200.

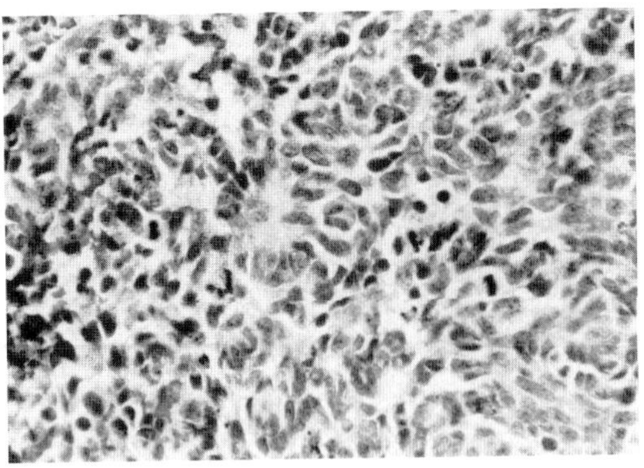

Figure 7–4. The primitive cells in a pineoblastoma have high nuclear/cytoplasmic ratios resembling neuroblastomas and medulloblastomas. Hematoxylin and eosin, ×200.

Clinical Presentation

In a population-based study from Manitoba, Canada (1980–1989), comprising all ages, pineal parenchymal tumors accounted for 1% of 315 cases (Sutherland et al., 1987). Pineal parenchymal tumors constituted 3.4% (8/234) of tumors in a large institutional survey of pediatric brain tumors in the Children's Hospital of Philadelphia series. Three pineocytomas and five pineoblastomas together comprised 32% (8/25) of the pineal region tumors from the same pediatric series (Packer et al., 1984). The incidence of pineal parenchymal tumors in a large, predominantly adult, series of 154 patients from the New York Neurologic Institute at Columbia University was 17% (Bruce and Stein, 1995).

Pineal parenchymal tumors present in a fashion similar to germ cell tumors with predominant symptoms related to aqueductal obstruction (raised intracranial pressure) and midbrain compression (Parinaud's syndrome). The malignant pineal parenchymal tumors (pineoblastoma or primitive neuroectodermal tumor) tend to arise in children with a median age of onset of 5 years (Packer et al., 1984). Pineocytomas arise predominantly in adults. The median age of onset of pineocytoma in an adult necropsy series of five cases was 51 years (Borit et al., 1980). The average duration of symptoms was 4 years.

Management

Because of the rarity of pineal parenchymal tumors, controversy surrounds their management. Pineocytomas in adults are, for the most part, locally aggressive and infrequently metastasize; optimum management consists of maximal surgical resection with or without involved-field RT. These tumors resemble an intraventricular neurocytoma, a relatively benign neuronal tumor that can be managed with radical surgical resection alone. Pineocytoma diagnosed in a child is problematic. Although the histologic diagnosis implies a relatively favorable prognosis, there have been a number of case reports of children with pineocytomas developing widespread CNS metastases (D'Andrea et al., 1987). Of six Children's Hospital of Philadelphia patients with pineocytomas, five received craniospinal RT and two received chemotherapy. Median progression-free survival rate was 2 years, and three patients died (D'Andrea et al., 1987). In an adult series, the median survival was 7 years, and at necropsy all had died of localized disease without evidence of metastases (Borit et al., 1980). Thus, pineocytomas may behave differently in adults than in children.

Pineoblastomas are managed in a similar fashion to primitive neuroectodermal tumors elsewhere in the CNS. Their prognosis relates, in part, to the same prognostic variables that govern the management of medulloblastoma. Standard-risk patients include those with gross total resections who have no metastases at diagnosis. High-risk patients consist of those with any of the following criteria: minimal resections, positive CSF cytology (M-1), diffuse leptomeningeal metastasis (M-2 or M-3), and diagnosis made when the patient is younger than 3 years. Infants and children under 3 years of age tend to be treated according to infant brain tumor protocols with intensive chemotherapy alone. Overall, they have a poor prognosis. In the Childrens Cancer Group protocol 921, eight infants younger than 2 years of age at diagnosis with pineoblastoma were treated only with the "8 drugs in 1 day" protocol. Under this schedule, all infants developed progressive disease and died. The median progression-free survival rate was 4 months (Jakacki et al., 1995), and this chemotherapy regimen was judged to be ineffective.

For children old enough to receive RT, multimodality therapy (surgery, RT, and chemotherapy) appears to be the preferred method. Chemotherapy may be given before and/or following RT, as in Childrens Cancer Group protocol—local; 36 Gy—craniospinal. Any measurable CNS metastases identified during the staging evaluation received additional RT. Results of a relatively large Childrens Cancer Group series (15 patients) treated on this randomized protocol are more favorable, with a 3-year progression-free survival rate of 61% (Jakacki et al., 1995). It is difficult to obtain comparative survival data from other large studies. Most prior publications are case reports, and patients were managed in a variety of ways (i.e., involved-field RT, craniospinal RT, and RT plus chemotherapy). Craniospinal RT appears to be the most effective treatment to date, and the added benefit of adjuvant chemotherapy can only be surmised from data concerning medulloblastoma clinical trials.

ASTROCYTOMAS

Astrocytomas are discussed briefly because they are one of the most common pineal region tumors. Astrocytomas are not pineal parenchymal tumors but arise in adjacent regions of the thalamus or midbrain. They are managed similarly to those arising elsewhere in the CNS, except they are more surgically inaccessible. Treatment guidelines are based on histologic grading. Because radical resections are difficult to perform in this region, the prognosis for high-grade fibrillary astrocytomas of the pineal region is poorer than the already dismal prognosis for high-grade astrocytomas elsewhere in the brain. The prognosis of low-grade astrocytomas is variable. The diffuse low-grade fibrillary astrocytoma behaves similarly to a brain stem glioma with a 3 year survival of less than 5% (Reardon et al., 1998). Low-grade juvenile pilocytic astrocytomas have a more favorable outcome. One variant, the tectal or midbrain glioma, appears to have a protracted course and may be managed with ventriculoperitoneal shunt and deferral of surgery or RT (Squires et al., 1994). For children or adults with radiographic and clinical progression from a midbrain or thalamic juvenile pilocytic astrocytoma, chemotherapy or RT may produce long-term palliation (Packer et al., 1993; Petronio et al., 1991).

CONCLUSIONS

It is clear that patients with symptomatic pineal region tumors benefit from a surgical procedure to establish a histologic diagnosis and control raised intracranial pressure. Modern multimodality therapy for these uncommon malignant tumors should involve participation in cooperative group clinical trials.

REFERENCES

Allen JC. 1987. Management of primary intracranial germ cell tumors of childhood. Pediatr Neurosci 13:152–157.

Allen JC. 1991. Controversies in the management of intracranial germ cell tumors. Neurol Clin 9:441–452.

Allen JC, DaRosso RC, Donahue B, Nirenberg A. 1994. A phase II trial of preirradiation carboplatin in newly diagnosed germinoma of the central nervous system. Cancer 74:940–944.

Allen JC, Kim JH, Packer RJ. 1987. Neoadjuvant chemotherapy for newly diagnosed CNS germ cell tumors of the central nervous system. J Neurosurg 67:65–70.

Balmaceda C, Heller G, Rosenblum M, et al. 1996. Chemotherapy without irradiation—a novel approach for newly diagnosed CNS germ cell tumors: results of an international cooperative trial. The First International Central Nervous System Germ Cell Tumor Study. J Clin Oncol 14:2908–2915.

Bamberg M, Kortmann R, Calaminus G, et al. 1999. Radiation therapy for intracranial germinoma: results of the German cooperative prospective trials MAKEI 83/86/89, J Clin Oncol 17:2585–2592.

Baranzelli MC, Patte C, Bouffet E, et al. 1998. An attempt to treat pediatric intracranial αFP and βHCG secreting germ cell tumors with chemotherapy alone. SFOP experience with 18 cases. Societe Francaise d'Oncologie Pediatrique. J Neurooncol 37:229–239.

Bjornsson J, Scheithauer BW, Leech RW. 1986. Primary intracranial choriocarcinoma: a case report. Clin Neuropathol 5:242–245.

Bjornsson J, Scheithauer BW, Okazaki H, Leech RW. 1985. Intracranial germ cell tumors: pathobiological and immunohistochemical aspects of 70 cases. J Neuropathol Exp Neurol 44:32–46.

Borit A, Blackwood W, Mair WG, et al. 1980. The separation of pineocytoma from pineoblastoma. Cancer 45:1408–1418.

Bouffet E, Baranzelli MC, Patte C, et al. 1999. Combined treatment modality for intracranial germinomas: results of a multicentre SFOP experience. Societe Francaise d'Oncologie Pediatrique. Br J Cancer 79:1199–1204.

Bruce J, Stein BM. 1993. Supracerebellar approaches in the pineal region. In: Apuzzo ML (ed), Brain Surgery: Complication Avoidance and Management. New York: Churchill-Livingstone, 511 pp.

Bruce J, Stein BM. 1995. Surgical management of pineal region tumors. Acta Neurochir (Wien) 134:130–135.

Buckner JC, Peethambaram PP, Smithson WA, et al. 1999. Phase II trial of primary chemotherapy followed by reduced-dose radiation for CNS germ cell tumors. J Clin Oncol 17:933–940.

Calaminus G, Andreussi L, Garre M, Kortmann RD, Schober R, Gobel U. 1997. Secreting germ cell tumors of the central nervous system (CNS). First results of the cooperative German/Italian pilot study (CNS sGCT). Klin Pediatr 209: 222–227.

Chandrasoma PT, Smith MM, Apuzzo MLJ. 1989. Stereotactic biopsy in the diagnosis of brain masses: comparison of results of biopsy and resected surgical specimen. Neurosurgery 24:160–165.

Chik K, Li C, Shing MM, Leung T, Yuen PM. 1999. Intracranial germ cell tumors in children with and without Down syndrome. J Pediatr Hematol Oncol 21:149–151.

D'Andrea AD, Packer RJ, Rorke LB, et al. 1987. Pineocytomas of childhood: a reappraisal of natural history and response to therapy. Cancer 59:1353–1357.

Dattoli MJ, Newall J. 1990. Radiation therapy for intracranial germinoma: the case for limited volume treatment. Int J Radiat Oncol Biol Phys 19:429–433.

Dearnaley DP, A'Hern RP, Whittaker S, Bloom HJ. 1990. Pineal and CNS germ cell tumors: Royal Marsden Hospital experience 1962–1987. Int J Radiat Oncol Biol Phys 18:773–781.

Dempsey PK, Kondziolka D, Lunsford LD. 1992. Stereotactic diagnosis and treatment of pineal region tumors and vascular malformations. Acta Neurochir (Wien) 116:14–22.

Edwards MS, Hudgins RJ, Wilson CB, Levin VA, Wara WM. 1988. Pineal region tumors in children. J Neurosurg 68: 689–697.

Felix I, Becker LE. 1990. Intracranial germ cell tumors in children: an immunohistochemical and electron microscopic study. Pediatr Neurosurg 16:156.

Ferrer E, Santamarta D, Garcia-Fructuoso G, Caral L, Rumia J. 1997. Neuroendoscopic management of pineal region tumors. Acta Neurochir (Wien) 139:12–20.

Fuller BG, Kapp DS, Cox R. 1994. Radiation therapy of pineal region tumors: 25 new cases and a review of 208 previously reported cases. Int J Radiat Oncol Biol Phys 28:229–245.

Glanzmann C, Seelentag W. 1989. Radiotherapy for tumors of the pineal region and suprasellar germinomas. Radiother Oncol 16:31–40.

Gonzalez-Crussi F. 1979. The human yolk sac and yolk sac (endodermal sinus) tumors: a review. Perspect Pediatr Pathol 5:179–215.

Goodman R. 1993. Magnetic resonance imaging-directed stereotactic endoscopic third ventriculostomy. Neurosurgery 32:1043–1047.

Haddock MG, Schild SE, Scheithauer BW, Schomberg PJ. 1997. Radiation therapy for histologically confirmed primary central nervous system germinoma. Int J Radiat Oncol Biol Phys 38:915–923.

Hardenbergh PH, Golden J, Billet A, et al. 1997. Intracranial germinoma: the case for lower dose radiation therapy. Int J Radiat Oncol Biol Phys 39:419–426.

Herrick MK, Rubinstein LJ. 1979. The cytological differentiating potential of pineal parenchymal neoplasms (true pinealomas): a clinicopathologic study of 28 tumors. Brain 102:289–320.

Hoffman HJ, Yoshida M, Becker LE, et al. 1983. Pineal region tumors in childhood: experience at the Hospital for Sick Children. In: Humphreys RP (ed), Concepts in Pediatric Neurosurgery, vol 4. Basel: S. Karger, 360 pp.

Jakacki RI, Zeltzer PM, Boyett JM. 1995. Survival and prognostic factors following radiation and/or chemotherapy for primitive neuroectodermal tumors of the pineal region in infants and children: a report of the Childrens Cancer Group. J Clin Oncol 13:1377–1383.

Jenkin D, Berry M, Chan H, et al. 1990. Pineal region germinomas in childhood: treatment considerations. Int J Radiat Oncol Biol Phys 18:541–545.

Jennings MT, Gelman R, Hochberg F. 1985. Intracranial germ-cell tumors: natural history and pathogenesis. J Neurosurg 63:155–167.

Lapras C, Patet JD. 1987. Controversies, techniques and strategies for pineal tumor surgery. In: Apuzzo MLJ (ed), Surgery of the Third Ventricle. Baltimore: Williams & Wilkins, p 649.

Legido A, Packer RJ, Sutton LN, et al. 1989. Suprasellar germinomas in childhood. A reappraisal. Cancer 63:340–344.

Linggood RM, Chapman PH. 1992. Pineal tumors. J Neurooncol 12:85–91.

Linstadt D, Wara WM, Edwards MS, Hudgins RJ, Sheline GE. 1988. Radiotherapy of primary intracranial germinomas: the case against routine craniospinal irradiation. Int J Radiat Oncol Biol Phys 15:291–297.

Malogolowkin MH, Mahour GH, Krailo M, Ortega JA. 1990. Germ cell tumors in infancy and childhood: a 45-year experience. Pediatr Pathol 10:231–241.

Merchant TE, Davis BJ, Sheldon JM, Leibel SA. 1998. Radiation therapy for relapsed CNS germinoma after primary chemotherapy. J Clin Oncol 16:204–209.

Midgley AR, Pierce GB. 1962. Immnohistochemical localization of human chorionic gonadotropin. Proc Soc Exp Biol Med 115:289–294.

Neuwelt EA, Glasberg M, Frenkel E, Clark WK. 1979. Malignant pineal region tumors. J Neurosurg 51:597–607.

Packer R, Lange B, Ater J. 1993. Carboplatin and vincristine for reccurent and newly diagnosed low-grade gliomas of childhood. J Clin Oncol 11:850–856.

Packer RJ, Sutton LN, Rosenstock JG, et al. 1984. Pineal region tumors of childhood. Pediatrics 74:97–102.

Peragut JC, Dupard T, Graziani N, Sedan R. 1987. [Prevention of risk in stereotaxic biopsy of various tumors of the pineal region. Apropos of 3 cases]. Neurochirurgie 33:23–27.

Petronio J, Edwards MS, Prados M, et al. 1991. Management of chiasmal and hypothalamic gliomas of infancy and childhood with chemotherapy. J Neurosurg 74:701–708.

Reardon D, Gajjar A, Sanford R, et al. 1998. Bithalamic involvement predicts poor outcome among children with thalamic glial tumors. Pediatr Neurosurg 29:29–35.

Rich TA, Cassady JR, Strand RD, Winston KR. 1985. Radiation therapy for pineal and suprasellar germ cell tumors. Cancer 55:932–940.

Robertson PL, DaRosso RC, Allen JC. 1997. Improved prognosis of intracranial non-germinoma germ cell tumors with multimodality therapy. J Neurooncol 32:71–80.

Rosenfeld JV, Murphy MA, Chow CW. 1990. Implantation metastasis of pineoblastoma after stereotactic biopsy. Case report. J Neurosurg 73:287–290.

Rubinstein LJ. 1970. Histological classification of pineal tumors. Tumors of the pineal region. In: Tumors of the Central Nervous System. Washington, DC: Armed Forces Institute of Pathology, 269 pp.

Rueda-Pedraza ME, Heifetz SA, Sesterhenn IA, Clark GB. 1987. Primary intracranial germ cell tumors in the first two-decades of life: a clinical, light-microscopic, and immunohistochemical analysis of 54 cases. Perspect Pediatr Pathol 10:160–207.

Russell DS, Rubinstein LJ. 1989. Tumors and tumor-like lesions of maldevelopmental origin. In: Russell DS, Rubinstein LJ (eds), Pathology of Tumours of the Nervous System. Baltimore: Williams & Wilkins, 664 pp.

Sano K. 1976. Diagnosis and treatment of tumours in the pineal region. Acta Neurochir (Wien) 34:153–157.
Schild SE, Scheithauer BW, Schomburg PJ, et al. 1993. Pineal parenchymal tumors. Clinical, pathologic and therapeutic aspects. Cancer 72:870–880.
Siffert J, Robertson P, Jakacki R, Hukin J, Domnahue B, Velasquez L, et al. 2000. Multiagent neoadjuvant chemotherapy followed by reduced dose radiotherapy for newly diagnosed central nervous system germinoma: preliminary results of a multi-institutional phase II pilot. J Neurooncol 2:294.
Squires LA, Allen JC, Abbott R, Epstein FJ. 1994. Focal tectal tumors: management and prognosis. Neurology 44:953–956.
Stein BM, Bruce JN. 1992. Surgical management of pineal region tumors (honored guest lecture). Clin Neurosurg 39:509–532.
Sung DI, Harisliadis L, Chang CH. 1978. Midline pineal tumors and suprasellar germinomas: highly curable by irradiation. Radiology 128:745–751.
Sutherland GR, Florell R, Louw D, Choi NW, Sims AA, et al. 1987. Epidemiology of primary intracranial neoplasms in Manitoba, Canada. Can J Neurol Sci 14:586–592.
Tien RD, Barkovich AJ, Edwards MS. 1990. MR imaging of pineal tumors. Am J Roentgenol 155:143–151.

8

Pituitary Tumors

IAN E. McCUTCHEON

Pituitary tumors are the most commonly occurring intracranial neoplasms. They are found in 8% to 24% of autopsied people, most of whom in life harbored small asymptomatic tumors that did not cause hormonal disturbance (Kovacs et al., 1980; Parent et al., 1981; Teramoto et al., 1994; Tomita and Gates, 1999). Pituitary tumors can, however, produce profound physiologic upset by secreting supraphysiologic amounts of hormones or, when large, by compressing critical neural structures adjacent to their typical location in the sella turcica.

The treatment of pituitary tumors has undergone a renaissance since the revival of transsphenoidal techniques by Guiot and Hardy 35 years ago. This process has been aided by the development of hormonal assaying techniques and radiographic imaging during the last three decades. Today, small pituitary tumors can be detected more easily and their hormonal activity can be assessed more accurately than has previously been possible. Medical therapy, particularly for prolactin-secreting adenomas, but also for acromegaly, has developed sufficiently so that surgery can be avoided in some patients who can be managed with drugs alone.

In general, pituitary tumors are diagnosed earlier and treated more effectively now than at any previous time. Nevertheless, a significant number of pituitary tumors deviate from the typical pattern of benign histology and slow growth.

Pituitary adenomas can be invasive and penetrate adjacent dura to enter the sphenoid sinus, cavernous sinuses, or other parts of the skull base. These tumors can grow to a significant size and cause neurologic damage by provoking cranial neuropathies or optic nerve dysfunction; engulfing the carotid arteries and their tributaries; or impinging on the brain. Such aggressive variants behave as malignant tumors of the skull base. Even small, benign tumors may produce a chronic, uncontrolled hypersecretion of pituitary hormone that causes profound physiologic changes over time. By any of these means, pituitary adenomas continue to pose an oncologic threat that warrants their inclusion in any list of clinically significant tumors of the central nervous system (CNS).

PATHOLOGY

Most pituitary gland tumors arise from the anterior portion of the gland known as the *adenohypophysis*. They are adenomas, tumors of the secretory elements, which in many cases produce and release one or more of the pituitary hormones produced by the anterior lobe. A pseudocapsule, sharply demarcating them from the adjacent normal gland, which may be compressed by tumor, usually encloses these lesions. Although preferred locations for each of the different secretory types have been described within the anterior lobe, in actual fact any of the different subtypes can arise anywhere within the anterior lobe. Rare cases have been reported of adenomas arising in the pars tuberalis, a small extension of the anterior lobe along the distal anterior portion of the stalk (Rothman et al., 1976), or of tumors arising within the sphenoid sinus, nasopharynx, or clivus from embryonic rests of the pharyngeal pituitary (Hori et al.,

1999). When less than 10 mm in diameter, these tumors are called *microadenomas;* when larger, they are called *macroadenomas.* A typical adenoma histologically shows loss of the normal acinar pattern and its intervening reticulin network. The cells are fairly uniform in appearance, with small nuclei and a small amount of cytoplasm (Fig. 8–1).

Older schemes of classification, which have relied on standard hematoxylin and eosin staining to produce an appearance of basophilic, acidophilic, or chromophobe staining, have little functional significance and are now obsolete. Current pathologic analysis of pituitary adenomas relies heavily on immunohistochemistry (Asa, 1998). The six major hormones of the anterior lobe (prolactin, growth hormone, thyrotropin [TSH], luteinizing hormone [LH], follicle-stimulating hormone [FSH], and adrenocorticotropin [ACTH]) can be detected by applying a polyclonal or monoclonal antiserum to tumor sections and then exposing the sections to a secondary antibody linked to reagents that give a colorizing reaction. The demonstration of hormonal *production* does not necessarily correlate with hormone *secretion,* and a number of clinically nonfunctional tumors, which produce no detectable rise in serum hormone levels, have been found to contain hormone, usually FSH or LH, that has been synthesized in small amounts but not secreted or secreted inefficiently (Black et al., 1987; Daneshdoost et al., 1993; Sano and Yamada, 1994). In addition, pituitary tumors in many cases produce hormones in a disorderly fashion, with an imbalance in the production of the α- and β-subunits, which (in the case of TSH, LH, and FSH) must link covalently to produce a bioactive molecule. Some tumors produce hormone that is detectable through conventional techniques but is biologically inactive (Katznelson et al., 1992; Trouillas et al., 1991) or hyperactive (Gesundheit et al., 1989). In most patients, however, a reasonable correlation exists between the clinical endocrine status of the patient, serum hormone levels, and the hormones demonstrated within the tumor through immunohistochemistry.

The spectrum of tumors that are truly inactive has narrowed greatly with the development of more sensitive hormone detection techniques. Such tumors are called *null-cell adenomas* (Kovacs et al., 1980). These tumors stain negatively for all hormones and contain none of the granules detected by electron microscopy in typical secretory tumors. It has been suggested that they arise from cells of gonadotrophic lineage, although their origin remains controversial. A subset of these tumors contains large numbers of mitochondria visible by electron microscopy, which are called *onocytomas* (Bauserman et al., 1978). Oncocytomas are typically large when diagnosed and affect males more frequently than females (Silbergeld et al., 1993).

It is now apparent that many of the tumors traditionally called *nonsecreting* actually do secrete hormone in amounts too small to be of clinical significance (Asa et al., 1992; Greenman et al., 1998), or they may produce the α-subunit or chromogranin (Nobels et al., 1993). These two secreted products, neither of which has hormonal activity, can be detected in the blood of some patients with clinically nonfunctional adenomas. The α-subunit is one of the

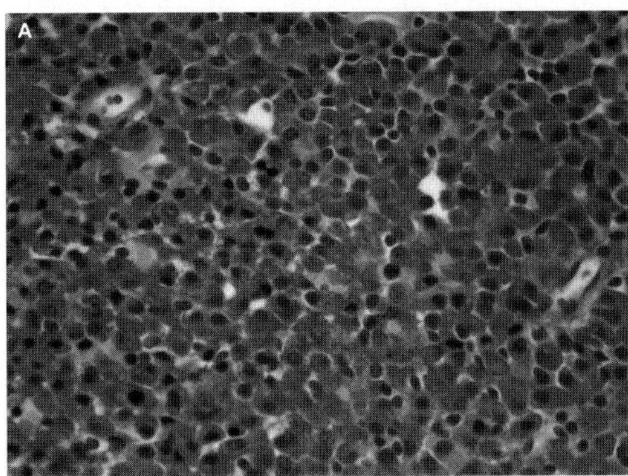

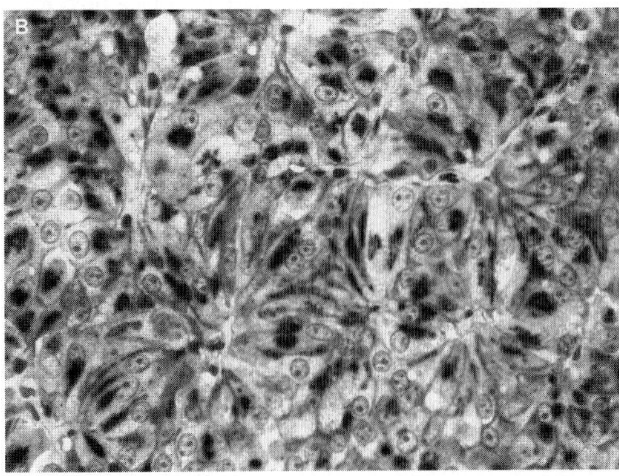

Figure 8–1. Hematotoxylin and eosin stained **(A)** prolactinoma demonstrating monomorphic population of cells with spherical nuclei and delicate rims of cytoplasm. The same tumor stained with prolactin **(B)** shows immunoreactivity in the paranuclear location corresponding to the Golgi apparatus.

two subunits necessary for hormonal activity in glycoprotein hormones; alone, however, the α-subunit has no hormonal function. Chromogranin is produced by a variety of neuroendocrine tumors, including most pituitary tumors. These two products may be the only molecular species available for surveillance after surgery or other types of therapy in patients with hormonally inactive adenomas. The most common nonfunctional adenomas in patients under 40 years of age are silent corticotropic and gonadotropic adenomas, and their oncocytic variants typically occur in patients over age 40 years.

NATURAL HISTORY

Although pituitary adenomas are rare in children and fairly common in elderly patients at autopsy, the true prevalence of pituitary tumors in the different decades of life is not known. One preliminary study found focal abnormality of the pituitary suggestive of tumor in 10% of asymptomatic adults undergoing high-resolution scans (Hall et al., 1994). The expected rate of change in small or large adenomas is also not known. Although one study of patients with prolactin-secreting microadenomas found that many do not change in size over time (March et al., 1981), its authors used now-outdated techniques for radiologic surveillance. Another survey that examined untreated hyperprolactinemia found a gradual increase in tumor size in only 20% of patients, but did not address the question of the rate of tumor growth (Schlechte et al., 1989). In patients with clinically nonfunctional tumors in whom a partial surgical removal has been achieved, careful radiographic surveillance of the tumor remnant has shown regrowth in one-third, with a mean time to detection of 5.4 years (Turner et al., 1999). However, another study showed only 6% of endocrine-inactive tumor remnants recurring within 5 years (Lillehei et al., 1998). As the odds of tumor progression weigh heavily on decisions to use (or withhold) postoperative radiotherapy, such information has great practical value. However, these determinations have never been addressed adequately for patients with other forms of pituitary tumor. Most therapeutic decisions in pituitary tumor algorithms are based on logical, although not clearly proven, assumptions that the tumor will enlarge over time and that present hormone levels predict future hormone levels in the untreated state.

CLINICAL PRESENTATION

Pituitary tumors cause a panoply of signs and symptoms that can be grouped into four categories: *(1)* compression of adjacent normal gland, *(2)* hormonal hypersecretion, *(3)* visual disturbance, and *(4)* headache.

Compression of Adjacent Normal Gland

Patients may present with hypopituitarism, that is, impairment of the normal function of the various hormonal axes subserved by the anterior pituitary. Particularly vulnerable is the pituitary-gonadal axis, in which minor disturbances of the cycling of FSH or LH can affect libido and fertility in both sexes and the menstrual cycle of women. Also vulnerable to local pressure effects are the pituitary-thyroid and pituitary-adrenal axes. Patients may therefore present with secondary hypothyroidism or a relative hypocortisolism predisposing them to addisonian crisis.

In adults, low levels of prolactin are not thought to be significant. Traditionally, the same assumption has been held regarding growth hormone. During the past decade, however, the clinical effects of growth hormone deficiency on body composition and bone metabolism—and the benefits of treating such deficiency—have become widely accepted. Diabetes insipidus caused by insufficient production of antidiuretic hormone rarely occurs, but, when it does, it heralds granulomatous involvement of the skull base (or a metastasis to the pituitary from a systemic cancer) rather than a pituitary adenoma in most patients who present with the disorder.

Hormonal Hypersecretion

Pituitary tumors may produce excess amounts of one or more pituitary hormones, which can induce symptoms relative to the specific hormone present in excess. Growth hormone–secreting tumors produce the syndrome of acromegaly, which is characterized by enlargement of the distal extremities and a coarsening of facial features from bony overgrowth in the skull. Patients with these tumors are prone to cardiac disease and diabetes mellitus and if untreated (or unsuccessfully treated) have a significantly shortened life expectancy, with an observed-to-expected mortality ratio of 1.6 to 3.3 (Wright et al., 1970; Holdaway and Rajasoorya, 1999).

Adrenocorticotropin-secreting tumors produce hypercortisolism and present with the findings of Cushing's disease. The protean nature of this disease reflects the importance of cortisol in many organ systems. Patients with Cushing's disease show changes in body habitus caused by excess fat deposits, giving them the classic "buffalo hump" and moon facies. Patients also tend to have abdominal striae, osteoporosis, and diabetes mellitus; show muscle weakness, particularly in the proximal distribution; and may exhibit psychiatric disturbances (McCutcheon and Oldfield, 1992).

The effects of ACTH-secreting tumors can be subtle in some patients and may present only as a tendency to arterial hypertension or as a very slow change in skin texture and facial contour. Patients with thyrotropin-secreting tumors have typical sequelae of the hyperthyroid state, including heat intolerance, nervousness, and cardiac dysrhythmias.

Prolactinomas cause galactorrhea in men and women and menstrual irregularity in women, which in many cases leads to infertility. A chronic, indirect suppression of estrogen caused by excess prolactin also predisposes the patient to osteoporosis. Men with prolactinomas may show a decreased sex drive and are prone to infertility. Gonadotropin-secreting tumors producing FSH, LH, or both, have a similar effect on the menstrual cycle, fertility, potency, and sex drive as do prolactinomas, but do not cause galactorrhea.

Visual Disturbance

Patients with suprasellar extension of a clinically nonfunctional tumor usually come to medical attention because of visual loss. Any pituitary tumor can cause decreasing vision if it grows large enough to compress the visual pathways. Typically a macroadenoma extending above the sella to the optic chiasm causes a defect in the bitemporal fields that begins in the upper quadrants and can progress to complete bitemporal hemianopia. Because of the anatomic variability in the placement of the chiasm relative to the pituitary stalk, a variety of presentations have been noted. Von Willebrandt's knee (where nerve tracts from the contralateral retina occupy part of the proximal optic nerve anterior to the chiasm) allows patients occasionally to present with a junctional scotoma, and some tumors are more eccentric to the right or left, thus causing a diversity of nonhomonymous field cuts. Long-standing compression of the optic nerves or chiasm can produce optic atrophy, with a resulting permanent loss of visual acuity. In addition, a tumor that extends into the cavernous sinus may, in its later phases of growth, cause disturbances of third, fourth, or sixth cranial nerve function, resulting in diplopia and ptosis.

Headache

Many patients with pituitary tumors present with headache. These patients often have chronic, refractory headaches that lead a physician to request a brain scan, which may disclose an unsuspected lesion in the pituitary fossa. Although headache is logical in patients with large tumors spilling out of the sella turcica and invading or compressing the pain-sensitive dura, its presence in patients with small, noninvasive tumors must be regarded as coincidental in the absence of any other logical explanation. Suggestions that such tumors cause headache by raising intrasellar pressure are intriguing but have not been proven sufficiently to gain general acceptance (Arafah et al., 2000). Occasionally, pituitary adenomas are found in patients who present with persistent headache after a minor head injury and in whom imaging performed once the headache begins reveals a small pituitary tumor that had been previously undetected.

In a few patients, headache indicates sudden changes in the size and structural integrity of the pituitary tumor. A small percentage of pituitary adenomas hemorrhage and produce an apoplectic syndrome of acute headache and sudden neurologic deterioration caused either by direct compression of the hypothalamus or its vascular supply or by diffuse effects of bleeding across the diaphragma sellae into the subarachnoid space (Randeva et al., 1999). In addition, such patients may show sudden hypopituitarism from acute compression of the normal gland. Occasionally, a patient with a clinically nonfunctional, previously unsuspected adenoma will present in this fashion and will experience diplopia, headache, and a sudden decrease in vision. Such patients require urgent surgical decompression if vision is to be recovered or preserved.

LABORATORY INVESTIGATIONS

The standard laboratory work-up for a patient suspected of having a pituitary tumor involves measurement of an array of hormones that provide direct and indirect indices of pituitary and tumor function (Table 8–1). The typical biochemical survey includes serum levels of prolactin, TSH, LH, and FSH. Growth hormone may also be measured, but this is only necessary if there is clinical evidence of acromegaly. If it is measured, then somatomedin-C (insulin-like growth factor-I) should also be determined because it provides a better picture of growth hormone secretion over time. Some endocrinologists have advocated measuring insulin-like growth factor binding proteins (most specifically IGFBP-3) as a measure of disease activity in acromegaly, but this remains controversial and has not gained widespread acceptance as a replacement for insulin-like growth factor-I surveillance (DeHerder et al., 1995; Paramo et al., 1997; Halperin et al., 1999). Normal levels of LH and FSH differ in men and women, and also differ in women during the various phases of the menstrual cycle. Measurement of thyrotropin levels should be accompanied by measurement of triiodothyronine and L-thyroxine so that elevations in TSH caused by primary pituitary hypersecretion can be distinguished from elevations caused by primary thyroid insufficiency.

Table 8–1. Laboratory Work-Up for Patients Suspected of Having a Pituitary Tumor

- Prolactin
- Thyrotropin
  - Triiodothyronine
  - L-thyroxine
- Luteinizing hormone
- Follicle-stimulating hormone
- Growth hormone, if clinical evidence of acromegaly
- Somatomedin-C (insulin-like growth factor-I)
- Cortisol
- Estradiol levels in women
- Prolactin
- Provocative hormonal tests (tailor to clinical situation: critical in Cushing's disease)
- Serum electrolytes (serum and urine osmolality, fluid intake and output, urine specific gravity when diabetes is suspected)
- Measurement of α-subunit for patients with clinically nonfunctional adenomas or those with a thyrotropin-secreting adenoma

Adrenocorticotropic hormone is not generally measured directly; rather, the activity of the pituitary-adrenal axis is determined by measurement of cortisol, one of the main adrenal hormones produced in response to adrenocorticotropic stimulation. Both cortisol and ACTH are heavily subject to diurnal rhythms, and it is generally considered best for coherent and consistent interpretation of serum cortisol levels to collect them at 8 AM, when they are relatively high. For women, estradiol levels are checked. These are fairly sensitive indices of gonadal failure but must be interpreted in conjunction with levels of FSH and LH.

Prolactin is measured for all patients. Elevations of prolactin may occur because of hypersecretion by tumor cells but can also be caused by anatomic distortion of the pituitary stalk by the tumor mass. This distortion results in inadequate flow through the portal-hypophyseal system of those dopaminergic factors that exert a tonic inhibition on prolactin production. When the stalk is compressed, this inhibition is released, and prolactin levels rise. Because the elevation caused by a prolactin-secreting tumor is usually significantly higher than that caused by a nonfunctional tumor disturbing the stalk, it is usually possible to distinguish between the two by a careful analysis of prolactin levels over time.

Other important information on the hormonal condition of the patient can be obtained by the use of provocative hormonal tests. In these tests, a synthetic stimulatory factor (such as the corticotrophin-releasing factor) is administered intravenously to the patient, and the hormonal response is evaluated over time. Such tests provide a dynamic indication of the ability of the gland to push hormone levels above baseline values. In subtle cases of hormone dysfunction, and particularly in patients with Cushing's syndrome where these tests can help with the differential diagnosis and localization of the hypersecretory source, the use of provocative tests may be considered. They also have value for the assessment of normal pituitary function in patients recovering from surgery for a pituitary tumor. In the postoperative setting, basal hormone values are remeasured after a suitable interval. This helps both to establish the presence or absence of continuing hypersecretion by residual tumor and to assess the adequacy of normal gland function, because such function may be damaged by the gentle manipulation required to separate a tumor from the adjacent normal gland. After surgery pre-existing hormone deficits will be restored in approximately 50% of patients, and 20% develop new deficits of anterior pituitary function (Webb et al., 1999).

The function of the posterior lobe is assessed by measurement of serum electrolytes and, in cases where there is a high suspicion of diabetes insipidus, by checking serum and urine osmolality and by recording fluid intake and output and urine specific gravity. It is exceedingly rare for a patient with a pituitary tumor to present with diabetes insipidus. If a sellar mass is seen on a scan and diabetes insipidus forms part of the clinical presentation, it is highly possible that the tumor is not a pituitary adenoma, but rather a metastatic tumor arising in the lung, breast, prostate, or another organ system. Diabetes insipidus occurs much more often in the postoperative period, when about 15% of patients show this phenomenon either transiently or permanently. The production of vasopressin by the pituitary is more sensitive than other hormonal axes to the trauma of surgery. Special vigilance is necessary during the first week after surgery, because patients with partial diabetes insipidus can become dehydrated and hypernatremic if the condition goes unrecognized and if no hormone supplementation is given. Surveillance for hyponatremia is also required during the first 2 weeks after surgery, as 2% (Hensen et al., 1999) to 21% (Olson et al., 1997) of patients develop a transient dysregulation of vasopressin release that can be clinically significant.

Measurement of the α-subunit has been considered experimental but is gaining acceptance. It is now recognized that some tumors are pure α-subunit–secreting adenomas (Ridgway et al., 1981). As a rule, this measurement should be taken for all patients with clinically nonfunctional adenomas (Warnet et al., 1994). The other group in whom the α-subunit has particular relevance is the occasional patient who presents with a TSH-secreting adenoma. Measurement of the α-subunit/TSH molar ratio in this instance is valuable in sorting out those patients with a "syndrome of inappropriate TSH secretion" who have a pituitary tumor from those who have pituitary resistance to the effects of TSH (Gesundheit et al., 1989; McCutcheon et al., 1990).

RADIOLOGIC EVALUATION

The preferred radiologic technique for pituitary tumor detection and follow up is magnetic resonance imaging (MRI). Magnetic resonance imaging has now supplanted previous methods of sellar tomography and computed tomography (CT), which are less sensitive and should only be used when MRI is unavailable (Webb et al., 1992). An occasional patient is still brought to medical attention by the incidental finding of erosion or enlargement of the sellar boundaries on a skull radiograph. Such patients generally have large nonfunctional tumors, and the most accurate way of defining the anatomic boundaries of the tumor is with a MRI scan. In years past, concerns about carotid artery aneurysms that masquerade as pituitary tumors led to the occasional use of angiograms for such patients. This too is now unnecessary, as standard MRI shows nicely the distinction between the flow void of the carotid artery within the cavernous sinus and the tumor within the sella and adjacent areas.

Tumors as small as 3 mm in diameter now represent the limits of detection of MRI scans enhanced by gadolinium (Lundin and Bergstrom, 1992). Pituitary tumors are generally seen on contrast scans as hypointense to isointense areas against a slightly hyperintense area of normal gland (Fig. 8–1). This situation is the reverse of that seen with glial tumors of the cerebral parenchyma, where enhancement is seen within the tumor and within adjacent areas of edematous brain with an impaired blood–brain barrier. There is no blood–brain barrier in the pituitary gland, and by virtue of this pattern of enhancement the vessels within the tumor would seem to be less immediately leaky to contrast than those of the normal gland. The best delineation is therefore seen in scans done early (i.e., from 2 to 5 minutes after gadolinium injection) (Hayashi et al., 1995).

There are still a number of patients in whom no distinct adenoma is seen but in whom biochemical tests suggest the presence of such a lesion. This circumstance is particularly relevant in Cushing's disease, where tumors may be very small, yet produce a profound physiologic upset because of the primacy of ACTH in a number of the physiologic processes relevant to homeostasis. Other secretory tumors tend to come to attention only when they are larger. Patients with Cushing's disease frequently have obvious hypercortisolism on biochemical and clinical examination, but can have a normal MRI of the sella turcica. Although a few such occult tumors become visible when dynamic scanning is performed during contrast infusion, this technique is not widely available (Bartynski and Lin, 1997). The possibility of misdiagnosis of ectopic secretion of ACTH for pituitary hypersecretion emphasizes the importance of rigorous biochemical testing, which should be able to distinguish between these two etiologies. In addition, even tumors larger than 3 mm in diameter can escape detection by scans if their signal characteristics are isointense to those of normal gland. The selection of patients for surgery who have been shown to secrete hormone in excess should be on the basis of biochemical evidence first and, second, on radiologic evidence.

TREATMENT

Rationale for Treatment

Determining the best way to treat pituitary adenomas depends on the predicted nature of the pathology. Hormonally active tumors usually require suppression by surgery, medical means, and/or radiation therapy to prevent the long-term sequelae of hypersecretion. In particular, patients with Cushing's disease or acromegaly rarely reach a normal life expectancy because of the deleterious effects that excess ACTH and growth hormone exert on a variety of organ systems, particularly the cardiovascular system. Patients with prolactinomas may require therapy to reverse the infertility imposed by such tumors and to prevent the accelerated osteoporosis that occurs in patients with chronically elevated prolactin levels (Klibanski et al., 1988). Those with TSH-secreting adenomas suffer an intractable form of hyperthyroidism with attendant cardiac irritability and also require definitive treatment. Clinically nonfunctional tumors often present because of chiasmal compression causing visual field defects. The presence of an increasing field cut is a strong indication for surgical decompression, a statement that applies equally to patients with secretory tumors of whatever type. For pituitary tumors as a group, statistics show a twofold excess mortality relative to the population at large, but the reason for this difference is unclear (Nilsson et al., 2000).

The goals of therapy for pituitary tumor include

- Elimination of hormonal excess by tumor section
- Prevention of optic nerve dysfunction caused by suprasellar extension of tumor
- Restoration or preservation of normal pituitary function
- Avoidance of therapeutic complications
- Long-term remission without biochemical or radiographic evidence for regrowth of tumor

Any treatment that is chosen must be judged by these standards in assessing its efficacy and suitability for a given patient.

Surgical Approaches

Entry to the sella turcica is achieved most safely by the transsphenoidal approach in patients with small tumors without extrasellar extension. This method allows the surgeon to avoid entering the intracranial compartment and has the advantage of midline trajectory that circumvents critical structures on either side of the gland (Hardy, 1969, 1991). The incision in such an operation can be made in the sublabial (below the lip) area over the maxilla just beneath the inferior extent of the pyriform apertures, a route that allows direct exposure of the virtual space between the cartilaginous nasal septum and the medial nasal mucosa (mucoperichondrium). A tunnel created within this virtual space leads directly to the vomer, sphenoid sinus, and sella. Alternatively, an endonasal route that avoids an external incision can be chosen, but this requires either a wide nasal cavity or incision of the nasal ala to allow room for a speculum within the nose (Griffith and Veerapen, 1987). In the endonasal approach, the incision is made in the nasal mucosa at the posterior edge of the cartilaginous septum where it meets the bony septum. Transsphenoidal approaches should be chosen for tumors confined to the sella, those with relatively minor suprasellar extension, or those that extend into the sphenoid sinus. Tumors with cavernous sinus extension are frequently excised by the transsphenoidal route, but complete resection should not be expected as the contents of the cavernous sinus usually elude full inspection.

The transcranial approach is reserved for patients with larger tumors that elevate the diaphragma sellae more than 2 cm above its normal level or that extend laterally from their intrasellar origin. Often, a pterional or combined pterional/subfrontal craniotomy is used, and a bone flap is fashioned that extends as close as possible to the floor of the anterior cranial fossa (Tindall and Tindall, 1987). The sylvian fissure is then split medially, the frontal lobe is elevated, the temporal lobe is slightly depressed with malleable retractors, and the suprasellar and sellar areas are visualized. The operating microscope is an essential tool in this small and anatomically complex region when transcranial and transsphenoidal procedures are performed. Intraoperative fluoroscopy is vital as well in transsphenoidal procedures and allows localization of the position of instruments relative to the bony landmarks of the skull base.

If cavernous sinus exploration or exenteration is desired, a fronto-orbito-zygomatic craniotomy can be performed. This procedure involves a more extensive bony removal that includes the orbital rim and roof, anterior clinoid, and malar eminence (Al-Mefty and Smith, 1990). The zygoma is usually cut free and allowed to fall down with the temporalis muscle, a tactic that grants the surgeon additional exposure over a fairly wide field of view. If carotid resection is planned, we prefer to expose the internal carotid artery in the neck in case a sudden rupture occurs requiring arterial tamponade; others unroof the petrous segment of the carotid instead. Before any cavernous sinus exploration is done, a preoperative carotid balloon occlusion test must be performed, which predicts the ability of the patient to tolerate carotid resection. This clinically qualitative test may be enhanced by the performance of single-photon emission CT or xenon-CT scans that measure cerebral blood flow in the ipsilateral and contralateral cerebral hemispheres (Origitano et al., 1994). These techniques continue to evolve and may offer hope for those patients with extensive disease in the cavernous sinus or skull base who, until recently, were offered radiation therapy as palliative treatment but for whom little other therapy was available (MacKay and Hosobuchi, 1978).

Other variations on these themes have been used over the years. The transethmoidal approach has had some proponents but is generally not used because it requires a facial incision and provides an angled, imperfect view that makes anatomic landmarks more difficult to identify than does the midline transsphenoidal approach (Kirchner, 1984). Endoscopic excision of pituitary tumors has been reported and is gaining increasing popularity as part of the trend in all surgical disciplines toward reducing incision size and the "invasiveness" of any given procedure. Although improvement in the quality of endoscopic instrumentation has fostered its use in pituitary surgery, and several medical centers have been enthusiastic in reporting its advantages (Jho, 1999; Sheehan et al., 1999; Jarrahy et al., 2000), no prospective comparison of its efficacy in achieving complete resection of adenomas, large or small, has yet been undertaken. Even though less disruption of the nasal septum occurs during endoscopic transsphenoidal surgery, patients are still subject to the risks of cerebrospinal fluid rhinorrhea and endocrine disturbance, so it is not clear why use of the endoscope should lead to shorter stays in hospital after operation, as some authors have proposed (Jho, 1999). It seems appropriate to use endoscopy as a tool for examining areas within the sella turcica that currently elude direct inspection by the surgeon. In particular, in many patients, the medial wall of the cavernous sinus is poorly seen or not seen at all, and adherent tumor can be left there after an otherwise successful operation. It is likely that endoscopy will become an additional, quite valuable tool for maximizing tumor resection, but that open procedures using the operative microscope will continue to be used for many patients (Jankowski et al., 1992).

Computer-assisted navigation has also been applied to pituitary surgery during the past 5 years. Such devices provide the surgeon with a pointer (typically tracked optically), the location of which is determined by a workstation and displayed on a screen showing the operative field on relevant multiplanar MRI slices. This technology is still evolving and is not yet ready to replace fluoroscopy as the standard localizing tool in transsphenoidal surgery (McCutcheon et al., 2001). However, it is quite useful in locating such surgically relevant structures as the carotid arteries and sphenoid septations, in planning the surgical trajectomy, and in locating lateral or inferior extensions of pituitary tumors invading the skull base (Sandeman and Moufid, 1998). Such tools, together with endoscopy, will become important aids to safer and more complete removal of pituitary tumors during the next decade.

SPECIFIC TUMOR TYPES

Table 8–2 summarizes specific types of pituitary tumors.

Prolactin-Secreting Adenomas

Approximately 40% of pituitary adenomas secrete prolactin, and such tumors are more common than any other type of pituitary neoplasm. In contrast to the reliance on surgery as the primary treatment for other forms of pituitary tumor, these tumors are usually treated medically before surgery is considered.

Drug Therapy

Various dopamine analogues that inhibit prolactin release are available, the most common being bromocriptine (Parlodel). About 70% to 80% of patients respond to this drug, but significant side effects occur in 20% to 30% of patients, which limits its use (Molitch et al., 1985). Side effects associated with bromocriptine include nausea, vomiting, orthostatic hypotension, and, in some patients, psychotic reactions. The drug may be stopped, therefore, because of a failure to arrest tumor growth and bring prolactin levels to normal or because the patient cannot tolerate the drug. An alternative long-acting dopamine agonist called quinagolide (or CV 205-502) has been developed. This agent has a higher affinity than bromocriptine for dopamine receptors. Approximately one-half of adenomas that resist bromocriptine therapy respond to quinagolide (Brue et al., 1992b). Quinagolide also invokes side effects and has caused weight loss and psychiatric breakdown in some patients, but has fewer side effects than bromocriptine (Glaser et al., 1994; Merola et al., 1994). Other long-acting bromocriptine analogues have also been studied that may lower the incidence of side effects (Brue et al., 1992a; Maraschini et al., 1991; Jamrozik et al., 1996); however, their role and that of quinagolide, in the clinical management of these patients has been eclipsed by cabergoline, another long-acting dopaminergic agent released for use in the United States in 1998.

Cabergoline (Dostinex) was developed as a D_2-receptor–specific agonist, by virtue of which it has less of a tendency to provoke side effects (operating through the D_1 as well as the D_2 receptor) than either bromocriptine or quinagolide. Because of this and because it is given once or twice weekly, patients are more likely to be compliant in taking the drug. It normalizes prolactin levels in 80% to 90% of patients and causes tumor shrinkage in two-thirds (Verhelst et al., 1999). In a series of patients resistant to bromocriptine, prolactin became normal in 70% of patients taking cabergoline; and, of patients intolerant of bromocriptine's side effects, 84% tolerated cabergoline and normalized their prolactin levels. Dose escalation improves these numbers even further (Colao et al., 2000). Comparison of cabergoline with quinagolide shows that the two drugs normalize prolactin in an equal proportion of patients, but that a greater chance of tumor shrinkage occurs with cabergoline (Di Sarno et al., 2000). Because of such results, cabergoline is now the drug of choice for medical treatment of prolactinomas, although bromocriptine remains a well-established (and significantly less expensive) alternative.

The response of patients with prolactinomas to medical therapy depends on tumor size and prolactin level. Patients with smaller tumors and lower prolactin levels respond best. If the prolactin level before treatment is greater than 1000 ng/ml, the levels usually fall with dopamine agonist therapy, but do not normalize (Hardy, 1984). Most tumors cause prolactin levels between 50 and 250 ng/ml. From 65% to 80% of patients taking bromocriptine in this range will normalize their prolactin levels, and over time tumor reduction occurs in 76% (Brue et al., 1992a; Maraschini et al., 1991). Cabergoline's statistics, alluded to above, are comparable or better.

The general assumption is that patients treated medically require life-long therapy to avoid regrowth of suppressed tumor; however, in some patients, the tumor disappears completely and does not recur when bromocriptine is stopped. After withdrawal of cabergoline, approximately 10% of patients exhibit this phenomenon, which appears to be confined to those with microadenomas (Di Sarno et al., 2000). Unfortunately, it is only possible to identify these pa-

Table 8–2. Specific Pituitary Tumor Types

Clinically nonfunctional adenomas (incidentalomas)
Gonadotropin-secreting adenomas
Growth hormone–secreting adenomas
Adrenocorticotropin-secreting adenomas
Thyrotropin-secreting adenomas

tients after the fact. This dilemma cannot be resolved fully at this time, but does suggest a clinical approach of stopping the drug at intervals and following hormone levels and scans for any sign of regrowth or return of hypersecretion. It is likely that the tumor will regain its activity in the majority of patients who are evaluated long enough and, in those patients, treatment must begin anew.

Surgery

Surgery is used only if medical treatment fails or if the patient cannot tolerate the side effects of the treatment. There has been some evidence to support the idea that pretreatment with bromocriptine enhances surgical results (Hubbard et al., 1987) and opposing evidence that it makes tumor excision more difficult by inducing fibrosis within the tumor (Bevan et al., 1987). Although patients may wish to temporize and avoid surgery, it is best not to continue trials of medical therapy for more than 1 year without declaring success or failure and deciding whether surgery will or will not be indicated.

The success of surgical treatment depends on tumor size and preoperative hormone level, both of which predict the invasiveness of the tumor in question. Microadenomas are more readily excised and generally show prolactin levels of 50 ng/ml to 100 ng/ml. In the series of Randall et al. (1983), prolactin levels normalized after surgery in 88% of those with preoperative levels less than 100 ng/ml, but in only 43% of those with levels greater than 100 ng/ml. Patients with prolactin levels greater than 350 ng/ml should be considered to have an invasive tumor, and all will harbor macroadenomas. In the very extensive series of Hardy (1984), the immediate remission rate was 86% for patients with levels less than 250 ng/ml but only 6% for those with levels greater than 1000 ng/ml.

Given the predominant role of medical therapy for prolactinomas, it is now uncommon to operate on patients with small tumors who have not received prior dopamine agonist therapy. It has been suggested that such pre-treatment compromises the success rate of surgical removal. In one surgical series in which all patients had been previously given bromocriptine, only 45% of patients with microadenomas and only 17% of those with macroadenomas had normal levels of prolactin postoperatively (Soule et al., 1996). Such results may reflect bromocriptine-induced fibrosis within the tumor, as well as a selection bias such that more difficult cases were more likely to be referred for surgery.

Despite initial success in most surgical series, a significant number of patients relapse when studied long-term after surgery (Hardy, 1984). Hardy's recurrence rate was 22% during the first 5 years after surgery. Others have shown recurrence rates of 17% to 50% during the first 2 years after surgery for microadenomas and 20% to 80% for macroadenomas during the same time period (Rodman et al., 1983; Serri et al., 1983). In Wilson's modern series, more than 90% of patients with microadenomas (and more than 80% of those with small macroadenomas) showed initial remission, as did 40% of those with prolactin levels above 200 ng/ml or with large, invasive tumors (Tyrrell et al., 1999). During 15 years of follow up, about 15% of those in remission relapsed to hyperprolactinemia.

In Adams' surgical series of microprolactinomas with a mean follow-up period of 70 months, only 1 of 32 patients recurred. It is certainly possible to normalize prolactin in most patients with a small, encapsulated tumor and to expect a sustained remission, but the persistence of remission has not been sufficiently studied for periods longer than 5 years. Because many patients in surgical series are between 25 and 40 years old and may be expected to live for several decades, more data on long-term rates of recurrence are needed. Tumor reactivation may occur for several reasons, including the regrowth of residual microscopic clusters of tumor cells, the presence of an underlying genetic mutation predisposing to tumor growth, or the presence of a mechanism of hypothalamic overdrive that continues unabated after tumor excision.

Radiation Therapy

Radiation therapy is useful for patients in whom such regrowth recurs and who wish to avoid further surgery. It is also a valuable adjunct for patients in whom a complete excision cannot be achieved because tumor has infiltrated adjacent dura, neural structures, or the cavernous sinus. Usually a fractionated dose of 45 to 50 Gy is given over 4 to 5 weeks by a limited-field technique that excludes structures outside a 4 cm window centered on the sella turcica. The drawbacks of radiotherapy are its gradual effect and its ability to damage parapituitary structures contained within the field as well as late effects that can occur. Several years usually pass before maximum tumor regression occurs, and 2 to 10 years may be required for normalization of prolactin levels. The success rate of sellar irradiation within this time frame has been reported to be as low as 30% (Sheline et al., 1984; Williams et al., 1994), although others have reported an 83% rate of local control over 10 years (Sasaki et al., 2000). Larger prolactinomas (i.e., with volume >30 cm^3), however, show particularly poor local control rates and may require specialized techniques or repeat surgery (Isobe et al., 2000).

New methods of irradiation include one that links beam delivery with stereotactic localization, allowing delivery of a highly concentrated, accurately focused dose of radiation to an intracranial target. Although the name "radiosurgery" has been applied to this method, no surgical incision is involved. Rather, this method involves attachment of a stereotactic ring to the patient's head by a neurosurgeon who assists a radiotherapist in planning the isodose contours, a complicated process that requires specialized computers and precise three-dimensional representation of the target. Either a standard radiotherapy gantry with a stationary target (LINAC) or multiple stationary sources of irradiation all focused simultaneously on the target (gamma knife) may be used. In theory, this method reduces the risk of radiation damage to adjacent structures, particularly the medial temporal lobes and the optic chiasm, while maximizing radiation dose. The pituitary gland is still included in the radiation field because of its intimate relation with any intrasellar tumor. In addition, if the cavernous sinus is included within the radiation field, 10% to 15% of patients will develop a cranial neuropathy within 3 years of radiosurgical treatment (Tishler et al., 1993).

The function of the normal gland is at risk with both stereotactic and conventional radiation techniques, and as many as 100% of patients treated conventionally show pituitary insufficiency when studied for 10 years (Littley et al., 1989). The administration of a stereotactic dose of 40 to 70 Gy by charged particle beam (no longer much used since the advent of the gamma knife) yielded a 10% to 30% incidence of post-treatment hypopituitarism, and 60% of patients with prolactin-secreting tumors had normalized prolactin levels within 1 year after treatment (Levy et al., 1991). Although such techniques have been available for a number of years in Europe and North America and were widely used during the 1990s, good long-term statistics are still unavailable. Most treatment centers that perform radiosurgery for pituitary tumors use the gamma knife system in which the target (i.e., the tumor) is placed at the center of a fixed, spherical array of radiation sources. LINAC-based systems, which utilize a roving gantry arm to deliver the radiation beam, can also be employed. However, the gamma knife has a dosimetric advantage in treating pituitary adenomas, as it can achieve a greater conformity index than the LINAC in this anatomic region (Plowman and Doughty, 1999).

In one small series of patients with microprolactinomas, radiosurgery caused normalization of prolactin levels in 23%, and a decrease (but not normalization) in 62%, during 1 year of follow up (Kim et al., 1999). In a larger series, similar results were achieved but correction of endocrinopathy occurred more frequently in patients with acromegaly or Cushing's disease than in those with prolactin-secreting tumors (Pan et al., 1998). As radiosurgery can only be done in patients with microadenomas or tumors with lateral (rather than superior) extension, many patients do not qualify for it and must be treated surgically and/or with more conventional radiotherapeutic techniques. For some, fractionated conformal irradiation may offer increased accuracy of targeting, with reduction in the volume of normal tissue exposed to irradiation. However, only preliminary experience has been reported with its use for pituitary tumors, so it is impossible to conclude whether it will prove safer or more effective than conventional limited-field techniques (Jalali et al., 2000; Perks et al., 1999).

Summary of Therapeutic Approach

In our current practice, we treat patients with prolactinomas first with cabergoline, unless a trial of the drug shows side effects the patient cannot tolerate. In years past, such patients were offered quinagolide as an alternative or they chose surgery. Quinagolide has been withdrawn from use in clinical trials in the United States despite its published clinical utility; it remains available in Europe and in Canada. Patients with progressive visual loss are also treated with surgery, but those with a macroadenoma and visual field cut can sometimes be controlled with dopamine agonists, and surgery can thereby be avoided. Radiotherapy is reserved for the relatively few patients whose tumors regrow after surgery or whose tumors cannot be completely excised, as proven by persistent elevation of prolactin despite maximal removal of tumor.

No Treatment

Prolactinomas, gonadotropin-secreting adenomas, and clinically nonfunctional adenomas comprise the majority of pituitary tumors and do not generally provoke hormonal derangements affecting long-term survival. What are the chances that a small tumor in this group that does not affect chiasmal function will grow at all if simply left untreated? Patients with macroadenomas often require treatment to preserve or improve vision and to control (in prolactinomas) high levels of hormone secretion that impair fertility and menstruation. These conditions must be corrected in those patients who wish to conceive.

Microadenomas, however, have been shown in some instances not to change for as long as 20 years, and their ability to secrete excess hormone may fade or actually increase over time. Spontaneous involution of such tumors, sometimes as a result of an apoplectic event, may occasionally occur. In a study of 30 patients with small tumors in whom no treatment was given, 14 showed no change in prolactin levels over time; 6 showed a gradual increase; and 10 showed a decrease (Schlechte et al., 1989). For patients with prolactin-secreting microadenomas and for those with small nonfunctional tumors, it is reasonable to follow those in whom some menstruation is present and child-bearing is not desired, with intervention reserved for those in whom tumor growth or increased secretory activity occurs.

Clinically Nonfunctional Adenomas

The category of clinically nonfunctional adenomas has been redefined in recent years as techniques in pathologic analysis have become more powerful. It now includes patients with true null cell adenomas that secrete no hormone of any kind; those with α-subunit–secreting adenomas that produce no active hormone; and those with tumors that, although secretory, produce quantities of hormone too small to effect clinical change in endocrine function. Many of the patients in the last category have tumors that, by immunohistochemical analysis, produce FSH or LH (Asa et al., 1992; Young et al., 1996). These gonadotropin-secreting adenomas were previously thought to be quite rare. It is now recognized that a spectrum exists that, at its lower end, includes patients previously classified as nonsecreting and at its high end includes those with detectable elevations of FSH and/or LH in peripheral blood. Each category is addressed here.

About 25% to 33% of pituitary adenomas are clinically nonfunctional and produce symptoms only by compressing the pituitary and parasellar structures and, eventually, causing frank hypopituitarism. This condition often goes unrecognized, except in retrospect, until compression of the visual pathways leads to the diagnosis of a sellar lesion. Approximately one-half of all pituitary adenomas stain on immunocytochemistry for one or more of the glycoprotein hormones or their subunits (α or β) (Black et al., 1987; Daneshdoost et al., 1993; Sano and Yamada, 1994). They are not clinically active because of inefficient hormone release or because they produce hormonal species of low bioactivity. Between 20% and 30% of patients with endocrine-silent pituitary adenomas do have increased levels of serum α-subunit, which may be useful in some cases as a marker of tumor activity (Oppenheim et al., 1990; Nobels et al., 1993). Such hypersecretion of α-subunit is most common in larger tumors (Warnet et al., 1994).

As for any large pituitary tumor, treatment includes hormone replacement to correct deficiency of normal pituitary function. There is no available medical treatment that effectively suppresses the growth of these tumors. However, octreotide has been shown to cause improvement in visual field deficits in clinically nonfunctional macroadenomas, although it has no effect in 50% of such tumors (Warnet et al., 1997). Although nonfunctional tumors are quite common, only a few large surgical series have been published, and all such series include both null cell adenomas and weakly gonadotropin-secreting tumors under the "nonsecreting" or "nonfunctional" heading. Ebersold et al. (1986) reported results from the excision of 100 nonfunctioning adenomas, of which 82 were greater than 2 cm in diameter. Most of these patients had preoperative visual impairment that generally improved after surgery. Because of the high prevalence of invasive features in such tumors, 50% were incompletely resected and required postoperative radiotherapy. Regrowth occurred in 18% of those who received radiation after surgery and in 12% of those (presumably smaller tumors) treated with surgery alone. In Hardy's series of 126 patients treated over 25 years, vision improved in 75% of those who had visual impairment before surgery, and 21% regrew during a mean follow-up period of 6.4 years (Comtois et al., 1991). In addition, preoperative hypopituitarism (present in >75% overall) improved in 41% of those with deficits in the pituitary-adrenal axis and in 14% of those with hypogonadism.

As with prolactinomas, radiotherapy is generally recommended when obvious residual tumor remains after surgery or when regrowth occurs and such treatment has not previously been given. Halberg and Sheline (1987) administered radiotherapy to 140 patients with clinically nonfunctional tumors. Of these, 23 were poor surgical candidates who received irradiation alone, 37 were treated by surgery only, and 80 underwent combined treatment. A long follow-up period (up to 20 years) was achieved. All patients treated with irradiation alone showed arrested growth of tumor; tumor recurred in 75% of those treated with surgery and radiotherapy and in 100% of patients treated with surgery alone. Such results suggest that many tumors in this category are invasive and are incompletely resected.

An opposing school of more conservative bent has arisen during the past 10 years. The volume of residual tumor in patients undergoing incomplete resection may be small and sit well away from the optic nerves or chiasm and may be followed up accurately with MRI. One group evaluated such nonirradiated patients with serial imaging and found that tumor in only 6% regrew after 5 years (Lillehei et al., 1998). A second report by others showing a recurrence rate of 18% at 5 years and 44% at 10 years is more pessimistic even than their own earlier report, which had suggested a much lower incidence of recurrence (Bradley et al., 1994; Turner et al., 1999). In our practice we strive for maximum resection of intrasellar and suprasellar tumors and follow up nonfunctional tumors (even if they are grossly invasive) without further treatment unless atypical pathologic findings suggest anaplasia. If a tumor regrows, our first inclination is to operate if it is technically feasible and only to irradiate if a second instance of recurrence follows or if the pathologic appearance of the tumor has changed since the first resection. In this way we defer or avoid altogether the risks of delayed loss of pituitary function or of radiation-induced optic neuropathy (which is rare, but devastating and difficult to arrest when it happens).

Patients with small, clinically nonfunctional tumors confined to the sella are followed up clinically and radiographically; surgery is performed only if tumor growth is confirmed on serial MRI scans or if there is confusion about whether the tumor is truly nonfunctional. We prefer to avoid radiotherapy as a primary modality because of the high incidence of hypopituitarism after its use.

Patients with "incidentalomas," that is, clinically occult but radiologically detectable adenomas, generally discovered when patients are scanned after they complain of headache or suffer minor head trauma, are frequently seen in the neurosurgical clinic in this era of easily available MRI scans (Donovan and Corenblum, 1995). Although a minimalist approach has been suggested in which only screening for hyperprolactinemia is performed (King et al., 1997), longitudinal studies show that 15% of these patients have partial hypopituitarism and that 3% of incidentally discovered microadenomas and 26% of larger tumors grew during a mean follow-up period of 2.7 years (Feldkamp et al., 1999). We do a full endocrine screen on such patients and scan them yearly for several years, partly in response to the need to alleviate the patient's anxiety and partly to identify the minority with endocrine deficits and/or active tumors. Any patient with a tumor causing an asymptomatic visual field loss, however, is offered surgery.

Gonadotropin-Secreting Adenomas

Gonadotropin-secreting adenomas produce no specific clinical syndrome and are treated much like other clinically nonfunctional adenomas (Snyder, 1997). When large, they more often present because of visual impairment and hypopituitarism than endocrine excess. Hypogonadism in such patients may reflect impairment of normal pituitary function through mass effect or may relate to the elevation of FSH or, less commonly, LH produced by the tumor itself. Some tumors secrete gonadotropins in vitro but produce no detectable change in hormone levels in vivo except an occasional elevation of the α-subunit (Asa et al., 1992; Snyder et al., 1984). Others produce small but measurable increases in serum levels of LH, but not consistently enough to allow its use as a tumor marker (Greenman et al., 1998). In addition, tumor immunostaining does not correlate well with serum gonadotropin levels, which further weakens the utility of studying those levels for any clinical purpose (Ho et al., 1997).

The main reason for distinguishing this group from other nonfunctional tumors lies in the potential that medical therapy may prove effective against them. Because dopamine suppresses gonadotropin secretion in the normal gland, bromocriptine has been used with occasional success for patients who have gonadotropin-secreting adenomas (Lamberts et al., 1987). In addition, innovative therapy using LH-releasing hormone and its antagonists has been used for a few patients. LH-releasing hormone increases secretion in most patients, but inhibits it in a few, perhaps by desensitizing the tumor (Klibanski et al., 1989). Antagonists to LH-releasing hormone have yielded mixed results but may eliminate the presumptive hypothalamic stimulus to tumor growth. As mentioned above for clinically nonfunctional tumors, somatostatin analogues have also been used in this subset of patients to obtain clinical improvement, and less often tumor shrinkage. In general, most patients with gonadotropin-secreting tumors are treated like those with other clinically nonfunctional tumors.

Growth Hormone–Secreting Adenomas

Medical Treatment

The results of drug therapy in treating growth hormone–secreting adenomas are less predictable than those achieved in treating prolactinomas. Bromocriptine, cabergoline, short-acting somatostatin analogues (SMS 201-995, octreotide acetate), or long-acting analogues (lanreotide) have been used. Bromocriptine normalizes growth hormone levels in 20% of patients, but doses at the higher end of the accepted range (20 mg/day) are often necessary, producing a greater incidence of side effects (Wass et al., 1977). Most such tumors will not shrink with bromocriptine, although octreotide has been reported to induce tumor regression in 50% of patients and reduces growth hormone levels in a majority of cases (Barkan et al., 1988; Arosio et al., 1995; Newman et al., 1998). Because some patients achieve persistent biochemical and clinical improvement over long periods of time with chronic somatostatin therapy, this drug can be used as a medical alternative to surgery. Somatostatin has the disadvantages of a subcutaneous route of administration and causes gallstones and gastrointestinal upset in some patients.

We use octreotide occasionally as a preoperative adjunct because it will shrink tumor in 50% of patients to whom it is given, which may make complete surgical excision more feasible. Unlike bromocriptine for prolactinomas, octreotide does not cause histologic changes that impede tumor removal. Shrinkage occurs during the first 2 weeks of treatment, if it is to occur at all, so prolonged courses give no added benefit (Lucas-Morante et al., 1994). Pre-surgical treatment with octreotide does make more complete removal possible in some cases, but the data are not conclusive and studies have been published that both confirm (Stevenaert and Beckers, 1993; Lucas-Morante et al., 1994) and deny (Kristof et al., 1999) its utility before surgery for macroadenomas. We have not been impressed with the degree of shrinkage, however, and have become less inclined to pretreat patients unless lateral extension of tumor is present. Somatostatin may also be used to suppress growth hormone production in patients with residual tumor after surgery, a setting in which we are much more likely to apply it. The chance of biochemical normalization does not, however, depend on the dose chosen (Ezzat et al., 1995). These results can be improved by continuous infusion, but this is expensive and rarely used in most medical centers (Tamura et al., 1998).

If medical therapy is chosen, several alternatives to octreotide are available. Long-acting analogues of octreotide (lanreotide, somatostatin-LAR) are similarly efficacious, but may be better tolerated as they are given much less frequently (two to four times per month) (Verhelst et al., 2000). Although bromocriptine has limited utility, cabergoline is more effective and induces a degree of biochemical normalization and tumor shrinkage comparable with that achieved by the somatostatin analogues (Cozzi et al., 1998; Abs et al., 1998). As cabergoline is given orally, it may very well become more popular than octreotide or lanreotide. Data have not yet been accumulated on its use in the preoperative setting.

The newest drug applied to acromegaly is pegvisoment, a growth hormone analogue that binds to and blocks the action of the growth hormone receptor. In a major prospective randomized trial involving in-patients given pegvisoment for 12 weeks, IGF-I normalized in 89% of patients receiving the highest dose tested (20 mg/day subcutaneously) (Trainer et al., 2000). Although side effects seem minimal and these data are promising, it is not known whether it will be effective in long-term use or whether loss of negative feedback due to lower circulating levels of IGF-I will promote growth of the (otherwise untreated) adenoma responsible for the ongoing growth hormone excess. This drug will be further studied and is expected to join cabergoline and lanreotide as the medical therapies of choice in the future.

Surgery

Surgery is the primary mode of treatment for most patients with pituitary acromegaly. Success rates vary widely among series, and when examining their rates of induced remission, it is important to consider which biochemical criteria the authors used. The largest surgical series reported so far involved 254 patients treated at the University of California, San Francisco as described by Abosch et al. (1998). In that series, growth hormone levels less than 5 ng/ml were achieved in 76% of patients; 29% of patients required postoperative radiotherapy for residual tumor. In a previous paper, these authors compared their own statistics with those of 30 other surgical series involving a total of 1360 patients (Ross and Wilson, 1988). Overall growth hormone levels of less than 5 ng/ml were achieved in 60% of patients. Other series have based successful outcome on achieving growth hormone levels of less than 10 ng/ml (Laws et al., 1987), but the most vigorous modern definition of "cure" requires a level of ≤2.3 ng/ml (Melmed et al., 1998; Levitt et al., 1995). Only a few have followed up somatomedin-C levels, and none has applied provocative testing as a criterion for cure (Kao et al., 1992; Tindall et al., 1993; Abosch et al., 1998). In the series by Tindall et al. (1993), sustained postoperative levels less than 5 ng/ml were achieved in 88% of patients and in 82% when somatomedin-C levels were included in the analysis.

Other series have comparable results, particularly if a single, experienced surgeon has performed all included operations (Ahmed et al., 1999). About 90% of patients with microadenomas, and 40% to 50% of those with macroadenomas, achieve a postsurgical remission.

Sustained remission after surgery should be expected in 60% to 80% of patients overall. The size and location of the tumor affects the ease with which tumor excision is achieved. Fortunately, most of these tumors present as microadenomas and can be identified at surgery and selectively excised. Tumors with suprasellar extension can still be cured, but the chance for leaving residual tumor is greater in such cases. In patients with cavernous sinus tumor, residual tumor almost always remains, even when a transcranial approach is used together with skull-base techniques for cavernous sinus entry that have evolved over the past 10 years (Al-Mefty and Smith, 1990; Origitano et al., 1994). We currently enter the cavernous sinus rarely, with trepidation, and only if tumor mass within it must be debulked to decompress the optic nerve; the risk of cranial neuropathy is high, radiosurgery is available to control focal areas of tumor, and pituitary tumor within the cavernous sinus often goes for years without clinically significant alteration in carotid diameter or cranial nerve function.

Treatment failures should lead to the consideration of several possibilities. Some patients will, of course, have residual tumor. If a complete excision of a microadenoma has been done, however, the possibility of primary hypothalamic gangliocytoma secreting growth hormone–releasing hormone should be considered, as should the possibility that growth hormone or growth hormone–releasing hormone secretion is ectopic (usually from the pancreas) (Asa et al., 1987; Melmed et al., 1985). Although the great majority of patients with acromegaly have pituitary pathology, those who do not can be identified by measuring the plasma level of growth hormone–releasing hormone. If the level is greater than 300 ng/ml, an ectopic source of secretion is likely. In such patients, evidence of pituitary enlargement may appear on MRI scans, and the patient may undergo inappropriate transsphenoidal surgery. Patients in whom a somatotroph hyperplasia is found but no adenoma should have growth hormone–releasing hormone levels measured and, if elevated, the source should be identified by radiologic studies of the chest and abdomen.

Radiation Therapy

Radiation therapy has been used in the past for many patients as a primary treatment for acromegaly. The dose given is similar to that used for other forms of pituitary tumor, and the incidences of hypopituitarism, optic nerve damage, and cerebral radionecrosis are similar as well. Both conventional irradiation and proton-beam bombardment have been used and produce comparable results, although morbidity may be somewhat higher with the latter (Eastman et al., 1979; Kliman et al., 1987; Lüdecke et al., 1989). As with other tumors, the main drawback is the gradual effect of such therapy. In most patients, growth hormone levels decline slowly over the first year and may continue to do so for as long as 10 years after treatment. In 70% of irradiated patients, growth hormone levels less than 10 ng/ml are eventually reached in 5 years, although the response slips to 40% at 10 years (Clarke et al., 1993; Plataniotis et al., 1998; Kokubo et al., 2000). In normal individuals, growth hormone levels range from 0.25 to 0.7 ng/ml, and most authors now consider a level of 2.3 ng/ml or less as remission. A truly rigorous biochemical definition would include normalization of growth hormone and somatomedin-C levels as well as a normal oral glucose tolerance test and thyrotropin-releasing hormone stimulation test (Melmed, 1990; Melmed et al., 1998). These data are generally absent in reported series. Even these criteria are imperfect, as 40% of patients with persistently abnormal dynamic responses show no radiographic regrowth of tumor during the decade after surgery (Ross and Wilson, 1988).

Radiosurgery must also be considered in the array of options available for treating acromegaly. Data on its efficacy in this specific disease are buried within general series of pituitary tumors treated with this modality and are scanty. Two studies have been published that focus on its role in acromegaly. In one, 96% of 79 patients treated achieved normal growth hormone levels over 3 years after treatment (Zhang et al., 2000). Increasing tumor shrinkage was seen over the same time period. Follow up was insufficient in this study to allow conclusions about long-term control. In another study of 16 patients with recurrent acromegaly, growth hormone and IGF-I normalized after 1.4 years, on average; in a comparison group who received conventional fractionated irradiation, the mean time to normalization was 7.1 years (Landolt et al., 1998). Thus, radiosurgery may act more quickly, but the relative risks (over time) for radiosurgery versus fractionated radiation are not well understood. In addition, the interesting observation has been made that acromegalic patients taking octreotide during radiosurgery show a slower, less complete response to irradiation. Thus, octreotide may act as a radioprotectant (Landolt et al., 2000).

Preferred Treatment

At our institution, the general treatment schema for acromegaly includes the preoperative and postoperative measurement of growth hormone and somatomedin-C levels. We use provocative testing only in borderline cases. For a few patients (usually with tumors extending laterally or with large suprasellar components) a trial of somatostatin analogue therapy is given for up to 3 months, and the scans are repeated to check for tumor shrinkage. Half of those so treated show partial regression of the tumor and an unpredictable degree of correction in biochemical abnormalities. Only those in whom somatomedin-C and growth hormone levels normalize (or nearly so, as long as clinical symptoms substantially regress) are offered continuing medical therapy. The majority of patients undergo surgery at this point, and then radiotherapy is used with conventional limited-field techniques for any residual active tumor. Octreotide-LAR is used to control continuing hypersecretion while the patient waits for the irradiation to take effect.

Adrenocorticotropin-Secreting Adenomas

Approximately 4% to 10% of pituitary tumors secrete adrenocorticotropin, and another 5% produce the hormone but do not secrete it in significant amounts. Those in the former category develop Cushing's disease, the name for a hypercortisolism (Cushing's syndrome) of pituitary source. About 70% of adults with true hypercortisolism have such a pituitary tumor.

Much endocrinologic effort has been expended inventing and validating tests that identify hypercortisolism as present and identify its ultimate source as the pituitary gland, the adrenals, or an ectopic tumor secreting adrenocorticotropin, such as in the lung. A diagnosis of Cushing's disease is sometimes difficult to make, because MRI scans fail to show a tumor in 20% to 30% of patients who have an ACTH-secreting adenoma in the pituitary. In years past, as many as 10% of patients with Cushing's disease were treated with bilateral adrenalectomy as a measure of some desperation to eliminate the target organ on which ACTH acts and thereby eliminate the clinical effects of hypercortisolism. In this circumstance, the naturally occurring negative feedback exerted by cortisol on the normal gland (and on the pituitary tumor) is eliminated, and hypersecretion of ACTH increases dramatically. In the 15% to 25% of adrenalectomized patients in whom Nelson's syndrome develops, a dramatic growth of pituitary adenoma occurs, although it may be delayed for a number of years (Nelson et al., 1960; Moore et al., 1976; Nagesser et al., 2000). At least one case has now been reported in which this syndrome was successfully treated with cabergoline, suggesting that it may be as useful in a subset of patients with hypercortisolism as it is in those with prolactin-secreting tumors (Pivonello et al., 1999).

The biochemical assessment of patients with Cushing's disease must take into account the diurnal variation in levels both of ACTH and cortisol normally released by the pituitary gland. Although this episodic secretion still occurs when a pituitary adenoma is present, neoplastic corticotrophs are relatively insensitive to negative feedback from any glucocorticoid, whether endogenous or exogenous. Within the spectrum of tumor autonomy, only 33% have any real measure of hypothalamic control exerted on them (Van Cauter and Refetoff, 1985).

The bewildering array of diagnostic tests used to establish the presence and source of hypercortisolism in a patient suspected of having Cushing's syndrome is beyond the scope of this chapter. Several excellent reviews cover the diagnostic approach in detail and explain how to interpret test results (Kaye and Crapo, 1990; McCutcheon and Oldfield, 1992). In general, one recognizes cortisol excess by determining blood levels in relation to time of day or by collecting urine over 24 hours to eliminate diurnal variations. Even salivary sampling may be done when multiple measurements of cortisol are required (Mosnier-Pudar et al., 1995). If confusion persists (as it often does) even after several assays of blood and urine have been performed, provocative tests are used to clarify the presence of a true hypercortisolism; they also give clues to the etiology of the excess. The most popular of these is the dexamethasone suppression test, which has several variations and is accurate about 90% of the time (Liddle, 1960; Nieman et al., 1986). Stimulation tests using corticotrophin-releasing factor are frequently used and show a normal or excessive rise in ACTH in patients with Cushing's disease, but little response in patients with tumor of the adrenal gland or other sites. This test, like the dexamethasone suppression test, is misleading approximately 10% of the time (Nieman et al., 1986).

In the past 10 years, a great deal of attention has been given to bilateral sampling of the inferior petrosal sinus. In theory, this technique can detect central/peripheral gradients that confirm the presence of pituitary tumor and also can be used to lateralize the tumor within the gland to the right or left half. In practice, the test is useful for confirming the presence of a tumor within the pituitary gland, but intermixing between the two cavernous sinuses leads to numerous cases of inappropriate lateralization (Mamelak et al., 1996). It is now apparent that the rate of false lateralization approaches 40%. The use of corticotrophin-releasing factor stimulation with this test increases its diagnostic accuracy to nearly 100% when a central-to-peripheral ACTH gradient >3.0 is used as the criterion for diagnosis (Oldfield et al., 1991; Kaltsas et al., 1999). Direct sampling of hormone levels in cavernous sinus blood performed during surgery may also be used to localize occult microadenomas, but has practical limitations given the time required to perform the analyses; false negatives may still occur, especially in the absence of corticotrophin-releasing hormone stimulation (Doppman et al., 1995; Graham et al., 1999).

Surgery

Surgical excision is the most popular method of eradicating these tumors. Because many are microadenomas, transsphenoidal techniques have proven useful and can achieve a cure rate of 88%, as reported by Mampalam et al. (1988) from a series of 221 such patients. About 5% of these patients showed eventual recurrence of hypersecretion, with a mean time to recurrence of almost 4 years. Those in whom an intrasellar exploration showed no tumor were cured using biochemical criteria a little less than 50% of the time. Some of these patients had hemihypophysectomy based on petrosal sinus sampling, which as mentioned above is an imperfect method of determining tumor location within the gland. Others had complete hypophysectomy, which remains a valid treatment for patients with this ultimately life-threatening disease. The morbidity among all patients in this series was 9% with a mortality of 1%. Such statistics are fairly representative of those reported from other surgical series of ACTH-secreting pituitary tumors (Burke et al., 1990; Chandler et al., 1987; Bochicchio et al., 1995). Only two-thirds of patients with macroadenomas achieve remission after surgery, and they also tend to relapse sooner than those with smaller tumors (Blevins et al., 1998a).

Some patients in whom Cushing's disease is biochemically identified but in whom surgery fails to effect remission have been misdiagnosed and actually harbor other lesions causing cortisol excess. It is therefore important to review rigorously the evidence from which the diagnosis was made before performing surgery to re-explore the sella and perhaps to perform a complete hypophysectomy. Reoperation certainly has its place in the treatment of Cushing's disease and can raise the rate of remission by 20% or more (Ram et al., 1994). If surgery is redone in this setting and an adenoma is found that had previously been overlooked, it is still better to excise it selectively, together with a margin of adjacent normal pituitary, than to extirpate the entire gland. This approach results in remission of hypercortisolism in about half of these patients with much less risk of hypopituitarism.

Radiation and Other Therapy

Radiotherapy is not often used as the primary treatment as this tumor, like others, is slow to respond to it. This group of patients, however, needs a fairly quick and definitive elimination of the hormonal excess to correct physiologic derangement in multiple organ systems. Adrenal ablation is now reserved for patients for whom other attempts to ablate the source of adrenocorticotropin, either surgically or medically, have failed. When radiotherapy is used after incomplete surgical resection, 80% of patients achieve remission, most within 2 years (Estrada et al., 1997).

Preferred Treatment

Currently, we approach patients suspected of having Cushing's disease with a rigorous and lengthy endocrine evaluation before any treatment is considered. The work-up includes repeated sampling of blood and collection of 24 hour urine volumes to prove hypersecretion. Even if the first one or two samples fail to show any abnormality, patients with appropriate symptoms should be repeatedly studied because some will harbor a tumor that secretes cortisol episodically, which is easy to miss with a less than strenuous diagnostic work-up (Loh, 1999). Most patients have dexamethasone suppression testing and then petrosal sinus sampling before and after stimulation by corticotrophin-releasing factor. Only then is surgery considered.

In the great majority of patients, a transsphenoidal approach is used and the sella is explored vigorously. For patients with Cushing's disease, the frequency of cerebrospinal fluid leak and of intraoperative bleeding from the cavernous sinus should be higher than for other patients because a more aggressive exploration is often necessary to find and completely remove small tumors (or areas of corticotroph hyperplasia) that may lurk unseen in the far lateral areas of a normal-appearing gland. The concept that such tumors occur in the "central median wedge" of the gland and that a search for occult tumor should be directed first to the area of the middle third of the gland is somewhat erroneous. These tumors can occur in any part of the anterior lobe and have even been found in the posterior lobe or outside the gland (Pluta et al., 1999), and the stakes for the patient are high enough to make a higher incidence of (treatable) cerebrospinal fluid leakage acceptable. Patients who remain hypercortisolemic even after such a vigorous exploration and perhaps after excision of histologically confirmed tumor should be reviewed assiduously. If any doubt exists about the diagnosis, appropriate tests should be redone. If, despite these precautions, the pituitary is still thought to be the source of ACTH excess, reoperation may be needed with the intent to perform a hemihypophysectomy or more complete removal of the anterior lobe (Friedman et al., 1989). Only after two surgical procedures should radiotherapy, adrenalectomy, or medical suppression of the adrenals with ketoconazole or mitotane be entertained.

Thyroid-Stimulating Hormone Secreting Adenomas

Tumors that secrete TSH are rare and represent less than 1% of large series of pituitary tumors. Their rarity is probably exaggerated somewhat by the tendency of physicians to misdiagnose as primary hyperthyroidism, which is much more common, the hyperthyroid syndrome they typically produce. Patients with TSH-secreting adenomas are usually falsely diagnosed with primary thyroid disease for years and are often treated with thyroid ablation without success. This delay frequently allows TSH-secreting tumors to enlarge and makes surgical removal more difficult. In theory, the loss of negative homeostatic feedback caused by thyroid ablation in patients with such tumors might be expected to make the tumor more aggressive, as happens in the occasional case of Nelson's syndrome that develops after adrenal ablation in patients with Cushing's disease. Only small series of these patients have been reported, supporting the idea that these tumors are aggressive and that surgery for TSH-secreting adenomas carries a higher risk of perioperative death and/or neurologic morbidity than occurs with other tumor types (McCutcheon et al., 1990). The largest series currently on record are composed of 24 patients treated in Europe (Losa et al., 1999) and

25 patients followed up at the National Institutes of Health (Brucker-Davis et al., 1999). In these series, long-term remission was achieved by a combination of surgical and other therapy in 60% of patients, and only those with undetectable levels of TSH in the early postoperative period demonstrated remission after surgery alone.

If found when small, these tumors are as amenable to surgical cure as are other pituitary adenomas. When the tumor is large, incomplete resection is the rule, and radiotherapy is usually applied as it is with other forms of invasive pituitary adenoma. Although bromocriptine is of little value in controlling this kind of tumor, a somatostatin analogue (e.g., octreotide) can control excess secretion of TSH. In some patients, gross tumor shrinkage occurs after medical therapy begins, and visual field defects have improved in others who are treated medically (Comi et al., 1987; Warnet et al., 1989). Lanreotide, a somatostatin analogue with a longer duration of action than octreotide, also has been effective in normalizing TSH and α-subunit, but does not generally cause tumor shrinkage (Kuhn et al., 2000). The same drawbacks are associated with the use of somatostatin against TSH-secreting adenomas, but it is occasionally helpful for patients with unresectable tumors that do not respond well to radiotherapy.

Patients with these tumors who have been treated inappropriately with chemical or radiotherapeutic ablation of the thyroid gland may be hypothyroid rather than hyperthyroid, so obtaining a careful endocrine history is mandatory if TSH-secreting adenoma is suspected. Also, primary hypothyroidism may itself cause pituitary thyrotroph hyperplasia and adenohypophyseal enlargement that mimics an adenoma. Such patients respond to exogenous thyroxine and should not undergo transsphenoidal surgery, as they have no pituitary disease and pituitary enlargement disappears as a euthyroid state is restored (Young et al., 1999).

MALIGNANCY IN PITUITARY ADENOMAS

Pituitary tumors exhibit malignant behavior through a tendency toward invasion, proliferation, or metastasis. Invasive behavior, in particular dural invasion, which allows extension of tumor into the suprasellar areas, sphenoid sinus, or cavernous sinuses, is more common than generally believed. The true incidence of dural invasion in pituitary tumors has not been studied to a great extent, but Selman et al. (1986) reported a rate of 40% in patients from the Mayo Clinic. This figure describes patients with gross evidence of invasion; when microscopic verification is added, the incidence climbs to 85%. Because pituitary tumors are traditionally considered to be benign and well-circumscribed lesions with a plane dividing them from normal gland, and because most are slow growing, the high incidence of a phenomenon that indicates malignancy is surprising. In this sense, pituitary tumors behave most like meningiomas, which are able to invade dura and adjacent bone much more easily than brain.

This phenomenon is not confined to the tumor–dura interface, as microinvasion of normal gland by tumor also occurs frequently along the tumor's pseudocapsule (Shaffi and Wrightson, 1975). In pituitary adenomas, invasive features leading to incomplete surgical resection are commonly associated with TSH-secreting tumors, large prolactin-secreting tumors associated with very high serum prolactin levels, and acromegaly. In patients with growth hormone excess, invasive features are most often associated with an acidophilic stem cell adenoma, a relatively undifferentiated form of somatotropic tumor comprised from stem cells that can give rise either to prolactin-secreting or growth hormone–secreting cells (Horvath et al., 1981).

The most common form of invasion affects the floor of the sella turcica. As the tumor enlarges, the bony confines of the sella are eroded and appear thinned on lateral skull radiographs or MRI scans. Disappearance of the clinoid processes and a "double floor" sign are considered pathognomonic for an intrasellar tumor. As the tumor enlarges and extends into the suprasellar cistern, the diaphragma bulges upward and stretches, and in some patients allows a dumbbell-like extension through the fenestration provided for the pituitary stalk. Most suprasellar extensions occur in the midline and in severe cases fill the third ventricle and produce hydrocephalus. The adjacent optic chiasm and nerves are thus at high risk for compression in tumors that expand in this direction. Less frequently, lateral extension into one or both cavernous sinuses occurs (Fig. 8–2). In these

→

Figure 8–2, MRI of pituitary adenomas. **(A)** T_1-weighted coronal MRI, post-gadolinium contrast, with arrow pointing to an occult microadenoma in a patient with Cushing's disease shows an apparent signal abnormality in an otherwise normal gland (optic chiasm = C). **(B)** Another coronal image of the microadenoma on the right side of the gland's superior surface with associated stalk (S) deviation (carotid artery in cavernous sinus = C).

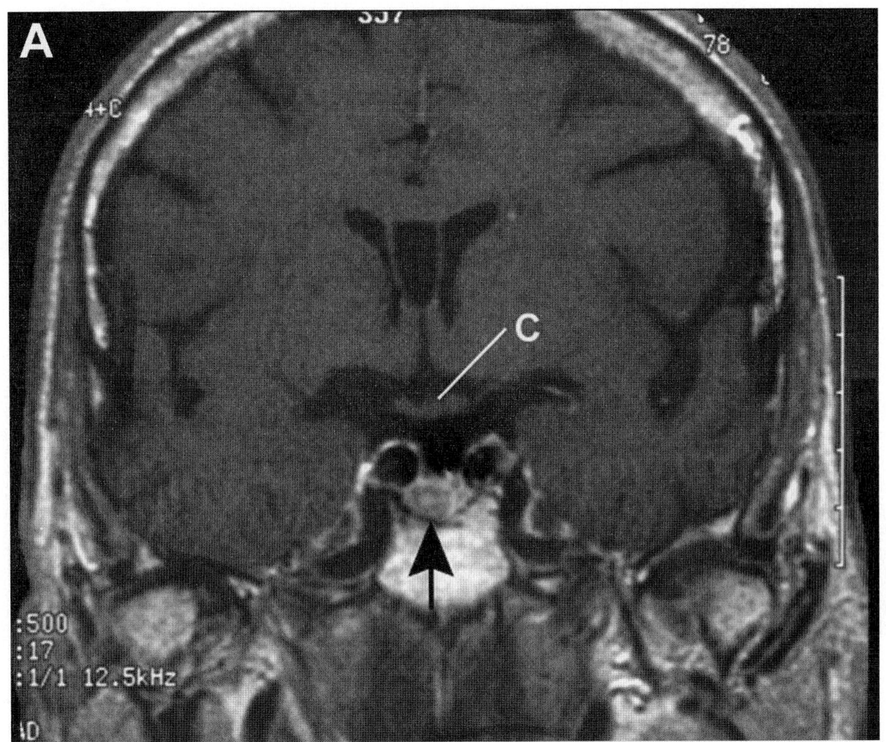
A
C
:500
:17
:1/1 12.5kHz

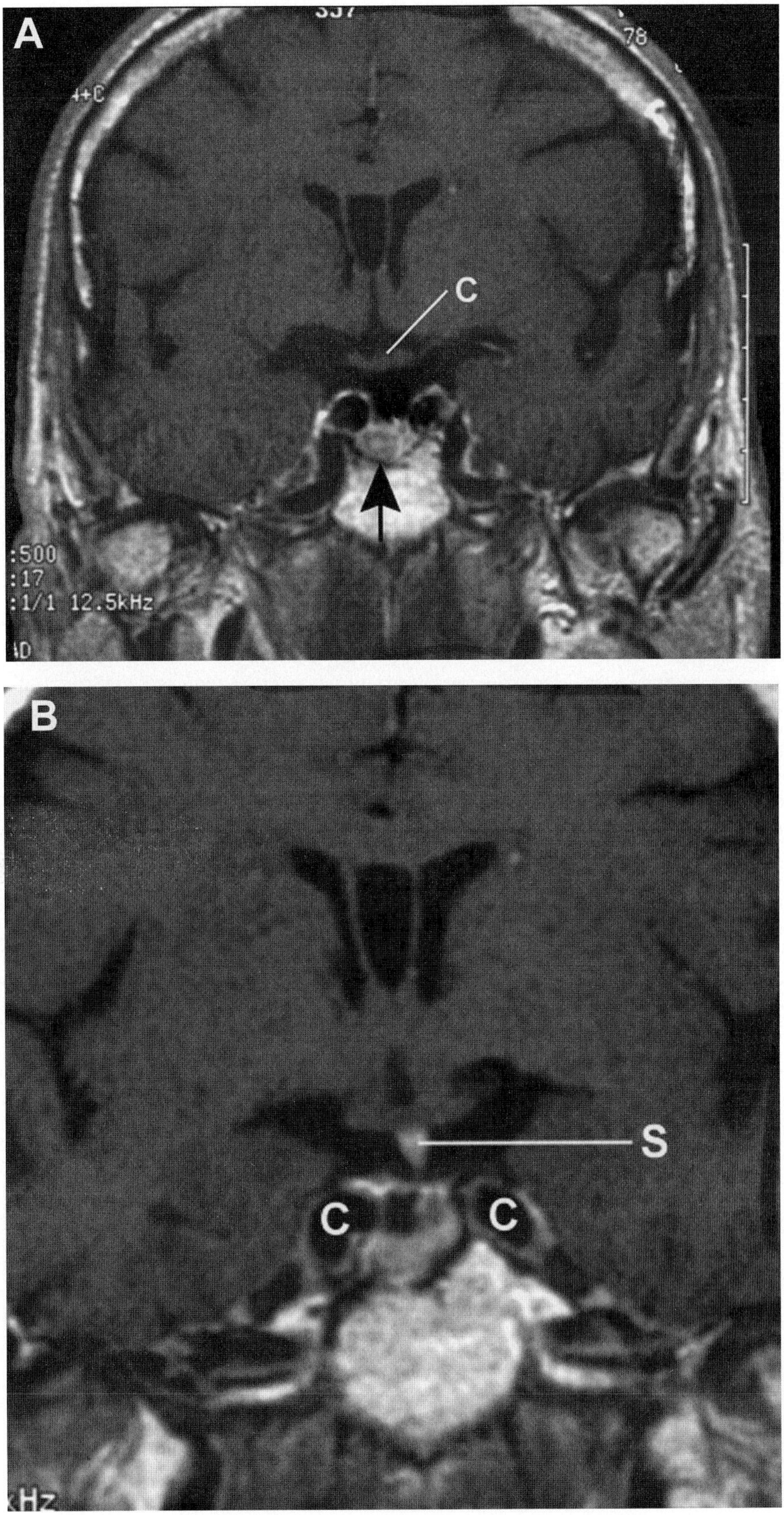

B
S
C
C

C
O
O
S
C
T
C

D
T
C
T
T
cs
400
10/Fr
1/1 16kHz

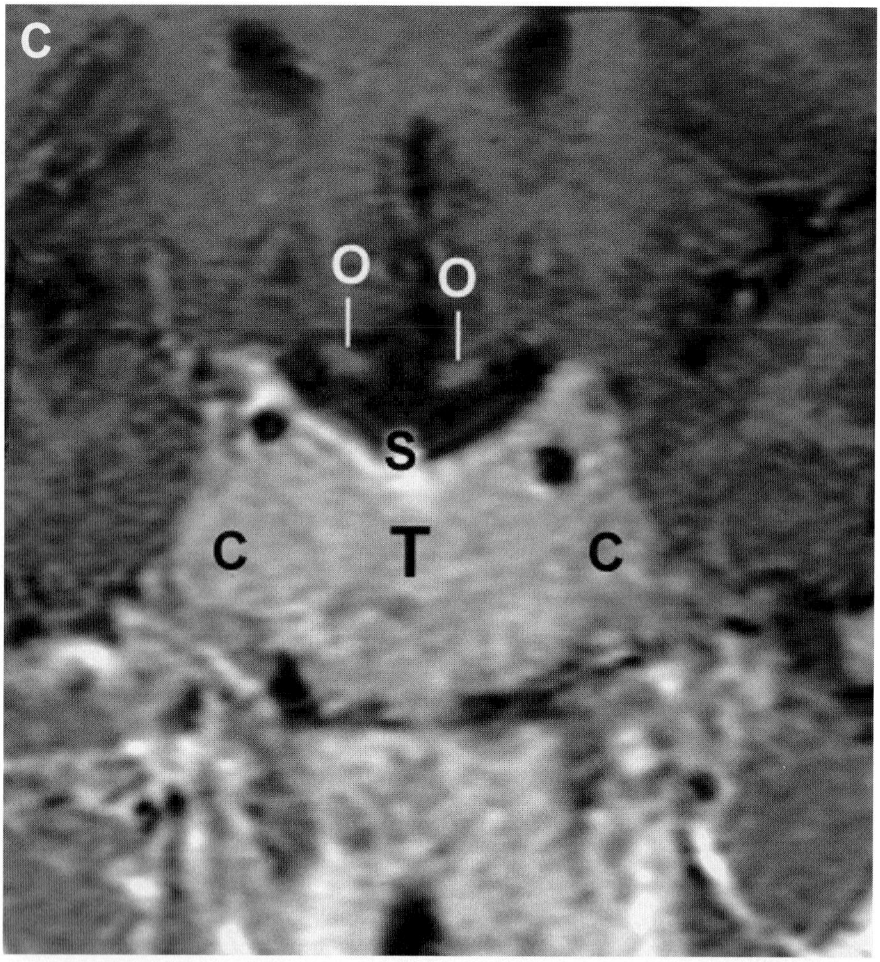

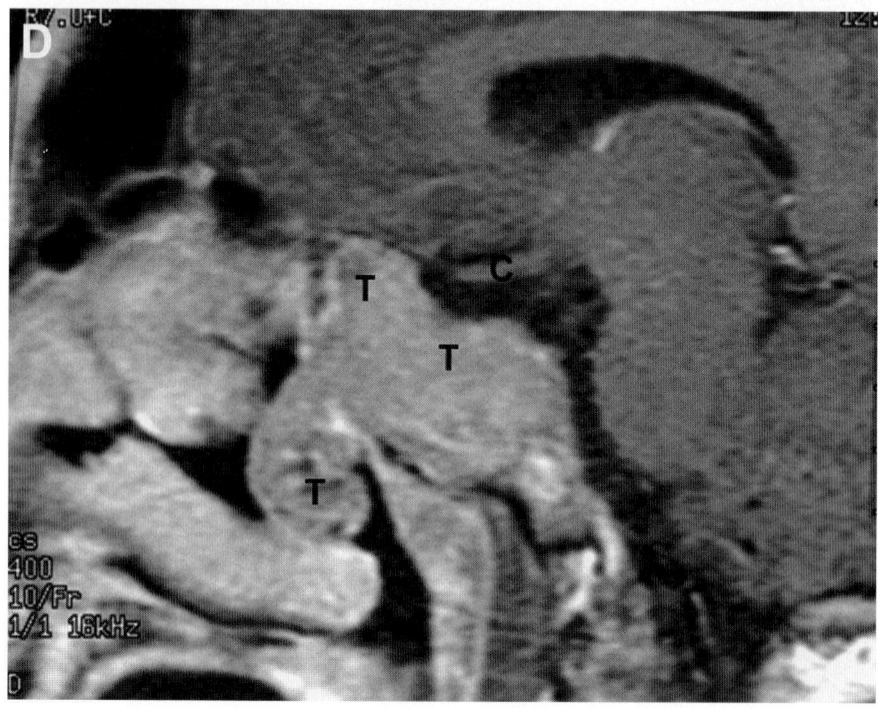

patients, the dura is physically breached by tumor, which gradually fills the venous sinus spaces and encases the carotid artery and cranial nerves. In some patients, tumor also breaches the lateral wall of the cavernous sinus and encroaches directly on the medial temporal lobe. Usually, it simply expands the cavernous sinus, and cranial nerve dysfunction occurs only in later stages of the disease. Narrowing of the carotid artery is seen as tumor progression occurs and can be devastating to patients with poor collateral flow through an anatomically incomplete circle of Willis. Such invasion, whether superiorly, inferiorly, or laterally directed, usually occurs in the absence of the cytologic hallmarks of malignancy. It may, however, correlate with alterations in p53 status, epidermal growth factor receptor activity, or protein kinase C activity; and proliferation indices (such as the MIB-1 labeling index) correlate well with the degree of invasiveness and are highest in frankly metastatic pituitary tumors (Blevins et al., 1998b).

A much smaller proportion of tumors represents the very rare phenomenon of metastasis, and these are considered true pituitary carcinomas. Such metastases have been reported in both cerebrospinal and extraneural sites. Approximately 120 cases have been described, which represent an infinitesimal fraction of all pituitary tumors. In about 50% of patients, tumors disseminate within the neural axis and on histologic examination generally exhibit the cytologic features of malignancy, including pleomorphism, nuclear atypia, and mitotic figures. Some patients demonstrate true leptomeningeal spread of tumor and have positive cytology on examination of cerebrospinal fluid (Ogilvy and Jakubowski, 1973). Most such patients have clinically nonfunctional tumors, although acromegaly, hypoprolactinemia, and Cushing's disease have all been reported in this setting (Ogilvy and Jakubowski, 1973; Petterson et al., 1992; Pernicone et al., 1997).

A similar number of patients with pituitary carcinoma have metastasis to extracranial and extraspinal sites. About 50% of these have ACTH-secreting tumors, and some are associated with Nelson's syndrome. Approximately 50% of pituitary carcinomas metastasize to the liver with lesser numbers metastasizing to bones, lungs, and lymph nodes (Mountcastle et al., 1989). It has been suggested that metastatic pituitary tumors that spread within the CNS tend to enlarge upward and laterally, whereas those that metastasize outside the CNS erode through the floor of the sella, thus gaining access to parasellar soft tissues, which permits lymphatic and/or hematogenous spread (Scheithauer, 1984).

Overall, pituitary carcinomas are nonfunctional about half the time and secrete ACTH in 22% of patients, growth hormone in 13%, and prolactin in 11% (Mountcastle et al., 1989). Nonfunctional and ACTH-secreting adenomas are thus overrepresented. Although TSH-secreting tumors are known for their clinical tenacity, only one has been reported with frank metastasis (McCutcheon et al., 1990). Because some patients were reported before the advent of prolactin assays or routine immunocytochemical staining, it is possible that nonfunctional cases have been overestimated and that some were actually prolactinomas or gonadotropin-secreting tumors (McCutcheon et al., 2000).

Many cases of pituitary carcinoma begin as histologically benign, slow-growing adenomas, then progress over a number of years to a more aggressive state. A few are diagnosed de novo as carcinomas. In Nelson's syndrome and in patients who have TSH-secreting tumors and have undergone thyroid ablation, pituitary carcinomas actually occur quite infrequently. This fact argues against the importance of release of feedback inhibition as a factor promoting malignancy in pituitary tumors. Although radiotherapy causes sarcomatous change in some patients with benign adenomas (Waltz and Brownell, 1966), more than 50% of patients with carcinomas have not had sellar exposure to irradiation, and its role as a transforming agent remains unclear.

Even with aggressive treatment, survival is short in these patients. Kaiser et al. (1983) reviewed 15 patients and found a mean survival time of 1.4 years after the discovery of metastasis; the longest survival time was 4.8 years. One reason these statistics are so dismal is that a true oncologic approach to these neoplasms has not been applied in most patients. By definition, such an approach would include radical resection of the primary site and of any surgically accessible metastatic sites followed by a combination of radiotherapy and cytotoxic chemotherapy. Because

Figure 8–2, (*continued*) **(C)** T_1-weighted coronal MRI, post-gadolinium contrast, showing macroadenoma (T) extending into the sphenoid sinus and obscuring normal pituitary gland (optic nerves = O, stalk = S, cavernous sinus = C). **(D)** T_1-weighted sagittal MRI, post-gadolinium contrast, showing an invasive macroadenoma (T) filling the sphenoid sinus and destroying the skull base and projecting into the nasopharynx (optic chiasm = C).

such patients are rare, chemotherapy protocols have not been developed for them. Isolated, temporary success has been reported in one patient who received 5-fluorouracil, adriamycin, and cyclophosphamide over two courses before tumor relapse occurred (Mixson et al., 1993). A patient with a prolactin-secreting pituitary carcinoma has also been reported in whom improvement of vision occurred with radiographic arrest of tumor growth during four cycles of combined lomustine, procarbazine, and etoposide (Petterson et al., 1992).

A combination of lomustine and 5-fluorouracil has been given to seven patients with aggressive pituitary tumors, four of whom had frank carcinoma (Kaltsas et al., 1998). Some temporary success was obtained in stabilizing symptoms or shrinking tumors, but all died of their disease from 3 to 65 months after starting treatment. Based on chromogranin positivity and a histologic similarity with paraganglioma, we have used a sarcoma regimen for such lesions with limited success (McCutcheon et al., 2000).

The development of skull-base approaches now makes resection of cavernous sinus disease feasible, and this approach might be used for young patients who can tolerate a radical cavernous sinus exenteration. If cavernous sinus exploration is done without carotid and cranial nerve excision, residual tumor is bound to remain, and regrowth will ineluctably occur. Given the dismal natural history of the disease, whenever possible patients with pituitary carcinoma should undergo as aggressive an operation as neurosurgical technical constraints permit.

PITUITARY APOPLEXY

Pituitary tumors can also do significant harm to patients when sudden expansion occurs because of intratumoral hemorrhage. This phenomenon, known as *pituitary apoplexy,* probably represents infarction and subsequent bleeding within a tumor whose angiogenic capacity is insufficient to keep pace with its proliferative capacity. Hemorrhage into the infarcted areas therefore occurs within tumor, not in the adjacent gland, and the gland may recover lost function due to this sudden compression if the tumor and clot are surgically excised without delay (Arafah et al., 1990). Patients who are not operatively treated usually fail to recover from hypopituitarism induced by acute compression, and their pituitary function may actually worsen with time. Some patients present with hemorrhage into a previously undiagnosed, clinically nonfunctional adenoma. In severe cases, bleeding breaks through into the subarachnoid space and produces a typical syndrome of subarachnoid hemorrhage. In that circumstance, the risk of vasospasm depends on the amount of blood in the basal cisterns, just as in patients with aneurysmal rupture that has caused a subarachnoid hemorrhage. These patients can be left with subtle neurophysiologic impairment from cerebral microinfarcts caused by vasospasm in small perforating vessels and should be treated prospectively with hyperdynamic therapy during the recovery phase after transsphenoidal decompression of the sellar contents.

For patients who have macroadenomas, pituitary apoplexy usually presents with the sudden onset of headache, nausea, visual loss, or diplopia. Some patients do not lose pituitary function, but in most patients two or more hormonal axes are impaired. One series reported 9 of 13 patients with hypopituitarism before surgery (Arafah et al., 1990). Surgery may correct endocrine and visual abnormalities in a significant percentage of patients. Long-term hormone replacement with corticosteroids (58%), thyroxine (45%), and testosterone (43% of males) was necessary in one recent series (Randeva et al., 1999). In most of these patients, decreasing vision demands relatively urgent surgical decompression (certainly, within a week of the ictus) in which the goal is to decompress parasellar structures, remove tumor, and restore pituitary function.

CONCLUSION

Pituitary tumors act malignantly if they produce a hormonal excess that promotes premature death in afflicted patients; if they invade or compress parasellar structures, particularly the visual pathways; or if they bleed or metastasize. Many are now detected, however, by MRI and by sensitive biochemical tests before they achieve symptomatic size. Although a general reclassification of these tumors according to hormonal production has been ongoing for the past 15 years, a true understanding of their pathogenesis has not been achieved. Medical, surgical, and radiobiologic approaches to treating these lesions have been greatly refined, but a significant number of them cannot be cured by currently available means. Although more aggressive surgery is now possible, it sometimes achieves its success at the expense of neurologic or pituitary function, and the real hope for future therapeutic advances lies in a better understanding of the molecular mechanisms that subserve the proliferative and invasive nature of these diverse neoplasms.

REFERENCES

Abosch A, Tyrrell JB, Lamborn KR, Hannegan LT, Applebury CB, Wilson CB. 1998. Transsphenoidal microsurgery for growth hormone-secreting pituitary adenomas: initial outcome and long-term results. J Clin Endocrinol Metab 83:3411–3418.

Abs R, Verhelst J, Maiter D, et al. 1998. Cabergoline in the treatment of acromegaly: a study of 64 patients. J Clin Endocrinol Metab 83:374–378.

Ahmed S, Elsheikh M, Stratton IM, Page RC, Adams CB, Wass JA. 1999. Outcome of transsphenoidal surgery for acromegaly and its relationship to surgical experience. Clin Endocrinol 50:561–567.

Al-Mefty O, Smith RR. 1990. Tailoring the cranio-orbital approach. Keio J Med 39:217–224.

Arafah BM, Harrington JF, Madhoun ZT, Selman WR. 1990. Improvement in pituitary function following surgical decompression for pituitary tumor apoplexy. J Clin Endocrinol Metab 71:323–328.

Arafah BM, Prunty D, Ybarra J, Hlavin ML, Selman WR. 2000. The dominant role of increased intrasellar pressure in the pathogenesis of hypopituitarism, hyperprolactinemia, and headaches in patients with pituitary adenomas. J Clin Endocrinol Metab 85:1789–1793.

Arosio M, Macchelli S, Rossi CM, Casati G, Biella O, Faglia G. 1995. Effects of treatment with octreotide in acromegalic patients: a multicenter Italian study—Italian Multicenter Octreotide Study Group. Eur J Endocrinol 133:430–439.

Asa SL. 1998. Tumors of the Pituitary Gland. Washington, DC: Armed Forces Institute of Pathology.

Asa SL, Cheng Z, Ramyar L, et al. 1992. Human pituitary null cell adenomas and oncocytomas in vitro: effects of adenohypophysiotropic hormones and gonadal steroids on hormonal secretion and tumor cell morphology. J Clin Endocrinol Metab 74:1128–1134.

Asa SL, Singer W, Kovacs K, et al. 1987. Pancreatic endocrine tumour producing growth hormone-releasing hormone associated with multiple endocrine neoplasia type 1 syndrome. Acta Endocrinol (Copenh) 115:331–337.

Barkan AL, Lloyd RV, Chandler WF, et al. 1988. Preoperative treatment of acromegaly with long-acting somatostatin analog SMS 201-995: shrinkage of invasive pituitary macroadenomas and improved surgical remission rate. J Clin Endocrinol Metab 67:1040–1048.

Bartynski WS, Lin L. 1997. Dynamic and conventional spin-echo MR of pituitary microlesions. AJNR Am J Neuroradiol 18:965–972.

Bauserman SC, Hardman JM, Schochet SS, Earle KM. 1978. Pituitary oncocytoma. Indispensable role of electron microscopy in its identification. Arch Pathol Lab Med 102:456–459.

Bevan JS, Adams CBT, Burke CW, et al. 1987. Factors in the outcome of transsphenoidal surgery for prolactinoma and non-functioning pituitary tumor, including pre-operative bromocriptine therapy. Clin Endocrinol (Oxf) 26:541–556.

Black PM, Hsu DW, Klibanski A, et al. 1987. Hormone production in clinically nonfunctioning pituitary adenomas. J Neurosurg 66:244–250.

Blevins LS, Christy JH, Khajavi M, Tindall GT. 1998a. Outcomes of therapy for Cushing's disease due to adrenocorticotropin-secreting pituitary macroadenomas. J Clin Endocrinol Metab 83:63–67.

Blevins LS, Verity DK, Allen G. 1998b. Aggressive pituitary tumors. Oncology (Huntingt) 12:1307–1312.

Bochicchio D, Losa M, Buchfelder M. 1995. Factors influencing the immediate and late outcome of Cushing's disease treated by transsphenoidal surgery: a retrospective study by the European Cushing's Disease Survey Group. J Clin Endocrinol Metab 80:3114–3120.

Bradley KM, Adams CB, Potter CP, Wheeler DW, Anslow PJ, Burke CW. 1994. An audit of selected patients with non-functioning pituitary adenoma treated by transsphenoidal surgery without irradiation. Clin Endocrinol (Oxf) 41:655–659.

Brucker-Davis F, Oldfield EH, Skarulis MC, Doppman JL, Weintraub BD. 1999. Thyrotropin-secreting pituitary tumors: diagnostic criteria, thyroid hormone sensitivity, and treatment outcome in 25 patients followed at the National Institutes of Health. J Clin Endocrinol Metab 84:476–486.

Brue T, Lancranjan I, Louvet JP, Dewailly D, Roger P, Jaquet P. 1992a. A long-acting repeatable form of bromocriptine as long-term treatment of prolactin-secreting macroadenomas: a multicenter study. Fertil Steril 57:74–80.

Brue T, Pellegrini I, Gunz G, et al. 1992b. Effects of the dopamine agonist CV 205-502 in human prolactinomas resistant to bromocriptine. J Clin Endocrinol Metab 74:577–584.

Burke CW, Adams CB, Esiri MM, Morris C, Bevan JS. 1990. Transsphenoidal surgery for Cushing's disease: does what is removed determine the endocrine outcome? Clin Endocrinol (Oxf) 33:525–537.

Chandler WF, Schteingart DE, Lloyd RV, McKeever PE, Ibarra-Perez G. 1987. Surgical treatment of Cushing's disease. J Neurosurg 66:204–212.

Clarke SD, Woo SY, Butler EB, et al. 1993. Treatment of secreting pituitary adenoma with radiation therapy. Radiology 188:759–763.

Colao A, Di Sarno A, Landi ML, et al. 2000. Macroprolactinoma shrinkage during cabergoline treatment is greater in naïve patients than in patients pretreated with other dopamine agonists: a prospective study in 110 patients. J Clin Endocrinol Metab 85:2247–2252.

Comi RJ, Gesundheit N, Murray L, Gorden P, Weintraub BD. 1987. Response of thyrotropin-secreting pituitary adenomas to a long-acting somatostatin analogue. N Engl J Med 317:12–17.

Comtois R, Beauregard H, Somma M, Serri O, Aris-Jilwan N, Hardy J. 1991. The clinical and endocrine outcome to transsphenoidal microsurgery of nonsecreting pituitary adenomas. Cancer 68:860–866.

Cozzi R, Attanasio R, Barausse M, et al. 1998. Cabergoline in acromegaly: a renewed role for dopamine agonist treatment? Eur J Endocrinol 139:516–521.

Daneshdoost L, Gennarelli TA, Bashey HM, et al. 1993. Identification of gonadotroph adenomas in men with clinically nonfunctioning adenomas by the luteinizing hormone beta subunit response to thyrotropin-releasing hormone. J Clin Endocrinol Metab 77:1352–1355.

De Herder WW, van der Lely AJ, Janssen JA, Uitterlinden P, Hofland LJ, Lamberts SW. 1995. IGFBP-3 is a poor parameter for assessment of clinical activity in acromegaly. Clin Endocrinol (Oxf) 43:501–505.

Di Sarno A, Landi ML, Marzullo P, et al. 2000. The effect of quinagolide and cabergoline, two selective dopamine receptor type 2 agonists, in the treatment of prolactinomas. Clin Endocrinol (Oxf) 53:53–60.

Donovan LE, Corenblum B. 1995. The natural history of the pituitary incidentaloma. Arch Intern Med 155:181–183.

Doppman JL, Nieman LK, Chang R, et al. 1995. Selective venous sampling from the cavernous sinuses is not a more reliable technique than sampling from the inferior petrosal sinuses in Cushing's syndrome. J Clin Endocrinol Metab 80:2485–2489.

Eastman RC, Gorden P, Roth J. 1979. Conventional supervoltage irradiation is an effective treatment for acromegaly. J Clin Endocrinol Metab 48:931–940.

Ebersold MJ, Quast LM, Laws ER, Scheithauer B, Randall RV. 1986. Long-term results in transsphenoidal removal of nonfunctioning pituitary adenomas. J Neurosurg 64:713–719.

Estrada J, Boronat M, Mielgo M, et al. 1997. The long-term outcome of pituitary irradiation after unsuccessful transsphenoidal surgery in Cushing's disease. N Engl J Med 336:172–177.

Ezzat S, Redelmeier DA, Gnehm M, Harris AG. 1995. A prospective multicenter octreotide dose response study in the treatment of acromegaly. J Endocrinol Invest 18:364–369.

Feldkamp J, Santen R, Harms E, Aulich A, Modder U, Scherbaum WA. 1999. Incidentally discovered pituitary lesions: high frequency of macroadenomas and hormone-secreting adenomas—results of a prospective study. Clin Endocrinol 51:109–113.

Friedman RB, Oldfield EH, Nieman LK. 1989. Repeat transsphenoidal surgery for Cushing's disease. J Neurosurg 71:520–527.

Gesundheit N, Petrick PA, Nissim M, et al. 1989. Thyrotropin-secreting pituitary adenomas: clinical and biochemical heterogeneity. Case reports and follow-up of nine patients. Ann Intern Med 111:827–835.

Glaser B, Nesher Y, Barziliai S. 1994. Long-term treatment of bromocriptine-intolerant prolactinoma patients with CV 205-502. J Reprod Med 39:449–454.

Graham KE, Samuels MH, Nesbit GM, et al. 1999. Cavernous sinus sampling is highly accurate in distinguishing Cushing's disease from the ectopic adrenocorticotropin syndrome and in predicting intrapituitary tumor location. J Clin Endocrinol Metab 84:1602–1610.

Greenman Y, Tordjman K, Somjen D, et al. 1998. The use of beta-subunits of gonadotrophin hormones in the follow-up of clinically non-functioning pituitary tumors. Clin Endocrinol (Oxf) 49:185–190.

Griffith HB, Veerapen R. 1987. A direct transnasal approach to the sphenoid sinus. Technical note. J Neurosurg 66:140–142.

Halberg FE, Sheline GE. 1987. Radiotherapy of pituitary tumors. Endocrinol Metab Clin North Am 16:667–684.

Hall WA, Luciano MG, Doppman JL, Patronas NJ, Oldfield EH. 1994. Pituitary magnetic resonance imaging in normal human volunteers: occult adenomas in the general population. Ann Intern Med 120:817–820.

Halperin I, Casamitjana R, Flores L, Fernandez-Balsells M, Vilardell E. 1999. The role of IGF binding protein-3 as a parameter of activity in acromegalic patients. Eur J Endocrinol 141:145–148.

Hardy J. 1969. Transsphenoidal microsurgery of the normal and pathological pituitary. Clin Neurosurg 16:185–217.

Hardy J. 1984. Transsphenoidal microsurgery of prolactinomas. In: Black PM, Zervas NT, Ridgway EC, et al. (eds), Secretory Tumors of the Pituitary Gland. New York: Raven Press, p 73.

Hardy J. 1991. Atlas of Transsphenoidal Microsurgery in Pituitary Tumors. New York: Igaku Shoin.

Hensen J, Henig A, Fahlbusch R, et al. 1999. Prevalence, predictors and patterns of postoperative polyuria and hyponatremia in the immediate course after transsphenoidal surgery for pituitary adenomas. Clin Endocrinol 50:431–439.

Hayashi S, Ito K, Shimada M, et al. 1995. Dynamic MRI with slow injection of contrast material for the diagnosis of pituitary adenoma. Radiat Med 13:167–170.

Ho DM, Hsu CY, Ting LT, Chiang H. 1997. The clinicopathological characteristics of gonadotroph cell adenoma: a study of 118 cases. Hum Pathol 28:905–911.

Holdaway IM, Rajasoorya C. 1999. Epidemiology of acromegaly. Pituitary 2:29–41.

Hori A, Schmidt D, Rickels E. 1999. Pharyngeal pituitary: development, malformation, and tumorigenesis. Acta Neuropathol (Berl) 98:262–272.

Horvath E, Kovacs K, Singer W, et al. 1981. Acidophil stem cell adenoma of the human pituitary: clinicopathological analysis of 15 cases. Cancer 47:761–771.

Hubbard JL, Scheithauer BW, Abboud CF, Laws ER. 1987. Prolactin-secreting adenomas: the preoperative response to bromocriptine treatment and surgical outcome. J Neurosurg 67:816–821.

Isobe K, Ohta M, Yasuda S. 2000. Postoperative radiation therapy for pituitary adenoma. J Neurooncol 48:135–140.

Jalali R, Brada M, Perks JR, et al. 2000. Stereotactic conformal radiotherapy for pituitary adenomas: technique and preliminary experience. Clin Endocrinol (Oxf) 52:695–702.

Jamrozik SI, Bennet AP, James-Deidier A, et al. 1996. Treatment with long acting repeatable bromocriptine (Parlodel-LAR*) in patients with macroprolactinomas: long-term study in 29 patients. J Endocrinol Invest 19:472–479.

Jankowski R, Auque J, Simon C, Marchal JC, Hepner H, Wayoff M. 1992. Endoscopic pituitary tumor surgery. Laryngoscope 102:198–202.

Jarrahy R, Berci G, Shahinian HK. 2000. Assessment of the efficacy of endoscopy in pituitary adenoma resection. Arch Otolaryngol Head Neck Surg 126:1487–1490.

Jho HD. 1999. Endoscopic pituitary surgery. Pituitary 2:139–154.

Kaiser FE, Orth DN, Mukai K, Oppenheimer JH. 1983. A pituitary parasellar tumor with extracranial metastases and high, partially suppressible levels of adrenocorticotropin and related peptides. J Clin Endocrinol Metab 57:649–653.

Kaltsas GA, Giannulis MG, Newell-Price JD, et al. 1999. A critical analysis of the value of simultaneous inferior petrosal sinus sampling in Cushing's disease and the occult ectopic adrenocorticotropin syndrome. J Clin Endocrinol Metab 84:487–492.

Kaltsas GA, Mukherjee JJ, Plowman PN, Monson JP, Grossman AB, Besser GM. 1998. The role of cytotoxic chemotherapy in the management of aggressive and malignant pituitary tumors. J Clin Endocrinol Metab 83:4233–4238.

Kao PC, Laws ER Jr, Zimmerman D. 1992. Somatomedin C/insulin-like growth factor 1 levels after treatment of acromegaly. Ann Clin Lab Sci 22:95–99.

Katznelson L, Alexander JM, Bikkal HA, Jameson JL, Hsu DW, Klibanski A. 1992. Imbalanced follicle-stimulating hormone beta-subunit hormone biosynthesis in human pituitary adenomas. J Clin Endocrinol Metab 74:1343–1351.

Kaye TB, Crapo L. 1990. The Cushing syndrome: an update on diagnostic tests. Ann Intern Med 112:434–444.

Kim MS, Lee SI, Sim JH. 1999. Gamma knife radiosurgery for functioning pituitary microadenoma. Stereotact Funct Neurosurg 72 (suppl 1):119–124.

King JT, Justice AC, Aron DC. 1997. Management of incidental pituitary microadenomas: a cost-effectiveness analysis. J Clin Endocrinol Metab 82:3625–3632.

Kirchner JA. 1984. Transethmoidal approach to the sella. In: Sasaki CT, McCabe BF, Kirchner JA (eds), Surgery of the Skull Base. Philadelphia: JB Lippincott, p 63

Klibanski A, Biller BM, Rosenthal DI, Schoenfeld DA, Saxe V. 1988. Effects of prolactin and estrogen deficiency in amenorrheic bone loss. J Clin Endocrinol Metab 67: 124–130.

Klibanski A, Jameson JL, Biller BM, et al. 1989. Gonadotropin and alpha-subunit responses to chronic gonadotropin-releasing hormone analog administration in patients with glycoprotein hormone-secreting pituitary tumors. J Clin Endocrinol Metab 68:81–86.

Kliman B, Kjellberg RN, Swisher B, Butler W. 1987. Long-term effects of proton beam therapy for acromegaly. In: Robbins RJ, Melmed S (eds), Acromegaly: a Century of Scientific and Clinical Progress. New York: Plenum, pp 221–228.

Kokubo M, Sasai K, Shibamoto Y, et al. 2000. Long-term results of radiation therapy for pituitary adenoma. J Neurooncol 47:79–84.

Kovacs K, Horvath E, Ryan N, Ezrin C. 1980. Null cell adenoma of the human pituitary. Virchows Arch A Pathol Anat Histol 387:165–174.

Kristof RA, Stoffel-Wagner B, Klingmuller D, Schramm J. 1999. Does octreotide treatment improve the surgical results of macro-adenomas in acromegaly? A randomized study. Acta Neurochir (Wien) 141:399–405.

Kuhn JM, Arlot S, Lefebvre H, et al. 2000. Evaluation of the treatment of thyrotropin-secreting pituitary adenomas with a slow release formulation of the somatostatin analog lanreotide. J Clin Endocrinol Metab 85:1487–1491.

Lamberts SW, Verleun T, Oosterom R, et al. 1987. The effects of bromocriptine, thyrotropin-releasing hormone, and gonadotropin-releasing hormone on hormone secretion by gonadotropin-secreting pituitary adenomas in vivo and in vitro. J Clin Endocrinol Metab 64:524–530.

Landolt AM, Haller D, Lomax N, et al. 1998. Stereotactic radiosurgery for recurrent surgically treated acromegaly: comparison with fractionated radiotherapy. J Neurosurg 88:1002–1008.

Landolt AM, Haller D, Lomax N, et al. 2000. Octreotide may act as a radioprotective agent in acromegaly. J Clin Endocrinol Metab 85:1287–1289.

Laws ER Jr, Carpenter SM, Scheithauer BW, et al. 1987. Long-term results of transsphenoidal surgery for the management of acromegaly. In: Robbins RJ, Melmed S (eds), Acromegaly: a Century of Scientific and Clinical Progress. New York: Plenum, pp 241–248.

Levitt NS, Ratanjee BD, Abrahamson MJ. 1995. Do "so-called" normal growth hormone concentrations (2–5 micrograms/l) indicate cure in acromegaly? Horm Metab Res 27:185–188.

Levy RP, Fabrikant JI, Frankel KA, et al. 1991. Heavy-charged particle radiosurgery of the pituitary gland: clinical results of 840 patients. Stereotact Funct Neurosurg 57:22–35.

Liddle GW. 1960. Test of pituitary-adrenal suppressibility in the diagnosis of Cushing's syndrome. J Clin Endocrinol Metab 20:1539–1560.

Lillehei KO, Kirschman DL, Kleinschmidt-DeMasters BK, Ridgway EC. 1998. Reassessment of the role of radiation therapy in the treatment of endocrine-inactive pituitary macroadenomas. Neurosurgery 43:432–439.

Littley MD, Shalet SM, Beardwell CG, Ahmed SR, Applegate G, Sutton ML. 1989. Hypopituitarism following external radiotherapy for pituitary tumours in adults. Q J Med 70:145–160.

Loh KC. 1999. Cyclical Cushing's syndrome—a trap for the unwary. Singapore Med J 40:321–324.

Losa M, Mortini P, Franzin A, Barzaghi R, Mandelli C, Giovanelli M. 1999. Surgical management of thyrotropin-secreting pituitary adenomas. Pituitary 2:127–131.

Lucas-Morante T, Garcia-Uria J, Estrada J, et al. 1994. Treatment of invasive growth hormone pituitary adenomas with long-acting somatostatin analog SMS 201-995 before transsphenoidal surgery. J Neurosurg 81:10–14.

Lüdecke DK, Lutz BS, Niedworok G. 1989. The choice of treatment after incomplete adenomectomy in acromegaly: proton versus high voltage radiation. Acta Neurochir (Wien) 96:32–38.

Lundin P, Bergstrom K. 1992. Gd-DTPA-enhanced MR imaging of pituitary macroadenomas. Acta Radiol 33:323–332.

MacKay A, Hosobuchi Y. 1978. Treatment of intracavernous extensions of pituitary adenomas. Surg Neurol 10:377–383.

Mamelak AN, Dowd CF, Tyrrell JB, McDonald JF, Wilson CB. 1996. Venous angiography is needed to interpret inferior petrosal sinus and cavernous sinus sampling data for lateralizing adrenocorticotropin-secreting adenomas. J Clin Endocrinol Metab 81:475–481.

Mampalam TJ, Tyrrell JB, Wilson CB. 1988. Transsphenoidal microsurgery for Cushing disease. A report of 216 cases. Ann Intern Med 109:487–493.

Maraschini C, Moro M, Masala A, et al. 1991. Chronic treatment with parlodel LAR of patients with prolactin-secreting tumours. Different responsiveness of micro- and macroprolactinomas. Acta Endocrinol (Copenh) 125:494–501.

March CM, Kletzky OA, Davajan V, et al. 1981. Longitudinal evaluation of patients with untreated prolactin-secreting pituitary adenomas. Am J Obstet Gynecol 139:835–844.

McCutcheon IE, Kitagawa RS, DeMasi PF, et al. 2001. Frameless stereotactic navigation in transsphenoidal surgery: comparison with fluoroscopy. Neurosurgery (in press).

McCutcheon IE, Oldfield EH. 1992. Cortisol: regulation, disorders, and clinical evaluation. In: Barrow DL, Selman WR (eds), Neuroendocrinology. Baltimore: Williams & Wilkins, pp 117–173.

McCutcheon IE, Pieper DR, Fuller GN, Benjamin RS, Friend KE, Gagel RF. 2000. Pituitary carcinoma containing gonadotropins: treatment by radical excision and cytotoxic chemotherapy: case report. Neurosurgery 46:1233–1240.

McCutcheon IE, Weintraub BD, Oldfield EH. 1990. Surgical treatment of thyrotropin-secreting pituitary adenomas. J Neurosurg 73:674–683.

Melmed S. 1990. Acromegaly. N Engl J Med 322:966–977.

Melmed S, Ezrin C, Kovacs K, Goodman RS, Frohman LA. 1985. Acromegaly due to secretion of growth hormone by an ectopic pancreatic islet-cell tumor. N Engl J Med 312:9–17.

Melmed S, Jackson I, Kleinberg D, Klibanski A. 1998. Current treatment guidelines for acromegaly. J Clin Endocrinol Metab 83:2646–2652.

Merola B, Sarnacchiaro F, Colao A, et al. 1994. Positive response to compound CV 205-502 in hyperprolactinemic patients resistant to or intolerant of bromocriptine. Gynecol Endocrinol 8:175–181.

Mixson AJ, Friedman TC, Katz DA, et al. 1993. Thyrotropin-secreting pituitary carcinoma. J Clin Endocrinol Metab 76:529–533.

Molitch ME, Elton RL, Blackwell RE, et al. 1985. Bromocriptine as primary therapy for prolactin-secreting macroadenomas: results of a prospective multicenter study. J Clin Endocrinol Metab 60:698–705.

Moore TJ, Dluhy RG, Williams GH, Cain JP. 1976. Nelson's syndrome: frequency, prognosis, and effect of prior pituitary irradiation. Ann Intern Med 85:731–734.

Mosnier-Pudar H, Thomopoulos P, Bertagna X, Fournier C, Guiban D, Luton JP. 1995. Long-distance and long-term follow-up of a patient with intermittent Cushing's disease by salivary cortisol measurements. Eur J Endocrinol 133:313–316.

Mountcastle RB, Roof BS, Mayfield RK, et al. 1989. Pituitary adenocarcinoma in an acromegalic patient: response to bromocriptine and pituitary testing: a review of the literature on 36 cases of pituitary carcinoma. Am J Med Sci 298:109–118.

Nagesser SK, van Seters AP, Kievit J, Hermans J, Krans HM, van de Velde CJ. 2000. Long-term results of total adrenalectomy for Cushing's disease. World J Surg 24:108–113.

Nelson DH, Meakin JW, Thorn GW. 1960. ACTH-producing tumors following adrenalectomy for Cushing's syndrome. Ann Intern Med 52:560–569.

Newman CB, Melmed S, George A, et al. 1998. Octreotide as primary therapy for acromegaly. J Clin Endocrinol Metab 83:3034–3040.

Nieman LK, Chrousos GP, Oldfield EH, Avgerinos PC, Cutler GB, Loriaux DI. 1986. The ovine corticotropin-releasing hormone stimulation test and the dexamethasone suppression test in the differential diagnosis of Cushing's syndrome. Ann Intern Med 105:862–867.

Nilsson B, Gustavasson-Kadaka E, Bengtsson BA, Jonsson B. 2000. Pituitary adenomas in Sweden between 1958 and 1991: incidence, survival, and mortality. J Clin Endocrinol Metab 85:1420–1425.

Nobels FR, Kwekkeboom DJ, Coopmans W, et al. 1993. A comparison between the diagnostic value of gonadotropins, alpha-subunit, and chromogranin-A and their response to thyrotropin-releasing hormone in clinically nonfunctioning, alpha-subunit–secreting, and gonadotroph pituitary adenomas. J Clin Endocrinol Metab 77:784–789.

Ogilvy KM, Jakubowski J. 1973. Intracranial dissemination of pituitary adenomas. J Neurol Neurosurg Psychiatry 36:199–205.

Oldfield EH, Doppman JL, Nieman LK, et al. 1991. Petrosal sinus sampling with and without corticotropin-releasing hormone for the differential diagnosis of Cushing's syndrome. N Engl J Med 325:897–905 (erratum in N Engl J Med 326:1172, 1992).

Olson BR, Gumowski J, Rubino D, Oldfield EH. 1997. Pathophysiology of hyponatremia after transsphenoidal pituitary surgery. J Neurosurg 87:499–507.

Oppenheim DS, Kana AR, Sangha JS, Klibanski A. 1990. Prevalence of alpha-subunit hypersecretion in patients with pituitary tumors: clinically nonfunctioning and somatotroph adenomas. J Clin Endocrinol Metab 70:859–864.

Origitano TC, Al-Mefty O, Leonetti JP, DeMonte F, Reichman OH. 1994. Vascular considerations and complications in cranial base surgery. Neurosurgery 35:351–363.

Pan L, Zhang N, Wang E, Wang B, Xu W. 1998. Pituitary adenomas: the effect of gamma knife radiosurgery on tumor growth and endocrinopathies. Stereotact Funct Neurosurg 70:119–126.

Paramo C, Andrade O MA, Fluiters E, Luna R, de la Fuente J, Garcia-Mayor RV. 1997. Comparative study of insulin-like growth factor-I (IGF-I) and IGF-binding protein-3 (IGFBP-3) level and IGF-I/IGFBP-3 ratio measurements and their relationship with an index of clinical activity in the management of patients with acromegaly. Metabolism 46:494–498.

Parent AD, Bebin J, Smith RR. 1981. Incidental pituitary adenomas. J Neurosurg 54:228–231.

Perks JR, Jalali R, Cosgrove VP, et al. 1999. Optimization of stereotactically-guided conformal treatment planning of sellar and parasellar tumors, based on normal brain dose volume histograms. Int J Radiat Oncol Biol Phys 45:507–513.

Pernicone PJ, Scheithauer BW, Sebo TJ, et al. 1997. Pituitary carcinoma: a clinicopathologic study of 15 cases. Cancer 79:804–812.

Petterson T, MacFarlane IA, MacKenzie JM, Shaw MD. 1992. Prolactin secreting pituitary carcinoma. J Neurol Neurosurg Psychiatry 55:1205–1206.

Pivonello R, Faggiano A, Di Salle F, et al. 1999. Complete remission of Nelson's syndrome after 1-year treatment with cabergoline. J Endocrinol Invest 22:860–865.

Plataniotis GA, Kouvaris JR, Vlahos L, Papavasiliou C. 1998. Radiation therapy alone for growth hormone–producing pituitary adenomas. Acta Oncol 37:97–99.

Plowman PN, Doughty D. 1999. Stereotactic radiosurgery, X: clinical isodosimetry of gamma knife versus accelerator X-knife for pituitary and acoustic tumours. Clin Oncol (R Coll Radiol) 11:321–329.

Pluta RM, Nieman L, Doppman JL, et al. 1999. Extrapituitary parasellar microadenoma in Cushing's disease. J Clin Endocrinol Metab 84:2912–2923.

Ram Z, Nieman LK, Cutler GB, Chrousas GP, Doppman JL, Oldfield EH. 1994. Early repeat surgery for persistent Cushing's disease. J Neurosurg 80:37–45.

Randall RV, Laws ER, Abboud CF, Ebersold MJ, Kao PC, Scheithauer BW. 1983. Transsphenoidal microsurgical treatment of prolactin-producing pituitary adenomas: results in 100 patients. Mayo Clin Proc 58:108–121.

Randeva HS, Schoebel J, Byrne J, Esiri M, Adams CB, Wass JA. 1999. Classical pituitary apoplexy: clinical features, management and outcome. Clin Endocrinol (Oxf) 51:181–188.

Ridgway EC, Klibanski A, Ladenson PW, et al. 1981. Pure alpha-secreting pituitary adenomas. N Engl J Med 304:1254–1259.

Rodman EF, Molitch ME, Post KD, Biller BJ, Reichlin S. 1983. Long-term follow-up of transsphenoidal selective adenomectomy for prolactinoma. JAMA 252:921–924.

Ross DA, Wilson CB. 1988. Results of transsphenoidal microsurgery for growth hormone–secreting pituitary adenoma in a series of 214 patients. J Neurosurg 68:854–867.

Rothman LM, Sher J, Quencer RM, Tenner MS. 1976. Intracranial ectopic pituitary adenoma. Case report. J Neurosurg 44:96–99.

Sandeman D, Moufid A. 1998. Interactive image-guided pituitary surgery. An experience of 101 procedures. Neurochirurgie 44:331–338.

Sano T, Yamada S. 1994. Histologic and immunohistochemcial study of clinically non-functioning pituitary adenomas: special reference to gonadotropin-positive adenomas. Pathol Int 44:697–703.

Sasaki R, Murakami M, Okamoto Y, et al. 2000. The efficacy of conventional radiation therapy in the management of pituitary adenoma. Int J Radiat Oncol Biol Phys 47:1337–1345.

Scheithauer BW. 1984. Surgical pathology of the pituitary: the adenomas. Part I. Pathol Annu 19:317–374.

Schlechte J, Dolan K, Sherman B, Chapler F, Luciano A. 1989. The natural history of untreated hyperprolactinemia: a prospective analysis. J Clin Endocrinol Metab 68:412–418.

Selman WR, Laws ER, Scheithauer BW, Carpenter SM. 1986. The occurrence of dural invasion in pituitary adenomas. J Neurosurg 64:402–407.

Serri O, Rasio E, Beauregard H, Hardy J, Somma M. 1983. Recurrence of hyperprolactinemia after selective transsphenoidal adenomectomy in women with prolactinoma. N Engl J Med 309:280–283.

Shaffi OM, Wrightson P. 1975. Dural invasion by pituitary tumors. NZ Med J 81:386–390.

Sheehan MT, Atkinson JL, Kasperbauer JL, Erickson BJ, Nippoldt TB. 1999. Preliminary comparison of the endoscopic transnasal vs. the sublabial transseptal approach for clinically non-functioning pituitary macroadenomas. Mayo Clin Proc 74:661–670.

Sheline GE, Grossman A, Jones AE, Besser GM. 1984. Radiation therapy for prolactinomas. In: Black PM, Zervas NT, Ridgway EC, Martin JB (eds), Secretory Tumors of the Pituitary Gland. New York: Raven Press, pp 93–108.

Silbergeld DL, Mayberg MR, Berger MS, Ali-Osman F, Kelly WA, Shaw CM. 1993. Pituitary oncocytomas: clinical features, characteristics in cell culture, and treatment recommendations. J Neurooncol 16:39–46.

Snyder PJ. 1997. Gonadotroph and other clinically nonfunctioning pituitary adenomas. Cancer Treat Res 89:57–72.

Snyder PJ, Bashey HM, Kim SU, Chappel SC. 1984. Secretion of uncombined subunits of luteinizing hormone by gonadotroph cell adenomas. J Clin Endocrinol Metab 59:1169–1175.

Soule SG, Farhi J, Conway GS, Jacobs HS, Powell M. 1996. The outcome of hypophysectomy for prolactinomas in the era of dopamine agonist therapy. Clin Endocrinol (Oxf) 44:711–716.

Stevenaert A, Beckers A. 1993. Presurgical octreotide treatment in acromegaly. Acta Endocrinol (Copenh) 129:18–20.

Tamura M, Yokoyama N, Abe Y, et al. 1998. Preoperative treatment of growth hormone-producing pituitary adenoma with continuous subcutaneous infusion of octreotide. Endocr J 45:269–275.

Teramoto A, Hirakawa K, Sanno N, Osamura Y. 1994. Incidental pituitary lesions in 1,000 unselected autopsy specimens. Radiology 193:161–164.

Tindall GT, Oyesiku NM, Watts NB, Clark RV, Christy JH, Adams DA. 1993. Transsphenoidal adenomectomy for growth hormone-secreting pituitary adenomas in acromegaly: outcome analysis and determinants of failure. J Neurosurg 78:205–215.

Tindall GT, Tindall SC. 1987. Pterional approach. In: Apuzzo MLJ (ed), Surgery of the Third Ventricle. Baltimore: Williams & Wilkins, p. 440–461.

Tishler RB, Loeffler JS, Lunsford LD, et al. 1993. Tolerance of cranial nerves of the cavernous sinus to radiosurgery. Int J Radiat Oncol Biol Phys 27:215–221.

Tomita T, Gates E. 1999. Pituitary adenomas and granular cell tumors. Incidence, cell type, and location of tumor in 100 pituitary glands at autopsy. Am J Clin Pathol 111:817–825.

Trainer PJ, Drake WM, Katznelson L, et al. 2000. Treatment of acromegaly with the growth hormone–receptor antagonist pegvisomant. N Engl J Med 342:1171–1177.

Trouillas J, Sassolas G, Loras B, et al. 1991. Somatotropic adenomas without acromegaly. Pathol Res Pract 187:943–949.

Turner HE, Stratton IM, Byrne JV, Adams CB, Wass JA. 1999. Audit of selected patients with nonfunctioning pituitary adenomas treated without irradiation—a follow-up study. Clin Endocrinol 51:281–284.

Tyrrell JB, Lamborn KR, Hannegan LT, Applebury CB, Wilson CB. 1999. Transsphenoidal microsurgical therapy of prolactinomas: initial outcomes and long-term results. Neurosurgery 44:254–261.

Van Cauter E, Refetoff S. 1985. Evidence for two subtypes of Cushing's disease based on the analysis of episodic cortisol secretion. N Engl J Med 312:1343–1349.

Verhelst J, Abs R, Maiter D, et al. 1999. Cabergoline in the treatment of hyperprolactinemia: a study in 455 patients. J Clin Endocrinol Metab 84:2518–2522.

Verhelst JA, Pedroncelli AM, Abs R, et al. 2000. Slow-release lanreotide in the treatment of acromegaly: a study in 66 patients. Eur J Endocrinol 143:577–584.

Waltz TA, Brownell B. 1966. Sarcoma: a possible late result of effective radiation therapy for pituitary adenoma. Report of two cases. J Neurosurg 24:901–907.

Warnet A, Harris AG, Renard E, Martin D, James-Deidier A, Chaumet-Riffaud P. 1997. A prospective multicenter trial of octreotide in 24 patients with visual defects caused by non-functioning and gonadotropin-secreting pituitary adenomas. French Multicenter Octreotide Study Group. Neurosurgery 41:786–797.

Warnet A, Porsova-Dutoit I, Lahlou N, et al. 1994. Glycoprotein hormone alpha-subunit secretion in prolactinomas and in non-functioning adenomas: relation with the tumour size. Clin Endocrinol (Oxf) 41:177–184.

Warnet A, Timsit J, Chanson P, et al. 1989. The effect of somatostatin analogue on chiasmal dysfunction from pituitary macroadenomas. J Neurosurg 71:687–690.

Wass JAH, Thorner MO, Morris DV, et al. 1977. Long-term treatment of acromegaly with bromocriptine. BMJ 1:875–878.

Webb SM, Rigla M, Wagner A, Oliver B, Bartumeus F. 1999. Recovery of hypopituitarism after neurosurgical treatment of pituitary adenomas. J Clin Endocrinol Metab 84:3696–3700.

Webb SM, Ruscalleda J, Schwarzstein D, et al. 1992. Computerized tomography versus magnetic resonance imaging: a comparative study in hypothalamic-pituitary and parasellar pathology. Clin Endocrinol (Oxf) 36:459–465.

Williams M, van Seters AP, Hermans J, Leer JW. 1994. Evaluation of the effects of radiotherapy on macroprolactinomas using the decline rate of serum prolactin levels as a dynamic parameter. Clin Oncol (R Coll Radiol) 6:102–109.

Wright AD, Hill DM, Lowy C, Fraser TR. 1970. Mortality in acromegaly. Q J Med 39:1–16.

Young M, Kattner K, Gupta K. 1999. Pituitary hyperplasia resulting from primary hypothyroidism mimicking macroadenomas. Br J Neurosurg 13:138–142.

Young WF, Scheithauer BW, Kovacs KT, Horvath E, Davis DH, Randall RV. 1996. Gonadotroph adenoma of the pituitary gland: a clinicopathological analysis of 100 cases. Mayo Clin Proc 71:649–656.

Zhang N, Pan L, Wang EM, Dai JZ, Wang BJ, Cai PW. 2000. Radiosurgery for growth hormone-producing pituitary adenomas. J Neurosurg 93:6–9.

Part III

Genetics and Epidemiology of Primary Tumors

9

Genetic and Molecular Basis of Primary Central Nervous System Tumors

C. DAVID JAMES, JUSTIN S. SMITH, AND ROBERT B. JENKINS

Our understanding of the genetic etiology of nervous system tumors has advanced considerably during the last decade. During this time, investigators studying genetic alterations in these tumors were able to make several successful transitions from cytogenetic observations to the identification of specific genes that are targeted for mutation. The new information associated with the results of their investigations will benefit patients with nervous system cancer in at least two ways. One benefit involves the predictive value associated with the identification of specific gene alterations, that is, it is clear that certain mutations are consistently associated with specific clinical behaviors. A second benefit concerns the ability of molecular genetics to provide insights into the fundamental mechanisms associated with tumor development and, in so doing, provide information about potential therapeutic targets. In the near future, it seems likely that concepts that have evolved from this area of study will allow for the application of individualized treatments that will extend the length and quality of life for people afflicted with nervous system cancer.

MOLECULAR AND CYTOGENETIC METHODS

Cytogenetics

Cytogenetic studies provided the earliest clues concerning the genomic locations of genes whose alterations are associated with nervous system tumor development. Many of the karyotypic abnormalities described in the literature are based on the study of glioblastoma multiforme, the most common and malignant central nervous system tumor. Anomalies that occur frequently in glioblastoma include gain of chromosome 7, loss of chromosomes 10 and 22, and structural alterations of chromosomes 1p, 9p, 11p, 12q, and 13q (Bigner et al., 1984). In addition, double-minute chromosomes are often observed in these tumors; their presence suggests the occurrence of gene amplification (Bigner et al., 1987). Alterations associated with other types of glial tumors include loss of chromosomal arms 1p and 19q in tumors with oligodendroglial differentiation (Ransom et al., 1992) and loss of chromosome 22 in ependymomas (Ransom et al., 1992; Weremovicz et al., 1992).

Whereas the most frequent chromosomal anomalies in gliomas involve numerical deviations, medulloblastomas exhibit predominantly structural chromosomal abnormalities that often involve chromosomes 1, 3, 6, 10, 17, and 20 (Bigner et al., 1988; Biegel et al., 1989); among these, isochromosome 17q, with associated 17p loss, appears to be the most frequent. With regard to mesodermal tumors, loss of chromosome 22 occurs frequently in meningiomas and has also been reported in a significant proportion of schwannomas (Zang, 1982; Stenman et al., 1991).

Fluorescence In Situ Hybridization

In the past few years, molecular techniques have been combined with conventional cytogenetic methods to develop new procedures for identifying chromosomal alterations in brain tumors. The resulting molecular cytogenetic procedures have not only helped to make infrequently used archival material amenable to genetic analysis, but have also provided information leading to the identification of novel gene alterations. The first of these to be discussed is referred to as FISH (fluorescence in situ hybridization). Although FISH was initially applied to the study of chromosome structure in 1986 by Pinkel et al., the widespread use of this technique in a clinical setting has not been achieved until recently.

The FISH method involves the fluorescent labeling, either directly or indirectly (e.g., biotin labeling followed by fluorescence-labeled avidin detection), of relatively large segments of cloned human DNA. The cloned DNA segments, each of which has been previously determined to contain known genes from specific chromosomal regions, can be hybridized to either isolated metaphase chromosomes or to intact interphase nuclei. In many instances the probes can be used to find their target sequence in cells that have been embedded and preserved in paraffin (Color Fig. 9–1). By labeling different probes with different fluorochromes it is possible to examine multiple chromosomes for alterations, and, in fact, there is a derivative of FISH known as spectral karyotyping (SKY) (Schrock et al., 1997) in which 23 chromosome-specific probes, each labeled with a different fluorochrome or combination of fluorochromes, are simultaneously hybridized to metaphase preparations. Although yet to be extensively applied to the study of brain tumors, this technique may prove useful for the analysis of complex karyotypes that are typical of many nervous system malignancies.

Comparative Genomic Hybridization

An additional molecular cytogenetic method that has been efficacious in identifying chromosomal and gene alterations in solid tumors is comparative genomic hybridization (CGH) (Kallioniemi et al., 1992). This method is based on the competition between two different DNAs, one from a tumor and one from a normal tissue, for hybridization to normal metaphase chromosomes. Before hybridization, the normal and tumor DNAs are labeled with different fluorochromes (usually red and green, respectively), and as a result most regions of hybridized metaphase chromosomes show a fluorescence color combination that is equally balanced between the two labeled DNAs. When the tumor DNA shows either a gain or loss of genetic material, there is either an increase or decrease in green fluorescence, respectively, at points on the normal chromosomes where the gene alteration has occurred (Color Fig. 9–2).

This technique has provided information beyond that available through conventional cytogenetics for a variety of brain tumors (Kim et al., 1995; Reardon et al., 1997; Weber et al., 1997) and has suggested several chromosomal locations of genetic alterations for which there are no established mutation targets. Findings obtained through the application of this technique have provided an effective springboard from which to launch positional cloning projects and/or from which to examine databases containing the chromosomal locations for thousands of genes so that candidate sequences associated with specific chromosomal alterations can be examined.

Molecular Genetics

Linkage Analysis

Linkage analysis, as studied with molecular genetic methods, relies on subtle DNA sequence variations (called *polymorphisms*) between chromosome homologues that allow one to "track" the segregation pattern of a disease-predisposing locus (gene) through multiple generations of an affected family (White and Lalouel, 1988). In the study of such families, the chromosomal proximity of a DNA marker (probe) to a cancer-predisposing gene is indicated by the consistency of the marker's co-segregation with the occurrence of cancer within the family. This approach has been useful in identifying and/or associating tumor suppressor genes (TSGs) such as *TP53, NF2,* and *VHL* with their respective cancer syndromes: Li-Fraumeni, neurofibromatosis type 2, and von Hippel-Lindau.

Loss of Heterozygosity (LOH) Analysis

DNA polymorphisms have also been utilized to locate TSGs in sporadic tumors through a process known as *deletion mapping.* A chromosomal deletion map is obtained through the application of loss of heterozygosity (LOH) analysis (Lasko et al., 1991) in which the patterns of restriction enzyme or polymerase chain reaction (PCR) DNA fragments are compared in a patient's normal and tumor DNAs. Loss of a restriction or PCR fragment-length allele in a tumor DNA sample is indicative of a genetic alteration directed at the deletion of a TSG. By applying a battery of mapped probes (markers) from a chromosome of interest, one can limit the chromosomal location of a TSG by determining the smallest common region of deletion among a panel of similar tumors. This type of analysis has been applied extensively to brain tumors and has revealed several associations between detectable alterations and tumor histopathology.

GENES IMPORTANT TO NERVOUS SYSTEM TUMORS

Classification of Cancer Genes

As in all human cancers, two families of genes appear to be involved in the pathogenesis of brain tumors: oncogenes and tumor suppressor genes (Nagane et al., 1997). The protein products of oncogenes promote cell proliferation, and oncogenes can be activated by increasing the synthesis of their corresponding protein, in its normal form, or by alteration of corresponding protein function through gene mutation. In general, oncogene alterations only involve one of the two copies of a specific oncogene within a cell. In contrast, both copies of a specific tumor suppressor gene (TSG) must be inactivated through deletion or mutation for a cell to gain a growth advantage. As might be suspected from their name, proteins encoded by TSGs inhibit cell growth. Table 9–1 summarizes the oncogene and TSG alterations important to the development of various types of nervous system tumors, and following are brief discussions of specific genes that are frequently altered during the development of specific types of tumors.

Table 9–1. Gene and Chromosomal Alterations Associated with the Development of Central Nervous System Tumors

Tumor Types	*Genes/Chromosomes*	*Frequency*
Gliobastoma and anaplastic astrocytoma	EGFR (a, m)*	30%–40% (GBM)
		10%–15% (AA)
	CDK4 (a)	10%–15%
	MDM2 (a)	5%–10%
	TP53 (d, m)*	20%–30% (GBM)
		30%–40% (AA)
	CDKN2A (d)	30%–40%
	PTEN (d, m)	25%–30% (GBM)
		10% (AA)
	RB (d, m)	10%–15%
Astrocytoma	TP53 (d, m)	30%–40%
Oligodendroglioma	Chromosome 1p (d)	40%–90%
	Chromosome 19q (d)	50%–80%
Ependymoma	Chromosome 22 (d)	25%–50%
Medulloblastoma	MYCN (a)	5%–10%
	CMYC (a)	5%–10%
	PTCH (d, m)	10%–20%
	Chromosome 17p (d)	30%–50%
Pilocytic astrocytoma	Chromosome 17q (d)	20%–30%
Meningioma and schwannoma	NF2 (d, m)	50%–60%
Hemangioblastoma	VHL (d, m)	10%–20%

Type of gene alterations: a, amplification; d, deletion; m, mutation. Chromosome arms are listed in instances where the corresponding gene alteration is yet to be identified. GBM, gliobastoma multiforme; AA, anaplastic astrocytoma.

*Frequency in glioblastoma series strongly influenced by proportion of primary and secondary tumors.

Oncogenes

EFGR. In nervous system tumors, specifically gliomas, oncogene activation appears to exclusively result from gene amplification. Gene amplification causes an increase in number of a specific gene within a cell and invariably results in a corresponding increased expression of the gene's encoded protein. The vast majority of brain tumor gene amplifications occur in astrocytomas, and of the oncogenes involved the most frequently amplified is the epidermal growth factor receptor *(EGFR)* gene (Libermann et al., 1985; Wong et al., 1987; Ekstrand et al., 1991). The *EGFR* gene encodes a transmembrane tyrosine kinase that is activated by its binding of the growth factors epidermal growth factor (EGF) and transforming growth factor-α. With regard to cytogenetics, this gene alteration is manifested as double-minute chromosomes that contain the amplified genes and are observed in nearly 40% of glioblastomas (Bigner et al., 1987). *EGFR* amplification occurs much less frequently in lower grade gliomas and has not been reported in nervous system tumors other than gliomas.

In approximately 50% of the patients having *EGFR* amplification, the amplified genes undergo intragene deletion rearrangements that result in the overexpression of a mutant receptor that lacks a portion of the extracellular domain (Sugawa et al., 1990). This mutant has been shown to have constitutive tyrosine kinase activity, as well as an extended half-life, that stimulates cell proliferation and enhances the tumorigenicity of human glioma cells in nude mice (Ekstrand et al., 1994; Nishikawa et al., 1994; Ekstrand et al., 1995). Gene alterations affecting the receptor's intracellular domain have also been reported (Eley et al., 1998).

EGFR amplification and/or overexpression have been evaluated as prognostic indicators in multiple glioma series, and the majority of these studies indicate that increased *EGFR* gene expression and gene dosage are not predictive of patient survival once tumor grade is taken into account (Olson et al., 1998). However, a recent report suggests that analysis of this gene alteration may be a useful prognostic variable if also considered in the context of patient age (Smith et al., 2001). The associated study showed that *EGFR* amplification was significantly correlated with shorter survival among glioblastoma patients younger than 40 years of age, while in patients aged 60 years or more amplification was associated with extended survival.

Other Oncogenes. Additional oncogenes whose amplification have been observed in patients with malignant gliomas include *MYCN* (Bigner et al., 1987), *CDK4* and *MDM2* (Reifenberger et al., 1994a; He et al., 1994), *CCND1* (He et al., 1994), *PDGFRA* (Fleming et al., 1992), and *MET* (Fischer et al., 1995), the latter two of which, like *EGFR,* are members of the family of tyrosine kinase growth factor receptors. The reported amplification frequencies for these genes are lower than that for *EGFR,* with the highest being 10% to 15% for *CDK4* in anaplastic astrocytomas and glioblastomas. There is a positive correlation between amplification and increasing glial tumor malignancy grade for each of the genes mentioned above.

Tumor Suppressor Genes (TSGs)

TP53. Loss of heterozygosity analysis was instrumental in identifying the TSG whose inactivation is most frequently involved in tumor development. The gene, *TP53,* is at chromosomal location 17p13.1, a site that is often deleted in astrocytomas (James et al., 1989). The remaining copy of *TP53* in an affected cell is usually inactivated by a subtle mutation, most of which results in amino acid substitutions that occur in four "hot spots" in exons 5 through 8 (Hollstein et al., 1991). No type of brain tumor other than those with predominant astrocytic differentiation have been shown to have appreciable *TP53* mutation rates, and studies in which large series of astrocytomas have been examined for *TP53* mutations indicate that similar mutation rates are observed in grade II and grade III tumors, while a decreased mutation rate occurs in the glioblastomas (grade IV). Although *TP53* mutations have most often been observed in sporadic astrocytomas, inherited mutations of the *TP53* gene have been identified in the majority of brain tumor patients with Li-Fraumeni syndrome, an inherited condition that additionally confers an elevated risk for the development of sarcomas, breast cancer, and leukemia (Malkin, 1993).

Normal p53 protein induces the transcription of genes that promote cell cycle arrest and apoptosis, including p21 and bax, respectively. Because of p53's role in regulating these cell responses, the loss of p53 function has been shown, in independent studies, to promote the accelerated growth and malignant transformation of astrocytes (Bogler et al., 1995; Yahamada et al., 1995). In these investigations, primary cortical astrocytes isolated from mice bred to lack any p53 function (−/−), but not from mice homozygous for normal p53 (+/+), were shown to grow rapidly in culture and with limited contact inhibition. With continued passaging, p53 null (−/−) astrocytes exhibited a multistep progression to a transformed phenotype indicated by their ability to form large, well-vascularized tumors in nude mice. Cells heterozygous (+/−) for wild-type p53 generally did not grow well in culture, but on occasion would form colonies that expanded rapidly. In such instances it was determined that these colonies had arisen from cells that had inactivated their single, normal *TP53* gene, causing them to become p53 (−/−). These results, which suggest p53 inactivation as an early event in astrocytoma development, may be consistent with clinical data indicating that constitutional (germline) *TP53* mutations predispose individuals to the development of astrocytic tumors at a relatively young age (Chen et al., 1995).

Results from a few studies suggest that *TP53* mutation status is of prognostic relevance to astrocytoma patients. In a study of 66 similarly treated anaplastic astrocytomas (Smith et al., 2001), *TP53* mutations were a strong univariate predictor of increased survival. In another study, the analysis of p53 expression in a series of 51 astrocytic gliomas, most of which were glioblastoma, showed a statistically significant association between increased p53 expression and disease-free survival (Korkolopoulou et al., 1997). In the majority of investigations, however, *TP53* mutations have not been shown to correlate with survival regardless of whether the gene alterations are examined with respect to tumor histologic grade.

CDKN2A. Identification of a second TSG whose inactivation is important to glioma development stemmed from both cytogenetic and LOH studies, which indicated that the short arm of chromosome 9 was frequently deleted in these tumors. Although the 9p loss was initially localized to a relatively large region that generally included the centromere-proximal end of the interferon-α gene cluster (Ichimura et al., 1994; James et al., 1994), it is now clear that the *CDKN2A* gene, which resides close to the interferon gene cluster, represents the primary chromosome 9p deletion target. There are, however, additional genes within as well as near *CDKN2A* that may also have a growth-suppressive function. Deletions of *CDKN2A* occur in a variety of cancers, including malignant gliomas (Kamb et al., 1994; Nobori et al., 1994). Among the gliomas, deletions of *CDKN2A* have been demonstrated in primary glioblastomas as well as in glioblastoma xenografts and cell lines (He et al., 1994; Jen et al., 1994; Schmidt et al., 1994).

In addition to *CDKN2A* inactivation by gene deletion, the p16 protein, which is encoded by *CDKN2A,* is not expressed in a significant fraction of gliomas having intact *CDKN2A* genes, indicating that loss of p16 expression can occur in the absence of a corresponding gene alteration. In at least a small proportion of such cases, this appears to be associated with *CDKN2A* gene hypermethylation (Nishikawa et al., 1995). As opposed to *TP53* mutations, which are observed at a decreasing frequency with increasing astrocytoma malignancy, *CDKN2A*-inactivating mutations occur more frequently with increasing glial tumor malignancy grade.

PTEN/MMAC1. Genetic changes resulting in inactivation of the *PTEN* gene (also referred to as *MMAC1*), residing at chromosomal location 10q23, represents the TSG alteration most highly associated with advanced-stage glial tumor malignancy (Li et al., 1997; Steck et al., 1997). *PTEN* has been shown to be inactivated in as many as 44% of all glioblastomas and in 60% of glioblastomas having 10q deletions (Wang et al., 1997). These results are consistent with *PTEN* being the primary target of inactivation associated with the loss of chromosome 10 that was originally observed in glioblastoma multiforme by cytogenetic analysis.

Although the encoded protein of *PTEN,* Tep1, has been shown to have a dual-specificity phosphatase activity (tyrosine and serine) (Myers et al., 1997), recent evidence suggests that its biologically relevant targets include inositol phospholipids as well as proteins. Among the phospholipid substrates is phosphoinositol triphosphate (Maehama and Dixon, 1998), which promotes the activity of Akt, a serine/threonine kinase that is an important regulator of cell survival and cell proliferation (Cantley and Neel, 1999). Tep1 additionally modulates cell migration and invasion by negatively regulating the signals generated at the focal adhesions (Tamura et al., 1998) through the direct dephosphorylation and inhibition of focal adhesion kinase (FAK). Finally, Tep1 negatively regulates receptor tyrosine kinase (RTK) signaling through its inhibition of the adaptor protein Shc (Gu et al., 1998).

Results from two recent studies suggest that the genetic status of *PTEN* is an important prognostic variable in malignant glioma. Lin et al. (1998) used LOH analysis to examine the *PTEN* locus in 110 such tumors and showed that *PTEN* LOH was a significant predictor of shorter survival. A similar conclusion was reached from the analysis of *PTEN* mutations in pediatric malignant astrocytomas (Raffel et al., 1999).

NF1. Inheritance of a mutated *NF1* gene predisposes to type 1 neurofibromatosis, a syndrome characterized by the development of neurofibromas, café-au-lait spots, and an increased risk for pheochromocytomas, schwannomas, neurofibrosarcomas, and primary brain tumors such as optic gliomas and pilocytic astrocytomas (Pollack and Mulvihill, 1997). Pilocytic astrocytomas occurring in the absence of *NF1* syndrome may also be due to *NF1*-inactivating mutations as deletions of this gene have been found in as many as 20% of such tumors (von Deimling et al., 1993). *NF1* encodes a GTPase-activating protein, neurofibromin, which has been shown to downregulate the activity of ras, an important effector of RTK signaling (Martin et al., 1990).

NF2. Localized to chromosomal region 22q12, the *NF2* gene is responsible for neurofibromatosis type 2, an autosomal dominant disease characterized by bilateral acoustic neuromas, meningiomas, and spinal schwannomas (Pollack and Mulvihill, 1997). Somatic mutations of the gene are seen in as many as 60% of sporadic (non-*NF2*–associated) meningiomas and schwannomas (Ruttledge et al., 1994; Sainz et al., 1994). The *NF2* gene product, merlin/schwannomin, is a cytoskeleton-associated protein whose function is important to the regulation of cell adhesion (Gonzalez-Agosti et al., 1996).

VHL. The *VHL* gene is located at chromosome 3p25–26, and its germline mutation is responsible for the von Hippel-Lindau syndrome (Decker et al., 1997), characterized by predisposition to the development of hemangioblastomas of the central nervous system and retina, as well as to other malignancies (renal cell carcinomas, pheochromocytomas). Somatic mutations of the *VHL* gene are seen in as many as 40% of sporadic hemangioblastomas (Tse et al., 1997). Functional analyses have indicated that the *VHL* gene product is an inhibitor of transcription elongation (Duan et al., 1995). In addition, the VHL protein has been implicated in controlling the expression of VEGF (Gnarra et al., 1996), a potent angiogenesis factor.

PTCH. The identification of tumor suppressor genes whose inactivation are involved with medulloblastoma development has been an area of active research for several years and only recently has yielded a viable candidate. The gene, *PTCH,* was discovered as a result of the association of its mutation with predisposition to nevoid basal cell carcinoma (NBCC) syndrome, an inherited condition in which there is occasional development of medulloblastoma in addition to the more commonly occurring nevoid basal cell carcinomas (Hahn et al., 1996). The *PTCH* gene has now been shown to be inactivated in approximately 20% of cases of sporadic medulloblastoma, and this gene alteration may be primarily associated with the desmoplastic subtype (Raffel et al., 1997; Wolter et al., 1997). Additional investigations have been conducted to determine whether genes that encode proteins that interact with the *PTCH* gene product, a transmembrane receptor (Marigo et al., 1996), are also altered in medulloblastoma. However, their associated results have failed to indicate that these genes are important mutational targets in this nervous system tumor (Reifenberger et al., 1998).

Chromosomal Regions Harboring Putative Tumor Suppressor Genes

Chromosome 19q. Allelic loss of 19q occurs in approximately 50% to 80% of oligodendroglial tumors and, with rare exception, involves the entire 19q chromosomal arm (von Deimling et al., 1992; Reifenberger et al., 1994a; Bello et al., 1995; Kraus et al., 1995; Smith et al., 1999). However, multiple investigations have progressively narrowed the chromosome 19q deletion region to an interval within 19q13.3 (Rosenberg et al., 1996; Smith et al., 1999), allowing for several candidate genes within the region to be examined for mutation. The incidence of 19q deletion is not significantly different between low- and high-grade oligodendrogliomas, suggesting that this alteration is an early event in the neoplastic development of these tumors (Reifenberger et al., 1994b; Bello et al., 1995; Kraus et al., 1995), a finding that contrasts with the 19q loss observed in astrocytic gliomas that is generally restricted to the high-grade cases (Smith et al., 1999).

Chromosome 1p. Deletion of chromosome 1p is another frequent event in oligodendrogliomas, occurring in 40% to 90% of these tumors (Bello et al.,

1994; Reifenberger et al., 1994b; Kraus et al., 1995; Smith et al., 1999). Interestingly, nearly all cases of oligodendroglioma studied with deletion of 1p also exhibit deletion of 19q, suggesting that inactivation of one or more genes on each of these chromosomal arms is an important event in oligodendroglioma oncogenesis. Data from a recent report showed two distinct deletion regions on 1p, D1S76-D1S253 at 1p36.3 and D1S482-D1S2743 at 1p34-35, that contain potential TSGs whose inactivation may be important to the development of these tumors (Husemann et al., 1999).

Evaluation of chromosomal arms 1p and 19q are of prognostic utility for the oligodendroglioma patient. Cairncross et al. (1998) examined 39 anaplastic oligodendroglioma patients, 37 of whom had received PCV chemotherapy. Allelic loss of 1p was a statistically significant predictor of chemosensitivity, and combined loss of 1p and 19q was significantly associated with both chemosensitivity and longer recurrence-free survival following chemotherapy. Moreover, Smith et al. (2001) have demonstrated that the association of 1p and 19q loss with prolonged survival is also evident in low-grade oligodendroglioma patients, and that this association may be independent of PCV chemotherapy.

CANCER GENE ALTERATIONS AND CELL CYCLE DYSFUNCTION

p53–MDM2–p14^{ARF}–p21

The mammalian cell cycle is divided into four distinct phases: G1, S, G2, and M. Unrestricted cell multiplication represents a hallmark feature of cancer, and this process is associated with continued cell cycle progression, a process that is usually kept under control by a complex system of positive and negative regulators that constitute a series of cell cycle checkpoints. One of the most important of these checkpoints involves the p53, MDM2, p14^{ARF}, and p21 proteins, which regulate the progression of cells through the G1 cell cycle phase.

Initially this checkpoint was thought to be abrogated only by inactivation of p53 through gene deletion or mutation. However, a considerable amount of information has emerged during the past few years concerning the regulation of p53 function by other cellular proteins. Important among the relevant studies are those dealing with MDM2, which binds to, destabilizes, and inactivates p53 (Oliner et al., 1993). Significantly, amplification of the *MDM2* gene has been demonstrated as an alternative mechanism to inactivating mutations of *TP53* in astrocytomas (Reifenberger et al., 1993). *MDM2* gene amplification has been reported in as many as 10% of anaplastic astrocytomas lacking *TP53* mutations, and the combined frequency of *TP53* and *MDM2* gene alterations indicates the inactivation of p53 function in approximately one-half of these tumors (Reifenberger et al., 1993).

MDM2-mediated destabilization of p53 is inhibited by p14^{ARF} (Pomerantz et al., 1998), whose gene resides partly within the coding sequence of the gene for p16 (Mao et al., 1995), *CDKN2A*. Because of its overlapping localization with *CDKN2A*, both copies of the *p14^{ARF}* gene are often deleted in astrocytomas. Consequently the 9p alterations that are so common in these tumors contribute to aberrant p53 function by promoting increased interaction between p53 and MDM2 (Fig. 9–3).

The activity of wild-type p53 is known to promote the synthesis of the universal cyclin–cdk inhibitor p21 (el-Deiry et al., 1994), and this is thought to prevent the replication of altered DNA in normal cells that have incurred DNA damage (Di Leonardo et al., 1994). Because the synthesis of p21 is stimulated by wild-type p53 activity, *TP53* gene inactivation, *MDM2* amplification, or *p14^{ARF}* gene deletion could contribute to reduced p21 synthesis and thus promote the accumulation of gene alterations in tumor cells due to the reduced function of a checkpoint preventing the synthesis of damaged DNA. Although reduced p21 expression appears to play an important role in tumor development, thus far there is no evidence that the p21 gene itself is mutated in human cancers (Shiohara et al., 1994; Tenan et al., 1995).

p16–cdk4–pRb–cyclin D

Another important G1 checkpoint is constituted by the p16, pRb, cdk4, and cyclin D proteins. The protein encoded by the *CDKN2A* gene, p16, acts as a negative regulator of cell growth and proliferation through its binding to cdk4 protein kinase and preventing it from forming an activated complex with cyclin D proteins (Serrano et al., 1993). The primary substrate of this complex is the retinoblastoma protein (Lukas et al., 1995), pRb. In its hypophosphorylated form, pRb

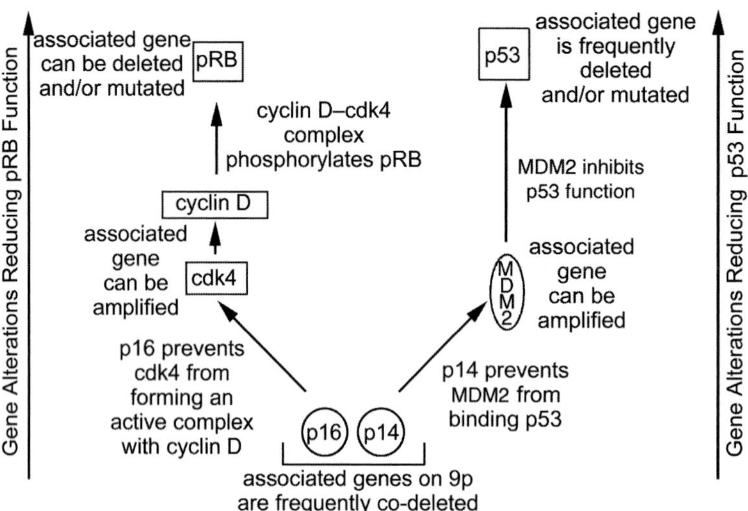

Figure 9–3. Gene alterations reducing pRb- and p53-associated cell cycle regulation.

arrests cells at the G1/S cell cycle checkpoint. This checkpoint is abrogated when pRb is phosphorylated, and cyclin D1–cdk4 has been shown to phosphorylate most retinoblastoma sites in vitro that are phosphorylated in vivo during late G1.

In association with the proposed model relating the activities of these proteins, one might anticipate the existence of at least three tumor-associated mechanisms for suppression of retinoblastoma function (Fig. 9–3): *(1)* inactivation of the positive upstream regulator p16; *(2)* increased expression of the negative upstream regulator cdk4; or *(3)* inactivation of the retinoblastoma protein through mutation of its gene. Consistent with this hypothesis, *CDK4* gene amplification and associated overexpression of cdk4 protein has been determined to occur in gliomas with intact and expressed *CDKN2A* genes (He et al., 1994; Schmidt et al., 1994). Furthermore, it has been shown that loss of pRb expression, in association with inactivating *RB* gene mutations, generally occurs in glial tumors and cell lines for which there is no evidence of *CDKN2A* or *CDK4* gene alterations (He et al., 1995; Ueki et al., 1996).

Although there are inconsistencies between the results of studies that examined the prognostic significance of detecting *CDKN2A, CDK4,* or *RB* gene alterations, it is generally thought that a member of this pathway is altered during the malignant transformation of nearly every astrocytoma (Ichimura et al., 1996). Interestingly, the results of investigations that support this concept show a genetic change to one and only one member of the *CDKN2A–CDK4–RB* triad in each malignant astrocytoma studied, suggesting that a single alteration within this pathway is sufficient to disrupt its regulatory function. Although the prognostic significance of this checkpoint's alteration in malignant astrocytoma is unclear, a recent study indicates that detection of *CDKN2A* deletions in tumors from patients with oligodendroglial tumors, albeit an infrequent event in oligodendroglioma, is significantly associated with decreased survival. Additionally, these deletions occur in tumors having intact copies of chromosomes 1 and 19 (Cairncross et al., 1998).

Because the activity of cdk4 depends on its binding to D-type cyclins, one might predict that increased cyclin D synthesis would contribute to oncogenesis by promoting the formation of active cyclin D–cdk4 complexes. Increased cyclin D1 expression in association with gene amplification has been reported in a number of cancers (Peters, 1994), but is uncommon in gliomas. However, it has been shown that cyclin D1 expression is increased by stimulating receptor tyrosine kinase activity (Sherr, 1995), and on this basis it is reasonable to speculate that the increased receptor tyrosine kinase activity that commonly occurs in malignant gliomas, usually in association with *EGFR* gene amplification or alteration, may play an important role in promoting cyclin D expression and thereby contribute to pRb protein inactivation.

HIGH-GRADE MALIGNANCY: SPONTANEOUS VERSUS DEVELOPMENT FROM A LOW-GRADE PRECURSOR

Much has been written and discussed during the past several years concerning the genetic etiology of malignant astrocytoma. The most common hypothesis considers two types of malignant brain tumor: one occurring spontaneously in full-blown malignancy and the other arising through a series of steps, with each step conferring an additional, incremental growth advantage. The former group of tumors appear to be characterized by the more frequent occurrence of *EGFR* amplification, whereas in the latter *TP53*-inactivating mutations are more common (Ng and Lam, 1998). In one study, for instance, it was shown that the incidence of *TP53* mutations was approximately six-fold less in de novo glioblastomas than in recurrent glioblastomas, which had displayed malignant progression (Watanabe et al., 1996).

The significance of the debate involving primary and progressive glioblastoma is related to potential differences in clinical behavior between the two groups of tumors, and their accurate genetic classification will continue to be of interest. Regardless of one's position on this issue, it is possible to construct a reasonably detailed model that describes the molecular genetic changes that are associated with different stages of malignant astrocytoma (Fig. 9–4). It is because of these associations between specific gene alterations and astrocytoma malignancy, as well as cellular differentiation, that genetic analysis will play an increasingly important role in the diagnosis and treatment of these tumors.

THE FUTURE OF CANCER GENETICS RESEARCH

It is anticipated that within the next few months to, at most, the next few years it will be possible to perform comprehensive analyses of gene expression patterns in human tissues and thereby obtain extensive detail regarding the identities of genes that are consistently overexpressed or underexpressed in specific types of tumors (DeRisi et al., 1996). This will result from combining microarray technological advances (Brown and Botstein, 1999) with by-products of the Human Genome Project (Sinsheimer, 1990).

Microarrays represent solid support templates on which single-stranded DNAs, representing coding sequences of thousands of different genes, can be placed. These arrays or "chips" are used for competitive hybridizations of normal-tumor cDNA or ge-

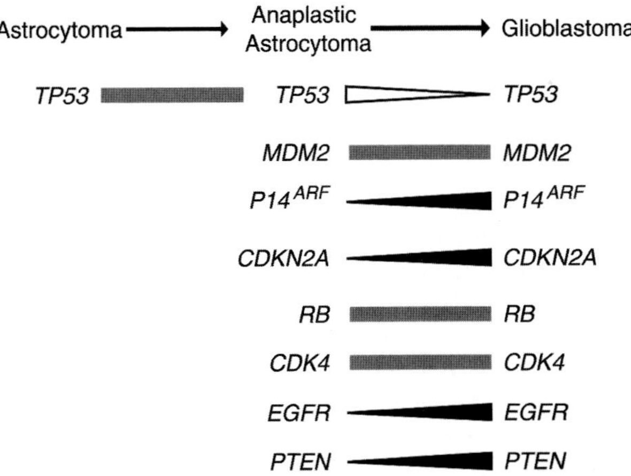

Figure 9–4. Gene alterations associated with astrocytoma malignancy stages. Gray, horizontal bars indicate that there are similar frequencies of alteration in different stages of malignancy. Black and white sloped bars indicate increasing and decreasing alteration frequencies, respectively, in association with increasing malignancy grade. This model, suggesting an accumulation of gene alterations with increasing astrocytoma malignancy, may be applicable to other types of nervous system tumors, but for all other tumor types there are insufficient data with which to propose specific gene alterations as associated with specific stages of malignant progression.

nomic DNA pairs that have been labeled with different fluorochromes. The principle on which this works is entirely analogous to that described previously for comparative genomic hybridizations (Fig. 9–2). Overrepresentation of the tumor cDNA or genomic DNA fluorochrome at a specific coordinate on the array indicates overexpression or overrepresentation, respectively, of the gene whose nucleotide sequence was spotted onto that coordinate. From a time-cost perspective the potential efficiency of this process for providing extensive information on gene expression patterns in tumors is astounding and will allow for the development of databases containing expression profiles for all common cancers. Such databases are already being developed (Kuska, 1996). Microarray technology is being extended to the detection of gene sequence alterations, and a first generation model for *TP53* mutation detection has already been marketed (Ahrendt et al., 1999). Chips for the detection of gene amplification and gene deletion are also being developed.

Developments in microarray technology have been largely driven by the progress and imminent completion of the Human Genome Project. In 1989 The Department of Energy and the National Institutes of Health began funding this project, whose purpose is to provide a series of linked datasets containing the genetic and physical locations of all genes on each human chromosome, plus the complete nucleotide sequence of the genome for humans. This initiative now appears to be entering its final phase and will result, as early as 2002, in a complete and accurate whole genome DNA sequence representing the genetic blueprint of the human species. With respect to the gene identification and localization aspect of this initiative, the most recent report indicates that more than 30,000 genes have been localized to specific chromosomal regions with a high degree of accuracy (Deloukas et al., 1998).

The total gene content within our cells is not currently known but most estimates place it at approximately 50,000. The map that currently exists can already be applied to the identification and isolation of genes that either directly cause human ailments or increase our susceptibility to disease. It is obvious that this initiative when combined with emerging technologies, some of which have been described here, will allow for the rapid and in many cases complete diagnosis of specific genetic lesions in individual brain tumors.

THERAPEUTIC IMPLICATIONS

The characterization of the genetic mechanisms associated with malignant transformation has opened the way to test novel molecular therapeutic modalities such as the delivery of small molecules that target disrupted growth-regulatory pathways. Examples of small molecules that may be useful in targeting unbalanced pathways include cdk4 inhibitors (Sausville et al., 1999), farnesyltransferase inhibitors (Ferrante et al., 1999), and inhibitors of EGF receptor-associated tyrosine kinase activity (Fry, 1999). Knowing whether a tumor has a gene alteration that would affect the function of a protein that is being used as a therapeutic target could be critical to determining the success of the agent. For example, it is clear that p53 function is critically important to ascertain the manner in which cells respond to radiation-induced DNA damage (Kuerbitz et al., 1992). Consequently, information regarding a tumor's *TP53* gene status may help determine a patient's response to radiation treatment; a recent report suggests this is the case for glioblastoma patients (Tada et al., 1998).

The identification of specific genetic lesions in combination with exciting new therapeutic strategies that depend on the knowledge of tumor genotypes should greatly facilitate the development of effective, individualized therapies for patients with nervous system tumors. It is reasonable to suspect that knowledge of tumor genotypes will soon play an important part in the clinical decision-making process for all cancer patients and that this information will result in improved patient care.

REFERENCES

Ahrendt SA, Halachmi S, Chow JT, et al. 1999. Rapid p53 sequence analysis in primary lung cancer using an oligonucleotide probe array. Proc Natl Acad Sci USA 96: 7382–7387.

Bello MJ, Leone PE, Vaquero J, et al. 1995. Allelic loss at 1p and 19q frequently occurs in association and may represent early oncogenic events in oligodendroglial tumors. Int J Cancer 64:207–210.

Bello MJ, Vaquero J, de Campos JM, et al. 1994. Molecular analysis of chromosome 1 abnormalities in human gliomas reveals frequent loss of 1p in oligodendroglial tumors. Int J Cancer 57:172–175.

Biegel JA, Rorke LB, Packer RJ, et al. 1989. Isochromosome 17q in primitive neuroectodermal tumors of the central nervous system. Genes Chromosomes Cancer 1:139–147.

Bigner SH, Mark J, Mahaley MS, Bigner DD. 1984. Patterns of

the early gross chromosomal changes in malignant human gliomas. Hereditas 101:103–113.

Bigner SH, Mark J, Friedman HS, Biegel JA, Bigner DD. 1988. Structural chromosomal abnormalities in human medulloblastoma. Cancer Genet Cytogenet 30:91–101.

Bigner SH, Wong AJ, Mark J, et al. 1987. Relationship between gene amplification and chromosomal deviations in malignant human gliomas. Cancer Genet Cytogenet 29:165–170.

Bogler O, Huang HJ, Cavenee WK. 1995. Loss of wild-type p53 bestows a growth advantage on primary cortical astrocytes and facilitates their in vitro transformation. Cancer Res 55:2746–2751.

Brown PO, Botstein D. 1999. Exploring the new world of the genome with DNA microarrays. Nat Genet 21:33–37.

Cairncross JG, Ueki K, Zlatescu MC, et al. 1998. Specific genetic predictors of chemotherapeutic response and survival in patients with anaplastic oligodendrogliomas. J Natl Cancer Inst 90:1473–1479.

Cantley LC, Neel BG. 1999. New insights into tumor suppression: PTEN suppresses tumor formation by restraining the phosphoinositide 3-kinase/AKT pathway. Proc Natl Acad Sci USA 96:4240–4245.

Chen P, Iavarone A, Fick J, Edwards M, Prados M, Israel MA. 1995. Constitutional p53 mutations associated with brain tumors in young adults. Cancer Genet Cytogenet 82:106–115.

Decker HJ, Weidt EJ, Brieger J. 1997. The von Hippel-Lindau tumor suppressor gene. A rare and intriguing disease opening new insight into basic mechanisms of carcinogenesis. Cancer Genet Cytogenet 93:74–83.

Deloukas P, Schuler GD, Gyapay G, et al. 1998. A physical map of 30,000 human genes. Science 282:744–746.

DeRisi J, Penland L, Brown PO, et al. 1996. Use of a cDNA microarray to analyse gene expression patterns in human cancer. Nat Genet 14:457–460.

Di Leonardo A, Linke SP, Clarkin K, Wahl GM. 1994. DNA damage triggers a prolonged p53-dependent G1 arrest and long-term induction of Cip1 in normal human fibroblasts. Genes Dev 8:2540–2551.

Duan DR, Pause A, Burgess WH, et al. 1995. Inhibition of transcription elongation by the VHL tumor suppressor protein. Science 269:1402–1406.

Ekstrand AJ, James CD, Cavenee WK, Seliger B, Petterson RF, Collins VP. 1991. Genes for epidermal growth factor receptor, transforming growth factor alpha, and epidermal growth factor and their expression in human gliomas in vivo. Cancer Res 51:2164–2172.

Ekstrand AJ, Liu L, He J, et al. 1995. Altered subcellular location of an activated and tumour-associated epidermal growth factor receptor. Oncogene 10:1455–1460.

Ekstrand AJ, Longo N, Hamid ML, et al. 1994. Functional characterization of an EGF receptor with a truncated extracellular domain expressed in glioblastomas with EGFR gene amplification. Oncogene 9:2313–2320.

el-Deiry WS, Harper JW, O'Connor PM, et al. 1994. WAF1/CIP1 is induced in p53-mediated G1 arrest and apoptosis. Cancer Res 54:1169–1174.

Eley G, Frederick L, Wang XY, Smith DI, James CD. 1998. 3′ end structure and rearrangements of EGFR in glioblastomas. Genes Chromosomes Cancer 23:248–254.

Ferrante K, Winograd B, Canetta R. 1999. Promising new developments in cancer chemotherapy. Cancer Chemother Pharmacol 43:S61–68.

Fischer U, Muller HW, Sattler HP, Feiden K, Zang MD, Meese E. 1995. Amplification of the MET gene in glioma. Genes Chromosomes Cancer 12:63–65.

Fleming TP, Saxena A, Clark WC, et al. 1992. Amplification and/or overexpression of platelet-derived growth factor receptors and epidermal growth factor receptor in human glial tumors. Cancer Res 52:4550–4553.

Fry DW. 1999. Inhibition of the epidermal growth factor receptor family of tyrosine kinases as an approach to cancer chemotherapy: progression from reversible to irreversible inhibitors. Pharmacol Ther 82:207–218.

Gnarra JR, Zhou S, Merrill MJ, et al. 1996. Post-transcriptional regulation of vascular endothelial growth factor mRNA by the product of the VHL tumor suppressor gene. Proc Natl Acad Sci USA 93:10589–10594.

Gonzalez-Agosti C, Xu L, Pinney D, et al. 1996. The merlin tumor suppressor localizes preferentially in membrane ruffles. Oncogene 13:1239–1247.

Gu J, Tamura M, Yamada KM. 1998. Tumor suppressor PTEN inhibits integrin- and growth factor–mediated mitogen-activated protein (MAP) kinase signaling pathways. J Cell Biol 143:1375–1383.

Hahn H, Wicking C, Zaphiropoulous PG, et al. 1996. Mutations of the human homolog of *Drosophila* patched in the nevoid basal cell carcinoma syndrome. Cell 85:841–851.

He J, Allen JR, Collins VP, Allalunis-Turner MJ, Godbout R, Day RS 3rd, James CD. 1994. CDK4 amplification is an alternative mechanism to p16 gene homozygous deletion in glioma cell lines. Cancer Res 54:5804–5807.

He J, Olson JJ, James CD. 1995. Lack of p16INK4 or retinoblastoma protein (pRb) or amplification-associated overexpression of cdk4 is observed in distinct subsets of malignant glial tumors and cell lines. Cancer Res 55:4833–4836.

Hollstein M, Sidransky D, Vogelstein B, Harris CC. 1991. p53 mutations in human cancers. Science 253:49–53.

Husemann K, Wolter M, Büschges R, Boström J, Sabel M, Reifenberger G. 1999. Identification of two distinct deleted regions on the short arm of chromosome 1 and rare mutation of the CDKN2C gene from 1p32 in oligodendroglial tumors. J Neuropathol Exp Neurol 58:1041–1050.

Ichimura K, Schmidt EE, Goike HM, Collins VP. 1996. Human glioblastomas with no alterations of the CDKN2A (p16INK4A, MTS1) and CDK4 genes have frequent mutations of the retinoblastoma gene. Oncogene 13:1065–1072.

Ichimura K, Schmidt EE, Yamaguchi N, James CD, Collins VP. 1994. A common region of homozygous deletion in malignant human gliomas lie between the IFN-alpha/omega gene cluster and the D9S171 locus. Cancer Res 54:3127–3130.

James CD, Carlbom E, Nordenskjold M, Collins VP, Cavenee WK. 1989. Mitotic recombination of chromosome 17 in astrocytomas. Proc Natl Acad Sci USA 86:2858–2862.

James CD, He J, Collins VP, Allalunis-Turner MJ, Day RS 3d. 1993. Localization of chromosome 9p homozygous deletions in glioma cell lines with markers constituting a continuous linkage group. Cancer Res 53:3674–3636.

Jen J, Harper JW, Bigner SH, et al. 1994. Deletion of p16 and p15 genes in brain tumors. Cancer Res 54:6353–6358.

Kallioniemi A, Kallioniemi OP, Sudar D,, et al. 1992. Comparative genomic hybridization for molecular cytogenetic analysis of solid tumors. Science 258:818–821.

Kamb A, Gruis NA, Weaver-Feldhaus J, et al. 1994. A cell cycle regulator potentially involved in the genesis of many tumor types. Science 264:436–440.

Kim DH, Mohapatra G, Bollen A, Waldman FM, Feuerstein BG. 1995. Chromosomal abnormalities in glioblastoma multiforme tumors and glioma cell lines detected by comparative genomic hybridization. Int J Cancer 60:812–819.

Korkolopoulou P, Christodoulou P, Kouzelis K, et al. 1997. MDM2 and p53 expression in gliomas: a multivariate survival analysis including proliferation markers and epidermal growth factor receptor. Br J Cancer 75:1269–1278.

Kraus JA, Koopman J, Kaskel P, et al. 1995. Shared allelic losses on chromosomes 1p and 19q suggest a common origin of oligodendroglioma and oligoastrocytoma. J Neuropathol Exp Neurol 54:91–95.

Kuerbitz SJ, Plunkett BS, Walsh WV, Kastan MB. 1992. Wild-type p53 is a cell cycle checkpoint determinant following irradiation. Proc Natl Acad Sci USA 89:7491–7495.

Kuska B. 1996. Cancer genome anatomy project set for take-off. J Natl Cancer Inst 88:1801–1803.

Lasko D, Cavenee W, Nordenskjold M. 1991. Loss of constitutional heterozygosity in human cancer. Annu Rev Genet 25:281–314.

Li J, Yen C, Liaw D, et al. 1997. PTEN, a putative protein tyrosine phosphatase gene mutated in human brain, breast, and prostate cancer. Science 275:1943–1947.

Libermann TA, Nusbaum HR, Razon N, et al. 1985. Amplification, enhanced expression and possible rearrangement of EGF receptor gene in primary human brain tumours of glial origin. Nature 313:144–147.

Lin H, Bondy ML, Langford LA, et al. 1998. Allelic deletion analyses of MMAC/PTEN and DMBT1 loci in gliomas: relationship to prognostic significance. Clin Cancer Res 4:2447–2454.

Lukas J, Parry D, Aagaard L, et al. 1995. Retinoblastoma-protein–dependent cell-cycle inhibition by the tumour suppressor p16. Nature 375:503–506.

Maehama T, Dixon JE. 1998. The tumor suppressor, PTEN/MMAC1, dephosphorylates the lipid second messenger, phosphatidylinositol 3,4,5-trisphosphate. J Biol Chem 273:13375–13378.

Malkin D. 1993. p53 and the Li-Fraumeni syndrome. Cancer Genet Cytogenet 66:83–92.

Mao L, Merlo A, Bedi G, et al. 1995. A novel p16INK4A transcript. Cancer Res 55:2995–2997.

Marigo V, Davey RA, Zuo Y, Cunningham JM, Tabin CJ. 1996. Biochemical evidence that patched is the Hedgehog receptor. Nature 384:176–179.

Martin GA, Viskochil D, Bollag G, et al. 1990. The GAP-related domain of the neurofibromatosis type 1 gene product interacts with ras p21. Cell 63:843–849.

Myers MP, Stolarov JP, Eng C, et al. 1997. P-TEN, the tumor suppressor from human chromosome 10q23, is a dual-specificity phosphatase. Proc Natl Acad Sci USA 94:9052–9057.

Nagane M, Huang HJ, Cavenee WK. 1997. Advances in the molecular genetics of gliomas. Curr Opin Oncol 9:215–222.

Ng HK, Lam PY. 1998. The molecular genetics of central nervous system tumors. Pathology 30:196–202.

Nishikawa R, Furnari FB, Lin H, et al. 1995. Loss of p16INK4 expression is frequent in high grade gliomas. Cancer Res 55:1941–1945.

Nishikawa R, Ji XD, Harmon RC, et al. 1994. A mutant epidermal growth factor receptor common in human glioma confers enhanced tumorigenicity. Proc Natl Acad Sci USA 91:7727–7731.

Nobori T, Miura K, Wu DJ, Lois A, Takabayashi K, Carson DA. 1994. Deletions of the cyclin-dependent kinase-4 inhibitor gene in multiple human cancers. Nature 368:753–756.

Oliner JD, Pietenpol JA, Thiagalingam S, Gyuris J, Kinzler KW, Vogelstein B. 1993. Oncoprotein MDM2 conceals the activation domain of tumor suppressor p53. Nature 362: 857–860.

Olson JJ, Barnett D, Yang J, Assietti R, Cotsonis G, James CD. 1998. Gene amplification as a prognostic factor in primary brain tumors. Clin Cancer Res 4:215–222.

Peters G. 1994. The D-type cyclins and their role in tumorigenesis. J Cell Sci Suppl 18:89–96.

Pinkel D, Straume T, Gray JW. 1986. Cytogenetic analysis using quantitative, high-sensitivity, fluorescence hybridization. Proc Natl Acad Sci USA 83:2934–2938.

Pollack IF, Mulvihill JJ. 1997. Neurofibromatosis 1 and 2. Brain Pathol 7:823–836.

Pomerantz J, Schreiber-Agus N, Liegeois NJ, et al. 1998. The Ink4a tumor suppressor gene product, p19Arf, interacts with MDM2 and neutralizes MDM2's inhibition of p53. Cell 92:713–723.

Raffel C, Frederick L, O'Fallon JR, et al. 1999. Analysis of oncogene and tumor suppressor gene alterations in pediatric malignant astrocytomas reveals reduced survival for patients with PTEN mutations. Clin Cancer Res 5:4085–4090.

Raffel C, Jenkins RB, Frederick L, et al. 1997. Sporadic medulloblastomas contain PTCH mutations. Cancer Res 57: 842–845.

Ransom DT, Ritland SR, Kimmel DW, et al. 1992. Cytogenetic and loss of heterozygosity studies in ependymomas, pilocytic astrocytomas, and oligodendrogliomas. Genes Chromosomes Cancer 5:348–356.

Reardon DA, Michalkiewicz E, Boyett JM, et al. 1997. Extensive genomic abnormalities in childhood medulloblastoma by comparative genomic hybridization. Cancer Res 57: 4042–4047.

Reifenberger G, Liu L, Ichimura K, Schmidt EE, Collins VP. 1993. Amplification and overexpression of the MDM2 gene in a subset of human malignant gliomas without p53 mutations. Cancer Res 53:2736–2739.

Reifenberger G, Reifenberger J, Ichimura K, James CD, Wechsler W, Collins VP. 1994a. Amplification of multiple genes from chromosomal region 12q13–14 in human malignant gliomas: preliminary mapping of the amplicons shows preferential involvement of CDK4, SAS, and MDM2. Cancer Res 54:4299–4303.

Reifenberger J, Reifenberger G, Liu L, et al. 1994b. Molecular genetic analysis of oligodendroglial tumors shows preferential allelic deletions on 19q and 1p. Am J Pathol 145:1175–1190.

Reifenberger J, Wolter M, Weber RG, et al. 1998. Missense mutations in SMOH in sporadic basal cell carcinomas of the skin and primitive neuroectodermal tumors of the central nervous system. Cancer Res 58:1798–1803.

Rosenberg JE, Lisle DK, Burwick JA, Ueki K, Mohrenweiser A, Louis DN. 1996. Refined deletion mapping of the chromosome 19q glioma tumor suppressor gene to the D19S412-STD interval. Oncogene 13:2483–2485.

Ruttledge MH, Sarrazin J, Rangaratnam S, et al. 1994. Evidence for the complete inactivation of the NF2 gene in the majority of sporadic meningiomas. Nat Genet 6:180–184.

Sainz J, Huynh DP, Figueroa K, Ragge NK, Baser ME, Pulst SM. 1994. Mutations of the neurofibromatosis type 2 gene and lack of the gene product in vestibular schwannomas. Hum Mol Genet 3:885–891.

Sausville EA, Zaharevitz D, Gussio R, et al. 1999. Cyclin-dependent kinases: initial approaches to exploit a novel therapeutic target. Pharmacol Ther 82:285–292.

Sherr CJ. 1995. D-type cyclins. Trends Biochem Sci 20:187–190.

Schmidt EE, Ichimura K, Reifenberger G, Collins VP. 1994. CDKN2 (p16/MTS1) gene deletion or CDK4 amplification occurs in the majority of glioblastomas. Cancer Res 54:6321–6324.

Schrock E, Veldman T, Padilla-Nash H, et al. 1997. Spectral karyotyping refines cytogenetic diagnostics of constitutional chromosomal abnormalities. Hum Genet 101:255–262.

Serrano M, Hannon GJ, Beach D. 1993. A new regulatory motif in cell-cycle control causing specific inhibition of cyclin D/CDK4. Nature 366:704–707.

Shiohara M, el-Deiry WS, Wada M, et al. 1994. Absence of WAF1 mutations in a variety of human malignancies. Blood 84:3781–3784.

Sinsheimer RL. 1990. Human genome initiative. Science 249:1359.

Smith JS, Alderete B, Minn Y, et al. 1999. Localization of common deletion regions on 1p and 19q in human gliomas and their association with histological subtype. Oncogene 18:4144–4152.

Smith JS, Perry A, Borell TJ, et al. 2000. Alterations of chromosome arms 1p and 19q as predictors of survival in oligodendrogliomas, astrocytomas, and mixed oligoastrocytomas. J Clin Oncol 18:636–645.

Smith JS, Tachibana I, Passe SM, Huntley BK, Borell TJ, et al. 2001. PTEN mutation, EGFR amplification, and outcome in patients with anaplastic astrocytoma and glioblastoma multiforme. J Natl Cancer Inst 93:1246–56.

Steck PA, Pershouse MA, Jasser SA, et al. 1997. Identification of a candidate tumour suppressor gene, MMAC1, at chromosome 10q23.3 that is mutated in multiple advanced cancers. Nat Genet 15:356–362.

Stenman G, Kindblom LG, Johansson M, Angervall L. 1991. Clonal chromosome abnormalities and in vitro growth characteristics of classical and cellular schwannomas. Cancer Genet Cytogenet 57:121–131.

Sugawa N, Ekstrand AJ, James CD, Collins VP. 1990. Identical splicing of aberrant epidermal growth factor receptor transcripts from amplified rearranged genes in human glioblastomas. Proc Natl Acad Sci USA 87:8602–8606.

Tada M, Matsumoto R, Iggo RD, et al. 1998. Selective sensitivity to radiation of cerebral glioblastomas harboring p53 mutations. Cancer Res 58:1793–1797.

Tamura M, Gu J, Matsumoto K, Aota S, Parsons R, Yamada KM. 1998. Inhibition of cell migration, spreading, and focal adhesions by tumor suppressor PTEN. Science 280:1614–1617.

Tenan M, Carrara F, DiDonato S, Finocchiaro G. 1995. Absence of mutations and identification of two polymorphisms in the SSCP and sequence analysis of p21CK1 gene in malignant gliomas. Int J Cancer 62:115–117.

Tse JY, Wong JH, Lo KW, Poon WS, Huang DP, Ng HK. 1997. Molecular genetic analysis of the von Hippel-Lindau disease tumor suppressor gene in familial and sporadic cerebellar hemangioblastomas. Am J Clin Pathol 107:459–466.

Ueki K, Ono Y, Henson JW, Efird JT, von Deimling A, Louis DN. 1996. CDKN2/p16 or RB alterations occur in the majority of glioblastomas and are inversely correlated. Cancer Res 56:150–153.

von Deimling A, Louis DN, von Ammon K, Petersen I, Weistler OD, Seizinger BR. 1992. Evidence for a tumor suppressor gene on chromosome 19q associated with human astrocytomas, oligodendrogliomas, and mixed gliomas. Cancer Res 52:4277–4279.

von Deimling A, Louis DN, Menon AG, et al. 1993. Deletions on the long arm of chromosome 17 in pilocytic astrocytoma. Acta Neuropathol 86:81–85.

Wang SI, Puc J, Li J, et al. 1997. Somatic mutations of PTEN in glioblastoma multiforme. Cancer Res 57:4183–4186.

Watanabe K, Tachibana O, Sata K, Yonekawa Y, Kleihues P, Ohgaki H. 1996. Overexpression of the EGF receptor and p53 mutations are mutually exclusive in the evolution of primary and secondary glioblastomas. Brain Pathol 6:217–223.

Weber RG, Bostrom J, Wolter M, et al. 1997. Analysis of genomic alterations in benign, atypical, and anaplastic meningiomas: toward a genetic model of meningioma progression. Proc Natl Acad Sci USA 94:14719–14724.

Weremovicz S, Kupsky WJ, Morton CC, Fletcher JA. 1992. Cytogenetic evidence for a chromosome 22 tumor suppressor gene in ependymoma. Cancer Genet Cytogenet 61:193–196.

White R, Lalouel JM. 1988. Chromosome mapping with DNA markers. Sci Am 258:40–48.

Wolter M, Reifenberger J, Sommer C, Ruzicka T, Reifenberger G. 1997. Mutations in the human homologue of the Drosophila segment polarity gene patched (PTCH) in sporadic basal cell carcinomas of the skin and primitive neuroectodermal tumors of the central nervous system. Cancer Res 57:2581–2585.

Wong AJ, Bigner SH, Bigner DD, Kinzler KW, Hamilton SR, Vogelstein B. 1987. Increased expression of the epidermal growth factor receptor gene in malignant gliomas is invariably associated with gene amplification. Proc Natl Acad Sci USA 84:6899–6903.

Yahamada AM, Bruner JM, Donehower LA, Morrison RS. 1995. Astrocytes derived from p53-deficient mice provide a multistep in vitro model for development of malignant gliomas. Mol Cell Biol 15:4249–4259.

Zang KD. 1982. Cytological and cytogenetical studies on human meningioma. Cancer Genet Cytogenet 6:249–274.

10

Epidemiology of Brain Tumors

RANDA EL-ZEIN, ANN YURIKO MINN, MARGARET WRENSCH,
AND MELISSA L. BONDY

Brain cancer accounts for approximately 1.4% of all cancers and 2.3% of all cancer-related deaths. The tumors are particularly deleterious in that they can interfere with the normal brain function that is essential for life (American Cancer Society, 2000). The American Cancer Society estimated that 16,800 individuals would be diagnosed with malignant brain tumors in 1999 and that 13,100 of those individuals would die from their disease (American Cancer Society, 2000). Despite their high degree of lethality and inescapable traumatic impact, brain tumors rarely metastasize beyond the central nervous system (CNS).

Although there has been a recent increase in the number of epidemiologic studies of brain cancer, little consensus exists regarding the nature and magnitude of the risk factors contributing to its development. In addition to the differences in methods and eligibility criteria used and in the representativeness of the patients studied, other confounding factors exist. These include the variable use of proxies to report information about case subjects; differences of control groups selected; substantial heterogeneity of primary brain tumors; inconsistencies in histologic diagnoses, definitions and groupings; and difficulties inherent in retrospective analyses.

ETIOLOGY AND RISK FACTORS OF BRAIN TUMORS

Ionizing Radiation

There is reasonable consensus from ongoing research that therapeutic ionizing radiation is a strong risk factor for intracranial tumors (Bondy et al., 1994; Hodges et al., 1992). Even the comparatively low doses (averaging 1.5 Gy) used to treat ringworm of the scalp (tinea capitis) have been associated with relative risks of 18, 10, and 3 for nerve sheath tumors, meningiomas, and gliomas, respectively (Bondy et al., 1994; Hodges et al., 1992). Other studies showed a high (17%) prevalence of prior therapeutic radiation among patients with glioblastoma or glioma and increased risk of brain tumors in children after radiation for acute lymphoblastic leukemia.

Diagnostic radiation, on the other hand, does not seem to play a role in glioma; three case–control studies of exposure to dental X-rays reported relative risks of 0.4, 1.2, and 3.0. The evidence is slightly stronger for meningioma, for which three of four studies have shown relative risks exceeding 2 after exposure to dental X-rays. Because the studies with positive findings were all conducted in Los Angeles (Hodges et al., 1992), they should be replicated in other geographic areas to test the validity of existing data.

The role of prenatal exposure to radiation in the etiology of childhood brain tumors is unclear. Japanese studies of individuals exposed in utero to atomic bomb radiation revealed no increased incidence of brain tumors (Hodges et al., 1992). Other studies that reported increased relative risks of 1.2 to 1.6 for those exposed prenatally were statistically insignificant because of their small sample sizes. Furthermore, relative risks of this low magnitude associated with a comparatively uncommon exposure cannot account for most childhood brain tumors. Parental exposure to ionizing radiation before conception of the affected child has not been shown to be a risk factor for childhood brain tumors (Hodges et al., 1992).

Occupational risk findings from atomic energy and airline employees are equivocal. A small but statistically significant elevated risk of 1.2 for the occurrence of brain tumors in nuclear facility employees and nuclear materials production workers has been reported (Hodges et al., 1992; Loomis and Wolf, 1996). However, the confounding effect modification by chemical exposures complicates interpretation of causality. One study reported increased mortality from brain tumors among airline pilots, possibly implicating exposure to cosmic radiation at high altitudes in brain tumor risk. Conversely, another study of airline pilots found no excess of brain tumor deaths (Bondy et al., 1994), a finding substantiated by a more recent population-based cohort study, which demonstrated that although malignant melanoma and skin cancer were found in excess in cockpit crew members with a long flying history, there was no increased risk of brain cancer in pilots (Gundestrup and Storm, 1999).

Electromagnetic Fields

The debate on the impact of electromagnetic fields on brain cancer continues despite largely negative findings, and it has been prolonged by methodologic difficulties with some study designs. Wertheimer and Leeper (1979) first reported an increased risk of cancer and later (1987), an increased risk of brain tumors and leukemia in children living in homes in Denver near high-current versus low-current wiring. This report triggered widespread public and scientific interest in the potential health effects caused by electromagnetic fields. One meta-analysis revealed a 50% increased risk of childhood brain tumors in children living in high versus low wire-coded homes (Meinert and Michaelis, 1996). In a meta-analysis of 29 studies of adult brain tumors related to occupational exposures to electric and magnetic fields, Kheifets and colleagues (1995) found a significantly (10% to 20%) increased risk for brain cancer among electrical workers but found no evidence for a consistent dose–response relationship between disease and jobs considered to have higher versus lower exposures.

A recent case–cohort analysis of brain cancer and leukemia in electric utility workers found that magnetic field exposure remained unrelated to leukemia mortality but was positively associated with brain cancer mortality on the basis of both cumulative and average magnetic field indices gathered from a refined magnetic field job-exposure matrix. Increased risk of brain cancer was found in relation to career exposure, with risk ratios of 1.8 (95% CI = 0.7–4.7) and 2.5 (95% CI = 1.0–6.3) in the uppermost categories for cumulative and average exposure, strongest for exposure 2 to 10 years past (Savitz et al., 2000). Another epidemiologic study of adult brain tumors (reviewed by Wrensch et al., 2000) and a recent large population-based study of adult glioma in the San Francisco Bay area provided no strong support for the hypothesis that high electromagnetic fields in homes may increase the risk of brain tumors (Wrensch et al., 1999). In the San Francisco study, 492 adults with glioma and 463 controls were equally likely to have lived in homes with high wire-codes during the 7 years before diagnosis. Spot measurements taken in homes also showed no correlation with controls (Wrensch et al., 1999).

Although a recent study found that exposure to 60 Hz magnetic fields stimulated proliferation of human astrocytoma cells in vitro (Wei et al., 2000), a study of childhood brain tumors and residential electromagnetic fields by Kheifets et al. (1999) found no support for an overall association between electromagnetic fields and childhood brain cancer. This lack of support applied to all surrogates of past magnetic fields, including wire code, distance, measured or calculated fields, and use of appliances by either child or mother. Mutnik and Muscat (1997) in a case–control study similarly found no increased risk of brain cancer with exposure to the use of common household appliances, including personal computers, electric heaters, electric hair dryers, and electric razors. The difficulty with many of the studies in this area, diverse as they are, is that conclusions may have been based on a sample size insufficient to detect small, elevated risks, skewing their results. Furthermore, most epidemiologic studies do not present quantitative exposure or data on the specific frequencies of electromagnetic fields (Blettner and Schlehofer, 1999).

The fact that measurements of electromagnetic fields are not precise also confounds interpretation of existing data. Wire codes of electrical distribution to homes and spot measurements of electromagnetic fields in and around homes can lead to incorrect exposure estimates (EMF Science Review Symposium, 1998). Wire codes also do not reflect exposures from internal wiring or household appliances. Spot measurements change over time and do not reflect the actual measurement in homes. Furthermore, the spot measurements may be made in places where the occupants spend little or no time. Such assessments also neglect exposures outside the home, which may exceed those in the home.

A positive Swedish study of adult leukemia and CNS tumors found increased risks in those exposed both residentially and occupationally, but not in those with no exposure or with only residential or only occupational exposure (EMF Science Review Symposium, 1998). The Swedish study was able to calculate residential magnetic field exposures over time because of detailed information available from Swedish power suppliers. Such data are not available in United States (Floderus et al., 1994). Finally, McKean-Cowdin et al. (1998) found that children of fathers employed as electrical workers were at increased risk of developing brain tumors of any histologic type (OR, 2.3; 95% CI, 1.3–4.0).

Aside from the lack of precise information about total electromagnetic field exposure and its duration, an even more basic limitation in assessing relative risk has been the failure, thus far, to show that electromagnetic fields induce mutations, which in turn might promote tumorigenesis and the development of brain tumors (Gurney and van Wijnagaarden, 1999).

Cellular Telephones

The use of cellular telephones has grown remarkably over the last decade, and it is estimated that more than 500 million individuals worldwide use hand-held cellular devices. The telephones contain a small transmitter that emits low-energy radio frequency radiation next to the head. This led to public concern that individuals exposed to radiation emitted from wireless communication technologies might have an increased risk of developing tumors of the brain and nervous system. To date, six papers have been published (Rothman et al., 1996; Dreyer et al., 1999; Hardell et al., 1999; Muscat et al., 2000; Inskip et al., 2001; Johansen et al., 2001), and none of the studies supports an association between use of these telephones and tumors of the brain or other cancers.

The first study by Rothman and colleagues (1996) reviewed mortality among more than 250,000 customers of a large cellular phone operator in the United States and did not find an increased risk after follow up of only 1 year. The numbers of brain cancers (n = 6) and of leukemias (n = 15) were small, and there were no statistically significant associations with number of minutes of phone use per day or years of phone ownership found in a study 3 years later (Dreyer et al., 1999). The third study, a case–control study from Sweden by Hardell and colleagues (1999), reported a statistically nonsignificant increased risk for brain tumors on the side of the head on which cellular telephones were used. However, the risk for brain tumors overall was not increased, and there were methodologic concerns related to ascertainment of cases. The fourth report was a case–control study from five academic institutions in the United States that reported 469 patients with primary brain cancer and 422 matched controls between 18 and 80 years of age (Muscat et al., 2000). They found no association with brain cancer by duration of use (p = 0.54) and an inconsistent association with side of the head where cellular telephones had been used that led them to conclude that it "is not associated with risk of brain cancer." The fifth study was a hospital-based case– control study conducted by investigators at the National Cancer Institute (Inskip et al., 2001). They included 782 patients and 799 controls. The relative risks associated with cellular phone use for more than 100 hours was 0.9 for gliomas (95% CI, 0.5–1.6), 0.7 for meningioma (95% CI, 0.3–1.7), and 1.4 for acoustic neuroma (95% CI, 0.6–3.0). There was no evidence of higher risks among persons who used cellular phones for more than 5 years or of more tumors on the side of the head where the phone was typically used.

The sixth study was a retrospective cohort study of cancer incidence conducted in Denmark using subscriber lists from the two Danish operating companies (Johansen et al., 2001). Investigators identified 420,095 cellular telephone users during the period from 1982 through 1995 and linked the list with the Danish Cancer Registry. They observed 3391 cancers overall and expected 3825 cases (SIR, 0.89; 95% CI, = 0.86–0.92), and the risk of cancers of the brain or nervous system was also lower than expected (SIR, 0.95; 95% CI, 0.81–1.12).

In addition, a large occupational cohort mortality study among 195,775 employees of Motorola, a manufacturer of wireless communication products, did not support an association between occupational radio frequency exposure and brain cancers or lymphoma/leukemia (Morgan et al., 2000).

To date, the studies all seem to support the hypothesis that there is no association between use of these telephones and tumors of the brain or other cancers.

FOOD AND DIETARY FACTORS

Several observations have led to studies of diet and brain tumors. In experimental animal studies, N-nitroso compounds have been clearly identified as neurocarcinogens (Koestner et al., 1972; Swenberg et al., 1975a,b; Preston-Martin, 1988). Other investigations have identified several mechanisms involving DNA damage through which N-nitroso compounds might cause brain tumors (Kleihues et al., 1979; Magnani et al., 1994; Bondy et al., 1994). N-nitroso compounds can initiate carcinogenesis in the CNS through both prenatal and postnatal exposure, with more tumors in animals resulting from fetal rather than postnatal exposures (Koestner et al., 1972; Swenberg et al., 1975a,b). Because there is a substantial lag between exposure and tumor formation it is likely that childhood exposure produces tumors in adults. Animal studies have shown that a wide variety of primates and other mammals are susceptible to chemically induced brain tumors (Preston-Martin, 1988).

For humans, the ubiquity of N-nitroso compounds has complicated their epidemiologic evaluation as carcinogens. About one-half of all human exposures in the digestive system occur when common amino compounds produced from fish, other foods, and drugs contact a nitrosating agent (such as nitrites in cured meats) in the right enzymatic milieu (Magnani et al., 1994). Equally common external exposures include agents such as tobacco smoke, cosmetics, auto interiors, and cured meats. Complicating matters further, some vegetables convert nitrates to nitrites but also contain a high enough level of vitamins to block formation of N-nitroso compounds. A meaningful assessment of risks from exposure to dietary and environmental compounds is thus difficult to achieve. Nevertheless, many studies have tried to examine major dietary sources of these chemicals and assess safeguards against formation of nitrosoureas presented by vitamins such as C and E, which are thought to inhibit N-nitroso formation.

There has been no consensus arising from the plethora of human studies. Diet and vitamin supplementation investigations have provided only limited support for the hypothesis that dietary N-nitroso compounds increase the risk of both childhood and adult brain tumors (Magnani et al., 1994; Berleur and Cordier, 1995). However, a verbal history of higher levels of consumption of foods cured with nitrosamines have been reported among brain tumor patients and mothers of brain tumor patients compared with control observers (Preston-Martin et al., 1996; Preston-Martin and Mack, 1996). Also, lower rates of N-nitroso compound formation after increased consumption of fruits and vegetables and vitamins that might block nitrosation or harmful effects of nitrosamines has been observed in some, but not all, studies.

Preston-Martin et al. (1998) uncovered a possible reduction in risk for pediatric brain tumors from maternal vitamin use during pregnancy. Their international case–control study examined data from 1051 cases and 1919 controls in eight geographic areas of Europe, Israel, and North America. Despite a huge international variation in the use of supplements by controls, combined results suggest that maternal supplementation for two trimesters may decrease the risk of brain tumor, with the greatest risk reduction among children diagnosed under 5 years of age whose mothers used supplements during all three trimesters of pregnancy.

Lee et al. (1997) found that adults with glioma were more likely than controls to consume diets high in cured foods and nitrites and low in fruits and vegetables rich in vitamin C. The effect was more pronounced in and only achieved statistical significance in men. Although this finding is compatible with the hypothesis that N-nitroso compounds might play a role in human neuro-oncogenesis, the observed patterns also support the hypothesis of nuclear and mitochondrial DNA damage caused by an increased level of N-nitroso compounds and the consequential oxidative burden versus antioxidant protection.

One comprehensive survey of nitrosamines in food and beverages found that beer contaminated with the nitrosamine derivative NDMA proved harmful, especially in Germany. The source of the contamination was traced to oxidation of malt (Mangino et al., 1982). Beer in several countries produced a major source of exposure to carcinogenic nitrosamines because of the very large quantities consumed. NDMA was also present in alcoholic beverages of various kinds, but at lower concentrations than in beer, therefore creating a lower cancer risk probably because of the smaller amounts consumed relative to beer. Despite much investigation, particularly in connection with pediatric brain tumors, alcoholic products have not been implicated as causing brain tumors (Wrensch et al., 1993).

Because tobacco smoke contains polycyclic aromatic hydrocarbons and nitroso compounds, many studies have attempted to establish a relationship between brain tumors and cigarette smoke. No significant effect has been found from smoking, although two studies report increased risk of adult glioma from smoking unfiltered, but not filtered, cigarettes (reviewed by Wrensch et al., 1993; Lee et al., 1997). A suspected role of secondary, or passive, smoke has more empirical support. Several studies found slightly increased relative risks, generally smaller than an order of magnitude associated with recognized hazards of exposure to passive smoking (1.2 to 1.3 for adult lung cancer and cardiovascular diseases) (Scheidt, 1997; Schwarz and Schmeiser-Rieder, 1996). Tumors most often associated with maternal smoking in pregnancy and passive smoke exposures are childhood brain tumors and leukemia/lymphoma, with risks as high as or greater than 2 in selected studies (Cordier et al., 1994; Filippini et al., 1994; Sasco and Vainio, 1999). Several studies have found elevated risk more closely associated with paternal rather than maternal smoking (Magnani et al., 1989).

INDUSTRY AND OCCUPATION

Attempts to link specific chemicals with human brain tumors in occupationally or industrially exposed groups have proved inconclusive. Thomas and Waxweiler (1986) published a comprehensive review of occupational risk factors for brain tumors and established a group of suspect chemicals and occupations. Additional studies in the intervening 14 years have not established a conclusive link between any of these factors and brain tumor risk. Many occupational and industrial studies focused on individuals exposed to carcinogenic and neurotoxic substances, including organic solvents, lubricating oils, acrylonitrile, formaldehyde, polycyclic aromatic hydrocarbons, phenols, and phenolic compounds, all of which are components of workplace exposures and induce brain tumors in experimental animals. Animal CNS carcinogenicity studies, mainly in rats, have shown that susceptibility is significantly influenced by strain, gestational age, and fetal versus adult status, factors that cannot be accounted for in or generalized to human occupational cohort exposure studies.

Animal studies assess exposures that cannot be tested in humans. For instance, some compounds such as polycyclic aromatic hydrocarbons generally induce brain tumors only through direct placental implantation, not through inhalation or dermal exposure as in worker populations. Workers are also rarely exposed to a single chemical but are exposed to many chemicals that probably interact to affect risk. Follow-up studies of occupationally induced brain cancer usually consist of too few affected subjects to permit pinpointing the causal chemicals, physical agents, work processes, interactions, or mechanisms involved.

There have been interesting occupational findings relating to motor vehicle operation with an associated increased risk for developing brain tumors. Kaplan et al. (1997) assessed occupationally related risk factors in a population-based, case–control study of 139 patients with primary brain tumors carried out in central Israel between 1987 and 1991. For each case, two control groups were matched by age (± 5 years), sex, and ethnic origin. Odds ratios for brain tumors showed a significantly increased risk among blue-collar workers, especially among those employed in the textile industry, and among drivers and motor vehicle operators. When tumor types were assessed separately, a significantly increased risk for malignant brain tumors was found among drivers and motor vehicle operator occupations, whereas for meningiomas there was an increased risk among weavers and tailors.

Other studies suggest that certain parental occupational exposures might be harmful to children (Cordier et al., 1997; Colt and Blair 1998). Data suggest that childhood nervous system tumors are increased if parents worked with solvents, polycyclic aromatic hydrocarbons, paints, and/or were employed in motor vehicle-related occupations. Results from a study by Cocco et al. (1998) to determine the risk of brain cancer and occupational exposure to lead lend some support to the hypothesis of an association between parental occupational exposure to lead and brain cancer risk in their children.

No definitive link has, however, been established between brain tumors and specific chemicals or strongly suspected carcinogens. Organochlorides, alkyl ureas, and copper sulfate compounds reliably induce cancer in laboratory animals, for example. Yet studies of agricultural workers using these chemicals have equally as often produced negative and positive findings with regard to brain tumor risk. Nor have all studies shown excess risk for workers involved in manufacturing pesticides or fertilizers. On the other hand, four of five studies of pesticide applicators found a nearly threefold elevated risk of developing brain tumors (Khuder et al., 1998). Viel et al. (1998) assessed the association between vineyard pesticides and brain cancer mortality among agricultural workers. A pesticide exposure index in vineyards was calculated for 89 French geographical units (1984 to 1986). Mortality from brain cancer among these farmers was significantly higher than mortality for the overall population. Univariate and multivariate analyses revealed a significant association between pesticide exposure in vineyards and brain cancer.

Daniels et al. (1997) critically reviewed 31 epidemiologic studies published between 1970 and 1996 to determine whether occupational or residential exposure to pesticides by either parents or children was related to increased risk of childhood cancer. The reported relative risk estimates were generally modest, although the highest risk estimates were found in those studies where pesticide exposure was measured in more detail. Frequent occupational exposure to pesticides or home pesticide use was more strongly associated with childhood leukemia and brain cancer than either professional exterminations or the use of garden pesticides. Occupational pesticide exposure was also associated with increased risk of Wilm's tumor, Ewing's sarcoma, and germ cell tumors. Residence on a farm, a proxy for pesticide exposure, was associated with increased risk of a number of childhood cancers. However, as in studies dealing with electromagnetic fields, methodologic limitations to many studies restrict the value of their conclusions. These limitations include indirect exposure classification, small sample size, and potential biases in control selection.

In a follow up of a population-based case–control study of pediatric brain tumors in Los Angeles County, California, involving mothers of 224 cases and 218 controls, Pogoda and Preston-Martin (1997) investigated the risk of household pesticide use from pregnancy to diagnosis. Particularly in subjects younger than 5 years of age, risk was significantly elevated for prenatal exposure to flea/tick pesticides (OR, 1.7; 95% CI, 1.1–2.6). Prenatal risk was highest for mothers who prepared, applied, or cleaned up tick/flea products themselves (OR, 2.2; CI, 1.1–4.2). A significant trend of increased risk with increased exposure was observed for number of pets treated ($p = 0.04$). Multivariate analysis of types of flea/tick products indicated that sprays/foggers were the only products significantly related to risk (OR, 10.8; CI, 1.3–89.1). Elevated risks were not observed for termite or lice treatments, pesticides for nuisance pests, or yard and garden insecticides, herbicides, fungicides, or snail killer. The findings indicate that chemicals used in flea/tick products may increase the risk of pediatric brain tumors and suggest that further research is warranted to determine the specific chemicals causing the most risk.

Kristensen et al. (1996) looked at the possible connections between parents working in agriculture in Norway and cancer in their children. Factors linked to horticulture and the use of pesticides are associated with cancer at an early age, whereas factors in animal husbandry, in particular poultry farming, are associated with cancers in later childhood and young adulthood. Risk factors were found for brain tumors, in particular nonastrocytic neuroepithelial tumors; for all ages pig farming tripled the risk. Indicators of pesticide use had an independent effect of the same magnitude in a dose–response fashion, strongest in children aged 0 to 14 years. Horticulture and pesticide indicators were associated with all cancers at ages 4 to 9 years, Wilm's tumor, non-Hodgkin's lymphoma, eye cancer, and neuroblastoma. Chicken farming was associated with common cancers of adolescence and was strongest for osteosarcoma and the mixed cellular type of Hodgkin's disease. The crude exposure indicators available limit this large cohort study, with the resulting misclassification likely to bias any true association toward unity.

Yeni-Komshian and Holly (2000) reviewed data from seven case–control studies published between 1979 and 1998 that considered a possible relationship between fetal or childhood exposure to farm animals or pets and childhood brain tumors. Five of the seven studies examined childhood residence or exposure of mother or child to farm animals or pets and childhood brain tumors. Four of these five studies reported elevated risk for childhood brain tumors with ORs ranging from 0.9 to 2.5 for maternal exposures and from 0.6 to 6.7 for children's exposures.

Later and larger studies subsequently examined histologic type and reported excess risk for primitive neuroectodermal tumors with farm residence prenatally (OR, 3.7; CI, 0.8–24) or in childhood (OR, 5.0; CI, 1.1–4.7). Increased risk of primitive neuroectodermal tumors was also associated with maternal exposure to pigs or poultry.

Because they involve production of many suspect carcinogens, synthetic rubber production and processing have received careful scrutiny by investigators who found a median increase in the occurrence of brain tumors of as much as 90% (Thomas and Waxweiler, 1986; Bohnen and Kurland, 1995). The by-products of synthetic rubber processing, such as coal tars, carbon tetrachloride, N-nitroso compounds, and carbon disulfide, might appear to account for the increased risk. In contrast, other studies showed no increased risk (Symons et al., 1982), or a decreased risk, of brain tumors caused by working in this industry, but studies have usually failed to show a link with a single chemical.

An association seems to exist between exposure to vinyl chloride and brain tumors. Vinyl chloride has been shown to induce brain tumors in rats, and 9 of 11 studies of polyvinyl chloride production workers have shown a median increased relative risk of dying of brain tumors that is twofold more than in the general population. A large European multicenter cohort study investigating the dose–response relationship between vinyl chloride and liver cancer, as well as assessing cancer risk for other sites, found no particular link between brain cancer and exposure (Simonato et al., 1991). Some argue, however, that the small number of brain tumor cases and statistical insignificance shown by most research cast doubt on the existence of any causal relationship (McLaughlin and Lipworth, 1999; Kielhorn et al., 2000). Another problem with the overall meaningfulness of results has been that, in general, epidemiologic studies have not followed individuals over a period of time adequate for cancer to become clinically manifest (Kalmaz and Kalmaz, 1984).

Formaldehyde is an additional long-suspected compound. The numbers derived from experimental data and retrospective review are greater than for other chemicals, but the conclusions are just as elusive. Formaldehyde produces cancer in laboratory animals, and nearly 2 million workers in the United States are occupationally exposed to it. Thirty epidemiologic studies of segments of this large group were evaluated by Blair and colleagues (1990). The unclear result was that elevated risk (approximately 50%) existed for those exposed in professional roles such as embalmers, pathologists, and anatomists. However, Blair et al. (1990) did not find a similar risk for industrial workers with formaldehyde exposure and therefore rejected a causal relationship between formaldehyde and human brain tumorigenesis. Other unknown cofactors may obscure the true risk in industrially exposed workers and create a skewed estimate of risk in associated occupational groups.

VIRUSES

Specific viruses, like chemicals, have been found to induce brain tumors in animal studies. As in the chemical studies, small numbers and negative findings hinder epidemiologic evaluation and conclusions. Performing aggressive studies of the role of viruses (and other infectious agents), in causing human brain tumors has been promulgated (Wrensch et al., 1993; Berleur and Cordier, 1995). The putative cancer–virus connection has been supported by several studies of animal tumor induction caused by viral exposure. Unfortunately, few epidemiologic studies have addressed the virus–tumor relationship probably because of the difficulties implicit in designing meaningful studies.

Between 1955 and 1963, 92 million U.S. residents received a Salk polio vaccine that may have been contaminated with simian virus 40 (SV40) (Shah, 1998). Levels of SV40 varied between lots and manufacturers. The vaccine was treated with formalin, but because SV40 is less susceptible to formalin inactivation than is poliovirus, the polio vaccine contained infectious SV40. Early cohort studies of cancer in SV40-contaminated poliovirus vaccine recipients demonstrated no clear association between SV40 exposure and cancer mortality among children in the United States (Fraumeni et al., 1970; Heinonen et al., 1973; Mortimer et al., 1981) and in Germany (Geissler, 1990). A recently published cohort study specifically examined the risk of ependymoma, osteosarcoma, and mesothelioma among Americans who as children received SV40-contaminated poliovirus vaccine (Strickler et al., 1999). There was no association between exposure and significantly increased rates of brain cancers, osteosarcomas, mesotheliomas, or medulloblastomas (Strickler et al.,

1999). Another study, one of the rare case–control studies of SV40 and cancer, showed no association with poliovirus immunization and childhood cancer among children in England, whereas yet another study showed a small association between poliovirus immunization and cancer in Australian children (Innis, 1968). Studies of maternal vaccination with SV40-contaminated vaccines have demonstrated an association with brain cancers in particular (Farwell et al., 1979; Heinonen et al., 1973). Interpreting these reports is difficult because of the small number of available cases and methodologic limitations. As with other brain tumor investigations, studies of SV40 are often case reports and follow ups, offering hints, clues, or perhaps merely coincidences that must be further tested and analyzed before any firm conclusions can be made.

Another virus investigated in a small number of studies is the human neurotropic polyomavirus JC virus, which is commonly excreted in urine, particularly by immunosuppressed, immunodeficient, and pregnant women. Khalili et al. (1999) recently detected JC virus in paraffin-embedded tissues from children with medulloblastoma. JC virus was also found in a rare case of pleomorphic xanthoastrocytoma (Martin et al., 1985) and in oligodendrogliomas (Rencic et al., 1996). However, JC virus exists in cancer-free subjects, and its connection, if any, to tumorigenesis is hypothetical at best.

Similarly, contradicting studies have found that more mothers of children with medulloblastoma than mothers of children without it were exposed to chicken pox, a herpes virus, during pregnancy. Wrensch and colleagues (1997b) found that adults with glioma in the San Francisco Bay area were significantly less likely to report having had either chicken pox or shingles than controls were. This observation was supported by serologic evidence that cases were less likely than controls to have antibody to varicella zoster virus, the agent that causes chicken pox and shingles. It is plausible that viruses and infectious agents explain the occurrence of brain tumors. However, as intriguing as this hypothesis is, further research is needed to clarify the role of viruses and any associations they may have with brain tumors. Linos et al. (1998) examined the hypothesis that exposure to influenza in pregnancy increased the risk of tumor in childhood. Ninety-four patients (ages ≤ 17 years) diagnosed in Greece with brain tumors or neuroblastomas from 1982 to 1993 were contrasted with 210 controls. The results show a significant association between influenza in pregnant women and occurrence of tumor in their children.

DRUGS AND MEDICATIONS

Few studies have examined the effects of medications and drugs on risk of adult brain tumors. A nonsignificant protective association was observed for headache, sleep, and pain medications (reviewed by Preston-Martin and Mack, 1996). Ryan and colleagues (1992) found that diuretics have a nonsignificant protective association with meningioma but have an opposite association with adult glioma, and they found essentially no association between antihistamine use and adult glioma, but a 60% increased relative risk for meningioma. Three studies have assessed childhood brain tumors and prenatal exposures to some or all of the following drugs: fertility drugs, oral contraceptives, sleeping pills or tranquilizers, pain medications, antihistamines, and diuretics. These studies have yielded few significant findings. Prenatal exposure to diuretics was 50% less common among children with brain tumors compared with controls in two studies but twice as common in one study. Prenatal exposure to barbiturates has not been consistently or convincingly linked with childhood brain tumors. Because nonsteroidal anti-inflammatory drugs are protective against certain cancers, the role of these drugs in inducing brain tumors, alone or with other factors, should be investigated.

SUSCEPTIBILITY TO BRAIN TUMORS

The most generally accepted current model of carcinogenesis is that cancers develop through an accumulation of genetic alterations that allow cells to grow out of the control of normal regulatory mechanisms and escape destruction by the immune system. Some inherited alterations in crucial cell cycle control genes, such as *P53*, as well as chemical, physical, and biologic agents that damage DNA, are therefore considered candidate carcinogens. Although rapid advances in molecular biology, genetics, and virology promise to help elucidate the molecular mechanisms behind the formation of human brain tumors, continued epidemiologic work is necessary to clarify the relative roles of different mechanisms in that process. Genetic and familial factors implicated in brain tumors have been the subject of many studies and were previously reviewed by Bondy et al. (1994).

Familial Aggregation

Because only a small proportion of brain tumors are heritable, most are likely due to an interaction between genes and the environment. Whereas findings of familial cancer aggregation may suggest a genetic etiology, such aggregations may be the result of common familial exposure to environmental agents. Some epidemiologic studies have compared family medical histories of patients with brain tumor with those of controls. Significantly increased family histories, of both brain tumors and other cancers, have been reported. Although few studies have been published, a family history of brain tumors was associated with a relative risk ranging from 1 to 9 (Bondy et al., 1994). Differences in study methodologies, sample size, which relatives are included, how cancers were ascertained and validated, and the country where the study was conducted might explain some of the disparities among the findings.

Supporting a genetic etiology for brain tumors are studies of siblings reporting a high frequency of brain tumors between them, although twin studies have not demonstrated a similar association. In a family study of 250 children with brain tumors, Bondy et al. (1994) showed by segregation analysis a low probability that familial aggregation supported multifactorial inheritance rather than chance alone. Segregation analyses of the families of more than 600 adults with glioma revealed that a polygenic environment–interactive model best explained the pattern of occurrence of brain tumors (de Andrade et al., 2001). Given the previously described complexities of environmental impact and multiplicity of possible heritable factors, more work is required to delineate the manner by which genetic susceptibility affects brain cancer risk.

Hereditary Syndromes

A few rare mutated genes and chromosomal abnormalities can greatly increase one's chance of developing brain tumors. Numerous case reports have associated CNS tumors, including medulloblastoma, and gross malformations with gastrointestinal and genitourinary system abnormalities. Ependymoma has been associated with multisystem abnormalities; astrocytoma with arteriovenous malformation of the overlying meninges; and glioblastoma multiforme with adjacent arteriovenous angiomatous malformation and pulmonary arteriovenous fistula. Central nervous system tumors may also be associated with Down's syndrome, which involves chromosome 21. Three epidemiologic studies have found that patients with brain tumor are two to five times more likely than controls to have a mentally retarded relative, although the result was statistically significant in only one study (reviewed by Bondy et al., 1994). The heritability of brain tumors is also suggested by many reports of individuals with hereditary syndromes such as tuberous sclerosis, neurofibromatosis types 1 and 2, nevoid basal cell carcinoma syndrome, and syndromes involving adenomatous polyps, developing tumors (reviewed by Bondy et al., 1994).

Although there is convincing evidence that genetics plays a role in most cancers, including brain tumors, inherited predisposition to brain tumors probably accounts for only a very small percentage (5% to 10%) of them (Narod et al., 1991). In a review of 16,564 cases of childhood cancers diagnosed between 1971 to 1983 and reported to the National Registry of Childhood Tumors in Great Britain, Narod et al. (1991) estimated that the heritable fraction of childhood brain tumors was about 2%. In a population-based study of nearly 500 adults with glioma, only 4 individuals (less than 1%), all of whom were diagnosed in their thirties, reported having a known heritable syndrome (3 had neurofibromatosis and 1 had tuberous sclerosis) (Wrensch et al., 1997a).

Another class of heritable conditions are the cancer family syndromes (such as the Li-Fraumeni syndrome [LFS]), so-called because individuals in affected families have an increased risk of developing certain types of cancers. Individuals with LFS have inherited at least one copy of a defective gene. In LFS, cancers that develop include brain tumors, sarcomas, breast cancer, and cancer of the adrenal gland.

In some families, LFS has been linked to a gene mutation in *P53* on chromosome 17p (Bondy et al., 1994). In addition, germline *P53* mutations were found to be more frequent in patients with multifocal glioma, glioma and another primary malignancy, and a family history of cancer. In a population-based study of malignant glioma, Li et al. (1998) reported that *P53* mutation-positive patients were more likely than normally to have a first-degree relative affected with cancer (58% versus 42%) or personal history of a previous cancer (17% versus 8%). Further research is necessary to determine the role of heredity, the frequency of *P53* mutations, and whether specific *P53* mutations correlate with specific exposures.

Metabolic Susceptibility

Genetic traits involved in susceptibility are common genetic alterations that influence oxidative metabolism, carcinogen detoxification, and DNA damage and repair. The role of genetic polymorphisms (alternative alleles) of genes established in the population in modulating susceptibility to carcinogenic exposures has been explored in some detail for tobacco-related neoplasms but much less so for other neoplasms, including gliomas. Due to rapid developments in genetic technology, an increasing number of potentially relevant polymorphisms are available for epidemiologic evaluation, including genes involved in carcinogen detoxification, oxidative metabolism, and DNA repair. The first study to report the role of metabolic polymorphisms in brain tumor risk found that the variants of cytochrome P450 2D6 *(CYP2D6)* and glutathione transferase *(GSTT1)* were significantly associated with increased risk of brain tumors (Elexpuru-Camiruaga et al., 1995). Kelsey et al. (1997) were unable to find an association between adult onset glioma with the *GSTT1*-null genotype or homozygosity for the *CYP2D6* variant, a poor-metabolizer genotype. However, when they stratified their data by histologic subtype, there was a significantly (threefold) increased risk for oligodendroglioma associated with the G*STT1*-null genotype. Trizna et al. (1998) found no statistically significant associations between the null genotypes of glutathione transferase-μ, *GSTT1,* and *CYP1A1* and risk of adult gliomas. However, they observed an intriguing pattern with *N*-acetyltransferase acetylation status, with a nearly twofold increased risk for rapid acetylation, but a 30% increased risk for intermediate acetylation.

It is unlikely that any single polymorphism is predictive of brain tumor risk. Therefore, a panel of relevant markers integrated with epidemiologic data should be assessed in a large number of study participants to clarify the relationship between genetic polymorphisms and brain tumor risk.

Mutagen Sensitivity

Cytogenetic assays of peripheral blood lymphocytes have been used extensively to determine response to genotoxic agents. The basis for these cytogenetic assays is that genetic damage is reflected by critical events in carcinogenesis in the affected tissue. To test this hypothesis, Hsu et al. (1989) developed a mutagen sensitivity assay in which the frequency of in vitro bleomycin-induced breaks in short-term lymphocyte cultures is used to measure genetic susceptibility. Bondy et al. (1996) modified the assay by using gamma radiation to induce chromosome breaks because radiation is a risk factor for brain tumors and can produce double-stranded DNA breaks and mutations. It is believed that mutagen sensitivity indirectly assesses the effectiveness of one or more DNA repair mechanisms. The following observations support this hypothesis. First, the relationship between chromosome instability syndromes and cancer susceptibility is well established (Busch, 1994). Patients with these syndromes also have defective DNA repair systems (Wei et al., 1996). Furthermore, patients with ataxia telangiectasia, who are extremely sensitive to the clastogenic effects of x-irradiation and bleomycin, differ from normal people in the speed with which aberrations induced by these agents are repaired, but not in the number of aberrations produced (Hittelman and Sen, 1988).

Gamma radiation-induced mutagen sensitivity is one of the few significant independent risk factors for brain tumors (Bondy et al., 1996). DNA repair capability and predisposition to cancer are hallmarks of rare chromosome instability syndromes and are related to differences in radiosensitivity. One in vitro study showed that individuals vary in lymphocyte radiosensitivity, which correlates with DNA repair capacity (Bondy et al., 1996). Therefore, it is biologically plausible that increased sensitivity to gamma radiation results in increased risk of developing brain tumors because of a genetic inability to repair radiation damage. However, this finding needs to be tested in a larger study to determine the roles of mutagen sensitivity and radiation exposure in the risk of developing gliomas. A positive mutagen sensitivity assay has been shown to be an independent risk factor for other cancers, including head and neck and lung, suggesting that the phenotype is constitutional (Cloos et al., 1996). The chromosome breaks are not affected by smoking or dietary factors (micronutrients) (Spitz et al., 1997).

Chromosome Instability

A number of chromosomal loci have been reported to play a role in brain tumorigenesis because of the numerous gains and losses observed in those loci. For example, Bigner et al. (1988), reported gain of chromosome 7 and loss of chromosome 10 in malignant gliomas and structural abnormalities involving chromosomes 1, 6p, 9p, and 19q. A more recent comparative genomic hybridization study revealed recurrent enhancements on chromosome 20 and also found gain of chromosome 7 and loss of chromosome 10 in several cases of astrocytoma. Partial or complete gains of chromosome 20 were found in six other tumors, suggesting that chromosome 20, and in particular 20p11.2p12, may harbor relevant genes for glioma progression (Brunner et al., 2000). Bello et al. (1994) reported involvement of chromosome 1 in oligodendrogliomas and meningiomas; and Magnani et al. (1994) demonstrated involvement of chromosomes 1, 7, 10, and 19 in anaplastic gliomas and glioblastomas.

Loss of heterozygosity for loci on chromosome 17p (Fults et al., 1989) and 11p15 (Sonoda et al., 1995) have also been reported. Indeed, deletions of 17p have consistently been reported in as many as 50% of medulloblastomas, and the major breakpoint interval has been localized to 17p11.2, a chromosome instability that has been linked to hypermethylation in this region in medulloblastomas but not with supratentorial primitive neuroectodermal tumors (Fruhwald et al., 2001).

Comparative genomic hybridization has been recently utilized to review chromosomal imbalances in a series of 20 adult and 8 childhood ependymomas. All tumors exhibited multiple genomic imbalances with loss of genetic material observed in chromosomes 22q (71%), 17 (46%), 6 (39%), 19q (32%), and 1p (29%), with overlapping regions of deletion. These findings suggest greater genomic imbalance in ependymomas than earlier recognized and confirmed previous findings of frequent losses of 17 and 22q and loss of chromosome 16 as recurrent genetic aberrations found in these tumors (Zheng et al., 2000). Similarly, fluorescence in situ hybridization uncovered deletion of 22q12–q13 in two intracerebral ependymomas (Rousseau-Merck et al., 2000).

There are few data regarding chromosomal alterations in the peripheral blood lymphocytes of patients with brain tumor. Such information might shed light on the pre-malignant changes that herald tumor development. Bondy et al. (1996) demonstrated that, compared with controls, glioma cases have less efficient DNA repair, as measured by increased chromosome sensitivity to gamma radiation in stimulated peripheral blood lymphocytes, and that was shown to be an independent risk factor for glioma. Recently, we investigated whether glioma patients have an increased chromosomal instability that could account for their heightened susceptibility to cancer (El-Zein et al., 1999). With fluorescence in situ hybridization methods, background instability in these patients was measured at hyper-breakable regions in the genome. Findings indicate that the human heterochromatin regions are frequently involved in stable chromosome rearrangements (Larizza et al., 1988; Doneda et al., 1989). Smith and Grosovsky (1993) and Grosovsky et al. (1996) reported that breakage affecting the centromeric and pericentromeric heterochromatin regions of human chromosomes could lead to mutations and chromosomal rearrangements and increase genomic instability.

A study performed by El-Zein et al. (1999) demonstrated that individuals with a significantly higher level of background chromosomal instability have a 15-fold increased risk of developing gliomas. A significantly higher level of hyperdiploidy was also detected. Chromosome instability leading to aneuploidy has been observed in many cancer types (Lengauer et al., 1997). Although previous studies have demonstrated the presence of chromosomal instability in brain tumor tissues (Arnoldus et al., 1992; Mohapatra et al., 1995; Wernicke et al., 1997; Rosso et al., 1997), our study was the first to investigate the role of background chromosomal instability in the peripheral blood lymphocytes of patients with gliomas (El-Zein et al., 1999). Our results suggest that accumulated chromosomal damage in peripheral blood lymphocytes may be an important biomarker for identifying individuals at risk of developing gliomas.

CONCLUSION

In summary, the etiology of brain tumors remains largely unknown. Biologically intensive studies incorporating new molecular genetic techniques have the potential to increase our understanding of the etiology of gliomas. Use of more consistently applied histopathologic classification systems, and greater understanding and use of molecular and genetic markers to classify tumors, should help to delineate the natural history and pathogenesis of brain tumors. It is well known that primary brain tumors have many causes; however, no single cause has yet been identified that can account for most cases. Many possibilities remain that will enable us to discover pertinent risk factors. Moreover, in the continuing search for explanations for this devastating disease, new concepts about neuro-oncogenesis will likely emerge, making the study of brain tumor epidemiology even more exciting.

REFERENCES

American Cancer Society. 2000. Cancer Facts and Figures. Washington, DC: American Cancer Society.

Arnoldus EP, Walters LB, Voormolen JH, et al. 1992. Interphase cytogenetics: a new tool for the study of genetic changes in brain tumors. J Neurosurg 76:997–1003.

Bello MJ, de Campos JM, Kusak ME, et al. 1994. Molecular analysis of chromosome 1 abnormalities in human gliomas reveals frequent loss of 1p in oligodendroglial tumors. Int J Cancer 57:172–175.

Berleur MP, Cordier S. 1995. The role of chemical, physical, or viral exposures and health factors in neurocarcinogenesis: implications for epidemiologic studies of brain tumors. Cancer Causes Control 6:240–256.

Bigner SH, Mark J, Burger PC, Mahaley MS Jr, Bullard DE, Muhlbaier LH, Bigner DD. 1988. Specific chromosomal abnormalities in malignant gliomas. Cancer Res 88:405–411.

Blair A, Saracci R, Stewart PA, Hayes RB, Shy C. 1990. Epidemiologic evidence on the relationship between formaldehyde exposure and cancer. Scand J Work Environ Health 16:381–393.

Blettner M, Schlehofer B. 1999. [Is there an increased risk of leukemia, brain tumors or breast cancer after exposure to high-frequency radiation? Review of methods and results of epidemiologic studies.] Med Klin 94:150–158.

Bohnen NI, Kurland LT. 1995. Brain tumor and exposure to pesticides in humans: a review of the epidemiologic data. J Neurol Sci 132:110–121.

Bondy M, Wiencke J, Wrensch M, Kyritsis AP. 1994. Genetics of primary brain tumors: a review. J Neurooncol 18:69–81.

Bondy ML, Kryitsis AP, Gu J, et al. 1996. Mutagen sensitivity and risk of gliomas: a case–control analysis. Cancer Res 56:1484–1486.

Brunner C, Jung V, Henn W, Zang KD, Urbschat S. 2000. Comparative genomic hybridization reveals recurrent enhancements on chromosome 20 and in one case combined amplification sites on 15q24q26 and 20p11p12 in glioblastomas. Cancer Genet Cytogenet 121:124–127.

Busch D. 1994. Genetic susceptibility to radiation and chemotherapy injury: diagnosis and management. Int J Radiat Oncol Biol Phys 30:997–1002.

Cloos J, Spitz MR, Schantz SP, Hsu TC, Zhang ZF, Tobi H, Braakhuis BJ, Snow GB. 1996. Genetic susceptibility to head and neck squamous cell carcinoma. J Natl Cancer Inst 88:530–535.

Cocco P, Dosemeci M, Heineman EF. 1998. Brain cancer and occupational exposure to lead. J Occup Environ Med 40:937–942.

Colt JS, Blair A. 1998. Parental occupational exposures and risk of childhood cancer. Environ Health Perspect 106:909–925.

Cordier S, Iglesias MJ, Le Goaster C, Guyot MM, Mandereau L, Hemon D. 1994. Incidence and risk factors for childhood brain tumors in the Ile de France. Int J Cancer 59:776–782.

Cordier S, Lefeuvre B, Filippini G, et al. 1997. Parental occupation, occupational exposure to solvents and polycyclic aromatic hydrocarbons and risk of childhood brain tumors (Italy, France, Spain). Cancer Causes Control 8:688–697.

Daniels JL, Olshan AF, Savitz DA. 1997. Pesticides and childhood cancers. Environ Health Perspect 105:1068–1077.

de Andrade M, Barnholtz JS, Amos CI, Adatto P, Spencer C, Bondy M. 2001. Segregation analysis of cancer in families of glioma patients. Genet Epidemiol 20:258–270.

Doneda L, Ginelli E, Agresti A, Larizza L. 1989. In situ hybridization analysis of interstitial C-heterochromatin in marker chromosomes of two human melanomas. Cancer Res 49:433–438.

Dreyer NA, Loughlin JE, Rothman KJ. 1999. Cause-specific mortality in cellular telephone users. JAMA 282:1814–1816.

Elexpuru-Camiruaga J, Buxton N, Kandula V, et al. 1995. Susceptibility to astrocytoma and meningioma: influence of allelism at glutathione S-transferase (GSTT1 and GSTM1) and cytochrome P-450 (CYP2D6) loci. Cancer Res 55: 4237–4239.

El-Zein R, Bondy ML, Wang LE, et al. 1999. Increased chromosomal instability in peripheral lymphocytes and risk of human gliomas. Carcinogenesis 20:811–815.

EMF Science Review Symposium. 1998. Breakout Group Reports for Epidemiological Research Findings. January 12–14, 1998. Symposium, San Antonio, TX. Research Triangle, NC: National Institute of Environmental Health Sciences, National Institutes of Health, p. 121.

Farwell JR, Dohrmann GJ, Marrett LD, Meigs JW. 1979. Effect of SV40 virus–contaminated polio vaccine on the incidence and type of CNS neoplasms in children: a population-based study. Trans Am Neurol Assoc 104:261–264.

Filippini G, Farinotti M, Lovicu G, Maisonneuve P, Boyle P. 1994. Mothers' active and passive smoking during pregnancy and risk of brain tumours in children. Int J Cancer 57:769–774.

Floderus B, Tornqvist S, Stenlund C. 1994. Incidence of selected cancers in Swedish railway workers, 1961–79. Cancer Causes Control 5:189–194.

Fraumeni JF Jr, Stark CR, Gold E, Lepow ML. 1970. Simian virus 40 in polio vaccine: follow-up of newborn recipients. Science 167:59–60.

Fruhwald MC, O'Dorisio MS, Dai Z, et al. 2001. Aberrant hypermethylation of the major breakpoint cluster region in 17p11.2 in medulloblastomas but not supratentorial PNETs. Genes Chromosomes Cancer 30:38–47.

Fults D, Tippets RH, Thomas GA, Nakamura Y, White R. 1989. Loss of heterozygosity for loci on chromosome 17p in human malignant astrocytoma. Cancer Res 49:6572–6577.

Geissler E. 1990. SV40 and human brain tumors. Prog Med Virol 37:211–222.

Grosovsky AJ, Parks KK, Giver CR, Nelson SL. 1996. Clonal analysis of delayed karyotypic abnormalities and gene mutations in radiation-induced genetic instability. Mol Cell Biol 16: 6252–6262.

Gundestrup M, Storm HH. 1999. Radiation-induced acute myeloid leukaemia and other cancers in commercial jet cockpit crew: a population-based cohort study. Lancet 354:2029–2031.

Gurney JG, van Wijnagaarden E. 1999. Extremely low frequency electromagnetic fields (EMF) and brain cancer in adults and children: review and comment. Neuro-Oncology 1:212–220.

Hardell L, Nasman A, Pahlson A, Hallquist A, Hansson Mild K. 1999. Use of cellular telephones and the risk for brain tumours: a case–control study. Int J Oncol 15:113–116.

Heinonen OP, Shapiro S, Monson RR, Hartz SC, Rosenberg L, Slone D. 1973. Immunization during pregnancy against poliomyelitis and influenza in relation to childhood malignancy. Int J Epidemiol 2:229–235.

Hittelman WN, Sen P. 1988. Heterogeneity in chromosome damage and repair rates after bleomycin in ataxia telangiectasia cells. Cancer Res 48:276–279.

Hodges LC, Smith JL, Garrett A, Tate S. 1992. Prevalence of glioblastoma multiforme in subjects with prior therapeutic radiation. J Neurocsci Nurs 24:79–83.

Hsu TC, Johnston DA, Cherry LM, et al. 1989. Sensitivity to genotoxic effects of bleomycin in humans: possible relationship to environmental carcinogenesis. Int J Cancer 43:403–409.

Innis MD. 1968. Oncogenesis and poliomyelitis vaccine. Nature 219:972–973.

Inskip PD, Tarone RE,, et al. 2001. Cellular-telephone use and brain tumors. N Engl J Med 344:79–86.

Johansen C, Boice J Jr, McLaughlin J, Olsen J. 2001. Cellular telephones and cancer—a nationwide cohort study in Denmark. J Natl Cancer Inst 93:203–207.

Kalmaz EE, Kalmaz GD. 1984. Carcinogenicity and epidemiological profile analysis of vinyl chloride and polyvinyl chloride. Regul Toxicol Pharmacol 4:13–27.

Kaplan S, Etlin S, Novikov I, Modan B. 1997. Occupational risks for the development of brain tumors. Am J Ind Med 31:15–20.

Kelsey KT, Wrensch M, Zuo ZF, Miike R, Wiencke JK. 1997. A population-based case–control study of the CYP2D6 and GSTT1 polymorphisms and malignant brain tumors. Pharmacogenetics 7:463–468.

Khalili K, Krynska B, Del Valle L, Katsetos CD, Croul S. 1999. Medulloblastomas and the human neurotropic polyomavirus JC virus. Lancet 353:1152–1153.

Kheifets LI, Afifi AA, Buffler PA, Zhang SW. 1995. Occupational electric and magnetic field exposure and brain cancer: a meta analysis. J Occup Environ Med 37:1327–1341.

Kheifets LI, Sussman SS, Preston-Martin S. 1999. Childhood brain tumors and residential electromagnetic fields (EMF). Rev Environ Contam Toxicol 159:111–129.

Khuder SA, Mutgi AB, Schaub ES. 1998. Meta-analysis of brain cancer and farming. Am J Ind Med. 34:252–260.

Kielhorn J, Melber C, Wahnschaffe U, Aitio A, Mangelsdorf I. 2000. Vinyl chloride: still a cause for concern. Environ Health Perspect 108:579–588.

Kleihues P, Doerjer G, Swenberg JA, Hauenstein E, Bucheler J, Cooper HK. 1979. DNA repair as regulatory factor in the organotropy of alkylating carcinogens. Arch Toxicol Suppl 2:253–261.

Koestner A, Swenberg JA, Wechsler W. 1972. Experimental tumors of the nervous system induced by resorptive N-nitrosourea compounds. Prog Exp Tumor Res 7:9–30.

Kristensen P, Andersen A, Irgens LM, Bye AS, Sundheim L. 1996. Cancer in offspring of parents engaged in agricultural activities in Norway: incidence and risk factors in the farm environment. Int J Cancer 65:39–50.

Larizza L, Doneda L, Ginelli E, Fossati G. 1988. C-heterochromatin vartiation and transposition in tumor progression. In: Prodi G et al. (eds), Cancer Metastasis: Biological and Biochemical Mechanisms and Clinical Aspects. New York: Plenum, pp 309–318.

Lee M, Wrensch M, Miike. 1997. Dietary and tobacco risk factors for adult onset glioma in the San Francisco Bay Area. Cancer Causes Control 8:13–24.

Lengauer C, Kinzler KW, Vogelstein B. 1997. Genetic instability in colorectal cancers. Nature 386:623–627.

Li Y, Millikan RC, Carozza S, et al. 1998. p53 mutations in malignant gliomas. Cancer Epidemiol Biomarkers Prev 7:303–308.

Linos A, Kardara M, Kosmidis H, et al. 1998. Reported influenza in pregnancy and childhood tumour. Eur J Epidemiol 14:471–475.

Magnani I, Guerneri S, Pollo B, et al. 1994. Increasing complexity of the karyotype in 50 human gliomas: progressive evolution and de novo occurrence of cytogenetic alterations. Cancer Genet Cytogenet 75:77–89.

Magnani C, Pastore G, Luzzatto L, Carli M, Lubrano P, Terracini B. 1989. Risk factors for soft tissue sarcomas in childhood cancer: a case–control study. Tumori 75:396–400.

Mangino MM, Libbey LM, Scanlan RA. 1982. Nitrosation of *N*-methyltyramine and *N*-methyl-3-aminomethylindole, two barley malt alkaloids. IARC Sci Publ 41:57–69.

Martin JD, King DM, Slauch JM, Frisque RJ. 1985. Differences in regulatory sequences of naturally occuring JC virus variants. J Virol, 53:306–311.

McKean-Cowdin R, Preston-Martin S, Pogoda JM, Holly EA, Mueller BA, Davis RL. 1998. Parental occupation and childhood brain tumors: astroglial and primitive neuroectodermal tumors. J Occup Environ Med 40:332–340.

McLaughlin JK, Lipworth L. 1999. A critical review of the epidemiologic literature on health effects of occupational exposure to vinyl chloride. J Epidemiol Biostat 4:253–275.

Meinert R, Michaelis J. 1996. Meta-analysis of studies on the association between electromagnetic fields and childhood cancer. Radiat Environ Biophys 35:11–18.

Mohapatra G, Kim DH, Feuerstein BG. 1995. Detection of multiple gains and losses of genetic material in ten glioma cell lines by comparative genomic hybridization. Genes Chromosomes Cancer 13:86–93.

Morgan RW, Kelsh MA, Zhao K, Exuzides KA, Heringer S, Negrete W. 2000. Radiofrequency exposure and mortality from cancer of the brain and lymphatic/hematopoietic systems. Epidemiology 11:118–127.

Mortimer EA Jr, Lepow ML, Gold E, Robbins FC, Burton GJ, Fraumeni JF Jr. 1981. Long-term follow-up of persons inadvertently inoculated with SV40 as neonates. N Engl J Med 305:1517–1518.

Muscat JE, Malkin MG, Thompson S, et al. 2000. Handheld cellular telephone use and risk of brain cancer. JAMA 284:3001–3007.

Mutnick A, Muscat JE. 1997. Primary brain cancer in adults and the use of common household appliances: a case–control study. Rev Environ Health 12:59–62.

Narod SA, Stiller C, Lenoir GM. 1991. An estimate of the heritable fraction of childhood cancer. Br J Cancer 63:993–999.

Pogoda JM, Preston-Martin S. 1997. Household pesticides and risk of pediatric brain tumors. Environ Health Perspect 105:12214–1220.

Preston-Martin S. 1988. Epidemiological studies of perinatal carcinogeneis. In Napalkov NP, Rice JM, Tomatis L, et al. (eds), Perinatal and Multigeneration Carcinogenesis. Lyon: IARC Sci Publ (96), pp 289–314.

Preston-Martin S, Mack WJ. 1996. Neoplasms of the nervous system. In: Schottenfeld D, Fraumeni JF (eds), Cancer Epidemiology and Prevention, 2nd ed. New York: Oxford University Press, pp 1231–1281.

Preston-Martin S, Pogoda JM, Mueller BA, et al. 1998. Prenatal vitamin supplementation and pediatric brain tumors: huge international variation in use and possible reduction in risk. Childs Nerv Syst 14:551–557.

Preston-Martin S, Pogoda JM, Mueller BA, Holly EA, Lijinsky W, Davis RL. 1996. Maternal consumption of cured meats and vitamins in relation to pediatric brain tumors. Cancer Epidemiol Biomarkers Prev 5:599–605.

Rencic A, Gordon J, Otte J, et al. 1996. Detection of JC virus DNA sequence and expression of the viral oncoprotein, tumor antigen, in brain of immunocompetent patients with oligoastrocytoma. Proc Natl Acad Sci USA 93:7352–7357.

Rosso SM, Van Dekken H, Krishnadath KK, Alers JC, Kros JM. 1997. Detection of chromosomal changes by interphase cytogenetics in biopsies of recurrent astrocytomas and oligodendrogliomas. J Neuropathol Exp Neurol 56:1125–1131.

Rothman KJ, Loughlin JE, Funch DP, Dreyer NA. 1996. Overall mortality of cellular telephone customers. Epidemiology 7:303–305.

Rousseau-Merck M, Versteege I, Zattara-Cannoni H, et al. 2000. Fluorescence in situ hybridization determination of 2wq12–q13 deletion in two intracerebral ependymomas. Cancer Genet Cytogenet 121:223–227.

Ryan P, Lee MW, North JB, McMichael AJ. 1992. Risk factors for tumors of the brain and meninges: results from the Adelaide Adult Brain Tumor Study. Int J Cancer 51:20–27.

Sasco AJ, Vainio H. 1999. From in utero and childhood exposure to parental smoking to childhood cancer: a possible link and the need for action. Hum Exp Toxicol 18: 192–201.

Savitz DA, Cai J, van Wijngaarden E, et al. 2000. Case–cohort analysis of brain cancer and leukemia in electric utility workers using a refined magnetic field job-exposure matrix. Am J Ind Med 38:417–425.

Scheidt S. 1997. Changing mortality from coronary hear disease among smokers and nonsmokers over a 20-year interval. Prev Med 26:441–446.

Schwarz B, Schmeiser-Rieder A. 1996. [Epidemiology of health problems caused by passive smoking.] Wien Klin Wochenschr 108:565–569.

Shah KV. 1998. SV40 infections in simians and humans. Dev Biol Stand 94:9–12.

Simonato L, L'Abbe KA, Andersen A, et al. 1991. A collaborative study of cancer incidence and mortality among vinyl chloride workers. Scand J Work Environ Health 17:159–169.

Smith LE, Grosovsky AJ. 1993. Genetic instability on chromosome 16 in a human B lymphoblastoid cell line. Somat Cell Mol Genet 19:515–527.

Sonoda Y, Iizuka M, Yasuda J, et al. 1995. Loss of heterozygosity at 11p15 in malignant glioma. Cancer Res 55: 2166–2168.

Spitz MR, McPherson RS, Jiang H, et al. 1997. Correlates of mutagen sensitivity in patients with upper aerodigestive tract cancer. Cancer Epidemiol Biomarkers Prev 6:687–692.

Strickler HD, Rosenberg PS, Devesa SS, Fraumeni JF Jr, Goedert JJ. 1999. Contamination of poliovirus vaccine with SV40 and the incidence of medulloblastoma. Med Pediatr Oncol 32:77–78.

Swenberg JA, Clendenon N, Denlinger R, Gordon WA. 1975a. Sequential development of ethylnitrosourea-induced neurinomas: morphology, biochemistry, and transplantability. J Natl Cancer Inst 55:147–152.

Swenberg JA, Koestner A, Wechsler W, Brunden MN, Abe H. 1975b. Differential oncogenic effects of methylnitrosourea. J Natl Cancer Inst 54:89–96.

Symons MJ, Andjelkovich DA, Spirtas R, Herman DR. 1982. Brain and central nervous system cancer mortality in U.S. rubber workers. Ann NY Acad Sci 281:146–159.

Thomas TL, Waxweiler RJ. 1986. Brain tumors and occupational risk factors. Scand J Work Environ Health 12:1–15.

Trizna Z, de Andrade M, Kryitsis AP, et al. 1998. Genetic polymorphisms in glutathione S-transferase μ and O *N*-acetyltransferase, and CYP1A1 and risk of gliomas. Cancer Epidemiol Biomarkers Prev 7:553–555.

Viel JF, Challier B, Pitard A, Pobel D. 1998. Brain cancer mortality among French farmers: the vineyard pesticide hypothesis. Arch Environ Health 53:65–70.

Wei M, Guizzetti M, Yost M, Costa LG. 2000. Exposure to 60 Hz magnetic fields and proliferation of human astrocytoma cells in vitro. Toxicol Appl Pharmacol 162:166–176.

Wei Q, Spitz MR, Gu J, et al. 1996. DNA repair capacity correlates with mutagen sensitivity in lymphoblastoid cell lines. Cancer Epidemiol Biomarkers Prev 5:199–204.

Wernicke C, Thiel G, Lozanova T, Vogel S, Witkowski R. 1997. Numerical aberrations of chromosomes 1, 2, and 7 in astrocytomas studied by interphase cytogenetics. Genes Chromosomes Cancer 19:6–13.

Wertheimer N, Leeper E. 1979. Electrical wiring configurations and childhood cancer. Am J Epidemiol 109:273–84.

Wertheimer N, Leeper E. 1987. Magnetic field exposure related to cancer subtypes. Ann NY Acad Sci 502:43–54.

Wrensch M, Bondy ML, Wiencke J, Yost M. 1993. Environmental risk factors for primary malignant brain tumors: a review. J Neurooncol 17:47–64.

Wrensch M, Lee M, Mike R, et al. 1997a. Family and personal medical history of cancer and nervous system conditions among adults with glioma and controls. Am J Epidemiol 145:581–593.

Wrensch M, Minn Y, Bondy ML. 2000. Epidemiology. In: Bernstein M, Berger M (eds), Neuro-oncology: The Essentials. New York: Thieme, pp 1–17.

Wrensch M, Weinberg A, Wiencke J, Masters H, Mike R, Lee M. 1997b. Does prior infection with varicella-zoster virus influence risk of adult glioma? Am J Epidemiol 145: 594–597.

Wrensch M, Yost M, Mike R, Lee G, Touchstone J. 1999. Adult glioma in relation to residential power frequency electromagnetic filed exposures in the San Francisco Bay area. Epidemiology 10:523–527.

Yeni-Komshian H, Holly EA. 2000. Childhood brain tumours and exposure to animals and farm life: a review. Paediatr Perinat Epidemiol 14:248–256.

Zheng PP, Pang JC, Hui AB, Ng HK. 2000. Comparative genomic hybridization detects losses of chromosomes 22 and 16 as the most common recurrent genetic alterations in primary ependymomas. Cancer Genet Cytogenet 122:18–25.

Part IV

Intracranial Extra-Axial Primary Tumors

11

Meningiomas

MICHAEL W. McDERMOTT, ALFREDO QUINONES-HINOSA,
GREGORY N. FULLER, AND CHARLES B. WILSON

In 1614, the Swiss physician Felix Plater provided the first documented account of a meningioma (Netsky and Lapresle, 1956). In the eighteenth century, Antoine Louis, from France, presented a series of patients with "fungueuses de la dure-mere" (Louis, 1771) or "fungating mass of the dura matter." In the United States, W.W. Keen successfully resected a meningioma in 1887 (Bingham and Keen, 1986). Years later, Harvey Cushing coined the term "meningioma" to describe any primary discrete mass attached to the meninges (Cushing, 1922; Cushing and Eisenhardt, 1938).

The classic publication of Cushing and Eisenhardt's 32 chapter book in 1938 did much to bring together the classic neurology with which these tumors can present. Even today this book is an essential review for all those who deal on a regular basis with patients harboring these tumors. Cushing thought that meningiomas were a formidable problem and that the "prognosis hinges on the surgeon's wide experience with the problem in all its many aspects than is true of almost any other operation that can be named."

A recent update on the surgical management of meningiomas by Al-Mefty (1991) indicates that many of the challenges presented by these tumors cannot be overcome even with modern-day technology. Yet only in the last 15 years has the true long-term clinical problem of meningiomas come to be appreciated, largely because of the availability of magnetic resonance imaging (MRI). This imaging modality allows us to see with great detail small residual or recurrent tumors on the convexity and at the skull base.

Meningiomas can be found throughout the central nervous system, from the optic nerve sheath to the spinal cord but rarely, however, below the thoracic spine region. Their biologic behavior is almost always one of continuous slow growth, with metastases occurring only with the malignant form of the disease. These tumors affect women more commonly than men and are mostly found in the fifth and sixth decades of life (Burger et al., 1991; Martuza et al., 1985; Russell and Rubinstein, 1989). The expression of steroid hormone receptors on meningiomas has been used to try to explain this predilection for the female sex and has been the center of numerous studies (Carroll et al., 1997; Halper et al., 1989; Schwartz et al., 1984; Smith and Cahill, 1994).

Recently, new discoveries about the molecular biology of brain tumors have changed the way in which we view them; for example, techniques for their diagnosis have evolved and now include everything from minimally invasive image-directed biopsy to extensive craniofacial exposures for total removal of the tumor and dural attachments, aided by cytologic, chromosomal, genetic, and molecular studies. The insights provided by these sophisticated analytical laboratory tools provide the basis for the rapid translation of new discoveries from the bench to the bedside. This chapter reviews the current understanding of the basic biology of meningiomas and the current standards of clinical management.

INCIDENCE

Meningiomas account for 20% of all primary intracranial neoplasms and 25% of all intraspinal tumors (Burger and Vogel, 1991; Carroll et al., 1993, 1995a,b, 1997, 1999). In the original surgical series of Cushing (1938), meningiomas accounted for 13.4% of more than 2000 brain tumor patients he had treated. The incidence of meningiomas in the general population varies between 2 and 15 per 100,000 people, the incidence increasing with age (Young, 1981; Kurland et al., 1982). The 1997 report of the Central Brain Tumor Registry of the United States shows that for the period 1990 to 1994, meningiomas accounted for 24% (4989) of primary brain tumors, with an incidence ranging from 0.08 (ages 0 to 19 years) to 13.72 (ages 75 to 84 years) per 100,000 population.

Two recent studies from the Kumamoto Prefecture in Japan (Kuratsu and Ushio, 1996a; Kuratsu et al., 2000) (population 1.85 million) have provided a longitudinal follow up from 5 to 7 years regarding the incidence of meningiomas. The first report (Kuratsu and Ushio, 1996a) found that the age-adjusted incidence of meningiomas in males and females was 1.56 and 3.95 per 100,000, respectively. Overall, meningiomas were the most common primary brain tumor in this population group, with an age-adjusted incidence of 2.76 per 100,000, with the highest incidence of 13.02 per 100,000 among women aged 70 to 79 years. A subsequent study from the same group, which included two more years of data, showed that meningiomas accounted for 32% of all primary tumors and that 39% of these tumors were asymptomatic (Kuratsu et al., 2000). Meningiomas tended to be asymptomatic most often in females and in particular those over the age of 70 years.

Other epidemiologic observations also note that intracranial and intraspinal meningiomas afflict women twofold and nearly ninefold as often as men, respectively (Earle and Richany, 1969; McDermott, 1996; Schmidek, 1991). Studies performed during the past two decades have demonstrated that meningiomas express estrogen (infrequently), progesterone, and androgen hormone receptors, leading to the hypothesis that steroid sex hormones may contribute to their growth, which could explain the higher incidence of meningiomas in women (Black et al., 1996; Black, 1993, 1997).

Race may also be important, as a higher percentage of all brain tumors are meningiomas in African countries. In one study of brain tumors in Los Angeles County, the male and female meningioma tumor rates were highest in the black population (Preston-Martin, 1989).

In children, meningiomas are uncommon, comprising only 1% to 4% of all brain tumors and with no female preponderance. In the recent review by Erdincler and colleagues (1998), 62% of pediatric patients presented between the ages of 10 to 15 years, and 41% had associated neurofibromatosis.

LOCATION

Meningiomas can occur anywhere along the course of the intracranial arachnoid and dura, but tend to cluster along sites where arachnoid granulations return cerebrospinal fluid to the venous system, that is, the convexity and basal venous sinuses. Larger clinical series with more than 500 patients document that the three most common locations for intracranial meningiomas are all supratentorial: parasagittal, convexity, and sphenoid wing. In the surgical series of Cushing (1922), 8% of meningiomas were in the posterior fossa, and they occurred along the tentorium, in the cerebellopontine angle, and at the foramen magnum, in decreasing order of frequency. A modern series that included patients treated surgically as well as those simply observed revealed convexity, falcine, sphenoid wing, and tentorium as the four most common locations. In the first two decades of life, Germano (1994) found that 67% of meningiomas were supratentorial and 14.4% were infratentorial. Intraventricular meningiomas are most commonly within the lateral ventricle (80%) near the atrium and most often on the left side of the brain. Three-fourths of the remaining 20% of intraventricular meningiomas occur in the third ventricle, and the rest occur in the fourth ventricle.

ETIOLOGY

Exogenous and Endogenous Factors Associated with Meningiomas

Meningiomas are thought to mainly arise from cap cells of the arachnoid layer around the major sinuses and large cerebral veins where arachnoid granulations are most prominent (Kida et al., 1988; O'Rahilly and Muller, 1986). Cushing pointed out that meningiomas are almost always attached to the dura even though they do not arise from it. Exogenous and endogenous factors acting alone or in combination are thought to account for the tumorigenesis of meningiomas. Trauma, viral infection, and prior brain irradiation are some of the exogenous factors implicated in the development of meningiomas (Harrison et al., 1991; McDermott, 1996; Musa et al., 1995; Ron et al., 1988a,b). Presently, studies of radiation therapy for tinea capitis in childhood present the strongest and most convincing epidemiologic evidence linking ionizing radiation to the occurrence of meningiomas (Ron et al., 1988a,b). There are numerous other etiologic risk factors reported in the literature, including head trauma, cigarette smoking, nitrite consumption, and even elevated cholesterol levels (Longstreth et al., 1993).

Endogenous factors associated with meningiomas include progestins (McDermott et al., 1996), estrogen (Carroll et al., 1999), prolactin (Black, 1996), glucocorticoids (Carroll et al., 1993), dopamine, somatostatin (Black, 1993) and growth factors, including platelet-derived growth factor (PDGF) (Black et al., 1994) and epidermal growth factor (EGF) (Carroll et al., 1997).

The Role of Hormones and Growth Factors

The finding that meningiomas occur twice as often in females than in males raises the question of the possible role of estrogen and progestins in their growth (Black, 1997). Donnell and colleagues (1979) showed in the 1970s that estrogen binding sites were preserved in the cytosol of meningiomas. More recently, with highly sensitive detection methods, at least two isotypes of estrogen receptors have been found in meningiomas (Carroll et al., 1999). Many groups have investigated the potential role of estrogen, progesterone, and androgen on the growth of meningiomas (Carroll et al., 1993, 1999; Halper et al., 1989; Hsu et al., 1997; Martuza and Eldridge, 1988; Martuza et al., 1981; Martuza et al., 1981, 1985; Maxwell et al., 1990, 1993, 1998; Schwartz et al., 1984; Tilzer et al., 1982). The function of estrogen receptors in meningiomas, however, is still unclear (Table 11–1).

There appears to be a consensus in the literature that most meningiomas are progesterone receptor

Table 11–1. Tumor Suppressor Genes, Proto-oncogenes, and Receptors Identified in Meningiomas

Tumor Suppressor Genes	*Merlin* *p53 (rarely involved)*
Proto-oncogenes	c-myc
	N-myc
	c-sys
	IGF-I
	IGF-II
Receptors	Androgens
	Dopamine
	Endothelin A
	Epidermal growth factor
	Fibroblast growth factor receptor-1
	Glucocorticoids
	Interferon-α
	Interleukin 6
	Neurotensin
	Platelet-derived growth factor-β
	Progesterone
	Somatostatin
	Transforming growth factor-β_1

positive and some are estrogen receptor positive (Blankenstein et al., 1995; Bouillot et al., 1994; Carroll et al., 1999). In one study 33 meningiomas were examined for the presence of the progesterone receptor by Northern blot analysis, and 11 of these were analyzed by immunohistochemistry (Carroll et al., 1993). In this analysis the progesterone receptor mRNA was expressed in 81% of tumors and the progesterone receptor was found in the nucleus in 40% of meningiomas (Carroll et al., 1993). By transfecting a construct with a progesterone-responsive element and a reporter sequence into primary cultures of meningiomas, it was later shown that endogenously expressed progesterone receptors were activated in these tumors (Black, 1997; Carroll et al., 1993). The precise function of progesterone receptors in vivo is, however, unknown.

The antiprogesterone agent medroxyprogesterone acetate (MPA) has been used in an attempt to exploit the known positive progesterone receptor status of most meningiomas. MPA failed to decrease tumor size in four of five patients treated for 17 to 29 weeks (Markwalder et al., 1987; Olson et al., 1987). The antiprogesterone agent mifepristone (RU-486) has also been used with only modestly better results. Grunberg and colleagues (1991) studied the effects of long-term oral RU-486 therapy in 14 patients with unresectable meningiomas. Five patients showed some signs of reduced tumor measurement on computerized tomography (CT) scan, MRI, or improved visual field examination. Three patients experienced improved extraocular muscle function or relief from headache. Lamberts and colleagues (1992) examined mifepristone treatment of meningiomas. In this study, 6 of 10 patients were said to be responsive to the therapy, and 3 of them experienced tumor shrinkage. Although these studies suggest that long-term therapy with mifepristone may be effective in cases of unresectable benign meningiomas, the extremely small sample size and nonblinded methodology make the significance of the results difficult to determine.

In the mid-1980s, Weisman and colleagues demonstrated the enhancing effect of EGF on DNA synthesis and cell growth in primary cultures of meningioma cells (Weisman et al., 1986, 1987). Subsequently, they characterized the EGF receptor (EGFR) in meningiomas and suggested the involvement of this growth factor in the proliferation and/or differentiation of meningioma cells (Weisman et al., 1986, 1987). More recent studies demonstrate that the EGFR is expressed in human meningioma specimens and that the EGFRs are activated in some meningiomas (Carroll et al., 1997).

Several studies suggest that the growth of meningiomas may also be mediated by PDGF (Black et al., 1994, 1996; Shamah et al., 1997; Todo et al., 1996; Zhang et al., 1996). The PDGF ligand is found in two subunits, A and B, and there are two isoforms of the receptors, α and β. The role of PDGF has been evaluated in 20 meningiomas, and it has been observed that PDGF-A, PDGF-B, and PDGF-β-R are expressed in meningiomas (Black et al., 1994). This analysis suggests that the β-receptor is functionally involved in meningioma growth. When activated, c-fos levels were increased, and an increase in meningioma cell division was observed in response to addition of PDGF-BB. These findings support the hypothesis that PDGF acts as a growth factor in meningiomas (Black et al., 1994, 1996).

Meningioma and Pregnancy

Some have noted that the growth of meningiomas is accelerated during the luteal phase of the menstrual cycle and during pregnancy (Narayansingh et al., 1992; Roelvink et al., 1987; Saitoh et al., 1989; Wan et al., 1990). A literature review of 62 cases of pregnancy-related symptomatic meningiomas by Roelvink and colleagues (1991), however, failed to support a cause and effect relationship between pregnancy and meningiomas. They indicated that that if a causal relationship between pregnancy and meningiomas existed, the number of cases reported in the literature up to 1991 should have been greater than 62 with a higher incidence in the reproductive years. In reality, however, the incidence of meningiomas is highest during the fifth, sixth, and seventh decades of a woman's life (McCarthy et al., 1998), when progestins and estradiol are low, if not absent. Interestingly, it has been noted that while progestins and estradiol are no longer being produced by the female reproductive system of older women, peripheral tissues such as adipose cells are still producing progesterone.

Relationships with Breast Cancer

A positive correlation between meningiomas and breast cancer has been reported (Rachlin et al., 1991; Rubinstein et al., 1989; Schoenberg et al., 1975, 1977). This finding, however, has since been called into question. In a study of 238 patients with meningiomas, after a person-year method from age- and sex-matched cancer incidence, Jacobs and colleagues (1992) found that the number of breast cancers in the meningioma group was not significantly higher than predicted for age and sex.

In direct support of the correlation between meningiomas and breast cancer, Sulman and colleagues (1998) found that 34% had a loss of heterozygosity in the short arm of chromosome 1p32 region. Loss of heterozygosity in the same region, 1p32, has been reported for breast carcinoma, melanoma, and other cancers (Sulman et al., 1998). Other studies, however, have failed to find a genetic link between meningiomas and breast cancer. For instance, the putative tumor suppressor genes *BRCA1* and *BRCA2,* associated with familial and sporadic forms of breast and ovarian cancer, do not appear to share a common pathogenic pathway with meningiomas (Kirsch et al., 1997). Lauge and colleagues (1999) searched for germline mutations in the *PTEN* gene, known to be affected in Cowden's disease, a genetic condition associated with increased risk of breast cancers, but found no evidence for germline *PTEN* mutations in families with breast cancer and meningiomas. The issue of the responsiveness of meningiomas to hormones, in analogy to breast cancer, is still unresolved.

ANGIOGENESIS

Meningiomas, while most often benign, can grow to a large size before being detected, can encircle critical structures, and can even be accompanied by peritumoral edema (Bitzer et al., 1997; Bradac et al., 1986; New et al., 1980). Any of these occurrences can cause distortion of local structures and, if left untreated, can cause life-threatening mass effect. Meningiomas can also cause diffuse elevation of intracranial pressure, with a subsequent decrease in cerebral blood flow, leading to a slowing of metabolism in nearby cells (Al-Mefty, 1991; Al-Mefty et al., 1994; Black, 1993). A small subset of meningiomas exhibits very aggressive behavior and can invade and destroy adjacent brain; these rare tumors are malignant.

Several groups have studied the role of peritumoral vasogenic edema in meningiomas and its complications (Bitzer et al., 1997, 1998; Black, 1993; Bradac et al., 1986; Kalkanis et al., 1996; Kondziolka et al., 1998; Park et al., 2000; Provias et al., 1997; Tsai et al., 1999; Vuorinen et al., 1996). The source of such edema is not well known but is thought to result from increased microvascular permeability and extravasation of proteinaceous and plasma fluid into the adjacent peritumoral space (Bradac et al., 1986; Kalkanis et al., 1996). Several studies have confirmed the importance of vascular endothelial growth factor (VEGF) production, a 40 to 46 kDa protein that is 10,000 to 50,000 times more potent than histamine in increasing vascular permeability (Guha, 1998), in tumorigenesis, neovascularization, and edema production of some tumors (Bielenberg et al., 1999; Cao et al., 1996; Folkman and Shing, 1992; Goto et al., 1993; Kenyon et al., 1996; Miller et al., 1994; Rosenthal et al., 1994; Shima et al., 1995), including meningiomas (Bitzer et al., 1998; Kalkanis et al., 1996; Park et al., 2000; Provias et al., 1997; Tsai et al., 1999).

To demonstrate the strong link between VEGF mRNA expression and peritumoral edema in meningiomas, 31 meningioma specimens were subjected to Northern blot analysis, hybridization with a complementary DNA VEGF probe, and laser densitometry to determine the relative levels of VEGF mRNA expression (Kalkanis et al., 1996). Magnetic resonance imaging was used in a double-blind fashion to correlate the neuropathologic tissue samples with the presence of preoperative peritumoral edema. Of 31 patients studied, 14 exhibited no edema and 17 exhibited some level of peritumoral fluid accumulation. The results demonstrated that meningiomas with peritumoral edema exhibited 3.4 times the level of VEGF mRNA as those without edema. These data indicate that VEGF expression is an important factor in the etiology of edema around meningiomas (Kalkanis et al., 1996).

Regulation of the expression of VEGF by meningiomas has been studied by means of an enzyme-linked immunosorbent assay of CH-157MN meningioma cell supernatants (Tsai et al., 1999). Tsai and colleagues (1999) demonstrated that epidermal and basic fibroblast growth factors similarly induce VEGF secretion by CH-157MN meningioma cells to 160% above baseline constitutive secretion. The sex hormones estradiol, progesterone, and testosterone did not stimulate or inhibit VEGF secretion in CH-157MN meningioma cells. Dexamethasone in this study was shown to decrease VEGF secretion to 32% of baseline constitutive secretion, thus providing a potential explanation for the effect of corticosteroids in alleviating peritumoral brain edema in meningiomas. The results from this study suggest that growth factors and corticosteroids, but not sex hormones, may regulate VEGF secretion (Tsai et al., 1999).

Recent evidence suggests that both mitogenic signals and angiogenic signals (via induction of VEGF) share a common link by activation of the ras signaling pathway (Feldkamp et al., 1999a,b; Guha, 1998). Consequently, inhibition of ras activity may lead to control of both tumor cell and tumor angiogenic growth. The relevance of the ras pathway in meningioma proliferation was recently studied by Shu and colleagues (1999) using nine primary meningioma cell cultures infected with the recombinant adenovirus Ad-rasN17, encoding the dominant negative ras protein or control adenovirus Ad-pAC. Ras-N17 is a ras mutant protein that inhibits function of all endogenous cellular ras proteins. The results demonstrated that infection of meningioma cells with Ad-rasN17 increased the expression levels of the ras-N17 mutant protein and inhibited phosphorylation of the mitogen-activated protein kinases. Suppression of ras proteins inhibited proliferation of all exponentially growing and growth-arrested meningioma cells stimulated with serum, suggesting that proliferation of primary meningioma cells depends on the presence of functional ras proteins. Inhibiting the ras pathway may be of great value in preventing growth factor–stimulated meningioma proliferation (Shu et al., 1999).

APOPTOSIS

Studies with 20 different low passage meningioma cell cultures and the addition of hydroxyurea resulted in a decrease in cell proliferation and arrested cell growth in the S phase in vitro. Characteristic signs of apoptosis, including DNA fragmentation, detected by in situ DNA strand break labeling, and discrete oligonucleosomal fragments (DNA ladder) were observed (Schrell et al., 1997). In vivo studies showed that when tissues from five different meningiomas were transplanted into mice followed by treatment with hydroxyurea, in situ DNA fragmentation was observed in all hydroxyurea-treated meningioma transplants, providing evidence that hydroxyurea can cause apoptosis in tumor cells (Schrell et al., 1997).

Recent reports indicate that preoperative embolization of intracranial meningiomas, used for selected patients to reduce tumor vascularity and blood loss during surgery, may produce ischemic changes consistent with apoptosis (Matyja et al., 1999; Nakasu et al., 1997, 1998). Alterations of *p53, bcl-2,* and *bax* expression, genes involved in an apoptotic death pathway, have been observed in embolized meningiomas (Nakasu et al., 1998). *p53* and its downstream effector p21 accumulated mainly in perinecrotic areas, where apoptosis was also observed (Nakasu et al., 1997, 1998). *bcl-2* was often expressed in the areas distant from necrosis, whereas *bax* was immunostained more intensely in the perinecrotic areas (Nakasu et al., 1998). Matyja and colleagues (1999), in addition to finding similar results in four biopsy specimens of embolized meningiomas with *p53* and *bcl-2,* also found that the anti-CD-68 immunostained cells were distributed around or within the necrotic foci. These results are consistent with the hypothesis that cell injury by preoperative tumor embolization correlates with the expression of apoptosis-related proteins (Matyja et al., 1999).

Apoptotic cell death in some meningiomas and schwannomas has been associated with the use of gamma knife radiosurgery. Indeed, radiation-induced apoptosis is thought to contribute to the low-dose effects of gamma knife radiosurgery (Tsuzuki et al., 1996).

CYTOGENETICS AND MOLECULAR GENETICS

As early as the 1960s, monosomy of chromosome 22 was reported in meningiomas (Zang and Singer, 1967), a feature found in 40% to 80% of these tumors (Collins et al., 1990; Dumanski et al., 1990). There also seems to be an association with partial or total loss of chromosomes 14 (Katsuyama et al., 1986) and 17 (Maltby et al., 1988) and with the Y chromosome (Maltby et al., 1988). Abnormalities of chromosomes 1, 3, 6, 7, 8, 10, 12, 18, and X have also been reported in meningiomas (Arnoldus et al., 1992; Smith and Cahill, 1994; Vagner-Capodano et al., 1993).

In the mid-1980s, several groups described partial losses such as the terminal deletion of chromosome 22 (Dumanski et al., 1987, 1990; Seizinger et al., 1987a–d). With restriction fragment-length polymorphisms (RFLP), a tumor suppressor gene involved in meningiomas has been narrowed to a locus on the long arm of chromosome 22 (Dumanski et al., 1987, 1990; Lekanne Deprez et al., 1991; Rouleau et al., 1987; Seizinger et al., 1987a–d) between the myoglobin locus and the 22q12.3-qter (Dumanski et al., 1990; Leon et al., 1994; Peyrard et al., 1999).

TUMOR SUPPRESSOR GENES PROTO-ONCOGENES

The concept of tumor suppressor genes originated in the late 1960s when Harris and colleagues (1969) demonstrated that normal cells contain genes that can suppress neoplastic growth via inhibition of cell division and cell proliferation. In meningiomas, the *p53* tumor suppressor gene has been studied for point mutations, but such mutations were rarely found (Mashiyama et al., 1991; Ohgaki et al., 1993). In contrast, the putative tumor suppressor gene mapping to chromosome 22 has more often been implicated in the tumorigenesis of meningiomas (Arnoldus et al., 1992; Black, 1993; Collins et al., 1990; Dumanski et al., 1987; Gutmann et al., 1997; Kazumoto et al., 1990; Merel et al., 1995a,b; Parry et al., 1996; Rouleau et al., 1987, 1989; Ruttledge et al., 1994; Seizinger et al., 1987a,b; Sulman et al., 1998; Trofatter et al., 1993; Twist et al., 1994).

The *NF1* gene resides on chromosome 17. Its product, neurofibromin, is a large protein of 2818 amino acids. The protein acts as a negative regulator in the ras signal transduction pathway and might also act downstream of ras (Sundaram et al., 1997; Zwarthoff, 1996). A 360 amino acid region of neurofibromin shows significant homology to the catalytic domain of the mammalian p21 ras-specific 120 kDa GTPase-activating protein. In the cell types that are affected in NF1 patients, the absence of neurofibromin leads to increased proliferation, resulting in benign, and in some cases malignant, tumors. A study by Sundaram and colleagues (1997) analyzed the expression and functional status of neurofibromin in established human leptomeningeal LTAg2B cells, in 17 sporadic meningiomas, and in a meningioma from a patient affected by NF2. The expression of neurofibromin was determined via immunoblotting and immunoprecipitation with antineurofibromin antibodies, whereas its functional status was determined through its ability to stimulate the intrinsic GTPase activity of p21 ras. This study showed for the first time that neurofibromin is expressed at high levels in leptomeningeal cells and in sporadic meningiomas, and diminished GAP activity of neurofibromin was found in approximately 28% of the tumors analyzed. These results suggested also for the first time that decreased levels of neurofibromin in these tumors might contribute to their tumorigenesis (Sundaram et al., 1997).

Another tumor suppression gene, known as *NF2,* merlin, or schwannomin, is found to be mutated in most sporadic meningiomas, and it has been recently implicated in their tumorigenesis (Gutmann et al., 1997; Kimura et al., 1998; Lee et al., 1997). Schwannomin is a member of the band 4.1 superfamily of proteins that have been shown to play important roles in linking cell membrane proteins with the cytoskeleton, a site of activation of tumor suppressor genes in humans (Rouleau et al., 1993). Lee and colleagues (1997) used immunoblotting and immunoprecipitation experiments to determine the size and subcellular distribution of normal schwannomin in rabbit and human brain tissue, and established human leptomeningeal LTAg2B cells. Subsequently, they used similar techniques to determine the expression level of schwannomin in 14 human sporadic meningiomas. Their results showed that schwannomin is a protein of approximately 66 kDa predominantly expressed in the Triton X-100–insoluble fraction of the brain and LTAg2B cells. The expression of schwannomin was severely reduced in almost 60% of primary sporadic meningiomas, which raises the issue that this may be an important factor in the tumorigenesis of meningiomas. The development of meningotheliomatous meningiomas is probably linked to alterations in other oncogenes or tumor suppressor genes as results showed that all six tumors with normal schwannomin expression were of this type (Lee et al., 1997).

Proto-oncogenes, or genes that stimulate cell division, can become oncogenes when mutated. Oncogenes encode proteins that stimulate proliferation and sometimes mediate biologic activities that contribute to invasion. In a study of 19 meningiomas, Kazumoto and colleagues (1990) found that there was at least a fivefold expression of the *sis* oncogene and of the *c-myc* oncogene in a great percentage of these tumors. The *n-myc* gene has also been found to be involved in meningiomas (Detta et al., 1993; McDonald and Dohrmann, 1988; Tanaka et al., 1989). IGF-I and IGF-II have been found in a large number of meningiomas and may play an important role in tumor growth and cell division of meningiomas (Antoniades et al., 1992; Friend et al., 1999; Glick et al., 1997; Nordqvist et al., 1997).

PATHOLOGY

In the classic monograph by Cushing and Eisenhardt (1938), meningiomas were divided into 9 major morphologic types; 7 of these categories were further divided into a total of 20 subtypes. Subsequent recognition of the lack of associated prognostic significance for most of these subtypes led to a widely adopted simplified scheme of three commonly encountered "classic" patterns: meningothelial, fibrous (fibroblastic), and transitional (mixed) (Fig. 11–1). In addition to these three basic patterns, the newly revised World Health Organization (WHO) classification (Kleihues and Cavenee, 2000) includes six additional morphologically distinct variants of low-grade meningioma (WHO grade I): psammomatous, angiomatous, microcystic, secretory, lymphoplasmacyte rich, and metaplastic. There is no prognostic difference between these morphologic variants and those that exhibit a "classic" pattern; the formal codification and morphologic description of these entities is provided in acknowledgment of the importance of recognizing them as meningiomas despite their unusual phenotypic appearance.

Four specific meningeal tumor morphologies recognized by the WHO classification are associated with a greater likelihood of recurrence and/or aggressive behavior and thus warrant brief comment: the clear cell, chordoid, rhabdoid, and papillary variants. Clear cell and chordoid meningiomas are classified as WHO grade II tumors, and rhabdoid and papillary meningiomas are classified as WHO grade III. Papillary meningiomas were originally described as an aggressive variant characterized by a high rate of recurrence and distant metastases (Ludwin et al., 1975). This description was subsequently confirmed by other investigators (Pasquier et al., 1986) and is currently recognized in the WHO classification (Fig. 11–2). Any discussion of aggressive meningeal tumors includes the issue of meningeal hemangiopericytoma. The meningeal hemangiopericytoma is a morphologically distinct neoplasm (Fig. 11–3) that historically has been variously considered as either an aggressive variant of meningioma (Russell and Rubinstein, 1989) or as the meningeal equivalent of systemically occurring hemangiopericytomas (Burger et al., 1991). The current WHO schema classifies meningeal hemangiopericytoma as a malignant mesenchymal neoplasm of nonmeningotheliomatous origin. It is agreed by all investigators that these tumors exhibit a generally more aggressive behavior than "typical" meningiomas and therefore must be distinguished from them.

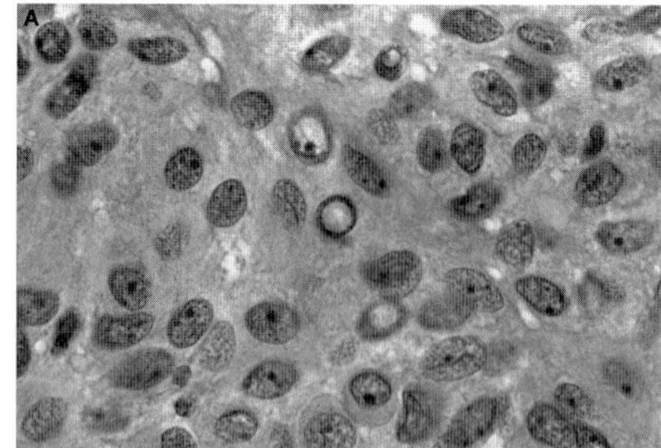

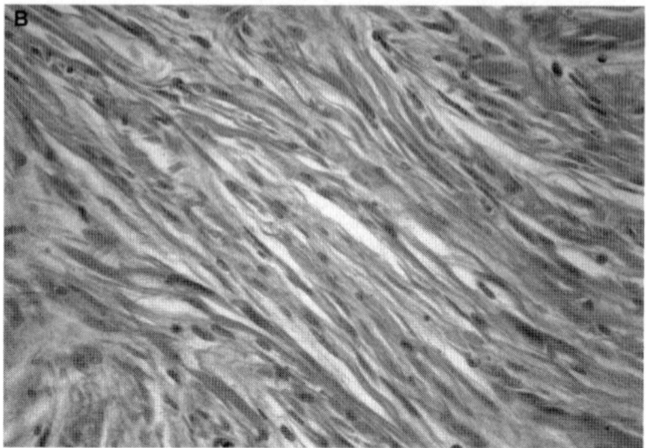

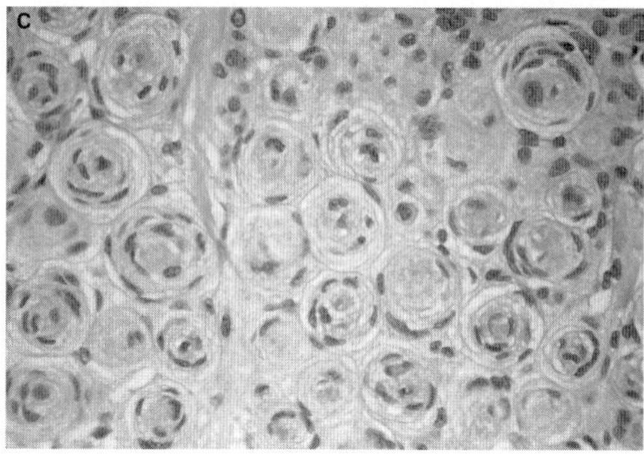

Figure 11–1. Meningioma. The three "classic" histologic patterns of meningioma are meningothelial **(A)**, fibrous **(B)**, and transitional **(C)**.

Any of the various subtypes of meningiomas discussed above may exhibit morphologic features asso-

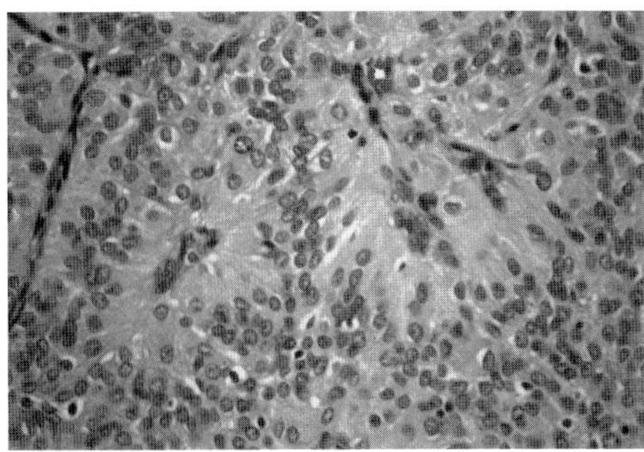

Figure 11–2. Papillary meningioma. This unusual variant is characterized by prominent perivascular arrangement of meningothelial cells, often with distinctive perivascular anuclear zones that resemble the perivascular pseudorosettes of ependymoma. Separation of adjacent angiocentric phalanges gives rise to the pseudopapillae that typify the lesion.

ciated with aggressive clinical behavior and warrant upgrading to either atypical (WHO grade II) or anaplastic (WHO grade III) meningioma. Morphologic criteria for atypical meningioma include either increased mitotic activity (defined as greater than or equal to 4 mitoses per 10 high power fields), brain invasion (invasion of the dura and cranial bone does not by itself constitute an indication of atypicality), or at least three of the following five features: dense cellularity, small cell formation, prominent nucleoli, patternless or sheet-like growth, and foci of tumor necrosis. Criteria for anaplastic meningioma (WHO grade III; WHO terminology prefers the term *anaplastic* over *malignant*) include either a very high mitotic rate (defined as 20 or more mitotic figures per 10 high power fields) or morphologic features far in excess of those seen in atypical meningiomas, which would include appearances similar to sarcoma, carcinoma, or melanoma. Frank brain invasion may be seen in low-grade, atypical, or anaplastic meningiomas. When present in an ordinary low-grade meningioma, this feature was previously used as a criterion that warranted a diagnosis of anaplastic (or malignant) meningioma; however, recent studies have shown that the clinical behavior of otherwise ordinary meningiomas that show brain invasion is much closer to that of atypical meningiomas than to truly anaplastic (malignant) meningiomas (Perry et al., 1999), and current WHO criteria recommend classification as such. Much research effort is currently directed toward the evaluation of proliferation markers, such as MIB-1 (a monoclonal antibody that recognizes the Ki-67 antigen in routinely processed formalin-fixed, paraffin-embedded tissue), as potentially powerful prognostic indicators of aggressive behavior.

CLINICAL PRESENTATION BY LOCATION

In general, meningiomas present with the usual triad of symptoms of brain tumors in an adult patient, namely, headache, seizures, progressive focal neurologic deficit, and/or change in personality. Given that many of these tumors grow slowly, the onset of symptoms can be insidious. Those symptoms caused by delayed effects of chronic increased intracranial pressure, such as deteriorating vision from papilledema, or double vision from sixth nerve palsies, are uncommon today.

Supratentorial Meningiomas

Olfactory groove meningiomas arise in the midline adjacent to the crista galli and the planum sphenoidale. As they enlarge, they compress the inferior frontal lobe, elevating it, and posteriorly displace the

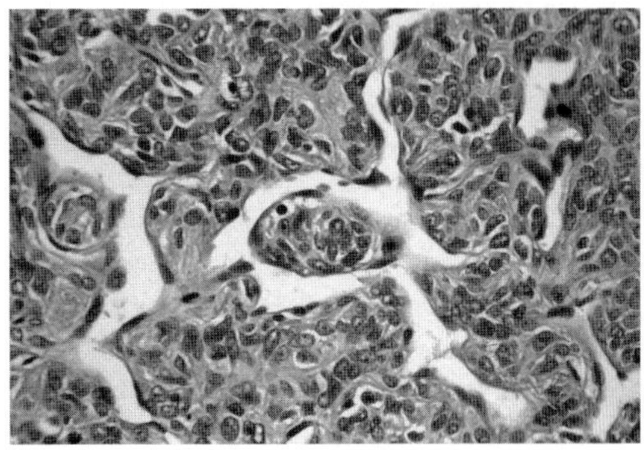

Figure 11–3. Meningeal hemangiopericytoma. Distinctive features of this aggressive tumor include the densely packed, disorganized cellularity and characteristic angular, branching vasculature ("staghorn" pattern). Meningeal hemangiopericytomas also differ from meningiomas immunohistochemically (lack of epithelial membrane antigen expression), ultrastructurally (presence of basement membrane-like material and lack of abundant intercellular desmosomal attachments), and in incidence between the sexes (equal frequency for hemangiopericytomas compared with a definite female predilection for meningiomas).

optic apparatus. Typically these patients have slow onset of change in mental status, depressed mood, and impaired insight, judgment, and motivation. It is rare for patients to complain of a loss of the sense of smell. Family members usually notice a change in personality first; late in the course of their disease, patients may complain of headaches and reduced vision. The rare syndrome described by Foster and Kennedy of anosmia, unilateral optic atrophy, and contralateral papilledema was originally attributed to tumors in this location.

Immediately behind the olfactory grove is another location where meningiomas develop, the *tuberculum sellae.* This is the bone on the anterior aspect of the sella turcica, and most patients with tumors in this location have progressive visual loss, which is usually asymmetric. Changes in personality and mental status are uncommon because the patients come to medical attention with their visual disturbance before their tumors become large. They occur more commonly in women than in men and typically present in the fifth and sixth decades of life. Visual field findings may resemble those of pituitary adenoma with a bitemporal field defect.

The *sphenoid wing* is one of the most common locations for an intracranial, supratentorial meningioma. These tumors typically arise anywhere along the course of the sphenoid wing, from the anterior clinoid medially to the pterion laterally. Symptomatology is related to location along the sphenoid wing. Those patients with medial clinoid meningiomas usually have slow progressive unilateral visual loss, headaches, and seizures. Middle-third sphenoid wing meningiomas present with headaches, seizures, and mild proptosis, without prominent visual disturbance. Lateral sphenoid meningiomas present with headaches, seizures, and swelling in the region of the temporal fossa. A type of meningioma in this location that occurs much more commonly in women is the hyperostosing "en plaque" meningioma. The typical chronology is "a middle-aged women who for long periods has slowly had increasing unilateral exophthalmos with ultimate impairment of vision and with palpable swelling in the temporal region," as described by Cushing and Eisenhardt (1938). Edema of the inferior lid may be prominent in these patients. An impairment of lateral gaze may also be present due to involvement of lateral periorbital and/or lateral rectus muscle.

Cavernous sinus meningiomas are a difficult clinical problem. Typically, patients with these tumors present with double vision, facial numbness, and, later in their course, headache and reduced visual acuity. Seizures are uncommon and usually occur only if there is a large exophytic middle fossa component to the tumor. These symptoms make sense anatomically given the presence of the third, fourth, fifth, and sixth cranial nerves within the cavernous sinus compartment.

Parasagittal meningiomas fill the angle between the convexity dura and the midline falx. The classic clinical presentation is a patient with a headache and focal motor or sensory seizures, beginning with symptoms in the lower extremity progressing up into the body, arm, and face. Frequently these patients will have unilateral upper motor neuron signs or cortical sensory disturbance. Papilledema is relatively uncommon except in the largest tumors.

Meningiomas that arise truly from the *falx* are covered on their superior aspects by cortical tissue of the frontal, parietal, or occipital lobes. Clinical signs or symptoms depend partly on where along the falx these tumors grow. Anatomically these tumors are defined as occurring in the anterior, middle, or posterior third of the falx. Anterior-third falx meningiomas may present with headache, seizure, and mental status change. Middle-third falx meningiomas present with headache, seizures, and focal motor sensory deficit. Posterior-third falx meningiomas present with headache and visual loss, or irritative visual phenomenon with visual hallucinations. It is rare for a large bilateral dumbbell-shaped falx tumor to present with a spastic paraparesis.

Convexity meningiomas arise in the dura over the frontal, temporal, parietal, or occipital lobes. Frequently these tumors are asymptomatic and are discovered on imaging carried out for another reason. However, when the tumors are large, they present with headache, seizures, and focal neurologic deficit depending on whether the tumor is on the right or left side and over speech, motor, sensory, or occipital cortex. These tumors are the most favorable for surgical treatment.

Patients with *intraventricular* meningiomas have protean manifestations. In the series of Cushing and Eisenhardt (1938), tumors within the atrium of the lateral ventricle typically presented with headache, nausea, vomiting, seizures, and speech disturbance. Patients with large tumors may also have a hemianopsia and unilateral sensorimotor deficit. Third-ventricular meningiomas present with nonspecific symptoms, which are predominantly from increased intracranial pressure.

Posterior Fossa Meningiomas

Tentorial meningiomas present most often with headache, extremity or gait ataxia, nausea, and vomiting. Seizures and mental status changes are uncommon because of their posterior fossa location. Common clinical findings include evidence of cranial nerve III, IV, V, and VI deficits and appendicular cerebellum disturbance. The more medial and anterior the location of the tentorial meningioma, the more likely the patients are to have extraocular muscle disturbance. Tentorial meningiomas that have a significant component extending up into the inferior temporal or occipital lobes may cause seizure or visual disturbance. A peculiar and surgically unfavorable type of meningioma involving the tentorium is the falcotentorial meningioma, which involves the junction of the falx cerebri and tentorium, usually including the straight sinus. These patients typically present with symptoms of increased intracranial pressure without focal neurologic deficit.

Petroclival meningiomas usually have an insidious onset of headache, gait disturbance, double vision, reduced hearing, and vertigo. Common clinical signs include cranial neuropathy, particularly involving nerves IV, V, VI, and VIII, along with papilledema, ataxia, and cerebellar dysmetria. For meningiomas that arise along the posterior petrous bone within the CP angle, Sami and Ammarati (1988) distinguished symptoms of those tumors arising anterior to the internal auditory canal (IAC) from those arising posterior to it. Anteriorly placed lesions usually present with facial pain, facial numbness, and reduced hearing. With tumors posterior to the IAC, cerebellar signs are predominant and gait disturbance is common. It is not infrequent for a tumor in this location to be confused with a vestibular schwannoma. Meningiomas of the *cerebellar convexity* usually present with symptoms and signs of increased intracranial pressure, hydrocephalus, or cerebellar dysfunction ipsilateral to the tumor. Papilledema, appendicular, and truncal ataxia are common.

Foramen magnum meningiomas are difficult to diagnose clinically and, before MR imaging, were frequently confused with demyelinating disorders. Most patients have a history of neck and suboccipital pain that is worse with flexion and Valsalva maneuvers. Motor and sensory deficits usually develop first in the arm and then in the legs and may involve all extremities to the point of spastic quadraparesis. The so-called crural palsy, with atrophy in the intrinsic muscles of the hand, trapezius, and shoulder, can be particularly confusing for the clinician. Secondary damage from increased venous pressure in the cervical spinal cord may be the cause for some of these symptoms and signs. In a clinical series from the Mayo Clinic, 94% of patients complained of upper extremity dysesthesia; 75% of suboccipital or neck pain; 49% of upper extremity weakness; 47% of gait disturbance; and 42% of clumsiness of their hands. Problems with lower cranial nerve function may lead to complaints of dysarthria and dysphasia. Differential diagnosis in these patients can also include syringomyelia and intramedullary cervical spinal cord tumors.

Meningiomas occurring near the *torcular of Herophilus,* or confluence of the superior sagittal, straight, transverse, and occipital sinuses, present with symptoms of increased intracranial pressure. The patients of Cushing and Eisenhardt (1938) complained of visual impairment related to papilledema, headaches, and neck pain. The authors noted that lower quadrants of the visual field appeared to be affected before the upper quadrant of the visual field, and recovery of these fields postoperatively proceeded in a reverse direction. The last location for meningiomas of the posterior fossa is the fourth ventricle. Despite the abundance of critical nuclei immediately below the pial surface of the floor of the ventricle, these tumors usually present only with symptoms of obstructive hydrocephalus and increased pressure.

IMAGING STUDIES

Plain X-Rays

For the most part the use of plain radiographs for the diagnosis of intracranial meningiomas is of historic interest only. In the past, evidence of intracranial calcification, hyperostosis of the sphenoid wing or calvarium, displacement of the pineal gland or enlarged vascular channels were used as indirect supportive evidence of the presence of a long-standing, vascular tumor attached to the dura and/or invading the bone. Computed tomography followed by MR imaging have become standards of imaging for the diagnosis and follow up of intracranial meningiomas. Sometimes, when only MR imaging has been done and the patient has a history of prior craniotomy or craniectomy, plain X-rays are helpful in delineating the extent of bone removal, which may assist with preoperative planning and intraoperative cranial pin fixation.

Computed Axial Tomography

Computed tomography is inferior to MRI for delineating soft tissue details of both the meningioma under investigation and the surrounding brain. It is superior to MRI for defining the extent of bony hyperostosis, a key point in the consideration of basal and convexity meningiomas with associated hyperostosis. Pathologic studies have demonstrated that hyperostotic bone contains meningiothelial cells, and failure to remove this involved bone may lead to later recurrence of a soft tissue tumor or progression primarily within bone. Thin-cut CT imaging may now be used with image-guided surgical systems primarily for the purpose of helping the surgeon define the bony margins of tumor intraoperatively. In these circumstances, image fusion technologies allow the surgeon to use MRI data to determine the soft tissue margins of the tumor adjacent to brain (e.g., determining the distance to the medial or deep aspect of the tumor) and then switch to CT-based images for the resection of tumor-involved bone.

On non-contrast CT imaging, meningiomas appear isodense to slightly hyperdense. Calcification within the tumor can be punctate or confluent and is easily seen. Optic nerve sheath meningiomas may show the traditional "tram track" linear calcification outlining the orbital course of the optic nerve. When hyperostosis of the calvarium is extensive the bone can have a mottled to radiating starburst appearance. Meningiomas along the sphenoid wing produce dense sclerotic hyperostosis of the greater wing and pterion producing associated exophthalmos. These tumors are characteristically seen in women. With the administration of iodinated contrast, meningiomas usually enhance homogenously and intensely. The "dural tail" so often referred to with MRI is not well visualized with CT as it is thinly opposed to the underlying bone.

Mantle et al. (1999) reported on the use of quantifying peritumoral brain edema on CT scanning for predicting the probability for meningioma recurrence. Between 1980 and 1998, 135 patients were evaluated. Edema grade was linearly related to edema volume by digitizing the CT scans. The completeness of resection was the most powerful predictor of recurrence, followed by edema grade and brain invasion. The chance of recurrence within 10 years after complete resection was exponentially related to the maximum linear dimension of surrounding peritumoral edema. The chance of recurrence increased by approximately 10% for each centimeter grade increase in the amount of edema. The authors also found that the histopathologic documentation of brain invasion increased by 20% per centimeter of edema thickness on the actual CT scan. Thus, valuable information can be derived by this simple imaging study, which may influence treatment and outcome. Furthermore, Kuratsu and colleagues (2000) in evaluating the clinical features of asymptomatic meningiomas found that patients with evidence of tumoral calcification on CT scans had a significantly lower likelihood of tumor growth after longer than a 1 year follow up ($p = 0.008$).

One disadvantage of CT is that multiplanar imaging is limited. Direct coronal imaging without much artifact is limited to the anterior and middle cranial fossa. Direct sagittal images cannot be achieved. On the other hand, bony foramina within the skull base are clearly seen, and three-dimensional reconstructions available from image-guided system workstations give bony spatial resolution and detail superior to that obtained from MRI.

Magnetic Resonance Imaging

As originally described by Cushing, meningiomas are typically dural-based lesions when seen on MR scans. Approximately 60% of these tumors are isointense and 30% hypointense on T_1-weighted images (Fig. 11–4A,B). On T_2-weighted imaging studies, intensities may vary anywhere between hypointense to hyperintense, and there may be a correlation between pathologic type and T_1/T_2 imaging features. On the T_2-weighted images, a hypointense signal that surrounds the edge of a meningioma may represent the compressed, but preserved arachnoid plane between brain and tumor (Fig. 11–4C).

Hypointensity within the tumor may relate to cystic change or intratumoral calcification, such as is seen with psammomatous meningiomas. The so-called "dural tail" is an imaging feature thought to be

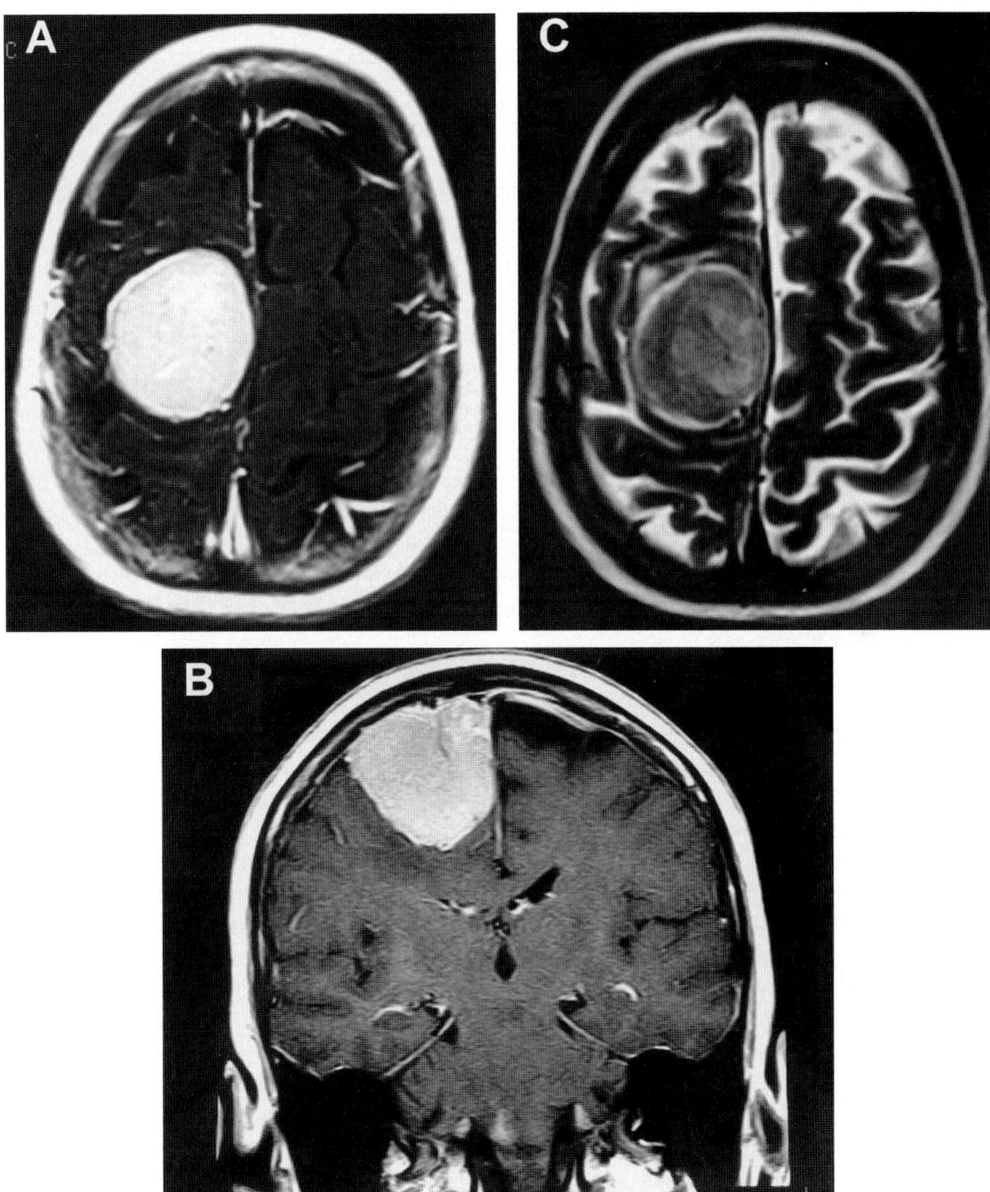

Figure 11–4. **(A)** Axial T_1-weighted MRI scan of right frontoparietal parasagittal meningioma with homogenous enhancement typical of benign meningioma. **(B)** Coronal T_1-weighted MRI showing meningioma filling the angle between falx and convexity dura, characteristic of parasagittal meningioma. Signal flow void near midline is consistent with patent superior sagittal sinus. Note relative lack of mass effect given large size of tumor, suggesting slow tumor growth over a long interval of time. **(C)** Axial T_2, second echo image showing no edema in surrounding brain and thin rim of hyperintensity between tumor edge and brain, consistent with preserved arachnoid plane.

characteristic of meningiomas. This tail typically extends several millimeters from the edge of the tumor and is thought to represent hypervascularity rather than tumor infiltration. Magnetic resonance imaging is the preferred modality for deriving a volumetric study for the use of image-guided surgical systems, and these systems help with planning skin flaps, bony openings, and extent of removal as surgery proceeds.

Paleologos et al. (2000) evaluated the use of image-guided surgical systems in 100 patients treated surgically for meningiomas. This group was compared with 170 patients operated on without the use of intraoperative navigational systems. Although the study was not randomized, surgical times were shorter for the image-guided group, and blood loss and mean hospital days spent were less for the image-guided group. Importantly, surgical complications, either permanent neurologic deficit or those complications requiring an additional surgical procedure, were significantly less in the image-guided group. There are technical considerations with the use of image-guided systems for skull-based neoplasms, such as the type of imaging, imaging sequence, and convenience issues referable to the type of image guidance system, either light-emitting diode or passive mechanical arm, to be used. At our institution, The University of California, San Francisco, image-guided surgical systems are the standard for operations on large convexity or skull-based meningiomas, and we prefer an older passive arm system because it avoids problems with line of sight when the operating microscope is in position.

Magnetic resonance imaging has been reported to be of value in predicting the relationship between peritumoral edema as evidenced by hyperintensity on T_2-weighted images and the cleavage plane between tumor and surrounding brain. In the study by Ildan et al. (1989) increasing degrees of peritumoral edema on T_2 images correlated significantly with worsening of surgical cleavage plane between tumor and surrounding brain. On angiographic studies, those tumors with pial arterial supply were much more likely to demonstrate significant peritumoral edema. The authors proposed that MRI findings might predict the difficulty of microsurgical dissection for the surgeon before operation.

In another study of cystic meningioma, Zee et al. (1995) evaluated the MRI features of 15 cystic meningiomas classifying them into three different types. Type I cystic meningiomas were those with cysts wholly within tumor. Type II were those with cysts at the periphery, but still within margins of the tumor, and type III were cysts peripheral to the tumor in adjacent brain. Enhancement of cyst walls was seen in type II cystic meningiomas, but not in type III. The authors suggested that this pattern of enhancement required surgical excision of the enhancing wall. They also found that the pathology in these cystic meningiomas tended to be more aggressive.

Functional MRI techniques are also useful in predicting the location of visual, motor, sensory, and speech language cortex relative to meningiomas. Presuming that the meningiomas do not invade the adjacent brain, information about the adjacent cortex may nonetheless be important for predicting temporary neurologic disability that may result after removal of large meningiomas.

Cerebral Angiography

Conventional cerebral angiography is still useful in the management of patients with meningiomas despite the advent of MR angiography and MR venography. Whereas the blood supply for the variety of tumor locations is predictable based on anatomy, this information can still assist the surgeon with planning a surgical approach, and embolization of very hypovascular tumors may assist with surgical removal. Angiographic information about tumor blood supply and the displacement of major arteries and their positions relative to the margins of the tumor are important. On the venous phase of these studies, the positions of draining cortical veins are critical as well because these must be preserved. The later phase of angiography, which gives information about venous anatomy, is still the gold standard for determining whether or not a major venous sinus is still patent (Fig. 11–5).

Bendszus et al. (2000) recently tried to evaluate the benefit of preoperative embolization of meningiomas. Their perspective was drawn from a nonrandomized, noncontrolled study of 60 consecutive patients in two different neurosurgical centers who were operated on and followed up. In Center A, no embolization was performed. In Center B, all patients underwent embolization. Mean tumor sizes and mean blood losses with surgery did not differ between groups, but, in the subgroup of patients who had subtotal devascularization in more than 90% of the tumor, blood loss was significantly less than in patients who were not embolized ($p < 0.05$). There were no differences in surgeons' observations regarding hemostasis, tumor consistency or intratumoral necrosis. There was one new permanent neurologic deficit related to embolization (3%).

At our institution, preoperative embolization is reserved for the largest meningiomas even if the external carotid supply can be accessed easily during the opening (Fig. 11–6). A variety of embolic agents may

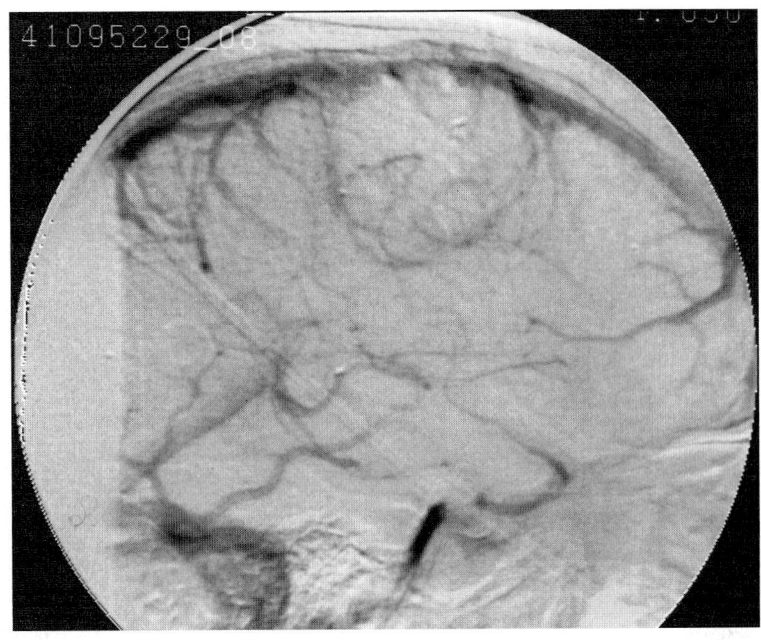

Figure 11–5. Sagittal, venous phase of cerebral angiogram in same tumor as in Figure 11–1. Study confirms patency of superior sagittal sinus and displacement of draining veins.

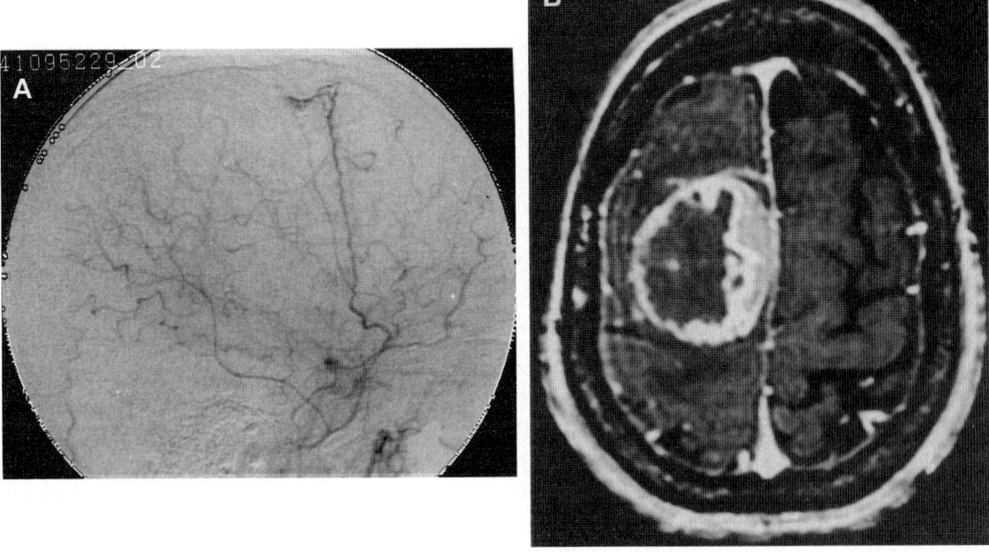

Figure 11–6. **(A)** Lateral external carotid injection of middle meningeal artery supplying tumor. **(B)** Preoperative T_1-weighted MRI with contrast (for image-guided system) showing dramatic effect of embolization on central blood supply to tumor. Persistent medial enhancement is due to supply from falcine artery originating off the anterior ethmoid arteries, not suitable for embolization.

get into the smallest blood vessels supplying tumors. We have used a combination of gelfoam powder, polyvinyl alcohol foam, and platinum coils. It has been our practice to embolize these large meningiomas the day before operation without waiting for further thrombosis to occur. In the principal author's experience there have been no problems with this approach in more than 100 surgical cases. If embolization is performed, a surgeon must remember that compromise of the blood supply to the scalp may have occurred and consider this when planning skin incisions.

OPTIONS FOR TREATMENT

Observation

Not every patient with an intracranial meningioma requires surgical intervention, and many factors, patient and tumor related, are involved in the decision to recommend surgery. One of the first questions to ask when a tumor is found on imaging studies is whether the imaged tumor is responsible for the patient's symptoms and signs. If not, and the imaging features are consistent with a benign tumor (homogeneous enhancement, smooth rounded margins, no associated brain edema, no satellite lesions), a period of observation is recommended. More and more asymptomatic meningiomas are discovered on imaging studies done for some other reason.

Olivero et al. (1995) followed 57 patients with symptomatic meningiomas over an average of 32 months (range 6 months to 15 years). None of the patients became symptomatic from their enlarging tumor during follow up, and tumor growth was observed in only 10 of 45 patients (22%) imaged. The average growth rate in these patients was a 0.24 cm increase in maximum diameter per year. In another study, Kuratsu et al. (2000) studied 109 patients. Of these, 63 (57.7%) had imaging follow ups of more than 1 year. Thirty-one percent of this subgroup showed tumor growth over an average follow-up period of 27.8 months (range, 12 to 87 months). While the average age in the two groups of patients, with and without tumor growth, was similar (67.5 versus 66.0 years), tumors that did not grow were more likely to be calcified on CT or hypointense on T_2-weighted MRI, consistent with intratumoral calcification. Clearly, then, not all tumors grow under observation, and it is our policy to recommend 6 month interval follow-up imaging with MRI for 2 years and then once a year if tumors are stable and the patient remains asymptomatic.

Surgery

A discussion of the specific surgical approach for each tumor location is beyond the scope of this text, but some general comments can be made. First, for symptomatic meningiomas, surgery is the mainstay of diagnosis and is the first step in treatment. With surgical removal there is no delay in "tumor response" as with other forms of therapy. Symptoms related to increased intracranial pressure or those related to local compression of brain can be improved quickly. Chozick et al. (1996) found that 39.9% of 158 patients with meningiomas had preoperative seizures and 88.9% of these patients had complete control of seizures postoperatively following tumor removal.

The surgeon must consider the indications for, risks associated with, reasonable goals of, and projected outcomes for expected or unexpected pathologies associated with surgery. These issues must be reviewed frankly with patients but without frightening them. Patient factors such as age, life expectancy, neurologic condition, and associated medical conditions should be taken into account. A determination of the resectability of the tumor should also be made. In some skull-base locations, such as cavernous sinus, complete removal of all microscopic tumor tissue is very difficult, if not impossible. Larson et al. (1995), in their experience with 36 patients who had cavernous sinus meningiomas, documented microscopic invasion into cranial nerves by tumor. Sen and Hague (1997) examined six patients with benign meningiomas of the cavernous sinus at autopsy. There was a tendency for infiltration of the carotid artery, the pituitary gland, and the connective tissue between fascicles of nerves. The trigeminal nerve and ganglion were particularly prone to invasion. These pathologic studies, as well as clinical experience, have prompted a conservative surgical approach with these tumor locations, treating residual or recurrent disease with radiotherapy.

The degree of surgical removal is also related to the risk of recurrence. This was outlined in the seminal paper of Donald Simpson (1957) (Table 11–2). Tumor-infiltrated bone left behind increases the risk of recurrence as does simple coagulation rather than

Table 11–2. Simpson Grade by Extent of Tumor, Dura, and Bone/Venous Sinus Excision

Grade	*Tumor Removal*			*Dural Attachment*		*Bone/ Sinus Excised*
	Complete	*Partial*	*Biopsy*	*Excised*	*Coagulated*	
I	X			X		X
II	X				X	X
III	X					
IV		X				
V			X			

excision of the tumor's dural attachment (Fig. 11–7). Surgical decision-making during the operation with respect to the degree of tumor removal attempted and the length of the operation may also affect outcome. Condra et al. (1997) classified "total excision" (TE) as a Simpson grade I, II, or III excision and found that of the 174 of 229 (76%) patients with this degree of excision, local control rates were 93%, 80%, and 76% at 5, 10, and 15 years, respectively. In contrast, the "subtotal excision" (SE; Simpson grade IV) results for equivalent time periods were 53%, 40%, and 30%, with cause-specific survival results mirroring local control for the TE and SE groups. Condra et al. (1997) thought that SE alone was inadequate therapy. In contrast, Jung et al. (2000), in reporting their results for the removal of 38 petroclival meningiomas, found that the median progression-free survival (PFS) was 66 months after SE and that the growth rate was slow (0.37 cm/year). The mean tumor doubling time was 8 years. These authors thought that subtotal resection, with or without radiation, was an option for patients with petroclival meningiomas. Similarly, Couldwell et al. (1996) reported their experience with 109 patients with petroclival meningiomas, many of who had subtotal resection of the posterior cavernous sinus component. In 69%, gross total tumor resection was achieved with a recurrence rate of only 13% over a 6.1 year mean follow up. In the 20 patients with known subtotal resection of the cavernous sinus component, 12 (60%) demonstrated radiographic progression and went on to further treatment.

Whether complications result from surgery for meningiomas depends on a number of factors, with patient age and tumor location as major considerations. In the series of Kuratsu et al. (2000), asymptomatic meningiomas that underwent surgical removal had a perioperative morbidity of 23.3% for those over the age of 70 years and 3.5% for those younger. The neurologic, medical, and surgical morbidity rates in the entire group were 6.9%, 3.4%, and 2.3%, respectively. For supratentorial meningiomas, a parietal location is a risk factor for the development of postoperative seizures. Infratentorial and skull-base meningiomas present challenges for cranial nerve preservation. In the series of Couldwell et al. (1996), of 109 petroclival meningiomas, permanent new cranial nerve deficits developed in 33% and the mortality rate was 3.7%. Modern neurosurgical series also reveal that neurologic morbidity after operation is site dependent.

At open operation, meningiomas are attached to the dura, and displacing the adjacent arachnoid and brain maintaining the "arachnoid plane" assists the surgeon with dissection. Two common principles employed during meningioma surgery are *(1)* to debulk the tumor centrally, first folding the thinned-out walls back into the cavity created rather than retracting brain to define the tumor margin; and *(2)* to respect the arachnoid membranes, which help separate tumor from the adjacent brain, blood vessels, and cranial nerves. A variety of instruments are now used routinely to assist with the surgical removal of these tumors, including the operating microscope, neurophysiologic monitoring, image-guided surgical navigation systems, ultrasonic aspirators, and, more recently, intraoperative MRI. For many of the complex skull-base tumors, especially those in the middle and posterior fossa, a team approach is taken, combining the skills of neurosurgeons and neuro-otologists. For very long operations this method allows co-surgeons to share the workload, with a rest between operative sessions of 2 to 4 hours helping to maintain their concentration and stamina. Without going into

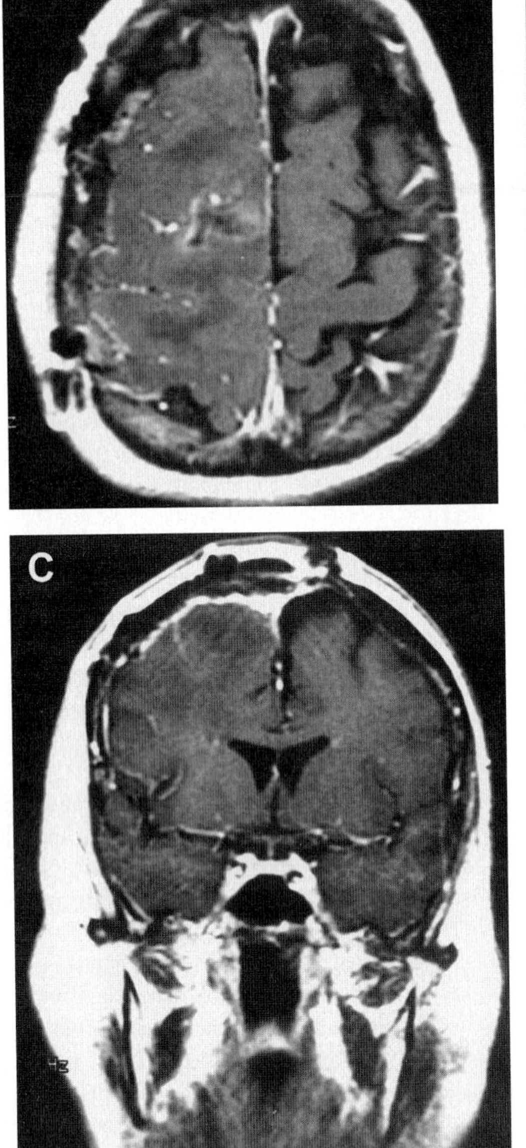

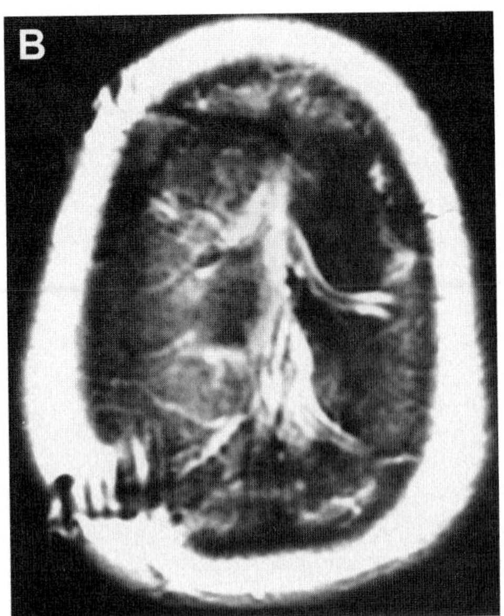

Figure 11–7. Postoperative axial **(A,B)** and coronal **(C)** T_1-weighted MRIs taken postoperatively confirm gross tumor resection of the same tumor as in Figures 11–4 to 11–6. Inferior two-thirds of falx giving rise to a portion of the tumor base was also excised. Intraoperative and imaging findings consistent with Simpson grade II removal as the lateral wall of the superior sagittal sinus was coagulated, not excised.

exhaustive detail, a few specific comments can be made about the most common tumor locations.

Supratentorial

Common locations in the supratentorial compartment include convexity, falx/parasagittal, sphenoid wing, and parasellar. Convexity meningiomas, when small, are straightforward. Image-guided surgical systems can be used to map out the location of the tumor and then to plan a margin of normal dural excision. Al-Mefty (1991) has coined the term "grade zero" excision for tumors in these locations to include a cuff of 2 cm of normal dura around the tumor base. When the tumors are very large, the most medial surface may have a poor brain–tumor interface even with benign pathology.

For falx/parasagittal meningiomas, preoperative assessments of the venous sinuses and parasagittal draining veins with MR venography or angiography will help the surgeon decide whether total excision is possible and which is the best route for avoiding important veins. Use of surgical navigational systems has become almost routine for the approach to these tumors. When the superior sagittal sinus is occluded on the preoperative angiogram, the point along the sinus where flow is present or not can be determined with a small intraoperative Doppler probe.

For sphenoid wing and parasellar tumors, the increased use of skull-base approaches limits the amount of brain retraction needed, reducing early and late complications. Orbitozygomatic osteotomies, combined with removal of the roof, lateral walls of the orbit, and the pterion, can be performed before the dura is opened for tumor removal. Similarly, for large olfactory groove, planum sphenoidale, and tuberculum meningiomas, a bifrontal, extended frontal (bilateral supraorbital osteotomy) craniotomy provides excellent exposure with the least brain retraction. Microdissection of the olfactory nerves back to the optic nerves can be done to preserve smell.

Infratentorial

Medial anterior tentorial tumors with extension into Meckel's cave or the posterior cavernous sinus and petroclival tumors are best approached with a retrolabyrinthine petrosal craniotomy. An incision in the dura along the temporal floor, crossing the superior petrosal sinus and then down in front of the sigmoid sinus, is combined with incision of the tentorium to its medial free edge. Care is taken to avoid injury to the vein of Labbe entering the tentorium and to the fourth nerve at its free edge. This provides the shortest route to the center of the tumor without significant cerebellar retraction and, when combined with physiologic monitoring, hearing is not inadvertently affected.

For foramen magnum meningiomas, the far lateral transcondylar approach provides a corridor to the tumor without spinal cord or brain retraction. After suboccipital craniotomy and C-1 hemilaminectomy, the posterior one-third of the occipital condyle is drilled off and the dura is opened in a curvilinear fashion just medial to the entry of the vertebral artery into the posterior fossa dura. With intraoperative monitoring of cranial nerves IX to XII, internal debulking of the tumor allows displacement of the capsule away from the nerves, brain stem, and upper spinal cord. Arnautovic et al. (2000) reported gross total resection in 12 of 18 patients using this approach.

RADIATION THERAPY

External Beam Irradiation

It seems somewhat paradoxical that a form of treatment implicated in the development of meningiomas would be recommended for benign residual or recurrent disease. Radiation therapy for residual benign meningiomas is still somewhat controversial, although there is good evidence that subtotal excision plus radiotherapy produces local control and overall survival that is superior to subtotal removal alone. For surgeons the problem of arachnoid scarring created by radiotherapy makes reoperation for recurrence much more difficult. This concern needs to be balanced against the risk of earlier recurrence. Modern series of external irradiation (XRT) using three-dimensional treatment planning limits the amount of dose delivered to surrounding normal brain compared with bilateral opposed fields. The advent of intensity-modulated radiation therapy (IMRT) provides for even greater dose conformity, although clinical experience with this technology is in its early stages.

Radiation affects tumor cells (reproductive and apoptotic cell death) and tumor vasculature by both direct and indirect means. The indirect form of DNA damage that results from the ionization of water and production of free radical species accounts for approximately 80% of the observed clinical effect. This effect is observed following a latent interval characterized by slowly proliferating tumors, which take longer to shrink after radiation than quickly proliferating tissues (e.g., lymphoma). Several studies since 1990 document the effectiveness of this treatment (Table 11–3). McCarthy et al. (1998), in an evaluation of factors associated with meningioma patient survival from the National Cancer Data Base, found that radiation was a significant factor associated with improved survival for both benign ($N = 8891$; $p < 0.0001$) and malignant ($N = 771$; $p < 0.001$) meningiomas. No details about treatment were given.

Table 11–3. Results of External Irradiation for Meningiomas Since 1990

Author	*Pathology*	*No. Patients*	*Dose (Gy)*	*Control Rate*
Glaholm et al. (1990)	Benign	177	50–55 (range)	84% 5 yr 74% 10 yr
Miralbell et al. (1992)	Primary Recurrent	17 16	54 (median) 54 (median)	88% 8 yr 78% 8 yr
Goldsmith et al. (1994)	Benign	117	54 (median)	89% 5 yr 77% 10 yr
	Malignant	23	54 (median)	48% 5 yr
Maire et al. (1995)	Mixed*	91	50.9 (mean)	91% 5 yr† 72% 10 yr
Milosevic et al. (1996)	Atypical Malignant	17 42	50 (40–60)	51%† 27%†
Condra et al. (1997)	Benign	21	53.3 (median)	87% 15 yr 86% 15 yr†
Maguire et al. (1999)	Mixed*	28	53.1 (median)	81% 8 yr
Nutting et al. (1999)	Benign	82	55–60 (range)	92% 5 yr 83% 10 yr

*Majority of cases benign; see reference for details.

†Cause-specific survival.

At the University of California, San Francisco, the 5 and 10 year PFSs for residual benign meningiomas treated with XRT were 89% and 77%, respectively (Goldsmith et al., 1994). Frontal and olfactory locations had slightly higher recurrence rates, and the risk of recurrence increased 2.2-fold for every 100 cm^2 increase in tumor size. A dose–response effect on tumor control was observed for benign and malignant tumors: For benign tumors doses >52 Gy and for malignant tumors doses >53 Gy were associated with significantly improved local control.

Condra et al. (1997) analyzed the experience with 262 patients at the University of Florida, dividing them into treatment groups of total excision (TE), subtotal excision (SE), and subtotal excision plus radiotherapy (SE + RT). The median follow up for the entire group was 8.2 years, and in this time no radiation-induced malignancy was reported as a complication of treatment. Of the 25 patients with SE alone who recurred, salvage therapy of any type was less successful in regaining long-term tumor control. Local control (LC) and cause-specific survival (CSS) at 15 years were significantly reduced after SE alone (30% LC/51% CSS) compared with TE (76% LC/88% CSS) or SE + RT (87% LC/86% CSS) ($p = 0.0001$ LC; $p = 0.0003$ CSS). Multivariate analysis confirmed the prognostic importance of treatment selection, with SE alone inferior to others ($p = 0.0001$). Atypical pathologic features and Karnofsky performance score were also predictive of CSS.

Radiosurgery has been used most often for small, well-defined meningiomas, residual or recurrent, that are commonly seen in skull-base locations. Nutting et al. (1999) published their results with fractionated XRT, proposing these as a baseline for the evaluation of new treatment strategies such as radiosurgery and skull-base surgery. There were 82 patients with histologically confirmed benign meningiomas, with a median follow up of 9 years included in the study. The 5 and 10 year rates of freedom from progression were 92% and 83%, respectively. Sphenoid ridge tumor locations had a higher recurrence rate than parasellar locations (31% versus 10%). There were no cases of secondary tumor development, and only one patient had radiation retinopathy.

Complications of XRT with current delivery methods are few. Toxicity is usually described in terms of the time interval from treatment as acute (hours to days), early delayed (weeks to months), and late delayed (months to years). Goldsmith et al. (1994) provided a detailed account of complications in their series. Of 140 patients, 5 (3.6%) had permanent (late-delayed) complications of treatment. Three patients had sudden blindness 20 to 22 months after the completion of radiation therapy, and 2 patients developed cerebral necrosis at 13 and 30 months after treatment. In the series of Nutting et al. (1999) of cavernous sinus meningiomas, 61 of 82 patients were available for long-term follow up. Six patients had visual impairment (9.8%), five due to cataracts and one due to retinopathy. Three patients developed hypopituitarism (4.9%), and four had impairment of short-term memory (6.5%).

Radiosurgery

The technique of radiosurgery delivers a high dose of radiation to a defined intracranial target using stereotactic methods in a single treatment session. Typically, a stereotactic frame is applied to the patient's skull under local anesthesia. Relocatable frames using straps and dental bite blocks are used for fractionated stereotactic radiotherapy. Radiosurgical treatments can be delivered with a specially adapted linear accelerator or gamma knife unit. Each relies on a steep dose gradient outside the edge of the target to limit normal tissue effects. Published results are now maturing, and there appear to be good data that this treatment is an effective form of therapy for small, well-defined tumors that are more than 4 mm from the optic nerve or chiasm (Table 11–4).

For meningiomas located outside the cranial base, complete excision of the tumor and dural attachments is the goal. For parasagittal meningiomas, achieving this goal is problematic due to involvement of the superior sagittal sinus and draining veins. Kondziolka and colleagues (1998) in a multicenter study of radiosurgery for benign parasagittal meningiomas collected 203 cases with a median follow up of 3.5 years. The mean tumor volume was 10 cc. The 5 year overall tumor control rate was 67% ± 8.77% for the entire series. Considering just the "in-field" control rate for the targeted lesion, it was 85% ± 6.2% at 5 years. Patients who had radiosurgery as the primary mode of therapy had a better control rate than those who had undergone prior resection (93% versus 60%; $p = 0.08$). In multivariate analysis, predictors of tumor progression were pre-existing neurologic deficit and tumor volume greater than 7.5 cc. A marginal dose of 15 Gy or greater, or the maximum dose, did not improve tumor control. The 3 and 5 year actuarial rate of symptomatic edema was 16% ± 3.8%. This is similar to the 14.8% rate of symptomatic edema reported by Singh et al. (2000). Outcomes were also dependent on neurologic status at the time of treatment. For those with deficit before radiosurgery 65% were improved or stable compared with a rate of 83% for those without deficit before treatment. A follow-up article on perspectives of 99 patients who underwent radiosurgery for meningiomas

Table 11–4. Radiosurgery Results for Meningiomas Based on Selected Series Published Since 1990

Author	*Pathology*	*No. Patients*	*Min./Max. Dose (Gy)*	*Control Rate*
Engenhart et al. (1990)	Benign	17	29 (mean max.), LN	76% at 3.3 yr
Kondziolka and Lundsford (1992)	Benign	50	16.9 (mean marginal), GK	96% at 2 yr
Duma et al. (1993)	Benign	34	16 (median marginal), GK	100% at 2.2 yr
Valentino et al. (1993)	Benign	72	37 (median max.), LN	94% at 2.5–8 yr
Chang et al. (1998)	Benign	55	18.3 (median marginal), LN	98% at 2 yr
Kondziolka et al. (1998)	Benign	185	15 (median marginal), GK	85% at 5 yr
Hakim et al. (1998)	Benign	106	15 (median marginal), LN	89% at 5 yr
Subach et al. (1998)	Benign	62	15 (mean marginal), GK	87% at 8 yr
Shafron et al. (1999)	Benign	38	12.7 (mean marginal), LN	100% at 2 yr
Iwai et al. (1999)	Benign	24	10.6 (median marginal), GK	100% at 1.5 yr
Morita et al. (1999)	Benign	88	16 (median marginal), GK	95% at 5 yr
Roche et al. (2000)	Benign	92	15 (median marginal), GK	93% at 5 yr
Ojemann et al. (2000)	Malignant	22	15.5 (median marginal), GK	48% at 2 yr

LN, linear accelerator; GK, Gamma knife

revealed that 5 to 10 years after treatment 96% of those surveyed believed that radiosurgery provided a satisfactory outcome and 93% had required no further treatment (Kondziolka et al., 1999).

Hakim et al. (1998) reported similar results in 127 patients with 155 meningiomas treated using a linear accelerator, 52.9% of which were categorized as being located in the skull base. Their median tumor volume was 4.1 cc, and median follow up was 31 months. Of the tumors studied, 106 were benign, 26 atypical, and 18 malignant. The 1, 2, 3, 4, and 5 year tumor control rates for benign meningiomas outside versus within the cranial base were 100/100%, 92.0/93.8%, 92.0/88.9%, 92.0/88.9%, and 92.0/88.9%, respectively. The median time to progression for atypical and malignant meningiomas was 24.4 and 13.9 months, respectively. When death from intercurrent disease was excluded, the 2 and 4 year survivals for benign, atypical, and malignant meningiomas following radiosurgery were 94.8/91%, 83.3/83.3%, and 64.6/21.5%, respectively. Six patients (4.7%) developed permanent complications, including two deaths, one from cerebral infarction and a second from hypothalamic dysfunction.

For many skull-base meningiomas with extension into the cavernous sinus complete surgical removal would seem to be the exception rather than the rule. Radiosurgery for residual or progressive disease is effective and with acceptable risks. Conformal treatment plans are a must to keep complication rates low. Chang et al. (1998) reported preliminary results with radiosurgery for 55 patients with skull-base meningiomas. The 2 year actuarial control rate was 98%, with 29% of tumors decreasing in size and 69% remaining stable. Twenty-seven percent of patients had improvement in neurologic status, and 22% (12) developed new cranial nerve deficits 6 to 12 months after treatment (transient in 10, permanent in 2). Roche et al. (2000) reported the largest series of 80 cavernous sinus meningiomas treated with radiosurgery with a minimum 1 year follow up. The mean patient age was 49 years, and mean tumor volume was 5.8 cc (range 0.9 to 18.6 cc). The mean maximum prescription dose was 28 Gy (range 12 to 50 Gy) delivered with a median planning isodose line of 50% (range 30% to 70%). With a median follow up of 30.5 months (range 12 to 79 months) the actuarial 5 year PFS was 92.8%. No new oculomotor deficit was observed.

Morita et al. (1999) reported that in their series of 88 skull-base meningiomas treated with radiosurgery, the risk of trigeminal neuropathy was associated with doses of 19 Gy or more, and the optic apparatus appeared to tolerate doses greater than 10 Gy. If lower doses to cranial nerves are associated with reduced side effects, the question is what effect lowering the dose will have on tumor control rates. Iwai et al. (1999) achieved similar control rates to other series over a shorter term of follow up (median 17.1 months) with a much lower marginal median prescription dose of 10.6 Gy. Only one patient in their series (1/24) developed worsening of a preexisting cranial nerve deficit, and no patient had any new deficit.

Brachytherapy

Interstitial brachytherapy is an irradiation technique that is not commonly used for newly diagnosed or recurrent meningiomas. Permanent ^{125}I-sources can be implanted either at open craniotomy or stereotactically. These low-activity implants have a half-life of 60 days and produce low-energy photons (27 to 35 keV) with a half value in tissue of 20 mm. Continuous low-dose irradiation has many theoretical biologic advantages for tumor control and protects the surrounding normal brain tissue. One additional method of protecting the brain stem from high doses is to place a small amount of sterile gold foil between the implant site and surrounding neural tissue.

Gutin et al. (1987) reported one of the first series of interstitial brachytherapy for recurrent skull-base tumors, six of which were meningiomas: three benign and three malignant. Five to 36 sources were implanted at open operation, delivering 80 to 150 Gy to the periphery of the tumors over the lifetime of the sources. Two patients recurred outside the implanted volume, surviving only 8 and 9 months, respectively. The remaining four patients were stable at follow up from 2+ to 54+ months. At last review, 13 patients had been treated in a similar manner, with 8 stable at a median follow up of 10.5 months (range 5 months to 6.5 years). Kumar et al. (1993) treated 15 patients with primary and recurrent skull-base meningiomas using stereotactic implantation of ^{125}I-sources with a median follow up of 29 months. They reported an impressive 73% complete radiographic response rate and stabilization of tumors in the remaining patients (100% control). No patients were reported to have developed early or late delayed radiation toxicity.

Vuorinen et al. (1996) published the largest experience with interstitial brachytherapy for 25 parasellar-clival meningiomas and 19 globoid meningiomas in elderly patients. The dose to the margin of the tumors ranged from 100 to 150 Gy, with sources implanted using stereotactic methods. In 2 of the 44 cases, sources were found on postoperative imaging studies to lie on the surface of the tumor. In the parasellar-clival group, studied for a median of 19 months, 16% were moderately smaller, 52% slightly smaller, and 20% were stable in size. Of the 17 patients with III, V, VI cranial neuropathy before treatment, 36% showed improvement. One patient suffered a third nerve injury with the implant procedure, and facial numbness developed or increased in 47% of patients. There was no serious bleeding and no procedural mortality. Even this small amount of data may indicate a role for brachytherapy for recurrent meningiomas undergoing reoperation where the residual tumor, or involved cranial base dura, can be implanted at the same sitting.

CHEMOTHERAPY

Cytotoxic Chemotherapy

The treatment of recurrent benign or malignant meningiomas with standard alkylating agents, while used in a number of cancer centers since the 1980s, did not appear in the medical literature until the mid-1990s. Wilson (1994) reported an experience with cyclophosphamide, adriamycin, and vincristine for malignant meningiomas recurrent after surgery and radiation therapy. In 11 patients, 73% had progression at 1 year and 100% at 2 years. Chamberlain (1996) reported prospective results giving the same agents to 14 patients. Patients who had gross total tumor resection received three cycles of chemotherapy, and those with subtotal removal received six cycles of treatment. Four patients required dose reductions for neutropenia, and for three the planned course of treatment could not be completed. There were 3 partial responses, and 11 patients had stable disease. The median time to tumor progression was 4.6 years, and the median survival was 5.3 years.

Other reports documenting the use of intra-arterial or intravenous use of drugs such as cisplatin, doxorubicin, and/or dacarbazine have not produced dramatic results. Schrell et al. (1997) reported on four patients with 15% to 74% reductions in tumor volumes who received 1000 to 1500 mg per day of hydroxyurea over a period of 5 to 24 months. Despite this report, there are no other published data documenting a similar experience, and so the search for a well-tolerated, effective form of therapy is ongoing.

Biologic Therapy

The largest series of immunomodulatory therapy for recurrent benign and malignant meningiomas involves the use of interferon-α_{2B}. This leukocyte-produced cytokine may have two mechanisms of action: one tumor antiproliferative effect and a second antiangiogenic effect. Kaba et al. (1997) reported on the use of this agent by six patients at a dosage of 4 mU/m^2 per day, 5 days per week. Patients were treated for 4 to more than 14 months, and side effects were limited. Five of six patients showed radiographic response, four had stabilization of disease, and one had slight tumor reduction. One of the responding patients had progression of his tumor on two occasions after stopping treatment. Further investigations with this agent and other biologic response modifiers seem to be indicated.

Hormone Receptor Antagonists

As previously mentioned, because meningiomas are more common in women than in men, and some tumors become symptomatic during pregnancy, a role for female sex hormones has been suggested in their development. Laboratory work has shown that estrogen receptors are present at reduced levels compared with progesterone receptors. Clinical trials of the antiestrogen agent tamoxifen have not been encouraging. Markwalder et al. (1987) studied six patients with recurrent inoperable meningiomas treated with tamoxifen over a 6 to 12 month period. One patient appeared to show an initial tumor response; two had stabilization of tumor; and three others had disease progression at follow up.

The Southwest Oncology Group (Goodwin et al., 1993) studied 21 patients, and, after a median follow up of 15.1 months, 32% of patients had no tumor growth and 53% had disease progression on imaging studies. In subsequent studies with the antiprogestational agent medroxyprogesterone acetate (MPA), the drug could reduce the level of tumor progesterone receptor compared with historic controls, but it did not reduce tumor size in four of five women who took the drug once a week for 17 to 29 weeks. As noted at the beginning of this chapter, another antiprogestational drug, RU-486, mifepristone, was given to 14 patients with recurrent and unresectable meningiomas, and 4 had a minor decrease in tumor size on imaging studies. Another patient had an improved visual field examination. Lamberts et al. (1992), using the same dosage of 200 mg per day, noted that of 12 patients 3 had transient tumor regression and 1 had a sustained regression (70% volume reduction). A recent case report by Oura et al. (2000) also showed a volume reduction (73%) in a presumed meningioma after 2 years of treatment with MPA. Clearly, there may be some role for the treatment of benign recurrent meningiomas with antiprogesterone agents, and it is hoped that responses can be correlated with progesterone receptor status derived from surgical specimens.

MALIGNANT MENINGIOMA

Malignant meningiomas generally account for less than 10% of all meningiomas and deserve separate mention as they are one of the most difficult primary brain tumors to control. Survivals from a number of clinical series range from 2 to 9 years (Table 11–5). In the recent series of Palma et al. (1997), 8.6% of intracranial meningiomas were atypical or malignant, and in the personal series of Wilson (1994) the incidence was 12%. Unlike benign meningiomas, there does not appear to be the same predominance of female sex, and, in fact, the ratio may be reversed. Younis et al. (1995) found that 67% of malignant meningiomas occurred in males.

The most common presenting symptoms are headache, seizures, personality change, and painless subcutaneous scalp lumps. The duration of symptoms is shorter than with benign meningiomas. Spread of tumor outside the nervous system has been documented in as many as 24% of patients before death, and common sites for metastases are lung, liver, and bone. On imaging studies, these tumors reflect their aggressive nature with irregular borders, surrounding

Table 11–5. Malignant and Anaplastic Meningioma Recurrence Rates and Survivals in Selected Series Since 1990

Author	*Pathology*	*No. Patients*	*Recurrence Rate*	*Survival*
Maier et al. (1992)	Anaplastic	14	73%	na
Mahmood et al. (1993)	Atypical	20	50% at 5 yr	5.95 yr
	Anaplastic	5	33% at 5 yr	8.75 yr
Goldsmith et al. (1994)	Malignant	23	52% at 5 yr	58% at 3.3 yr
Wilson (1994)	Malignant	24	na	2.0 yrs. (median)
Younis et al. (1995)	Atypical	6	67% at 2 yr	50% at 5 yr
	Malignant	12	44% at 2 yr	62% at 5 yr
Milosevic et al. (1996)	Atypical	17	66%	28% at 5 yr
	Malignant	42	(all patients)	(all patients)
Palma et al. (1997)	Atypical	42	52% at 5 yr	95% at 5 yr
	Malignant	29	84% at 5 yrs.	64.3% at 5 yr
Hakim et al. (1998)	Atypical	26	24.4 mo. PFS	83.3% at 4 yr
	Malignant	18	13.9 mo. PFS	21.5% at 4 yr
Hug et al. (2000)	Atypical	15	62% at 5 yr	93%
	Malignant	16	48% at 5 yrs.	38% (mean 59 mo.)
Ojemann et al. (2000)	Malignant	22	68% at 2 yr	75% at 2 yr
			74% at 5 yr	40% at 5 yr

na, Not available; PFS, progression-free survival.

edema, and nonhomogeneous contrast enhancement. "Mushrooming" is also a feature of these tumors, where the main body of the dural-based tumor pushes off nodules of tumor into the dura adjacent to it. In one series where both CT and MRI had been used in diagnostic imaging, 50% of tumors showed indistinct margins, 41% "mushrooming," 33% had soft tissue involvement, and none exhibited intratumoral calcification.

The mainstay of therapy for these tumors is surgical removal. As expected, time to recurrence and overall survival are shorter in those with partial resections versus complete resection. Palma et al. (1997) found that for atypical meningiomas, those with a Simpson grade I excision did significantly better than those with Simpson grade II or III ($p <$ 0.0071). Tumor location in the convexity was strongly related to grade I surgical excision ($r = 0.75$). For malignant meningiomas, even though a grade I excision was not significantly associated with improved survival versus grade II resection, patients with tumors of the convexity did significantly better than those with basal/parasagittal malignant tumors. In multivariate analysis, convexity location proved to be a positive factor for survival.

Radiotherapy has been shown in most series to lengthen time to recurrence and survival. Goldsmith et al. (1994) found a dose–response relationship for XRT with a 5 year PFS of 63% for those receiving a dose of ≥53 Gy versus 17% for those whose dose was <53 Gy. Milosevic et al. (1996) also found a significant relationship between cause-specific survival and dose above or below 50 Gy ($p = 0.0005$). Boosting the tumor site with additional photon or proton radiation may improve local control. At the Harvard proton therapy unit, significantly improved local control was achieved for both atypical and malignant meningiomas with the addition of a proton boost for total doses ≥60 Gy. Actuarial 5 and 8 year survival rates for malignant meningioma were significantly improved with proton over photon therapy and doses >60 Gy.

Radiosurgery has been used to treat malignant meningioma immediately following XRT as a boost, but more often for recurrent disease. Hakim et al. (1998) treated 26 atypical and 18 malignant meningiomas with radiosurgery in an overall series of 127 patients of whom 51% were being treated for recurrence. The median time to progression (TTP) for atypical and malignant meningioma was 24.4 and 13.9 months, respectively. Five year disease-free survivals were 83.3% and 21.5% for atypical meningiomas and malignant meningiomas. Ojemann et al. (2000) recently reported the results of radiosurgery for malignant meningioma in 22 patients, 3 of whom were treated in a boost setting. The median prescription dose was 15.5 Gy (range 12 to 18 Gy), and the median target volume was 7.35 cc (range 0.59 to 35.0 cc). Nineteen patients were treated for recurrence and had 37 lesions treated in 30 sessions. For the 31 malignant meningioma tumors treated, the 2 and 5 year PFS rates were 48% and 34%, respectively. On multivariate analysis of factors affecting time to progression, age <50 years ($p = 0.0003$) and tumor volume <8 cc ($p < 0.05$) were significant. A number of patient and treatment factors were also analyzed for effect on overall survival, but no significant relationships were found. Five of the 22 patients treated (23%) developed radiation necrosis as a complication of treatment with a median time to onset of 77 weeks after treatment (range 15 to 120 weeks). Given its effectiveness for recurrent malignant meningioma, the role and timing of radiosurgery in the management of malignant meningioma requires further evaluation.

CONCLUSION

Despite their benign histology in the majority of cases, meningiomas located around the venous sinuses and base of the skull can be difficult to control and at times impossible to eradicate. Whereas selected series reporting the results of specific therapies show favorable outcomes, population-based data have suggested otherwise. The availability of cytogenetic and molecular techniques for the identification of exogenous and endogenous factors associated with meningiomas will improve our understanding of the basic mechanisms involved in tumorigenesis and provide for new methods of treatment. At present, it is not clear what roles hormones, growth factors, and oncogenes, as well as tumor suppressor genes, play in the development of meningiomas. These tumors remain a clinical problem to be best solved by the combined approaches of basic scientists and those clinicians who treat patients suffering from these tumors. Cushing and Eisenhardt (1938) were correct more than 60 years ago when they said that "the ultimate prognosis hinges more on the surgeon's wide experience with the problem in all its many aspects than is true of almost any other operation that can be named."

REFERENCES

Al-Mefty O.1991. Meningiomas. New York: Raven Press, p 630.

Al-Mefty O, Origitano T. 1994. Meningiomas. In: Regachary S, Wilkins R (eds), Principles of Neurosurgery. London: Wolfe Publishing, pp 28.21–28.12

Antoniades HN, Galanopoulos T, Neville-Golden J, Maxwell M. 1992. Expression of insulin-like growth factors I and II and their receptor mRNAs in primary human astrocytomas and meningiomas; in vivo studies using in situ hybridization and immunocytochemistry. Int J Cancer 50:215–222.

Arnautovic K I, Al-Mefty O, et al. 2000. Ventral foramen magnum meninigiomas. J Neurosurg 92:71–80.

Arnoldus EP, Wolters LB, Voormolen JH, et al. 1992. Interphase cytogenetics: a new tool for the study of genetic changes in brain tumors. J Neurosurg 76:997–1003.

Bendszus M, Rao G, Burger R, et al. 2000. Is there a benefit of preoperative meningioma embolization? Neurosurgery 47:1306–1312.

Bielenberg DR, Bucana CD, Sanchez R, Mulliken JB, Folkman J, Fidler IJ. 1999. Progressive growth of infantile cutaneous hemangiomas is directly correlated with hyperplasia and angiogenesis of adjacent epidermis and inversely correlated with expression of the endogenous angiogenesis inhibitor, IFN-beta. Int J Oncol 14:401–408.

Bingham WF. 1986. W. W. Keen and the dawn of American neurosurgery. J Neurosurg 64:705–712.

Bitzer M, Opitz H, Popp J, et al. 1998. Angiogenesis and brain oedema in intracranial meningiomas: influence of vascular endothelial growth factor. Acta Neurochir 140:333–340.

Bitzer M, Wockel L, Luft AR, et al. 1997. The importance of pial blood supply to the development of peritumoral brain edema in meningiomas. J Neurosurg 87:368–373.

Black P, Carroll R, Zhang J. 1996. The molecular biology of hormone and growth factor receptors in meningiomas. Acta Neurochir Suppl (Wien) 65:50–53.

Black PM. 1997. Hormones, radiosurgery and virtual reality: new aspects of meningioma management. Can J Neurol Sci 24:302–306.

Black PM. 1993. Meningiomas. Neurosurgery 32:643–657.

Black PM, Carroll R, Glowacka D, Riley K, Dashner K. 1994. Platelet-derived growth factor expression and stimulation in human meningiomas. J Neurosurg 81:388–393.

Blankenstein MA, Koehorst SG, van der Kallen CJ, et al. 1995. Oestrogen receptor independent expression of progestin receptors in human meningioma—a review. J Steroid Biochem Mol Biol 53:361–365.

Bouillot P, Pellissier JF, Devictor B, et al. 1994. Quantitative imaging of estrogen and progesterone receptors, estrogen-regulated protein, and growth fraction: immunocytochemical assays in 52 meningiomas. Correlation with clinical and morphological data. J Neurosurg 81:765–773.

Bradac GB, Ferszt R, Bender A, Schorner W. 1986. Peritumoral edema in meningiomas. A radiological and histological study. Neuroradiology 28:304–312.

Burger PC, Scheithauer F, Vogel FS. 1991. Surgical Pathology of the Nervous System and its Coverings, 3rd ed. New York: Churchill Livingstone, p 737.

Cao Y, Linden P, Shima D, Browne F, Folkman J. 1996. In vivo angiogenic activity and hypoxia induction of heterodimers of placenta growth factor/vascular endothelial growth factor. J Clin Invest 98:2507–2511.

Carroll RS, Black PM, Zhang J, et al. 1997. Expression and activation of epidermal growth factor receptors in meningiomas. J Neurosurg 87:315–323.

Carroll RS, Glowacka D, Dashner K, Black PM. 1993. Progesterone receptor expression in meningiomas. Cancer Res 53:1312–1316.

Carroll RS, Zhang J, Black PM. 1999. Expression of estrogen receptors alpha and beta in human meningiomas. J Neurooncol 42:109–116.

Carroll RS, Zhang J, Dashner K, Black PM. 1995a. Progesterone and glucocorticoid receptor activation in meningiomas. Neurosurgery 37:92–97.

Carroll RS, Zhang J, Dashner K, Sar M, Wilson EM, Black PM. 1995b. Androgen receptor expression in meningiomas. J Neurosurg 82:453–460.

Chamberlain MC. 1996. Adjuvant combined modality therapy for malignant meningiomas. J Neurosurg 84:733–736.

Chang SD, Adler JR, Martin DP. 1998. LINAC radiosurgery for cavernous sinus meningiomas. Stereotact Funct Neurosurg 71:43–50.

Chozick BS, Reinert SE, Greenblatt SH, et al. 1996. Incidence of seizures after surgery for supratentorial meningiomas: a modern analysis. J Neurosurg 84:382–386.

Collins VP, Nordenskjold M, Dumanski JP. 1990. The molecular genetics of meningiomas. Brain Pathol 1:19–24.

Condra KS, Buatti JM, Mendenhall WM, Friedman WA, Marcus RB, Rhoton AL, et al. 1997. Benign meningiomas: primary treatment selection affects survival. Int J Radiat Oncol Biol Phys 39:427–436.

Couldwell WT, Fukushima T, Giannotta SL, Weiss MH. 1996. Petroclival meningiomas: surgical experience in 109 cases. J Neurosurg 84:20–28.

Cushing H. 1922. The meningiomas (dural endotheliomas): their souce, and favoured seats of origin. Brain 45: 282–316.

Cushing H, Eisenhardt L. 1938. Meningiomas: Their Classification, Regional Behavior, Life History and Surgical End Results. Springfield, IL: Thomas, p 785.

Detta A, Kenny BG, Smith C, Logan A, Hitchcock E. 1993. Correlation of proto-oncogene expression and proliferation and meningiomas. Neurosurgery 33:1065–1074.

Donnell MS, Meyer GA, Donegan WL. 1979. Estrogen-receptor protein in intracranial meningiomas. J Neurosurg 50:499–502.

Duma CM, Lunsford LD, Kondziolka D, et al. 1993. Stereotactic radiosurgery of cavernous sinus meningiomas as an addition or alternative to microsurgery. Neurosurgery 32: 699–705.

Dumanski JP, Carlbom E, Collins VP, Nordenskjold M. 1987.

Deletion mapping of a locus on human chromosome 22 involved in the oncogenesis of meningioma. Proc Natl Acad Sci USA 84:9275–9279.

Dumanski JP, Rouleau GA, Nordenskjold M, Collins VP. 1990. Molecular genetic analysis of chromosome 22 in 81 cases of meningioma. Cancer Res 50:5863–5867.

Earle KM, Richany SF. 1969. Meningiomas. A study of the histology, incidence, and biologic behavior of 243 cases from the Frazier-Grant collection of brain tumors. Med Ann Dist Columbia 38:353–356 passim.

Engenhart R, Kimmig BN, Hover KH, et al. 1990. Stereotactic single high dose radiation therapy of benign intracranial meningiomas. Int J Radiat Oncol Biol Phys 19:1021–1026.

Erdincler P, Lena G, Sarioglu AC, Kuday C, Choux M. 1998. Intracranial meningiomas in children: review of 29 cases. Surg Neurol 49:136–140.

Feldkamp MM, Lau N, Guha A. 1999a. Growth inhibition of astrocytoma cells by farnesyl transferase inhibitors is mediated by a combination of antiproliferative, proapoptotic and anti-angiogenic effects. Oncogene 18:7514–7526.

Feldkamp MM, Lau N, Rak J, Kerbel RS, Guha A. 1999b. Normoxic and hypoxic regulation of vascular endothelial growth factor (VEGF) by astrocytoma cells is mediated by Ras. Int J Cancer 81:118–124.

Folkman J, Shing Y. 1992. Control of angiogenesis by heparin and other sulfated polysaccharides. Adv Exp Med Biol 313:355–364.

Friend KE, Radinsky R, McCutcheon IE. 1999. Growth hormone receptor expression and function in meningiomas: effect of a specific receptor antagonist. J Neurosurg 91:93–99.

Germano IM, Edwards MSB, Davis RL, Schiffer D. 1994. Intracranial meningiomas of the first 2 decades of life. J Neurosurg 80:447–453.

Glaholm J, Bloom HJG, Crow JH. 1990. The role of radiotherapy in the management of intracranial meningiomas: The Royal Marsden Hospital experience with 186 patients. Int J Radiat Oncol Biol Phys 18:755–761.

Glick RP, Lichtor T, Unterman TG. 1997. Insulin-like growth factors in central nervous system tumors. J Neurooncol 35:315–325.

Goldsmith BJ, Wara WM, Wilson CB, Larson DA. 1994. Postoperative irradiation for subtotally resected meningiomas—a retrospective analysis of 140 patients treated from 1967 to 1990 [published erratum appears in J Neurosurg 1994 Apr; 80(4):777]. J Neurosurg 80:195–201.

Goodwin JW, Crowley J, Eyre HJ, Stafford B, Jaeckle KA, Townsend JJ. 1993. A phase II evaluation of tamoxifen in unresectable or refractory meningiomas: a Southwest Oncology Group study. J Neurooncol 15:75–77.

Goto F, Goto K, Weindel K, Folkman J. 1993. Synergistic effects of vascular endothelial growth factor and basic fibroblast growth factor on the proliferation and cord formation of bovine capillary endothelial cells within collagen gels. Lab Invest 69:508–517.

Grunberg SM, Weiss MH, Spitz IM, et al. 1991. Treatment of unresectable meningiomas with the antiprogesterone agent mifepristone. J Neurosurg 74:861–866.

Guha A. 1998. Ras activation in astrocytomas and neurofibromas. Can J Neurol Sci 25:267–281.

Gutin PH, Leibel SA, Hosobuchi Y, et al. 1987. Brachytherapy of recurrent tumors of the skull base and spine with iodine-125 sources. Neurosurgery 20:938–945.

Gutmann DH, Giordano MJ, Fishback AS, Guha A. 1997. Loss of merlin expression in sporadic meningiomas, ependymomas and schwannomas. Neurology 49:267–270.

Hakim RH, E. Alexander E 3d, Loeffler JS, et al. 1998. Results of linear accelerator-based radiosurgery for intracranial meningiomas. Neurosurgery 42:446–454.

Halper J, Colvard DS, Scheithauer BW, et al. 1989. Estrogen and progesterone receptors in meningiomas: comparison of nuclear binding, dextran-coated charcoal, and immunoperoxidase staining assays. Neurosurgery 25:546–552; discussion, 552–543.

Harris H, Miller OJ, Klein G, Worst P, Tachibana T. 1969. Suppression of malignancy by cell fusion. Nature 223:363–368.

Harrison MJ, Wolfe DE, Lau TS, Mitnick RJ, Sachdev VP. 1991. Radiation-induced meningiomas: experience at the Mount Sinai Hospital and review of the literature. J Neurosurg 75:564–574.

Hsu DW, Efird JT, Hedley-Whyte ET. 1997. Progesterone and estrogen receptors in meningiomas: prognostic considerations. J Neurosurg 86:113–120.

Hug EB, Devries A, Thornton AF, et al. 2000. Management of atypical and mailgnant meningiomas: role of high-dose, 3D-conformal radiation therapy. J Neurooncol 48:151–160.

Ildan F, Tuna A, Gocer AI, et al. 1999. Correlation of the relationships of brain-tumor interfaces, magnetic resonance imaging, and angiographic findings to predict cleavage of meningiomas. J Neurosurg 91:384–390.

Iwai Y, Yamanaka K, Yasui T, et al. 1999. Gamma knife surgery for skull base meningiomas—the effectiveness of low-dose treatment. Surg Neurol 52:40–45.

Jacobs DH, Holmes FF, McFarlane MJ. 1992. Meningiomas are not significantly associated with breast cancer. Arch Neurol 49:753–756.

Jung HW, Yoo H, Paek SH, Choi KS. 2000. Long-term outcome and growth rate of subtotally resected petroclival meningiomas—experience with 38 cases. Neurosurgery 46:567–575.

Kaba SE, DeMonte F, Bruner JM, et al. 1997. The treatment of recurrent unresectable and malignant meningiomas with interferon alpha-2B. Neurosurgery 40:271–275.

Kalkanis SN, Carroll RS, Zhang J, Zamani AA, Black PM. 1996. Correlation of vascular endothelial growth factor messenger RNA expression with peritumoral vasogenic cerebral edema in meningiomas. J Neurosurg 85:1095–1101.

Katsuyama J, Papenhausen PR, Herz F, Gazivoda P, Hirano A, Koss LG. 1986. Chromosome abnormalities in meningiomas. Cancer Genet Cytogenet 22:63–68.

Kazumoto K, Tamura M, Hoshino H, Yuasa Y. 1990. Enhanced expression of the sis and c-myc oncogenes in human meningiomas. J Neurosurg 72:786–791.

Kenyon BM, Voest EE, Chen CC, Flynn E, Folkman J, D'Amato RJ. 1996. A model of angiogenesis in the mouse cornea. Invest Ophthalmol Vis Sci 37:1625–1632.

Kida S, Yamashima T, Kubota T, Ito H, Yamamoto S. 1988. A light and electron microscopic and immunohistochemical study of human arachnoid villi. J Neurosurg 69:429–435.

Kimura Y, Koga H, Araki N, et al.1998. The involvement of calpain-dependent proteolysis of the tumor suppressor NF2 (merlin) in schwannomas and meningiomas. Nat Med 4:915–922.

Kirsch M, Zhu JJ, Black PM. 1997. Analysis of the BRCA1 and BRCA2 genes in sporadic meningiomas. Genes Chromosomes Cancer 20:53–59.

Kleihues P, Cavenee WK. 2000. Pathology and Genetics of Tumours of the Nervous System. Lyon: IARC Press.

Kondziolka D, Flickinger JC, Perez B. 1998. Judicious resection and/or radiosurgery for parasagittal meningiomas: outcomes from a multicenter review. Gamma Knife Meningioma Study Group. Neurosurgery 43:405–413; discussion, 413–404.

Kondziolka D, Levy EI, Niranjan A, Flickinger JC, Lunsford LD. 1999. Long-term outcomes after meningioma radiosurgery: physician and patient perspectives. J Neurosurg 91:44–50.

Kondziolka D, Lunsford LD. 1992. Radiosurgery of meningiomas. Neurosurg Clin North Am 3:219–230.

Kumar PP, Patil AA, Leibrock LJ, et al. 1993. Continuous low dose rate brachytherapy with high activity iodine-125 seeds in the management of meningiomas. Int J Radiat Oncol Biol Phys 25:325–328.

Kuratsu J, Ushio Y. 1996a. Epidemiological study of primary intracranial tumors: a regional survey in Kumamoto Prefecture in the southern part of Japan. J Neurosurg 84: 946–950.

Kuratsu J, Ushio Y. 1996b. Epidemiological study of primary intracranial tumors in childhood. A population-based survey in Kumamoto Prefecture, Japan. Pediatr Neurosurg 25:240–247.

Kuratsu J, Kochi M, Ushio Y. 2000. Incidence and clinical features of asymptomatic meningiomas. J Neurosurg 92: 766–770.

Kurland LT, Schoenberg BS, Annegers JF, Okazaki H, Molgaard CA. 1982. The incidence of primary intracranial neoplasms in Rochester, Minnesota, 1935–1977. Ann NY Acad Sci 381:6–16.

Lamberts SW, Tanghe HL, Avezaat CJ, et al. 1992. Mifepristone (RU 486) treatment of meningiomas. J Neurol Neurosurg Psychiatry 55:486–490.

Larson JJ, van Loveren HR, Balko MG, Tew JM. 1995. Evidence of meningioma infiltration into cranial nerves: clinical implications for cavernous sinus meningiomas. J Neurosurg 83:596–599.

Lauge A, Lefebvre C, Laurent-Puig P, et al. 1999. No evidence for germline PTEN mutations in families with breast and brain tumours. Int J Cancer 84:216–219.

Lee JH, Sundaram V, Stein DJ, Kinney SE, Stacey DW, Golubic M. 1997. Reduced expression of schwannomin/merlin in human sporadic meningiomas. Neurosurgery 40:578–587.

Lekanne Deprez RH, Groen NA, van Biezen NA, et al. 1991. A t(4;22) in a meningioma points to the localization of a putative tumor-suppressor gene. Am J Hum Genet 48: 783–790.

Leon SP, Zhu J, Black PM. 1994. Genetic aberrations in human brain tumors. Neurosurgery 34:708–722.

Longstreth WT Jr, Dennis LK, McGuire VM, Drangsholt MT, Koepsell TD. 1993. Epidemiology of intracranial meningioma. Cancer 72:639–648.

Louis A. 1771. Memoire sur les Tumeurs Fongueuses de la Dure-Mere. In: Memoires de L'Academie Royale de Chirurgie, vol 5. Paris: P.F. Didot le Jeune, pp 1–59.

Ludwin SK, Rubinstein LJ, Russell DS. 1975. Papillary meningioma: a malignant variant of meningioma. Cancer 36:1363–1373.

Maguire PD, Clough R, Friedman AH, Halperin EC. 1999. Fractionated external-beam radiation therapy for meningiomas of the cavernous sinus. Int J Radiat Oncol Biol Phys 44:75–79.

Mahmood A, Caccamo DV, Tomecek FJ, Malik GM. 1993. Atypical and malignant meningiomas: a clinicopathological review. Neurosurgery 33:955–963.

Maier H, Ofner D, Hittmair A, Kitz K, Budka H. 1992. Classic, atypical, and anaplastic meningioma: three histopathological subtypes of clinical relevance. J Neurosurg 77:616–623.

Maire JP, Caudry M, Guerin J, et al. 1995. Fractionated radiation therapy in the treatment of intracranial meningiomas: local control, functional efficacy, and tolerance in 91 patients. Int J Radiat Oncol Biol Phys 33:315–321.

Maltby EL, Ironside JW, Battersby RD. 1988. Cytogenetic studies in 50 meningiomas. Cancer Genet Cytogenet 31:199–210.

Mantle RE, Lach B, Delgado MR, Baeesa S, Belanger G. 1999. Predicting the probability of meningioma recurrence based on the quantity of peritumoral brain edema on computerized tomography scanning. J Neurosurg 91:375–383.

Markwalder TM, Waelti E, Konig MP. 1987. Endocrine manipulation of meningiomas with medroxyprogesterone acetate. Effect of MPA on receptor status of meningioma cytosols. Surg Neurol 28:3–9.

Martuza RL, Eldridge R. 1988. Neurofibromatosis 2 (bilateral acoustic neurofibromatosis). N Engl J Med 318:684–688.

Martuza RL, MacLaughlin DT, Ojemann RG. 1981. Specific estradiol binding in schwannomas, meningiomas, and neurofibromas. Neurosurgery 9:665–671.

Martuza RL, Miller DC, MacLaughlin DT. 1985. Estrogen and progestin binding by cytosolic and nuclear fractions of human meningiomas. J Neurosurg 62:750–756.

Mashiyama S, Murakami Y, Yoshimoto T, Sekiya T, Hayashi K. 1991. Detection of p53 gene mutations in human brain tumors by single-strand conformation polymorphism analysis of polymerase chain reaction products. Oncogene 6:1313–1318.

Matyja E, Taraszewska A, Marszalek P. 1999. Necrosis and apoptosis of tumor cells in embolized meningiomas: histopathology and P53, BCL-2, CD-68 immunohistochemistry. Folia Neuropathol 37:93–98.

Maxwell M, Galanopoulos T, Hedley-Whyte ET, Black PM, Antoniades HN. 1990. Human meningiomas co-express platelet-derived growth factor (PDGF) and PDGF-receptor genes and their protein products. Int J Cancer 46:16–21.

Maxwell M, Galanopoulos T, Neville-Golden J, Antoniades HN. 1993. Expression of androgen and progesterone receptors in primary human meningiomas J Neurosurg 78:456–462.

Maxwell M, Shih SD, Galanopoulos T, Hedley-Whyte ET, Cosgrove GR. 1998. Familial meningioma: analysis of expression of neurofibromatosis 2 protein Merlin. Report of two cases. J Neurosurg 88:562–569.

McCarthy BJ, Davis FG, Freels S, et al. 1998. Factors associated with survival in patients with meningioma. J Neurosurg 88:831–839.

McDermott M, Wilson C. 1996. Meningiomas. In: Youmans JR (ed), Neurological Surgery: A Comprehensive Reference Guide to the Diagnosis and Management of Neurosurgical Problems, 4th ed. Philadelphia: Saunders, pp 2782–2825.

McDermott MW. 1996. Current treatment of meningiomas. Curr Opin Neurol 9:409–413.

McDonald JD, Dohrmann GJ. 1988. Molecular biology of brain tumors. Neurosurgery 23:537–544.

Merel P, Haong-Xuan K, Sanson M, et al. 1995a. Predominant occurrence of somatic mutations of the NF2 gene in meningiomas and schwannomas. Genes Chromosomes Cancer 13:211–216.

Merel P, Khe HX, Sanson M, et al. 1995b. Screening for germline mutations in the NF2 gene. Genes Chromosomes Cancer 12:117–127.

Miller JW, Adamis AP, Shima DT, et al. 1994. Vascular endothelial growth factor/vascular permeability factor is temporally and spatially correlated with ocular angiogenesis in a primate model. Am J Pathol 145:574–584.

Milosevic MF, Frost PJ, Laperriere NJ, Wong CS, Simpson WJ. 1996. Radiotherapy for atypical or malignant intracranial meningioma. Int J Radiat Oncol Biol Phys 34:817–822.

Miralbell R, Linggood RM, de la Monte S, Vonvery K, Munzenrider JE, Mirimanoff RO. 1992. The role of radiotherapy in the treatment of subtotally resected benign meningiomas. J Neurooncol 13:157–164.

Morita A, Coffey RJ, Foote RL, Schiff D, Gorman D. 1999. Risk of injury to cranial nerves after gamma knife radiosurgery for skull base meningiomas: experience in 88 patients. J Neurosurg 90:42–49.

Musa BS, Pople IK, Cummins BH. 1995. Intracranial meningiomas following irradiation—a growing problem? Br J Neurosurg 9:629–637.

Nakasu S, Nakajima M, Nakazawa T, Nakasu Y, Handa J. 1998. Alteration of bcl-2 and bax expression in embolized meningiomas. Brain Tumor Pathol 15:13–17.

Nakasu S, Nakajima M, Nakazawa T, Nakasu Y, Handa J. 1997. p53 accumulation and apoptosis in embolized meningiomas. Acta Neuropathol (Berl) 93:599–605.

Narayansingh GV, Ramsewak S, Cross JN, Adam RU, Kissoon W. 1992. Worsening neurological status in late pregnancy: consider meningioma. Postgrad Med J 68:486.

Netsky M, Lapresle J. 1956. The first account of a meningioma. Bull Hist Med 30:465–468.

New PF, Aronow S, Hesselink JR. 1980. National Cancer Institute study: evaluation of computed tomography in the diagnosis of intracranial neoplasms. IV. Meningiomas. Radiology 136:665–675.

Nordqvist AC, Peyrard M, Pettersson H, et al. 1997. A high ratio of insulin-like growth factor II/insulin-like growth factor binding protein 2 messenger RNA as a marker for anaplasia in meningiomas. Cancer Res 57:2611–2614, 1997.

Nutting C, Brada M, Brazil L, et al. 1999. Radiotherapy in the treatment of benign meningioma of the skull base. J Neurosurg 90:823–827.

Ohgaki H, Eibl RH, Schwab M, et al. 1993. Mutations of the p53 tumor suppressor gene in neoplasms of the human nervous system. Mol Carcinog 8:74–80.

Ojemann SG, Sneed PK, Larson DA, et al. 2000. Radiosurgery for malignant meningioma: results in 22 patients. J Neurosurg 93:62–67.

Olivero WC, Lister JR, Elwood PW. 1995. The natural history and growth rate of asymptomatic meningiomas: a review of 60 patients. J Neurosurg 83:222–224.

Olson JJ, Beck DW, Schlechte JA, Loh PM. 1987. Effect of the antiprogesterone RU-38486 on meningioma implanted into nude mice. J Neurosurg 66:584–587.

O'Rahilly R, Muller F. 1986. The meninges in human development. J Neuropathol Exp Neurol 45:588–608.

Oura S, Sakurai T, Yoshimura G, et al. 2000. Regression of a presumed meningioma with the antiestrogen agent mepitiostane. Case report. J Neurosurg 93:132–135.

Paleologos TS, Wadley JP, Kitchen ND, Thomas DG. 2000. Clinical utility and cost-effectiveness of interactive image-guided craniotomy: clinical comparison between conventional and image-guided meningioma surgery Neurosurgery 47:40–48.

Palma L, Celli P, Franco C, Cervoni L, Cantore G. 1997. Long-term prognosis for atypical and malignant meningiomas: a study of 71 surgical cases. J Neurosurg 86:793–800.

Park K, Kim JH, Nam DH, et al. 2000. Vascular endothelial growth factor expression under ischemic stress in human meningiomas. Neurosci Lett 283:45–48.

Parry DM, MacCollin MM, Kaiser-Kupfer MI, et al. 1996. Germline mutations in the neurofibromatosis 2 gene: correlations with disease severity and retinal abnormalities. Am J Hum Genet 59:529–539.

Pasquier B, Gasnier F, Pasquier D, Keddari E, Morens A, Couderc P. 1986. Papillary meningioma. Clinicopathologic study of seven cases and review of the literature. Cancer 58:299–305.

Perry A, Scheithauer BW, Stafford SL, Lohse CM, Wollan PC. 1999. "Malignancy" in meningiomas. A clinicopathologic study of 116 patients, with grading implications. Cancer 85:2046–2056.

Peyrard M, Seroussi E, Sandberg-Nordqvist AC, et al. 1999. The human LARGE gene from 22q12.3–q13.1 is a new, distinct member of the glycosyltransferase gene family. Proc Natl Acad Sci USA 96:598–603.

Provias J, Claffey K, delAguila L, Lau N, Feldkamp M, Guha A. 1997. Meningiomas: role of vascular endothelial growth factor/vascular permeability factor in angiogenesis and peritumoral edema. Neurosurgery 40:1016–1026.

Preston-Martin S. 1989. Descriptive epidemiology of primary tumors of the brain, cranial nerves and cranial meninges in Los Angeles County. Neuroepidemiology 8:283–295.

Rachlin J, Rosenblum M. 1991. Etiology and biology of meningiomas. In: Al-Mefty O (ed), Meningiomas. New York: Raven Press, pp 27–36.

Roche PH, Regis J, Dufour H, et al. 2000. Gamma knife radiosurgery in the management of cavernous sinus meningiomas. J Neurosurg 93:68–73.

Roelvink NC, Kamphorst W, August H, van Alphen M, Rao BR. 1987a. Literature statistics do not support a growth stimulating role for female sex steroid hormones in haemangiomas and meningiomas. J Neurooncol 11:243–253.

Roelvink NC, Kamphorst W, van Alphen HA, Rao BR. 1987b. Pregnancy-related primary brain and spinal tumors. Arch Neurol 44:209–215.

Ron E, Modan B, Boice JD Jr. 1988a. Mortality after radiotherapy for ringworm of the scalp. Am J Epidemiol 127:713–725.

Ron E, Modan B, Boice JD Jr,, et al. 1988b. Tumors of the brain and nervous system after radiotherapy in childhood. N Engl J Med 319:1033–1039.

Rosenthal RA, Moses MA, Shintani Y, Megyesi JF, Langer R, Folkman J. 1994. Purification and characterization of two collagenase inhibitors from mouse sarcoma 180 conditioned medium. J Cell Biochem 56:97–105.

Rouleau GA, Haines JL, Bazanowski A, et al. 1989. A genetic linkage map of the long arm of human chromosome 22. Genomics 4:1–6.

Rouleau GA, Merel P, Lutchman M, et al. 1993. Alteration in a new gene encoding a putative membrane-organizing protein causes neuro-fibromatosis type 2. Nature 363: 515–521.

Rouleau GA, Wertelecki W, Haines JL, et al. 1987. Genetic linkage of bilateral acoustic neurofibromatosis to a DNA marker on chromosome 22. Nature 329:246–248.

Rubinstein AB, Schein M, Reichenthal E. 1989. The association of carcinoma of the breast with meningioma. Surg Gynecol Obstet 169:334–336.

Russell DS, Rubinstein LJ. 1989. Pathology of Tumours of the Nervous System, 5th ed. Baltimore: Williams & Wilkins, p 1012.

Ruttledge MH, Sarrazin J, Rangaratnam S, et al. 1994. Evidence for the complete inactivation of the NF2 gene in the majority of sporadic meningiomas. Nat Genet 6:180–184.

Saitoh Y, Oku Y, Izumoto S, Go J. 1989. Rapid growth of a meningioma during pregnancy: relationship with estrogen and progesterone receptors—case report. Neurol Med Chir (Tokyo) 29:440–443.

Samii M, Ammirati M. 1988. The combined supra-infratentorial pre-sigmoid sinus avenue to the petro-clival region. Surgical technique and clinical applications. Acta Neurochir (Wien) 95:6–12.

Schmidek HH. 1991. Meningiomas and their Surgical Management. Philadelphia: Saunders, p 557.

Schoenberg BS. 1977. Multiple primary neoplasms and the nervous system. Cancer 40:1961–1967.

Schoenberg BS, Christine BW, Whisnant JP. 1975. Nervous system neoplasms and primary malignancies of other sites. The unique association between meningiomas and breast cancer. Neurology 25:705–712.

Schrell UM, Rittig MG, Anders M, et al. 1997. Hydroxyurea for treatment of unresectable and recurrent meningiomas. I. Inhibition of primary human meningioma cells in culture and in meningioma transplants by induction of the apoptotic pathway. J Neurosurg 86:845–852.

Schwartz MR, Randolph RL, Cech DA, Rose JE, Panko WB. 1984. Steroid hormone binding macromolecules in meningiomas. Failure to meet criteria of specific receptors. Cancer 53:922–927.

Seizinger BR, de la Monte S, Atkins L, Gusella JF, Martuza RL. 1987a. Molecular genetic approach to human meningioma: loss of genes on chromosome 22. Proc Natl Acad Sci USA 84:5419–5423.

Seizinger BR, Martuza RL, Rouleau G, Breakefield XO, Gusella JF. 1987b. Models for inherited susceptibility to cancer in the nervous system: a molecular-genetic approach to neurofibromatosis. Dev Neurosci 9:144–153.

Seizinger BR, Rouleau G, Lane AH, et al. 1987c. DNA linkage analysis in von Recklinghausen neurofibromatosis. J Med Genet 24:529–530

Seizinger BR, Rouleau G, Ozelius LJ, et al. 1987d. Common pathogenetic mechanism for three tumor types in bilateral acoustic neurofibromatosis. Science 236:317–319.

Sen C, Hague K. 1997. Meningiomas involving the cavernous sinus: histological factors affecting the degree of resection. J Neurosurg 87:535–543.

Shafron DH, Friedman WA, Buatti JM, Bova FJ, Mendenhall WM. 1999. Linac radiosurgery for benign meningiomas. Int J Radiat Oncol Biol Phys 43:321–327.

Shamah SM, Alberta JA, Giannobile WV, et al. 1997. Detection of activated platelet-derived growth factor receptors in human meningioma. Cancer Res 57:4141–4147.

Shima DT, Adamis AP, Ferrara N, et al. 1995. Hypoxic induction of endothelial cell growth factors in retinal cells: identification and characterization of vascular endothelial growth factor (VEGF) as the mitogen. Mol Med 1:182–193.

Shu J, Lee JH, Harwalkar JA, Oh-Siskovic S, Stacey DW, Golubic M. 1999. Adenovirus-mediated gene transfer of dominant negative Ha-Ras inhibits proliferation of primary meningioma cells. Neurosurgery 44:579–587; discussion, 587–578.

Simpson D. 1957. The recurrence of intracranial meningiomas after surgical treatment. J Neurol Neurosurg Psychiatry 20:22–39.

Singh VP, Kansai S, Vaishya S, Julka PK, Mehta VS. 2000. Early complications following gamma knife radiosurgery for intracranial meningiomas. J Neurosurg 93(suppl 3):57–61.

Smith DA, Cahill DW. 1994. The biology of meningiomas. Neurosurg Clin North Am 5:201–215.

Subach BR, Lunsford LD, Kondziolka D, Maltz AH, Flickinger JC. 1998. Management of petroclival meningiomas by stereotactic radiosurgery. Neurosurgery 42:437–445.

Sulman EP, Dumanski JP, White PS, et al. 1998. Identification of a consistent region of allelic loss on 1p32 in meningiomas: correlation with increased morbidity. Cancer Res 58:3226–3230.

Sundaram V, Lee JH, Harwalkar JA, et al. 1997. Reduced expression of neurofibromin in human meningiomas. Br J Cancer 76:747–756.

Tanaka K, Sato C, Maeda Y, et al. 1989. Establishment of a human malignant meningioma cell line with amplified c-myc oncogene. Cancer 64:2243–2249.

Tilzer LL, Plapp FV, Evans JP, Stone D, Alward K. 1982. Steroid receptor proteins in human meningiomas. Cancer 49:633–636.

Todo T, Adams EF, Fahlbusch R, Dingermann T, Werner H. 1996. Autocrine growth stimulation of human meningioma cells by platelet-derived growth factor. J Neurosurg 84:852–858; discussion, 858–859.

Trofatter JA, MacCollin MM, Rutter JL, et al. 1993. A novel

moesin-, ezrin-, radixin-like gene is a candidate for the neurofibromatosis 2 tumor suppressor [published erratum appears in Cell 1993 Nov 19;75(4):826]. Cell 72:791–800.

Tsai JC, Hsiao YY, Teng LJ, et al. 1999. Regulation of vascular endothelial growth factor secretion in human meningioma cells. J Formos Med Assoc 98:111–117.

Tsuzuki T, Tsunoda S, Sakaki T, et al. 1996. Tumor cell proliferation and apoptosis associated with the Gamma Knife effect. Stereotact Funct Neurosurg 66:39–48.

Twist EC, Ruttledge MH, Rousseau M, et al. 1994. The neurofibromatosis type 2 gene is inactivated in schwannomas. Hum Mol Genet 3:147–151.

Vagner-Capodano AM, Grisoli F, Gambarelli D, Sedan R, Pellet W, De Victor B. 1993. Correlation between cytogenetic and histopathological findings in 75 human meningiomas. Neurosurgery 32:892–900; discussion, 900.

Valentino V, Schinaia G, Raimondi AJ. 1993. The results of radiosurgical management of 72 middle fossa meningiomas. Acta Neurochir (Wien) 122:60–70.

Vuorinen V, Heikkonen J, Brander A, et al. 1996. Interstitial radiotherapy of 25 parasellar/clival meningiomas and 19 meningiomas in the elderly. Analysis of short-term tolerance and responses. Acta Neurochir (Wien) 138: 495–508.

Wan WL, Geller JL, Feldon SE, Sadun AA. 1990. Visual loss caused by rapidly progressive intracranial meningiomas during pregnancy. Ophthalmology 97:18–21.

Weisman AS, Raguet SS, Kelly PA. 1987. Characterization of the epidermal growth factor receptor in human meningioma. Cancer Res 47:2172–2176.

Weisman AS, Villemure JG, Kelly PA. 1986. Regulation of DNA synthesis and growth of cells derived from primary human meningiomas. Cancer Res 46:2545–2550.

Wilson CB. 1994. Meningiomas: genetics, malignancy, and the role of radiation in induction and treatment. The Richard C. Schneider Lecture. J Neurosurg 81:666–675.

Young JL Jr, Percy CL, Asire AJ. 1981. Surveillance, epidemiology, and end results: incidence and mortality data, 1973–1977. Prepared by Demographic Analysis Section, Division of Cancer Cause and Prevention, National Cancer Institute.

Younis GA, Sawaya R, DeMonte F, Hess KR, Albrecht S, Bruner JM. 1995. Aggressive meningeal tumors: review of a series. J Neurosurg 82:17–27.

Zang KD, Singer H. 1967. Chromosomal consitution of meningiomas. Nature 216:84–85.

Zee CS, Chen T, Hinton DR, Tan M, Segall HD, Apuzzo ML. 1995. Magnetic resonance imaging of cystic meningiomas and its surgical implications. Neurosurgery 36:482–488.

Zhang ZJ, Muhr C, Wang JL. 1996. Interferon-alpha inhibits the DNA synthesis induced by PDGF and EGF in cultured meningioma cells. Anticancer Res 16:717–723.

Zwarthoff EC. 1996. Neurofibromatosis and associated tumour suppressor genes. Pathol Res Pract 192:647–657.

12

Skull Base Tumors

MIKHAIL CHERNOV AND FRANCO DEMONTE

Skull base tumors arise from the cranial base or reach it, either from an intracranial or extracranial origin. A diverse group, these tumors present unique management challenges because of their relative rarity, typically deep location, close proximity to critical neurovascular structures, and extension beyond classically taught anatomic and specialty boundaries. Management outcomes for skull base tumors are maximized when their treatment is approached in a multidisciplinary fashion, utilizing the knowledge base of varied medical, surgical, and radiotherapeutic specialists.

CLASSIFICATION

Skull base tumors may originate from the neurovascular structures of the base of the brain and the basal meninges (e.g., meningioma, pituitary adenoma, schwannoma, paraganglioma), the cranial base itself (e.g., chordoma, chondrosarcoma), or the subcranial structures of the head and neck (e.g., paranasal sinus carcinomas). A unified classification system does not exist for the plethora of pathologies, some quite rare, that may affect this area of the brain (Table 12–1).

Classifications based on location are useful for clinicopathologic correlation due to the relatively constant constellation of signs and symptoms produced by tumors located in specific regions of the skull base and due to the propensity for certain tumor pathologies to have a regional specificity (Table 12–2). Tumor location is also the prime determinant of the surgical approach that is selected.

Whereas location is the most important consideration for surgical planning, the tumor's biologic behavior dictates the need for, and order of, the various available therapies needed to optimize patient outcome. Some tumors, such as meningiomas and schwannomas, may require complete surgical excision only to optimize patient outcome. Pathologies such as paranasal sinus carcinomas may, however, require induction chemotherapy, surgical excision, and radiation therapy (RT) to achieve local control and possibly cure (Table 12–3).

In general, the outcome of surgery for basal tumors depends on the type, size, and location of the neoplasm, patient's age and general medical status, and extent of preoperative neurologic disability (Lang et al., 1999). Large tumor size, encasement of major cerebral arteries, invasion of the cavernous sinus and severe brain stem compression can necessitate incomplete tumor resection, whereas older age and low preoperative Karnofsky score have been associated with increased risk of stroke and longer hospital stay (Holmes et al., 1995).

MENINGIOMA

Meningiomas (see Chapter 11) occur with an incidence of 2.6 per 100,000 persons per year and account for 20% of all intracranial tumors. Forty percent of all meningiomas arise from the base of the anterior, middle, or posterior fossa and are the most common skull base tumors. Sphenoid wing meningiomas make up almost half of these tumors; tuber-

Table 12–1. Tumors of the Skull Base

Site of Tumor Origin	*Tumor Pathology*
Basal neurovascular structures and meninges	Meningioma Schwannoma Pituitary adenoma Craniopharyngioma Paraganglioma Hemangiopericytoma
Cranial base	Chordoma Chondrosarcoma Osteosarcoma Plasmacytoma Metastasis
Subcranial with upward extension	Sinonasal carcinomas Olfactory neuroblastoma Juvenile angiofibroma Nasopharyngeal carcinoma Adenoid cystic carcinoma Primary sarcomas

Table 12–2. Classification of Skull-Base Tumors Based on Location

Location	*Clinical Features*	*Common Pathologies*
Anterior skull base	Anosmia, frontal lobe dysfunction, increased intracranial pressure, nasal obstruction, epistaxis, visual changes	Meningioma, olfactory neuroblastoma, sinonasal malignancies
Middle skull base		
Central	Pituitary hypo- or hyperfunction, optic neuropathy (nerve and chiasm)	Pituitary adenoma, meningioma, craniopharyngioma, sphenoid sinus carcinoma
Paracentral	Optic neuropathy, sphenocavernous syndrome	Meningioma, schwannoma, adenoid cystic carcinoma, nasopharyngeal carcinoma
Lateral	Proptosis, facial dysesthesia and pain, trismus, epistaxis	Meningioma, schwannoma, juvenile nasal angiofibroma, adenoid cystic carcinoma, sarcoma
Posterior skull base		
Cerebellopontine angle	Hearing loss, facial numbness or weakness, dysmetria, ataxia, lower cranial nerve dysfunction, brain stem signs, increased intracranial pressure	Acoustic neuroma, meningioma, epidermoid, trigeminal neuroma, cholesterol granuloma
Clival	Abducens palsy, bilateral cranial neuropathies, brain stem signs	Chordoma, meningioma, paraganglioma, nasopharyngeal carcinoma, schwannoma, chondrosarcoma
Jugular foramen	Palsies of cranial nerves 9,10,11 (Vernet's syndrome), 9,10,11,12 (Collet-Sicard syndrome), 9,10,11,12, and sympathetics (Villaret's syndrome)	Paraganglioma, schwannoma, meningioma, metastasis
Foramen magnum	Suboccipital neck pain (C2 dermatome), ipsilateral dysesthesias, contralateral dissociated sensory loss, progressive weakness, wasting of intrinsic hand muscles	Meningioma, schwannoma, chordoma, intramedullary tumor

Table 12–3. Classification of Skull-Base Tumors by Biologic Behavior

Benign	Meningioma, schwannoma, paraganglioma, pituitary adenoma, dermoid, epidermoid, juvenile angiofibroma, cholesterol granuloma, osteoma
Low-grade malignancy	Chordoma, chondrosarcoma, adenoid cystic carcinoma, desmoid, low-grade fibrosarcoma, olfactory neuroblastoma, low-grade sarcomas, hemangiopericytoma
High-grade malignancy	Carcinomas, high-grade sarcomas (e.g., rhabdomyosarcoma, Ewing's sarcoma, osteogenic), lymphoma, metastases

culum sella tumors and olfactory groove tumors comprise the other half. Meningiomas of the posterior and middle fossa are less common, with incidences of 8% and 4%, respectively.

PITUITARY ADENOMA

In 2.6% to 15% of cases pituitary adenomas (see Chapter 8) may attain giant size (more than 4 to 5 cm in any direction) and exhibit extensive invasion of the skull base and paranasal sinuses (Pia et al., 1985; Majos et al., 1998). These are mainly endocrinologically inactive tumors in the elderly and prolactinomas in the young. Clinical and imaging features of giant pituitary adenomas differ from tumors that are smaller in size.

SCHWANNOMA

Intracranial nerve sheath tumors represent only 4% to 8% of intracranial neoplasms with the most common being vestibular schwannomas, followed by trigeminal nerve tumors. These neoplasms can arise, although infrequently, from other cranial nerves, both intra- and extracranially. Although schwannomas can develop as an isolated disease process, most intracranial nonvestibular tumors and 5% of vestibular schwannomas are associated with neurofibromatosis type 2 (NF2).

Pathology and Pathogenesis

Schwannomas are typically globoid, ovoid, or dumbbell-shaped, well-circumscribed tumors. They arise from Schwann cells, which form the myelin sheaths surrounding peripheral nerves. Tumors may have small or large cystic components and can be moderately vascular. The cellular components of schwannomas are typically organized into densely packed hypercellular areas of spindly cells ("Antoni type A") with intervening hypocellular zones composed of loosely organized stellate cells ("Antoni type B"). The compact Antoni type A tissue often, but not invariably, exhibits prominent nuclear palisading (Verocay bodies). Cytologically, no differences are found between spontaneous and familial tumors; however, on histologic examination approximately 40% of the NF2 neoplasms appear to have grapelike clusters that can infiltrate the fibers of the individual nerves. Growth fraction varies from 0.36% to 3.15% (Lesser et al., 1991).

Diagnosis and Treatment

Vestibular Schwannomas

Vestibular schwannomas represent nearly 6% of all intracranial tumors. The tumors arise at the transitional zone between the central and peripheral myelin sheaths of the nerve. The majority of neoplasms originate within the internal auditory canal; however, more medially located tumors constitute 10% to 15% of cases. Whereas tumors in the more typical location compress the adjacent auditory nerve early in their growth, the medial tumors may grow to a significant size without causing hearing loss. Clinical features, as well as treatment strategy and prognosis, are greatly influenced by the size and extension of the tumor.

Unilateral hearing loss occurs in more than 90% of patients and is often accompanied by tinnitus. Cochlear nerve dysfunction usually is the most long-standing symptom followed by vestibular disturbances, which may have an intermittent course. Imbalance is encountered in 50% of cases and vertigo in 19%. Trigeminal nerve signs are the third most common symptom, with 50% of patients reporting facial numbness (Pitts et al., 1996). Larger tumors can cause facial weakness, signs of brain stem compression, and obstructive hydrocephalus. The average duration of symptoms is 3.7 years (Matthies and Samii, 1997). By the time of diagnosis 63% to 80% of vestibular schwannomas already fill the cerebellopontine cistern with or without compression of the brain stem (Matthies and Samii, 1997; Gormley et al., 1997) (Fig. 12–1).

Management alternatives include observation, microsurgical removal, and stereotactic radiosurgery. Currently, the ideal treatment for symptomatic patients with vestibular schwannoma is complete microsurgical excision of the tumor. Concomitant goals include preservation of facial nerve function, low morbidity and mortality, and, when possible, preservation of hearing.

The choice of surgical approach needs to take into account the size and the amount of extension of the tumor into the internal auditory canal (IAC) as well as the patient's hearing ability and experience of the surgical team. Every attempt should be made to preserve useful hearing, although it must be realized that when the tumor is greater than 2 cm in size or when it fills the fundus of the IAC this goal is not often realized. Total tumor removal can be accomplished in most patients, with less than a 1% mortality and excellent long-term tumor control. Hearing preservation is possible in 48% of small tumors, 25% of medium, and only occasionally in cases of large neoplasms. Similarly, facial nerve function can be preserved in 96% of small tumors, 74% of medium, and 38% of large tumors (Gormley et al., 1997).

Stereotactic radiosurgery is the principal alternative to microsurgical resection of vestibular schwan-

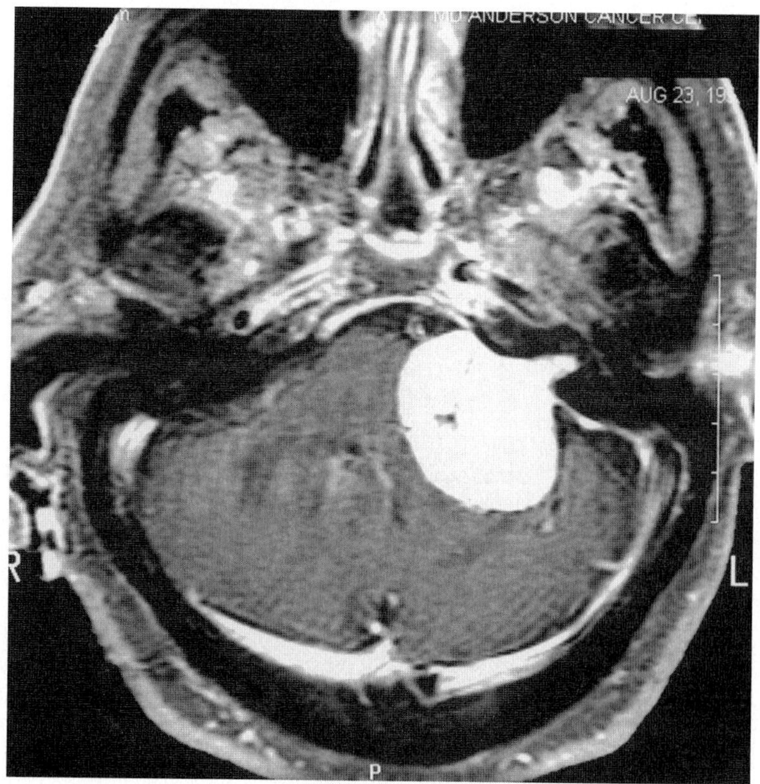

Figure 12–1. Axial post-contrast T_1-weighted MRI reveals a giant left-sided acoustic neuroma. Note the extension of the tumor to the lateral end of the internal auditory canal and the marked brain stem compression.

nomas. The goals of radiosurgical treatment are prevention of tumor growth, maintenance of neurologic function, and prevention of new neurologic deficits (Kondziolka et al., 1998). The rate of tumor control (shrinkage or stabilization of the neoplasm) is 96.9% at 3 and 5 years (Fig. 12–2). Ogunrinde et al. (1994) reported facial nerve function of grade I or II in 100% of patients post-treatment, dropping to 95% at 2 year follow up. Two years after radiosurgery 25% of patients still had mild residual trigeminal nerve sensory symptoms. The incidence of hearing preservation is typically 100% immediately following treatment but drops to 50% at 6 months and to 45% at both 1 and 2 years following treatment (Ogunrinde et al., 1994). A trend of improved rates of hearing preservation with smaller tumor diameters was noted.

During the first 4 years after radiosurgical treatment 2% to 3% of patients required microsurgical removal of tumors (Pollock et al., 1998; Sims et al., 1999; Shirato et al., 1999).

Trigeminal Nerve Schwannomas

Schwannomas of the trigeminal nerve account for 0.07% to 0.36% of intracranial tumors and 0.8% to 8% of intracranial Schwann cell tumors (McCormick et al., 1988; Pollack et al., 1989). One-half of these tumors are primarily located in the middle fossa arising from the ganglionic segment of the trigeminal nerve (Jefferson's type A tumors [Jefferson, 1955]).

Trigeminal schwannomas of the ganglionic segment result in facial numbness or pain and corneal hypesthesia in 80% to 90% of patients, which are the initial complaints in about 60% of these patients. A few patients (10% to 20%), however, never develop trigeminal dysfunction. Tumors of the ganglionic segment are more frequently associated with facial pain (52%) than those of the trigeminal root (28%) (McCormick et al., 1988). Diplopia is the initial symptom in about 15% of patients, but is present in 50% by the time of diagnosis and is usually due to an abducens palsy. Facial weakness and hearing loss are rare symptoms of this lesion. When they occur the presumptive mechanisms are through involvement of the greater superficial petrosal nerve, facial nerve, and eustachian tube or cochlea in the temporal bone.

Tumors of the trigeminal root account for 20% to 30% of trigeminal schwannomas and are usually confined to the posterior fossa (Jefferson's type B tumors). The clinical presentation is usually a combination of hearing loss, tinnitus, and facial nerve and cerebellar dysfunction. Early trigeminal symptomatology may imply the diagnosis, but as many as 10% of patients with vestibular schwannomas initially present with trigeminal nerve dysfunction. As a corollary, 6% of patients with trigeminal schwannomas initially complain of hearing loss.

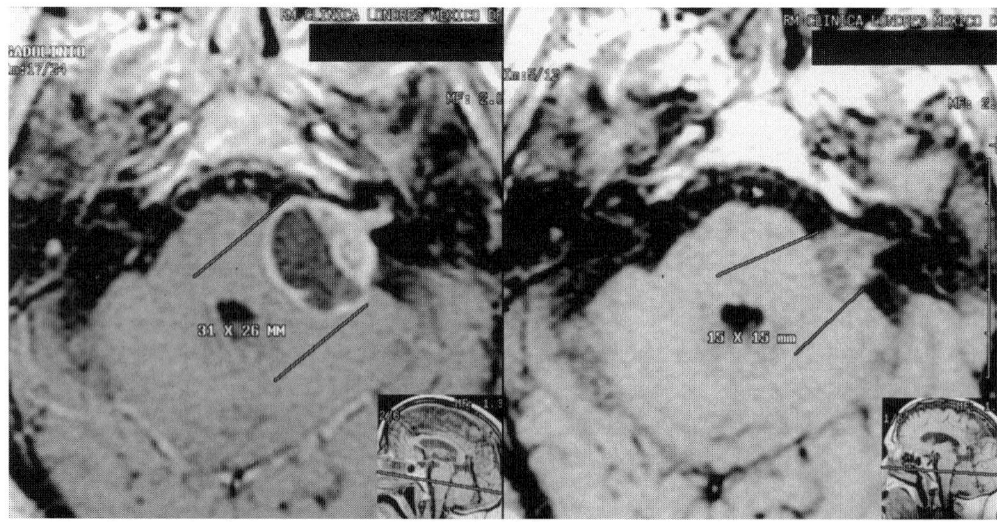

Figure 12–2. Pretreatment (left) and post-treatment (right) axial T_1-weighted MRIs demonstrate a marked reduction in size of a cystic acoustic neuroma treated by gamma knife radiosurgery. The post-treatment scan was performed without contrast.

Impairment of lower cranial nerve function and long tract signs are noted at diagnosis in 30% to 50% of patients.

Dumbbell-shaped tumors, which occupy both the middle and posterior fossae, make up 15% to 25% of all trigeminal schwannomas (Jefferson's type C tumors). Their clinical presentation is a composite of the symptoms and signs of tumors occurring in the ganglionic segment and in the posterior fossa (Fig. 12–3).

Complete excision, as for vestibular schwannomas, nearly always results in cure and is the goal of each surgical procedure. When results from five recent surgical reports were combined, 72 of 93 patients had a gross total tumor excision (GTR), 9 of 93 had a near total excision (NTR), and 12 of 93 had a subtotal or partial resection (STR). One recurrence was noted following GTR. Tumor progression occurred in 6 of 9 of near-total resections and in 5 of 12 subtotal resections (Bordi et al., 1989; Dolenc, 1994; McCormick et al., 1988; Pollack et al., 1989; Samii et al., 1995a). Tumors of the trigeminal root were generally approached through a retrosigmoid craniectomy, whereas a variety of approaches were necessary for the middle fossa or dumbbell-shaped tumors. These approaches included the standard subtemporal approach (Bordi et al., 1989; McCormick et al., 1988), the frontotemporal epidural approach (Dolenc, 1994), and combined approaches such as the petrosal (Samii et al., 1995b), supra- and infratentorial approach (McCormick et al., 1988), or subtemporal and infratemporal approaches (Pollack et al., 1989).

Before 1970, a mortality rate of 25% had been reported for patients with these tumors. In the recent surgical series noted above there was only one instance of operative mortality reported. Morbidity consisted mainly of new or worsened trigeminal deficits in 43 of 93 patients (46%), although instances of improvement occurred. Other morbidity included ab-

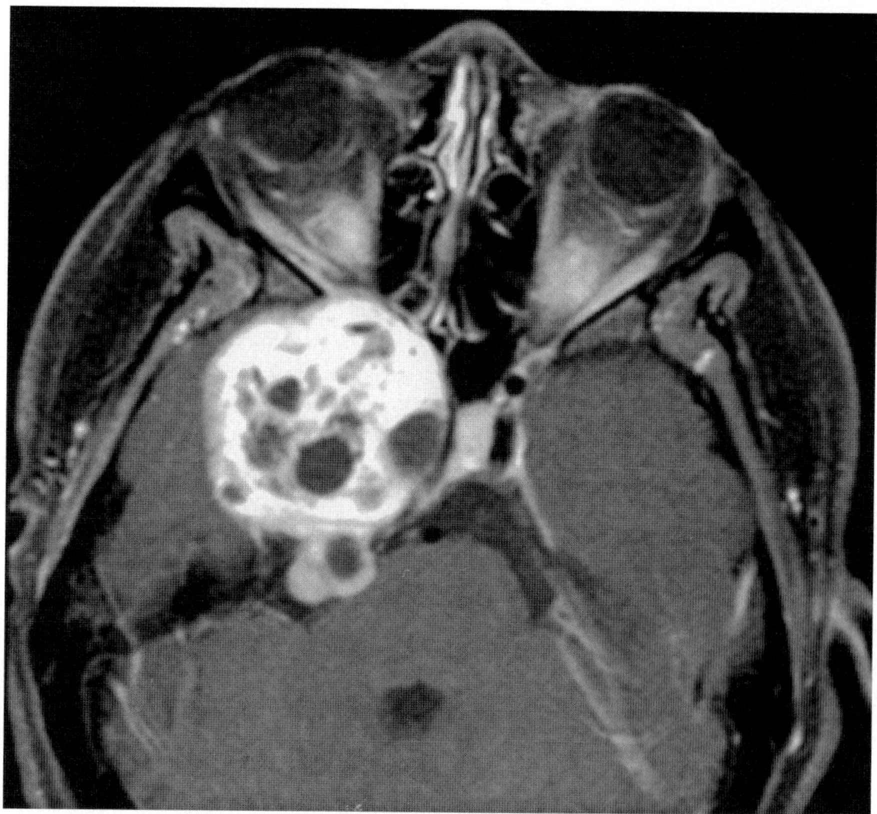

Figure 12–3. Axial post-contrast T_1-weighted MRI reveals a dumbbell-shaped trigeminal schwannoma predominately involving the right middle fossa with extension through Meckel's cave into the posterior fossa.

ducens nerve palsies in two, facial palsy in two, and hearing loss in three patients.

Radiosurgical treatment of a group of 16 patients with trigeminal schwannomas achieved a tumor control rate of 100%, improvement of neurologic symptoms in 5 patients, and absence of any new neurologic deficits during the evaluation period (follow-up, 44 months; Huang et al., 1999).

Facial Nerve Schwannomas

Slowly progressive facial weakness is the typical clinical presentation of a facial nerve schwannoma. Although sudden facial weakness occurs in approximately 11% of cases, 27% of patients with facial nerve schwannomas never manifest facial weakness. Facial spasm has been reported in as many as 17% of patients. Hearing loss of a conductive, sensorineural, or mixed nature occurs in approximately 50% of patients. Facial schwannomas located in the middle ear may cause conductive hearing loss, whereas tumors in the labyrinth and internal auditory channel usually result in cochlear or retrocochlear hearing dysfunction, respectively. Tinnitus and vertigo, or dizziness, occur in 13% and 10%, respectively. External manifestations of the tumor such as a mass, pain, or otorrhea occur in 30% or more of patients (Lipkin et al., 1987).

These tumors are rare, accounting for only 1.5% of cerebellopontine angle tumors (Baker and Ojemann, 1993). Schwannomas of the facial nerve involve the tympanic or vertical segments in most patients (58% and 48%, respectively) and multiple segments are almost always affected.

Facial schwannomas may appear as a soft tissue mass in the tympanomastoid compartment, cerebellopontine angle, or middle fossa, accompanied by destruction of the fallopian canal and/or widening of the IAC, in which case differentiation from vestibular schwannomas may be a challenge (O'Donoghue et al., 1989). Imaging features specific for facial neuromas include enlargement of the labyrinthine segment of the fallopian canal associated with a middle fossa mass; erosion of the anterosuperior aspect of the internal auditory canal; and contrast enhancement of the geniculate ganglion and distal facial nerve in the case of cerebellopontine angle tumor (Inoue et al., 1987; Parnes et al., 1991).

Rarely, the tumor, if small, may be separable from the nerve, but in most cases resection and facial nerve grafting are required (Dort and Fisch, 1991; King and Morrison, 1990; O'Donoghue et al., 1989). At best, a House grade 3 facial weakness can be expected following facial nerve grafting. Complete excision is curative.

Schwannomas of the Jugular Foramen (Nerves IX, X, XI)

Although it is difficult, if not impossible, to identify the specific nerve of origin (Pluchino et al., 1975), the clinical presentation and surgical management of jugular foramen schwannomas are more a function of anatomic location than specific nerve origin (Franklin et al., 1989; Horn et al., 1985; Kaye et al., 1984; Samii et al., 1995a; Tan et al., 1990). Jugular foramen tumors comprise 2.9%–4% of intracranial schwannomas. Marked cystic degeneration is not rare. Kaye et al. (1984) classified these tumors into three types (A, B, C) based on their location. Type A tumors are primarily intracranial masses with only minor extension into the foramen. Tumors within the bony foramen with or without an intracranial component are classified as type B (Fig. 12–4). Type C tumors are primarily extracranial with only minor extension into the bony foramen or the posterior fossa.

Patients with type B and C tumors present with various forms of the jugular foramen syndrome (Table 12–2), but hoarseness is usually the initial symptom. Type A tumors may not cause dysfunction of the lower cranial nerves and may cause a clinical syndrome indistinguishable from that of a vestibular schwannoma.

Type A tumors are generally removed through a standard retrosigmoid suboccipital craniectomy, whereas type B and C tumors usually require combined approaches, such as the combined posterior fossa–infratemporal fossa approach or the infratemporal approaches of Fisch (Franklin et al., 1989). Postoperative cranial nerve morbidity rates of 38% have been reported (Samii et al., 1995a).

Radiosurgery can be a good alternative for the treatment of small jugular foramen schwannomas. Pollock et al. (1993) reported five patients with jugular foramen schwannomas treated with the gamma knife. With a mean follow-up period of 10 months, tumor control was attained in three patients without an increase of cranial nerve deficits.

The management of lower cranial nerve dysfunction is by far the most important aspect of the pa-

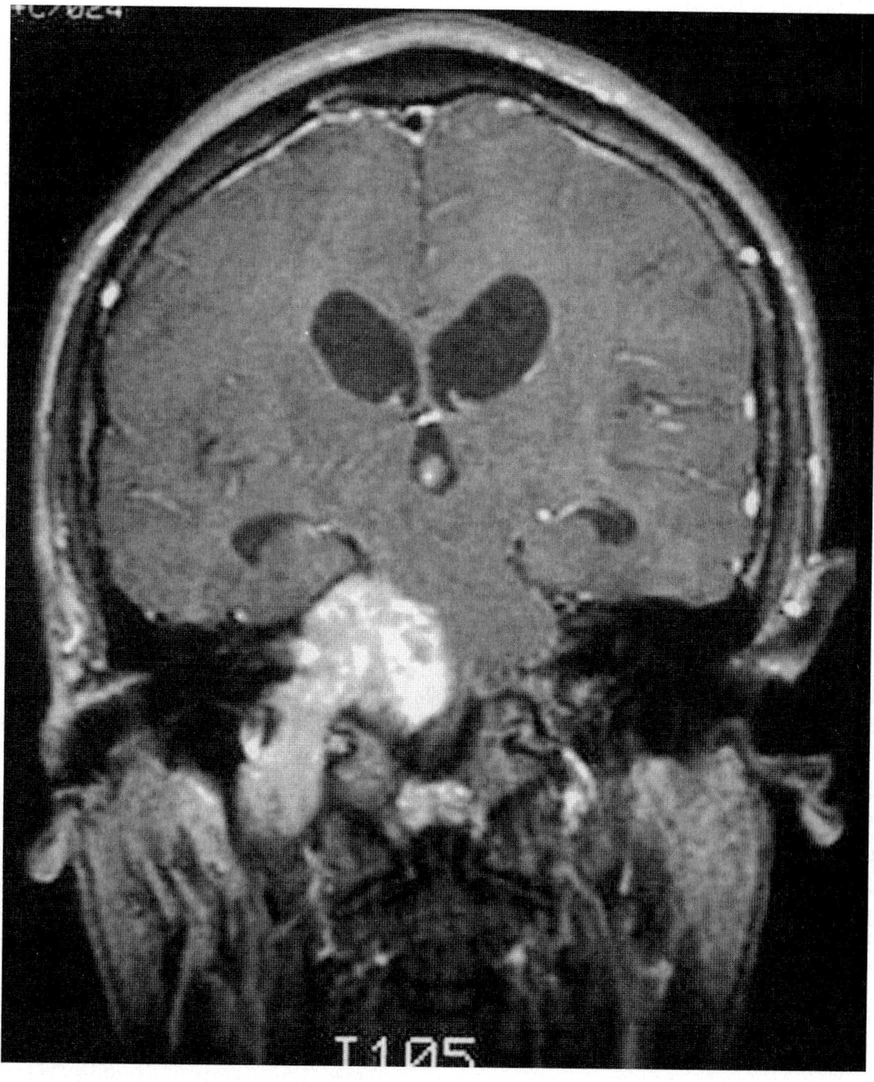

Figure 12–4. Coronal post-contrast T_1-weighted MRI identifies the jugular foramen component of this type B jugular foramen schwannoma.

tients' care. If extensive jugular foramen dissection is necessary, early tracheostomy may be warranted to avoid aspiration pneumonitis. Patients must be kept NPO until definite objective evidence of an adequate swallowing mechanism without aspiration is obtained.

A modified barium swallow, consultation with a speech pathologist, and laryngoscopy should be arranged. Pooling of secretions, a dysfunctional swallowing mechanism, or aspiration may be seen, thus identifying those patients who require further rehabilitative maneuvers.

Schwannomas of Cranial Nerves III, IV, VI, and X

Schwannomas of the cranial nerves subserving extraocular muscle function are extremely rare. Clinical presentation usually involves diplopia due to dysfunction of the tumor's nerve of origin, but may include decreased visual acuity, hemiparesis, ataxia of gait, paresthesias, and symptoms of intracranial hypertension (Celli et al.,1992; Jackowski et al., 1994; Tung et al., 1991). Treatment is surgical resection, which may occasionally be associated with functionally normal eye movements (Schultheiss et al., 1993).

Hypoglossal schwannomas, when they occur, are usually located entirely within the intracranial compartment or, less commonly, have a dumbbell-shaped appearance with both intra- and extracranial components (Odake, 1989). Purely extracranial tumors can also occur. Unilateral lingual atrophy, deviation, and fibrillation are nearly universal findings. Intracranial hypertension, long tract signs, ataxia, and dysfunction of the other lower cranial nerves may occur. Surgical removal is best accomplished via a transcondylar approach, either alone or in combination with an anterior transcervical approach. Purely extracranial tumors can be removed via an anterior transcervical approach alone.

Schwannomas of the Nasal Cavity and Paranasal Sinuses

Schwannomas of the nasal cavity and paranasal sinuses arise from the ophthalmic or maxillary branches of the trigeminal nerve and autonomic ganglia and constitute only 4% of schwannomas in the head and neck region. Identification of the nerve of origin is rarely possible. In the majority of cases multiple paranasal sinuses are involved.

The clinical presentation is typical for tumors of the nasal cavity and paranasal sinuses. Nasal obstruction, epistaxis, mucopurulent rhinorrhea, hyposmia, localized facial swelling, facial or orbital pain, and proptosis are usual manifestations. Deficits of the extraocular nerves can develop with sphenoidal tumors.

Surgical excision is the preferred treatment modality for schwannomas of the paranasal sinuses. En bloc excision should be performed in cases of malignancy.

NEUROFIBROMATOSIS

Treatment of tumors of patients with either form of NF usually consists of surgical removal of neoplasms, although irradiation may be helpful. Surgical management must have a clear goal, such as the relief of pain, prevention of compression, or decompression of critical nervous tissue, including brain, brain stem, or spinal cord (Pitts et al., 1996). Overall, the chances of anatomic and functional nerve preservation in NF2 patients are lower than in unilateral tumors (Samii et al., 1997).

A good outcome is best achieved when surgery is performed early and when there is good preoperative hearing function. Welling (1998) recommends early removal of small neoplasms if hearing is useable binaurally. The smallest tumor is removed first to maximize hearing preservation opportunity. If hearing is preserved and the second tumor is smaller than 1.5 cm, it is removed 3 to 6 months later. If hearing is not preserved, the second tumor is followed expectantly until either hearing is lost or brain stem encroachment requires removal.

Radiosurgical treatment can be effective in NF2 patients with vestibular schwannomas. Subach et al. (1999) reported a 98% tumor control rate over a median follow up of 3 years. Useful hearing was preserved in 43% of patients and normal facial nerve function in 81%.

CHONDROSARCOMA

Chondrosarcoma is a tumor of cartilaginous origin with nonuniform biologic behavior. It represents 0.15% of all cranial space-occupying lesions. Nearly one-half of these are located in the cranial base and constitute 6% of skull base neoplasms (Hassounah et al., 1985; Korten et al., 1998). The middle cranial fossa is affected in 64% of cases, middle and posterior fossae in 14%, anterior cranial fossa in 14%, and posterior cranial fossa in 7% (Kveton et al., 1986).

Chondrosarcomas may develop at any age with an average of 37 years (Evans et al., 1977). Overall there is no sex predominance. Tumor growth may be bulky, permeative, or mixed. Dural invasion is present in 30% of cases (Korten et al., 1998). The majority of tumors are nearly avascular; however, in about 30% the vascularity can be significant (Hassounah et al., 1985). Distant metastases from skull base chondrosarcomas are reported in 10% of cases (Hassounah et al., 1985).

Pathology

It is assumed that chondrosarcomas originate from remnants of embryonal cartilage or from metaplasia of meningeal fibroblasts. Typically, the tumor is composed of multiple, interconnecting lobules of varying size with chondroid or myxoid consistency, which can contain central necrosis. Several tumor subtypes have been described: conventional (grades I to III), myxoid, clear cell, dedifferentiated, and mesenchymal (Barnes and Kapadia, 1994).

Conventional chondrosarcomas represent 62% of chondrosarcomas of the cranial base (Korten et al., 1998). Microscopically they are composed of hypercellular hyaline cartilage, which contains cytologically atypical chondrocytes within lacunae. On the basis of differences in nuclear size, cellularity, mitotic rate, and frequency of lacunae with multiple nuclei, these tumors are graded in a three-tier system. The exclusive presence or marked preponderance of small, densely staining nuclei is a typical sign of grade I (well-differentiated) neoplasms. Multiple nuclei within one lacuna are easily found. Dense cellularity, presence of significant numbers of moderately sized or larger nuclei, and rare mitotic figures are features of grade II (moderately differentiated) chondrosarcoma. The presence of 2 or more mitoses per 10 higher power fields indicates a grade III (poorly differentiated) neoplasm. Overall 5 year survival rates for grades I, II, and III chondrosarcomas are 90%, 81%, and 43%, respectively (Evans et al., 1977).

Mesenchymal chondrosarcomas constitute 30% of skull-base chondrosarcomas and represent a distinct clinicopathologic entity (Stapleton et al., 1993). This tumor arises from primitive multipotential mesenchymal cells, usually manifests at a young age (10 to 30 years), and is most typically seen in females (Hassounah et al., 1985). Microscopically, this tumor is characterized by a bimorphic pattern of small or large islands of relatively well-differentiated cartilage and sheets of primitive undifferentiated round or spindle-shaped cells (the presence of the latter is the most typical sign). The stroma is rich in collagen fibrils. Well-developed vascularity is typical. Mesenchymal chondrosarcoma has a high frequency of dural and cerebral invasion, local recurrence, and systemic metastases (Hassounah et al., 1985; Korten et al., 1998).

Diagnosis

The clinical manifestations of chondrosarcoma are mainly related to its preferred location at the skull base. The most common signs and symptoms are dysfunction of extraocular movement with diplopia (51%), headache (31%), hearing loss, dizziness and tinnitus (21%), and sensory disturbances of the face (21%). The median period between presentation and diagnosis is 15 months (Korten et al., 1998).

Computed tomography (CT) most commonly reveals bone destruction and tumoral calcification, the latter being encountered in 56% of tumors (Hassounah et al., 1985). On T_1-weighted magnetic resonance imaging (MRI), chondrosarcomas have a low to intermediate signal intensity and are isointense or hypointense to gray matter. On proton density and T_2-weighted images they have a high signal intensity and are hyperintense to gray matter (Korten et al., 1998). Contrast enhancement is typically heterogeneous. The radiologic distinction of chondrosarcoma and chordoma is usually not possible.

Treatment

If possible, gross total tumor removal in a one-stage operation is advocated for chondrosarcoma, as repeated surgical interventions risk tumor progression, development of scar tissue, and secondary spread of tumor cells (Hassounah et al., 1985; Korten et al., 1998) (Fig. 12–5). Macroscopically complete removal of intracranial chondrosarcomas has been accomplished in 5% to 47% of cases (Stapleton et al., 1993; Gay et al., 1995; Rosenberg et al., 1999). Sixty percent of patients have been reported to experience at least transient deterioration of function immediately after surgery. The most common postoperative complications are cerebrospinal fluid (CSF) leak (30%) with secondary meningitis (10%) and permanent cranial nerve palsy (Gay et al., 1995). Local recurrence after surgery is 53% with a mean recurrence-free period of 3 years. Risk of recurrence is greater among patients who were already operated on and in cases of partial resection. Recurrence-free survival rates at 2, 3, and 5 years are 67%, 56%, and 43%, respectively (Korten et al., 1998).

In general, chondrosarcomas are considered to be refractory to conventional radiation therapy (RT). Local control rates of 78% and survival rates of 83% have been reported 5 years following proton irradiation (Castro et al., 1994). Despite the high rates of local success of charged particle radiotherapy, complication rates have been considerable (27%). Tumor volume influences control rate. In one series all tumors with volumes of 25 cc or less remained locally controlled, whereas only a 56% control rate was found for larger neoplasms (Hug et al., 1999). Subtotal tumor resection with preservation of functionally

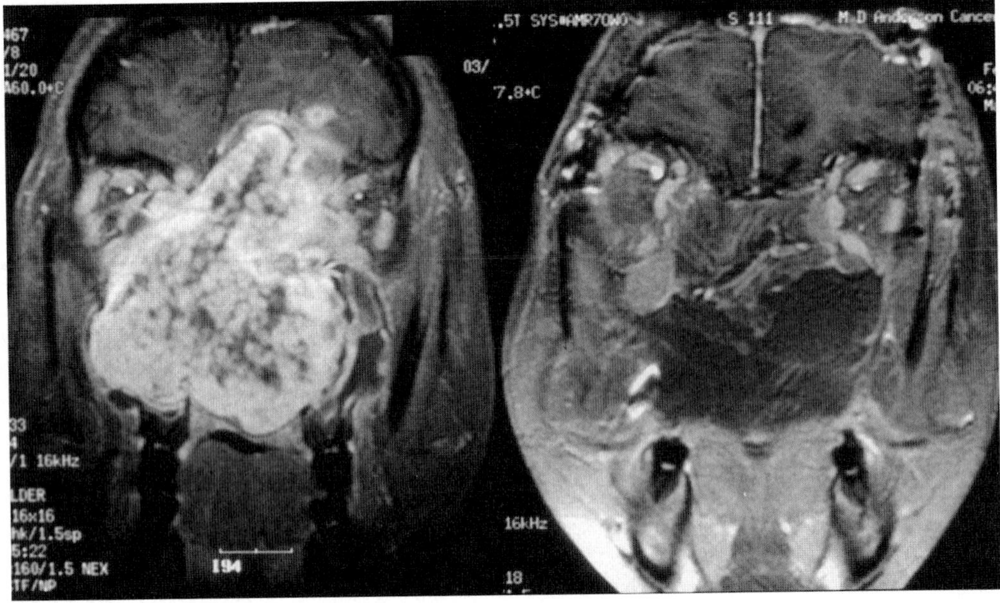

Figure 12–5. Coronal post-contrast T_1-weighted MRIs reveal complete removal of this massive midfacial, skull base chondrosarcoma. A one-stage en bloc resection with free tissue transfer reconstruction was performed.

important structures and improvement of the tumor–normal tissue configuration to allow better targeting geometry for postoperative proton beam irradiation has been advocated. Such an approach resulted in 99% 5 year local control and disease-specific survival rates for conventional chondrosarcoma (Rosenberg et al., 1999).

CHORDOMA

Chordomas are slowly growing, locally aggressive, malignant tumors derived from embryonic remnants of the notochord. Nearly 35% of these neoplasms arise from the skull base, and these constitute 0.1% to 0.2% of primary intracranial tumors. The male/female ratio in chordomas is 1.5:1, with a mean age of patients of 46 years (Forsyth et al., 1993).

In 79% of cases, chordomas are located in the posterior fossa with not uncommon extension into the sphenoid sinus, parapharyngeal space, nasopharynx, suprasellar cistern, and middle cranial fossa. Although typically considered as midline tumors of the clivus, nearly one-third of intracranial chordomas have eccentrically positioned extensions. Cavernous sinus involvement is encountered in 65% of cases, whereas encasement of the internal carotid or basilar artery occurs in 36%. By the time of surgery one-third of tumors exhibit dural erosion (Maira et al., 1996).

Pathology

Macroscopically chordoma is usually a lobulated, soft gelatinous mass that destroys bone. It commonly calcifies, may show areas of hemorrhage and necrosis, and usually grossly appears somewhat demarcated.

Three subtypes of chordomas have been identified pathologically (Barnes and Kapadia, 1994). The most common variant shows no evidence of cartilaginous or additional mesenchymal components. It is composed of cells arranged in cords with eosinophilic cytoplasm lying in a mucinous background. Cytoplasmic vacuolation is common. Lobules of tumor cells are separated by fibrovascular septa. Mitotic figures, nuclear pleomorphism, areas of necrosis, hemorrhage, and calcification may be present without prognostic significance. A defining feature of classic chordomas is their immunopositivity for markers of epithelial differentiation, specifically keratins. Reactivity for epithelial membrane antigen is common, whereas carcinoembryonic staining is less frequently seen (Mitchell et al., 1993). Chondroid chordoma contains both chordomatous and cartilaginous components in a highly variable ratio. The cartilaginous component may appear either histologically benign or malignant. The vast majority of these tumors arise from the cranial base. Dedifferentiated chordomas are rare. They contain areas of conventional chordoma as well as malignant mesenchymal components. In these cases, prognosis is poor and most patients are dead of disease within 6–12 months.

Metastases can develop, with the most common sites of distant spread being the lungs, bones, lymph nodes, liver, and skin.

Diagnosis

Clinical presentation depends on the site of origin and direction of growth. The most typical symptoms are diplopia (49%), headache (24%), and ataxia (4%). Palsy of the sixth nerve is encountered in 57% of cases, lower cranial nerves in 36%, sensory fifth in 27%, third in 22%, and optic neuropathy in 12%. The median time from symptom onset to diagnosis has been reported as 10 months (Forsyth et al., 1993).

Radiographic assessment reveals a midline soft tissue mass associated with osteolytic bone destruction and occasional calcifications. The typical CT appearance of an intracranial chordoma is of a well-defined extra-axial mass, with both hyperdense and hypodense areas associated with bone destruction, foci of calcification, and varying degrees of encroachment of adjacent neural structures (Brown et al., 1990). On T_1-weighted MRI, chordomas exhibited low to intermediate signal intensity with a typically hyperintense signal on T_2-weighted images. Heterogeneous enhancement with gadolinium is seen (Meyers et al., 1992) (Fig. 12–6).

Treatment

Skull base chordomas are locally aggressive tumors, and surgery in conjunction with postoperative RT is the standard form of treatment. Staged surgeries using different approaches may be needed for removal of the tumor (Gay et al., 1995). Gross total resection of the tumor is the surgical goal. Even in the best of circumstances, however, this can be accomplished in only 67% of patients due to involvement of critical neurovascular structures (Maira et al., 1996). Because of the invasive nature of the tumor, local recurrences are the rule and most of these appear within 3 years of treatment with the mean interval to the first recurrence being 12.5 months. Despite various salvage treatments, stabilization of disease at the time of recurrence is uncommon (Hug et al., 1999).

For improvement of local control and survival in the cases of incomplete tumor resection a radiotherapeutic dose of at least 55 Gy of fractionated RT is necessary. This still achieves only a 39% to 51% 5 year survival and an 18% to 35% 10 year survival

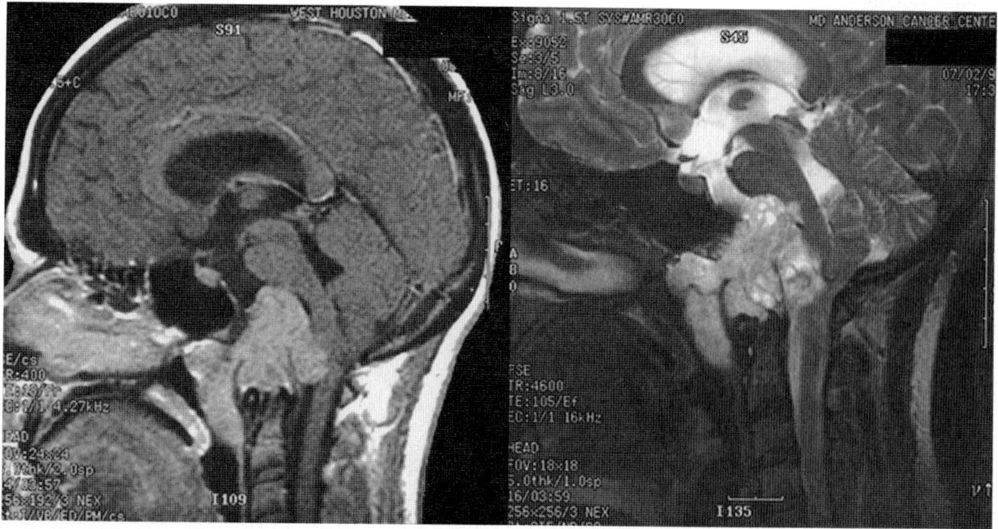

Figure 12–6. Sagittal post-contrast T_1-weighted (left) and T_2-weighted (right) MRI of a patient with a clival chordoma. Note the increased signal seen on the T_2-weighted images. The tumor extends from the posterior nasopharynx to compress the brain stem.

(Fuller and Bloom, 1988; Forsyth et al., 1993). The most common cause of death is uncontrolled local disease progression. Proton beam irradiation resulted in a 59% to 63% 5 year local control rate and a 72% to 79% 5 year survival (Castro et al., 1994; Hug et al., 1999). The 10 year survival rate for these patients is still only 45% (Rosenberg et al., 1999). Older age, female gender, high proliferative index, and large intracranial tumor volume are negative prognostic factors, and in these cases more aggressive management is warranted (Forsyth et al., 1993; Matsuno et al., 1997; Terahara et al., 1999). Several, mainly unsuccessful, chemotherapeutic attempts have been made to treat patients with chordoma. Use of vincristine alone or in combination with methotrexate resulted in a degree of symptomatic improvement (Harwick and Miller, 1979; Fuller and Bloom, 1988).

PARAGANGLIOMA

Paragangliomas are the most common tumors of the middle ear and, after acoustic neuromas, are the most common tumors of the temporal bone. These tumors have a distinct predilection for females, who make up more than 80% of patients in the series of tympanic, jugular, and vagal paragangliomas. Most of these tumors occur in the sixth decade of life.

Paragangliomas are slow-growing tumors that extend along anatomic planes of least resistance (along blood vessels and mastoid air-cell tracts and through cranial nerve foraminae). Malignancy occurs in 10% of cases, and catecholamine secretion is detected in another 5%.

Hearing loss occurs in 90% of patients with glomus tympanicum tumors and in 70% of patients with glomus jugulare tumors, but only rarely in patients with glomus vagale tumors. The hearing loss is more often conductive than sensorineural. Pulsatile tinnitus, an audible bruit, or spontaneous aural bleeding can be seen in 60% to 70% of patients with tympanicum or jugulare tumors and in 30% of those with vagale paragangliomas.

Involvement of the facial nerve occurs in approximately 20% of patients with tympanicum or jugulare tumors. The vertical mastoid segment is the usual site of compression, although compression in the soft tissue of the stylomastoid foramen may also occur.

Dysfunction of the lower cranial nerves occurs in 13% of patients with glomus jugulare tumors and in 70% of patients with glomus vagale tumors. A change in voice may precede other symptoms by 2 to 3 years in patients with glomus vagale tumors. Vocal cord paralysis is the usual finding on examination. If present, hypoglossal paresis denotes tumor extension into the hypoglossal canal or high in the neck.

Pathology

Macroscopically, paragangliomas have a beefy red brown to gray appearance, with hemorrhage or fibrosis. They may have a thin capsule and are composed of round or polygonal epithelioid cells. Histologically, the tumor is composed of two cell types: chief cells (type I) arranged in compact cell nests laden with neurosecretory granules; and sustentacular (type II) or modified Schwann cells found peripheral to the chief cells (Barnes and Kapadia, 1994). Nuclei are centrally located with finely clumped chromatin and a moderate amount of eosinophilic, granular cytoplasm. Immunohistochemical stains confirm the neuroendocrine nature of the chief cells, which are diffusely and strongly positive for neuron-specific enolase, synaptophysin, and chromogranin. In contrast, the sustentacular cells may show positivity for S-100 protein, glial fibrillary acidic protein, and nerve growth factor receptor. Nuclear pleomorphism, necrosis, mitoses, and even vascular or neural invasion, may be seen in benign tumors and are not sufficient criteria for the diagnosis of malignancy, which is encountered in 2% to 13% of cases.

Diagnosis

The tumor is usually isointense to muscle on T_1-weighted MRI and hyperintense on T_2-weighted images. Multiple punctuate and serpiginous areas of signal void due to high velocity flow in tumor vessels are frequently seen, resulting in the classic "salt-and-pepper" heterogeneity seen on T_2-weighted images (Olsen et al., 1987) (Fig. 12–7A). Angiography confirms the hypervascular nature of the tumor (Fig. 12–7B). "Bone window" CT is invaluable for the detection of bone erosion and can be helpful in the clinical staging of lateral skull-base paragangliomas (Table 12–4).

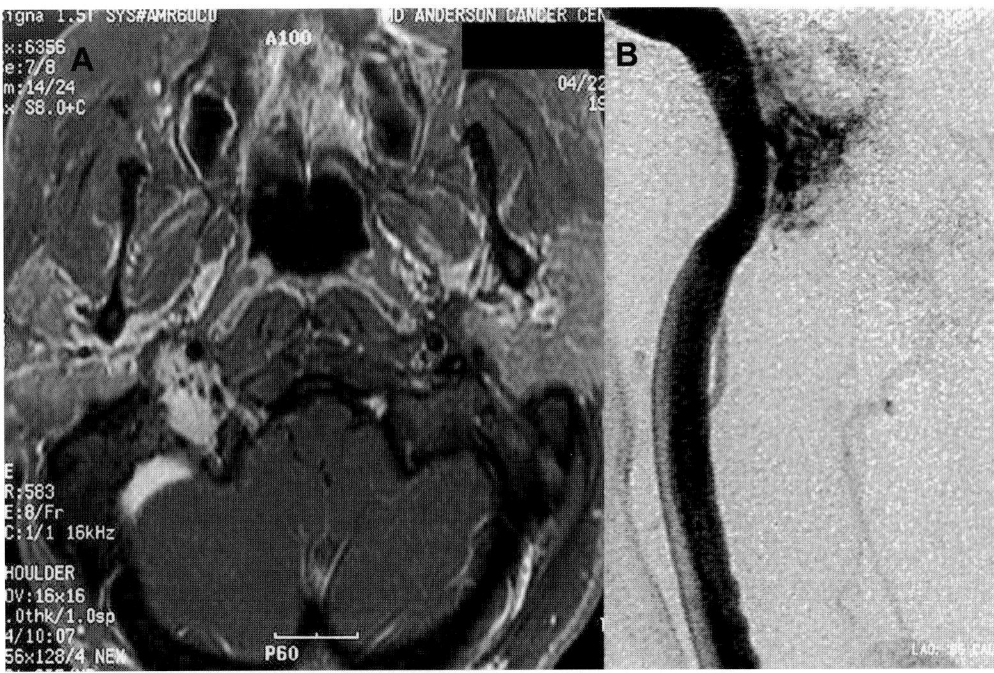

Figure 12–7. **(A)** Axial post-contrast T_1-weighted MRI reveals signal voids within the contrast-enhancing tumor in the right jugular foramen. **(B)** Right lateral internal carotid angiogram confirms the hypervascular nature of this paraganglioma.

Treatment

Surgical excision is generally considered the method of choice in the treatment of paragangliomas. Tumor control rates of 90% to 100% have been reported following gross total resection. Whereas surgical excision can be safely performed in small localized lesions, in extensive neoplasms it can be accompanied by serious morbidity. The risk of postoperative lower cranial nerve deficit is approximately 30% (Jackson, 1993). Upper aerodigestive tract procedures may be required in as many as 19% of patients (Anand et al., 1990; Green et al., 1994). Reported perioperative mortality varies from 0% to 5% (Green et al., 1994; Gjuric et al., 1996). Subtotal resection with preservation of functional cranial nerves with subsequent RT may be a valuable treatment alternative for selected patients. Gjuric et al. (1996) reported a 67% long-term tumor control rate with this approach

Radiation therapy is an accepted primary treatment modality for paragangliomas. It may be recommended when there is demonstrable involvement of

Table 12–4. Fisch Classification of Glomus Jugulare Tumors

Type A	Tumors confined to middle ear cleft (tympanicum)
Type B	Tumors limited to the tympanomastoid area with no bone destruction in the infralabyrinthine compartment of the temporal bone
Type C	Tumors involving the infralabyrinthine compartment with extension into the petrous apex
Type D	Tumors with intracranial extension less than 2 cm in diameter
Type E	Tumors with intracranial extension greater than 2 cm in diameter

Source: Fisch U, Fagan P, Valavanis A. 1984. The infratemporal fossa approach for the lateral skull base. Otolaryngol Clin North Am 17:513–552.

the internal carotid artery in patients who fail a balloon occlusion test; in bilateral tumors with contralateral deficits of the lower cranial nerves or concerns of venous return; in patients with poor medical condition or refusal of surgery; and in cases with contralateral sensorineural hearing loss (Anand et al., 1993). With a mean follow up of 10.5 years, Konefal et al. (1987) achieved long-term control in all patients with localized paragangliomas treated with radiation (minimum dose 46 Gy). In seven patients with massive disease, radiation was able to control tumor in five. Carrasco and Rosenman (1993) reviewed 24 series of patients treated with RT and found an overall 90% rate of survival, with only 5% of patients dying of their disease. Sims et al. (1999) reported good results in four patients with skull-base paragangliomas treated by linac-based radiosurgery with a single marginal doses of 15 to 17.5 Gy. Despite a possible decrease in blood and urine norepinephrine levels, radiation may not completely control the secretory activity of the tumor (Pluta et al., 1994).

OLFACTORY NEUROBLASTOMA

Olfactory neuroblastoma, also known as esthesioneuroblastoma, is an uncommon malignant neoplasm of neuroectodermal origin, arising from the olfactory neuroepithelium of the superior third of the nasal septum, cribriform plate, and superior turbinates. The mean age of patients is 45 years, with a nearly equal distribution between males and females (Levine et al., 1999). Orbital invasion is encountered in 17% of cases, whereas intracranial extension is identified in 25%.

Pathology

On gross examination, the tumor is polyploid, soft, pink to red brown, and hemorrhagic. Microscopically it is composed of discrete nests or lobules of small round cells with hyperchromatic nuclei and sparse cytoplasm. The stroma is pink, delicate, neurofibrillary, or edematous and well vascularized. Mitoses are rare. Homer-Wright pseudorosettes are seen in 30% to 50% of olfactory neuroblastomas. Flexner true rosettes are infrequent. Necrosis, dystrophic calcification, and vascular or lymphatic invasion are not uncommon. According to Hyams, four grades of olfactory neuroblastomas can be delineated (Table 12–5).

Immunohistochemistry can reveal staining of the tumor cells for neuron-specific enolase (100%), synaptophysin (65%), and chromogranin.

Diagnosis

Unilateral nasal obstruction and epistaxis are typical manifestations of olfactory neuroblastoma. In 20% of patients, rhinoscopy can disclose a red–gray mass, located high in the nasal cavity. Other symptoms include headache, periorbital swelling, hyposmia, and visual disturbances. Nearly 6% of patients present with cervical metastases.

Radiographs usually reveal an intranasal soft tissue density sometimes with bone erosion, septal deviation away from the involved side, occasional calcifications, and pacification of the paranasal sinuses. The imaging appearance of olfactory neuroblastoma does not allow differentiation from other sinonasal malignancies, but is invaluable in tumor staging. On CT, olfactory neuroblastoma is usually seen as a homogeneous iso- or slightly hyperdense lesion, with homogeneous and moderate contrast enhancement.

Table 12–5. Hyams' Grading System of Olfactory Neuroblastomas

Feature	*Grade I*	*Grade II*	*Grade III*	*Grade IV*
Architecture	Lobular	Lobular	Nearly lobular	Nearly lobular
Mitotic activity	Absent	Present	Prominent	Marked
Nuclear pleomorphism	Absent	Moderate	Prominent	Marked
Fibrillary matrix	Prominent	Present	Minimal	Absent
Rosettes	Homer-Wright	Homer-Wright	Flexner	Absent
Necrosis	Absent	Absent	Present	Common

Source: Hyams VJ, Batsakis JG, Micheals L. 1988. Tumors of the Upper Respiratory Tract and Ear. Washington, DC: Armed Forces Institute of Pathology, p 343.

"Direct" coronal images can be useful for delineation of tumor extension into the orbits and through the cribriform plate (Eustace et al., 1995). On T_1-weighted MRI, olfactory neuroblastoma is usually hypointense. (Fig. 12–8)

Treatment

En bloc craniofacial resection of the tumor, cribriform plate, and overlying dura is the preferred treatment for olfactory neuroblastoma (Biller et al., 1990; Morita et al., 1993). Whereas localized tumors can be treated successfully with excellent long-term results, management of advanced disease is much more challenging. Preoperative RT (average dose, 51.1 Gy) with or without chemotherapy (cyclophosphamide, vincristine, adriamycin) can result in a 50% reduction in tumor volume in nearly one-half of patients, which can facilitate surgical removal (Polin et al., 1998). Platinum-based chemotherapy can be effective for advanced high-grade tumors (McElroy et al., 1998).

The estimated survival rates of patients with olfactory neuroblastoma are 97% at 1 year, 74% to 87% at 5 years, and 54% to 60% at 10 years (Dulguerov and Calcaterra, 1992; Polin et al., 1998). Recurrences following therapy are encountered in 30% to 70% of patients. In the series of Levine et al. (1999),

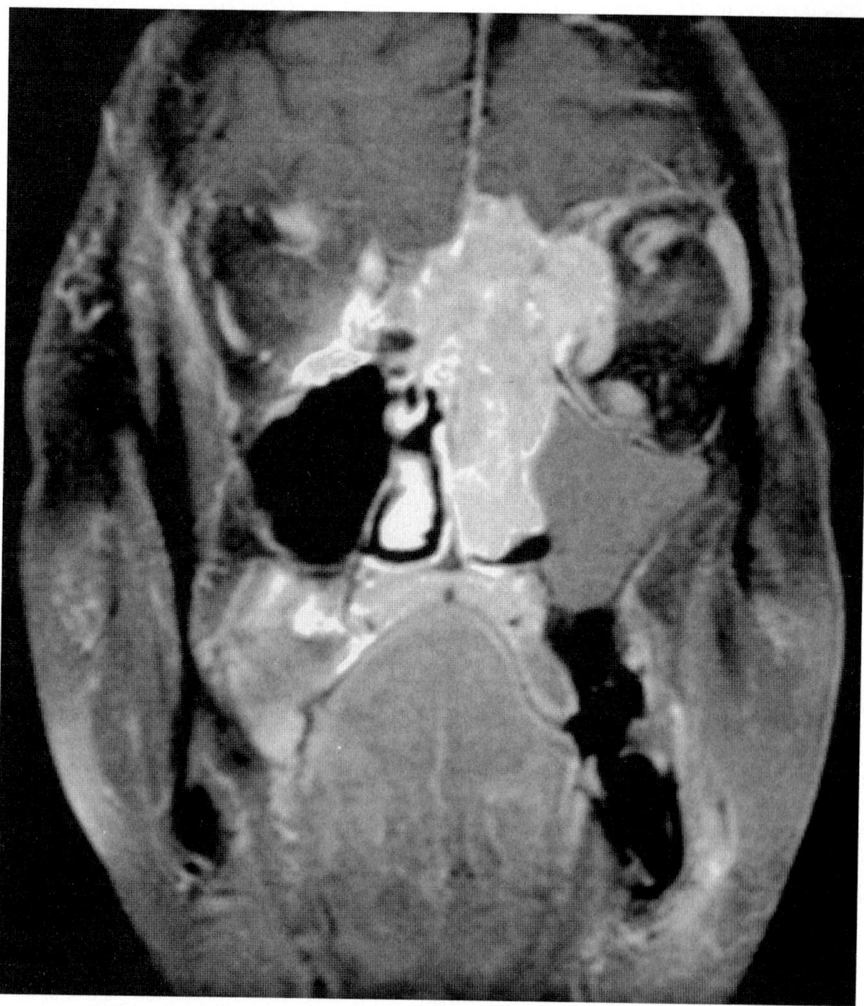

Figure 12–8. Coronal post-contrast T_1-weighted MRI of a patient with a large olfactory neuroblastoma. Note the extension of this tumor intracranially and into the left orbit.

the longest duration for the presentation of the first recurrence was 13.3 years. Cervical lymph node metastases may develop in 10% to 40% of cases. The lungs and bones are common sites of distant metastases. Salvage rates for olfactory neuroblastoma are far superior to those of other superior nasal vault malignancies, with a 82% 5 year survival rate after salvage treatment for local recurrence (Morita et al., 1993).

The histologic grade is an important prognostic indicator. In the series of McElroy et al. (1998) the mean survival from the time of initial diagnosis was 139.5 months for low-grade and 32.25 months for high-grade tumors. Advanced Kadish stage is associated with a higher rate of disease-related mortality and characterized by aggressive clinical behavior, independently of tumor grade (Polin et al., 1998; Levine et al., 1999). Three year disease-free survival is 100% for Kadish stage A patients, 80% for stage B, and 40% for stage C (Kadish et al., 1976). Involvement of the brain is a poor prognostic sign. Advanced aged is also predictive of a decreased probability of disease-free survival.

CARCINOMAS OF THE ANTERIOR SKULL BASE

Carcinomas of the anterior skull base may arise from the nasal cavity, paranasal sinuses, pharynx, or the major and minor salivary glands of the upper aerodigestive tract. The anterior skull base is most frequently affected due to direct extension of the neoplasm with erosion of the bone.

Diagnosis

Disease presentation is often nonspecific and depends on the site of origin of the tumor. Sinonasal tumors can grow to a large size before causing significant symptoms. The most frequently encountered signs and symptoms include nasal obstruction, loss of the sense of smell, epistaxis, rhinorrhea, serous otitis media, diplopia, exophthalmos, and facial hypoesthesia, swelling, or pain. Approximately 10% of patients do not have symptoms of tumor. Fewer than 10% of patients have cervical lymphadenopathy, and fewer than 7% have distant metastases. Second malignancies are discovered in 10% to 20% of patients.

Pathology

Squamous cell carcinoma is the most common tumor of the paranasal sinuses, accounting for 50% of most surgical series. The maxillary sinus is the most common site of origin. Adenocarcinoma most frequently occurs in the upper nasal cavity or in the ethmoid sinuses. The grade of this tumor is highly correlated with prognosis. Adenoid cystic carcinomas arise from the major and minor salivary glands and characteristically infiltrate diffusely, especially along perineural pathways, contributing to a high rate of recurrence and late metastasis. Neuroendocrine carcinomas are malignancies of the exocrine glands found in the normal nasal and paranasal mucosa. Differentiation from olfactory neuroblastoma is important as these tumors are exquisitely chemosensitive and are primarily treated without need for extensive surgery (Table 12–6) (Perez-Ordonez et al., 1998).

Table 12–6. Criteria for Differential Diagnosis Between High-Grade Olfactory Neuroblastoma and Small Cell Neuroendocrine Carcinoma

Criteria	*High-Grade Olfactory Neuroblastoma*	*Neuroendocrine Carcinoma*
Lobular architecture	+/−	−
Neurofibrillary stroma	+/−	−
Rosette formation	+/−	−
Cell sizes	Large	Small
Nucleoli	Conspicuous	Not found
Immunohistochemistry		
S-100	Slightly positive	Negative
NF	Positive	Negative
Keratin	Uncommon	Diffuse
Mean proliferative index	7.4%	67%

Data are from Perez-Ordonez et al. (1998).

Sinonasal undifferentiated carcinoma is an extremely aggressive tumor with a high rate of early metastatic spread. Affected patients rarely live beyond 2 years. Other less common tumors of the nasal cavity and paranasal sinuses include mucoepidermoid carcinoma, melanoma, plasmacytoma, lymphoma, and various sarcomas.

Treatment

Tumor pathology and extent, the availability and potential success rates of adjuvant therapies, as well as the potential for functional impairment and esthetic deformity are all important parameters to consider when planning the best management options for a patient with anterior skull base malignancy. In most cases, surgery and radiation are employed as a combined treatment modality, but other adjuvant therapies such as radiosurgery, brachytherapy, and chemotherapy may be indicated.

Patient outcome is variable and depends on the tumor pathology, primary site and any extensions, and completeness of surgical excision. Several recent surgical series have reported survival rates of 47% to 70% at 5 years and 41% to 48% at 10 years for all types of malignancies. McCutcheon et al. (1996) reported median survival times of 20 months for squamous cell carcinoma, 26 months for adenocarcinoma, and 40 months for olfactory neuroblastoma.

REFERENCES

Al-Mefty O. Management of glomus jugulare tumors. 1988. Contemp Neurosurg 10:1–6.

Anand VK, Leonetti JP, Al-Mefty O. 1993. Neurovascular considerations in surgery of glomus tumors with intracranial extensions. Laryngoscope 103:722–728.

Baker FG, Ojemann RG. 1993. Surgical approaches to tumors of the posterior fossa cranial nerves (excluding acoustic neuromas). In: Barrow DL (ed), Surgery of the Cranial Nerves of the Posterior Fossa. AANS Publications Committee. Park Ridge, NJ: American Association of Neurological Surgeons, 322 pp.

Barnes L, Kapadia SB. 1994. The biology and pathology of selected skull base tumors. J Neurooncol 20:213–240.

Berger MS, Edwards MS, Bingham WG. 1982. Hypoglossal neurilemmoma: case report and review of the literature. Neurosurgery 10: 617–620.

Biller HF, Lawson W, Sachdev VP, Som P. 1990. Esthesioneuroblastoma: surgical treatment without radiation. Laryngoscope 100:1199–1201.

Bordi L, Compton J, Symon L. 1989. Trigeminal neuroma. A report of eleven cases. Surg Neurol 31:272–276.

Brown RV, Sage MR, Brophy BP. 1990. CT and MR findings in patients with chordomas of the petrous apex. Am J Neuroradiol 11:121–124.

Cantu G, Solero CL, Mariani L, et al. 1999. Anterior craniofacial resection for malignant ethmoid tumors—a series of 91 patients. Head Neck 21:185–191.

Carrasco V, Rosenman J. 1993. Radiation therapy of glomus jugulare tumors. Laryngoscope 103(suppl 60):23–27.

Castro JR, Linstadt DE, Bahary JP, et al. 1994. Experience in charged particle irradiation of tumors of the skull base: 1977–92. Int J Radiat Oncol Biol Phys 29:647–655.

Celli P, Ferrante L, Acqui M, Mastronardi L, Fortuna A, Palma L. 1992. Neurinoma of the third, fourth, and sixth cranial nerves: a survey and report of a new fourth nerve case. Surg Neurol 38:216–224.

Day JD, Fukushima T. 1998. The surgical management of trigeminal neuromas. Neurosurgery 42:233–241.

Dolenc VV. 1994. Frontotemporal epidural approach to trigeminal neurinomas. Acta Neurochir (Wien) 130:55–65.

Dort JC, Fisch U. 1991. Facial-nerve schwannomas. Skull Base Surg 1:51–56.

Dulguerov P, Calcaterra T. 1992. Esthesioneuroblastoma: the UCLA experience 1970–1990. Laryngoscope 102:843–849.

Eustace S, Suojanen J, Buff B, McEniff N, Janvario J, Norris C. 1995. Preoperative imaging of esthesioneuroblastoma. Clin Radiol 50:639–643.

Evans HL, Ayala AG, Romsdahl MM. 1977. Prognostic factors in chondrosarcoma of bone: a clinicopathologic analysis with emphasis on histologic grading. Cancer 40:818–831.

Farrior JB 3rd, Hyams VJ, Benke RH, Farrior JB. 1980. Carcinoid apudoma arising in a glomus jugulare tumor: review of endocrine activity in glomus jugulare tumors. Laryngoscope 90:110–119.

Franklin DJ, Moore GF, Fisch U. 1989. Jugular foramen peripheral nerve sheath tumors. Laryngoscope 99: 1081–1087.

Forsyth PA, Cascino TL, Shaw EG, et al. 1993. Intracranial chordomas: a clinicopathological and prognostic study of 51 cases. J Neurosurg 78:741–747.

Fuller DB, Bloom JG. 1988. Radiotherapy for chordoma. Int J Radiat Oncol Biol Phys 15:331–339.

Gay E, Sekhar LN, Rubinstein E, et al. 1995. Chordomas and chondrosarcomas of the cranial base: results and follow-up of 60 patients. Neurosurgery 36:887–897.

Gjuric M, Rudiger Wolf S, Wigand ME, Weidenbecher M. 1996. Cranial nerve and hearing function after combined-approach surgery for glomus jugulare tumors. Ann Otol Rhinol Laryngol 105:949–954.

Gormley WB, Sekhar LN, Wright DC, Kamerer D, Schessel D. 1997. Acoustic neuromas: results of current surgical management. Neurosurgery 41:50–60.

Green JD Jr, Brackmann DE, Nguyen CD, Arriaga MA, Telischi FF, De la Cruz. 1994. Surgical management of previously untreated glomus jugulare tumors. Laryngoscope 104: 917–921.

Harwick RD, Miller AS. 1979. Craniocervical chordomas. Am J Surg 138:512–516.

Hassounah M, Al-Mefty O, Akhtar M, Jinkins JR, Fox JL. 1985. Primary cranial and intracranial chondrosarcoma: a survey. Acta Neurochir (Wien) 78:123–132.

Holmes B, Sekhar L, Sofaer S, Holmes KL, Wright DC. 1995. Outcomes analysis in cranial base surgery—preliminary results. Acta Neurochir (Wien) 134:136–138.

Horn KL, House WF, Hitselberger WE. 1985. Schwannomas of the jugular foramen. Laryngoscope 95:761–765.

Huang CF, Kondziolka D, Flickinger JC, Lunsford LD. 1999. Stereotactic radiosurgery for trigeminal schwannomas. Neurosurgery 45:11–16.

Hug EB, Loredo LN, Slater JD, et al. 1999. Proton radiation therapy for chordomas and chondrosarcomas of the skull base. J Neurosurg 91:432–439.

Inoue Y, Tabuchi T, Hakuba A, et al. 1987. Facial nerve neuromas: CT findings. J Comput Assist Tomogr 11:942–947.

Jackowski A, Weiner G, O'Reilly G. 1994. Trochlear nerve schwannomas: a case report and literature review. Br J Neurosurg 8:219–223.

Jackson CG, Cueva RA, Thedinger BA, Glassock ME 3rd. 1991. Cranial nerve preservation in lesions of the jugular fossa. Otolaryngol Head Neck Surg 105:687–693.

Jefferson G. 1955. The trigeminal neurinomas with some remarks on malignant invasion of the gasserian ganglion. Clin Neurosurg 1:11–54.

Kamerer DB, Hirsch BE. 1987. Paragangliomas ("glomus tumors") of the temporal bone. In: Sekar LN, Schramm VL Jr (eds), Tumors of the Cranial Base. Diagnosis and Treatment. Mount Kisco, NY: Futura Press, pp 641–654.

Kadish S, Goodman M, Wang CC. 1976. Olfactory neuroblastoma. A clinical analysis of 17 cases. Cancer 37:1571–1576.

Kaye AH, Hahn JF, Kinney SE, Hardy RW Jr, Bay JW. 1984. Jugular foramen schwannomas. J Neurosurg 60:1045–1053.

King TT, Morrison AW. 1990. Primary facial nerve tumors within the skull. J Neurosurg 72:1–8.

Kondziolka D, Lunsford LD, McLaughlin MR, Flickinger JC. 1998. Long-term outcomes after radiosurgery for acoustic neuromas. N Engl J Med 339:1426–1433.

Konefal JB, Pilepich MV, Spector GJ, Perez CA. 1987. Radiation therapy in the treatment of chemodectomas. Laryngoscope 97:1331–1335.

Korten AG, ter Berg HJ, Spincemaille GH, van der Laan RT, Van de Wel AM. 1998. Intracranial chondrosarcoma: review of the literature and report of 15 cases. J Neurol Neurosurg Psychiatry 65:88–92.

Kveton JF, Brackmann DE, Glasscock ME 3rd, House WF, Hitselberger WE. 1986. Chondrosarcoma of the skull base. Otolaryngol Head Neck Surg 94:23–32.

Lang DA, Neil-Dwyer G, Garfield J. 1999. Outcome after complex neurosurgery: the caregiver's burden is forgotten. J Neurosurg 91:359–363.

Lesser THJ, Janzer RC, Kleihues P, Fisch U. 1991. Clinical growth rate of acoustic schwannomas: correlation with the growth fraction as defined by the monoclonal antibody Ki-67. Skull Base Surg 1:11–15.

Levine PA, Gallagher R, Cantrell RW. 1999. Esthesioneuroblastoma: reflections of a 21-year experience. Laryngoscope 109:1539–1543.

Lipkin AF, Coker NJ, Jenkins HA, Alford BR. 1987. Intracranial and intratemporal facial neuroma. Otolaryngol Head Neck Surg 96:71–79.

Lund VJ, Howard DJ, Wei WI, Cheesman AD. 1998. Craniofacial resection for tumors of the nasal cavity and paranasal sinuses—a 17-year experience. Head Neck 20:97–105.

Majos C, Coll S, Aguilera C, Acebes JJ, Pons LC. 1998. Imaging of giant pituitary adenomas. Neuroradiology 40:651–655.

Maira G, Pallini R, Anile C, et al. 1996. Surgical treatment of clival chordomas: The transsphenoidal approach revisited. J Neurosurg 85:784–792.

Mariniello G, Horvat A, Dolenc VV. 1999. En bloc resection of an intracavernous oculomotor nerve schwannoma and grafting of the oculomotor nerve with sural nerve. Case report and review of the literature. J Neurosurg 91: 1045–1049.

Matthies C, Samii M. 1997. Management of 1000 vestibular schwannomas (acoustic neuromas): clinical presentation. Neurosurgery 40:1–10.

McCormick PC, Bello JA, Post KD. 1988. Trigeminal schwannoma: surgical series of 14 cases with review of the literature. J. Neurosurg 69:850–860.

McCutcheon IE, Blacklock JB, Weber RS, et al. 1996. Anterior transcranial (craniofacial) resection of tumors of the paranasal sinuses: surgical techniques and results. Neurosurgery 38:471–479.

McElroy EA Jr, Buckner JC, Lewis JE. 1998. Chemotherapy for advanced esthesioneuroblastoma: the Mayo Clinic experience. Neurosurgery 42:1023–1028.

Meyers SP, Hirsch WL Jr, Curtin HD, Barnes L, Sekhar LN, Sen C. 1992. Chordomas of the skull base: MR features. Am J Neuroradiol 13:1627–1636.

Mitchell A, Scheithauer BW, Unni KK, Forsyth PJ, Wold LE, McGivney DJ. 1993. Chordoma and chondroid neoplasms of the spheno-occiput. An immunohistochemical study of 41 cases with prognostic and nosologic implications. Cancer 72:2943–2949.

Morita A, Ebersold MJ, Olsen KD, Foote RL, Lewis JE, Quast LM. 1993. Esthesioneuroblastoma: prognosis and management. Neurosurgery 32:706–715.

Odake G. 1989. Intracranial hypoglossal neurinoma with extracranial extension: review and case report. Neurosurgery 24:583–587.

O'Donoghue GM, Brackmann DE, House JW, Jackler RK. 1989. Neuromas of the facial nerve. Am J Otol 10:49–54.

Ogunrinde OK, Lunsford LD, Flickinger JC, Kondziolka D. 1994. Stereotactic radiosurgery for acoustic nerve tumors in patients with useful preoperative hearing: results at 2-year follow-up examination. J Neurosurg 80:1011–1017.

Olsen WL, Dillon WP, Kelly WM, Norman D, Brant-Zawadzki M, Newton JH. 1987. MR Imaging of paragangliomas. AJR Am J Roentgenol 148:201–204.

Parnes LS, Lee DH, Peerless SJ. 1991. Magnetic resonance imaging of facial nerve neuromas. Laryngoscope 101: 31–35.

Perez-Ordonez B, Caruana SM, Huvos AG, Shah JP. 1998. Small cell neuroendocrine carcinoma of the nasal cavity and paranasal sinuses. Hum Pathol 29:826–832.

Pia HW, Grote E, Hildebrandt G. 1985. Giant pituitary adenomas. Neurosurg Rev 8:207–220.

Pitts LH, Jackler RK, Fuller GN. 1996. Intracranial nerve sheath tumors. In: Levin VA (ed), Cancer in the Nervous System, 1st ed. New York: Churchill Livingstone, pp 199–210.

Pluchino F, Crivelli G, Vaghi MA. 1975. Intracranial neurinomas of the nerves of the jugular foramen. Report of 12 cases. Acta Neurochir (Wien) 31:201–221.

Pluta RM, Ram Z, Patronas NJ, Keiser H. 1994. Long-term effects of radiation therapy for a catecholamine-producing glomus jugular tumor. Case report. J Neurosurg 80:1091–1094.

Polin RS, Sheehan JP, Chenelle AG, et al. 1998. The role of preoperative adjuvant treatment in the management of esthesioneuroblastoma: the University of Virginia experience. Neurosurgery 42:1029–1037.

Pollock BE, Lunsford LD, Kondziolka D, et al. 1998. Vestibular schwannoma management. Part II. Failed radiosurgery and the role of delayed microsurgery. J Neurosurg 89:949–955.

Pollock IF, Sekhar LN, Jannetta PJ, Janecka IP. 1989. Neurilemomas of the trigeminal nerve. J Neurosurg 70:737–745.

Pollock BE, Kondziolka D, Flickinger JC, Maitz A, Lunsford LD. 1993. Preservation of cranial nerve function after radiosurgery for nonacoustic schwannomas. Neurosurgry 33 :597–601.

Rosenberg AE, Nielsen GP, Keel SB, et al. 1999. Chondrosarcoma of the base of the skull: a clinicopathologic study of 200 cases with emphasis on its distinction from chordoma. Am J Surg Pathol 23:1370–1378.

Samii M, Babu RP, Tatagiba M, Sepehrnia A. 1995a. Surgical treatment of jugular foramen scwannomas. J Neurosurg 82:924–932.

Samii M, Migliori MM, Tatagiba M, Babu R. 1995b. Surgical treatment of trigeminal schwannomas. J Neurosurg 82: 711–718.

Samii M, Matthies C, Tatagiba M. 1997. Management of vestibular scwannomas (acoustic neuromas): auditory and facial nerve function after resection of 120 vestibular scwannomas in patients with neurofibromatosis 2. Neurosurgery 40:696–706.

Schultheiss R, Kristof R, Schramm J. 1993. Complete removal of an oculomotor nerve neurinoma without permanent functional deficit. German J Ophthalmol 2:228–233.

Sen CN, Sekhar LN. 1993. Complications of cranial base surgery. In: Post KD, Friedman ED, McCormick P (eds), Postoperative Complications in Intracranial Neurosurgery. New York: Thieme Medical Publishers, pp 111–131.

Shah JP, Kraus DH, Bilsky MH, Gutin PH, Harrison LH, Strong EW. 1997. Craniofacial resection for malignant tumors involving the anterior skull base. Arch Otolaryngol Head Neck Surg 123:1312–1317.

Shirato H, Sakamoto T, Sawamura Y, et al. 1999. Comparison between observation policy and fractionated stereotactic radiotherapy (SRT) as an initial management for vestibular schwannoma. Int J Radiation Oncol Biol Phys 44:545–550.

Sims E, Doughty D, Macaulay E, et al. 1999. Stereotactically delivered cranial radiation therapy: a ten-year experience of linac-based radiosurgery in the UK. Clin Oncol (R Coll Radiol) 11:303–320.

Spector GJ, Druck NS, Gado M. 1976. Neurologic manifestations of glomus tumors in head and neck. Arch Neurol 33:270–274.

Stapleton SR, Wilkins PR, Archer DJ, et al. 1993. Chondrosarcoma of the skull base: a series of eight cases. Neurosurgery 32:348–356.

Subach BR, Kondziolka D, Lunsford LD, Bissonette DJ, Flickinger JC, Maitz AH. 1999. Stereotactic radiosurgery in the management of acoustic neuromas associated with neurofibromatosis type 2. J Neurosurg 90:815–822.

Tan LC, Bordi L, Symon L, Cheesman AD. 1990. Jugular foramen neuromas: a review of 14 cases. Surg Neurol 34:205–211.

Terahara A, Niemierko A, Goitein M, et al. 1999. Analysis of the relationship between tumor dose inhomogeneity and local control in patients with skull base chordoma. Int J Radiat Oncol Biol Phys 45:351–358.

Tung H, Chen T, Weiss MH. 1991. Sixth nerve schwannomas. Report of two cases. J Neurosurg 75:638–641.

Welling DB. 1998. Clinical manifestations of mutations in the neurofibromatosis type 2 gene in vestibular schwannomas (acoustic neuromas). Laryngoscope 108:178–189.

Woods CI, Strasnick B, Jackson CG. 1993. Surgery for glomus tumors: The Otology Group experience. Laryngoscope 103(Suppl 2):65–70.

Part V

Cancer Metastatic to the Central Nervous System

13

Intracranial Metastases

W.K. ALFRED YUNG, LARA J. KUNSCHNER, RAYMOND SAWAYA, ERIC L. CHANG, AND GREGORY N. FULLER

Tumors that metastasize to the brain and intracranial space are very common, occurring in approximately 10% to 15% of patients with systemic cancers (Posner and Chernik, 1978; Cairncross and Posner, 1983; Walker et al., 1985). In contrast to the 17,500 new primary brain tumors that are expected to occur annually, more than 150,000 new cases of metastatic brain tumors occur each year in the United States (Posner, 1992). Moreover, the occurrence of metastasis to the brain is increasing as cancer patients live longer because of improved treatment and because the incidences of lung cancer and malignant melanoma continue to rise (Galicich et al., 1980a). The following are systemic cancers with a high incidence of metastasis to the brain

- Lung carcinoma
- Breast carcinoma
- Malignant melanoma
- Renal cell carcinoma
- Colorectal carcinoma

Lung carcinoma, especially small cell carcinoma and adenocarcinoma, is the most common type of cancer to metastasize to the brain, often with no evidence of systemic relapse (Figlin et al., 1988). The increase in the number of women and teenagers who smoke cigarettes and the increased rate of cigarette consumption has undoubtedly accounted for the increased number of young patients developing lung carcinoma and subsequent metastases to the brain.

Approximately 50% of patients with tumors metastatic to the brain present with single lesions, whereas the other 50% have two or more lesions (Delattre et al., 1988). A significant number of patients are found to have asymptomatic metastasis to the brain at the time of presentation with lung carcinoma (Salbeck et al., 1990).

Breast cancer is the second most common type of cancer to metastasize to the brain, occurring in approximately 10% of patients with advanced breast cancer (DiStefano et al., 1979). Some studies report that as many as 30% of patients experience concurrent systemic metastasis involving other organs, including the lung, bone, and liver (Tsukada et al., 1983). Younger patients and premenopausal patients are more prone to develop metastasis to the brain than are older, postmenopausal patients.

Malignant melanoma represents the third most common type of cancer having a high incidence of metastasis to the brain. An estimated 30% to 40% of patients with malignant melanoma will develop intracranial disease, including parenchymal and meningeal metastases (Byrne et al., 1983). In the brain, melanoma metastases are often hemorrhagic and multiple. The increasing incidence of melanoma metastasis to the brain may be the result of better control of extracranial disease through aggressive chemotherapy and biologic therapies.

Renal cell carcinoma and colorectal carcinoma are the fourth and fifth most common sources of brain metastases, respectively. Renal cell metastases, like melanoma metastases, tend to be highly vascular and prone to hemorrhage. They produce single lesions more frequently than do lung cancer and melanoma and exhibit a rare, but well-documented, potential for producing late brain metastases that sometimes present more than a decade after resection of the primary renal tumor (Radley et al., 1993). The brain is one of the least frequent sites of metastasis from colorectal carcinoma; these metastases occur in approximately 5% of patients (compared with approximately 30% to 40% of melanoma patients, 35% of lung carcinoma patients, and 10% to 30% of breast carcinoma patients) (Cascino et al., 1983). Among patients who have solitary colorectal carcinoma metastases to the brain, it has also been shown that a disproportionately large percentage (approximately 50%) of metastases occur in the posterior fossa (cerebellar) (Delattre et al., 1988).

These five types of metastatic tumors account for approximately 85% of all metastases to the brain (Delattre et al., 1988). A large number of other systemic neoplasms may produce central nervous system (CNS) metastases, including hematologic malignancies (leukemia, lymphoma), a wide spectrum of systemic carcinomas, and, in small numbers but with increasing frequency, some varieties of sarcoma (Lewis, 1988).

PATHOLOGY

Intracranial metastatic disease may involve any of the three principal morphologic compartments: the dura, leptomeninges (subarachnoid space), or brain parenchyma. Metastases that initially involve only one compartment frequently invade other compartments as they grow. This is particularly true of parenchymal lesions located either very superficially in the gray matter or subjacent to the ventricular system. These lesions may secondarily breach the pia or ependyma, which allows them access to the ventricular system or subarachnoid space, and subsequently to disseminate widely via the cerebrospinal fluid pathways. Alternatively, tumors located primarily in the subarachnoid space (leptomeningeal carcinomatosis) often track centrally via the perivascular Virchow-Robin spaces (Fig. 13–1), with ultimate expansion into the brain parenchyma.

By far, the most commonly encountered site of metastasis from carcinoma and sarcoma is within the brain parenchyma. In contrast, metastasis resulting from leukemia preferentially involves the leptomeninges. Breast carcinoma tends to produce isolated dural metastases (Fig. 13–2) in addition to parenchymal lesions. Prostate carcinoma more commonly metastasizes to the skull and vertebrae than to

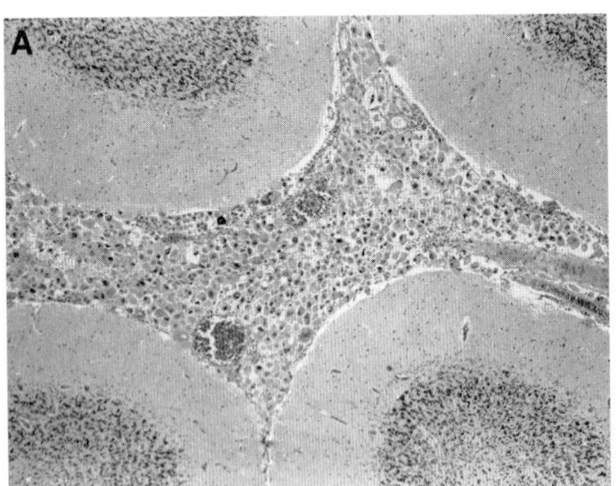

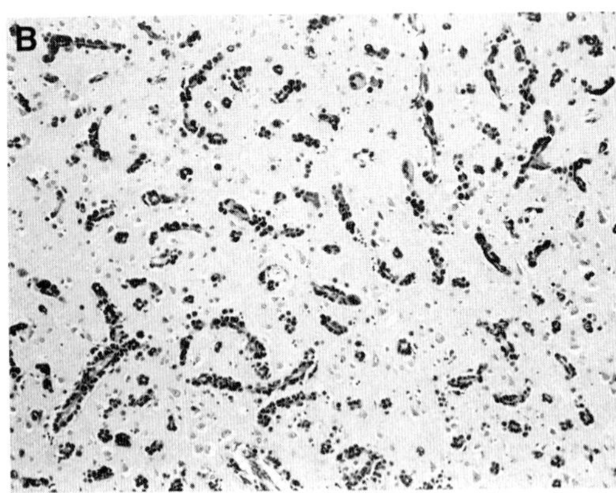

Figure 13–1. Leptomeningeal dissemination of tumor with secondary spread into brain parenchyma along perivascular (Virchow-Robin) spaces. **(A)** Melanoma cells fill the subarachnoid space. Once access to this strategic compartment has been gained, metastatic tumors can rapidly disseminate throughout the cerebrospinal fluid pathways of the neuraxis and may secondarily involve various anatomic constituents of the subarachnoid space such as blood vessels and cranial nerve rootlets or **(B)** may spread into the brain substance along the perivascular spaces of penetrating blood vessels. This is a common pattern of dissemination for melanoma and can also be seen with breast and other metastatic carcinomas. Diffuse leptomeningeal involvement is also frequently seen with the leukemias.

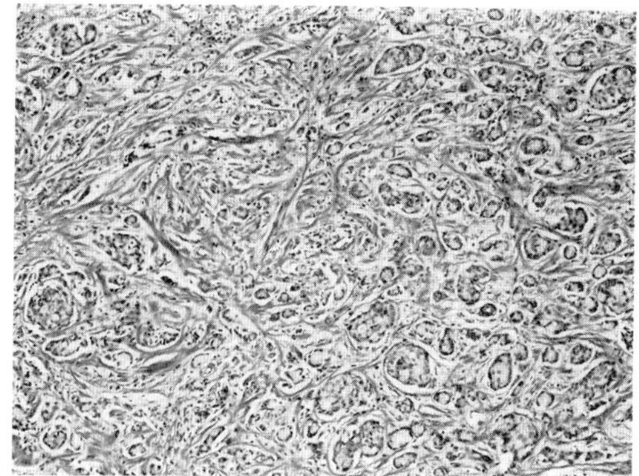

Figure 13–2. Dural metastasis. Breast carcinoma has a recognized tendency to produce dural metastases, as noted in this case in which cords and nests of infiltrating tumor cells are seen dissecting through the dense connective tissue of the dura. Such metastases from breast, prostate, lung, or other carcinomas can on occasion produce dural-based masses that mimic meningioma on neuroimaging studies.

the brain parenchyma, although intra-axial lesions may also occur. As in other locations, prostatic metastases to bone may be osteoblastic; in the cranium, such lesions may stimulate meningioma with hyperostosis.

Although parenchymal lesions may occur in any region of the CNS, several generalizations can be made:

1. Most metastases to the brain are supratentorial, the most common location being the cerebral hemispheres, where tumor emboli tend to lodge in the vascular gray matter, particularly at the gray matter–white matter interface where penetrating vessels narrow in caliber (Fig. 13–3).
2. Cortical hemispheric metastases are most frequently found in the vascular distribution territory of the middle cerebral arteries, particularly in the arterial border zones.
3. Metastases also occur frequently in the deep cerebral gray nuclei and white matter, as well as in the cerebellum.
4. Brain stem and spinal cord lesions occur far less frequently, but metastases may involve virtually any anatomic locus within the CNS, including such specialized organs as the choroid plexus, pineal gland, and pituitary.

In rare cases, systemic neoplasms may metastasize to a pre-existing primary brain tumor. The vast majority of such cases involve metastasis of a primary lung or breast carcinoma to a meningioma; very rarely, the host tumor is a schwannoma or glioma (Schmitt, 1984).

Microscopic Features

Intraparenchymal metastases tend to expand as roughly spherical masses and establish a well-defined interface with the surrounding brain parenchyma (Fig. 13–4). This sharp circumscription stands in contradistinction to the diffusely infiltrating margins of most primary brain tumors and can be of considerable practical importance to the surgical patholo-

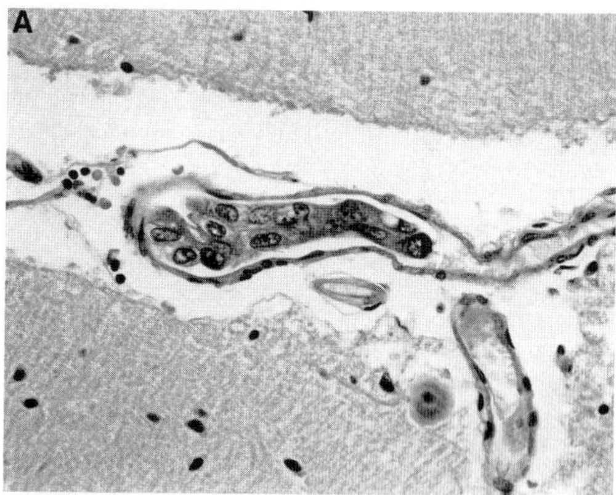

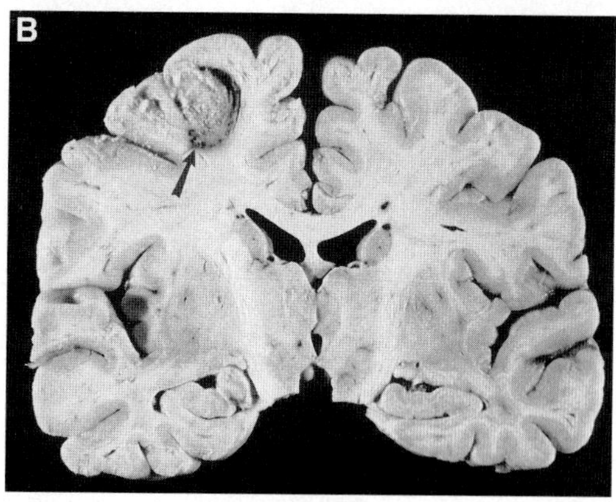

Figure 13–3. Parenchymal metastasis. **(A)** Most metastases originate by hematogenous dissemination of tumor emboli. **(B)** As illustrated in this case of metastatic lung adenocarcinoma, parenchymal metastases are commonly supratentorial, cortical in location, centered around the gray–white junction, and most frequently lie in the vascular distribution territory of the middle cerebral artery, particularly in the parasagittal arterial boundary zones.

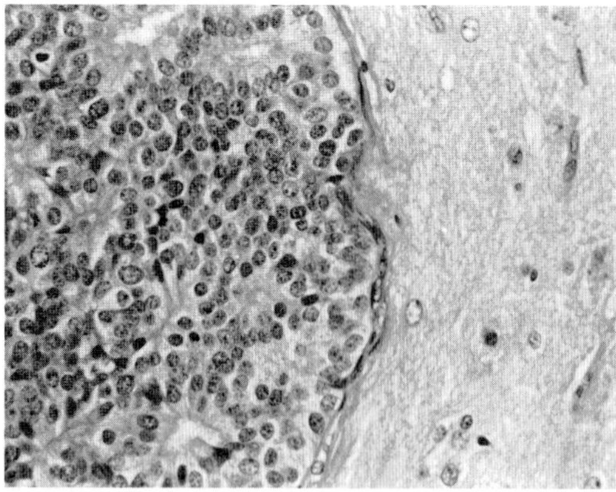

Figure 13–4. Interface of metastatic tumor with brain parenchyma. Sharp macroscopic (as in Fig. 13–3B) and microscopic circumscription is the rule for most metastatic tumors; for the surgical pathologist this is a useful diagnostic feature, and for the neurosurgeon it often permits total excision of the neoplasm. A notable exception to this rule is metastatic lymphoma, which, like primary CNS lymphoma, diffusely infiltrates nervous tissue from angiocentric foci.

gist, especially when dealing with small biopsy specimens of tumors that occur in the absence of a known primary systemic neoplasm.

As discussed, the overwhelming majority of tumors that give rise to CNS metastases are carcinomas; however, a variety of sarcomas may also metastasize to the CNS (Lewis, 1988). For all types of tumors, the morphology of the metastatic lesion in many cases recapitulates that of the primary neoplasm with great fidelity (Fig. 13–5). The degree of differentiation exhibited ranges from the metastatic lesion being almost pathognomonic of the primary organ of origin to being so poorly differentiated that only a diagnosis of metastatic carcinoma or metastatic malignant neoplasm can be made based on morphologic criteria. The brain parenchyma surrounding most metastatic lesions typically exhibits a robust reactive astrogliosis, a fact that must be considered when interpreting needle biopsy specimens obtained from this vicinity.

Immunostaining may be helpful in the diagnosis of some cases, particularly in distinguishing metastatic carcinoma from the other two major types of malignant neoplasms that involve the CNS parenchyma of older individuals: glioblastoma and primary CNS lym-

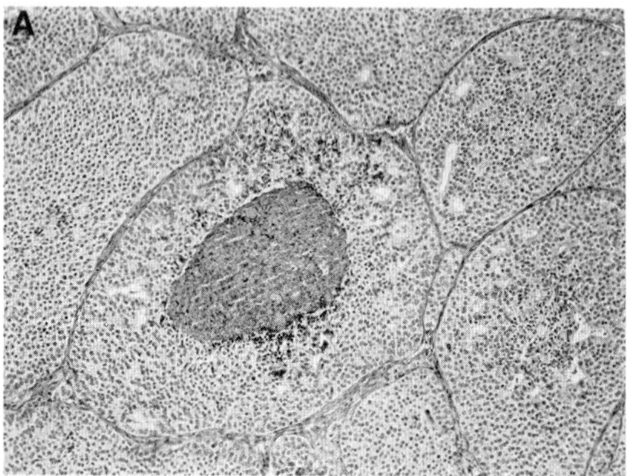

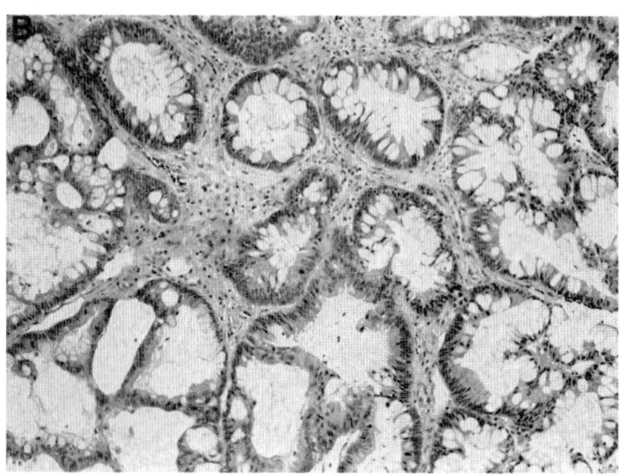

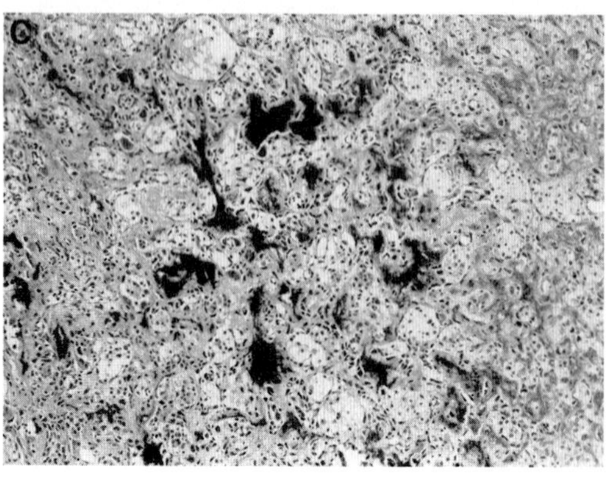

Figure 13–5. Histology of metastases. Many metastatic tumors closely recapitulate the morphology of the primary neoplasm, as illustrated here with **(A)** metastatic breast carcinoma, **(B)** mucinous colon carcinoma, and **(C)** osteosarcoma. Frequently, however, metastases are poorly differentiated and lack suggestive histologic features. Often, in the clinical setting of an unknown primary tumor, only a diagnosis of metastatic carcinoma or adenocarcinoma can be rendered in such cases, along with a list of the most likely primary sites.

phoma. In small and/or poorly preserved biopsy specimens, all three of these tumor types may appear quite similar on hematoxylin and eosin (H&E)–stained tissue sections: they are all high-grade pleomorphic tumors that show large atypical tumor cells, mitotic figures, and tumor necrosis. The basic panel of immunostains typically used in this situation is *(1)* glial fibrillary acidic protein (GFAP), which is positive only in gliomas; *(2)* a mixture of low- and high-molecular-weight keratin antibodies ("keratin cocktail") for metastatic carcinoma; and *(3)* the lymphoma markers CD45 (leukocyte common antigen), CD3 (a T-cell marker), and CD20cy (L26, a B-cell marker), either separately or combined as a "CNS lymphoma cocktail." This panel will usually permit separation of the three tumor types and definitive identification of metastatic carcinoma when present.

One important caveat is that many glioblastomas will show cross-reactivity with keratin antibodies; however, the GFAP immunostain will only be positive in glioblastomas, not in carcinomas or lymphoma. Once a diagnosis of metastatic carcinoma has been made, it is sometimes, but not always, possible to confirm the primary site of origin. If the patient has a known primary, a tentative diagnosis of metastatic carcinoma consistent with the primary can be rendered and immunostaining may not be necessary. If there is no known primary, a thorough clinical evaluation of the patient is required. For metastatic carcinomas in patients in whom no primary site can be identified after clinical work-up, a number of antibodies can be used to help identify tumor-specific phenotypic features. Unfortunately, many of the antibodies currently used in immunopathology are not uniformly as specific as one would like, and, therefore, both positive and negative antibody immunostaining must be interpreted with caution and in the context of the patient's clinical history. Nevertheless, antibody studies can be helpful. Useful antibodies include estrogen and progesterone receptor antibodies for breast carcinoma; thyroid transcription factor 1 (TTF-1) for lung and thyroid carcinomas; prostatic acid phosphatase (PAP) and prostate-specific antigen (PSA) for prostate carcinoma; and thyroglobulin (as well as TTF-1) for thyroid carcinoma. Again, it must be stressed that all these antibodies may show positivity in other carcinomas, and the results should not be considered absolute.

Another approach that has been taken is the use of several keratin antibodies of differing molecular weight together with other markers in large panels; diagnostic algorithms are then used to give estimates of the most likely primary site(s) based on the particular pattern of reactivity seen. Again, as with the use of individual antibodies, panel results can be helpful in directing attention to primary sites that should be investigated further clinically, but findings should be interpreted with caution. Brief mention must also be made of metastatic melanoma. Heavily pigmented lesions are easy to diagnose; however, up to a one-third of brain metastases appear amelanotic on H&E-stained slides, and melanoma may initially present as a CNS metastasis from an unknown primary tumor. Immunomarkers usually employed in this situation are S-100 protein, HMB-45, and MART-1.

PATHOPHYSIOLOGY

It is generally accepted that most metastatic brain tumors arise as a result of the hematogenous spread of cancer cells to the brain. Because brain microvessels are structured differently from systemic microvessels, cells destined to metastasize to the brain first adhere to and then penetrate the blood–brain barrier (BBB) formed by endothelial cells. Cells must penetrate the basement membrane and astrocytic foot processes before reaching the "soil" that allows their proliferation in brain parenchyma (Nicolson, 1982).

This process is thought to be nonrandom, as proposed by the "seeds" and "soil" hypothesis for cancer metastasis (Paget, 1989). The properties of the tumor cells, or "seeds," that determine the preferential development of brain metastasis from certain types of cancer include the quantitative expression of specific adhesive molecules that allow preferential adhesion to brain endothelial cells (Nicolson, 1988a,b) and the increased production of certain degradative enzymes, such as type IV collagenase and heparinase, that may enable tumor cells to penetrate the endothelial junction and the basement membrane (Liotta et al., 1991). Once the metastatic cells have penetrated the BBB, they proliferate in the appropriate microenvironment, or "soil," indigenous to brain parenchyma. Certainly, locally produced growth factors may stimulate the growth of specific metastatic tumor cells (Cavanaugh and Nicolson, 1991). In the brain, fibroblast growth factor, which has been found in high levels in the normal brain, may have such an effect (Rodeck et al., 1991).

Metastatic brain tumors, as opposed to primary malignant gliomas, usually grow as well-demarcated, spherical masses that are often amenable to total excision by surgery. Another difference between metastatic tumors and primary malignant gliomas is that brain metastases generally grow more rapidly and exhibit a high bromodeoxyuridine labeling index, often in the range of 20% to 25%, indicating a large proliferating fraction of tumor cells (Cho et al., 1988). Most gliomas, on the other hand, have lower labeling indices. Metastatic tumors are solid or cystic as a result of central necrosis; some tumors, such as metastases from melanoma, choriocarcinoma, and testicular carcinoma, are often hemorrhagic and tend to invade the vascular wall (Pullar et al., 1985).

CLINICAL PRESENTATION

The clinical presentation of patients with metastases to the brain depends on the number and location of the metastases. Multiple metastases frequently occur in lung carcinoma, breast carcinoma, and malignant melanoma; single metastases more commonly occur in patients with colorectal and renal cell carcinoma (Delattre et al., 1988). The common presenting symptoms in patients with metastases to the brain are listed in Table 13–1. Most patients present with complaints secondary to an increase in intracranial pressure (headache, mental change, or somnolence) or with focal (complex partial) or generalized seizures.

Patients with a single metastasis usually develop focal symptoms and signs in addition to headache and change in mental status. These may include *(1)* cranial nerve palsies, usually involving nerves VI and VII; *(2)* dysphasia; *(3)* visual deficits; *(4)* hemiparesis; or *(5)* hemisensory loss. Patients with multiple brain metastases can also present with diffuse, nonlocalized symptoms, such as generalized weakness and bowel and bladder incontinence. Surprisingly, many patients have few or no obvious symptoms and signs; thus, a physician should have a high index of suspicion for patients at risk of developing brain metastases.

Table 13–1. The Most Common Presenting Symptoms in Patients With Metastases to the Brain

Symptoms	*Relative Frequency at Diagnosis (%)*
Headache	71
Seizures	54
Mental change	52
Hemiparesis	43
Vomiting	32
Dysphasia	27
Impaired consciousness	25
Visual change	25

IMAGING

The diagnosis of brain metastasis is confirmed with computed tomography (CT) or magnetic resonance imaging (MRI) when the patient's history and neurologic examination raise the possibility of this diagnosis. Magnetic resonance imaging with gadolinium contrast enhancement represents the most sensitive diagnostic tool used to detect the presence of single or multiple metastases. Cerebrospinal fluid examination is only helpful in the presence of meningeal metastasis.

The presence of a single lesion seen on a CT or MRI scan in a patient with progressive systemic cancer is not an unequivocal indication of brain metastasis. The possibility that the lesion may be a cerebral abscess, a malignant glioma, or a meningioma must be considered and carefully ruled out. This will often require surgical biopsy or, preferably, excision of the lesion.

In patients who present with neurologic symptoms and whose CT or MRI results show a contrast-enhancing mass suggestive of a metastatic lesion, the primary cancer must be located before the brain lesion can be treated. The most common primary site will be the lung in men and the lung or breast in women. Once a brain metastasis has been discovered, the recommended techniques for screening systemic tumors are anteroposterior and lateral chest radiographs, chest CT scan if chest radiograph results are negative, mammogram (in women), bone scan, urinalysis, and stool guaiac test for occult blood (Voorhies et al., 1980). If these tests fail to identify a primary tumor site, surgical resection of the cerebral lesion can often provide the pathologic diagnosis. Frequently, however, metastatic adenocarcinomas do not exhibit pathognomonic morphologic features, and only a diagnosis of metastatic adenocarcinoma can be rendered. Not surprisingly, in one recent study, 85% of adenocarcinomas of unknown origin were ultimately found to have originated in the lung (Mrak, 1993). If there is more than one lesion in the brain, the largest or the most symptomatic lesion should be chosen first for surgical resection.

TREATMENT

General Considerations

The first stage of treatment for patients with single or multiple metastases to the brain is to stabilize acute neurologic symptoms caused by increased intracranial pressure and, in some patients, status epilepticus. Headache, nausea and vomiting, and change in mental status are the most common signs and symptoms of increased intracranial pressure. Patients with these symptoms should begin steroid treatment immediately (Cairncross and Posner, 1981). The typical starting bolus is 10 to 20 mg, followed by 16 mg/day in divided doses. The antiedema effect of steroids can often provide dramatic relief of symptoms such as headache and mental confusion. If the CT or MRI scan shows a marked increase in cerebral edema and evidence of impending herniation, the steroid dose can be increased to 24 or 30 mg/day with an initial loading dose as high as 100 mg, if necessary.

In patients showing signs of cerebral herniation, steroids usually do not take effect fast enough to reverse the rapid progression of neurologic dysfunction and impending death. Hyperventilation and intravenous hyperosmotic agents such as mannitol must be initiated immediately in addition to steroid therapy. Endotracheal intubation may be required to achieve adequate hyperventilation in obtunded or comatose patients. A pCO_2 level of 20 to 25 should be maintained to achieve optimal vasoconstriction. Mannitol should be given as a 20% solution at a dose of 1 to 2 g/kg body weight every 6 hours after an initial dose of 50 to 100 g administered intravenously over 20 to 30 minutes. The subsequent dose of mannitol can be adjusted according to the patient's level of consciousness and be tapered off when the patient's condition stabilizes with steroids (Ravussin et al., 1988).

Generalized or partial seizures are the presenting symptoms in 15% to 25% of patients with metastasis to the brain and are most common in patients with superficial lesions near the cortical gray matter. Status epilepticus can be lethal if allowed to continue for a prolonged period and should be eliminated with intravenous diazepam, lorazepam, or phenytoin, depending on the preference of the treating physician. Maintenance therapy should be initiated for long-term treatment. Phenytoin remains the most commonly used anticonvulsant, but carbamazepine and sodium valproate should also be considered. Unfortunately, there has been no study to compare the efficacy of these three drugs in this group of patients. However, several studies have reported fluctuation of phenytoin levels in patients receiving systemic chemotherapy (Grossman et al., 1989). Thus, the necessary anticonvulsant level should be monitored more frequently to maintain adequate control of seizures. Moreover, the issue of prophylactic anticonvulsant therapy in patients with metastasis to the brain or a primary brain tumor without seizures as a presenting symptom has not been resolved (Cohen et al., 1988). Despite the use of prophylactic anticonvulsants, the incidence of seizures with a later onset is the same as in patients not receiving prophylactic anticonvulsants. Nevertheless, it is advisable to start the patient on an anticonvulsant if the lesion is located in an epileptogenic area.

Radiation Therapy

The benefit of administering external-beam radiation therapy to patients afflicted with metastatic deposits of cancer in the brain was first reported by Chao and colleagues (1954) and subsequently by Chu and Hilaris (1961). Since that time, intermediate-dose whole-brain irradiation delivered in daily fractionation over 1 to 4 weeks has been considered the standard therapeutic approach for such patients (Coia et al., 1988). In numerous prospective and retrospective series, the value of cranial irradiation in preventing or delaying progression of neurologic deficits, restoring function, and decreasing steroid dependency has been well documented (Order et al., 1968; Borgelt et al., 1980; West and Maor, 1980; Kurtz et al., 1981).

The Radiation Therapy Oncology Group (RTOG) conducted several large phase III randomized trials in the 1970s evaluating the efficacy of myriad cranial irradiation fractionation schedules that varied radiation fraction sizes, total radiation doses, and times of treatment. The first two studies evaluated five one-fraction-per-day fractionation schemes: *(1)* 20.0 Gy in five 4.0-Gy fractions over 1 week; *(2)* 30.0 Gy in 10 3.0-Gy fractions over 2 weeks; *(3)* 30.0 Gy in 15 2.0-Gy fractions over 3 weeks; *(4)* 40.0 Gy in 15 2.67-Gy fractions over 3 weeks; and *(5)* 40.0 Gy in 20 2.0-Gy fractions over 4 weeks (Borgelt et al., 1980). No differences in survival time (less than 26 weeks), time to neurologic progression (12 to 19 weeks), or frequency of neurologic improvement were observed among these treatment arms.

From 1976 to 1979, the RTOG evaluated two radiation schedules for 255 patients whose distant metastases were limited to the brain and whose primary tumor was controlled or absent. The patients were randomized to receive 30.0 Gy in 10 3.0-Gy fractions over 2 weeks or 50.0 Gy in 20 2.5-Gy fractions over 4 weeks (Kurtz et al., 1981). No differences in palliative results or survival were observed. As a result of reports from these studies, 30.0 Gy in 10 3.0-Gy fractions has become the most commonly administered radiation regimen in the United States for patients with brain metastases, although the use of more protracted fractionation schemes should be considered in certain instances and is discussed later.

Patient factors are important in the evaluation of treatment response and outcome in clinical trials. Diener-West and coworkers (1989) used multivariate analysis to identify favorable subgroups of patients for future protocols and showed that four factors were associated with improved survival: having a Karnofsky performance scale (KPS) score of 70 or more, having an absent or controlled primary tumor, being younger than 60 years old, and having metastatic disease limited to the brain. Patients with all four favorable characteristics had a predicted 200 day survival of 52%. Those with none of the favorable factors had a predicted survival of 1.8 months (Diener-West et al., 1989). These prognostic factors were again identified by recursive partitioning analysis of a database from three consecutive RTOG trials. Three classes of patients were proposed: Class 1 included patients with a KPS score of ≥70 who were <65 years of age and who had a controlled primary tumor but no extracranial metastases; class 3 included those with a KPS score of <70; class 2 included all remaining patients (Gaspar et al., 1997).

An RTOG phase I/II trial of accelerated fractionation in patients with brain metastases prescribed whole-brain radiation of 1.6 Gy twice daily separated by 4 to 8 hours delivered for 5 days a week to 48 to 70.4 Gy. Analysis of the results suggested that dose escalation was tolerated without excessive toxicity and might improve survival in patients receiving 54 Gy or greater (Sause et al., 1993). In the follow-up RTOG phase III study, 445 unresected patients were randomized to receive either accelerated hyperfractionation of 1.6 Gy b.i.d. to 54.4 Gy or accelerated fractionation of 30 Gy in 10 fractions. Unfortunately, this trial failed to demonstrate any improvement in survival with 54.4 Gy (Murray et al., 1997).

Radiation sensitizers such as misonidazole and bromodeoxyuridine have been investigated by the RTOG. Randomized studies of patients with brain metastases have failed to show any statistically significant survival benefit with the administration of either compound along with whole-brain radiation therapy (WBRT) (Komarnicky et al., 1991; Phillips et al., 1995). Motexafin gadolinium texaphyrin (XCYTRIN), a drug that comes from a family of ring-shaped molecules adapted from porphyrin molecules, is being investigated as a radiation sensitizer in the treatment of brain metastases. The results from the phase I and II studies found that it was well tolerated when administered daily with WBRT (Viala et al., 1999; Mehta et al., 2000). A randomized phase III trial has been initiated.

Patchell and coworkers (1990) demonstrated a survival advantage for selected patients with resectable, single brain metastases randomized to receive resection and cranial irradiation over patients given cranial radiation alone, and this trial established surgery and postoperative irradiation as the standard approach for such patients. The study was limited to patients with a KPS score of 70 or greater and confirmed the benefit of resecting solitary lesions that had been previously suggested in nonrandomized study reports (Galicich et al., 1980a; Sause et al., 1990). The postoperative cranial radiation was delivered in 12 3.0-Gy fractions to a total dose of 36.0 Gy.

Several retrospective studies have examined the role of postoperative radiation therapy for patients with brain metastases (Dosoretz et al., 1980; DeAngelis et al., 1989b; Hagen et al., 1990; Smalley et al., 1992; Armstrong et al., 1994; Skibber et al., 1996). The majority of these studies do not demonstrate a survival benefit from adding WBRT after surgery. A prospective randomized study by Patchell and coworkers (1998) is the only one that addresses this issue. Ninety-five patients with a single metastasis to the brain were treated with complete surgical resection and were then randomized either to treatment with postoperative WBRT or to observation. Recurrence of metastases in the brain was less frequent in the radiation group (18%) than in the observation group (70%) ($p < 0.001$). Postoperative radiotherapy prevented brain metastasis recurrence at both the site of the original lesion (10% versus 46% for the untreated group; $p < 0.001$) and at other sites in the brain (14% versus 37%, respectively; $p < 0.01$). Deaths from neurologic causes were also reduced by administration of WBRT (14% versus 44% for untreated patients; $p = 0.003$). This reduction in neurologic deaths was seen only in those patients receiving WBRT immediately after surgery and not at the time of recurrence. No significant difference in overall survival was observed for untreated or irradiated patients. On the basis of randomized data demonstrating the reduction of neurologic deaths in patients receiving postoperative WBRT, it is reasonable to recommend its routine use.

Stereotactic radiosurgery was introduced in 1951 by the Swedish neurosurgeon Lars Leksell as a technique designed "to destroy" the target lesion with a single large dose of radiation delivered with a series of narrow radiation beams. Stereotactic radiation techniques exhibit rapid dose fall-off at the target edges, permitting significant sparing of normal brain tissue (Phillips et al., 1994). Numerous reports from different institutions support the use and effectiveness of radiosurgery for brain metastases (Wen and Loeffler, 1999). A multi-institutional outcome and prognostic factor analysis of radiosurgery for resectable single brain metastases showed that radiosurgery in conjunction with WBRT for a single brain metastasis can produce a substantial functional survival time of 56 weeks from the date of radiosurgery in patients with good performance status and who lack extracranial metastases. The comparability of these results to surgical series suggested that a randomized comparison of radiosurgery with surgery for brain metastasis treatment would be of great interest (Shaw, 1999). Such a trial is concurrently open to patients with a single brain metastasis at The University of Texas M. D. Anderson Cancer Center (M. D. Anderson). There are apparent advantages to either radiosurgery or surgery, depending on the clinical scenario. Surgery provides immediate resolution of mass effect and tissue for pathologic diagnosis if needed and poses no risk of radiation necrosis (Loeffler and Alexander, 1993). With radiosurgery, there are decreased risks of hemorrhage, infection, and tumor seeding as well as reduced costs produced, in part, by not requiring hospitalization.

The question has been raised by the results of the multi-institutional radiosurgery series as to whether radiosurgical treatment can improve survival beyond that produced by WBRT alone. This question was addressed by a study from the University of Pittsburgh in which 27 patients who had 2 to 4 metastases (<25 mm in diameter) were randomized to initial management with WBRT or with WBRT plus radiosurgery (Kondziolka et al., 1999). Local failure of tumor control was 100% in those receiving WBRT alone but was only 8% in those who received a radiosurgery boost. The median time to local failure was 6 months after WBRT alone and 36 months after WBRT plus radiosurgery ($p = 0.0005$). The median time to any local control failure in the brain was improved in the radiosurgery arm of the study (34 months) relative to the WBRT-alone arm (5 months; $p = 0.002$). Patients in the radiosurgery arm had a median survival time of 11 months versus 7.5 months in the WBRT-alone arm, but this difference was not statistically significant. The RTOG 95-08 trial, which is nearing completion, compares WBRT with or without a radiosurgery boost and stratifies patients as having a single metastasis or two to three metastases.

The role of WBRT after radiosurgery has been examined in a retrospective study by the group at the University of California at San Francisco, which reported on 106 patients with single or multiple brain metastases that were managed initially with radiosurgery or radiosurgery plus WBRT (Sneed et al., 1999). In the two treatment groups, both median survival and 1 year freedom from progression were similar at 11.3 months versus 11.1 months and 71% versus 79%, respectively. However, freedom from tumor progression in the brain at 1 year was significantly worse for the group treated by radiosurgery alone (28%) than for the group receiving radiosurgery plus WBRT (69%). The authors analyzed the results further by allowing for successful salvage of the first failure and found that if this was allowed, local control of tumor growth within the brain at 1 year was not significantly different for the two study arms (62% versus 73% at 1 year; $p = 0.56$) (Sneed et al., 1999). The group at the University of Heidelberg reported on a series of 311 brain metastases in 236 patients, each of whom had one to three brain metastases (Pirzkall et al., 1998). One hundred fifty-eight patients received radiosurgery only to a median dose of 20 Gy. The remaining 78 patients received a median radiosurgical dose of 15 Gy, followed by WBRT. Overall median survival time for patients was 5.5 months, and CNS disease control was achieved in 92% of treated brain metastases. Results were not significantly different for patients who did or did not receive WBRT, but there was a trend toward improved local control at 2 years (86% with WBRT versus 72% without it; $p = 0.13$). Interestingly, for patients without extracranial disease, there was a trend toward increased survival in patients receiving WBRT (15.4 months) relative to those not receiving it (8.3 months) ($p = 0.08$) (Pirzkall et al., 1998). The role of WBRT after radiosurgery warrants further study in a randomized trial that should include patient survival, freedom from progression, and a validated quality of life questionnaire component as endpoints to be evaluated.

Metastases from renal cell carcinoma and melanoma are described as "radioresistant" because of their lack of response to conventional radiotherapy. These histologic types deserve special attention and discussion. A review of the experience at M. D. Anderson with brain metastases from renal cell carcinoma described 119 patients who were treated with WBRT alone (Wronski et al., 1997). Overall median survival time of patients with the diagnosis of brain metastases was 4.4 months, and the cause of death was neurologic in 76% of patients and systemic in 16%. The authors suggest more aggressive approaches that include surgery or radiosurgery because of these unsatisfying results. A report from the University of Pittsburgh described the treatment of 35 patients who had 52 renal cell carcinoma metastases that were treated with radiosurgery over a 9 year period (Mori et al., 1998b). WBRT was given to 28 patients, and their median survival was 11 months after radiosurgical treatment. A 90% local control rate was achieved (21% disappearance, 44% tumor regression, 26% stable disease). The addition of WBRT did not improve survival or reduce distant failure (development of remote tumors) within the brain. However, local failure was only observed in the radiosurgery-alone arm of the study, leading the authors to hypothesize that WBRT might contribute to local control of tumor growth. The number of local control failures is small in this study, making it difficult to draw firm conclusions about the ability of WBRT to improve local control (Mori et al., 1998b).

The Harvard University group reported that melanoma and renal cell carcinoma metastases can be controlled just as easily with radiosurgery as tumors having "radiosensitive" histologies (Alexander et al., 1995). The University of California at San Francisco reported the use of gamma knife radiosurgery to treat brain metastases from melanoma in a series of 55 patients, including 16 treated for recurrence, 11 of whom received radiosurgery as a boost to WBRT, and 28 treated with radiosurgery alone as initial management (Seung et al., 1998). Median patient survival time was 35 weeks, and the only significant factor in multivariate analysis of survival was target volume of the tumor. No significant difference was seen in actuarial freedom from development of intracranial progression by log-rank analysis ($p = 0.85$), comparing patients treated with radiosurgery alone, radiosurgery plus WBRT, or radiosurgery for recurrence. Thus, the role of WBRT and how best to integrate it with radiosurgery in the management of melanoma and renal cell carcinoma, remains to be defined.

A series of patients who had single brain metastases from melanoma was also reported from the University of Pittsburgh, and the authors concluded that radiosurgery alone was appropriate because WBRT did not improve survival or local tumor control. New brain metastases developed less frequently with the addition of WBRT, but this was not statistically significant (Mori et al., 1998a). A multi-institutional report of the use of radiosurgery for single brain metastases demonstrated that tumor control improved significantly for melanoma and renal cell carcinoma relative to other tumor types ($p = 0.0006$) (Flickinger et al., 1994). Radiosurgery is thus an apparently effective modality for treating the so-called "radioresistant" tumor histologies such as solitary brain metastases from renal cell carcinoma and melanoma.

The subject of re-irradiation often arises when patients who have already received WBRT develop new, persistent, or recurrent brain metastases. Loeffler and co-workers (1990) treated 18 patients who had 21 recurrent or persistent brain metastases with radiosurgery. Patient eligibility requirements for treatment were having a KPS score that was ≥70 and having stable systemic disease. With a reported median patient follow up of 9 months, all tumors in the radiosurgery field were controlled, and no cases of symptomatic radiation necrosis occurred despite previous radiation treatment (Loeffler et al., 1990). A study to determine the maximum tolerable dose of single-fraction radiosurgery in patients with previously irradiated primary brain tumors or brain metastases was carried out by the RTOG study 90-05 (Shaw et al., 1996). There were 156 analyzable patients, 36% of whom had recurrent primary brain tumors (median prior dose = 60 Gy) and 64% of whom had recurrent brain metastases (median prior dose = 30 Gy), lesions that were all less than or equal to 40 mm in maximum diameter. Initially, patients were entered into arms of the study based on the maximum diameter of their recurrent lesion: tumors of 20 mm or less received 18 Gy; tumors ranging from 21 to 30 mm received 15 Gy; and those ranging from 31 to 40 mm received 12 Gy. Dose escalation was later carried out such that tumors smaller than 20 mm received 21 Gy; tumors between 21 and 30 mm received 18 Gy; and those between 31 and 40 mm received 15 Gy. Unacceptable acute toxicity secondary to cerebral edema was observed in 0%, 7%, and 5% of patients, respectively, in the first group. In the second, dose escalation, group, no unacceptable acute toxicity was seen. Multivariate analysis showed that maximum tumor diameter was one variable associated with significantly increased risk to patients with grade 3, 4, or 5 neurotoxicity. Specifically, patients with tumors of 21 to 40 mm in diameter were 7 to 16 times more likely to develop grade 3 to 5 neurotoxicity than those who had tumors less than 20 mm in diameter. Radiosurgery dose to the tumor was also associated with neurotoxicity. The actuarial incidence of radionecrosis was 5%, 8%, 9%, and 11% at 6, 12, 18, and 24 months after radiosurgery, respectively (Shaw et al., 1996, 2000). These results should be used as guidelines for dose selection to minimize unacceptable toxicities from radiosurgery.

Of note, in the final report of this study, a comparison between linear-accelerator–based radiosurgery and gamma knife radiosurgery results was made. The results, while interesting, cannot be meaningfully interpreted because of differences in the characteristics of the two groups of patients and the fact that this study was not originally designed to compare radiosurgical treatment units (Buatti et al., 2000).

The largest published series on external beam re-irradiation of brain metastases included 86 patients from the Mayo Clinic (Wong et al., 1996). The first course of radiation that was employed provided a median dose of 30 Gy, followed by 20 Gy for re-treatment. Patient median survival time after re-irradiation was 4 months; 27% of patients showed total symptom resolution; 43% experienced partial resolution; and 29% showed no change or had worsening of neurologic symptoms. There was no significant toxicity related to re-irradiation in the majority of patients. The only factor associated with improved survival on multivariate analysis was the absence of extracranial disease.

Another series, from New York University, included 52 patients selected for re-irradiation of recurrent cerebral metastases who were in relatively good medical condition, had an interval of at least 4 months from the initial course of radiation, and were experiencing a renewed deterioration in neurologic condition. Patients had initially been prescribed a dose of 30 Gy in 10 fractions over 2 weeks, whereas re-irradiation consisted of 25 Gy in 10 fractions. There was a 42% response rate to re-irradiation, and survival after the second treatment averaged 5 months (Cooper et al., 1990). If eligible, patients with recurrent brain metastases should be offered radiosurgery as the treatment of choice. If radiosurgery is not feasible, then whole brain re-irradiation may be carefully considered for patients who are highly motivated and have selection criteria of age, KPS status, absence of extracranial disease, and time interval between treatments in their favor.

Prophylactic cranial radiation therapy (PCI) should be considered for patients with limited-stage small cell lung cancer in complete remission because there is a 20% to 25% incidence of developing brain metastases subsequent to initial diagnosis (Ihde et al., 1997). Debate over PCI relates to concern that the treatment may itself directly cause neurologic deficits. The endpoints to be measured are quality of life and survival. The Prophylactic Cranial Irradiation Overview Collaboration Group published a meta-analysis of 987 patients with small cell lung cancer in complete remission based on seven trials that randomized patients to receive PCI or no PCI (Auperin et al., 1999). The relative risk of death in the treatment group compared with the control groups was 0.84, corresponding to a 5.4% increase in the rate of survival at 3 years—from 15.3% in the control group to 20.7% in the treatment group. Prophylactic cranial irradiation decreased the cumulative incidence of brain metastasis with a relative risk of 0.46 ($p <$ 0.001). Addressing the concern of neurocognitive impairment in patients who have undergone PCI, the investigators of the two largest trials included in the meta-analysis performed neuropsychological testing on most patients before and after treatment. Neurocognitive impairment was often detected at diagnosis, but no deterioration was found after PCI (Arriagada et al., 1995; Gregor et al., 1997). The meta-analysis makes a strong case that PCI should be included as standard care for all patients with small cell lung cancer in complete remission. Prophylactic cranial irradiation should not be given concurrently with chemotherapy, to avoid increased neurotoxicity.

The acute side effects of WBRT can include mild fatigue, reversible hair loss, and mild scalp erythema as well as hyperpigmentation. Of greater concern is the development of somnolence syndrome, described as persistent fatigue, anorexia, and irritability (especially in children), which may occur 3 to 10 weeks after treatment but may resolve within 6 weeks (Littman et al., 1984). Long-term survivors may be at risk of developing the late effects of WBRT. Progressive dementia, ataxia, and urinary incontinence were reported 5 to 36 months after WBRT in a series of 12 patients (DeAngelis et al., 1989a). Correlative CT findings identified cortical atrophy and hypodense white matter changes in these patients. Analysis of this study reveals that large radiation fractions (3 to 6 Gy) may have contributed to an increased incidence of late toxicities associated with WBRT. Based on this report, smaller fraction sizes of 1.8 to 2.5 Gy should be considered for patients who are expected to live longer than average because of favorable prognostic factors.

In conclusion, the effectiveness of WBRT in palliating brain metastases has been established by multiple RTOG trials. Prognostic factors identified by the RTOG that predict a greater life expectancy should be used to select patients for more aggressive treatments than WBRT alone, such as radiosurgery and surgery. This is important because control of neurologic disease is likely to impact overall survival. Also, long-term survivors are at increased risk of realizing the sequelae of radiation therapy, so that a patient belonging to the most favorable risk group should be given a more protracted course of radiation using smaller fraction sizes. Additional randomized trials that address quality of life in addition to traditional endpoints will be necessary to further evaluate the respective roles of radiosurgery and surgery and to determine the best way to combine these therapies with WBRT to maximize neurologic survival and quality of life. We hope that the data presented will help the reader make evidence-based decisions in the complex management of brain metastasis, the most common tumor type afflicting the brain.

Surgery

Although radiation therapy is frequently employed in the treatment of brain metastases, surgical removal of the tumor mass, whether single or multiple, may be the most effective palliation, especially for tumors from radioresistant diseases such as melanoma and carcinomas of the kidney and colon (Galicich and Arbit, 1990; Lang and Sawaya, 1996; Lang and Sawaya, 1998; Sawaya et al., 2000). Modern neurosurgical techniques and perioperative care have changed surgeons' perception of surgery for brain metastases over the past 30 years. With the potential for increased benefit that surgical resection offers, this treatment has become a routine consideration for certain patients.

Series examining heterogeneous groups of patients have revealed median survival times extending from 10 to 14 months for patients treated surgically for a single metastasis (Decker et al., 1984; Sundaresan and Galicich, 1985b; Ferrara et al., 1990; Patchell et al., 1990; Bindal et al., 1993). Previously, surgery for multiple metastases had not been considered as an option (Young and Patchell, 1990; Patchell, 1991), but one study of patients treated surgically for multiple metastases showed that the median survival extended to 10 months (Bindal et al., 1993). Because resection eliminates the neoplasm and the source of brain edema, surgery should be considered for large, symptomatic tumors, whereas removal of smaller asymptomatic lesions may be delayed until they become symptomatic or show rapid growth that would predict the onset of symptoms.

Numerous retrospective studies have confirmed that surgery with WBRT is more effective than WBRT alone. With the combined treatment, recurrence at the original site of metastasis occurs significantly less frequently and functional independence is significantly longer. Reports show that for patients with no other detectable evidence of disease at the time of craniotomy, the median survival after surgery is significantly increased (Galicich et al., 1980b). In a study of 33 patients who underwent surgical resection and postoperative WBRT for solitary brain metastases, Galicich and co-workers (1980a) found a low incidence of recurrence, a median survival time of 8 months, and a 1 year survival rate of 44%. A larger study of 78 patients conducted by the same group showed a median survival of 6 months, with a 1 year survival rate of 29% (Galicich et al., 1980b).

In two other studies, patients with cancer and a single brain metastasis were prospectively randomized to receive either surgery followed by WBRT or WBRT alone (Patchell et al., 1990; Vecht et al., 1993). In the study by Patchell and co-workers, the group undergoing surgery had fewer instances of recurrence (20% versus 52%, respectively), a significantly longer median survival (40 versus 15 weeks, respectively), and longer functional independence (38 versus 8 weeks, respectively). Similarly, Vecht's group demonstrated that surgery plus WBRT was superior to WBRT alone for the treatment of patients with single brain metastases (Vecht et al., 1993). More recently, Patchell and co-workers (1998) revealed that patients undergoing complete surgical resection of single brain metastases who also receive postoperative radiotherapy are subject to fewer tumor recurrences in the brain and die less frequently of neurologic causes than similar patients not receiving such radiotherapy; however, survival was not extended for patients receiving radiotherapy in addition to surgery.

Surgery is also beneficial for *(1)* controlling neurologic symptoms for patients with a functional status that dictates further treatment, *(2)* confirming a diagnosis that is questionable, *(3)* providing immediate palliation, *(4)* offering increased tolerance to and physician flexibility in using alternative treatments, *(5)* providing more durable local control, and *(6)* confirming or ascertaining the presence of metastases.

Patchell and co-workers (1990) noted that 6 of 54 patients initially considered to have brain metastases based on results from CT or MRI scans were found at surgery (or biopsy) to have other lesions, and 3 had no neoplastic disorder at all. These errors cannot always be precluded by diagnostic imaging and can be detected only by microscopic examination of tissue (Patchell et al., 1990).

Surgical considerations are based mainly on accessibility and resectability. Accessibility has been defined as "the risk and extent of neurologic injury the patient is willing to accept" (Moser and Johnson, 1989). The location of the lesion affects potential postoperative complications: lesions located in or near the motor cortex and Broca's speech area require particular care to avoid paresis or dysphasia; lesions located in the visual cortex can produce temporary or permanent visual deficits. For some of these lesions, techniques such as cortical mapping can be useful in minimizing damage to motor, sensory, and speech areas (Landy and Egnor, 1991), but careful pre- and intraoperative localization is vital, and each lesion must be considered individually. Lesions located deep within the brain parenchyma have traditionally been considered unresectable, but modern techniques, mainly intraoperative ultrasonography and stereotactic approaches, now allow access to these lesions (Kelly et al., 1988; Lange et al., 1990).

A factor that plays a significant role in considering resectability is the number of metastases. As late as 1990, most neuro-oncologists and neurosurgeons considered surgery for multiple metastases justified in only rare instances. The consensus was that the presence of multiple lesions strongly contraindicated surgery and that the circumstances precipitating the rare decisions to operate on patients with multiple metastases were limited to *(1)* a life-threatening mass effect on the brain stem (associated with an asymptomatic or relatively radiosensitive supratentorial lesion); *(2)* a large, life-threatening radiosensitive supratentorial lesion; or *(3)* two or more lesions that could be removed through a single cranial opening (Young and Patchell, 1990). Modern technology, however, is expanding surgical options.

At M. D. Anderson, we evaluated the results of surgery in patients with multiple lesions and found that surgery can play a very important role in managing these patients (Bindal et al., 1993). Fifty-six patients who underwent surgery for multiple brain metastases were divided into two groups: group A, those patients who had one or more lesions remaining after surgery (N = 30); and group B, those patients who had all lesions removed (N = 26). Patients in group B were matched by type of primary tumor, presence or absence of systemic disease, and time from first diagnosis of cancer to diagnosis of brain metastases to a third group of patients (group C, N = 26), undergoing surgery for a single lesion. Median survival times were 6, 14, and 14 months for patients in groups A, B, and C, respectively. Besides the significant difference in survival between groups A and B ($p = 0.003$) and between groups A and C ($p = 0.012$) there was a significant correspondence in recurrence or neurologic improvement rates between groups B and C, indicating that surgery for patients with multiple metastatic lesions that can all be removed is as effective as surgery for a single lesion. Although the results appear intuitively correct, a larger study may be required to confirm and expand these findings.

Patients with multiple brain metastases in whom all lesions cannot be surgically excised may also be candidates for surgery if resection of one or more highly symptomatic, debilitating, or life-threatening lesions will result in greater, more rapid palliation of symptoms than might be achieved by irradiation alone.

Although the microsurgical techniques used for the removal of brain metastases are largely the same as those used for the removal of other intracranial lesions, surgery is complicated by the generally small size of the tumors and the tendency of a cerebral metastasis to cause extensive edema with resulting neurologic symptoms, a factor that accounts for early diagnosis but contributes to the difficulty in locating metastases if they are not superficial. Modern imaging techniques allow for more efficacious treatment of asymptomatic tumors that may be discovered at the time that systemic cancers are first diagnosed and that, consequently, may still be quite small. Computer-assisted stereotactic and/or intraoperative ultrasound techniques *(1)* allow surgeons to precisely locate the tumor before making the cortical incision; *(2)* provide a direct route to the tumor that avoids eloquent areas of the brain; *(3)* aid surgeons in placing the bone flap precisely over the tumor location; and *(4)* eliminate the need to extensively probe for an elusive tumor, which can result in neurologic damage.

For patients experiencing considerable mass effect from the tumor, repeated preoperative CT scans help monitor the edema, which can be reduced in most cases by administering steroids. The preoperative administration of corticosteroids for a minimum of 48 hours helps prevent transdural herniation when the tumor is exposed. Administration of diuretics should be undertaken with caution because they reduce the extracellular volume and induce hyponatremia and vasoconstriction. Effective control of edema during surgery can be achieved by using a proper, safe anesthesiologic procedure (Gambardella et al., 1990). Surgery is limited by the functional importance of the brain tissue to be traversed. Another major consideration is the expected quality of survival, a subjectively determined factor. For one patient, a few months of restored neurologic function might be very important, whereas it might be of minimal significance for another patient.

Surgery and imaging technology came together in 1986 in the first successful removal of a lesion metastatic to the tectum of the midbrain (Tobler et al., 1986). Although metastasis to this site is a very rare occurrence (1% to 3% of brain metastases) and was previously considered an inoperable location, the tumor was vaporized with a carbon dioxide laser beam (up to 20 watts) and removed by a central coring technique. For patients with systemic cancer that cannot be controlled, management decisions for asymptomatic brain tumors are moot.

As noted previously, early neurosurgical attempts met with high rates of complications due to unsophisticated radiographic methods and a limited ability to control brain herniation. Modern advances, including the use of corticosteroids and modern anesthesia, the advent of CT and MRI, the use of the surgical microscope, and the development of intraoperative ultrasound, stereotactic localization, and cortical mapping, have significantly reduced operative mortalities and morbidities (Sawaya et al., 1998). Postoperative mortality is most often due to uncontrolled systemic cancer, but comparisons of results from gross total removal and partial removal of brain metastases indicate that the former yields the lowest rate of operative mortality and that the 30 day mortality risk may be doubled in cases of partial removal (Haar and Patterson, 1972). A recent study of neurosurgical outcomes in a series of 400 craniotomies performed for removal of brain metastases (48%) or gliomas (52%) (Sawaya et al., 1998) determined that gross total resection of most tumors (73%) did not lead to more major neurologic deficits than were observed for patients undergoing subtotal or partial resection. Nonfatal complications such as hematomas, wound infections, and pseudomeningocele formations, which occur in 8% to 9% of all craniotomies for brain metastases (Bindal et al., 1993), as well as surgically induced neurologic impairments, are usually transient events. Clinically evident thromboembolic complications, such as deep vein thrombosis or pulmonary embolism, occur in an estimated 10% of patients (Constantini et al., 1991; Sawaya et al., 1992). Mortality and morbidity rates have been reduced to 3% or less and 5% or less, respectively (Sundaresan and Galicich, 1985a; Brega et al., 1990; Patchell et al., 1990; Bindal et al., 1993).

Chemotherapy

Systemic chemotherapy has historically been considered ineffective in the treatment of brain metastases, with several reasons being given for this presumed failure (Buckner, 1991). The BBB has been assumed to be a major restriction to the CNS entry of many cytotoxic drugs that are large polar or hydrophobic compounds. Unlike normal brain capillaries, tumor capillaries are variably disrupted in patients who have brain metastases (and high-grade primary brain tumors). Evidence that the tumor capillaries in most metastatic tumors are disrupted is shown by the fact that virtually all metastatic tumors in the brain are contrast enhancing, reflecting the leakage of contrast material from the tumor vasculature to the interstitium. Drugs (cisplatin, etoposide, nimustine, and aziquinone) administered before surgery and measured in tumor samples removed at surgery have consistently demonstrated pharmacologically relevant levels in these tissues, suggesting that these agents are able to penetrate the tumor tissue in the brain when delivered systemically (Stewart et al., 1979; Stewart et al., 1982; Savaraj et al., 1983, 1984). Most animal studies, however, have shown lower capillary permeability and lower drug concentrations in brain tumors than in subcutaneous tumors for systemically administered chemotherapy (Stewart, 1994).

Lipophilic drugs such as nitrosoureas or other semisynthetic agents may be able to deliver even higher levels of drugs to the tumor periphery where the BBB may remain relatively intact (Levin et al., 1975, 1976). Some drugs may, however, inadequately penetrate tumor regions and will achieve subtherapeutic levels intracellularly (Levin et al., 1980). The observation of CNS relapse before relapse at other sites in acute leukemia and small cell lung cancer is often cited as evidence of the importance of the BBB in inhibiting the effectiveness of chemotherapy. Blood–brain barrier disruption with hyperosmolar agents, to increase chemotherapy delivery to brain, has been developed for primary brain tumors but has not yet been investigated for brain metastasis treatment.

The routine use of corticosteroids, which are capable of re-establishing disrupted BBB function, for symptomatic brain metastasis may provide an additional protective effect against cytotoxic agents (Weller et al., 1997; Mariotta et al., 1999) and may further limit drug delivery into CNS tumors (Nakagawa et al., 1987).

Cancers that most frequently metastasize to the brain, such as non–small cell lung cancer and malignant melanoma, are often inherently insensitive to systemic chemotherapy. Many patients develop brain metastases in the face of widespread systemic relapse and/or after failure of several prior treatment regimens, including radiotherapy and chemotherapy. While long-duration chemotherapy treatment can increase the frequency of acquired resistance to chemotherapy agents for brain tumor metastases because of increased expression of efflux pumps such as the P-glycoprotein, encoded by the multidrug-resistance-1 gene, nonetheless, the intact BBB already has functioning efflux pumps such as the P-glycoprotein, raising the question whether this is truly an acquired mechanism or a common de novo mechanism for drug failure of tumors in the brain.

Several lines of evidence suggest that a number of different chemotherapy regimens may be at least palliative with respect to some brain metastases (Greig, 1984). An increasing number of clinical trials have demonstrated response rates for brain metastases that are in keeping with those seen for systemic metastases using the same regimens, especially for breast and lung carcinomas.

Several clinical trials have reported the activity of single-agent and combination chemotherapy in some types of brain metastases. Breast carcinomas, in general, are considered chemosensitive tumors. Patients with extracranial metastatic breast carcinomas who have not had prior chemotherapy can achieve 50% to 70% response rates with combination chemotherapy, but only 20% to 30% of patients who failed prior chemotherapy will respond to second-line salvage chemotherapy. Rosner and coworkers (1986) demonstrated a response rate of >50% using cyclophosphamide, 5-fluorouracil, and prednisone in 100 breast cancer patients with cerebral metastasis. The best result reported to date has been with a five-drug combination—cyclophosphamide, methotrexate, fluorouracil, vincristine, and prednisone (CMFVP) with which Rosner and colleagues (1986) found 10% complete and 40% partial response rates for patients not receiving prior chemotherapy. There were some long-term survivors, but the median duration of response was only 7 months, and survival was similarly quite short. Several points should be emphasized in this study: *(1)* patients with brain metastases responded to combination chemotherapy at a rate similar to that experienced by patients treated for extracranial metastases; *(2)* patients who failed initial chemotherapy did respond, albeit at a lower rate, to second- or third-line regimens; *(3)* all patients received prednisone, an antiedema agent that may interfere with the response interpretation because of a prednisone-mediated decrease in edema and mass effect as visualized on neuroimaging studies; and *(4)* the high response rates have not been reproduced by other investigators (Flowers and Levin, 1993).

Other drug regimens, including etoposide and cisplatin (Cocconi et al., 1990; Franciosi et al., 1999) and CAF (cyclophosphamide, doxorubicin, and fluorouracil) have shown similar activities for breast carcinoma brain metastases with response rates in the range of 40% to 50%. A multidrug combination called TPDC-FuHu (6-thioguanine, procarbazine, dibromodulcitol, lomustine, fluorouracil, and hydroxyurea) that focused on overcoming nitrosourea resistance and potentiating nitrosourea tumor cell kill demonstrated similar results for patients with brain metastases from breast and non–small cell lung carcinoma and considerably better results for patients with small cell lung carcinoma who failed prior radiation therapy for these metastases. For patients with brain metastases from breast, non–small cell and small cell lung carcinoma, response rates were 36%, 26%, and 67%, respectively. The corresponding disease-free survival periods for these responding patient subgroups were 27, 21, and 133 weeks, respectively (Kaba et al., 1997).

Among the various lung cancers, small cell carcinoma is the most sensitive to chemotherapy. Lee and co-workers (1989) reported the use of cyclophosphamide, doxorubicin, vincristine, and etoposide as primary chemotherapy for 15 patients with small cell lung cancer who presented with brain metastases. Nine of 11 evaluable patients (82%) showed complete or partial responses. In another study, Twelves and co-workers (1990) treated 14 patients who had brain metastases from small cell lung cancer at presentation with cyclophosphamide, vincristine, and etoposide. Nine patients (64%) responded. In contrast, results from small studies in which chemotherapy combinations with etoposide and cisplatin (Croisile et al., 1992), fotemustine plus cisplatin (Cotto et al., 1996), and lomustine, carboplatin, vinorelbine, and fluorouracil (Colleoni et al., 1997) were used to treat brain metastases from non–small cell lung carcinoma (a less chemosensitive tumor type) were much less impressive. Response rates for patients in these studies were 0%, 14%, and 33%, respectively, to chemotherapy. Robinet and colleagues (1991) reported a 50% response rate using fluorouracil and cisplatin; however, this result has not yet been duplicated. These results suggest that the response of cerebral metastases to chemotherapy may depend on the inherent chemosensitivity of the primary cancer type.

Historically, malignant melanoma has been shown to be extremely insensitive to chemotherapy, with brain metastases from melanoma being no exception. However, a meeting abstract in 1996 reported that use of cisplatin combined with interleukin-2 and interferon-α_{2a} to treat brain metastases from melanoma had shown improved results with a response rate of 39% and a median survival time of 32 weeks (Mousseau et al., 1996).

Several studies of brain metastases from other systemic chemosensitive cancers, such as choriocarcinoma and germinoma, have demonstrated high response rates to combination chemotherapy regimens that are deemed active for the systemic cancers. In one study, 13 of 18 (72%) patients with choriocarcinoma and brain metastasis responded to primary chemotherapy with etoposide, methotrexate, dactinomycin, vincristine, cyclophosphamide, and cisplatin (Rustin et al., 1989), whereas in another study, 8 of 10 patients (80%) diagnosed with germinoma and brain metastases achieved complete response to cisplatin, vincristine, methotrexate, bleomycin, etoposide, dactinomycin, and cyclophosphamide (Rustin et al., 1986). In gestational trophoblastic disease metastatic to the brain, combination chemotherapy with etoposide, methotrexate, vincristine, actinomycin-D, and cyclophosphamide as sole therapy can be curative.

The role of chemotherapy in the overall management of patients with brain metastases remains under investigation. Chemotherapy should be considered for chemosensitive tumors, keeping in mind that surgery and radiotherapy remain the primary treatment modalities. There is insufficient positive experience to support the general use of chemotherapy in patients with brain metastases; therefore, chemotherapy should be considered as palliative and should be given under the auspices of appropriately designed clinical trials. The choice of the drug or drug combination should be guided by the chemosensitivity profile of the primary systemic cancer. Future treatment approaches may involve pre-radiation chemotherapy for patients who have minimal neurologic symptoms, which may reduce the tumor burden in the brain, allowing more prolonged control after radiation therapy and, perhaps, decreased radiation neurotoxicity, if the radiation dose can be reduced.

The role of the BBB in restricting drug entry into brain regions adjacent to a tumor probably plays some role in the efficacy of chemotherapy for brain metastases. The use of corticosteroids by these patients should be carefully limited as much as possible to allow maximal benefit from chemotherapeutic agents while maintaining neurologic function. Adjustments in steroid dose must be taken into consideration in clinical trial design, as the dose and the timing of steroid administration may partially rectify a leaky tumor vasculature and falsely produce a response on CT or MRI scans.

REFERENCES

Alexander E 3rd, Moriarty TM, Davis RB, et al. 1995. Stereotactic radiosurgery for the definitive, noninvasive treatment of brain metastases. J Natl Cancer Inst 87:34–40.

Armstrong JG, Wronski M, Galicich J, Arbit E, Leibel SA, Burt M. 1994. Postoperative radiation for lung cancer metastatic to the brain. J Clin Oncol 12:2340–2344.

Arriagada R, Le Chevalier T, Borie F, et al. 1995. Prophylactic cranial irradiation for patients with small-cell lung cancer in complete remission. J Natl Cancer Inst 87:183–190.

Auperin A, Arriagada R, Pignon JP, et al. 1999. Prophylactic cranial irradiation for patients with small-cell lung cancer in complete remission. Prophylactic Cranial Irradiation Overview Collaborative Group. N Engl J Med 341:476–484.

Bindal RK, Sawaya R, Leavens ME, Lee JJ. 1993. Surgical treatment of multiple brain metastases. J Neurosurg 79:210–216.

Borgelt B, Gelber R, Kramer S, et al. 1980. The palliation of brain metastases: final results of the first two studies by the Radiation Therapy Oncology Group. Int J Radiat Oncol Biol Phys 6:1–9.

Brega K, Robinson WA, Winston K, Wittenberg W. 1990. Surgical treatment of brain metastases in malignant melanoma. Cancer 66:2105–2110.

Buatti JM, Friedman WA, Meeks SL, Bova FJ. 2000. RTOG 90-05: the real conclusion. Int J Radiat Oncol Biol Phys 47:269–271.

Buckner JC. 1991. The role of chemotherapy in the treatment of patients with brain metastases from solid tumors. Cancer Metastasis Rev 10:335–341.

Byrne TN, Cascino TL, Posner JB. 1983. Brain metastasis from melanoma. J Neurooncol 1:313–317.

Cairncross JG, Posner JB. 1981. Neurological complications of systemic cancer. In: Yarbro JW, Bornstein RS (eds), Oncologic Emergencies. New York: Grune & Stratton, p 73.

Cairncross JG, Posner JB. 1983. The management of brain metastases. In: Walker MD (ed), Oncology of the Nervous System. Boston: Martinus Nijhof, p. 341–377.

Cascino TL, Leavengood JM, Kemeny N, Posner JB. 1983. Brain metastases from colon cancer. J Neurooncol 1:203–209.

Cavanaugh PG, Nicolson GL. 1991. Lung-derived growth factor that stimulates the growth of lung-metastasizing tumor cells: identification as transferrin. J Cell Biochem 47:261–271.

Chao J, Phillips R, Nickson J. 1954. Roentgen-ray therapy of cerebral metastases. Cancer 7:682–689.

Cho KG, Hoshino T, Pitts LH, Nomura K, Shimosato Y. 1988. Proliferative potential of brain metastases. Cancer 62:512–515.

Chu FCH, Hilaris BB. 1961. Value of radiation therapy in the management of intracranial metastases. Cancer 14:577.

Cocconi G, Lottici R, Bisagni G, et al. 1990. Combination therapy with platinum and etoposide of brain metastases from breast carcinoma. Cancer Invest 8:327–334.

Cohen N, Strauss G, Lew R, Silver D, Recht L. 1988. Should prophylactic anticonvulsants be administered to patients with newly-diagnosed cerebral metastases? A retrospective analysis. J Clin Oncol 6:1621–1624.

Coia LR, Hanks GE, Martz K, Steinfeld A, Diamond JJ, Kramer S. 1988. Practice patterns of palliative care for the United States 1984–1985. Int J Radiat Oncol Biol Phys 14: 1261–1269.

Colleoni M, Graiff C, Nelli P, et al. 1997. Activity of combination chemotherapy in brain metastases from breast and lung adenocarcinoma. Am J Clin Oncol 20:303–307.

Constantini S, Kornowski R, Pomeranz S, Rappaport ZH. 1991. Thromboembolic phenomena in neurosurgical patients operated upon for primary and metastatic brain tumors. Acta Neurochir (Wien) 109:93–97.

Cooper JS, Steinfeld AD, Lerch IA. 1990. Cerebral metastases: value of reirradiation in selected patients. Radiology 174:883–885.

Cotto C, Berille J, Souquet PJ, et al. 1996. A phase II trial of fotemustine and cisplatin in central nervous system metastases from non–small cell lung cancer. Eur J Cancer 32A:69–71.

Croisile B, Trillet-Lenoir V, Catajar JF, et al. 1992. Cerebral metastasis disclosing primary bronchogenic cancers. Rev Neurol (Paris) 148:488–492.

DeAngelis LM, Delattre JY, Posner JB. 1989a. Radiation-induced dementia in patients cured of brain metastases. Neurology 39:789–796.

DeAngelis LM, Mandell LR, Thaler HT, et al. 1989b. The role of postoperative radiotherapy after resection of single brain metastases. Neurosurgery 24:798–805.

Decker DA, Decker VL, Herskovic A, Cummings GD. 1984. Brain metastases in patients with renal cell carcinoma: prognosis and treatment. J Clin Oncol 2:169–173.

Delattre JY, Krol G, Thaler HT, Posner JB. 1988. Distribution of brain metastases. Arch Neurol 45:741–744.

Diener-West M, Dobbins TW, Phillips TL, Nelson DF. 1989. Identification of an optimal subgroup for treatment evaluation of patients with brain metastases using RTOG study 7916. Int J Radiat Oncol Biol Phys 16:669–673.

DiStefano A, Yong Yap Y, Hortobagyi GN, Blumenschein GR. 1979. The natural history of breast cancer patients with brain metastases. Cancer 44:1913–1918.

Dosoretz DE, Blitzer PH, Russell AH, Wang CC. 1980. Management of solitary metastasis to the brain: the role of elective brain irradiation following complete surgical resection. Int J Radiat Oncol Biol Phys 6:1727–1730.

Ferrara M, Bizzozzero L, Talamonti G, D'Angelo VA. 1990. Surgical treatment of 100 single brain metastases. Analysis of the results. J Neurosurg Sci 34:303–308.

Figlin RA, Piantadosi S, Feld R. 1988. Intracranial recurrence of carcinoma after complete surgical resection of stage I, II, and III non–small-cell lung cancer. N Engl J Med 318:1300–1305.

Flickinger JC, Kondziolka D, Lunsford LD, et al. 1994. A multi-institutional experience with stereotactic radiosurgery for solitary brain metastasis. Int J Radiat Oncol Biol Phys 28:797–802.

Flowers A, Levin VA. 1993. Management of brain metastases from breast carcinoma. Oncology 7:21–26.

Franciosi V, Cocconi G, Michiara M, et al. 1999. Front-line chemotherapy with cisplatin and etoposide for patients with brain metastases from breast carcinoma, nonsmall cell lung carcinoma, or malignant melanoma: a prospective study. Cancer 85:1599–1605.

Galicich J, Arbit E. 1990. Metastatic brain tumors. In: Youmans JR (ed), Neurological Surgery. Philadelphia: WB Saunders, pp 3204–3222.

Galicich JH, Sundaresan N, Arbit E, Passe S. 1980a. Surgical treatment of single brain metastasis: factors associated with survival. Cancer 45:381–386.

Galicich JH, Sundaresan N, Thaler HT. 1980b. Surgical treatment of single brain metastasis. Evaluation of results by computerized tomography scanning. J Neurosurg 53:63–67.

Gambardella G, Santamaria LB, Toscano SG, et al. 1990. Brain metastases: surgical versus conservative treatment. J Neurosurg Sci 34:309–314.

Gaspar L, Scott C, Rotman M, et al. 1997. Recursive partitioning analysis (RPA) of prognostic factors in three Radiation Therapy Oncology Group (RTOG) brain metastases trials. Int J Radiat Oncol Biol Phys 37:745–751.

Gregor A, Cull A, Stephens RJ, et al. 1997. Prophylactic cranial irradiation is indicated following complete response to induction therapy in small cell lung cancer: results of a multicentre randomised trial. United Kingdom Coordinating Committee for Cancer Research (UKCCCR) and the European Organization for Research and Treatment of Cancer (EORTC). Eur J Cancer 33:1752–1758.

Greig NH. 1984. Chemotherapy of brain metastases: current status. Cancer Treat Rev 11:157–186.

Grossman SA, Sheidler VR, Gilbert MR. 1989. Decreased phenytoin levels in patients receiving chemotherapy. Am J Med 87:505–510.

Haar F, Patterson RH Jr. 1972. Surgery for metastatic intracranial neoplasm. Cancer 30:1241–1245.

Hagen NA, Cirrincione C, Thaler HT, DeAngelis LM. 1990. The role of radiation therapy following resection of single brain metastasis from melanoma. Neurology 40:158–160.

Ihde DC, Pass HI, Glatstein E. 1997. Small cell lung cancer. In: DeVita VT, Hellman S, Rosenberg SA (eds), Cancer: Principles and Practice of Oncology. Philadelphia: Lippincott-Raven, pp 911–949.

Kaba SE, Kyritsis AP, Hess K, et al. 1997. TPDC-FuHu chemotherapy for the treatment of recurrent metastatic brain tumors. J Clin Oncol 15:1063–1070.

Kelly PJ, Kall BA, Goerss SJ. 1988. Results of computed tomography-based computer-assisted stereotactic resection of metastatic intracranial tumors. Neurosurgery 22:7–17.

Komarnicky LT, Phillips TL, Martz K, Asbell S, Isaacson S, Urtasun R. 1991. A randomized phase III protocol for the evaluation of misonidazole combined with radiation in the treatment of patients with brain metastases (RTOG-7916). Int J Radiat Oncol Biol Phys 20:53–58.

Kondziolka D, Patel A, Lunsford LD, Kassam A, Flickinger JC. 1999. Stereotactic radiosurgery plus whole brain radiotherapy versus radiotherapy alone for patients with multiple brain metastases. Int J Radiat Oncol Biol Phys 45:427–434.

Kurtz JM, Gelber R, Brady LW, Carella RJ, Cooper JS. 1981. The palliation of brain metastases in a favorable patient population: a randomized clinical trial by the Radiation Therapy Oncology Group. Int J Radiat Oncol Biol Phys 7:891–895.

Landy HJ, Egnor M. 1991. Intraoperative ultrasonography and cortical mapping for removal of deep cerebral tumors. South Med J 84:1323–1326.

Lang FF, Sawaya R. 1996. Surgical management of cerebral metastases. Neurosurg Clin North Am 7:459–484.

Lang FF, Sawaya R. 1998. Surgical treatment of metastatic brain tumors. Semin Surg Oncol 14:53–63.

Lange OF, Scheef W, Haase KD. 1990. Palliative radio-chemotherapy with ifosfamide and BCNU for breast cancer patients with cerebral metastases. A 5-year experience. Cancer Chemother Pharmacol 26:S78–80.

Lee JS, Murphy WK, Glisson BS, Dhingra HM, Holoye PY, Hong WK. 1989. Primary chemotherapy of brain metastasis in small-cell lung cancer. J Clin Oncol 7:916–922.

Leksell L. 1951. The stereotaxic method and radiosurgery of the brain. Acta Chir Scand 102:316.

Levin VA, Freeman-Dove M, Landahl HD. 1975. Permeability characteristics of brain adjacent to tumors in rats. Arch Neurol 32:785–791.

Levin VA, Landahl HD, Freeman-Dove MA. 1976. The application of brain capillary permeability coefficient measurements to pathological conditions and the selection of agents which cross the blood-brain barrier. J Pharmacokinet Biopharm 4:499–519.

Levin VA, Patlak CS, Landahl HD. 1980. Heuristic modeling of drug delivery to malignant brain tumors. J Pharmacokinet Biopharm 8:257–296.

Lewis AJ. 1988. Sarcoma metastatic to the brain. Cancer 61:593–601.

Liotta LA, Steeg PS, Stetler-Stevenson WG. 1991. Cancer metastasis and angiogenesis: an imbalance of positive and negative regulation. Cell 64:327–336.

Littman P, Rosenstock J, Gale G, et al. 1984. The somnolence syndrome in leukemic children following reduced daily dose fractions of cranial radiation. Int J Radiat Oncol Biol Phys 10:1851–1853.

Loeffler JS, Alexander E, 3rd. 1993. Radiosurgery for the treatment of intracranial metastases. In: Alexander E, 3rd, Loeffler JS, Lunsford LD (eds), Stereotactic Radiosurgery. New York: McGraw-Hill, pp 197–206.

Loeffler JS, Kooy HM, Wen PY, et al. 1990. The treatment of recurrent brain metastases with stereotactic radiosurgery. J Clin Oncol 8:576–582.

Mariotta M, Perewusnyk G, Koechli OR, et al. 1999. Dexamethasone-induced enhancement of resistance to ionizing radiation and chemotherapeutic agents in human tumor cells. Strahlenther Onkol 175:392–396.

Mehta MP, Meyers CA, Curran WJ, et al. 2000. XCYTRIN™ (motexafin gadolinium) and whole brain radiation for patients with brain metastases: lead-in phase to randomized trial—final results. Int J Radiat Oncol Biol Phys 48: 3S:204:A184.

Mori Y, Kondziolka D, Flickinger JC, Kirkwood JM, Agarwala S, Lunsford LD. 1998a. Stereotactic radiosurgery for cerebral metastatic melanoma: factors affecting local disease control and survival. Int J Radiat Oncol Biol Phys 42:581–589.

Mori Y, Kondziolka D, Flickinger JC, Logan T, Lunsford LD. 1998b. Stereotactic radiosurgery for brain metastasis from renal cell carcinoma. Cancer 83:344–353.

Moser RP, Johnson ML. 1989. Surgical management of brain metastases: how aggressive should we be? Oncology 3:123–128.

Mousseau M, Nerson F, Khayat D, et al. 1996. Sequential chemoimmunotherapy with cisplatin (CddP), interleukin 2 (IL2) and interferon alpha 2 a (IFNa) for melanoma brain metastasis (MBM). In: Sixth International Congress on Anti-cancer Treatment, p 108. Paris, France.

Mrak RE. 1993. Origins of adenocarcinomas presenting as intracranial metastases. An ultrastructural study. Arch Pathol Lab Med 117:1165–1169.

Murray KJ, Scott C, Greenberg HM, et al. 1997. A randomized phase III study of accelerated hyperfractionation versus standard in patients with unresected brain metastases: a report of the Radiation Therapy Oncology Group (RTOG) 9104. Int J Radiat Oncol Biol Phys 39:571–574.

Nakagawa H, Groothuis DR, Owens ES, Fenstermacher JD, Patlak CS, Blasberg RG. 1987. Dexamethasone effects on [125I]albumin distribution in experimental RG-2 gliomas and adjacent brain. J Cereb Blood Flow Metab 7:687–701.

Nicolson GL. 1982. Cancer metastasis. Organ colonization and the cell-surface properties of malignant cells. Biochim Biophys Acta 695:113–176.

Nicolson GL. 1988a. Cancer metastasis: tumor cell and host organ properties important in metastasis to specific secondary sites. Biochim Biophys Acta 948:175–224.

Nicolson GL. 1988b. Organ specificity of tumor metastasis: role of preferential adhesion, invasion and growth of malignant cells at specific secondary sites. Cancer Metastasis Rev 7:143–188.

Order SE, Hellman S, Von Essen CF, Kligerman MM. 1968. Improvement in quality of survival following whole-brain irradiation for brain metastasis. Radiology 91:149–153.

Paget S. 1989. The distribution of secondary growths in cancer of the breast. Cancer Metastasis Rev 8:98–101.

Patchell RA. 1991. Brain metastases. Neurol Clin 9:817–824.

Patchell RA, Tibbs PA, Regine WF, et al. 1998. Postoperative radiotherapy in the treatment of single metastases to the brain: a randomized trial. JAMA 280:1485–1489.

Patchell RA, Tibbs PA, Walsh JW, et al. 1990. A randomized trial of surgery in the treatment of single metastases to the brain. N Engl J Med 322:494–500.

Phillips MH, Stelzer KJ, Griffin TW, Mayberg MR, Winn HR. 1994. Stereotactic radiosurgery: a review and comparison of methods. J Clin Oncol 12:1085–1099.

Phillips TL, Scott CB, Leibel SA, Rotman M, Weigensberg IJ. 1995. Results of a randomized comparison of radiotherapy and bromodeoxyuridine with radiotherapy alone for brain metastases: report of RTOG trial 89-05. Int J Radiat Oncol Biol Phys 33:339–348.

Pirzkall A, Debus J, Lohr F, et al. 1998. Radiosurgery alone or in combination with whole-brain radiotherapy for brain metastases. J Clin Oncol 16:3563–3569.

Posner JB. 1992. Management of brain metastases. Rev Neurol (Paris) 148:477–487.

Posner JB, Chernik NL. 1978. Intracranial metastases from systemic cancer. Adv Neurol 19:579–592.

Pullar M, Blumbergs PC, Phillips GE, Carney PG. 1985. Neoplastic cerebral aneurysm from metastatic gestational choriocarcinoma. Case report. J Neurosurg 63:644–647.

Radley MG, McDonald JV, Pilcher WH, Wilbur DC. 1993. Late solitary cerebral metastases from renal cell carcinoma: report of two cases. Surg Neurol 39:230–234.

Ravussin P, Abou-Madi M, Archer D, et al. 1988. Changes in CSF pressure after mannitol in patients with and without elevated CSF pressure. J Neurosurg 69:869–876.

Robinet G, Gouva S, Clavier J, et al. 1991. Chemotherapy with cisplatin and 5-fluorouracil in inoperable brain metastases of bronchopulmonary cancers. Bull Cancer (Paris) 78:831–837.

Rodeck U, Becker D, Herlyn M. 1991. Basic fibroblast growth factor in human melanoma. Cancer Cells 3:308–311.

Rosner D, Nemoto T, Lane WW. 1986. Chemotherapy induces regression of brain metastases in breast carcinoma. Cancer 58:832–839.

Rustin GJ, Newlands ES, Bagshawe KD, Begent RH, Crawford SM. 1986. Successful management of metastatic and primary germ cell tumors in the brain. Cancer 57:2108–2113.

Rustin GJ, Newlands ES, Begent RH, Dent J, Bagshawe KD. 1989. Weekly alternating etoposide, methotrexate, and actinomycin/vincristine and cyclophosphamide chemotherapy for the treatment of CNS metastases of choriocarcinoma. J Clin Oncol 7:900–903.

Salbeck R, Grau HC, Artmann H. 1990. Cerebral tumor staging in patients with bronchial carcinoma by computed tomography. Cancer 66:2007–2011.

Sause WT, Crowley JJ, Morantz R, et al. 1990. Solitary brain metastasis: results of an RTOG/SWOG protocol evaluation surgery + RT versus RT alone. Am J Clin Oncol 13:427–432.

Sause WT, Scott C, Krisch R, et al. 1993. Phase I/II trial of accelerated fractionation in brain metastases RTOG 85-28. Int J Radiat Oncol Biol Phys 26:653–657.

Savaraj N, Lu K, Feun LG, et al. 1983. Intracerebral penetration and tissue distribution of 2,5-diaziridinyl 3,6-bis(carboethoxyamino) 1,4-benzoquinone (AZQ, NSC-182986). J Neurooncol 1:15–19.

Sawaya R, Bindal RK, Lang FF, Abi-Said D. 2000. Metastatic brain tumors. In: Kaye AH, Laws ER (eds), Brain Tumors: An Encyclopedic Approach. Edinburgh: Churchill Livingstone, pp 3–30.

Sawaya R, Hammoud M, Schoppa D, et al. 1998. Neurosurgical outcomes in a modern series of 400 craniotomies for treatment of parenchymal tumors. Neurosurgery 42:1044–1056.

Sawaya R, Zuccarello M, Elkalliny M, Nishiyama H. 1992. Postoperative venous thromboembolism and brain tumors: part I. Clinical profile. J Neurooncol 14:119–125.

Schmitt HP. 1984. Metastases of malignant neoplasms to intracranial tumours: the "tumour-in-a-tumour" phenomenon. Virchows Arch 405:155–160.

Seung SK, Sneed PK, McDermott MW, et al. 1998. Gamma knife radiosurgery for malignant melanoma brain metastases. Cancer J Sci Am 4:103–109.

Shaw EG. 1999. Radiotherapeutic management of multiple brain metastases: "3000 in 10" whole brain radiation is no longer a "no brainer." Int J Radiat Oncol Biol Phys 45:253–254.

Shaw E, Scott C, Souhami L, et al. 1996. Radiosurgery for the treatment of previously irradiated recurrent primary brain tumors and brain metastases: initial report of radiation therapy oncology group protocol (90-05). Int J Radiat Oncol Biol Phys 34:647–654.

Shaw E, Scott C, Souhami L, et al. 2000. Single dose radiosurgical treatment of recurrent previously irradiated primary brain tumors and brain metastases: final report of RTOG protocol 90-05. Int J Radiat Oncol Biol Phys 47:291–298.

Skibber JM, Soong SJ, Austin L, Balch CM, Sawaya RE. 1996. Cranial irradiation after surgical excision of brain metastases in melanoma patients. Ann Surg Oncol 3:118–123.

Smalley SR, Laws ER Jr, O' Fallon JR, Shaw EG, Schray MF. 1992. Resection for solitary brain metastasis. Role of adjuvant radiation and prognostic variables in 229 patients. J Neurosurg 77:531–540.

Sneed PK, Lamborn KR, Forstner JM, et al. 1999. Radiosurgery for brain metastases: is whole brain radiotherapy necessary? Int J Radiat Oncol Biol Phys 43:549–558.

Stewart DJ. 1994. A critique of the role of the blood–brain barrier in the chemotherapy of human brain tumors. J Neurooncol 20:121–139.

Stewart DJ, Benvenuto JA, Leavens M, et al. 1979. Penetration of 3-deazauridine into human brain, intracerebral tumor, and cerebrospinal fluid. Cancer Res 39:4119–4122.

Stewart DJ, Benvenuto JA, Leavens M, et al. 1983. Human central nervous system pharmacology of pentamethylmelamine and its metabolites. J Neurooncol 1:357–364.

Stewart DJ, Leavens M, Maor M, et al. 1982. Human central nervous system distribution of cis-diamminedichloroplatinum and use as a radiosensitizer in malignant brain tumors. Cancer Res 42:2474–2479.

Stewart DJ, Richard MT, Hugenholtz H, et al. 1984. Penetration of teniposide (VM-26) into human intracerebral tumors. Preliminary observations on the effect of tumor type, rate of drug infusion and prior treatment with amphotericin B or oral glycerol. J Neurooncol 2:315–324.

Sundaresan N, Galicich JH. 1985a. Surgical treatment of brain metastases. Clinical and computerized tomography evaluation of the results of treatment. Cancer 55:1382–1388.

Sundaresan N, Galicich JH. 1985b. Surgical treatment of single brain metastases from non–small-cell lung cancer. Cancer Invest 3:107–113.

Tobler WD, Sawaya R, Tew JM Jr. 1986. Successful laser-assisted excision of a metastatic midbrain tumor. Neurosurgery 18:795–797.

Tsukada Y, Fouad A, Pickren JW, Lane WW. 1983. Central nervous system metastasis from breast carcinoma. Autopsy study. Cancer 52:2349–2354.

Twelves CJ, Souhami RL, Harper PG, et al. 1990. The response of cerebral metastases in small cell lung cancer to systemic chemotherapy. Br J Cancer 61:147–150.

Vecht CJ, Haaxma-Reiche H, Noordijk EM, et al. 1993. Treatment of single brain metastasis: radiotherapy alone or combined with neurosurgery? Ann Neurol 33:583–590.

Viala J, Vanel D, Meingan P, Lartigau E, Carde P, Renschler M. 1999. Phases IB and II multidose trial of gadolinium texaphyrin, a radiation sensitizer detectable at MR imaging: preliminary results in brain metastases. Radiology 212:755–759.

Voorhies RM, Sundaresan N, Thaler HT. 1980. The single supratentorial lesion. An evaluation of preoperative diagnostic tests. J Neurosurg 53:364–368.

Walker AE, Robins M, Weinfeld FD. 1985. Epidemiology of brain tumors: the national survey of intracranial neoplasms. Neurology 35:219–226.

Weller M, Schmidt C, Roth W, Dichgans J. 1997. Chemotherapy of human malignant glioma: prevention of efficacy by dexamethasone? Neurology 48:1704–1709.

Wen PY, Loeffler JS. 1999. Management of brain metastases. Oncology 13:941–954.

West J, Maor M. 1980. Intracranial metastases: behavioral patterns related to primary site and results of treatment by whole brain irradiation. Int J Radiat Oncol Biol Phys 6:11–15.

Wong WW, Schild SE, Sawyer TE, Shaw EG. 1996. Analysis of outcome in patients reirradiated for brain metastases. Int J Radiat Oncol Biol Phys 34:585–590.

Wronski M, Maor MH, Davis BJ, Sawaya R, Levin VA. 1997. External radiation of brain metastases from renal carcinoma: a retrospective study of 119 patients from the M. D. Anderson Cancer Center. Int J Radiat Oncol Biol Phys 37:753–759.

Young DF, Patchell RA. 1990. Surgery for a single brain metastasis. In: Wilkins RH, Rengachary SS (eds), Neurosurgery Update I: Diagnosis, Operative Technique, and Neuro-oncology. New York: McGraw-Hill, pp 473–476.

14

Spinal Axis Metastases

RICHARD G. PERRIN, NORMAND J. LAPERRIERE, D. ANDREW LOBLAW, AND ADRIAN W. LAXTON

Secondary spinal tumors represent an ominous extension of systemic cancer and commonly present as a neurologic emergency. Advances in diagnostic imaging techniques, clarification of the relative benefits provided by radiation therapy and surgery, and refinement in surgical approaches and techniques have all contributed to improve the outlook for patients with spinal metastases (Maranzano et al., 1991; Perrin and McBroom, 1987; Rosenthal et al., 1996; Siegal and Siegal, 1985; Sundaresan et al., 1990, 1991).

CLASSIFICATION AND PATHOLOGY

Spinal tumors are classified by anatomic location (Table 14–1). Extradural metastases account for approximately 95% of secondary spinal tumors. These lesions arise through blood-borne spread of cancerous cells or by direct extension of the primary tumor. Most extradural tumors are metastatic to the vertebral bodies, but some lymphomas and tumors from Hodgkin's disease may occur in the epidural space without bone involvement. Metastatic spinal tumors seldom breach the dura. Intradural extramedullary metastases are uncommon and represent tertiary spread from cerebral secondary sites (Perrin et al., 1982). Intradural extramedullary metastases are transmitted through the cerebrospinal fluid and typically become entangled among the nerve roots of the cauda equina. Intramedullary tumors are rare, comprising approximately 3.5% of spinal metastases (Bruner and Tien, 1998). Intramedullary metastases arise through hematogenous spread.

Spinal tumors are also classified according to the level of the spine involved (cervical, thoracic, lumbosacral). Autopsy studies have shown that the distribution of spinal metastases parallels the bulk of the vertebrae; thus, the lumbosacral spine is most often afflicted, followed by the thoracic and cervical segments (Willis, 1973). Clinically, however, *symptomatic* spinal metastases most often involve the thoracic spine (49%) followed by the lumbosacral (40%) and cervical (11%) segments (Table 14–2).

Spinal tumors most often originate from primary tumors of breast, lung, and prostate, which reflects both the prevalence of these cancers and their propensity to metastasize to bone (Table 14–3). Primary tumors less commonly reported to metastasize to the spine include leukemia, schwannoma, mesothelioma, Merkel's tumor, plasmacytoma, teratoma, as well as basal cell, parotid, nasopharyngeal, laryngeal, esophageal, gall bladder, pancreas, ovarian, endometrial, and urinary bladder tumors (Helweg-Larsen, 1996; Kovner et al., 1999).

As many as 10% of patients with symptomatic spinal metastases present with no known primary lesion (Botterell and Fitzgerald, 1959; Livingston and Perrin, 1978; MacDonald, 1990).

INCIDENCE

Most patients with systemic cancer develop skeletal metastases, and the spine is most commonly involved (Willis, 1973). As many as 30% of all cancer patients develop secondary spinal tumors (Bach et al., 1990;

Table 14–1. Relative Frequencies of Spinal Metastases According to Location of Spinal Involvement

		Extradural		*Intradural Extramedullary*		*Intramedullary*	
Author	*Total*	*No.*	*%*	*No.*	*%*	*No.*	*%*
Rogers and Heard (1958)	17	16	94	1	6	—	—
Barron et al. (1959)	125	123	98	—	—	2	1.6
Edelson et al. (1972)	175	169	97	—	—	6	3.4
Perrin et al. (1982)	200	189	94	10	5	1	0.5

Gomez, 1955). Approximately 18,000 new cases of spinal metastases are diagnosed in North America each year (Gokaslan et al., 1998). Spinal metastases occur 20 times more commonly than primary tumors of the spine.

SYMPTOMS AND SIGNS

Symptomatic spinal metastases produce a characteristic clinical syndrome. Typically, local back or neck pain is followed by weakness, sensory loss, and sphincter dysfunction (Table 14–4) (Botterell and Fitzgerald, 1959; Helweg-Larsen and Sorensen, 1994; Livingston and Perrin, 1978; MacDonald, 1990).

Local back or neck pain is the earliest and most prominent feature in 90% of patients. Palpation or percussion over the posterior spine at an involved level usually elicits local tenderness. Associated radicular pain distribution indicates segmental root irritation and is an especially common symptom among patients with lumbar spine metastases (Helweg-Larsen and Sorensen, 1994). When local back or neck pain is aggravated by movement and relieved by immobility, spinal instability should be suspected (Perrin and Livingston, 1980). If the pain has a severe, burning, dysesthetic quality, intradural extramedullary metastases should be considered (Perrin et al., 1982). Pain caused by spinal metastases may be present for up to 1 year and is often initially attributed to arthritis, back strain, or a slipped disc (Goodkin et al., 1987). Correct diagnosis of spinal metastatic pain is often delayed until more blatant manifestations of spinal cord compromise are manifest. It is axiomatic that *new-onset back or neck pain in a cancer patient means spinal metastasis until proven otherwise.*

Spinal metastases may be the first manifestation of malignancy in 20% or more of patients (Schiff et al., 1997). By the time treatment is initiated, however, only about 2% of spinal metastases are of unknown origin.

Motor weakness is usually manifest after the onset of pain and is especially common in patients with tho-

Table 14–2. Relative Frequencies of Spinal Metastases According to Level of Spinal Involvement

		Cervical		*Thoracic*		*Lumbrosacral*	
Author	*Total*	*No.*	*%*	*No.*	*%*	*No.*	*%*
Sorensen et al. (1994)*	57	3	5	33	58	21	37
Helweg-Larsen (1996)	153	7	4.6	102	66.7	44	28.7
Tatsui et al. (1996)	695	106	15.3	203	29.2	386	55.5
Maranzano et al. (1997)	49	2	4	25	51	22	45
Schiff et al. (1998)	337	33	10	206	61	98	29
Brown et al. (1999)	40	5	12.5	13	32.5	22	55
Khaw et al. (1999)*	160	11	7	123	77	26	16
Kovner et al. (1999)	85	7	8	45	53	33	39
Rompe et al. (1999)*	106	9	8	76	72	21	20
Totals	1682	183	11	826	49	673	40

*In these studies, totals in the lumbosacral column refer to lumbar involvement only.

Table 14–3. Relative Frequencies of Various Primary Tumors Metastasizing to the Spine

Author	*Breast*	*Lung*	*Prostate*	*Kidney*	*Myeloma*	*Lymphoma*	*Colorectal*	*Cervix*	*Stomach*	*Sarcoma*	*Liver*	*Thyroid*	*Melanoma*	*Other**	*Unknown*	*Total*
Sorensen et al. (1994)	34	3	5	1	—	—	6	—	—	4	—	1	2	1	—	57
Akeyson and McCutcheon (1996)	4	8	—	5	—	—	—	1	—	3	—	—	—	3	1	25
Helweg-Larsen (1996)	56	27	43	—	—	—	—	—	—	—	—	—	—	27	—	163
Tatsui et al. (1996)	114	149	59	29	—	—	—	46	28	—	—	—	—	—	—	425
Maranzano et al. (1997)	3	12	11	5	4	—	9	—	—	—	—	—	—	5	—	49
Schiff et al. (1997)	64	58	81	15	23	25	13	—	1	15	3	6	5	—	15	324
Katagiri et al. (1998)	15	19	11	3	10	7	4	—	8	3	9	1	—	5	—	95
Khaw et al. (1999)	18	18	25	6	1	2	7	—	—	—	—	—	1	—	1	70
Kim et al. (1999)	3	18	1	—	17	5	1	—	4	1	2	2	1	3	2	60
Kovner et al. (1999)	28	9	12	—	—	9	2	—	—	—	—	—	—	17	2	79
Rompe et al. (1999)	31	20	6	16	8	—	—	—	—	—	—	5	—	16	4	184
Solberg and Bremnes (1999)	9	11	30	6	5	—	3	—	—	—	—	—	—	16	6	86
Van der Sande et al. (1999)	56	5	9	—	6	8	—	—	—	5	—	—	—	14	—	103
Wise et al. (1999)	18	11	6	6	13	9	—	—	—	8	—	—	—	4	5	80
Chen et al. (2000)	3	12	—	1	—	—	10	1	1	1	9	7	1	1	1	48
Totals	456	380	299	93	87	65	55	48	42	40	23	22	10	112	37	1846
%	26	22	17	5.2	5	3.7	3	2.7	2.4	2.3	1.3	1.2	0.6	6.3	2	100

*Includes leukemia, schwannoma, mesothelioma, Merkel's tumor, plasmacytoma, teratoma, as well as basal cell, parotid, nasopharyngeal, laryngeal, esophageal, gall bladder, pancreas, ovarian, endometrial, and urinary bladder tumors.

Table 14–4. Clinical Presentation of Spinal Metastases

Local back or neck pain (±radiculopathy)
Weakness
Sensory loss (including paresthesia)
Sphincter dysfunction

racic metastases (Helweg-Larsen and Sorensen, 1994). A Brown-Séquard syndrome may occur and is more common among patients with intramedullary rather than epidural metastases (Schiff and O'Neill, 1996).

The rate at which spinal cord compression develops varies. However, once established, weakness, sensory loss, and sphincter dysfunction will progress to complete and irreversible paraplegia unless timely treatment is undertaken (Botterell and Fitzgerald, 1959).

RADIOLOGIC INVESTIGATIONS

Radiologic investigations are conducted to determine the location and extent of spinal metastases. Such data form the basis for management strategies.

Plain Films

Plain radiographs of the spine demonstrate abnormalities in 90% of patients with symptomatic spinal metastases (Helweg-Larsen et al., 1997). Osteoblastic or osteosclerotic alteration may occur, especially with metastases originating from carcinoma of the prostate (Fig. 14–1). The majority of features on plain film, however, predominantly reflect osteolytic changes. Common findings on plain film include pedicle erosion ("winking owl" sign), paraspinal soft tissue shadow, compression fracture (vertebral collapse), and pathologic fracture dislocation (Fig. 14–2).

Myelography

Before the development of magnetic resonance imaging (MRI), lumbar myelography was the "gold standard" for determining the level of spinal cord compression by demonstrating a block to the flow of contrast. In addition, characteristics of the myelographic block ("paint brush," meniscus, or "fat cord") provides information concerning the anatomic location of the spinal lesion (extradural, intradural, extramedullary, or intramedullary) (Fig. 14–3). When the level of a complete lumbar myelographic block does not correspond to the clinical localization of the tumor or when multiple levels of involvement are suspected, a combination of lumbar and high cervical myelography may be used to delineate the extent of disease.

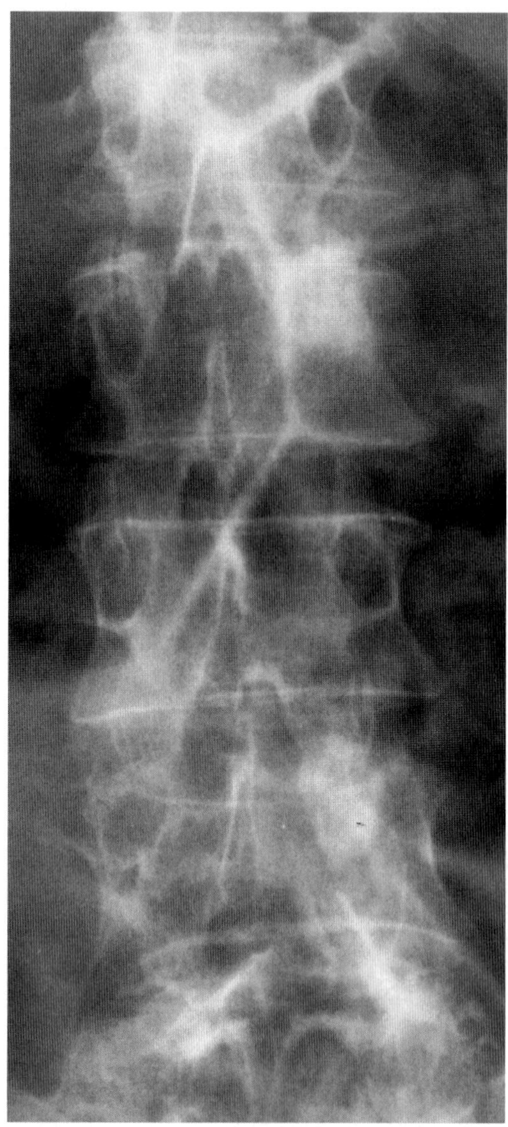

Figure 14–1. Common bone X-ray of osteosclerotic metastasis (pedicles) from prostatic cancer.

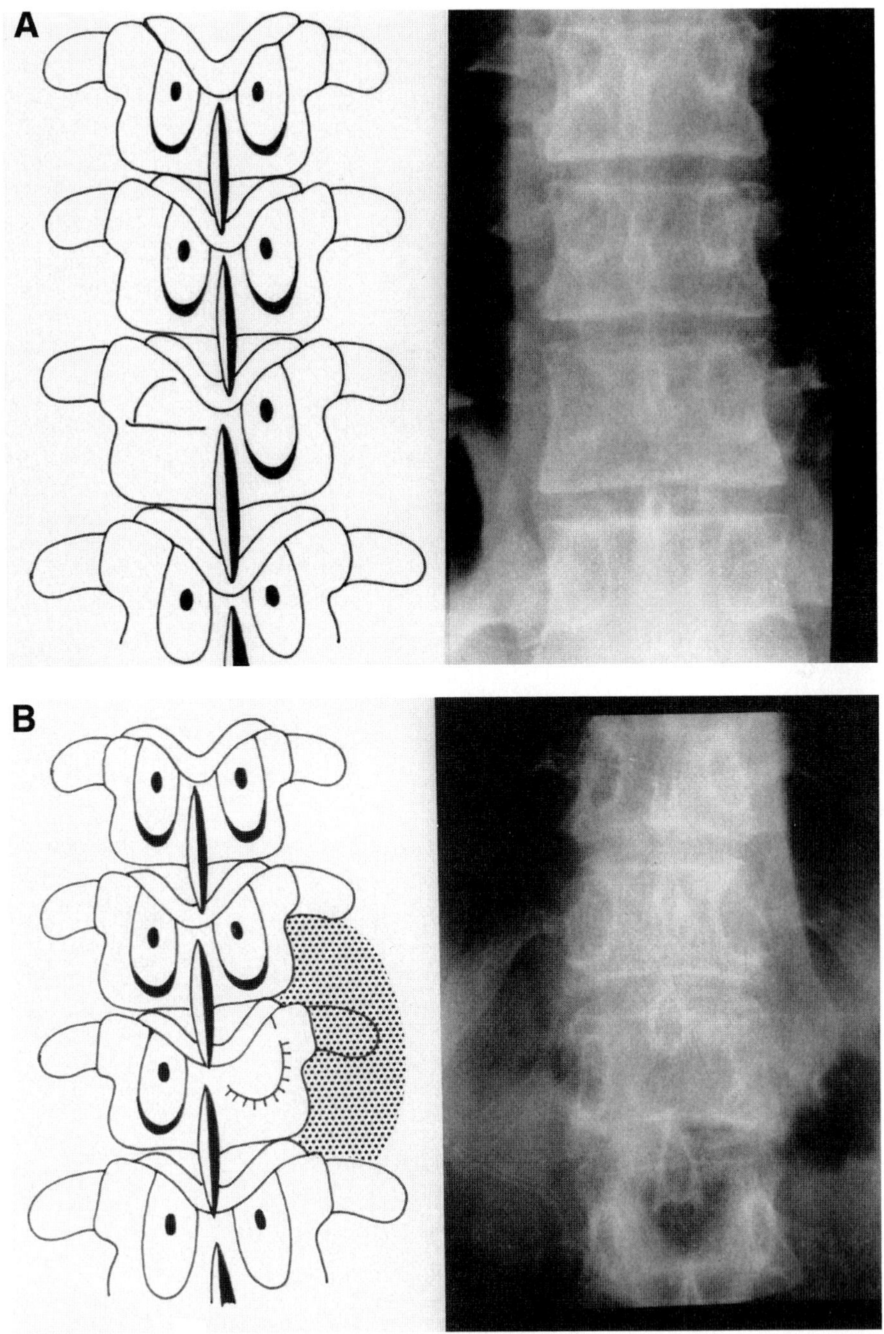

Figure 14–2. Common bone X-rays of **(A)** pedicle erosion producing "winking owl" sign; **(B)** paraspinal soft tissue shadow (with "winking owl"); **(C)** compression fracture (vertebral collapse); and **(D)** pathologic fracture dislocation. (*continued*)

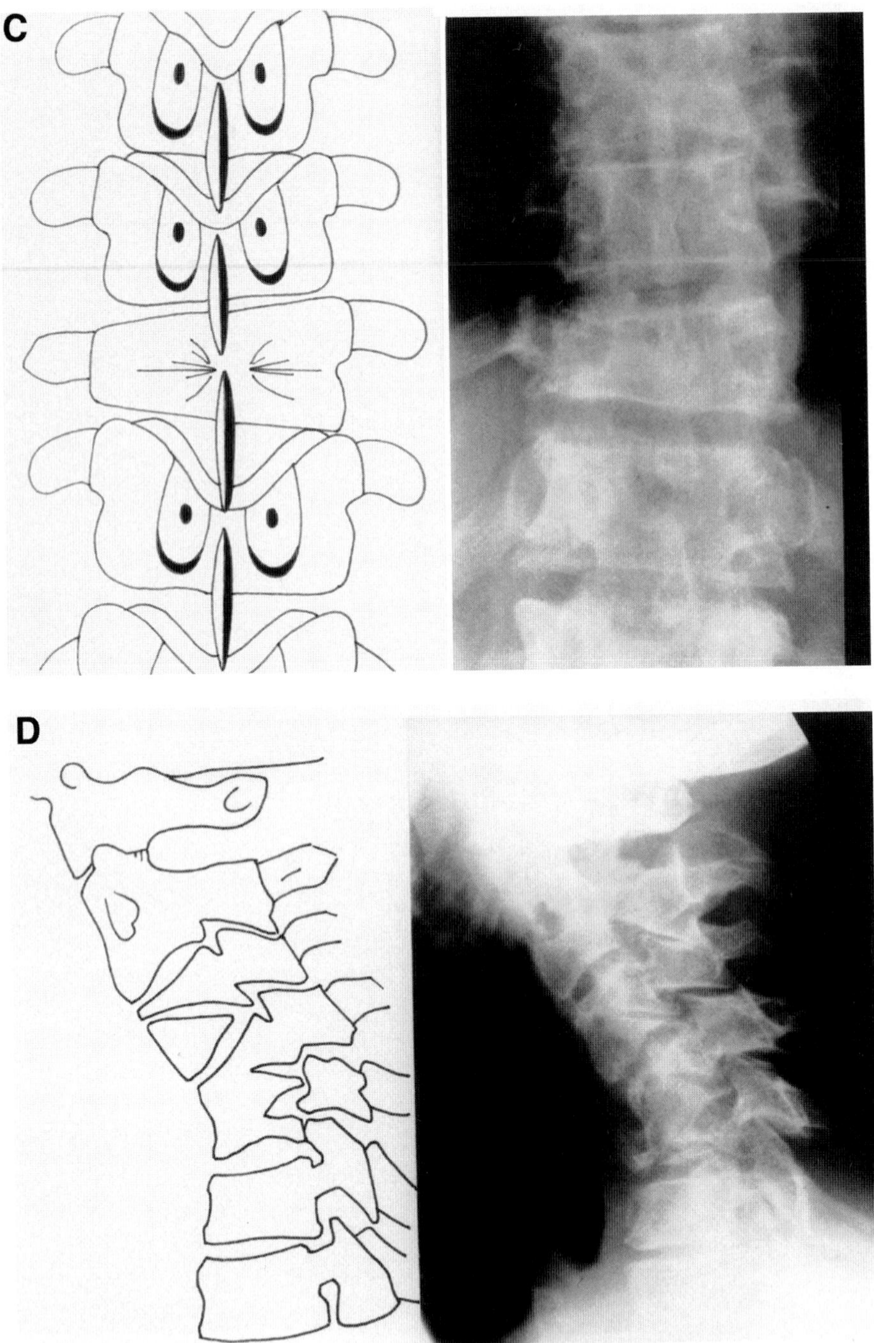

Figure 14–2. (*Continued*)

Computed Tomography

Computed tomography (CT) is useful for showing the disposition of spinal tumors by demonstrating vertebral destruction and paraspinal extension in transverse sections (Helweg-Larsen et al., 1997) (Fig. 14–4A). Computed tomography scans performed in conjunction with and following myelography are particularly valuable for displaying the degree of displacement of the dural sac and its contents (O'Rourke

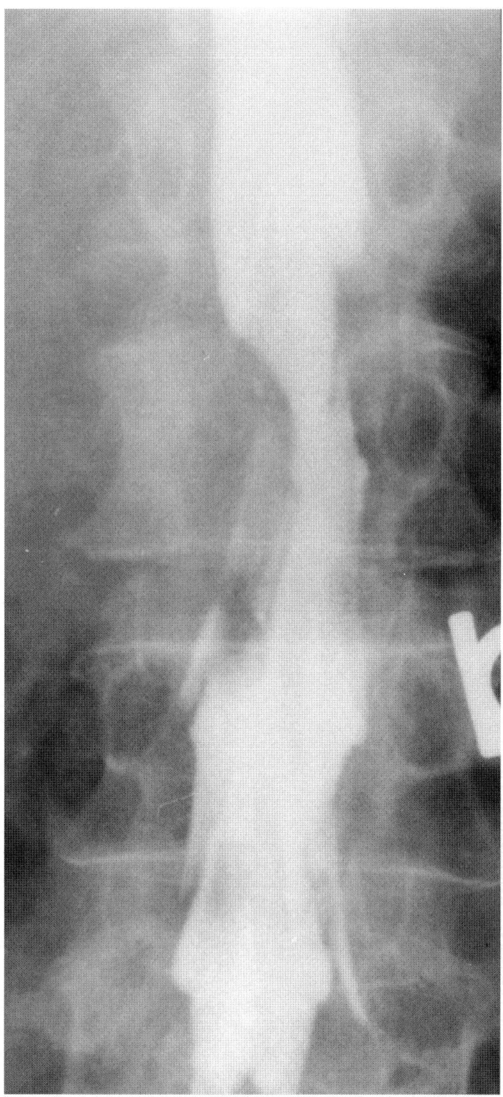

Figure 14–3. Extradural metastasis causing pedicle erosion ("winking owl") and myelographic block.

et al., 1986; Redmond et al., 1984) (Fig. 14–4B). However, CT scanning is effectively limited to transverse representations; coronal and sagittal reconstructions with this imaging method are less exact.

Magnetic Resonance Imaging

Magnetic resonance imaging is the imaging modality of choice for spinal tumors, including spinal metastases (Berenstein and Graeb, 1982; Jaeckle, 1991; Khaw et al., 1999; Markus, 1996; Schiff et al., 1998; Sze, 1991). The spine may be evaluated in various planes, and the entire spinal column can be visualized in sagittal cross sections. Patterns of extradural metastases can be identified, including an isolated level of focal disease, multiple levels of contiguous involvement, or multiple, noncontiguous levels of tumor foci (Fig. 14–5).

Magnetic resonance imaging with gadolinium enhancement permits identification of intradural extramedullary "drop" metastases typically found along the cauda equina nerve roots. Gadolinium-enhanced MRI will also delineate intramedullary spinal metastases.

Coronal, sagittal, and transverse reconstructions from MRI provide important information concerning the location, multiplicity, and geometry of secondary spinal tumors and demonstrate the degree of bony integrity at adjacent vertebral levels, all essential parameters for planning an optimal treatment.

MANAGEMENT

Rationale

Treatment of patients with spinal metastases is undertaken to relieve pain and preserve or restore neurologic function. Cancer patients do not die of spinal metastases per se (Table 14–5). Rather, they succumb to infection, organ failure, infarction, carcinomatosis, and hemorrhage (Inagaki et al., 1974). Morbidity from spinal metastases can increase a cancer patient's susceptibility to various complications, thereby reducing life expectancy. Morbidity is generally lessened if the diagnosis is made and treatment initiated before significant neurologic or functional disability has developed (Bilsky et al., 1999; Helweg-Larsen, 1996; Kovner et al., 1999). Relief from pain and preservation or restoration of neurologic function contribute immeasurably to the quality of remaining life and reduce the burden of care (Weigel et al., 1999).

Radiation Therapy Versus Surgery

Therapeutic irradiation and surgery are complementary treatment modalities for spinal metastases. Response to radiation depends on the primary histology and volume of disease. Complete response to radiation therapy for spinal cord compression is achieved

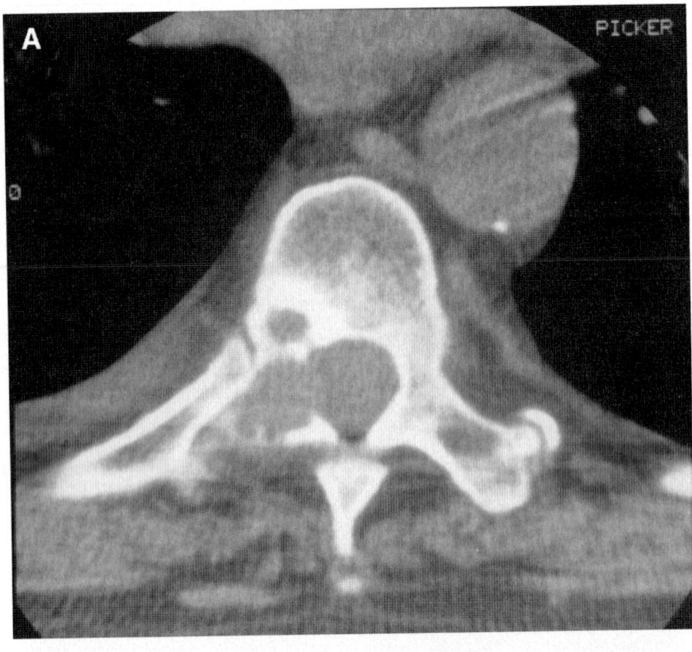

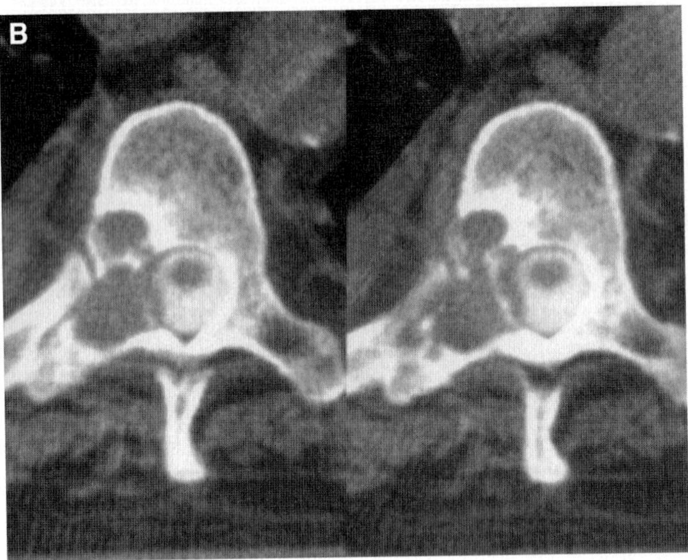

Figure 14–4. **(A)** Plain CT scan showing pedicle destruction. **(B)** CT scan following myelography showing compression of dural sac.

in 30% of patients with all types of tumors, including those with breast cancer and malignant melanoma (Leviov et al., 1993). Radiosensitive tumors, such as lymphoproliferative malignancies, multiple myelomas, and germ cell tumors, provide an exception; 77% of patients with these tumors achieve a complete response to irradiation alone.

Of patients with spinal metastases, 80% respond to radiation therapy alone. Improvement of motor dysfunction occurs in 49%, and stabilization of the clinical status occurs in an additional 31% of cases (Maranzano et al., 1991).

Due to irreversible spinal cord injury, patients presenting with a complete spinal cord block generally

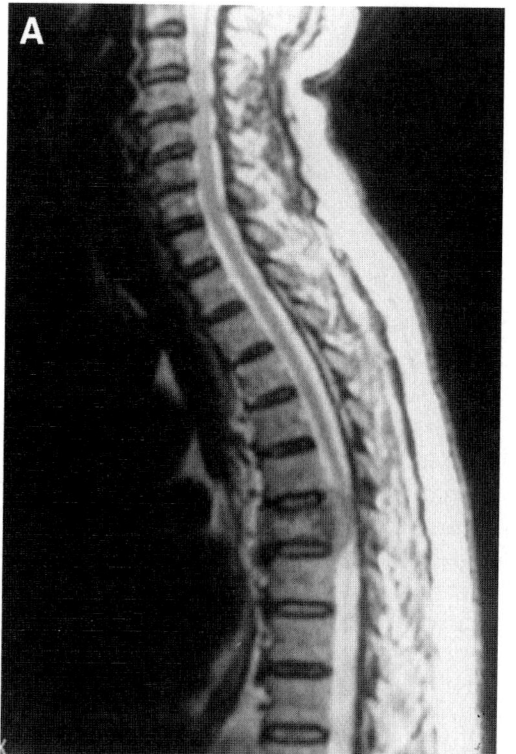

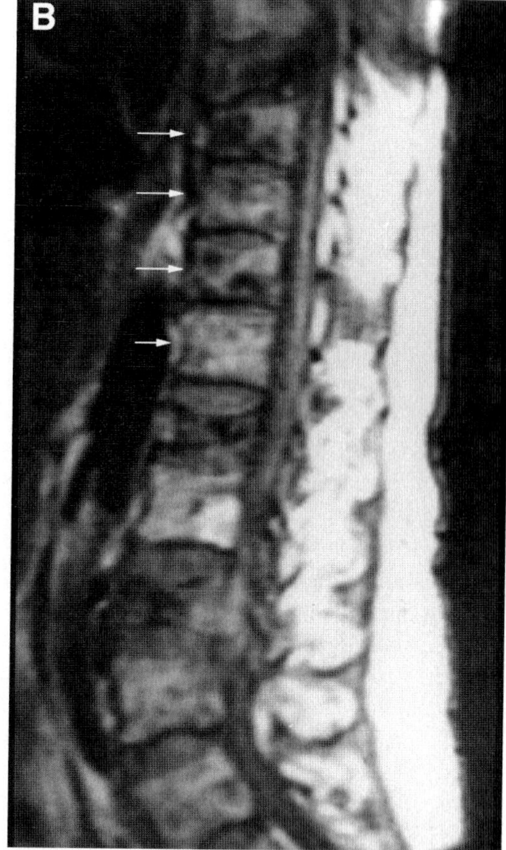

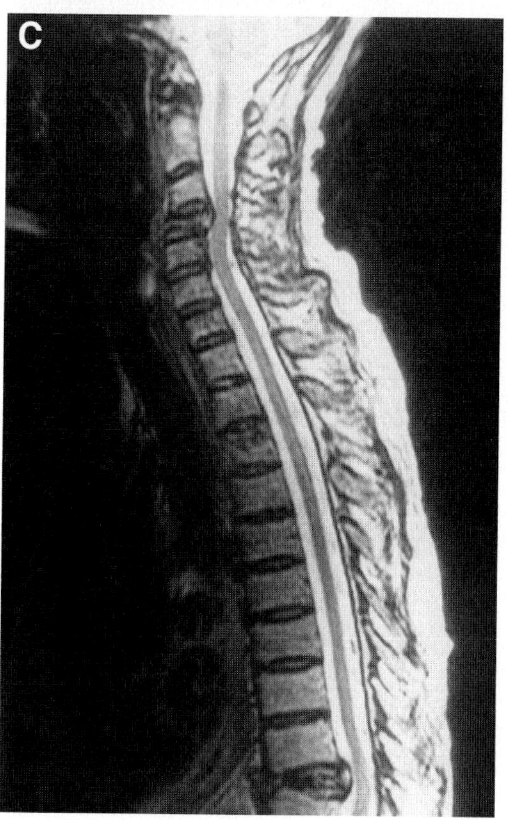

Figure 14–5. Saggital MRI of spine showing **(A)** isolated level of focal disease; **(B)** multiple levels of contiguous involvement; and **(C)** multiple noncontiguous levels of tumor foci.

Table 14–5. Causes of Death in Cancer Patients

Cause	%
Infection	47
Organ failure	25
Infarction	11
Carcinomatosis	10
Hemorrhage	7

have greater residual neurologic impairment after radiation therapy than those with a partial block (Boogerd and van der Sande, 1993). Approximately 20% of patients with epidural spinal cord compression will have an associated paravertebral mass (Kim et al., 1993; Turner et al., 1993). Radiation therapy is less effective when epidural spinal cord compression is associated with a paravertebral mass because of the large tumor burden. In these cases, surgical resection, followed by radiation therapy, has been suggested as a way to improve functional outcome (Kim et al., 1993). Moreover, Schiff et al. (1998) have identified surgical intervention as a favorable prognostic factor associated with survival among patients with epidural spinal metastases.

Radiation therapy has traditionally been the initial treatment of choice for most cases of spinal cord compression because no overall difference in the neurologic outcome has been observed when patients are treated by either radiation therapy alone or surgery with radiation therapy (Byrne, 1992; Young et al., 1980). Recent refinements in surgical strategies, including elaboration of posterolateral, anterior, and endoscopic approaches for spinal decompression, together with the evolution of spinal stabilization procedures, have improved the outcome for patients undergoing surgery for spinal metastases. Such improvement has, in turn, lent support to the concept of de novo surgery for secondary spinal tumors. Furthermore, operating on spinal metastasis before applying radiation minimizes the risk of wound complications, which can be as high as 30% with surgery through an irradiated tissue bed. Clarification of the relative roles of radiation and surgery (or a combination of these modalities) requires an appropriate prospective randomized trial.

RADIATION THERAPY

Traditional indications for radiation therapy are summarized in Table 14–6. Radiation therapy is generally delivered to an area that incorporates at least one to two vertebral levels above and below the known sites of spinal cord compression. Radiation is administered via a direct posterior field with dose specified at a depth of 5 to 8 cm. Occasionally the field length is adjusted to incorporate adjacent vertebral bodies involved by metastases but which are not causing spinal cord compression. The width of the field is usually 2 to 3 cm wider than the width of the vertebral body, but would be increased in situations where there exists a paraspinal mass. Doses on the order of 2000 to 3000 centigray (cGy) in 5 to 10 fractions are generally delivered once a day, but the range of published experiences extends from 1500 cGy in 5 fractions to 4000 cGy in 20 fractions per day. There is accumulating evidence that short-course, low-dose radiotherapy may be as effective as longer, higher dose regimens, but with fewer and less severe side effects (Maranzano et al., 1997; Tombolini et al., 1994).

When patients present with total paraplegia of several days duration, 800 cGy in one fraction is an acceptable alternative approach in an effort to minimize pain when there is no realistic prospect of neurologic recovery. Occasionally, when spinal cord compression occurs as a result of direct extension, rather than from hematogenous spread, and represents the initial manifestation of cancer, a potentially curative approach incorporating surgery, chemotherapy, and high-dose, localized radiation therapy might be appropriately considered depending on the histologic type of tumor.

Table 14–6. Indications for Radiation Therapy as the Initial Management of Spinal Metastases

Patients with radiation-sensitive tumors in the absence of any indications for surgery (i.e., lymphoma, multiple myeloma, small cell lung carcinoma, seminoma of testes)
Life expectancy of 3 months or less
More than one level of simultaneous spinal cord compression
Patients with paraplegia of greater than 12 to 24 hours duration
Co-morbid conditions that preclude surgery

The most common acute toxicities associated with radiation are nausea and vomiting, which occur as a direct result of the exit beam through the epigastrium in cord compression of the distal thoracic and proximal lumbar spine. This is usually most pronounced with the first two to three fractions and can generally be controlled with various antiemetics. Radiation esophagitis may occur 1 to 2 weeks following completion of treatment for an upper to midthoracic cord compression, but is usually mild and resolves within 1 week. The most important late toxicity is radiation myelopathy, but this is a rare event with the usual dosages quoted above and is only occasionally seen in the setting of re-treatment of the spine with a second or third course of irradiation (Wong et al., 1994).

Treatment of spinal cord compression involves a delicate balance between delivering a dose of radiation sufficient to kill the tumor and not injuring the spinal cord further. A ceiling of response, defined as maintaining the pretherapeutic level of ambulation and motor function, is considered to be 80% with radiation alone (Leviov et al., 1993). This is particularly true in patients with extensive tumor burdens, such as spinal cord compression associated with a paravertebral mass, which require high doses of radiation to achieve local control and may achieve little functional improvement after irradiation alone (Kim et al., 1993).

Table 14–7 summarizes the reported outcomes associated with radiation therapy for spinal metastases in a number of recent studies. Improvement or stabilization in patients' functional status occurred in 73% of cases following radiation therapy. Furthermore, whereas 49% of patients were able to walk before radiation therapy, 53% were able to walk after radiation therapy. These results suggest that radiation therapy is an appropriate and effective treatment for many patients with spinal metastases.

INDICATIONS FOR SURGERY

Indications for surgery in patients with symptomatic spinal metastases are listed in Table 14–8 (Botterell and Fitzgerald, 1959; Dunn et al., 1980; Gilbert et al., 1978; Perrin et al., 1982; Perrin and Livingston, 1980; Perrin and McBroom, 1990).

Table 14–7. Outcomes Following Radiation Therapy for Spinal Metastases

			Global Rating[†]		*Ambulatory*		
Author	*N*	*Dosage** *(cGy)*	*Good*	*Poor*	*Pre*	*Post*	*Mortality*[‡]
Sorensen et al. (1994)	57	2800	41	16	36	34	6
Tombolini et al. (1994)	103	Varied	60	43	—	—	—
Helweg-Larsen (1996)	153	2800	—	11	60	54	4
Schiff and O'Neill (1996)	35	3000	34	1	—	—	4
Maranzano et al. (1997)	53	1600	31	22	23	31	5
Katagiri et al. (1998)[§]	101	4000	67	33	73	75	10
Brown et al. (1999)	35	3000	31	4	21	18	4.1
Kovner et al. (1999)	79	3000	75	4	23	39	2
Solberg and Bremnes (1999)	58	Varied	—	—	—	—	3.3
Totals	674		339	134	236	251	$M = 4.8$
%		73	22	49	53		

*Median total dose.

[†]For global ratings, good outcomes are those in which functional or neurologic status either stabilized or improved following treatment, and poor outcomes are those in which further deterioration occurred following treatment.

[‡]Median total dose.

[‡]Median or mean survival for cohort in months.

[§]Sixty-two of these patients also received chemotherapy.

Table 14–8. Indications for Surgery in the Management of Spinal Metastases

Failed radiation therapy
Uncertain diagnosis
Pathologic fracture dislocation
Rapid progression or advanced paralysis

Failure of Radiation Therapy

Given the common practice of administering therapeutic radiation as the initial treatment for spinal metastases, the most common indication for surgical intervention for patients with symptomatic spinal metastases is failure of radiation to stop the spread of disease. Characteristically, symptoms persist or recur during or after radiation therapy. Surgical intervention is then indicated to relieve pain and to preserve or restore neurologic function.

Uncertain Diagnosis

Surgical intervention is indicated if it is suspected that a cancer patient's pain and neurologic dysfunction are due to disc extrusion, epidural abscess, hematoma, or some pathologic cause other than spinal metastasis. Approximately 10% of patients with symptomatic spinal metastases present without a known primary tumor. In such instances, spinal decompression may be diagnostic as well as therapeutic.

Pathologic Fracture Dislocation

Pathologic fracture dislocation occurs in approximately 10% of patients with symptomatic spinal metastases. In this circumstance, compression of the spinal cord and nerve roots by the tumor mass is compounded by distortion of the dural sac and its contents due to malalignment of the spine. Surgical intervention is required to restore alignment of the spine, to decompress the spinal cord and nerve roots, and to stabilize the spinal column.

Rapidly Progressing or Far-Advanced Paraplegia

Rapidly progressing or far-advanced paraplegia represents a neurosurgical emergency. Complete and irreversible spinal cord injury might supervene before the benefits of therapeutic radiation are manifest. Surgical decompression is indicated to provide prompt and effective decompression of the spinal cord and nerve roots.

SURGICAL STRATEGIES

Treatment for spinal metastases must ensure both decompression of the spinal cord and nerve roots and stabilization of the spinal column. Spinal instability may already have occurred at the time of clinical presentation or may be precipitated during the course of surgical decompression. In either case, appropriate spinal reconstruction must be carried out.

The surgical approach to spinal metastases may be from the front (anterior or anterolateral) or from behind (posterior or posterolateral). Each avenue has its place, and neither is always applicable (Perrin and McBroom, 1987). Because the surgical strategies must achieve both decompression of the neural elements and stabilization of the vertebral column, the optimal approach is based on a number of interrelated factors (Table 14–9).

Tumor Within the Dural Sac

Spinal metastases occurring within the dural sac are generally best approached from behind through a wide laminectomy. Occasionally, extradural spinal metastases involve only the posterior elements (Fig. 14–6), and, in these cases, decompression through a wide laminectomy is most appropriate. More often, however, spinal cord compression results from an anteriorly or laterally located extradural tumor mass or collapsed bone (Fig. 14–7; see also Fig. 14–5A). In such circumstances, adequate decompression may best be achieved through an anterior or anterolateral approach and vertebral corpectomy.

Table 14–9. Factors Determining the Optimal Surgical Approach for the Treatment of Spinal Metastases

Tumor location
Spinal level
Extent of the tumor
Bony integrity
Degree of debility

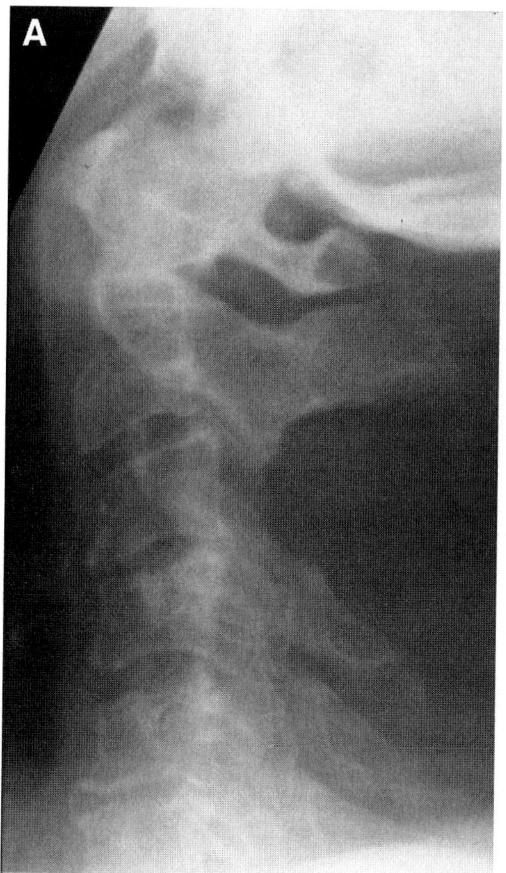

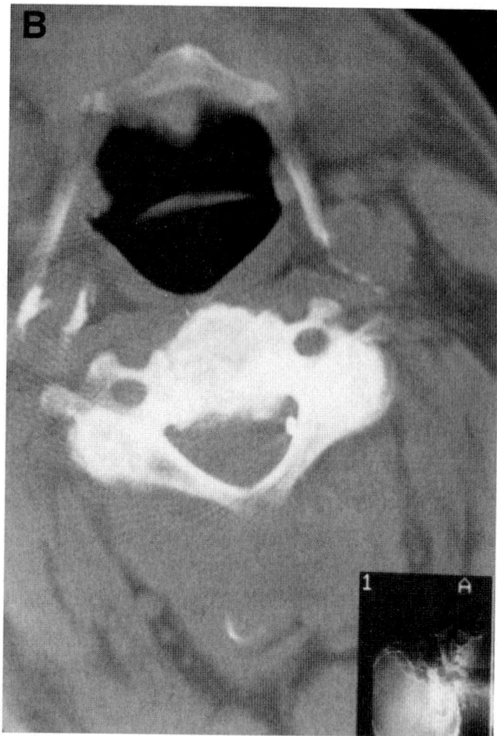

Figure 14–6. Spinal metastasis involving posterior elements, as shown by **(A)** plain film and **(B)** CT scan.

Tumor at Ends of Vertebral Column

Spinal metastases at the rostral and caudal ends of the vertebral column represent a particular challenge. Adequate anterior decompression at the craniocervical junction may be achieved through transoral and mandible-splitting exposures. However, the associated morbidity and lengthy postoperative convalescence is not in keeping with the intended palliation of a cancer patient who has a limited life expectancy. Even if adequate spinal decompression were achieved through an anterior approach at the rostral or caudal extremes of the spinal column, anterior spinal reconstruction at these levels poses an enormous technical challenge. Therefore, extradural metastases at the craniocervical and lumbosacral junctions are initially best approached from behind.

Extradural Tumor

Extradural metastases occurring anteriorly or anterolaterally and involving one or two contiguous levels are best approached from the front. The anterior (anterolateral) avenue provides direct access to the compressing mass. Furthermore, an anteriorly applied reconstruction device is biomechanically most effective. Anterior decompression (corpectomy) involving three or more contiguous segments is not impossible; however, fixation of an anteriorly applied prosthesis spanning three or more segments becomes tenuous, at best. Consequently, in such cases, posterolateral decompression and posterior fixation may be more appropriate. If vertebral corpectomy extending across three segments is undertaken, it is advisable to reinforce an anteriorly applied reconstruction prosthesis with posterior fixation.

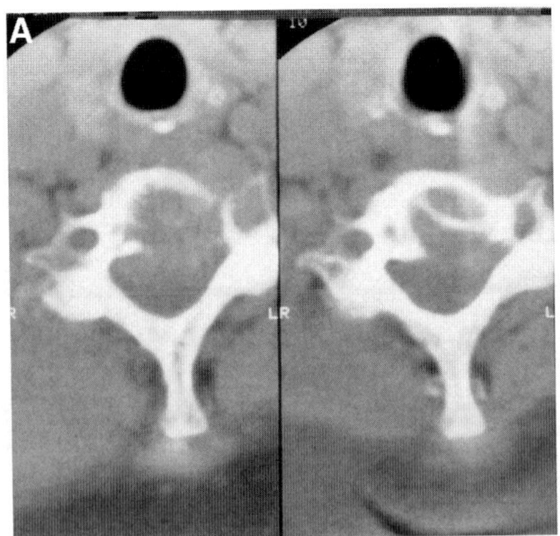

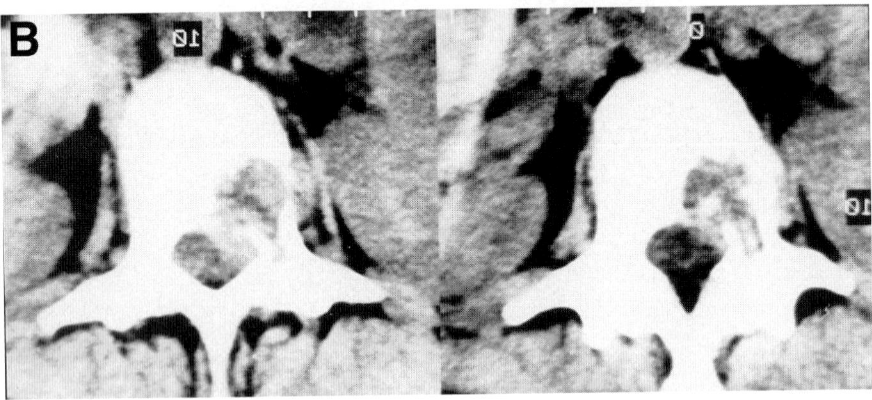

Figure14– 7. Spinal metastasis located **(A)** anteriorly and **(B)** laterally.

Integrity of Vertebral Bone

The bony integrity of vertebrae adjacent to a decompressed segment must be adequate to accept and anchor a prosthetic construct. When it is anticipated that an anteriorly applied reconstruction apparatus cannot be adequately anchored in place, it may be preferable to proceed with posterolateral decompression secured with sublaminar wires at several levels above and below the decompressed segment (see Fig. 14–5B).

Degree of Debility

The optimal surgical approach may be dictated by local and systemic factors. The anterior approach through an irradiated neck poses increased risk of tracheoesophageal perforation and associated consequences. By the same token, lengthy spinal procedures performed from behind in the thoracolumbar region with a midline incision through radiation-saturated skin in a cancer patient with impaired immunity and compromised nutrition carries a high risk of wound healing complications. On the other hand, the patient in the advanced stages of systemic cancer may be too debilitated to tolerate a transthoracic or thoracoabdominal operation.

SURGICAL APPROACHES

Preoperative Embolization

Metastases arising from thyroid and renal cell carcinoma are notoriously vascular. Catastrophic blood loss may occur unless preoperative embolization is undertaken to reduce tumor vascularity before direct surgical intervention (Bhojraj et al., 1992; Roscoe et al., 1989; Soo et al., 1982). Preoperative embolization greatly decreases intraoperative blood loss and has thus been found to allow for more complete tumor resection (Hess et al., 1997).

Posterior (Posterolateral) Decompression and Stabilization

Simple laminectomy is inadequate or inappropriate surgical treatment for all but a few patients with secondary spinal tumors. Laminectomy generally permits adequate exposure for intradural metastases and may also suffice in the uncommon event that extradural metastases involve only the posterior elements (e.g., Fig. 14–6). Most patients, however, require a wide laminectomy with posterolateral resection of the tumor-destroyed elements, which, in turn, permits excavation of the tumor-destroyed vertebral body (Fig. 14–8). Such posterolateral decompression, applied bilaterally, enables effective circumferential decompression of the dural sac and its contents (Akeyson and McCutcheon, 1996; Bauer, 1997; Perrin and McBroom, 1990; Rompe et al., 1999; Tomita et al., 1994).

Posterior spinal stabilization can be achieved with bone struts (when bony arthrodesis is anticipated in patients with prolonged life expectancy), steel rods (Harrington rods, Luque rods, or rectangle), or molded methyl methacrylate. The suitable struts are secured with sublaminar wires at a minimum of two levels above and two levels below the decompressed segment. Table 14–10 lists the variety of materials and methods described to secure spinal stabilization following posterior (posterolateral) decompression.

Anterior (Anterolateral) Decompression and Stabilization

Decompression from the front involves vertebral corpectomy. The approach is directly anterior in the cer-

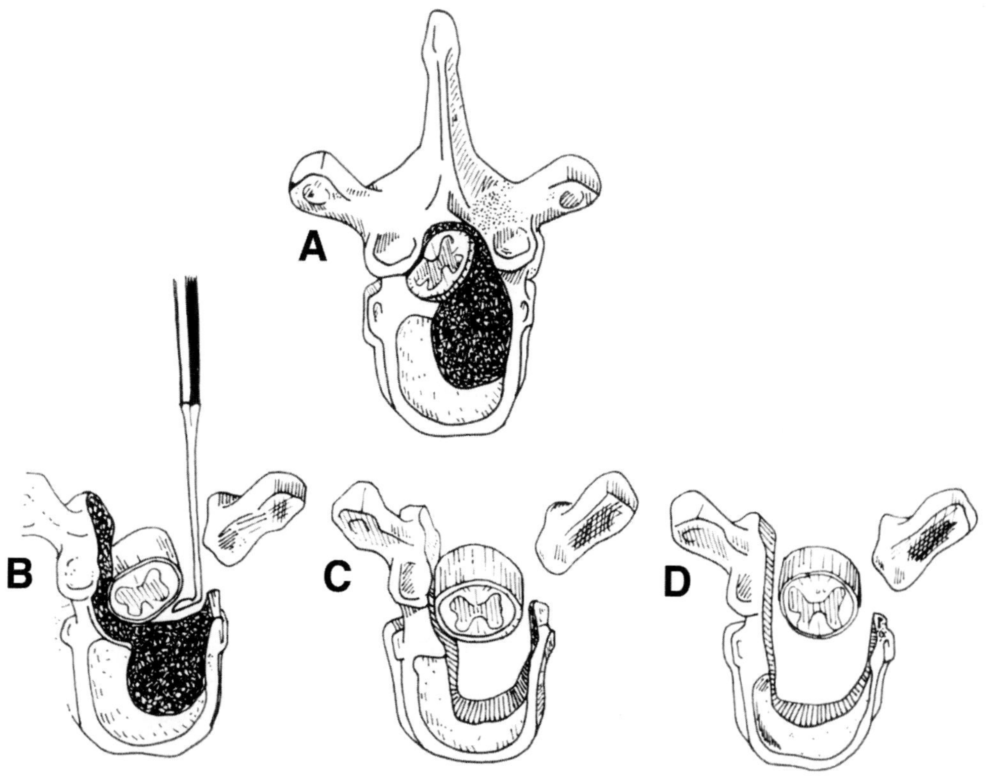

Figure 14–8. **(A)** Anterolaterally disposed extradural tumor. **(B)** Wide laminectomy with posterolateral access to vertebral body. **(C)** Posterolateral excavation of vertebral body. **(D)** Posterolaberal decompression, bilaterally.

Table 14–10. Posterior Spine Stabilization

Author	*Technique*
Rogers (1942)	Interspinous wiring
Robinson and Smith (1955)	Posterolateral facet fusion
Roy-Camille et al. (1976)	Roy-Camille plates
Livingston and Perrin (1978)	Rib struts
Perrin and Livingstone (1980)	Methylmethacrylate and sublaminar wiring
Holness et al. (1984)	Halifax clamp
Harrington (1984)	Harrington rods
Davey et al. (1985)	Dewar procedure
White et al. (1986)	San Francisco system
Krag et al. (1986)	Vermont system
Steffee et al. (1986)	Variable spine plating
Luque (1986)	Luque rods/rectangle
Ellis and Findlay (1994)	Contoured luque
Tomita et al. (1994)	En bloc spondylectomy stabilized with Cotrel-Dubousset instrumentation; vertebral reconstruction with apatite-wollastonite vertebral spacer supported by allograft bone
Akeyson and McCutcheon (1996)	Spondylectomy with posterior fixation using Luque rectangles and sublaminar cables and reconstruction with methylmethacrylate
Bauer (1997)	Wide decompression followed by stabilization without bone grafting using Cotrel-Dubousset instrumentation
Rompe et al. (1999)	Decompression and stabilization with Cotrel-Dubousset instrumentation
Weigel et al. (1999)	Laminectomy or hemilaminectomy and stabilization with titanium implants
Wise et al. (1999)	Decompression followed by autograft or allograft bone and instrumentation

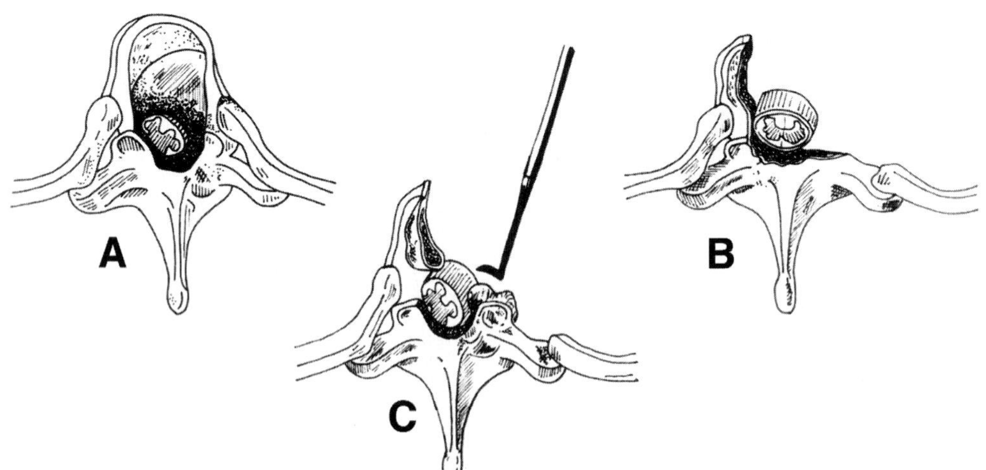

Figure 14–9. **(A)** Anterolaterally disposed extradural tumor. **(B)** Anterior decompression (corpectomy). **(C)** Anterolateral decompression.

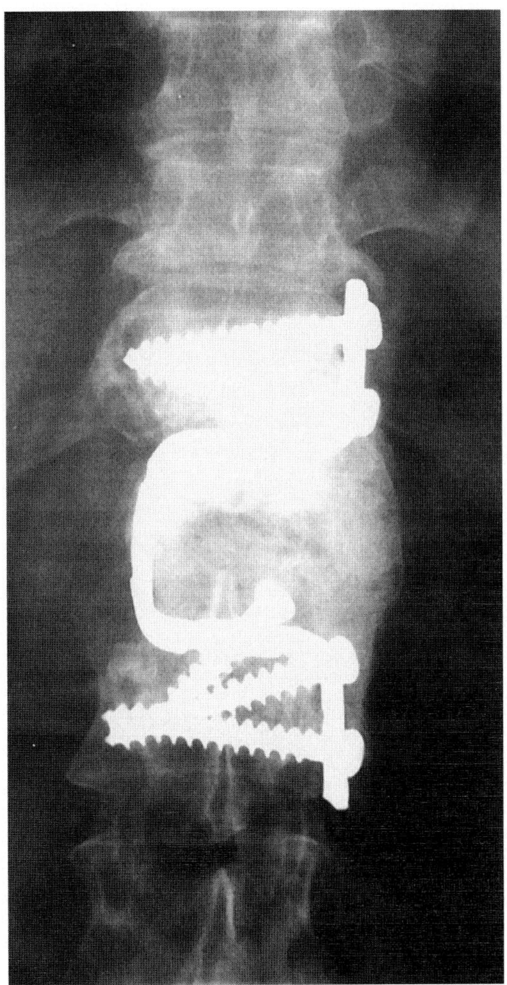

Figure 14–10. Anterior reconstruction "U"-shaped plate and methylmethacrylate (Wellesley wedge).

vical and lower lumbar regions and anterolateral in the thoracic (transthoracic avenue) and thoracolumbar (thoracoabdominal access) segments. The anterior (anterolateral) approach permits decompression under direct vision of approximately two-thirds of the dural sac circumference. When the approach is anterolateral (transthoracic and thoracoabdominal), the contralateral root sleeves are hidden from view and cannot be safely decompressed (Fig. 14–9) (Perrin and McBroom, 1994; Siegal and Siegal, 1985; Sundaresan et al., 1985).

Anterior spinal reconstruction can be achieved by means of a bone graft, with or without a plate, or with various prosthetic devices (Fig. 14–10) (Chen et al., 2000; Gokaslan et al., 1998; Perrin and McBroom, 1994). Table 14–11 lists the variety of materials and methods described to achieve spinal stability following anterior (anterolateral) decompression procedures. Because of the wide range of cervical spine mobility, if more than two vertebral segments are spanned, or when the integrity of the bone adjacent to the decompressed interval is insufficient to provide secure fixation, then supplemental stabilization with an apparatus applied from the back may be advisable.

Microsurgical endoscopic techniques provide a promising variation of anterior decompression surgery. Endoscopic surgery has been found to achieve adequate decompression and stabilization, but with a reduction in surgical trauma, postoperative pain, and postoperative hospitalization (Rosenthal et al., 1996).

Table 14–12 summarizes the outcomes associated with surgery in a number of recent studies. Improvement or stabilization of functional status occurred in 86% of cases following surgery. Whereas 68% of patients were able to walk before surgery, 85% were ambulatory after surgery. In addition to functional status, improvements have been reported in patients' quality of life following surgical treatment for spinal metastases (Weigel et al., 1999). These results suggest that, under the appropriate circumstances, surgery is an effective treatment option for many patients with spinal metastases.

CONCLUSION

The management of spinal metastases continues to pose a controversial challenge. Early diagnosis and prompt remedy are the cornerstones of treatment. Radiation and surgery constitute complimentary therapeutic modalities. Given the multiplicity of variables involved, it is impossible to critically compare reported series. In general, however, the outcomes for patients with spinal metastases depend on a number of factors, including the degree of deficit, speed of onset, culpable primary tumor burden (local and systemic), tumor location, and treatment technique (Table 14–13).

Optimal management of patients with spinal metastases involves multidisciplinary collaboration among specialists in neurology, oncology, radiation therapy, neurosurgery and orthopedics.

Table 14–11. Anterior Spine Stabilization

Author	*Technique*
Robinson and Smith (1955)	Smith-Robinson approach
Cloward (1958)	Cloward
Scoville et al. (1967)	Pins/methylmethacrylate
Cross et al. (1971)	Methylmethacrylate
Ono and Tada (1975)	Metal prosthesis
Fielding et al. (1979)	Corpectomy/iliac crest
Raycroft et al. (1978)	Corpectomy/tibia
Conley et al. (1979)	Corpectomy/fibula
Sundaresan et al. (1984)	Double K-wire/methylmethacrylate
Harrington (1984)	Knodt rods/methylmethacrylate
Perrin and McBroom (1988)	Wellesley wedge
Rosenthal et al. (1996)	Microsurgical endoscopic decompression, reconstruction with polymethylmethacrylate and plating for stabilization
Bauer (1997)	Decompression with Zielke instrumentation and cement
Gokaslan et al. (1998)	Transthroracic vertebrectomy with methylmethacrylate reconstruction and stabilization with locking plate and screw constructs
Weigel et al. (1999)	Screw fixation of the dense axis; corpectomy stabilized with titanium mesh cage filled with polymethylmethacrylate cement and titanium implants
Wise et al. (1999)	Decompression with autograft or allograft bone plus instrumentation or cement plus instrumentation
Chen et al. (2000)	Corpectomy and reconstruction using methylmethacrylate plus fixation with Zielke instrumentation

Table 14–12. Outcomes Following Surgery for Spinal Metastases

			*Global Rating**		*Ambulatory*		
Author	*No.*	*Approach*	*Good*	*Poor*	*Preop*	*Postop*	*Mortality*
Tomita et al. (1994)	20	Posterior	18	2	10	16	9
Akeyson and McCutcheon (1996)	25	Posterior	23	2	13	18	—
Rosenthal et al. (1996)	28	Anterior	28	0	—	28	—
Schiff and O'Neill (1996)	5	N/A‡	4	1	5	4	8
Tatsui et al. (1996)	1	Anterior	1	—	0	1	7.8
Tatsui et al. (1996)	15	Posterior	9	—	0	9	18.7
Bauer (1997)	67	Posterior	57	10	41	57	6
Gokaslan et al. (1998)	72	Anterior	69	3	59	68	>12
Rompe et al. (1999)	106	Posterior	98	8	73	88	19.2
Scarrow et al. (1999)	1	Posterior	1	—	1	1	—
Solberg and Bremnes (1999)	28	Posterior	—	—	—	—	10.1
Weigel et al. (1999)	96	Ant./post./both	58	28	76	90	13.1
Wise et al. (1999)	88	Ant./post./both	78	10	71	78	15.9
Chen et al. (2000)	60	Anterior	60	0	29	40	6–12
Totals	612		504	64	378	498	$M = 11.7$
%		86	11	68	85		

*For global ratings, good outcomes are those in which functional or neurologic status either stabilized or improved following treatment and poor outcomes are those in which further deterioration occurred following treatment.

†Median or mean survival for cohort in months.

‡Information on surgical approach was not available.

Table 14–13. Factors Determining Outcome

Degree of deficit
Speed of onset
Culpable primary tumor
Tumor burden (local and systemic)
Tumor location
Treatment technique

REFERENCES

Akeyson EW, McCutcheon IE. 1996. Single-stage posterior vertebrectomy and replacement combined with posterior instrumentation for spinal metastasis. J Neurosurg 85: 211–220.

Bach F, Larsen BH, Rohde K, et al. 1990. Metastatic spinal cord compression: Occurrence, symptoms, clinical presentations and prognosis in 398 patients with spinal cord compression. Acta Neurochir (Wien) 107:37–43.

Barron KD, Hirano A, Araki S, Terry RD. 1959. Experiences with metastatic neoplasms involving the spinal cord. Neurology 9:91–106.

Bauer HC. Posterior decompression and stabilization for spinal metastases: Analysis of 67 consecutive patients. 1997. J Bone Joint Surg Am 79:514–522.

Berenstein A, Graeb D. 1982. Convenient preparation of ready-to-use particles in polyvinyl alcohol foam suspensions for embolization. Radiology 145:846.

Bhojraj SY, Dandawate AV, Ramakantan R. 1992. Preoperative embolisation, transpedicular decompression and posterior stabilization for metastatic disease of the thoracic spine causing paraplegia. Paraplegia 30:292–299.

Bilsky MH, Lis E, Raizer J, Lee H, Boland P. 1999. The diagnosis and treatment of metastatic spinal tumor. Oncologist 4:459–469.

Boogerd W, van der Sande JJ. 1993. Diagnosis and treatment of spinal cord compression in malignant disease. Cancer Treat Rev 19:129–150.

Botterell EH, Fitzgerald GW. 1959. Spinal cord compression produced by extradural malignant tumours. Can Med Assoc J 80:791–796.

Brown PD, Stafford SL, Schild SE, Martenson JA, Schiff D. 1999. Metastatic spinal cord compression in patients with colorectal cancer. J Neurooncol 44:175–180.

Bruner JM, Tien RD. 1998. Secondary tumors. In: Bigner DD, McLendon RE, Bruner JM (eds), Russell and Rubinstein's Pathology of Tumors of the Nervous System, 6th ed. London: Arnold, p 441.

Byrne TN. 1992. Spinal cord compression from epidural metastses. N Engl J Med 327:614–619.

Chen LH, Chen WJ, Niu CC, Shih CH. 2000. Anterior reconstructive spinal surgery with Zielke instrumentation for metastatic malignancies of the spine. Arch Orthop Trauma Surg 120:27–31.

Cloward RB. 1958. The anterior approach for removal of ruptured cervical discs. J Neurosurg 15:602–614.

Conley FK, Britt RH, Hanberry JW, Silverberg GD. 1979. Anterior fibular strut graft in neoplastic disease of the cervical spine. J Neurosurg 51:677–684.

Cross GO, White HL, White LP. 1971. Acrylic prosthesis of the fifth vertebra in multiple myeloma. Technical note. J Neurosurg 35:112–114.

Davey JR, Rorabeck CH, Bailey SI, Bourne RB, Dewar FP. 1985. A technique of posterior cervical fusion for instability of the cervical spine. Spine 10:722–728.

Dunn RC Jr, Kelly WA, Wohns RN, Howe JF. 1980. Spinal epidural neoplasia: A 15-year review of the results of surgical therapy. J Neurosurg 52:47–51.

Edelson RN, Deck MD, Posner JB. 1972. Intramedullary spinal cord metastases. Clinical and radiographic findings in nine cases. Neurology 22:1222–1231.

Ellis PM, Findlay IM. 1994. Craniocervical fusion with contoured Luque rod and autogenic bone graft. Can J Surg 37:50–54.

Fielding JW, Pyle RN, Fietti VG. 1979. Anterior cervical vertebral body resection and bone-grafting for benign and malignant tumors. J Bone Joint Surg Am 61:251–253.

Gilbert RW, Kin JH, Posner JB. 1978. Epidural spinal cord compression from metastatic tumor: diagnosis and treatment. Ann Neurol 3:40–51.

Gokaslan ZL, York JE, Walsh GL, et al. 1998. Transthoracic vertebrectomy for metastatic spinal tumors. J Neurosurg 89:599–609.

Gomez JAO. 1955. The incidence of vertebral body metastases. Int Orthop 19:309–311.

Goodkin R, Carr BI, Perrin RG. 1987. Herniated lumbar disc disease in patients with malignancy. J Clin Oncol 5:667–671.

Harrington KD. 1984. Anterior decompression and spinal stabilization for patients with metastatic lesions of the spine. J. Neurosurg 61:107–117.

Helweg-Larsen S. 1996. Clinical outcome in metastatic spinal cord compression. A prospective study of 153 patients. Acta Neurol Scand 94:269–275.

Helweg-Larsen S, Johnsen A, Boesen J, Sorensen PS. 1997. Radiologic features compared to clinical findings in a prospective study of 153 patients with metastatic spinal cord compression treated by radiotherapy. Acta Neurochir (Wien) 139:105–111.

Helweg-Larsen S, Sorensen PS. 1994. Symptoms and signs in metastatic spinal cord compression: a study of progression from first symptom until diagnosis in 153 patients. Eur J Cancer 30A:396–398.

Hess T, Kramann B, Schmidt E, Rupp S. 1997. Use of preoperative vascular embolisation in spinal metastasis resection. Arch Orthop Trauma Surg 116:279–282.

Holness RO, Huestis WS, Howes JW, Langille RA. 1984. Posterior stabilization with an interlaminar clamp in cervical injuries: technical note and review of the long term experience with the method. Neurosurgery 14:318–322.

Inagaki J, Rodriguez V, Bodey GP. 1974. Causes of death in cancer patients. Cancer 33:568–573.

Jaeckle KA. 1991. Neuroimaging for central nervous system tumors. Semin Oncol 18:150–157.

Katagiri H, Takahashi M, Inagaki J, et al. 1998. Clinical results of nonsurgical treatment for spinal metastases. Int J Radiat Oncol Biol Phys 42:1127–1132.

Khaw FM, Worthy SA, Gibson MJ, Gholkar A. 1999. The appearance on MRI of vertebrae in acute compression of the spinal cord due to metastases. J Bone Joint Surg Br 81: 830–834.

Kim HJ, Ryu KN, Choi WS, Choi BK, Choi JM, Yoon Y. 1999. Spinal involvement of hematopoietic malignancies and metastasis: Differentiation using MR imaging. Clin Imaging 23:125–133.

Kim RY, Smith JW, Spencer SA, Meredith RF, Salter MM. 1993. Malignant epidural spinal cord compression associated with a paravertebral mass: its radiotherapeutic outcome on radiosensitivity. Int J Radiat Oncol Biol Phys 27:1079–1083.

Kovner F, Spigel S, Rider I, et al. 1999. Radiation therapy of metastatic spinal cord compression: multidisciplinary team diagnosis and treatment. J Neurooncol 42:85–92.

Krag MH, Beynnon, BD, Pope MH, Frymoyer JW, Haugh LD, Weaver DL. 1986. An internal fixator for posterior application to short segments of the thoracic, lumbar, or lumbosacral spine. Design and testing. Clin Orthop 203:75–98.

Leviov M, Dale J, Stein M et al. 1993. The management of metastatic spinal cord compression: a radiotherapeutic success ceiling. Int J Radiat Oncol Biol Phys 27:231–234.

Livingston KE, Perrin RG. 1978. The neurosurgical management of spinal metastases causing cord and cauda equina compression. J Neurosurg 49:839–843.

Luque ER. 1986. Interpeduncular segmental fixation. Clin Orthop 203:54–57.

MacDonald DR. 1990. Clinical manifestations. In: Sundaresan N, Schmidek H, Schuller A (eds), Tumors of the Spine. Philadelphia: WB Saunders, Philadelphia, pp 6–21.

Maranzano E, Latini P, Checcaglini F. 1991. Radiation therapy in metastatic spinal cord compression. A prospective analysis of 105 consecutive patients. Cancer 67:1311–1317.

Maranzano E, Latini P, Perrucci E, Beneventi S, Lupattelli M, Corgna E. 1997. Short-course radiotherapy (8 Gyx2) in metastatic spinal cord compression: an effective and feasible treatment. Int J Radiat Oncol Biol Phys 38:1037–1044.

Markus JB. 1996. Magnetic resonance imaging of intramedullary spinal cord metastases. Clin Imaging 20:238–242.

Ono K, Tada K. 1975. Metal prostheses of the cervical vertebra. J Neurosurg 42:562–566.

O'Rourke T, George CB, Redmond J 3rd, et al. 1986. Spinal computed tomography and computed tomographic metrizamide myelography in the early diagnosis of metastatic disease. J Clin Oncol 4:576–583.

Perrin RG, Livingston KE. 1980. Neurosurgical treatment of pathological fracture-dislocation of the spine. J Neurosurg 52:330–334.

Perrin RG, Livingston KE, Aarabi R. 1982. Intradural extramedullary spinal metastasis. A report of 10 cases. J Neurosurg 56:835–837.

Perrin RG, McBroom RJ. 1987. Anterior versus posterior decompression for symptomatic spinal metastasis. Can J Neurol Sci 14:75–80.

Perrin RG, McBroom RJ. 1988. Spinal fixation after anterior decompression for symptomatic spinal metastasis. J Neurosurg 22:324–327.

Perrin RG, McBroom RJ. 1990. Surgical treatment for spinal metastases: the posterolateral approach. In: Sundaresan N, Schmidek H, Schiller A, Rosenthal A (eds), Tumors of the Spine. Philadelphia: WB Saunders, pp 305–315.

Perrin RG, McBroom RJ. 1994. Metastatic tumors of the spine. In: Rengachary SS, Wikins RH (eds), Principles of Neurosurgery. St. Louis: Wolfe Publishing, pp 37.1–37.32.

Raycroft JF, Hockman RP, Southwick WO. 1978. Metastatic tumors involving the cervical vertebrae: surgical palliation. J Bone Joint Surg Am 60:763–768.

Redmond J 3d, Spring DB, Munderloh SH, George SB, Mansour RP, Volk SA. 1984. Spinal computed tomography scanning in the evaluation of metastatic disease. Cancer 54:253–258.

Robinson RA, Smith GW. 1955. Anterolateral cervical disc removal and interbody fusion for instability of the cervical spine. Bull Johns Hopkins Hosp 96:223–224.

Rogers L, Heard G. 1958. Intrathecal spinal metastases (rare tumours). Br J Surg 45:317–320.

Rogers WA. 1942. Treatment of fracture-dislocation of the cervical spine. J Bone Joint Surg 24:245–258.

Rompe JD, Hopf CG, Eysel P. 1999. Outcome after palliative posterior surgery for metastatic disease of the spine—evaluation of 106 consecutive patients after decompression and stabilisation with the Cotrel-Dubousset instrumentation. Arch Orthop Trauma Surg 119:394–400.

Roscoe MW, McBroom RJ, St. Louis E, Grossman H, Perrin R. 1989. Preoperative embolization in the treatment of osseous metastases from renal cell carcinoma. Clin Orthop 238:302–307.

Rosenthal D, Marquardt G, Lorenz R, Nichtweiss M. 1996. Anterior decompression and stabilization using a microsurgical endoscopic technique for metastatic tumors of the thoracic spine. J Neurosurg 84:565–572.

Roy-Camille R, Saillant G, Berteaux D, Salsado V. 1976. Osteosynthesis of thoraco-lumbar spine fractures with metal plates screwed through the vertebral pedicles. Reconstr Surg Traumatol 15:2–16.

Scarrow AM, Colina JL, Levy EI, Welch WC. 1999. Thyroid carcinoma with isolated spinal metastasis: case history and review of the literature. Clin Neurol Neurosurg 101:245–248.

Schiff D, O'Neill BP. 1996. Intramedullary spinal cord metastases: clinical features and treatment outcome. Neurology 47:906–912.

Schiff D, O'Neill BP, Suman VJ. 1997. Spinal epidural metastasis as the initial manifestation of malignancy: clinical features and diagnostic approach. Neurology 49:452–456.

Schiff D, O'Neill BP, Wang CH, O'Fallon Jr. 1998. Neuroimaging and treatment implications of patients with multiple epidural spinal metastases. Cancer 83:1593–1601.

Scoville WB, Palmer AH, Samra K, Chong G. 1967. The use of acrylic plastic for vertebral replacement or fixation in metastatic disease of the spine: technical note. J Neurosurg 27:274–279.

Siegal T, Siegal T. 1985. Treatment of malignant epidural cord and cauda equina compression. Prog Exp Tumor Res 29:225–234.

Solberg A, Bremnes RM. 1999. Metastatic spinal cord compression: diagnostic delay, treatment and outcome. Anticancer Res 19:677–684.

Soo C, Wallace S, Chuang VP, Carrasco CH, Phillies G. 1982. Lumbar artery embolization in cancer patients. Radiology 145:655–659.

Sorensen S, Helweg-Larsen S, Mouridsen H, Hansen HH. 1994. Effect of high-dose dexamethasone in carcinomatous metastatic spinal cord compression treated with radiotherapy: a randomised trial. Eur J Cancer 30A:22–27.

Steffee AD, Biscup RS, Sitkowski DJ. 1986. Segmental spine plates with pedicle screw fixation. A new internal fixation device for disorders of the lumbar and thoracolumbar spine. Clin Orthop 203:45–53.

Sundaresan N, DiGiacinto GV, Hughes JE, Cafferty M, Vallejo A. 1991. Treatment of neoplastic spinal cord compression: results of a prospective study. Neurosurgery 29:645–650.

Sundaresan N, DiGiacinto GV, Krol G, Hughes JE. 1990. Complete spondylectomy for malignant tumors. In: Sundaresan N, Schmidek H, Schiller A, Rosenthal A (eds), Tumors of the Spine. Philadelphia: WB Saunders, Philadelphia, pp 438–445.

Sundaresan N, Galicich JH, Bains MS, Martini N, Beattie EJ. 1984. Vertebral body resection in the treatment of cancer involving the spine. Cancer 53:1393–1396.

Sundaresan N, Galicich JH, Lane JM, Bains MS, McCormack P. 1985. Treatment of neoplastic epidural cord comprssion by vertebral body resection and stabilization. J Neurosurg 63:676–684.

Sze G. 1991. Magnetic resonance imaging in the evaluation of spinal tumors. Cancer 67:1229–1241.

Tatsui H, Onomura T, Morishita S, Oketa M, Inoue T. 1996. Survival rates of patients with metastatic spinal cancer after scintigraphic detection of abnormal radioactive accumulation. Spine 21:2143–2148.

Tombolini V, Zurlo A, Montagna A, et al. 1994. Radiation therapy of spinal metastases: results with different fractionations. Tumori 80:353–356.

Tomita K, Kawahara N, Baba H, Tsuchiya H, Nagata S, Toribatake Y. 1994. Total en bloc spondylectomy for solitary spinal metastases. Int Orthop 18:291–298.

Turner S, Marosszeky B, Timms I, Boyages J. 1993. Malignant spinal cord compression: a prospective evaluation. Int J Radiat Oncol Biol Phys 26:141–146.

Van der Sande JJ, Boogerd W, Kröger, Kapelle AC. 1999. Recurrent spinal epidural metastases: a prospective study with a complete follow up. J Neurol Neurosurg Psychiatry 66:623–627.

Weigel B, Maghsudi M, Neumann, Kretschmer R, Muller FJ, Nerlich M. 1999. Surgical management of symptomatic spinal metastases: postoperative outcome and quality of life. Spine 24:2240–2246.

White AH, Zucherman JF, Hsu K. 1986. Lumbosacral fusions with Harrington rods and intersegmental wiring. Clin Orthop 203:185–190.

Willis RA. 1973. The Spread of Tumors in the Human Body, 3rd ed. London: Butterworths, 429 pp.

Wise JJ, Fischgrund JS, Herkowitz HN, Montgomery D, Kurz LT. 1999. Complication, survival rates, and risk factors of surgery for metastatic disease of the spine. Spine 24:1943–1951.

Wong CS, Van Dyk J, Milosevic M, Laperriere NJ. 1994. Radiation myelopathy following single courses of radiotherapy and retreatment. Int J Radiat Oncol Biol Phys 30:575–581.

Young RF, Post EM, King GA. 1980. Treatment of spinal epidural metastases. Randomized prospective comparison of laminectomy and radiotherapy. J Neurosurg 53:741–748.

15

Leukemia and Lymphoma Metastases

LISA M. DEANGELIS

Central nervous system (CNS) metastases can occur with any primary systemic cancer, but some primary cancers such as melanoma have a specific predilection for the CNS. Brain metastasis is the most common CNS metastasis, occurring in 15% of all cancer patients (Posner, 1995). Leptomeningeal metastasis is less common, 3% to 8%, and epidural metastasis occurs in approximately 5% of cases (Posner, 1995; Byrne and Waxman, 1990). Leukemias and lymphomas do metastasize to the nervous system but rarely involve brain parenchyma and more characteristically involve the leptomeninges. Although epidural metastases do not represent nervous system metastases because they occur outside of the CNS, they typically have a neurologic presentation and for that reason are considered here.

The overwhelming majority of CNS metastases are due to solid tumors rather than to lymphoreticular malignancies. Lymphoma accounts for only 10% of epidural metastases whereas solid tumors account for the remaining 90% (Posner, 1995; Byrne and Waxman, 1990); leukemia rarely causes epidural disease (Bower et al., 1997; Kataoka et al., 1995). In contradistinction, the lymphoreticular malignancies account for a preponderance of patients with leptomeningeal metastases. The overall incidence is difficult to ascertain because leukemias and lymphomas are often excluded from most series, but approximately 24% of patients with leptomeningeal metastasis have non-Hodgkin's lymphoma (NHL) (Olson et al., 1974). Therefore, the pattern of CNS metastases from lymphoma and leukemia is different from that of solid tumors, and the differential diagnosis of these entities is different for patients with lymphoreticular malignancies. For example, leptomeningeal metastasis can mimic vincristine peripheral neuropathy, which is common among patients with lymphoma or leukemia. Patients with lymphoreticular malignancies are particularly vulnerable to opportunistic infections, which can mimic metastasis. Finally, isolated CNS metastasis is far more common with lymphoma or leukemia than with solid tumors where CNS disease typically occurs in the setting of widespread systemic metastases.

Systemic therapy of leukemia and lymphoma can be highly effective and can eradicate extra-CNS disease. However, microscopic tumor within the CNS may be protected from circulating systemic chemotherapy by the blood–brain barrier. This disease can progress while the patient is in remission systemically, leading to an isolated CNS relapse. This pattern of recurrence is characteristic of the leukemias and lymphomas, making them different from the solid tumors and warranting special consideration.

EPIDURAL METASTASES

Epidural metastases are seen in 3% to 5% of patients with systemic NHL (Levitt et al., 1980; Mackintosh et al., 1982; Raz et al., 1984). Epidural lymphoma can be the presenting manifestation of disseminated NHL, or can be an isolated site of disease, which accounts for approximately 1% of patients with NHL (Lyons et al., 1992; Gilbert et al., 1978). Epidural tumor occurs primarily in those patients with intermediate- to high-grade subtypes and in those with advanced disease (i.e., stage III or IV). Occasionally, the development of a complication such as epidural metastasis heralds the transformation of a previously low-grade or indolent neoplasm into a higher grade malignancy or may be the initial manifestation of the illness. The development of epidural metastases tends to occur in those patients with bone metastases, particularly vertebral metastases, and in those who have paraspinal nodal involvement. It has also been associated with retroperitoneal adenopathy and, in some series, with bone marrow infiltration.

Epidural metastasis is a very rare complication of any type of leukemia. It can be seen as a consequence of paraspinal chloroma formation in patients with acute myeloblastic leukemia (AML). It has a presentation, diagnosis, and treatment identical to epidural metastasis from NHL, and the following discussion can be applied to these unusual patients.

Clinical Features

The clinical features of epidural metastasis from lymphoma are not substantially different from those seen in solid tumors and described in Chapter 14. The predominant clinical symptom is back or neck pain (Byrne and Waxman, 1990; Gilbert et al., 1978; Posner, 1987), which is present in 95% of patients with epidural metastasis. Usually the first symptom, it often predates the development of neurologic deficits by months. The pain is typically thoracic, an unusual site of pain due to degenerative disease, because 80% of epidural metastases are in the thoracic spine. Most patients with epidural metastasis from solid tumors present first with back pain, which may develop a radicular component as the disease progresses. This occurs because the metastasis initially originates in the bone, usually the vertebral body, and then grows outside of the bone to involve paraspinal structures and cause nerve root compression.

In contrast, NHL more commonly involves the epidural space by tumor growing from the paravertebral area directly through the intervertebral foramen, causing spinal cord compression. For this reason, there is less back pain from bone destruction. The pain more commonly has a radicular component or may even be referred within the dermatomal distribution of the compressed root, which can lead to misdiagnosis. Radicular pain down a limb or across the trunk may, in fact, be the first indication of an epidural tumor from NHL. Unlike solid tumors, NHL can occasionally metastasize directly to the epidural space without bone or paravertebral involvement. These lesions may be asymptomatic and initially detected on body CT scans done to completely stage the patient's NHL. If suggested on CT scan, a comprehensive evaluation with magnetic resonance imaging (MRI) (see below) is essential to establish the diagnosis.

In order of frequency pain is followed by leg weakness, which occurs in approximately 50% of patients, and may be accompanied by sensory dysfunction in a comparable proportion. Sphincter dysfunction is seen in about 20% of patients. The back pain of epidural cord compression is characterized by progressive severity as well as increased severity when the patient lies down, in contrast to pain from degenerative spinal disease, which characteristically improves upon recumbency. In addition, pain that intensifies with cough, sneeze, or Valsalva strongly indicates compression of the spinal cord, which is transiently intensified with the increase in intraspinal pressure that occurs with these maneuvers. Sometimes these features can alert the physician that the back pain is due to something more serious than the common, benign causes of back pain.

Diagnosis

The best and only test necessary to establish a diagnosis of epidural metastasis is a spinal MRI (Jordan et al., 1995). This should be done without intravenous contrast material (i.e., gadolinium), which can actually obscure the diagnosis and make it more difficult to see tumor. Magnetic resonance imaging can visualize the entire spine noninvasively and identify epidural tumor at any level (Fig. 15–1). It is particularly useful for patients with lymphoma in whom tumor can enter the epidural space via the intervertebral foramen and not involve or destroy bone. This is a major limitation of plain films and bone scans, which can only identify sites of bony destruction. Even if a bone metastasis is present, these techniques do not indicate whether or not the disease has progressed to involve the epidural space. Furthermore, they can be negative in the face of significant bone involvement with epidural tumor causing spinal cord compression. Any patient with NHL who has significant, progressive back pain should be considered for spinal MRI even in the absence of neurologic deficits.

Another feature of MRI is that it easily images the entire spine. This is essential as multilevel epidural

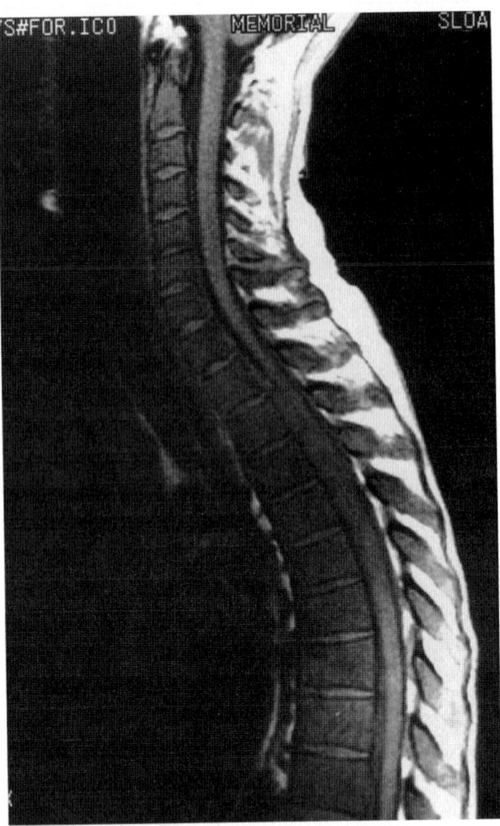

Figure 15–1. Magnetic resonance image of the spine demonstrating ventral epidural lymphoma extending from T2 to T5. Note the preserved vertebral bodies and absence of bone destruction.

disease occurs in about 5% of patients with an epidural metastasis. Consequently, if MR images are obtained, an epidural metastasis identified, and only a portion of the spinal column visualized, then the patient should return to the scanner to complete imaging of the remainder of the spine.

Some patients are unable to undergo MR imaging because they have a pacemaker or other device that prohibits them from being in a high magnetic field. A computed tomography (CT) myelogram should be performed for such patients. If a complete block is identified with dye introduced into the lumbar space, then a C1–C2 puncture should be performed to introduce dye from above to define the upper limit of the epidural tumor. This is particularly important in NHL in which the disease can grow extensively in the rostral caudal direction once it has reached the epidural space. Accurate identification of the full extent of tumor is critical for treatment planning.

Initial Management

Many patients with an epidural metastasis are easily identified clinically. They have severe progressive back pain accompanied by neurologic symptoms and signs suggestive of a myelopathy. For such patients, dexamethasone is often administered even before neuroimaging is obtained. Dexamethasone rapidly relieves the pain of spinal cord compression and may facilitate neurologic recovery. Experimental data and substantial but retrospective clinical data suggest a dose–response relationship between corticosteroids and control of back pain associated with epidural tumor (Posner, 1995). The pain can be substantially ameliorated within hours of drug administration, which can facilitate the patient's ability to tolerate any diagnostic procedure, especially an MRI scan. Typically, an intravenous bolus of dexamethasone is administered. Clinical data support the use of a very high initial dose, 100 mg, to rapidly relieve back pain (Loblaw and Laperriere, 1998). With the exception of patients with NHL, for those patients with known cancer, particularly solid tumors, this is a very reasonable approach.

Corticosteroids are a well-recognized, effective chemotherapeutic agent for the treatment of NHL. Because they can cause rapid cell lysis, tumor can disappear very quickly after their administration (Posner et al., 1977). Consequently, it is essential that neuroimages be obtained before the dispensation of any corticosteroids to NHL patients suspected of having epidural tumor. Their pain should be managed with narcotic analgesics to facilitate performing the necessary neuroimaging. Once the MRI scan is complete and an epidural metastasis has been identified, administration of dexamethasone is appropriate.

This approach is very straightforward for patients with known NHL, but it becomes more complicated for patients whose malignancy presents for the first time as an epidural mass. For such patients, MR images are obtained first, and there is usually no consideration given to administering corticosteroids before identification of an epidural mass. Once such a mass is seen on an MRI scan, however, corticosteroids are usually given immediately. If the mass is a lymphoma, one can see rapid resolution of the lesion. If tissue has not yet been obtained for diagnosis, the opportunity to confirm the diagnosis pathologically is thus lost, and appropriate treatment is deferred, resulting in a significant delay for the patient. Despite their clinical response to the corticosteroids, patients must be tapered off the drug to allow the disease to declare itself once again so that tissue can be obtained for biopsy. Not only does this delay definitive treatment, but also puts the patient at substantial risk of progressive neurologic compromise from recurrent epidural metastasis. It is essential that these issues be considered before "standard therapy" is administered on a routine basis.

Treatment

Once the diagnosis is established, treatment of epidural metastasis should be implemented as rapidly as possible. Treatment may involve any one of the three major anticancer therapeutic modalities: radiotherapy (RT), surgery, and chemotherapy. The choice of treatment, or combination of therapies, depends on the patient's clinical and neurologic condition, his or her prior treatment for the underlying lymphoma, and any prior therapy for epidural metastasis. Rapid institution of treatment is imperative as a patient's neurologic function can deteriorate precipitously. A general rule of thumb for most patients with spinal cord compression is that if they are ambulatory at diagnosis, they remain ambulatory after treatment, but if they are nonambulatory at diagnosis, they rarely regain the ability to ambulate independently (Posner, 1995).

Radiotherapy

Radiotherapy is the most common and effective modality for the treatment of epidural spinal cord compression (Maranzano et al., 1991; Bilsky et al., 1999). It is easily administered and highly effective, particularly for a radiosensitive primary tumor such as lymphoma. A complete spinal MRI will define the rostral caudal extent of the epidural metastasis. Typically, we administer radiotherapy to a port encompassing the area of tumor plus two vertebral bodies superior and inferior to the tumor margin. The usual course of treatment is 300 cGy for 10 fractions, for a total of 30 Gy. Patients should receive corticosteroids before and during RT to minimize exacerbation of neurologic problems from edema engendered by the treatment, but for select patients steroids are not required during RT (Maranzano et al., 1996).

Radiotherapy is particularly effective for NHL for two reasons: *(1)* Lymphoma is a highly radiosensitive neoplasm so that focal RT can be very effective in relieving a spinal cord compression from epidural metastasis; and *(2)* because lymphoma frequently involves the epidural space by growing through the intervertebral foramen, or metastasizing directly to the epidural compartment, bone destruction is a less prominent feature of epidural metastases from NHL. Epidural spinal cord compression is typically caused by the tumor itself and is a consequence of soft tissue compression rather than bone compression so that RT is more likely to relieve spinal cord compression in this circumstance.

Side effects from RT can include myelosuppression, particularly if the patient is heavily pretreated with chemotherapy or a long expanse of spine must be included in the port of RT. Patients can also develop gastrointestinal irritation from RT to the lower spine or mucositis from cervical RT.

Surgery

Surgery is rarely the first line of treatment for patients with spinal cord compression from lymphoma (Byrne and Waxman, 1990). It is used initially when a tissue diagnosis has not been made. Surgery can establish the diagnosis and also decompress the spinal cord. Even if gross total excision of the disease seems to have been accomplished in such patients, postoperative RT is appropriate to avoid local recurrence and subsequent recompression of the spinal cord.

Surgery may be appropriate for patients who are experiencing spinal cord compression in a previously irradiated location. For those patients who are not candidates for a second course of RT (Schiff et al.,1995), surgery may improve or at least maintain neurologic function (Bilsky et al.,1999; Sioutos et al., 1995; Klekamp and Samii, 1998). The surgical approach depends on the location of the tumor mass. If the tumor has arisen from a vertebral body metastasis and is compressing the cord anteriorly, a vertebrectomy from an anterior approach may be most appropriate. Data suggest that such patients who have severe neurologic impairment may regain sphincter control and leg strength when a complete decompression is achieved by anterior resection. However, disease that has arisen in the paravertebral location or more posteriorly may be more amenable to laminectomy, which would allow for tumor removal and direct decompression of the spinal cord. Laminectomy for patients with disease located anteriorly probably does not improve neurologic outcome and does not effectively treat the tumor.

Surgery should be reserved for patients in good preoperative condition who have systemic disease that is controlled or controllable and who do not have multilevel epidural tumor (Sioutos et al., 1995; Klekamp and Samii, 1998). Surgical complications include worsening neurologic deficit, wound dehiscence or infection (particularly in those who require sustained doses of corticosteroids), and delayed hardware disruption, which often heralds tumor regrowth.

Chemotherapy

Chemotherapy is rarely the first line of treatment for epidural metastasis. However, it has been shown to be effective for those patients whose epidural tumors were identified during their extent of disease evaluation at initial presentation (Lyons et al., 1992; Oviatt et al., 1982; Wong et al., 1996). These patients typically have an epidural site of disease identified on the initial body CT scan done to evaluate intrathoracic and intra-abdominal disease. Epidural tumor is then confirmed by spinal MRI; however, patients may be asymptomatic or have minimal neurologic symptomatology. These patients usually require combination chemotherapy as an initial treatment for systemic lymphoma. For such patients, chemotherapy can be administered and the epidural disease monitored closely. Typically, the epidural tumor responds in the same fashion as the rest of the systemic disease. For those patients whose epidural disease does not respond, focal RT can be administered.

Although epidural tumor presents with neurologic symptoms and signs referable to the spinal cord, it is important to remember that epidural disease exists outside of the CNS and is not behind the blood–brain barrier. Systemically administered chemotherapy is as effective against disease in this location as in any systemic location. The choice of drugs should be based on the optimal regimen likely to be effective against the systemic lymphoma.

Chemotherapy can also be used for patients whose disease has developed in a previously irradiated site or for whom surgery is not an option or has already failed. However, for such patients who have heavily pretreated disease and for whom prior chemotherapy has often been administered, the probability of an excellent response from such treatment is substantially less than at initial therapy.

LEPTOMENINGEAL METASTASES

Leptomeningeal metastases develop as a complication in 4% to 11% of patients with systemic NHL and in approximately 10% of patients with leukemia (Table 15–1) (Posner, 1995; Olson et al., 1974). In patients with NHL, the incidence is higher among those with high-grade and widespread disease. In leukemia patients, the incidence varies widely with type of leukemia, reaching a peak incidence of 56% at autopsy in those with acute lymphocytic leukemia (ALL). This was particularly true before the availability of prophylactic intrathecal chemotherapy (Price and Johnson, 1973). The development of vigorous systemic and CNS therapies has markedly decreased the incidence of meningeal leukemia in both ALL and acute myelocytic leukemia (AML) (Barcos et al., 1987). Currently, the incidence of CNS relapse is 2.2% in AML and 4.3% in ALL (Castagnola et al., 1997; Stark et al., 2000).

Clinical Features

The hallmark of leptomeningeal metastasis is multifocal involvement of the CNS (Wasserstrom et al., 1982; Balm and Hammack, 1996). The disease primarily involves three main regions of the CNS: cranial nerves, the cerebrum, and spinal compartment (Table 15–2). Patients may present with symptoms and signs involving one or all of these locations and

Table 15–1. Frequency of Leptomeningeal Metastasis

	No. of Autopsies	*No. of Metastases (%)*
Leukemia	287	28 (10)
ALL	87	21 (24)
AML	104	5 (5)
Lymphoma	309	15 (4)
Hodgkin's	119	2 (2)
Non-Hodgkin's	190	13 (7)

ALL, acute lymphocytic leukemia; AML, acute myelogenous leukemia.
Source: Adapted from Posner (1995).

Table 15–2. Symptoms and Signs of Leptomeningeal Metastases in Lymphoma

Radiculopathy	44%
Impaired mental function	42%
Cranial neuropathy	36%
Headaches	23%
Seizures	3%
None (positive CSF cytology only)	11%

Source: Adapted from Recht et al. (1998).

generally have more neurologic signs on examination than symptoms. This discrepancy is often the first clue that meningeal tumor is present.

Common symptoms are facial weakness, facial numbness and diplopia (Posner, 1995; Levitt et al., 1980). Radicular symptoms are most commonly observed in the legs, and numbness or weakness may be bilateral but is often asymmetric. Bowel and bladder disturbances are frequent. Cerebral symptoms are usually due to raised intracranial pressure and communicating hydrocephalus caused by tumor impairing absorption of cerebrospinal fluid (CSF) over the cerebral convexities. Headache and mental status changes are the most common cerebral symptoms. Seizures and ataxia are infrequent, occurring in fewer than 10% of patients. Lateralizing symptoms and signs, including hemiparesis, aphasia, or a visual field deficit, are not seen with leptomeningeal metastasis unless there is an accompanying parenchymal lesion, such as a brain metastasis; or leptomeningeal tumor has caused vascular occlusion leading to a stroke.

Pain is a variable accompaniment to leptomeningeal tumor. The cranial neuropathies are typically painless, except facial pain is reported occasionally. The radicular symptoms and signs may be painless, which is often a clue that the cause is leptomeningeal tumor rather than epidural tumor, which is almost always painful. However, radicular pain can be a prominent symptom of leptomeningeal metastasis and can be difficult to treat. When there is significant radicular, back, or neck pain, epidural tumor is the most important differential diagnostic consideration.

Diagnosis

The diagnosis of leptomeningeal lymphoma or leukemia has usually required the demonstration of tumor cells in the CSF, which are almost always abnormal in the presence of leptomeningeal metastasis. Positive cytology is, however, observed in only 50% of patients with documented leptomeningeal metastasis from solid tumors on the first lumbar puncture (Wasserstrom et al., 1982). Repeated spinal taps are frequently needed to demonstrate the presence of tumor cells, and positive cytology results can be obtained in 90% of patients with three lumbar punctures. However, with NHL leptomeningeal metastasis, the CSF yields a positive cytologic examination in 88% of patients with two lumbar punctures (Recht et al., 1988).

Routine studies of CSF are less helpful in patients with leukemia and NHL than in those with solid tumors (Posner, 1995; Wasserstrom et al., 1982; Recht et al., 1988). Cerebrospinal fluid protein concentration is elevated in approximately 60%, but rarely above 200 mg/dL. The CSF glucose level may be depressed, but only in a minority of patients. The CSF cell count is usually elevated and may be composed of tumor cells and reactive lymphocytes, making a cytologic distinction between the two very difficult in some patients. These abnormalities are seen in many patients with leptomeningeal lymphoma and leukemia, as they are in patients who have this complication from solid tumors. The exception is leptomeningeal leukemia, which can be present in otherwise completely normal CSF (Tubergen et al., 1994; Mahmoud et al., 1993). In particular, the cell count may be normal if patients are pancytopenic from either their disease or its treatment. Therefore, vigilance in the cytologic examination is essential for patients suspected of this process. Sending large volumes of CSF to the cytopathologist with rapid fixation of the specimen can increase the yield. In addition, sampling CSF from a location close to the area of clinical symptoms also improves yield. For example, patients with lumbar radicular symptoms have the highest incidence of positive cytology when CSF samples from a lumbar puncture are used (Rogers et al., 1992). However, those with cerebral symptoms or cranial neuropathies have a higher yield when CSF is obtained from a C1–C2 puncture or a ventricular sample when a ventricular reservoir is already in place.

Cerebrospinal fluid tumor markers can occasionally be helpful in identifying tumors (Schold et al., 1980; Oschmann et al., 1994; DeAngelis, 1998), but because there are no specific tumor markers for leukemia and lymphoma, they are more effective for identifying solid tumors. β_2 Microglobulin is often elevated in CSF in lymphoma and occasionally in leukemia, but is nonspecific and can be elevated in any inflammatory condition associated with a CSF pleocytosis. While this is also true of the nonspecific markers β-glucuronidase and LDH isoenzymes, these markers can nevertheless be useful in some patients (Lossos et al., 2000). Vascular endothelial growth factor has recently been shown to be predictive in patients with leptomeningeal metastasis from solid tumors; it may also prove valuable in hematologic malignancies (Stockhammer et al., 2000). Flow cytometry and molecular markers are helpful if adequate cells are available and the molecular phenotype is known (van Oostenbrugge et al., 1998; Cibas et al., 1987; Rhodes et al., 1996).

Demonstration of tumor cells in the CSF is not the only way to establish a diagnosis of leptomeningeal metastasis. Gadolinium-enhanced MRI of the neuraxis sometimes reveals findings that are so characteristic of leptomeningeal tumor as to be diagnostic (Rodesch et al., 1990; Freilich et al., 1995). Prominent enhancement and enlargement of cranial nerves due to tumor infiltration, nodules adherent to the cauda equina, large subarachnoid masses compressing the spinal cord, and prominent enhancement coating the surface of the brain extending deep into sulci are all definitive neuroradiologic features of tumor in the subarachnoid space in patients known to have cancer (Fig. 15–2). The presence of such findings, even in the absence of a positive CSF cytologic examination, can establish the diagnosis and be sufficient to initiate treatment.

These findings are not manifest in every patient who has leptomeningeal tumor. Normal neuroradiologic studies do not exclude leptomeningeal tumor, which is particularly problematic for patients with leukemia and lymphoma who have a lower incidence of neuroradiologic abnormalities than those with solid tumors. Furthermore, cranial imaging that reveals a pattern of miliary brain metastases with small lesions evident in the sulci of the brain, or superficially on the cortex, may suggest the presence of leptomeningeal tumor. These findings are exceedingly rare in lymphoma and leukemia. All patients suspected of having leptomeningeal tumor, and those in whom tumor has been confirmed on CSF cytologic examination, should undergo complete imaging of the neuraxis with gadolinium to delineate areas of focal or bulky disease, which may require focal RT as part of the treatment plan.

While the diagnosis of leptomeningeal tumor can be extremely difficult to make in any circumstance, the situation is particularly challenging for patients with leukemia and lymphoma. The tendency of these tumors to grow in sheets and not to form nodules makes diagnosis difficult because the incidence of

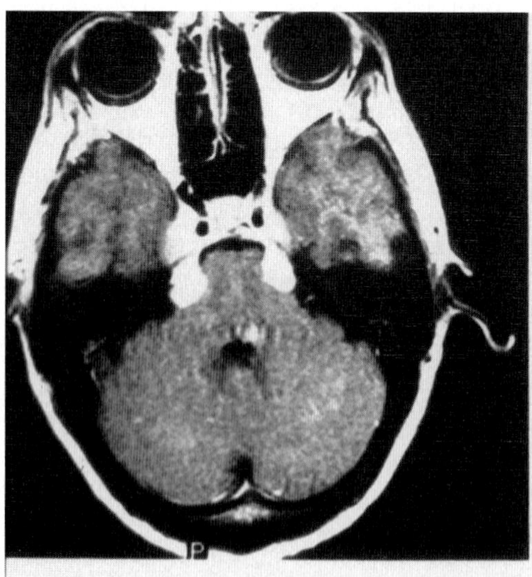

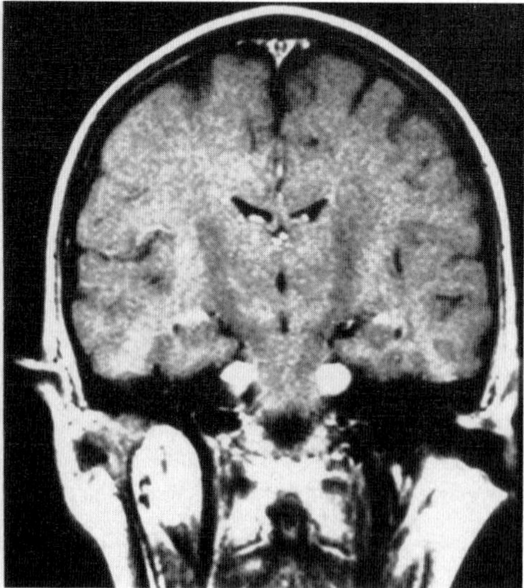

Figure 15–2. Gadolinium-enhanced MRI demonstrating bilateral enhancement and infiltration of the trigeminal nerves by lymphoma.

bulky disease, and, therefore, detectable disease on neuroimaging, is much lower. Furthermore, the incidence of leptomeningeal metastases is higher in these tumor types than in any other, making the need for recognition and aggressive treatment a common concern. Most importantly, vigorous treatment of leptomeningeal metastases in patients with leukemia and lymphoma can lead to prolonged remission and, sometimes, even cure. Consequently, it is imperative to diagnose these tumor types early.

When the diagnosis is not established on CSF analysis or neuroimaging, the clinician may deduce it by process of elimination. Imaging helps to exclude alternatives such as epidural or vertebral bone metastases, brachial or lumbosacral plexopathy, and parenchymal brain pathology. Laboratory work can exclude metabolic causes of lethargy or seizure. The medical history can usually indicate whether cranial neuropathies can be attributed to drugs such as vincristine. When all alternative diagnoses have been excluded and the patient has a characteristic presentation such as cranial neuropathy, some experienced clinicians will treat leukemia or lymphoma patients for leptomeningeal metastasis even in the absence of diagnostic confirmation.

Initial Management

Neurologic metastatic complications frequently lead the physician to initiate corticosteroid treatment immediately. Leptomeningeal metastasis from solid tumors rarely responds to corticosteroids unless the patient has markedly increased intracranial pressure. However, in lymphoma and to a lesser extent leukemia, corticosteroids can provide symptomatic relief, particularly from pain. This is because corticosteroids can function as a chemotherapeutic agent in lymphoma and cause tumor lysis, an important issue when the diagnosis is suspected but not yet confirmed. Premature administration of corticosteroids can give false-negative CSF cytologic examination and neuroimaging results. Corticosteroids should be reserved until the diagnosis has been established, at which time they may provide symptomatic relief. In the absence of clinical improvement, steroids should be rapidly tapered and then discontinued. Unlike brain or epidural metastases, corticosteroids are not required for irradiation of leptomeningeal tumor because there is no focal involvement or compression of the nervous system, inciting significant local edema or mass effect.

Treatment

Therapy should begin immediately after confirmation of the diagnosis of leptomeningeal metastasis. The goals of treatment are not only to prolong life but also to minimize neurologic disability. Rapid institution of therapy can halt the progression of neurologic dysfunction and, if the disease has not been long–standing, can often reverse some neurologic disability. Therapeutic choices include RT, systemic chemotherapy, and intrathecal chemotherapy. Which treatment is selected depends on the location and extent of leptomeningeal involvement as well as the patient's symptoms.

Radiotherapy

Radiotherapy can be a highly effective treatment, frequently causing rapid relief of pain and occasionally reversal of neurologic symptoms (Hanssens et al., 1998). It is usually delivered to focal areas of bulky disease seen on MRI and to symptomatic areas. For example, patients with lumbosacral radiculopathy would receive RT to the cauda equina, whereas those with cranial neuropathies would receive either whole brain or skull base RT. Radiotherapy is usually delivered in 300 cGy fractions for a total of 3000 cGy. Often, its effect can be substantial and durable, but it is not curative (Mackintosh et al., 1982; Hanssens et al., 1998; Gray and Wallner, 1990).

The major limitation of RT is that it is administered focally, leaving large areas of the subarachnoid space untreated. Because the CSF circulates along the neuraxis, tumor cells can be carried by bulk flow from one region to the other. Tumor cells can thus float in and out of the port of RT, never receiving a sufficient dose. Also, large areas of the neuraxis are untreated by focal RT. Neuraxis RT can treat the entire CSF compartment, but craniospinal RT is quite morbid, resulting in esophagitis and enteritis in many patients. In addition, treatment of the entire spinal axis often results in significant myelosuppression, particularly in heavily pretreated patients who previously received substantial chemotherapy. This sequela often causes interruption of treatment and, if severe, can necessitate transfusion or result in neutropenic infection or thrombocytopenic bleeding. Even focal spinal RT can occasionally result in depressed blood counts in some patients, although the condition is usually easily managed.

Intrathecal Chemotherapy

Intrathecal chemotherapy delivers drug into the subarachnoid space to treat the entire CSF compartment. Most systemically administered chemotherapeutic agents do not achieve sufficient concentration in the CSF to treat tumor cells, so drug must be instilled directly into the CSF. This is a safer method of treating the entire CSF than neuraxis RT. However, the number of drugs that can be safely administered directly into the CSF is limited, and the most commonly used agents are methotrexate, cytarabine, and thiotepa. These agents have a relatively narrow antitumor spectrum but can be effective in treating both lymphoma and leukemia. Other agents such as etoposide have been used experimentally with some efficacy but have not been adopted for routine use (van der Gaast et al., 1992; Champagne and Silver, 1992; Berg et al., 1992).

Intrathecal chemotherapy can be administered either by repeated lumbar punctures or by placement of a ventricular catheter with an Ommaya reservoir (Berweiler et al., 1998), which allows easy accessibility to the subarachnoid compartment and results in better disease control (Shapiro et al., 1975; Bleyer and Poplack, 1979). Use of a reservoir has three major advantages over repeated lumbar punctures. Drug delivered into a reservoir has better distribution throughout the CSF than drug introduced into the lumbar space (Shapiro et al., 1975). Even when a lumbar puncture is successful and the CSF is reached, injection of drug via a spinal needle results in instillation of the drug into the epidural space in approximately 10% of patients (Larson et al., 1971). Finally, the reservoir is much easier on the patient, and drug administration is less time consuming for staff.

However, the reservoirs can pose occasional difficulties and complications. They have a low incidence of infection, but, when infected, may require removal to clear infection, which is most commonly due to skin organisms such as coagulase-negative *Staphylococcus* or *Proprionibacterium* species. The reservoirs may become obstructed. If this develops, the reservoir should not be used as the drug may leak out of the reservoir catheter and into the surrounding brain, causing an area of focal encephalomalacia or a sterile abscess that can result in focal neurologic deficits. Patients with raised intracranial pressure are particularly vulnerable to this complication. In addition, patients with hydrocephalus or any impairment of CSF flow should not have a reservoir placed.

Drug is distributed along with the bulk flow of CSF. If there is obstruction to CSF flow, the drug will be trapped in one area of the neuraxis, leaving other regions untreated and causing neurotoxicity where the concentration is high for prolonged periods of time (Glantz et al., 1995; Mason et al., 1998). ^{111}Indium flow studies can ascertain with a high degree of accuracy whether the CSF flow is normal or not (Chamberlain, 1998). The ^{111}Indium should be administered by the same route as the drug, either via an Ommaya reservoir or by lumbar puncture. The patient is scanned for distribution of the ^{111}Indium throughout the neuraxis and for reabsorption over the cerebral convexities. Areas of bulky disease seen on MRI, such as large subarachnoid nodules in the spine, usually impair CSF flow at that level. The flow can occasionally be restored after focal RT has been administered to the area. There is controversy regarding obstructions, so-called physiologic obstruction, seen on ^{111}Indium studies where neuroimaging is negative (Glantz et al., 1995; Mason et al., 1998; Chamberlain, 1998). Some authors recommend radiating areas of reduced CSF flow; restoration of flow occasionally occurs. Others, however, remain unconvinced that this is a significant phenomenon and are concerned that RT can cause toxicity.

For drugs administered into the CSF, the doses are fixed and should not be calculated on a meter square basis. The volume of CSF is the same in all individuals over the age of 4 years, and it does not fluctuate with body size (Pfefferbaum et al., 1994). Doses of the commonly used agents are indicated in Table 15–3. When delivered into a reservoir, drug should be infused slowly because rapid administration can produce raised intracranial pressure and hypotension. If there is difficulty in removing CSF from the reservoir, placing the patient in the Trendelenburg position may facilitate CSF withdrawal.

When intrathecal methotrexate is used, oral leucovorin should be given for the following 4 days at a dose of 10 mg po b.i.d. This is to protect the gastrointestinal tract and the bone marrow from the chronic low-dose systemic exposure that results from

Table 15–3. Doses of Intrathecal Chemotherapy

Methotrexate	12 mg
Cytarabine	40–60 mg
Thiotepa	10 mg

reabsorption of drug from the subarachnoid space into the bloodstream.

The optimal duration and schedule of intrathecal treatments for leptomeningeal metastasis is unknown. The schedule has been derived largely from empiric information and from what is known about the pharmacokinetics of drug in the CSF (Mackintosh et al., 1982). Methotrexate is the best-studied agent. It rapidly achieves high concentrations after an intrathecal dose and maintains therapeutic concentrations in the CSF for at least 24 hours (Shapiro et al., 1975), which has led to initial treatment on a twice-a-week schedule so that the tumor receives therapeutic concentrations for a substantial period of time. If the patient appears to be responding to intrathecal drug, as assessed by improvement in the CSF and the absence of clinical deterioration, then after several weeks of giving the drug twice a week the frequency is reduced to once a week for an additional 3 to 4 weeks. This is followed by a further reduction to every other week and then a few months of monthly maintenance therapy, which is then discontinued.

An alternative approach is to use the concentration × time approach where small doses are given daily for 3 to 5 days (Moser et al., 1999), which produces sustained therapeutic concentrations in the CSF with a reduced total dose, possibly diminishing the risk of neurotoxicity. This is a superior approach but can be difficult to administer because of the requirement for daily injections. A new preparation of cytarabine addresses some of these issues. This liposomal preparation can be administered intrathecally once every 2 weeks (Glantz et al., 1999). This method releases drug slowly and can produce therapeutic concentrations of cytarabine in the CSF for more than 1 week in most patients. The consequent need for less frequent administration is an improvement in the patient's quality of life. This preparation may or may not represent a substantial therapeutic advantage over standard cytarabine or methotrexate but that remains to be ascertained.

Systemic Chemotherapy

Most systemic agents do not penetrate sufficiently into the subarachnoid space to treat leptomeningeal metastases. However, agents such as methotrexate and cytarabine when given in high doses can achieve therapeutic concentrations in the CSF (Glantz et al., 1998). This is particularly true when tumor involves the leptomeninges, which enhances drug penetration. The advantage of delivering chemotherapy systemically is that sufficient drug concentration can be achieved throughout the subarachnoid space because the drug does not have to circulate with the CSF to reach all areas of the subarachnoid compartment. In addition, systemically administered drug can reach and penetrate into nodules of tumor in the subarachnoid space and into neural structures infiltrated by tumor. Intrathecally administered drug can penetrate only 5 mm into the tumor and therefore cannot reach these areas of disease.

Other important agents in the treatment of lymphoma and leukemia such as anthracyclines, vincristine, and cyclophosphamide do not achieve sufficient penetration into the CSF to effectively treat leptomeningeal metastasis. Consequently, the options available for systemic chemotherapy are virtually the same drugs that can be administered directly into the CSF. Nevertheless, data suggest that patients do better when systemic chemotherapy is included in the therapeutic regimen of leptomeningeal metastasis (Siegal et al., 1994; Siegal, 1998).

OUTCOME

The prognosis for most patients with leptomeningeal metastasis is poor, with a median survival of 6 to 8 months for patients with NHL and 10 months for those with AML (Posner, 1995; Castagnola et al., 1997; Recht et al., 1988). It is difficult to control tumor in the CNS, and also, because leptomeningeal metastasis is usually a late complication of either lymphoma or leukemia, the systemic disease is often aggressive and refractory to treatment by the time metastasis is diagnosed, and death is related to progressive systemic tumor in most patients (Recht et al., 1988). Nevertheless, some patients do respond well to treatment and have prolonged survival (Siegal et al., 1994). Furthermore, for patients with isolated CNS relapse, control or remission of CNS disease can result in a sustained second remission so that vigorous treatment is warranted. Aggressive therapy can prevent neurologic dysfunction even if survival is not prolonged, which provides a substantial contribution to a patient's quality of life. Patients who do survive for 1 year or longer are, however, vulnerable to late neurotoxic effects of treatment (Siegal et al., 1994). Primarily restricted to the brain, this is a particular problem for patients who have received whole-brain RT in addition to chemotherapy.

NEUROTOXICITY

Combining cranial irradiation with systemic and/or intrathecal chemotherapy amplifies the potential of each modality to cause neurologic dysfunction. The risk rises with increasing doses of RT, a rising cumulative dose of systemic and/or intrathecal chemotherapy, and older age. The primary manifestation of neurotoxicity is memory impairment, which can progress to a severe dementia in adults or be a static learning deficit in children. Radiographically, a diffuse leukoencephalopathy is seen on MRI with increased signal throughout the periventricular white matter on T_2 or FLAIR images. Atrophy and ventricular dilatation are also common features. Occasionally, some patients may have amelioration of their symptoms with placement of a ventriculoperitoneal shunt, but improvement is usually incomplete and can be temporary. Once neurotoxicity develops, it is a permanent and irreversible condition. Considerable effort has been devoted to the development of efficacious, less toxic regimens for CNS prophylaxis, particularly for childhood ALL. Data show that vigorous systemic chemotherapy combined with extended triple intrathecal chemotherapy can produce control of CNS disease comparable to cranial RT plus drug (Stark et al., 2000). This type of regimen carries less risk of subsequent cognitive impairment.

PRIMARY CENTRAL NERVOUS SYSTEM LYMPHOMA

Clinical Features

Primary CNS lymphomas (PCNSL) represent 3.5% of primary brain tumors (Davis and Preston-Martin, 1999) and are usually large cell or immunoblastic lymphomas. There is a higher incidence of PCNSL in transplant recipients and patients with acquired immunodeficiency syndrome (AIDS), but these tumors are stimulated by latent Epstein-Barr virus infection whereas those in the immunocompetent population are not.

Diagnosis

PCNSL usually occurs in the fifth and sixth decades of life. Neurologic symptoms and signs depend on the site(s) of disease in the brain, but cognitive changes and lateralizing signs are common. PCNSL arises in the basal ganglia, corpus callosum, and periventricular regions. Following gadolinium administration, these tumors show intense and distinctive homogeneous enhancement on MR scans. Because glucocorticoids alone are sufficient to reverse vascular permeability of the tumor and lyse tumor cells, they must be withheld until tissue has been obtained to make a definitive diagnosis. An open or stereotactic biopsy is required to establish the diagnosis of PCNSL, but resection has no therapeutic role in this disease.

Initial Management

Radiation therapy alone is palliative with local control rates of 39% and a median survival of less than 1 year after 60 Gy (Nelson, 1999). Conventional systemic lymphoma drug combinations such as cyclophosphamide, doxorubicin, vincristine, and prednisone (CHOP) are ineffective (Mead et al., 2000). At present, high-dose methotrexate (HD-MTX) is the single most active agent for the treatment of PCNSL. HD-MTX combined with cranial irradiation yields a median survival of 60 months (Abrey, 2000), but has been associated with neurotoxicity in a significant proportion of patients, particularly those over the age of 60 at the time of treatment. Almost 100% of such patients develop severe dementia (Abrey, 1998).

Efforts to overcome CNS toxicity from irradiation has led to the use of chemotherapy alone, particularly in older patients. Using an HD-MTX based regimen, patients older than 60 years have the same median survival (32 months) as those treated with the same regimen plus cranial radiotherapy. However, no neurotoxicity was observed in those who only received chemotherapy. Intrathecal chemotherapy has not attained a defined role in PCNSL management as data indicate that treatment with HD-MTX alone produces comparable results in patients with a negative CSF cytologic examination at diagnosis. Those with a positive CSF cytology should receive concurrent intrathecal and systemic chemotherapy. Chemotherapy combined with blood-brain barrier disruption has been another approach; in one study, 74 patients had an estimated median survival of 40.7 months. Of 36 patients with a complete response lasting more than 1 year and available for study, none demonstrated evidence of cognitive loss in neuropsychologic tests and/or clinical examinations (McAllister et al., 2000).

Most neuro-oncologists agree that the optimal treatment for PCNSL has not yet been identified. In a recent review of published clinical trials, Ferreri and colleagues (Ferreri et al., 2000) found that chemotherapy followed by radiotherapy yielded a 5-year survival of 22%–40% compared with 3%–26% for irradiation only. In their review, HD-MTX was the most effective chemotherapy, producing response rates of 80%–90% and a 2-year survival rate of 60%–65%. To date, the addition of other drugs at conventional doses for treatment has not consistently improved outcome. With a few exceptions, any regimen without HD-MTX performed no better than RT alone.

REFERENCES

Abrey LE, DeAngelis LM, Yahalom J. 1998. Long-term survival in primary CNS lymphoma. J Clin Oncol 16:859–863.

Abrey LE, Yahalom J, DeAngelis LM. 2000. Treatment for primary CNS lymphoma: the next step. J Clin Oncol 18:3144–3150.

Balm M, Hammack J. 1996. Leptomeningeal carcinomatosis. Presenting features and prognostic factors. Arch Neurol 53:626–632.

Barcos M, Lane W, Gomez GA, et al. 1987. An autopsy study of 1206 acute and chronic leukemias (1958 to 1982).Cancer 60:827–837.

Berg SL, Balis FM, Zimm S, et al. 1992. Phase I/II trial and pharmacokinetics of intrathecal diaziquone in refractory meningeal malignancies. J Clin Oncol 10:143–148.

Berweiler U, Krone A, Tonn JC. 1998. Reservoir systems for intraventricular chemotherapy. J Neurooncol 38:141–143.

Bilsky MH, Lis E, Raizer J, Lee H, Boland P. 1999. The diagnosis and treatment of metastatic spinal tumor. Oncologist 4:459–469.

Bleyer WA, Poplack DG. 1979. Intraventricular versus intralumbar methotrexate for central-nervous-system leukemia: prolonged remission with the Ommaya reservoir. Med Pediatr Oncol 6:207–213.

Bower JH, Hammack JE, McDonnell SK, Tefferi A. 1997. The neurologic complications of B-cell chronic lymphocytic leukemia. Neurology 48:407–412.

Byrne TN, Waxman SG. 1990. Spinal Cord Compression: Diagnosis and Principles of Management. Philadelphia: FA Davis, 278 pp.

Castagnola C, Nozza A, Corso A, Bernasconi C. 1997. The value of combination therapy in adult acute myeloid leukemia with central nervous system involvement. Haematologica 82:577–580.

Chamberlain MC. 1998. Radioisotope CSF flow studies in leptomeningeal metastases. J Neurooncol 38:135–140.

Champagne MA, Silver HK. 1992. Intrathecal dacarbazine treatment of leptomeningeal malignant melanoma. J Natl Cancer Inst 84:1203–1204.

Cibas ES, Malkin MG, Posner JB, Melamed MR. 1987. Detection of DNA abnormalities by flow cytometry in cells from cerebrospinal fluid. Am J Clin Pathol 88:570–577.

Davis FG, Preston-Martin S. 1999. Epidemiology. Incidence and survival. In: Bigner DD, McLendon RE, Bruner JM (eds), Russell and Rubinstein's Pathology of Tumors of the Nervous System, London: Arnold, pp. 5–46.

DeAngelis LM. 1998. Current diagnosis and treatment of leptomeningeal metastasis. J Neurooncol 38:245–252.

Ferreri AJ, Reni M, and Villa E. 2000. Therapeutic management of primary central nervous system lymphoma: lessons from prospective trials. Ann Oncol 11:927–937.

Freilich RJ, Krol G, DeAngelis LM. 1995. Neuroimaging and cerebrospinal fluid cytology in the diagnosis of leptomeningeal metastasis. Ann Neurol 38:51–57.

Gilbert RW, Kim JH, Posner JB. 1978. Epidural spinal cord compression from metastatic tumor: diagnosis and treatment. Ann Neurol 3:40–51.

Glantz MJ, Cole BF, Recht L, et al. 1998. High-dose intravenous methotrexate for patients with nonleukemic leptomeningeal cancer: is intrathecal chemotherapy necessary? J Clin Oncol 16:1561–1567.

Glantz MJ, Hall WA, Cole BF, et al. 1995. Diagnosis, management, and survival of patients with leptomeningeal cancer based on cerebrospinal fluid-flow status. Cancer 75: 2919–2931.

Glantz MJ, LaFollette S, Jaeckle KA, et al. 1999. Randomized trial of a slow-release versus a standard formulation of cytarabine for the intrathecal treatment of lymphomatous meningitis. J Clin Oncol 17:3110–3116.

Gray JR, Wallner KE. 1990. Reversal of cranial nerve dysfunction with radiation therapy in adults with lymphoma and leukemia. Int J Radiat Oncol Biol Phys 19:439–444.

Hanssens PE, Lagerwaard FJ, Levendag PC. 1998. Principles of radiotherapy of neoplastic meningosis. J Neurooncol 38:145–150.

Jordan JE, Donaldson SS, Enzmann DR. 1995. Cost effectiveness and outcome assessment of magnetic resonance imaging in diagnosing cord compression. Cancer 75:2579–2586.

Kataoka A, Shimizu K, Matsumoto T, et al. 1995. Epidural spinal cord compression as an initial symptom in childhood acute lymphoblastic leukemia: rapid decompression by local irradiation and systemic chemotherapy. Pediatr Hematol Oncol 12:179–184.

Klekamp J, Samii H. 1998. Surgical results for spinal metastases. Acta Neurochir (Wien) 140:957–967.

Larson SM, Schall GL, DiChiro G. 1971. The influence of previous lumbar puncture and pneumoencephalography on the incidence of unsuccessful radioisotope cisternography. J Nucl Med 12:555–557.

Levitt LJ, Dawson DM, Rosenthal DS, Moloney WC. 1980. CNS involvement in the non-Hodgkin's lymphomas. Cancer 45:545–552.

Loblaw DA, Laperriere NJ. 1998. Emergency treatment of malignant extradural spinal cord compression: an evidence-based guideline. J Clin Oncol 16:1613–1624.

Lossos IS, Breuer R, Intrator O, Lossos A. 2000. Cerebrospinal fluid lactate dehydrogenase isoenzyme analysis for the diagnosis of central nervous system involvement in hematooncologic patients. Cancer 88:1599–1604.

Lyons MK, O'Neill BP, Marsh WR, Kurtin PJ. 1992. Primary spinal epidural non-Hodgkin's lymphoma: report of eight patients and review of the literature. Neurosurgery 30:675–680.

Mackintosh FR, Colby TV, Podolsky WJ, et al. 1982. Central nervous system involvement in non-Hodgkin's lymphoma: an analysis of 105 cases. Cancer 49:586–595.

Mahmoud HH, Rivera GK, Hancock ML, et al. 1993. Low leukocyte counts with blast cells in cerebrospinal fluid of children with newly diagnosed acute lymphoblastic leukemia. N Engl J Med 329:314–319.

Maranzano E, Latini P, Beneventi S, et al. 1996. Radiotherapy without steroids in selected metastatic spinal cord compression patients. A phase II trial. Am J Clin Oncol 19:179–183.

Maranzano E, Latini P, Checcaglini F, et al. 1991. Radiation therapy in metastatic spinal cord compression. Cancer 67: 1311–1317.

Mason WP, Yeh SDJ, DeAngelis LM. 1998. ^{111}Indium-diethylenetriamine pentaacetic acid cerebrospinal fluid flow studies predict distribution of intrathecally administered chemotherapy and outcome in patients with leptomeningeal metastases. Neurology 50:438–444.

McAllister LD, Doolittle ND, Guastadisegni PE, et al. 2000. Cognitive outcomes and long-term follow-up results after enhanced chemotherapy delivery for primary central nervous system lymphoma. Neurosurgery 46:51–60.

Mead GM, Bleehen NM, Gregor A, et al. 2000. A medical research council randomized trial in patients with primary cerebral non-Hodgkin lymphoma: cerebral radiotherapy with and without cyclophosphamide, doxorubicin, vincristine, and prednisone chemotherapy. Cancer 89:1359–1370.

Moser AM, Adamson PC, Gillespie AJ, Poplack DG, Balis FM. 1999. Intraventricular concentration times time ($C \times T$) methotrexate and cytarabine for patients with recurrent meningeal leukemia and lymphoma. Cancer 85:511–516.

Nelson DF. 1999. Radiotherapy in the treatment of primary central nervous system lymphoma (PCNSL). J Neurooncol 43:241–247.

Olson ME, Chernik NL, Posner JB. 1974. Infiltration of the leptomeninges by systemic cancer. Arch Neurol 30:122–137.

Oschmann P, Kaps M, Volker J, Dorndorf W. 1994. Meningeal carcinomatosis: CSF cytology, immunocytochemistry and biochemical tumor markers. Acta Neurol Scand 89:395–399.

Oviatt DL, Kirshner HS, Stein RS. 1982. Successful chemotherapeutic treatment of epidural compression of non-Hodgkin's lymphoma. Cancer 49:2446–2448.

Pfefferbaum A, Mathalon DH, Sullivan EV, Rawles JM, Zipursky RB, Lim KO. 1994. A quantitative magnetic resonance imaging study of changes in brain morphology from infancy to late adulthood. Arch Neurol 51:874–887.

Posner JB. 1987. Back pain and epidural spinal cord compression. Med Clin North Am 71:185–205.

Posner JB. 1995. Neurologic Complications of Cancer. Philadelphia: FA Davis, 482 pp.

Posner JB, Howieson J, Cvitkovic E. 1977. "Disappearing" spinal cord compression: oncolytic effect of glucocorticosteroids (and other chemotherapeutic agents) on epidural metastases. Ann Neurol 2:409–413.

Price RA, Johnson WW. 1973. The central nervous system in childhood leukemia: I. The arachnoid. Cancer 31:520–533.

Raz I, Siegal T, Siegal T, Polliack A. 1984. CNS involvement by non-Hodgkin's lymphoma. Response to a standard therapeutic protocol. Arch Neurol 41:1167–1171.

Recht L, Straus DJ, Cirrincione C, Thaler HT, Posner JB. 1988. Central nervous system metastases from non-Hodgkin's lymphoma: treatment and prophylaxis. Am J Med 84: 425–435.

Rhodes CH, Glantz MJ, Glantz L, et al. 1996. A comparison of polymerase chain reaction examination of cerebrospinal fluid and conventional cytology in the diagnosis of lymphomatous meningitis. Cancer 77:543–548.

Rodesch G. Van Bogaert P, Mavroudakis N, et al. 1990. Neuroradiologic findings in leptomeningeal carcinomatosis: the value interest of gadolinium-enhanced MRI. Neuroradiology 32:26–32.

Rogers LR, Duchesneau PM, Nunez C, et al. 1992. Comparison of cisternal and lumbar CSF examination in leptomeningeal metastasis. Neurology 42:1239–1241.

Schiff D, Shaw EG, Cascino TL. 1995. Outcome after spinal reirradiation for malignant epidural spinal cord compression. Ann Neurol 37:583–589.

Schold SC, Wasserstrom WR, Fleisher M, Schwartz MK, Posner JB. 1980. Cerebrospinal fluid biochemical markers of central nervous system metastases. Ann Neurol 8:597–604.

Shapiro WR, Young DF, Mehta BM. 1975. Methotrexate: distribution in cerebrospinal fluid after intravenous, ventricular and lumbar injections. N Engl J Med 293:161–166.

Siegal T. 1998. Leptomeningeal metastases: rationale for systemic chemotherapy or what is the role of intra-CSF-chemotherapy? J Neurooncol 38:151–157.

Siegal T, Lossos A, Pfeffer MR. 1994. Leptomeningeal metastases: analysis of 31 patients with sustained off-therapy response following combined-modality therapy. Neurology 44:1463–1469.

Sioutos PJ, Arbit E, Meshulam CF, Galicich JH. 1995. Spinal metastases from solid tumors. Analysis of factors affecting survival. Cancer 76:1453–1459.

Stark B, Sharon R, Rechavi G, et al. 2000. Effective preventive central nervous system therapy with extended triple intrathecal therapy and the modified ALL-BFM 86 chemotherapy program in an enlarged non-high risk group of children and adolescents with non-B-cell acute lymphoblastic leukemia: the Israel National Study report. Cancer 88: 205–216.

Stockhammer G, Poewe W, Burgstaller S, et al. 2000. Vascular endothelial growth factor in CSF. A biological marker for carcinomatous meningitis. Neurology 54: 1670–1676.

Tubergen DG, Cullen JW, Boyett JM, et al. 1994. Blasts in CSF with a normal cell count do not justify alteration of therapy for acute lymphoblastic leukemia in remission: a Childrens Cancer Group Study. J Clin Oncol 12:273–278.

van der Gaast A, Sonneveld P, Mans DR, Splinter TAW. 1992. Intrathecal administration of etoposide in the treatment of malignant meningitis: feasibility and pharmacokinetic data. Cancer Chemother Pharmacol 29:335–337.

Van Oostenbrugge RJ, Hopman AH, Ramaekers FC, Twijnstra A. 1998. In situ hybridization: a possible diagnostic aid in leptomeningeal metastasis. J Neurooncol 38: 127–133.

Wasserstrom WR, Glass JP, Posner JB. 1982. Diagnosis and treatment of leptomeningeal metastases from solid tumors: experience with 90 patients. Cancer 49:759–772.

Wong ET, Portlock CS, O'Brien JP, DeAngelis LM. 1996. Chemosensitive epidural spinal cord disease in non-Hodgkin's lymphoma. Neurology 46:1543–1547.

16

Leptomeningeal Metastases

LISA BOMGAARS, MARC C. CHAMBERLAIN,
DAVID G. POPLACK, AND SUSAN M. BLANEY

The leptomeninges are anatomically defined as the pia mater and the arachnoid, tissue envelopes that encase the brain and the spinal cord. Invasion of the leptomeninges or the cerebrospinal fluid (CSF) by cancer is called *leptomeningeal metastasis* or *neoplastic meningitis.* These are general terms that encompass

1. Carcinomatous meningitis (metastases caused by carcinoma such as lung and breast)
2. Meningeal gliomatosis (dissemination of CSF caused by malignant glial tumors)
3. Leptomeningeal metastases secondary to other underlying solid tumors (e.g., rhabdomyosarcoma, neuroblastoma, medulloblastoma, other primitive neuroectodermal tumors)
4. Lymphomatous meningitis (metastases caused by lymphoma)
5. Leukemic meningitis (metastases caused by leukemia) (Chamberlain, 1992; Grossman and Moynihan, 1991; Kaplan et al., 1990; Little et al., 1974; Olson et al., 1974; Packer et al., 1985; Shapiro et al., 1977; Theodore and Gendelman, 1981; Wasserstrom et al., 1982; Yung et al., 1980).

Leptomeningeal metastases are an increasingly common complication, estimated to occur in approximately 5% of all patients with cancer (Chamberlain, 1992; Grossman and Moynihan, 1991; Kaplan et al., 1990). The increasing incidence of leptomeningeal metastases in patients with solid tumors appears to be due to the increasing incidence of cancer in the general population and to the fact that cancer patients are living longer because of more effective treatment of their systemic cancer; the latter appears to lead to a paradoxical increase in central nervous system (CNS) metastases.

Leptomeningeal metastases resulting from solid tumors most often present in patients with advanced systemic or primary CNS cancer, and these metastases therefore coexist with active systemic bulk CNS parenchymal disease (Grossman and Moynihan, 1991; Kaplan et al., 1990; Posner and Chernik, 1978; Wasserstrom et al., 1982). In contrast, leukemic and lymphomatous meningitides frequently represent the first site of tumor recurrence without evidence of systemic disease (Kaplan et al., 1990). In approximately 5% to 10% of patients, leptomeningeal metastases are the initial presentation of cancer. In such cases, disease staging must be initiated to define the primary tumor and its pattern of metastases (Chamberlain, 1992; Grossman and Moynihan, 1991). This chapter discusses leptomeningeal metastases, with a primary emphasis on leptomeningeal metastases from solid tumors. It includes a review of the diverse clinical presentation of this disease entity, provides current information on diagnosis and management, and discusses new therapeutic options that are in preclinical or early clinical stages of development.

LEPTOMENINGEAL METASTASES BY CANCER TYPE

Reported histologic variability between series in organ-site tumors that lead to leptomeningeal metastasis reflects differences in hospital referral patterns. Solid tumors are disproportionately represented because of their overall greater prevalence and, in some series, because disseminated primary brain tumors and leukemic and lymphomatous meningitis are excluded. Of the solid tumors causing leptomeningeal metastases, those from breast occur in 30% of patients (range, 22% to 64%); lung in 16% (range, 10% to 26%); malignant melanoma in 11% (range, 7% to 15%); and the gastrointestinal tract in 6% (range, 4% to 14%). Carcinomas of an unknown primary origin constitute 1% to 7% of all cases of leptomeningeal metastases in most clinical series (Little et al., 1974; Theodore and Gendelman, 1981; Wasserstrom et al., 1982). The frequency of occurrence of primary brain tumors causing leptomeningeal metastases is from 10% to 32% depending on histology, patient age, and referral patterns (Chamberlain and Corey-Bloom, 1991; Kaplan et al., 1990; Shapiro et al., 1977; Wasserstrom et al., 1982). Lymphomatous meningitis associated with non-Hodgkin's lymphoma in patients with the acquired immunodeficiency syndrome (AIDS) is also an increasingly common cause of leptomeningeal metastases. This has been reported to occur in approximately 20% of patients with AIDS who have systemic non-Hodgkin's lymphoma and in 25% of those who have primary lymphoma of the CNS (Chamberlain and Kormanik, 1997; Chamberlain and Dirr, 1993).

Autopsy studies demonstrate an even higher incidence of leptomeningeal metastases than that established through clinical studies of patients with known leptomeningeal metastases. In the Memorial Sloan-Kettering Cancer Center experience, 8% of 2375 patients with cancer demonstrated leptomeningeal metastases at autopsy (Posner and Chernik, 1978). Similarly, in a National Institutes of Health study of patients with small cell lung cancer, 11% manifested leptomeningeal metastases while alive compared with a 25% incidence found at postmortem examination (Rosen et al., 1982).

CLINICAL PRESENTATIONS

Unlike other cancers that affect the CNS, the clinical signs and symptoms of leptomeningeal metastases are highly variable because they affect all levels of the neuraxis (Chamberlain and Corey-Bloom, 1991; Kaplan et al., 1990; Little et al., 1974; Olson et al., 1974; Theodore and Gendelman, 1981; Wasserstrom et al., 1982). The degree of clinical pleomorphism of leptomeningeal metastases is problematic as clinical recognition may be delayed because of unfamiliarity with the wide spectrum of associated signs and symptoms. As shown in Table 16–1, these signs and symptoms are traditionally referable to three broad domains encompassing the neuraxis, including the cerebral hemispheres, cranial nerves, spinal cord, and exiting nerve roots. Site-specific symptoms and signs are summarized in Table 16–2.

Symptoms referable to the cerebral hemispheres include, in decreasing order of frequency, headache, mental status change, nausea and vomiting, and hemibody weakness and seizures. Headache, the most common symptom of cerebral dysfunction caused by leptomeningeal metastases, may be the only symptom and usually involves the entire head or the occiput and the neck. Frequently, headache, like nausea and vomiting, is a consequence of raised intracranial pressure resulting from either obstructive or communicating hydrocephalus. Hydrocephalus is a common consequence of leptomeningeal metastases that results from an intraventricular tumor or from base-of-the-brain leptomeningeal infiltration (Kokkoris, 1983). Mental status changes range from slight slowing of thought processes (so-called *oligophrenia*) to depressed levels of consciousness. In late stages of leptomeningeal metastases, patients often manifest profound changes in mental status, referred to as *carcinomatous encephalopathy,* a process that is immediately progressive and contributes to death from leptomeningeal metastases. Seizures and hemibody weakness are uncommon manifestations of leptomeningeal metastases and often coexist with bulky intraparenchymal or subarachnoid tumor.

Table 16–1. Mean Frequency of Initial Symptoms and Signs of Leptomeningeal Metastasis

	Symptom (%)	Signs (%)
Cerebral hemisphere	46	41
Cranial nerves	37	58
Spinal cord and roots	50	69
Multiple site	32	47

Source: Data are from Chamberlain and Corey-Bloom (1991), Kaplan et al. (1990); Little et al. (1974), Olson et al. (1974); Theodore and Gendelman (1981), and Wasserstrom et al. (1982).

Table 16–2. Symptoms and Signs of Leptomeningeal Disease by Site and Decreasing Order of Frequency

	Symptom	*Signs*
Cerebral hemisphere	Headache	Mental status change
	Mental status change	Seizures
	Nausea/vomiting	Papilledema
	Hemibody weakness	Focal weakness
	Seizures	Hemiparesis
Cranial nerves	Diplopia	Ophthalmoplegia (VI,III,IV)
	Hearing loss	Facial weakness (VII)
	Facial numbness	Decreased hearing (VIII)
	Decreased vision	Facial neuropathy (V)
		Hypoglossal weakness (XII)
Spinal cord and roots	Limb weakness	Extremity weakness
	Pain	Dermatomal/segmental sensory loss
	Gait instability	Deep tendon reflex abnormality
	Bladder dysfunction	Nuchal rigidity (meningismus)
	Bowel dysfunction	Ataxia of gait
		Pain on straight leg raising

Signs referable to the cerebral hemispheres include, in decreasing order of frequency, mental status changes, seizures, papilledema, and hemiparesis. Mental status changes may manifest as dementia; in general, these signs are resistant to treatment. Papilledema, like headache, nausea, and vomiting, reflects raised intracranial pressure and, usually, hydrocephalus. Signs and symptoms of raised intracranial pressure caused by leptomeningeal metastases may transiently respond to combined treatment with whole-brain irradiation and intrathecal chemotherapy (Chamberlain, 1992; Chamberlain and Corey-Bloom, 1991).

Symptoms of cranial nerve involvement include, in decreasing order of frequency, double vision, hearing loss, facial numbness, and loss of vision. The most frequent signs of cranial nerve involvement include ophthalmoplegia (affecting, in order, cranial nerves VI, III, and IV); facial weakness (affecting cranial nerve VII); diminished hearing (affecting cranial nerve VIII); trigeminal neuropathy (affecting cranial nerve V); and hypoglossal weakness (affecting cranial nerve XII). A disturbance in eye movement with resultant diplopia or oscillopsia is frequently an early, and often isolated, sign of leptomeningeal metastases. Patients with cancer manifesting new onset of lateral rectus palsy (affecting cranial nerve VI) should be evaluated for possible leptomeningeal metastases following a negative neuroradiographic evaluation for intracranial tumor. Occasionally patients present with a disturbance of hearing (either unilateral or bilateral), facial weakness, or decreased facial sensation in a trigeminal distribution (trigeminal motor dysfunction, i.e., trouble opening or closing the jaw), although these findings occur more often in cases of advanced leptomeningeal metastases in which multiple cranial neuropathies coexist. As with altered mental status, multiple cranial nerve dysfunction, especially with rapid temporal evolution, is a poor prognostic sign. In addition, focal deficits such as cranial neuropathies respond poorly, if at all, to either radiotherapy (whole brain or base of brain) or intrathecal drug therapy. Cranial nerve dysfunction appears to reflect the tumor's preferential involvement at the base of the brain with the tumor infiltrating basal CSF compartments (Kokkoris, 1983).

Spinal cord and exiting root symptoms include those resulting from involvement of the spinal cord (cervical, thoracic, or lumbar); the conus medullaris (the caudal-most portion of the spinal cord proper); the cauda equina (nerve roots contained within the lumbosacral dural sac); the exiting nerve roots (contained within dural sleeves); and the spinal meninges. The most common of these symptoms are limb weakness or numbness, pain (i.e., meningismus), gait instability, and bladder and bowel dysfunction. Limb weakness usually manifests either as a polyradiculoneuropathy (involvement of multiple exiting nerve roots or cauda equina), in which lower motor neuron findings predominate (decreased limb tone, diminished or absent deep tendon reflexes, and dermatomal or root-referable sensory loss), or as a myelopathy (as with spinal cord or conus medullaris dysfunction), in which upper motor neuron findings predominate (increased limb tone, exaggerated deep tendon reflexes, extensor planar response, and segmental or fixed-level sensory loss). Bladder or bowel dysfunction in isolation is never a finding of leptomeningeal metastases but rather occurs early with spinal cord or conus medullaris dysfunction or late with cauda equina dysfunction in conjunction with other signs of neurologic disturbance. In a patient with cancer and spinal cord dysfunction, if spinal cord compression resulting from an epidural mass is ruled out by computed tomography (CT) myelography or contrast-enhanced magnetic resonance imaging (MRI) of the spine, then leptomeningeal metastases should be strongly considered. Pain, like epidural spinal cord compression, may be localized (e.g., neck, interscapular, or lumbar); radicular (conforming to a nerve root distribution); or referred (distant pain such as isolated knee pain). Gait instability is a common disorder of the spinal cord in patients with leptomeningeal metastases and often heralds tumor progression.

Common signs referable to the spine in patients who have leptomeningeal metastases include extremity weakness (lower or upper motor neuron pattern), dermatomal or segmental sensory loss, exaggerated or diminished to absent deep tendon reflexes, nuchal rigidity (meningismus), ataxia, and pain on raising a straightened leg. Spinal cord dysfunction is dominated by focal neurologic deficits that respond poorly to treatment, including limited-field spine irradiation or intrathecal fluid chemotherapy, whereas pain symptoms usually respond to treatment (Chamberlain, 1992; Kaplan et al., 1990).

With progression of leptomeningeal metastases, new signs and symptoms appear and pre-existing findings worsen. Patients with underlying solid tumors are more likely to present with spinal or radicular symptoms, whereas patients with hematologic malignancies more often present with cranial nerve dysfunction. Multifocal neurologic symptoms may be seen in two-thirds of patients and may be a sign of progressive leptomeningeal disease (Van Oostenbrugge and Twijnstra, 1999). Rapid progression of leptomeningeal metastases involving one or multiple CNS regions is invariably a poor prognostic sign.

APPROACH TO DIAGNOSIS

The diagnosis of leptomeningeal metastases is made by correlating physical signs and symptoms with laboratory findings and neuroimaging studies. In the past, the presence of malignant cells in the CSF was a prerequisite for diagnosing leptomeningeal disease. However, discrepancies may exist between clinical signs and symptoms and results of CSF examination(s). Improvements in neuroimaging technology, particularly the widespread availability of MRI, have increased the feasibility of establishing a diagnosis of leptomeningeal metastases using imaging techniques. In some instances the presence of typical clinical features coupled with appropriate neuroimaging abnormalities are adequate for making the diagnosis of leptomeningeal metastases (Freilich et al., 1995).

Cerebrospinal Fluid Examination

One of the most important diagnostic procedures for establishing the presence of leptomeningeal metastases is examination of the CSF (Table 16–3). Essential elements of the CSF laboratory evaluation include cell count and differential, cytology, and protein and glucose concentrations. In patients who have primary solid tumors, the finding of malignant cells in the CSF provides unequivocal evidence of leptomeningeal metastases. The initial lumbar puncture will show abnormalities in all but a minority of patients when opening pressure and CSF cell count, glucose protein levels and cytology are considered (Kaplan et al., 1990; Olson et al., 1974; Theodore and Gendelman, 1981; Wasserstrom et al., 1982). In approximately 50% of patients with leptomeningeal metastases, the CSF opening pressure will be elevated. Similarly, a majority of patients with leptomeningeal metastases have elevated protein levels, and increased CSF cell counts. A depressed CSF glucose level (so-called hypoglycorrhachia) is seen in a minority (<30%) of patients with leptomeningeal metastases. However, alone, such abnormal findings in the CSF are nonspecific and may be present in various neurologic disorders.

Until recently, the diagnosis of leptomeningeal metastases could not be made without finding malignant cells in the CSF. However, improvements in neuroimaging technology have increased the feasibility of establishing a radiographic diagnosis of leptomeningeal metastases. In a recent review, in 106

Table 16–3. Mean Findings at Lumbar Examination of the Cerebrospinal Fluid

Finding	*Initial Examination (%)*	*All Examinations (%)*
Pressure >150 mm of H_2O	46	66
WBC >4/mm^3	59	76
Protein >50 mg/dl	78	86
Glucose <40 mg/dl	43	60
Positive cytology	61	92

WBC, white blood cell count.

Source: Data are from Kaplan et al. (1990), Olson et al. (1974), Theodore and Gendelman (1981), and Wasserstrom et al. (1982).

consecutively diagnosed pediatric patients with medulloblastoma, spinal MRI and CSF cytology were evaluated for the presence of leptomeningeal metastases. Of these patients, 8.5% had positive MRI findings with negative CSF cytology; and 11.3% had positive CSF cytology with negative MRIs. Either CSF cytology or spinal MRI alone would have missed leptomeningeal disease in as many as 14% to 18% (Fouladi et al., 1999). Therefore, patients with a clinical syndrome or neuroradiographic findings compatible with a diagnosis of leptomeningeal metastases should be treated in a similar fashion to those patients with cytologically proven leptomeningeal metastases (Chamberlain, 1992).

Several series have demonstrated that, in some cases, serial CSF sampling via lumbar puncture or sampling from alternate sites (e.g., cisternal or ventricular) is required to detect malignant cells. The experience of Wasserstrom et al. (1982) in 90 patients with solid tumor leptomeningeal metastases revealed positive cytology in 55% of them after an initial lumbar puncture, increasing to 80% after a second lumbar puncture. Each subsequent lumbar puncture yielded positive cytology in approximately an additional 2% of patients per lumbar examination of CSF. An additional 5% of patients showed positive cytology only after cisternal or ventricular examination of CSF; 10% of patients showed persistently negative cytology for malignant cells in CSF regardless of site or number of examinations.

In a small series of patients with leptomeningeal metastases, Rogers et al. (1992) found that nearly 20% with leptomeningeal metastases demonstrated positive cytology only on cisternal examination of the CSF. In another study of 63 cases of cytologically confirmed leptomeningeal metastases, including solid tumors, leukemia, and lymphoma, Kaplan et al. (1990) reported positive cytologic findings in 71% of patients on the first lumbar puncture and in 21% on the second lumbar puncture; only 8% required more than two lumbar punctures to demonstrate positive cytology. In addition, Kaplan et al. (1990) emphasized that CSF cell count was a poor predictor of positive cytology because cell counts were normal in 29% of cases in which lumbar punctures yielded positive cytologic results.

Similarly, in a small number of patients with leptomeningeal metastases, Murray et al. (1983) emphasized marked variations in CSF composition, including cytologic specimens from different levels of the neuraxis (lumbar, cisternal, and ventricular CSF compartments) in the absence of an epidural block to the CSF flow. Harrison et al. (1998) also suggested that lumbar CSF samples correlate better with imaging findings when compared with ventricular CSF samples. Furthermore, in adults with leptomeningeal metastases, the initial CSF cytology was composed of malignant cells more often in patients with an underlying solid tumor versus those with hematologic malignancies that were predominantly non-Hodgkin's lymphomas (73% versus 53%) (Van Oostenbrugge and Twijnstra, 1999).

Results from these series suggest a practical approach to the examination of CSF in patients with solid tumors and clinically suspected leptomeningeal metastases: After two tumor-negative cytologic samples from lumbar puncture and negative neuroimaging studies (gadolinium-enhanced MRIs of the brain and spinal cord), examination of the CSF from alternate sites (e.g., cisternal or ventricular) should be considered. A minority of patients will have clinical presentations compatible with leptomeningeal metastases and negative evaluations for malignant cells from CSF along with negative neuroradiographic studies; in these patients treatment may be initiated, assuming there is a known history of an underlying malignancy and other diagnostic possibilities have been excluded (e.g., epidural spinal cord compression, paraneoplastic disorders, and toxic or metabolic complications of cancer therapy).

In patients with leptomeningeal metastases, measurement of CSF tumor markers such as carcinoembryonic antigen and α-glucuronidase may assist in diagnosis or evaluation after treatment (Chamberlain, 1998b; Schold et al., 1980; Twijnstra et al., 1989). Other biochemical markers for leptomeningeal metastases include α-fetoprotein, the β-subunit of human chronic gonadotropin, α_2-microglobulin, glucose-phosphate isomerase, immunoglobulin indices (either IgG or IgM), and oligoclonal bands (Ernerudh et al., 1987; Klee et al., 1986; Malkin and Posner, 1987; Newton et al., 1991; Schipper et al., 1988). Tumor markers should be simultaneously obtained from serum and CSF to determine if an elevation in a CSF marker is a result of passive diffusion or secondary to leptomeningeal disease (DeAngelis, 1998).

In addition to the specific biochemical markers noted above, other useful adjuncts to CSF cytology include flow cytometry, measurement of immunophenotype, fluorescence in situ hybridization, chromosomal analysis, and immunohistochemical studies. The underlying diagnostic utility of such studies largely depends on the underlying systemic malignancy. For example, lymphocytes in the CSF may not be readily identifiable as malignant by the cytopathologist, but a demonstration of monoclonality (lambda or kappa light chain–directed monoclonal antibody analysis), B-cell lineage, or a specific chromosomal abnormality may differentiate leukemic or lymphomatous meningitis from a normal or reactive T-cell population (Cibas et al., 1987; Coakham et al., 1984; Grossman and Moynihan, 1991; Recht, 1991; Walker, 1991). Glial fibrillary acidic protein histochemistry of CSF may also facilitate identification of malignant glial cells (Chamberlain, 1995a). Likewise, fluorescence in situ hybridization has been shown to be a feasible modality to aid in the diagnosis of leptomeningeal disease in breast cancer patients (Van Oostenbrugge et al., 1997).

Neuroradiographic Studies

Magnetic Resonance Imaging and Computed Tomography Scans

A variety of neuroradiographic studies may be helpful in establishing a diagnosis, defining the extent of disease (i.e., CNS staging), and following treatment response in patients who have leptomeningeal metastases. Abnormal neuroimaging is seen more commonly in patients with underlying solid malignancies than in those with underlying hematologic malignancies (Van Oostenbrugge and Twijnstra, 1999). As demonstrated by Chamberlain et al. (1990), gadolinium-enhanced imaging of the head and spine are the preferred neuroimaging studies for the diagnosis of leptomeningeal metastases, although contrast-enhanced CT studies may also demonstrate abnormalities. As shown in Table 16–4, gadolinium-enhanced MRI has both a higher specificity and a higher sensitivity than CT imaging.

Contrast-enhanced CT of the head reveals abnormalities in approximately 25% to 56% of patients with leptomeningeal metastases, including

1. Sulcal or cisternal enhancement
2. Ependymal and subependymal enhancement
3. Irregular tentorial enhancement
4. Cisternal or sulcal obliteration
5. Subarachnoid enhancing nodules
6. Intraventricular enhancing nodules
7. Communicating hydrocephalus

Table 16–4. Findings in Comparative MRI and CT Contrast-Enhanced Brain Imaging

Finding	*MRI Scan (%)*	*CT Scan (%)*
Parenchymal volume loss	93	93
Abnormal enhancement	71	29
Sulcal/dural	50	21
Cisternal	29	14
Tentorial	21	0
Ependymal	21	7
Nodules	43	36
Subarachnoid	36	29
Parenchymal	43	29
Hydrocephalus	7	7

Source: Adapted from Chamberlain et al. (1990).

In addition, as many as 60% of patients whose findings from contrast-enhanced CT suggest leptomeningeal metastases have coexistent parenchymal metastasis. All abnormalities detected on contrast-enhanced CT scans were detected through gadolinium-enhanced MRI, which also revealed additional lesions not otherwise seen. Despite the superiority of gadolinium-enhanced MRI, both modalities have a high incidence of false-negative results (30% for gadolinium-enhanced MRI and 58% for contrast-enhanced CT). Normal findings by either or both examinations do not exclude a diagnosis of leptomeningeal metastases. In the majority of patients with leptomeningeal metastases, gadolinium-enhanced MRI is also more useful than other imaging modalities in demonstrating bulky disease, a pattern of disease most responsive to radiotherapy. Kallmes et al. (1998) have suggested employing high-dose gadolinium-enhanced MRI to diagnose meningeal metastases when a strong clinical suspicion exists following a negative standard-dose gadolinium-enhanced MRI.

Kim et al. (1982) delineated the patterns seen in patients who had leptomeningeal metastases on CT myelography scans, including

1. Parallel longitudinal striations in the cauda equina caused by thickened nerve roots
2. Irregular intradural extramedullary filling defects with varying degrees of blockage resembling arachnoiditis
3. Multiple intradural nodular defects along nerve roots
4. Amputation of dural root sleeves
5. Focal enlargement of the spinal cord or conus
6. Intradural extramedullary blockage to contrast flow

Similar findings are noted on contrast-enhanced spinal MRI, which is superior in demonstrating intradural extramedullary nodules, focal spinal cord enlargement, clumping of nerve roots, and spinal cord pial enhancement, often termed "sugar coating" (Chamberlain, 1995b; Kramer et al., 1991; Lim et al., 1990; Sze et al., 1988). In a study by Chamberlain (1995a) that directly compared CT myelography with MR imaging of the spine, few discordant results were noted between these modalities. However, MRI is preferred because it is *(1)* comparable to CT myelography, *(2)* noninvasive, *(3)* has a low rate of procedure-related morbidity, and *(4)* is associated with greater patient acceptance (Chamberlain, 1995a,b).

The optimal contrast-enhanced MRI examination of the spine for evaluating intradural extramedullary disease seen in patients with leptomeningeal metastases includes T_1-weighted sagittal scans taken before and after gadolinium administration, with T_1-weighted axial images reserved for regions of interest that either are detected by sagittal imaging or exist in regions with clinically suspect disease (i.e., the cauda equina) (Sze et al., 1988). It is important to note that MRI changes may be seen following lumbar puncture or a neurosurgical procedure and include meningeal reaction appearing as leptomeningeal enhancement, which may occur at the level of the lumbar roots and extend as far rostral as the cranium. Linear enhancement may persist for weeks to months. To avoid neuroimaging artifacts it is therefore recommended that patients undergo spinal imaging before lumber puncture (DeAngelis, 1998; Mittl and Yousem, 1994). Similarly, for patients with primary CNS tumors, MR imaging of the spine should be performed before surgery or at a minimum of 14 to 21 days after surgery.

Cerebrospinal Fluid Flow Studies

Cerebrospinal fluid flow studies, using either ^{111}Indium-diethylenetriamine pentaacetic acid (DTPA), ^{99m}Technetium-DTPA, or ^{99m}Technetium-human serum albumin, are an invaluable tool in the evaluation and treatment of leptomeningeal metastases (Chamberlain, 1995b). Cerebrospinal fluid flow studies provide a safe physiologic assessment of the clinical anatomy of spaces in the CSF (Chamberlain and Corey-Bloom, 1991; Grossman et al., 1982). The CSF circulates through the ventricular system and subarachnoid space that surrounds both the brain and spinal cord (Lyons and Meyer, 1990). Normally, the CSF is elaborated by the choroid plexus of the lateral and fourth ventricles and flows from lateral ventricles through the foramen of Monro and into the third ventricle and then through the aqueduct of Sylvius into the fourth ventricle. Exit of the CSF from the fourth ventricle is directed into the dorsal spinal subarachnoid space through the foramen of Magendie and into the basal cisterns through the lateral foramina of Luschka. Passage of the CSF through the foramen of Magendie into the vallecula and the beginning of downward flow into the dorsal cervical subarachnoid space precedes the exit of CSF from the foramina of Luschka (Chiro et al., 1976). Cerebrospinal fluid then flows caudally through the dorsal spinal subarachnoid space, followed by its ascent into the ventral spinal subarachnoid space. Completion of the normal pattern of CSF circulation is by its ascent from the basal cisterns toward the superior sagittal sinus by way of migration over the cerebral convexities and along medial routes through the suprasellar and quadrigeminal cisterns.

Cerebrospinal fluid flow can be assessed following injection of the radionuclide via lumbar puncture or cisternal puncture or directly into the ventricles via an indwelling access device. Intraventricular and intralumbar routes of radionuclide administration reveal several of the same features of CSF flow. For instance, blockage to CSF flow that creates compartmentalization may affect the

1. Ventricular system
2. Basal cisterns or foramen magnum
3. Cervical subarachnoid space
4. Thoracic subarachnoid space
5. Lumbar subarachnoid space
6. Lateral cerebral convexity (sylvian cisterns)
7. High cerebral convexity (Chamberlain and Corey-Bloom, 1991; Grossman et al., 1982)

Radionuclide flow studies are superior for demonstrating interruption of the CSF flow versus contrast-enhanced CT, gadolinium-enhanced MRI, CT myelography, or contrast-enhanced MRI of the spine. This superiority in demonstrating CSF compartmentalization is independent of the route of radionuclide administration and may reflect the dynamic nature of the CSF flow, wherein radionuclide is passively carried by the CSF bulk flow. Usual times of the appearance of radionuclides in the CSF compartments following intraventricular administration are given in Table 16–5.

Cerebrospinal fluid flow studies should be performed for solid tumor patients with leptomeningeal metastases before administration of intrathecal therapy. Of patients with leptomeningeal metastases, approximately one-third in studies by Chamberlain (1995b, 1998a) have abnormal flow better demonstrated by radionuclide flow studies versus CT myelography or MRI. Clinicians should realize that alterations in CSF flow are not limited to patients with bulky leptomeningeal metastases. In fact, radionuclide imaging studies have shown that as many as 70% of adult patients with leptomeningeal metastases have ventricular outlet obstruction, abnormal flow in the spinal canal, or impaired flow over the cerebral convexities (Grossman et al., 1982). It is important to identify patients with CSF flow abnormalities prospectively, as they can affect the distribution of intrathecal chemotherapy, leading to decreased efficacy or severe toxicity (Chamberlain, 1992; Chamberlain and Corey-Bloom, 1991).

Other studies suggest that CSF flow abnormalities appear to correlate with response to treatment and prognosis. It seems likely that impaired flow is an indirect measure of tumor burden and that more extensive flow abnormalities are associated with worse disease and prognosis (Chamberlain, 1998a; DeAngelis, 1998; Glantz et al., 1995; Mason et al., 1996). Obstruction to CSF flow is best addressed by the administration of involved-field radiotherapy at the site of the block. Approximately 50% of base of the brain and 25% to 30% of spinal subarachnoid blocks re-

Table 16–5. Time of Appearance (Minutes) for ^{111}Indium-DTPA Following Intraventricular and Lumbar Spinal Administration

	Ventricular	*Basal Cisterns*	*Foramen Magnum*	*Cervical Cord*	*Thoracic Cord*	*Lumbar Cord*	*Cerebral Convexity*
Intraventricular							
Median	0	1	7.5	15	20	30	50
Range	0–2	0–2	5–15	5–20	10–20	25–50	35–90
Lumbar							
Median	1440	30	25	15	1	0	1440
Range	na	20–40	15–35	10–25	1	0–2	na

na, no intermediate times measured.

Source: Adapted from Chamberlain (1992).

spond to limited-field radiotherapy or intrathecal chemotherapy with restoration of CSF flow (Chamberlain and Corey-Bloom, 1991).

In summary, the following recommendations regarding neuroradiographic evaluation can be made for a patient with suspected leptomeningeal metastases from a solid tumor. Contrast-enhanced CT or, preferably, gadolinium-enhanced MRI should be performed to define both dural-based and intraparenchymal bulk disease and to document the presence or absence of hydrocephalus. Computed tomography myelography or, particularly, contrast-enhanced MRI of the spine should be performed to define bulk disease, including intradural extramedullary tumor nodules and extradural lesions that compress the epidural spinal cord. For patients for whom treatment with intrathecal chemotherapy is a consideration, radionuclide CSF flow studies, either by intralumbar or intraventricular routes, should be performed to determine whether there is evidence of CSF compartmentalization.

TREATMENT

The varied manifestations of the heterogeneous group of malignancies that may result in leptomeningeal metastases preclude recommendations in favor of a single treatment approach. The primary treatment modalities for either presymptomatic or overt leptomeningeal metastases include radiotherapy, intrathecal chemotherapy, and high-dose systemic chemotherapy. Factors to consider when making specific treatment recommendations include the histopathology of the primary malignancy, the age of the patient, any history of prior CNS-directed therapy, the extent of systemic disease at initial diagnosis, and the presence or absence of abnormal CSF flow.

Presymptomatic or "preventative" CNS-directed therapy is a standard component of the front-line treatment for most patients who have leukemia or lymphoma. In addition, children who have CNS tumors with a predisposition for dissemination to the neuraxis (e.g., childhood medulloblastoma) may also receive presymptomatic treatment for leptomeningeal metastases (Heideman et al., 1997). It may be difficult to accurately assess the durability of response to treatment of patients with overt leptomeningeal metastases, especially those with underlying solid tumors, as therapy directed at leptomeningeal disease is generally ineffective against the primary malignancy (Chamberlain et al., 1990; Glantz et al., 1995). Systemic cancer accounts for 50% to 60% of deaths of patients who have leptomeningeal metastases, and its treatment accounts for another 5% to 10% of deaths (Chamberlain, 1992; Grossman and Moynihan, 1991; Wasserstrom et al., 1982).

Response to treatment of leptomeningeal metastases is primarily evaluated by cytologic clearing of malignant cells from the CSF and secondarily by improvement of clinical signs or symptoms of leptomeningeal disease (Chamberlain, 1992; Grossman and Moynihan, 1991) and by lack of progression or improvement in neuroimaging studies. Given these considerations, treatment of leptomeningeal metastases from solid tumors is palliative and rarely curative, with a median patient survival of 4 to 6 months for those with overt disease (Chamberlain 1992, 1997; Grossman and Moynihan, 1991; Wasserstrom et al., 1982).

Radiotherapy

Treatment of leptomeningeal metastases with external beam radiotherapy is, with the exception of acute lymphocytic leukemia and some childhood brain tumors, directed at sites of symptomatic and bulky disease. This intervention is palliative, providing local control of and potential improvement in or resolution of neurologic deficits (DeAngelis, 1998; Grossman and Moynihan, 1991; Wasserstrom et al., 1982). External beam radiation to symptomatic sites, in either the cranium or spine, is often delivered to a total dose of 30 Gy in 10 fractions. This regimen is well tolerated, unlike whole neuraxis radiation, which results in significant morbidity with myelosuppression, and is not curative with the exceptions noted above. In addition to improvements in clinical signs and symptoms such as pain or weakness, directed radiotherapy may in some cases reduce or eliminate abnormalities in CSF flow. Restoration of CSF flow is a prerequisite for the safe administration of intrathecal chemotherapy.

Craniospinal irradiation alone or combined with intrathecal chemotherapy plus systemic chemotherapy may be curative for many children with hematologic malignancies. Craniospinal irradiation is also standard treatment for all patients with medulloblastoma. Craniospinal irradiation plus chemotherapy may be curative for some medulloblastoma patients who have subarachnoid dissemination at initial diagnosis (Heideman et al., 1997).

The primary drawback of radiotherapy is that it can be associated with both acute and long-term sequelae; although these effects sometimes are difficult to differentiate from the effects of other aspects of therapy or from manifestations of the disease itself. Craniospinal irradiation may cause significant myelosuppression, as a substantial portion of active bone marrow is irradiated (Kun et al., 1984). Cranial irradiation may result in the "somnolence syndrome," which consists of a prodrome of anorexia and irritability followed by a variable period of somnolence from which recovery is spontaneous (Freeman et al., 1973). Although this syndrome is more often reported in the pediatric population, it may occur in adults (Faithfull and Brada, 1998; Goldberg et al., 1992). Long-term complications of cranial and craniospinal irradiation include neuroendocrine sequelae such as hypothyroidism (Voorhess et al., 1986; Pasqualini et al., 1991) and disturbances in the secretion of growth hormone (Blatt et al., 1984); neuropsychological sequelae such as decreases in intellect and mild to severe leukoencephalopathy (Moss, 1981; Paolucci and Rosito, 1983; Poplack and Brouwers, 1985); and secondary malignancies (Walter et al., 1998). Crossen et al. (1994) report that the long-term neurobehavioral sequelae occurring in adults following radiotherapy may be underestimated, in contrast with the pediatric population, because children are evaluated routinely for neuropsychological sequelae. Because of the potential for severe long-term complications from radiotherapy, the identification and application of effective and less-toxic treatment strategies for patients with neoplastic meningitis is a high priority.

Chemotherapy

Penetration of most systemically administered antineoplastic agents into the CSF is limited because malignant cells within the CNS are protected from the cytotoxic effects of systemic chemotherapy by the blood–brain and the blood–CSF barriers. To overcome the limitations imposed by the blood–CSF barrier, several pharmacological approaches for treatment and prophylaxis of meningeal malignancy with chemotherapy have been developed. These include *(1)* high-dose systemic administration of chemotherapy, *(2)* regional direct administration of cytotoxic chemotherapeutic drugs into the CSF, and *(3)* pharmacokinetically guided dosing to achieve a target CSF drug exposure. Each approach has distinct advantages and disadvantages.

High-Dose Systemic Chemotherapy

The limited CSF penetration of some chemotherapeutic agents can be overcome by administering high doses of the drug systemically. Advantages of this approach include a more uniform distribution of the drug through the neuraxis and better penetration of cytotoxic concentrations of drug into the brain parenchyma and perivascular (Virchow-Robin) spaces. Protracted infusions may result in an equilibrium being reached between plasma and CSF drug levels, resulting in cytotoxic CSF drug concentrations for a prolonged period. In a retrospective study of high-dose methotrexate, Glantz and colleagues (1998) found that this strategy has limited application for the treatment of neoplastic meningitis from solid tumors. Conversely, it has been effectively employed using methotrexate and cytarabine in the treatment and prevention of CNS leukemias and lymphomas (Balis et al., 1985).

Although methotrexate penetration into the CSF is limited (CSF/plasma ratio of 0.03 [Bleyer et al., 1978]), the use of leucovorin calcium rescue along with the administration of very high doses can circumvent this poor penetration. With this approach, cytotoxic concentrations of methotrexate can be achieved within the CSF with doses as high as 33,600 mg/m^2 and tolerance of an infusion duration as long as 42 hours before administration of leucovorin (Balis et al., 1985). Whereas regimens using very high-dose systemic methotrexate have been effective, the optimal dose and schedule necessary for efficacious systemic therapy of CNS leukemia has not been clarified. A rational approach to dosing of this and other agents for the treatment of leptomeningeal metastases is to attain a CSF drug concentration and/or duration greater than the optimal in vitro concentration and/or duration. Because rescue agents are not available for many anticancer agents, this strategy is generally not feasible. However, the relative ease of autologous peripheral blood stem cell rescue technology has led to a resurgence of clinical trials that incorporate higher than standard doses of chemotherapy. The impact of this approach on efficacy and long-term sequelae is not yet known.

Cytarabine penetrates into the CSF more effectively than methotrexate and has a CSF/plasma ratio of 0.18 to 0.33 (Donehower et al., 1986). Following systemic infusion of cytarabine, the CSF drug concentration will eventually exceed that in plasma because cytarabine is not deaminated within the CSF but is rapidly deaminated in plasma (Lopez et al., 1985). High-dose regimens of 2 to 3 g/m^2 administered every 12 hours will result in persistent cytotoxic concentrations of cytarabine in the CSF. Although high-dose intravenous cytarabine has been shown to be efficacious in the treatment of meningeal leukemia (Frick et al., 1984), this approach is associated with significant systemic toxicity and may also be associated with neurotoxicity. Neurotoxicity, primarily in the form of severe and potentially irreversible cerebellar dysfunction, appears to occur in a dose-dependent manner, with an increased incidence in patients who receive total doses exceeding 24 g/m^2 (Herzig et al., 1985; Barnett et al., 1985).

Another approach to systemic therapy utilizes pharmacokinetic monitoring to adjust drug doses in individual patients in an attempt to achieve a target exposure duration threshold that has previously been defined in preclinical studies (Zamboni et al., 1998). An example of this approach is the studies performed by Zamboni et al. (1998) with topotecan, a topoisomerase I inhibitor with preclinical activity against medulloblastoma cell lines and xenografts (Houghton et al., 1995). In vitro studies in medulloblastoma cell lines were performed to define the optimal duration and extent of drug exposure required in vivo. Pharmacokinetic studies were then performed in nonhuman primates to determine the optimal dose and administration schedule required to achieve the desired exposure throughout the subarachnoid space.

On the basis of these results, a phase II clinical trial with children with high-risk medulloblastoma was initiated. Topotecan was administered as a 4 hour infusion for 5 consecutive days; the dosage was pharmacokinetically adjusted to attain the target concentration defined in preclinical studies. In addition, serial CSF samples were obtained to determine the length of time that drug exposure in the CSF exceeded the target concentration (Zamboni et al., 1998). The primary advantage of this approach is that it helps to ensure that an individual patient achieves the target drug exposure in both plasma and CSF, which may be very important for agents with marked interindividual differences in pharmacokinetic disposition. The primary disadvantage of this approach is that is requires numerous resources and may not be feasible in a multi-institutional, cooperative group setting, particularly for drugs that are chemically unstable. Further studies are required to determine the impact of this approach on therapeutic outcome.

Regional Cerebrospinal Fluid Therapy

Regional (intrathecal) administration of chemotherapy was one of the first approaches taken for the treatment of leptomeningeal metastases after the limitations of systemic chemotherapy were recognized. Direct administration of drugs into the CSF results in concentrations at the target site (the meninges) using relatively small doses because of the small volume of distribution (140 ml in CSF versus 3500 ml in plasma) and the relatively slow clearance of many drugs after intrathecal dosing (Poplack et al., 1980). As a result, cytotoxic concentrations may be attained in the CSF at a fraction of the dose that would have to be administered systemically to achieve the same concentration (Collins, 1987). Thus, systemic toxicity is rare when chemotherapy is delivered intrathecally.

In the treatment and prevention of leptomeningeal metastases secondary to leukemia or lymphoma, intrathecal drugs are most commonly administered via lumbar puncture. However, ventricular access devices, such as Ommaya reservoirs, are routinely employed for the treatment of leptomeningeal metastases secondary to an underlying primary CNS or solid tumor because of the limitations of intralumbar chemotherapy. In addition to the pain and inconvenience associated with lumbar punctures, radioisotope studies have demonstrated that in approximately 10% of intrathecal injections drug is not delivered into the subarachnoid space but rather into the subdural or epidural space (Larson et al., 1981). There may also be limited and variable drug distribution into the ventricular CSF after an intralumbar injection secondary to the unidirectional flow of the CSF or because of rapid elimination or metabolism of drug in the intrathecal space (Shapiro et al., 1975). Distribution may be further compromised because of alterations in CSF flow associated with disease (Poplack et al., 1980) or patient positioning (Blaney et al., 1995b).

Direct intraventricular administration of chemotherapy overcomes some of the limitations associated with intralumbar injections. Ventricular reservoirs circumvent the problems of local CSF leakage or epidural or subdural administration. Distribution of drug within the CSF is more complete because the drug no longer has to diffuse in an opposite direction from CSF bulk flow (Blasberg et al., 1977; Shapiro et al., 1975, 1977). Administration through a ventricular reservoir is also associated with less discomfort for patients and allows flexibility in dosing schedules such as the "concentration times time" ("C × T") approach. Repeated intraventricular administration of low-dose chemotherapy over a relatively short period increases the duration of CSF exposure to cytotoxic drug concentrations, an important determinant of cytotoxicity for cell cycle–specific agents such as methotrexate and cytarabine (Bleyer et al., 1978). In addition, the C × T approach may potentially reduce neurotoxicity by avoiding excessively high peak drug concentrations and reducing the total dose of administered drug (Bleyer et al., 1978). The obvious drawback of this method is that, because it requires surgical placement of an indwelling subcutaneous reservoir, there may be an increased risk of infection. In addition, no clinical studies have demonstrated a survival advantage for patients with leptomeningeal metastases who receive drugs into the CSF through the ventricular route compared with the lumbar route (Hitchins et al., 1987). Unfortunately, even regional delivery of cytotoxic drugs directly into the CSF via the intralumbar or intraventricular route has limitations because intrathecally administered drugs penetrate only very short distances into brain parenchyma and tumors. Drug penetration into nodules 2 to 3 mm in diameter is possible, but penetration of effective drug doses into 5 mm nodules is not feasible (Blasberg et al., 1977).

Intrathecal methotrexate therapy, developed nearly 30 years ago for the treatment of overt meningeal leukemia, remains the most commonly used intrathecal agent. The pharmacokinetic principle of age-based dosing rather than dosing based on body surface area for intrathecal agents was derived from early clinical studies involving intrathecal methotrexate. These studies demonstrated that CSF volume is an important factor in CSF drug distribution after intrathecal administration. In children, CSF volume increases much more rapidly than body surface area so that by the time a child is 3 years of age this volume is essentially equivalent to that of an adult (Fig. 16–1). Using age, rather than body surface area, to determine appropriate dosing of intrathecal methotrexate resulted in a reduced neurotoxicity and lower incidence of CNS relapse (Bleyer, 1977, 1983). Thus, because CSF volume increases much more rapidly than body surface area, dosages for all agents administered by the intrathecal route should be based on patient age (unlike systemic administration of chemotherapy).

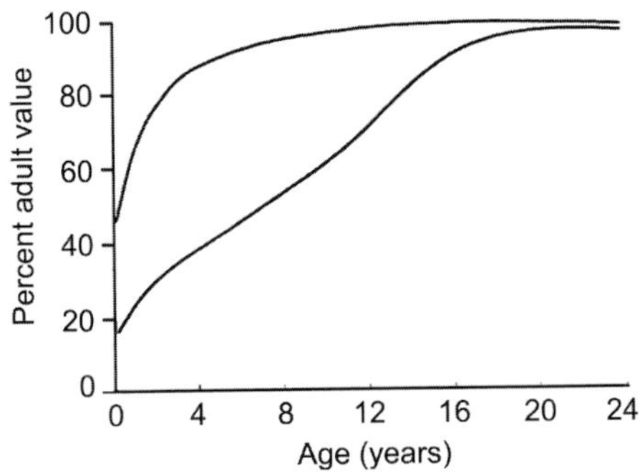

Figure 16–1. Relationship between CNS volume (upper curve) and body surface area (lower curve) as a function of age. CNS volume increases at a more rapid rate than body surface area, reaching the adult volume by 3 years of age. (Reproduced with permission from Bleyer, 1977.)

Other drugs routinely administered by the intrathecal route include cytarabine, hydrocortisone, and thiotepa. DTC101, a sustained-release formulation of cytarabine, has recently been approved by the Food and Drug Administration for the treatment of lymphomatous meningitis in adults (Glantz et al., 1999). It should be noted that the disposition and metabolism of drugs could vary after intrathecal versus systemic administration. For example, cytarabine is rapidly converted to the inactive metabolite uracil arabinoside (ara-U) by a ubiquitous enzyme, cytidine deaminase, after intravenous administration (Camiener and Smith, 1965). In contrast, after intrathecal injection, conversion to ara-U is negligible because of the significantly lower cytidine deaminase activity in the brain and CSF. This difference is partially responsible for the more prolonged half-life of cytarabine in the CSF versus in plasma. This and the fact that cytarabine clearance from the CSF is only slightly more rapid than bulk flow absorption from the CSF (Fulton et al., 1982; Zimm et al., 1984) favors the intrathecal route of cytarabine administration for leptomeningeal disease. Likewise, after systemic administration thiotepa is converted to the active metabolite TEPA. Both thiotepa and TEPA readily cross the blood–brain barrier, providing essentially identical drug exposure in the plasma and CSF. However, after intrathecal thiotepa administration drug is rapidly cleared from the CSF (nine times the rate of CSF bulk flow), which limits drug distribution throughout the neuraxis. In addition, TEPA is not detectable in the CSF following intrathecal administration (Strong et al., 1986).

The impact of regional therapy on the outcome of patients with leptomeningeal metastases is difficult to address because only a limited number of clinical trials have been performed with this patient population. Clinical trials for the treatment of leptomeningeal metastases are complicated by many factors, including the heterogeneous spectrum and inherent chemosensitivity of the underlying primary tumor; the advanced stage of many patients at presentation; and difficulties inherent in defining cytologic and radiographic response, especially in patients receiving concomitant systemic chemotherapy for the treatment of systemic or bulk CNS disease.

Intrathecal chemotherapy is associated with distinct toxic effects that may be acute, subacute, or delayed. Chemical arachnoiditis, an acute toxic effect common to both methotrexate and cytarabine, is characterized by headache, nuchal rigidity, vomiting, fever, and CSF pleocytosis occurring within hours to 1 to 2 days after administration of the drug (Pizzo et al., 1979). Less frequently, intrathecal cytarabine can result in acute neurotoxic effects consisting of seizures or paraplegia (Eden et al., 1978; Wolff et al., 1979). Within days or weeks after administration of intrathecal methotrexate, a subacute myelopathy or encephalopathy may occur that is sometimes irreversible (Pizzo et al., 1979; Bleyer, 1981). This syndrome is characterized by a weakness of limbs, cranial nerve palsies, ataxia, visual impairment, seizures, and coma. Leukoencephalopathy, a chronic, progressive demyelinating encephalopathy, is a delayed toxicity that can appear months to years after treatment with intrathecal methotrexate and cranial irradiation. The encephalopathy consists of dementia, spastic paralysis, seizures, and coma. Whereas arachnoiditis is noted to occur in adults, other acute, subacute, and delayed toxicities have been reported, primarily in the pediatric population.

Accidental intrathecal drug overdose, usually the result of inadvertent intrathecal injection of a higher dose appropriate for systemic administration, can produce severe and frequently lethal toxic effects. Extreme caution must therefore be exercised by clinicians administering drugs by this route. With the widespread use of intrathecal chemotherapy, however, the possibility of fatal dosing errors will continue to exist. In an effort to rescue patients who accidentally receive high doses of methotrexate intrathecally (the most frequent type of overdose), intrathecal administration of carboxypeptidase G2 ($CPDG_2$), a recombinant bacterial enzyme capable of rapidly inactivating methotrexate by cleaving its glutamate residue, has been studied in a nonhuman primate model (Adamson et al., 1991b). Administration of $CPDG_2$ following otherwise lethal doses of intrathecal methotrexate saved animals from death by decreasing the methotrexate concentration in CSF by more than 100-fold within 5 minutes of enzyme administration. The successful use of $CPDG_2$ in conjunction with ventriculolumbar perfusion for the treatment of inadvertent intrathecal methotrexate overdose in humans has also been reported (O'Marcaigh et al., 1996).

NEW PHARMACOLOGIC APPROACHES

The need to develop new approaches and combination therapy for the treatment of leptomeningeal metastases is an area of ongoing research. Evaluating the safety and effectiveness of chemotherapeutic agents administered intrathecally presents unique challenges not encountered in evaluating systemically administered drugs. For phase I (toxicity and dose-schedule trial) development of a new intrathecal agent, the classic approach, in which cohorts of patients receive progressively escalated doses until toxic effects are consistently observed, is not appropriate because the expected dose-limiting toxicity is neurologic. The wide experience with intrathecal methotrexate provides ample evidence for exercising extreme caution when escalating intrathecal doses of a drug. In studies of patients treated with doses of intrathecal methotrexate based on body surface area, neurotoxicity was found to correlate with an elevated concentration of the drug in the CSF (Bleyer et al., 1977). The manifestations of neurotoxic effects were often irreversible or fatal and included severe meningismus, sustained grand mal seizures, irreversible cerebellar dysfunction, quadriplegia, and fatal myelopathy.

Characteristics of an optimal intrathecal agent include:

1. Demonstration of cytotoxicity in in vitro and in vivo models
2. Absence of neurotoxicity following systemic administration
3. Novel mechanism of antitumor activity
4. Formulation suitable for intrathecal administration

Our laboratory has taken a three-step approach to the development of new intrathecal chemotherapeutic agents using a nonhuman primate model and in vitro cytotoxicity studies. Initially, a target cytotoxic concentration and schedule dependency of a drug is determined in vitro using human tumor cell lines. Next, the CSF and plasma pharmacokinetics of the drug following intrathecal dosing are determined in the nonhuman primate. When the intrathecal dose of a drug has been calculated to achieve or exceed the desired cytotoxic effect in the CSF and has been proven safe to administer in the nonhuman primate, a phase I trial in humans is initiated, with escalation of the dose to the target cytotoxic concentration of drug exposure. The pharmacokinetic parameters derived in the nonhuman primate predict human CSF pharmacokinetics, after known differences in CSF volume and bulk flow rate are corrected for, and are the basis for the starting dose in the phase I trial. Typically, the starting dose for phase I clinical trials is approximately 10% to 20% of the dose shown to exceed cytotoxic concentrations in nonhuman primates. Several agents that have been developed using this approach are summarized below.

Mafosfamide

Mafosfamide, a chemically stable thioethane sulfonic acid salt of cyclophosphamide, is a preactivated derivative of cyclophosphamide that, unlike cyclophosphamide, does not require activation by hepatic microsomal enzymes to express an antitumor effect. Mafosfamide has a spectrum of antitumor activity similar to cyclophosphamide, and an in vitro cytotoxic target concentration has been defined. Preclinical pharmacokinetic studies in a nonhuman primate model showed that, after intrathecal dosing, ventricular CSF mafosfamide concentrations in excess of in vitro cytocidal levels could be attained at doses that were not associated with systemic or neurologic toxicity.

On the basis of these results, a phase I study currently nearing completion was initiated with patients with leptomeningeal metastases (Blaney et al., 1992). In addition, the feasibility of administering intrathecal mafosfamide in infants and young children with newly diagnosed primary CNS embryonal tumors, tumors with a known predilection for leptomeningeal spread, is currently being evaluated in a Pediatric Brain Tumor Consortium study (SM Blaney is the PI).

Topotecan

Topotecan, a topoisomerase I inhibitor that has demonstrated promising evidence of antitumor activity against a broad spectrum of tumors, is another example of an agent with a novel mechanism of action that has entered clinical trials after initial evaluation in the nonhuman primate model. Preclinical studies in nonhuman primates revealed that intraventricular topotecan administration was safe and was not associated with either systemic or neurologic toxicity.

Following administration of a 0.1 mg intraventricular dose, the ventricular CSF drug exposure to the parent drug was 450-fold greater than following intravenous administration of a 40-fold higher dose (10 mg/m^2). In addition, peak lumbar levels approached 1 μM. Plasma levels of both the lactone and open-ring form were not measurable. Thus, compared with systemic topotecan administration, intrathecal administration resulted in a dramatic pharmacokinetic advantage of drug exposure in the CNS. Furthermore, there were no significant systemic or neurologic toxicities associated with intrathecal topotecan administration in nonhuman primates (Blaney et al., 1993, 1995a). A phase I study of intrathecal topotecan has recently been completed (Blaney et al., 1998), and a phase II study for children with leptomeningeal metastases has been initiated in the Children's Oncology Group.

Other Cytotoxic Agents

The same approach has been used in the development of several other intrathecal agents, including 6-mercaptopurine (Adamson et al., 1991a), diaziquone (Berg et al., 1992a), and sustained-release cytarabine (DTC101) (Kim et al., 1993). In addition, other agents were not brought to clinical trial after unexpected neurologic toxic effects were observed in the nonhuman primate. 5-Fluorouracil administered into the lumbar space resulted in significant injury to the spinal cord in a cohort of animals, and that drug was deemed unsafe for clinical trial (Berg et al., 1992b). Neuropathologic studies demonstrated local necrosis of the spinal cord at the level of intrathecal drug administration. Similarly, a series of other anticancer agents administered intrathecally to experimental animals resulted in paralysis or death (Table 16–6). Using a preclinical model has thus averted the testing of drugs that could result in severe or irreversible neurotoxic effects when administered intrathecally to patients.

Monoclonal Antibodies

Monoclonal antibodies have the theoretical advantage of selectively targeting malignant cells expressing specific antigens while sparing normal tissues that do not express the same epitopes (Berg and Poplack, 1995). Several preliminary studies have been performed in which tumor-specific monoclonal antibodies were conjugated to ^{131}Iodine isotope in doses from 25 to 160 mCi and administered intrathecally (Brown et al., 1996; Coakham and Kemshead, 1998; Pizer and Kemshead, 1994; Kemshead et al., 1998). Acute toxicities following intrathecal monoclonal antibody administration include aseptic meningitis and myelosuppression. A long-term follow-up report of 52 patients treated with ^{131}Iodine-labeled antibodies between 1984 and 1993 showed the best results in patients with primitive neuroectodermal tumors (n = 22) with 53% of evaluative cases having responses and 11% demonstrating stable disease. The mean survival of responders was 39 months compared with 4 months for nonresponders (Coakham and Kemshead, 1998). Additional studies are needed to better define the role of this therapy for leptomeningeal metastases.

Immunotoxins

Preclinical studies with animal models have evaluated the treatment of leptomeningeal metastases with intrathecal administration of monoclonal antibodies conjugated to myriad immunotoxins, including M6-ricin A-chain immunotoxin, B43 (anti CD19) pokeweed antiviral protein, and anti-CD7-ricin A-chain immunotoxin (Zovickian and Youle, 1988; Gunther et al., 1995; Herrlinger et al., 1998). Antitumor effects have been observed in these preclinical studies. Laske et al. (1997) reported the findings of a phase I study using intraventricular 454A12-rRA in patients with leptomeningeal spread of systemic neoplasm. In patients receiving 120 μg, toxicity with CSF inflammation resulting in transient headache, vomiting, and altered mental status was seen. The acute inflammation was responsive to steroids and CSF drainage. No systemic toxicity was identified. Four of the eight patients studied had a transient reduction in CSF tumor cell counts. Further clinical trials are needed to evaluate the utility of this therapeutic approach for patients with leptomeningeal metastases.

Gene Therapy

The feasibility of administering adenoviral gene vectors in rat models of leptomeningeal disease has been demonstrated (Ram et al., 1994; Rosenfeld et

Table 16–6. Antineoplastic Agents that Produced Unexpected Neurotoxicity When Administered to the Rhesus Monkey for Pharmacokinetic Evaluation

Drug	*Dose*	*Animals*	*Neurotoxicity (N)*
Melphalan (Berg et al., 1994)	1	3	Hind-limb paralysis (2/3); death (1/3)
5-Fluorouracil (Berg et al., 1992a)	10 1	2 1	Hind-limb paralysis (3/3)
6-Thioguanine (Poplack, 1992, personal communication)	1.5 0.5	1 1	Hind-limb dysfunction (2/2)
Cisplatin (Gormley et al., 1981)	0.5*	1	Death
CPE-C (Poplack, 1992, personal communication)	2	3	Hind-limb dysfunction (2/3)
Trimetrexate (Poplack, 1992, personal communication)	5*	2	Agitation and respiratory depression (1/2); irreversible respiratory depression (1/2)

Unless otherwise indicated, all drugs were administered into the lumbar space.

*Drug was only administered via a ventricular reservoir.

al., 1997). Recent studies have also described the distribution of adenoviral gene vectors and the pharmacokinetics of the antiviral drug ganciclovir in the nonhuman primate model (Driesse et al., 1999; Serabe et al., 1999). Preclinical studies to assess the feasibility and distribution after intralumbar injection of an adenoviral vector to nonhuman primates are in progress. This novel therapeutic approach may have potential application for the treatment of patients with leptomeningeal metastases; however, extensive preclinical and clinical studies are still required.

CONCLUSION

The successful treatment of leptomeningeal metastases continues to pose a significant challenge to the clinical oncologist. Research efforts to date have focused on the identification, dosage, and safety of new intrathecal and intraventricular chemotherapeutic agents or other treatment modalities as well as on methods to improve upon the use of currently available agents. While considerable progress has been made during the past several decades in the treatment and prevention of leptomeningeal leukemias and lymphomas, such progress has not been realized for patients with leptomeningeal metastases arising from and underlying solid or primary CNS tumors. Research using combination chemotherapy and other novel therapies, including monoclonal antibodies, immunotoxins, and gene therapy, must be pursued. Well-designed clinical trials that focus on efficacy, disease-free progression, and quality of life will be critical for evaluating the impact of these developments in patients with leptomeningeal metastases.

REFERENCES

Adamson PC, Balis FM, Arndt CA, et al. 1991a. Intrathecal 6-mercaptopurine: preclinical pharmacology, phase I/II trial, and pharmacokinetic study. Cancer Res 51:6079–6083.

Adamson PC, Balis FM, McCully CL, et al. 1991b. Rescue of experimental intrathecal methotrexate overdose with carboxypeptidase-G2. J Clin Oncol 9:670–674.

Balis FM, Savitch JL, Bleyer WA, Reaman GH, Poplack DG. 1985. Remission induction of meningeal leukemia with high-dose intravenous methotrexate. J Clin Oncol 3:485–489.

Barnett MJ, Richards MA, Ganesan TS, et al. 1985. Central nervous system toxicity of high-dose cytosine arabinoside. Semin Oncol 12(suppl 3):227–232.

Berg SL, Balis FM, McCully CL, Parker GA, Murphy RF, Poplack DG. 1992a. Intrathecal 5-fluorouracil in the rhesus monkey. Cancer Chemother Pharmacol 31:127–130.

Berg SL, Balis FM, Zimm S, et al. 1992b. Phase I/II trial and pharmacokinetics of intrathecal diaziquone in refractory meningeal malignancies. J Clin Oncol 10:143–148.

Berg S, Balis FM, McCully CL, Poplack DG. 1994. Re: toxicity of intrathecal melphalan. J Natl Cancer Inst 86:463.

Berg SL, Poplack DG. 1995. Advances in the treatment of meningeal cancers. Crit Rev Oncol Hematol 20:87–98.

Blaney SM, Balis F, Murphy R, et al. 1992. A phase I study of intrathecal mafosfamide (mf) in patients with refractory meningeal malignancies. Proc ASCO 11:113.

Blaney SM, Cole DE, Balis FM, Godwin K, Poplack DG. 1993. Plasma and cerebrospinal fluid pharmacokinetic study of topotecan in nonhuman primates. Cancer Res 53:725–727.

Blaney SM, Cole DE, Godwin K, McCully CL, Murphy R, Balis FM. 1995a. Intrathecal administration of topotecan in nonhuman primates. Cancer Chemother Pharmacol 36:121–124.

Blaney S, Heideman R, Cole D, et al. 1998. A phase I study of intrathecal topotecan. Proc Am Assoc Cancer Res 39:322.

Blaney SM, Poplack DG, Godwin K, McCully CL, Murphy R, Balis FM. 1995b. Effect of body position on ventricular CSF methotrexate concentration following intralumbar administration. J Clin Oncol 13:177–179.

Blasberg RG, Patlak CS, Shapiro WR. 1977. Distribution of methotrexate in the cerebrospinal fluid and brain after intraventricular administration. Cancer Treat Rep 61:633–641.

Blatt J, Bercu BB, Gillin JC, Mendelson WB, Poplack DG. 1984. Reduced pulsatile growth hormone secretion in children after therapy for acute lymphoblastic leukemia. J Pediatr 104:182–186.

Bleyer WA. 1977. Clinical pharmacology of intrathecal methotrexate. II. An improved dosage regimen derived from age related pharmacokinetics. Cancer Treat Rep 61: 1419–1425.

Bleyer WA. 1981. Neurologic sequelae of methotrexate and ionizing radiation: a new classification. Cancer Treat Rep 65:89–98.

Bleyer W. 1983. Central nervous system leukemia. In: Gunz FW, Henderson ES (eds), William Dameshek and Frederick Gunz's Leukemia, 4th ed. New York: Grune & Stratton, 865 pp.

Bleyer WA, Coccia PF, Sather HN, et al. 1983. Reduction in central nervous system leukemia with a pharmacokinetically derived intrathecal methotrexate dosage regimen. J Clin Oncol 1:317–325.

Bleyer W, Poplack D, Simon R. 1978. "Concentration × time" methotrexate via a subcutaneous reservoir: a less toxic regimen for intraventricular chemotherapy of central nervous system neoplasms. Blood 51:835–842.

Brown MT, Coleman RE, Friedman AH, et al. 1996. Intrathecal ^{131}I-labeled antitenascin monoclonal antibody 81C6 treatment of patients with leptomeningeal neoplasms or primary brain tumor resection cavities with subarachnoid communication: phase I trial results. Clin Cancer Res 2:963–972.

Camiener GW, Smith CG. 1965. Studies of the enzymatic deamination of cytosine arabinoside. I. Enzyme distribution and species specificity. Biochem Pharmacol 14:1405–1416.

Chamberlain MC. 1992. Current concepts in leptomeningeal metastasis. Curr Opin Oncol 4:533–539.

Chamberlain MC. 1995a. A review of leptomeningeal metastases in pediatrics. J Child Neurol 10:191–199.

Chamberlain MC. 1995b. Comparative spine imaging in leptomeningeal metastases. J Neurooncol 23:233–238.

Chamberlain MC. 1997. Pediatric leptomeningeal metastases: outcome following combined therapy. J Child Neurol 12:53–59.

Chamberlain MC. 1998a. Radioisotope CSF flow studies in leptomeningeal metastases. J Neurooncol 38:135–140.

Chamberlain MC. 1998b. Cytologically negative carcinomatous meningitis: usefulness of CSF biochemical markers. Neurology 50:1173–1175.

Chamberlain MC, Corey-Bloom J. 1991. Leptomeningeal metastases: ^{111}indium-DTPA CSF flow studies. Neurology 41:1765–1769.

Chamberlain MC, Dirr L. 1993. Involved field radiotherapy and intra-Ommaya methotrexate/cytarabine in patients with AIDS-related lymphomatous meningitis. J Clin Oncol 11: 1978–1984.

Chamberlain MC, Kormanik PA. 1997. Non-AIDS related lymphomatous meningitis: combined modality therapy. Neurology 49:1728–1731.

Chamberlain MC, Sandy AD, Press GA. 1990. Leptomeningeal metastasis: a comparison of gadolinium-enhanced MR and contrast-enhanced CT of the brain. Neurology 40:435–438.

Chiro GD, Hammock MK, Bleyer WA. 1976. Spinal descent of cerebrospinal fluid in man. Neurology 26:1–8.

Cibas ES, Malkin MG, Posner JB, Melamed MR. 1987. Detection of DNA abnormalities by flow cytometry in cells from cerebrospinal fluid. Am J Clin Pathol 88:570–577.

Coakham HB, Brownell B, Harper EI, et al. 1984. Use of monoclonal antibody panel to identify malignant cells in the cerebrospinal fluid. Lancet 1:1095–1098.

Coakham HB, Kemshead JT. 1998. Treatment of neoplastic meningitis by targeted radiation using (131)I-radiolabelled monoclonal antibodies. Results of responses and long term follow-up in 40 patients. J Neurooncol 38:225–232.

Collins J. 1987. Regional therapy: an overview. In: Poplack DG, Massimo L, Cornaglia-Ferraris P (eds), The Role of Pharmacology in Pediatric Oncology. Boston: Martinus Nijhoff Publishers, pp125–135.

Crossen JR, Garwood D, Glatstein E, Neuwelt EA. 1994. Neurobehavioral sequelae of cranial irradiation in adults: a review of radiation-induced encephalopathy. J Clin Oncol 12:627–642.

DeAngelis LM. 1998. Current diagnosis and treatment of leptomeningeal metastasis. J Neurooncol 38:245–252.

Donehower R, Karp JE, Burke PJ. 1986. Pharmacology and toxicity of high dose cytarabine by 72-hour continuous infusion. Cancer Treat Rep 70:1059–1065.

Driesse MJ, Kros JM, Avezaat CJ, et al. 1999. Distribution of recombinant adenovirus in the cerebrospinal fluid of nonhuman primates. Hum Gene Ther 10:2347–2354.

Eden OB, Goldie W, Wood T, Etcubanas E. 1978. Seizures following intrathecal cytosine arabinoside in young children with acute lymphoblastic leukemia. Cancer 42:53–58.

Ernerudh J, Olsson T, Berlin G, von Schenck H. 1987. Cerebrospinal fluid immunoglobulins and β_2-microglobulin in lymphoproliferative and other neoplastic diseases of the central nervous system. Arch Neurol 44:915–920.

Faithfull S, Brada M. 1998. Somnolence syndrome in adults following cranial irradiation for primary brain tumors. Clin Oncol 10:250–254.

Fouladi M, Gajjar A, Boyett JM, et al. 1999. Comparison of CSF cytology and spinal magnetic resonance imaging in the detection of leptomeningeal disease in pediatric medulloblastoma or primitive neuroectodermal tumor. J Clin Oncol 17:3234–3237.

Freeman J, Johnston PG, Voke JM. 1973. Somnolence after prophylactic cranial irradiation in children with acute lymphoblastic leukaemia. BMJ 4:523–525.

Freilich RJ, Krol G, DeAngelis LM. 1995. Neuroimaging and cerebrospinal fluid cytology in the diagnosis of leptomeningeal metastasis. Ann Neurol 38:51–57.

Frick J, Ritch PS, Hansen RM, Anderson T. 1984. Successful treatment of meningeal leukemia using systemic high-dose cytosine arabinoside. J Clin Oncol 2:365–368.

Fulton DS, Levin VA, Gutin PH, et al. 1982. Intrathecal cytosine arabinoside for the treatment of meningeal metastases from malignant brain tumors and systemic tumors. Cancer Chemother Pharmacol 8:285–291.

Glantz MJ, Cole BF, Recht L, et al. 1998. High-dose intravenous methotrexate for patients with nonleukemic leptomeningeal cancer: is intrathecal chemotherapy necessary? J Clin Oncol 16:1561–1567.

Glantz MJ, Hall WA, Cole BF, et al. 1995. Diagnosis, management, and survival of patients with leptomeningeal cancer based on cerebrospinal fluid-flow status. Cancer 75:2919–2931.

Glantz MJ, LaFollette S, Jaeckle KA, et al. 1999. Randomized trial of a slow-release versus a standard formulation of cytarabine for the intrathecal treatment of lymphomatous meningitis. J Clin Oncol 17:3110–3116.

Goldberg SL, Tefferi A, Rummans TA, Chen MG, Solberg LA, Noel P. 1992. Post-irradiation somnolence syndrome in an adult patient following allogeneic bone marrow transplantation. Bone Marrow Transplant 9:499–501.

Gormley PE, Gangji D, Wood JH, Poplack DG. 1981. Pharmacokinetic study of cerebrospinal fluid penetration of cis-diamminedichloroplatinum (II). Cancer Chemother Pharmacol 5:257–260.

Grossman SA, Moynihan TJ. 1991: Neoplastic meningitis. Neurol Clin 9:843–856.

Grossman SA, Trump CL, Chen DC, Thompson G, Murray K, Wharam M. 1982. Cerebrospinal fluid flow abnormalities in patients with neoplastic meningitis. An evaluation using 111indium-DTPA ventriculography. Am J Med 73:641–647.

Gunther R, Chelstrom LM, Tuel-Ahlgren L, Simon J, Myers DE, Uckan FM. 1995. Biotherapy for xenografted human central nervous system leukemia in mice with severe combined immunodeficiency using B43 (anti-CD19)-pokeweed antiviral protein immunotoxin. Blood 85:2537–2545.

Harrison SK, Ditchfield MR, Waters K. 1998. Correlation of MRI and CSF cytology in the diagnosis of medulloblastoma spinal metastases. Pediatr Radiol 28:571–574.

Heideman RL, Packer RJ, Albright A, et al. 1997. Tumors of the central nervous system. In: Pizzo Pa, Poplack DG (eds), Principles and Practice of Pediatric Oncology, 3rd ed. Philadelphia: Lippincott-Raven, pp 633–697.

Herrlinger U, Schmidberger H, Buchholz R, Wehrmann M, Vallera DA, Schabet M. 1998. Intrathecal therapy of leptomeningeal CEM T-cell lymphoma in nude rats with anti-CD7 ricin toxin A chain immunotoxin. J Neurooncol 40:1–9.

Herzig RH, Lazarus HM, Herzig GP, Coccia PF, Wolff SN. 1985. Central nervous system toxicity with high-dose cytosine arabinoside. Semin Oncol 12(suppl 3):233–236.

Hitchins RN, Bell DR, Woods RL, Levi JA. 1987. A prospective randomized trial of single-agent versus combination chemotherapy in meningeal carcinomatosis. J Clin Oncol 5:1655–1662.

Houghton PJ, Cheshire PJ, Hallman JD 2nd, et al. 1995. Efficacy of topoisomerase I inhibitors, topotecan and irinotecan, administered at low dose levels in protracted schedules to mice bearing xenografts of human tumors. Cancer Chemother Pharmacol 36:393–403.

Kallmes DF, Gray L, Glass JP. 1998. High-dose gadolinium-enhanced MRI for diagnosis of meningeal metastases. Neuroradiology 40:23–26.

Kaplan JG, DeSouza TG, Farkash A, et al. 1990. Leptomeningeal metastases: comparison of clinical features and laboratory data of solid tumors, lymphomas and leukemias. J Neurooncol 9:225–229.

Kemshead JT, Hopkins K, Pizer B,, et al. 1998. Dose escalation with repeated intrathecal injections of 131I-labelled MAbs for the treatment of central nervous system malignancies. Br J Cancer 77:2324–2330.

Kim KS, Ho SU, Weinberg PE, Lee C. 1982. Spinal leptomeningeal infiltration by systemic cancer: myelographic features. Am J Roentgenol 139:361–365.

Kim S, Khatibi S, Howell SB, McCully C, Balis FM, Poplack DG. 1993. Prolongation of drug exposure in cerebrospinal fluid by encapsulation into DepoFoam. Cancer Res 53:1596–1598.

Klee GG, Tallman RD, Goellner JR, Yanagihara T. 1986. Elevation of carcinoembryonic antigen in cerebrospinal fluid among patients with meningeal carcinomatosis. Mayo Clin Proc 61:9–13.

Kokkoris CP. 1983. Leptomeningeal carcinomatosis: how does cancer reach the pia-arachnoid? Cancer 51:154–160.

Kramer ED, Rafto S, Packer RJ, Zimmerman RA. 1991. Comparison of myelography with CT follow-up versus gadolinium MRI for subarachnoid metastatic disease in children. Neurology 41:46–50.

Kun LE, Camitta BM, Mulhern RK, et al. 1984. Treatment of meningeal relapse in childhood acute lymphoblastic leukemia. I. Results of craniospinal irradiation. J Clin Oncol 2:359–364.

Larson SM, Schall GL, Di Chiro G. 1981. The influence of previous lumbar puncture and pneumoencephalography on the incidence of unsuccessful radioisotope cisternography. J Nucl Med 12:555–557.

Laske DW, Muraszko KM, Oldfield EH, et al. 1997. Intraventricular immunotoxin therapy for leptomeningeal neoplasia. Neurosurgery 41:1039–1049.

Lim V, Sobel DF, Zyroff J. 1990. Spinal cord pial metastases: MR imaging with gadopentetate dimeglumine. Am J Roentgenol 155:1077–1084.

Little JR, Dale AJ, Okazaki H. 1974. Meningeal carcinomatosis: clinical manifestations. Arch Neurol 30:138–143.

Lopez JA, Nassif E, Vannicola P, et al. 1985. Central nervous system pharmacokinetics of high-dose cytosine arabinoside. J Neurooncol 3:119–124.

Lyons MK, Meyer FB. 1990. Cerebrospinal fluid physiology and the management of increased intracranial pressure. Mayo Clin Proc 65:684–707.

Malkin MG, Posner JB. 1987. Cerebrospinal fluid tumor markers for the diagnosis and management of leptomeningeal metastases. Eur J Cancer Clin Oncol 23:1–4.

Mason WP, DeAngelis LM, Yeh SDJ. 1996. ^{111}Indium-DTPA cerebrospinal fluid (CSF) studies in leptomeningeal metastases (LM) predict intrathecal methotrexate (MTX) distribution and response to therapy. Proc ASCO 15:155.

Mittl RL Jr, Yousem DM. 1994. Frequency of unexplained meningeal enhancement in the brain after lumbar puncture. Am J Neuroradiol 15:633–638.

Moss HA, Nannis ED, Poplack DG. 1981. The effects of prophylactic treatment of the central nervous system on the intellectual functioning of children with acute lymphocytic leukemia. Am J Med 71:47–52.

Murray JJ, Greco FA, Wolff SN, Hainsworth JD. 1983. Neoplastic meningitis: Marked variations of cerebrospinal fluid composition in the absence of extradural block. Am J Med 75:289–294.

Newton HB, Fleisher M, Schwartz MK, Malkin MG. 1991. Glucosephosphate isomerase as a CSF marker for leptomeningeal metastasis. Neurology 41:395–398.

Olson ME, Chernik NL, Posner JB. 1974. Infiltration of leptomeninges by systemic cancer: a clinical and pathologic study. Arch Neurol 30:122–137.

O'Marcaigh AS, Johnson CM, Smithson WA, et al. 1996. Successful treatment of intrathecal methotrexate overdose by using ventriculolumbar perfusion and intrathecal instillation of carboxypeptidase G_2. Mayo Clin Proc 71:161–165.

Packer RJ, Siegel KR, Sutton LN, Litmann P, Bruce DA, Schut L. 1985. Leptomeningeal dissemination of primary central nervous system tumors of childhood. Ann Neurol 18:217–221.

Paolucci G, Rosito P. 1983. Adverse sequelae of central nervous system prophylaxis in acute lymphoblastic leukemia. In: Mastrangelo R, Poplack D, Riccardi R (eds), Central Nervous System Leukemia. Boston: Martinus Nijhoff Publishers, pp 105–111.

Pasqualini T, McCalla J, Berg S, et al. 1991. Subtle primary hypothyroidism in patients treated for acute lymphoblastic leukemia. Acta Endocrinol 124:375–380.

Pizer BL, Kemshead JT. 1994. The potential of targeted radiotherapy in the treatment of central nervous system leukaemia. Leuk Lymphoma 15:281–289.

Pizzo P, Poplack DG, Bleyer WA. 1979. Neurotoxicities of current leukemia therapy. Am J Pediatr Hematol Oncol 1:127–140.

Poplack D, Bleyer W, Horowitz M. 1980. Pharmacology of antineoplastic agents in cerebrospinal fluid. In: Wood JH (ed), Neurobiology of Cerebrospinal Fluid, vol 11. New York: Plenum Press, pp 561–578.

Poplack DG, Brouwers P. 1985. Adverse sequelae of central nervous system therapy. In: Nesbit ME (ed), Clinics in Oncology. Philadeophia: WB Saunders, pp 263–285.

Posner JB, Chernik NL. 1978. Intracranial metastases from systemic cancer. Adv Neurol 19:579–592.

Ram Z, Walbridge S, Oshiro EM, et al. 1994. Intrathecal gene therapy for malignant leptomeningeal neoplasia. Cancer Res 54:2141–2145.

Recht LD. 1991. Neurologic complications of systemic lymphoma. Neurol Clin 9:1001–1015.

Rogers LR, Duchesneau PM, Nunez C, et al. 1992. Comparison of cisternal and lumbar CSF examination in leptomeningeal metastasis. Neurology 42:1239–1241.

Rosen ST, Aisner J, Makuch RW, et al. 1982. Carcinomatous leptomeningitis in small cell lung cancer: a clinicopathologic review of the National Cancer Institute experience. Medicine 61:45–53.

Rosenfeld MR, Bergman I, Schramm L, Griffin JA, Kaplitt MG, Meneses PI. 1997. Adeno-associated viral vector gene transfer into leptomeningeal xenografts. J Neurooncol 34:139–144.

Schipper HI, Bardosi A, Jacobi C, Felgenhauer K. 1988. Meningeal carcinomatosis: origin of local IgG production in the CSF. Neurology 38:413–416.

Schold SC, Wasserstrom WR, Fleisher M, Schwartz MK, Posner JB. 1980. Cerebrospinal fluid biochemical markers of central nervous system metastases. Ann Neurol 8: 597–604.

Serabe BM, Murry DJ, Dauser R, et al. 1999. Plasma and CSF pharmacokinetics of ganciclovir in nonhuman primates. Cancer Chemother Pharmacol 43:415–418.

Shapiro WR, Posner JB, Ushio Y, Chemik NL, Young DF. 1977. Treatment of meningeal neoplasms. Cancer Treat Rep 61:733–743.

Shapiro WR, Young DF, Mehta BM. 1975. Methotrexate: distribution in cerebrospinal fluid after intravenous, ventricular and lumbar injections. N Engl J Med 293:161–166.

Strong JM, Collins JM, Lester C, Poplack DG. 1986. Pharmacokinetics of intraventricular and intravenous N,N′,N″-triethylenethiophosphoramide (thiotepa) in rhesus monkeys and humans. Cancer Res 46:6101–6104.

Sze G, Abramson A, Krol G, et al. 1988. Gadolinium-DTPA in evaluation of intradural extramedullary spinal disease. Am J Roentgenol 150:911–921.

Theodore WH, Gendelman S. 1981. Meningeal carcinomatosis. Arch Neurol 38:696–699.

Twijnstra A, Ongerboer de Visser BW, van Zanten AP, Hart AA, Nooyen WF. 1989. Serial lumbar and ventricular cerebrospinal fluid biochemical marker measurements in patients with leptomeningeal metastases form solid and hematologic tumors. J Neurooncology 7:57–63.

Van Oostenbrugge RJ, Hopman AHN, Lenders MH, et al. 1997. Detection of malignant cells in cerebrospinal fluid using fluorescence in situ hybridization. J Neuropathol Exp Neurol 56:743–748.

Van Oostenbrugge RJ, Twijnstra A. 1999. Presenting features and value of diagnostic procedures in leptomeningeal metastases. Neurology 53:382–385.

Voorhess ML, Brecher ML, Glicksman AS, et al. 1986. Hypothalamic-pituitary function of children with acute lymphocytic leukemia after three forms of central nervous system prophylaxis. A retrospective study. Cancer 57: 1287–1291.

Walker RW. 1991. Neurologic complications of systemic cancer: neurologic complications of leukemia. Neurol Clin 9:989–999.

Walter AW, Hancock ML, Pui CH, et al. 1998. Secondary brain tumors in children treated for acute lymphoblastic leukemia at St Jude Children's Research Hospital. J Clin Oncol. 16:3761–3767.

Wasserstrom WR, Glass JP, Posner JB. 1982. Diagnosis and treatment of leptomeningeal metastases from solid tumors: experience with 90 patients. Cancer 49:759–772.

Wolff L, Zighelboim J, Gale RP. 1979. Paraplegia following intrathecal cytosine arabinoside. Cancer 43:83–85.

Yung WA, Horten BC, Shapiro WR. 1980. Meningeal gliomatosis: a review of 12 cases. Ann Neurol 8:605–608.

Zamboni WC, Gajjar AJ, Mandrell TD, et al. 1998. A four-hour topotecan infusion achieves cytotoxic exposure throughout the neuraxis in the nonhuman primate model: implications for treatment of children with metastatic medulloblastoma. Clin Cancer Res 4:2537–2544.

Zimm S, Collins JM, Miser J, Chatterji D, Poplack DG. 1984. Cytosine arabinoside cerebrospinal fluid kinetics. Clin Pharmacol Ther 35:826–830.

Zovickian J, Youle RJ. 1988. Efficacy of intrathecal immunotoxin therapy in an animal model of leptomeningeal neoplasia. J Neurosurg 68:767–774.

Part VI

Symptoms Secondary to Cancer and Its Treatment

17

Peripheral Neuropathy

ARTHUR FORMAN

Peripheral neuropathy in cancer patients causes significant morbidity and limits dose intensification of drugs such as vincristine, cisplatinum, paclitaxel (Taxol), and docetaxel (Taxotere). Considerable advances have been made in understanding the mechanisms of peripheral nerve disorders during the past 25 years, yet clinical oncologists are often frustrated in dealing with neuropathy, perhaps as a result of its protean manifestations, insidious symptomatology, and confusing classification.

INCIDENCE

Cancer patients are so frequently affected by peripheral nerve disorders that absent deep tendon ankle reflexes are almost considered routine on examination. In a series of lung cancer patients, 48% had clinically evident peripheral neuropathy, most of them before receiving chemotherapy (Teräväinen and Larsen, 1977). In another study of 195 Eastern Indian patients without other known causes of neuropathy and with untreated tumors of diverse types, neuromuscular signs were found in 30%; the highest incidence was in patients with cancers of bronchogenic, ovarian, or testicular origin (Paul et al., 1978). Only alcohol, nutritional deficiencies, and metabolic disturbances such as diabetes are acquired causes of peripheral neuropathy that occurs more frequently than in cancer. Peripheral neuropathies in cancer patients will become even more common as new treatments and longer survivals are achieved.

Confounding evaluation of neuropathy in a cancer patient are the multitude of injuries the peripheral nerves may acquire and the host of potential neuropathy risks to which patients are exposed. These include treatment with multiple cytotoxic drugs, deleterious drug interactions, pre-existing diabetes mellitus, and acquired nutritional and metabolic disturbances caused by the cancer as well as its treatment.

MORBIDITY

The clinical severity of neuropathy in cancer patients ranges from mild distal paresthesias, to ataxia severe enough to keep patients bed bound, to rare muscle-wasting syndromes sufficient to compromise breathing. It may be that most patients with peripheral neuropathy are not incapacitated enough to have decreased performance status, yet neuropathy remains a frequent reason that oncologists seek neurologic consultation. Peripheral neuropathy's consequences can be devastating; the morbidity associated with toxic treatment-related neuropathies certainly contributes to the suffering associated with cancer and can even be the limiting factor in the amount of therapy that can be given (Legha and Dimery, 1985). More patients suffer some morbidity from neuromuscular disease than are given the benefit of neurologic consultation, perhaps because the manifestations of neuropathy are mistaken for other conditions or because it is thought that little can be done to help.

Any understanding of peripheral nerve disorders in oncology must be grounded in a basic understanding of their general principles, a brief review of which follows.

CLINICAL FEATURES

Sensory

Peripheral sensory nerves have their cell bodies in the dorsal root ganglion, which lie outside the protective mechanisms of the central nervous system (CNS) and are therefore particularly susceptible to injury. Sensory complaints are often the first symptoms in cancer patients with neuropathy.

Neuropathic pain is a common symptom, more frequently seen in neuropathies predominantly affecting axons. The pain may have an electric or lancinating quality, but more often patients bitterly complain of chronic perversions of sensation such as "burning" or, oxymoronically, "painful numbness." Hyperpathia, increased sensitivity to stimuli so that mild stimuli (e.g., the weight of bed linens on legs) become noxious, is commonly experienced by patients with peripheral neuropathy. Acroparesthesia, or the stocking-glove distribution "tingling" numbness, is often the earliest and most persistent symptom. Great care must be exercised in distinguishing radicular or myelopathic paresthesiae from those due to neuropathy. Focusing on the quality of the symptoms, which unfortunately are not distinctive, yet are often the main concern of the patient, may lead to diagnostic errors. The symptom's distribution for cord or root disease will often have a characteristic anatomic pattern, whereas neuropathic symptoms typically have a stocking-glove and, with rare exception, distal appendicular predominance.

The clinical evaluation of sensation is the most exacting component of the neurologic examination, requiring both patience and skill on the part of the examiner. Complicating the examination is the heterogeneity of nerve fibers, with different-sized fibers having different functions and susceptibility to injury (Table 17–1). Proprioceptive axons and those serving the afferent limb of deep tendon reflex arcs are of similar size so that both functions are often lost concurrently. The clinical signs observed with large fiber dysfunction are reliable and can be quickly assessed so that these axons' physiology can usually be well documented. Romberg's sign, which is considered positive when a patient who is able to stand with feet together and eyes open loses balance when visual cues are taken away, indicates moderate to severe proprioceptive loss. When asked, patients with proprioceptive loss often note difficulty negotiating steps in the dark or shampooing their hair in the shower when closing their eyes.

Paradoxically, motor signs and symptoms are prominent in patients with relatively pure sensory neuropathies, and the degree to which sensory impairment contributes to reflex attenuation, weakness, or incoordination is often underestimated. Difficulty with walking can be the result of the loss of proprioceptive fibers; the loss of spindle afferents in the motor reflex arc causes loss of deep tendon reflexes independently from significant muscle wasting or weakness. Patients complaining of trouble tying shoes or buttoning buttons likely have proprioceptive loss, which causes their decreased fine motor control. The restless leg syndrome, in which patients with neuropathy complain of aching calves relieved by moving the limbs, may be caused by sensory fiber disease. These curiously compelling symptoms

Table 17–1. Size and Function Relationships in Peripheral Nerves

Conduction Fiber Size (μm)	*Fiber Type*	*Velocity (m/sec)*	*Function*
10–18	A	70	α-Motor neuron; first-degree spindle afferents
6–12	A	50	Touch and pressure afferents
4–8	A	30	γ-Efferents; second-degree spindle afferents
2–6	B	10	Autonomic; preganglionic
0.2–3	C	2	Temperature
			Nociception
			Autonomic; postganglionic

can be relieved by treatment with carisoprodol, vitamin E (Walton and Kolb, 1991), benzodiazepines (Horiguchi et al., 1992), carbamazepine, dopa agonists (Walters et al., 1988), gabapentin or opioids (Walters et al., 1993).

Motor

Neurogenic muscle atrophy is common in axonal neuropathies, often being evident in advance of weakness. As with sensory symptoms, the wasting due to neuropathy affects distal more than proximal musculature, with rare exceptions. Neuropathic disorders are best detected by neurophysiologic testing that can uncover abnormalities well before the appearance of symptomatic motor weakness.

Cramps, while occurring less frequently than muscle wasting, are not uncommon and at times are the source of bitter complaints in cancer patients suffering from neuropathy. Such pain is commonly the presenting symptom. Cramps consist of involuntary, paroxysmal, and painful muscle contraction. Typically, the cramp causes the patient to hold the affected limb in a fixed posture and can often be eased by stretching and massaging the cramped muscle. Patients complain of painful legs, often describing the pain as "spasms." While the physiologic mechanisms underlying cramping are incompletely understood, multiple experimental and clinical clues point to an origin from a lower motor neuron disturbance (Rowland, 1985). Examples can be an early complaint, particularly in vincristine neuropathy, in which cramping may occur acutely following or even during therapy. Besides mechanical therapy, cramps may respond to quinine, carbamazepine, or other agents that serve to raise the threshold of the motor neuron's action potential.

Small Fibers

Disturbance of small-diameter nerve fibers results in dysautonomia and/or in dysesthetic pain syndromes paradoxically associated with decreased pain and temperature sensation. Loss of small fiber afferent input causes the deafferentation pain syndrome. Such patients may have severe complaints despite having well-preserved reflexes and other negative tests of large fiber function, including nerve conduction studies. Dysautonomia causes complaints of dizziness, delayed gastric emptying, obstipation, impotence, and incontinence. Those affected may have cool, flushed, dry limbs with distal limb hair loss, easily damaged skin, and trophic nail changes.

Injury to small-diameter axons is the most difficult to clinically assess because of variability in the clinical expression of damage. Standard electrophysiologic studies measure only the fastest conducting fibers. Techniques presently exist to directly assay small fiber function, but these are too painful and laborious for use in routine clinical investigation. The use of thermal discrimination thresholds, in which a patient's ability to perceive changes in temperature is quantified, is one of the few painless and reproducible means of assessing small fiber function (Bertelsmann et al., 1985; Hanson et al., 1992).

Autonomic function can also be assessed by quantifying hemodynamic responses, Valsalva's maneuver, and, even more simply, by checking an electrocardiogram for sinus arrhythmia. A beat-to-beat variation of the heart occurs normally with changes in cardiac return during the respiratory cycle; attenuation of this variability indicates proximal loss of autonomic function. Loss of this beat-to-beat variation can be observed on the electrocardiogram. The galvanic skin response can be measured electrophysiologically, easily, and without undo discomfort. Whereas the thermal discrimination threshold correlates well with the galvanic skin response, it may not predict RR interval abnormality from neuropathy (Wieman et al., 1989), typical of the inhomogeneity of the autonomic nervous system.

Small fiber axon damage affects both autonomic and nociceptive functions; physicians treating patients with neuropathic deafferentation pain must regularly check for orthostatic hypotension. Patients taking tricyclic antidepressants, which ironically are a mainstay of treating neuropathic pain, are at increased risk of developing orthostatic hypotension. Volume depletion from diuresis, bleeding, or vomiting increases susceptibility to symptomatic orthostatic hypotension. The combination of hypotension, lack of proprioceptive function, and deadened reflexes is particularly treacherous, frequently producing subdural hematomas and falls resulting in fractured shoulders and hips.

The autonomic nervous system is very adaptable, and effector receptors become hypersensitive to neurotransmitters following postganglionic denervation (Cannon's rule). As long as the autonomic nervous system is not totally devastated, symptoms may wax and wane, and clinical improvement often occurs spontaneously. Accurate diagnosis using simple techniques permits rational management, which can lesson morbidity for symptomatic patients (Bannister and Mathias, 1988).

PATHOPHYSIOLOGY

Axons

Neural tissue has properties that make it unique in its responses to injury. The cell body, or soma, of peripheral nerves lies either in a ganglion, in sensory or autonomic peripheral nerves, or in the CNS, in motor and other effector neurons. The soma's axon may be as long as 1 m in humans, consequently giving the nerve an enormous surface area relative to the cell body. The distal ends of these cells have specialized structures, such as the synaptic terminal for motor fibers and the pacinian corpuscles for some sensory fibers.

The motor unit consists of the motor neuron soma in the gray matter of the spinal cord or brain stem, its dendrites and long axonal process, the muscle synaptic terminal, and the muscle fibers (extrafusal and intrafusal) themselves. This complex expresses injury as a whole.

Skeletal muscle, like peripheral nerve, is heterogeneous, composed of functionally different fibers most simply classified as type one, or slow-twitch, and type two, or fast-twitch, fibers, each with well-defined biochemical properties. Type one fibers are rich in oxidative metabolism enzymes, and type two fibers utilize anaerobic metabolic pathways. When peripheral nerve is damaged, surviving axons sprout new branches that reinnervate muscle fibers that have lost their nerve supply. The innervation of the individual fiber determines which metabolic type it will be by inducing the appropriate enzyme systems. Under experimental or clinical pathologic conditions producing axonal loss and subsequent reinnervation, the fibers change histochemical type. Determining fiber type grouping is one of the most reliable methods to diagnose an axonal neuropathy.

Myelin

Perhaps an even more intimate relationship than that between motor neuron and muscle exists between the peripheral nerve soma's axon and the supporting Schwann cells that accompany it along its lengthy path to its distal terminus. The Schwann cell, ubiquitous in peripheral nerves, envelops normal axons whether they are myelinated or not. The Schwann cell membrane forms the myelin surrounding peripheral nerve axons, but the fact that every unmyelinated axon carries with it an investiture of Schwann cell membrane portends that the Schwann cell plays a critical role in the maintenance of axons. With injury to the axon, the Schwann cells proliferate and play an important, yet presently inadequately understood, role in axonal regeneration. Although the Schwann cell shares with the CNS's oligodendroglia the function of myelinating axons, Schwann cells' rapid proliferation in axonal injury suggests a role analogous to the astrocytes' when axons are damaged in the CNS.

In pure axonal neuropathies, myelin damage occurs regularly and can range from trivial to profound. Myelin breakdown is a hallmark of Wallerian degeneration and occurs in classic axonal trauma, with the proliferating Schwann cells assuming a phagocytic role. In the less frequently seen predominantly demyelinating neuropathies, such as the Landry-Guillain-Barré-Strohl syndrome, the axon survives relatively unscathed, with symptomatology resulting from physiologic alterations in nerve conduction induced by segmental demyelination.

As opposed to axonal loss, which produces denervation, the pathophysiologic hallmark of demyelinating neuropathy is nerve-conduction velocity slowing. The deep tendon reflexes require that a synchronous afferent stimulus volley be generated to the motor neuron pool in the CNS. Because of the disturbance of individual fiber conduction velocity resulting from segmental myelin loss, the deep tendon reflexes are lost early in demyelinating neuropathies. Nerve conduction studies using conventional electrophysiologic technique are affected relatively early compared with the predominantly axonal neuropathies, in which muscle wasting can be profound without significant loss of deep tendon reflexes or decrease in nerve conduction velocity.

A late component of the compound muscle action potential is the F-wave, which is particularly useful in the neurophysiologic evaluation of demyelinating neuropathy. These are formed by an antidromic depolarization volley conducted along motor axons from the distal stimulus site toward the motor neuron pool in the spinal cord. The volley depolarizes a few motor neurons, which send an orthodromic volley down the same nerve, producing the F-wave, which always has a greater latency than the much larger compound action potential of the muscle caused by the initial orthodromic depolarization volley. Because the F-wave response reflects proximal as well as distal nerve conduction, the study is more sensitive in assessing neuropathies predominantly affecting proximal conduction velocity, such as in the Landry-Guillain-Barré-Strohl syndrome.

Axonal Transport

Protein synthesis in neurons resides in the perikaryon of the soma. The axon, unlike the soma, is virtually devoid of protein-synthesizing organelles; its volume, however, may be 1000-fold greater than that of its soma (Griffin and Watson, 1988). To what extent the Schwann cell serves to supplement the soma in maintaining the axon is uncertain, but the neuronal cell body's rich endowment of endoplasmic reticulum, as well as overwhelming experimental evidence, demonstrates that the nerve cell body plays the critical role, synthesizing proteins vital for the maintenance of its synaptic terminal or for specialized sensory receptor organs as diverse as the Golgi-Mazzoni corpuscles, involved in tactile sensation, and the muscle spindle axons providing the afferent limb of the stretch reflex.

Since the nineteenth century experiments of Augustus Waller (1852), it has been known that the axonal segment distal to a transection quickly degenerates, whereas the proximal segment, with its connection to the soma intact, survives and proliferates axonal sprouts essential to regeneration. The neuron's cell body synthesizes structural components, enzymes, and trophic factors critical for regenerative sprouting of axons when they are injured.

The soma, removed from the distal axon terminal by as much as 1 m, must have an elaborate transportation mechanism to communicate with its distant end. Multiple transport systems have been identified in the axon, with flow occurring in both the anterograde (away from the soma) and retrograde (toward the soma) directions. The axonal cytoskeleton's neurofilaments and microtubules form an important component of this vehicle for moving proteins, portions of membrane, and transmitters to and from the neuronal perikaryon to the periphery. Retrograde transport plays a critical role in maintaining the distal axon by continuously returning portions of neural membrane for recycling by the soma's synthetic apparatus, an economizing adaptation. The fast anterograde transport system and retrograde transport are intimately related, and most investigators believe they represent a single looping conveyance. Through retrograde transport from the distal axon terminus, viruses such as herpes simplex and rabies and noxious substances such as tetanus toxin and doxorubicin (Adriamycin) (Yamamoto et al., 1984) can gain access to the cell body.

Peripheral nerves have a limited number of ways of responding to injury, and, without doubt, insults can layer upon the vulnerable neuron, as in the well-known example of diabetics being highly susceptible to compressive neuropathies. Patients already compromised by peripheral neuropathy seem more susceptible to injury from neurotoxic agents. Even agents not commonly associated with causing neuropathic disease can act to potentiate neuropathy, as with the enhancement of vincristine neuropathy by the epipodophyllotoxins (Griffiths et al., 1986). Patients with dietary deficiency or diabetes and chemotherapeutic intoxication almost certainly express more severe neuropathic changes than do patients with any of these single insults alone.

CLINICAL SYNDROMES

The neuropathies associated with cancer have diverse etiologies and presentations. This section discusses the iatrogenic neuropathies associated with chemotherapy agents and the neuropathies associated with paraproteinemias. The paraneoplastic neuropathies are discussed in Chapter 19. Plexopathy resulting from tumor infiltration and irradiation are discussed in the next section.

Neuropathy Associated with Paraproteins

Paraproteinemia such as that occurring in multiple myeloma, Waldenstrom's macroglobulinemia, plasmacytoma, or lymphoproliferative disorders (in particular B-cell lymphoma, Hodgkin's disease, and angiofollicular hyperplasia) causes peripheral neuropathy with at least five distinct patterns (Table 17–2) (Gherardi et al., 1988). As with other paraneoplastic disorders, clinical recognition is critical,

Table 17–2. Neuropathic Manifestations of Paraproteins

IgM-associated chronic demyelinating sensorimotor polyneuropathy
IgG- or IgA-associated chronic and predominately demyelinating sensorimotor polyradiculoneuropathy
Amyloidosis neuropathy
Cryoglobulin neuropathy
Motor neuronopathy

as these neuropathies may be the presentation of a malignancy. The paraprotein-associated neuropathies are not uncommon disorders and may accompany the monoclonal gammopathy of uncertain significance syndrome. Monoclonal gammopathy of uncertain significance syndromes usually have a benign course, but in one study (Back et al., 1993) of 35 of these syndromes, 14% of patients evaluated over a 4-year period developed myeloma. In addition to the presence of bone lesions and myeloma protein levels (Dimopoulos et al., 1992), elevated levels of serum α_2-microglobins, neopterin, and interleukin-6 (Nachbaur et al., 1991) and circulating CD 38-lymphocyte percentages (Boccadoro et al., 1991) all have prognostic value.

The most common clinical pattern is a chronic demyelinating neuropathy, resembling a less severe form of chronic inflammatory demyelinating polyradiculoneuropathy (Simmons et al., 1993). Patients most frequently complain of appendicular ataxia and tremor but may have sensory or autonomic symptoms predominating early. IgM paraproteins with kappa light chains are most commonly expressed in these patients. An antimyelin-associated glycoprotein antibody has been implicated in the pathogenesis in some, but not all, cases (Latov et al., 1988; Nobile-Orazio et al., 1987; Pestronk et al., 1991) and may help make the diagnosis.

A second pattern of paraprotein neuropathy, a sensorimotor polyradiculoneuropathy, may be associated with the polyneuropathy, organomegaly (chiefly hepatic), endocrinopathy, serum myeloma protein, and skin changes (the POEMS, or Crow-Fukase, syndrome). IgG or IgA myeloma proteins with lambda light chains predominate in these patients. The cerebrospinal fluid may show a modest pleocytosis and elevated protein levels. Patients with POEMS syndrome have a demyelinating neuropathy associated with atrophic testes and gynecomastia as well as skin hyperpigmentation, hypertrichosis, and clubbing of the fingers and toes. For both of these paraprotein neuropathies, the neurophysiologic evaluation may strongly suggest the diagnosis: Nerve conduction velocities are greatly reduced, and there may be evidence of conduction block (Bleasel et al., 1993). Treatment may improve symptoms, particularly when the cause of the gammopathy is a solitary plasmacytoma.

Cryoglobulinemia is associated with an asymmetric, and often painful, axonal neuropathy; with exposure to cold, symptoms generally are increased. The IgM from these patients binds to a sulfated glycosphingolipid, sulfated glucuronic acid paragloboside, with the greatest binding affinity at 4°C (McGinnis et al., 1988), which explains the cold sensitivity of the symptoms. Neuropathy from cryoglobulins arises from two pathogenetic mechanisms. Distal cold-sensitive symptoms are caused by sludging of flow in the vasonervosum, whereas patients may develop mononeuritis multiplex from cryoglobulin-induced vasculitis (Garcia-Bragado et al., 1988). Rapid improvement of symptoms can be achieved with plasmapheresis (Bussel, 1993), but therapy directed at the source of the paraprotein is critical to long-term disease control.

Amyloid neuropathy occurs infrequently in patients with paraproteins. In the characteristic clinical picture, small fiber function bears the brunt of the insult. Presenting symptoms often consist of dysautonomia and dysesthetic pain (Tada et al., 1993; Zanusso et al., 1992) along with those typical of sensorimotor neuropathy. Peripheral nerve entrapments, especially of the median nerve at the carpal tunnel, are common in amyloid neuropathy. Unlike most neuropathic processes, proximal signs and symptoms may dominate the clinical presentation (Li et al., 1992). Unlike other paraprotein neuropathies, plasmapheresis does not reverse symptoms, although aggressive therapy of the primary disease should be undertaken.

A relatively pure motor neuropathy, distinguishable from amyotrophic lateral sclerosis by less prominent upper motor neuron or bulbar signs and a more indolent course, can be seen in rare cases in patients with paraproteinemia. The onset may be asymmetric, with cramping as an early sign. Neurophysiologic testing will demonstrate overt denervation of affected muscles, and, despite a lack of sensory symptoms, there may be slowing of sensory nerve conduction velocity (Bady et al., 1988). Nerve biopsy can help confirm the diagnosis, and immunohistochemical and ultrastructural techniques can demonstrate paraproteins deposited within nerve. As has been shown for the other paraprotein-mediated neuropathies, plasma exchange and treatment of the underlying disease may improve symptoms.

Overlap occurs in the paraneoplastic syndromes, and these areas are yet incompletely defined. In a large series of patients from India with cancer who were minimally treated or untreated with chemotherapy, approximately one-third had a neuromuscular syndrome with both neuropathic and myopathic features (Paul et al., 1978). Many patients with advanced (or rapidly advancing) tumors develop a muscle wasting–cachexia syndrome without clear cause. This syndrome likely has multiple etiologies, including malnutrition and circulating factors such as cytokines that affect metabolism.

Iatrogenic Neuropathies

Many chemotherapy agents can cause peripheral neuropathy. Table 17–3 lists agents used by cancer patients that can cause neuropathy; however, most of these infrequently cause symptomatic toxicity and are clinically important chiefly as their effects may be additive. The most common iatrogenic neuropathies occurring in cancer patients are those due to vinca and platinum compounds. Neuropathy from paclitaxel (Taxol) and its relatives has already become a concern. These agents offer unique advantages to the modern chemotherapeutic armamentarium, and understanding the natural history, pathogenesis, and therapy of the toxic neuropathies they produce will optimize their clinical use. Animal studies of nerve toxicology have come largely from the agriculture industry (chickens seem particularly susceptible [Moretto et al., 1991; Johnson et al., 1988; Anderson et al., 1988]) or the military (Egan al., 1980). Only recently have these techniques been widely applied to chemotherapeutic agents (Apfel et al., 1992). Despite the difficulties in the design of animal studies posed by oncologic therapy (Bradley, 1970), consideration of both clinical and experimental studies can be expected to improve patient care.

Table 17–3. Chemotherapy Drugs Associated with Peripheral Neuropathy

Vinca alkaloids (vincristine, vindesine, vinblastine)
Platinum compounds (cisplatin, carboplatin, iproplatin, ormaplatin)
Taxanes (paclitaxel, docetaxel)
Podophyllotoxins (etoposide, teniposide)
Azacytidine
Cytarabine
Bleomycin
Dapsone
Doxorubicin
Ethambutol
Fludarabine
Altretamine (hexamethylmelamine)
Isoniazid
Nitroimidazoles (metronidazole, misonidazole)
Phenytoin
Procarbazine
Pyridoxine
Suramin
Thalidomide

Vincristine

Of the Vinca alkaloids, vincristine has greatest use because of its efficacy and relative lack of myelosuppression, cardiac toxicity, or nephrotoxicity, but it is the most neurotoxic. The axonal neuropathy caused by vincristine, while usually recoverable and mild, may produce great morbidity and can limit the drug's use clinically. The earliest symptoms of vincristine neuropathy are usually myalgias, distal parathesiae, and decreases in ankle jerks (Rosenthal and Kaufman, 1974; Bradley et al., 1970b), although jaw pain and cramps and other muscle cramps (Haim et al., 1991) can occur shortly after its administration. The symptoms typically present insidiously, but patients with cranial neuropathies associated with vincristine intoxication often develop symptoms more rapidly. Ptosis and ophthalmoplegia causing visual disturbance may be of such abrupt onset as to mimic a brain stem stroke, particularly if these symptoms are accompanied by nausea and ataxia. Paralysis of the recurrent laryngeal nerve can occur, causing stridor, which reverses upon drug withdrawal (Annino et al., 1992). Symptomatic recovery of vincristine neuropathy may take as long as 40 months (Postma et al., 1993), but usually patients are not seriously affected if the total dose is kept under 12 mg.

The Vinca alkaloids frequently affect small fiber function, producing both painful parathesiae due to

C-fiber dysfunction and dysautonomia. The hemodynamic consequences of autonomic dysfunction appear dose related and consist primarily of orthostatic hypotension (Roca et al., 1985). It is plausible that a component of the syndrome of inappropriate antidiuretic hormone seen with vincristine stems from altered autonomic function. Other phenomena in patients affected by vincristine dysautonomia include reduced gastrointestinal motility, abdominal colic, impotence, and urinary retention (Legha, 1986). Abnormal cardiovascular reflexes are common in patients undergoing vincristine therapy (Hirvonen et al., 1989). Great care must be exercised when prescribing tricyclic antidepressants, neuroleptics, and diuretics, as these may worsen autonomic function.

Older patients are at greatest risk for developing symptomatic vincristine neuropathy, and individual doses higher than 2 mg are less well tolerated (Roca et al., 1985). How much pre-existing neuropathic conditions contribute to the severity of vincristine's neurotoxicity is hard to know with certainty, but evidence exists that severe vincristine neuropathy occurs in patients with the Landry-Guillain-Barré-Strohl syndrome (Norman et al., 1987), Charcot-Marie-Tooth disease (McGuire et al., 1989), or hepatic failure or in those who received concomitant isoniazid (Roca et al., 1985) or teniposide therapy (Yamamoto et al., 1984).

The Vinca alkaloids poison microtubules by interacting with the microtubular protein tubulin (Green et al., 1977), thereby inhibiting the mitotic spindle movements necessary for cellular reproduction. In vivo experiments have clearly demonstrated disruption of both neurofilament and microtubular physiology within hours of nerve exposure to vincristine (Sahenk et al., 1987). Given nature's parsimony, the microtubular system of peripheral nerve, essential to axonal transport, suffers injury from vincristine as an innocent bystander. The pace of the insult suffered by nerve has an important role in the expression of neuropathy. Unfortunately, no experimental studies for vincristine have been designed to determine optimal dose schedules to minimize neuropathic changes.

Taxanes

Recently two taxanes, paclitaxel (Taxol) and docetaxel (Taxotere), have been introduced for cancer chemotherapy. Like the Vinca alkaloids, the taxanes are plant-derived poisons of the mitotic spindle apparatus. In contradistinction to the Vinca drugs, the taxanes cause microtubular aggregation (Pazdur et al., 1993). Paclitaxel at doses of 200 mg/m^2 produces a mild to moderate sensorimotor neuropathy in most patients, but at higher doses the neuropathy can be severe (Rowinsky et al., 1993a,b). Severe orthostatic hypotension from autonomic neuropathy has occurred at this dose range (Jerian et al., 1993). When paclitaxel was combined with cisplatin in a careful study of patients with ovarian cancer, 95% developed dose-related sensorimotor axonal polyneuropathy (Chaudhry et al., 1994). Patients with pre-existing neuropathy were at greatest risk. In our experience, docetaxel may be less neurotoxic than paclitaxel. We, like others (Lipton et al., 1989), have found that sensory symptoms predominate early in taxane neuropathy.

Cisplatin

Cisplatin causes a peripheral neuropathy that was initially reported only in those patients receiving high doses of the drug. The minimal dose found to cause neuropathy progressively decreased as experience with the agent increased. The success of cisplatin in the therapy of certain solid tumors prompted the development of the related compounds iproplatin, ormaplatin, and carboplatin. Although there is less clinical experience with these drugs (van Glabbeke et al., 1988; Schilder et al., 1994), it is clear that carboplatin produces the least degree of neurotoxicity.

Sensory symptoms predominate early in the course of cisplatin neuropathy, with patients most frequently noting distal paresthesiae. Studies including detailed clinical and neurophysiologic testing found that symptoms of neuropathy were common at cumulative doses of approximately 300 mg/m^2 and virtually universal at cumulative doses of greater than 500 mg/m^2 (Roelofs et al., 1984; Thompson, 1984; van der Hoop et al., 1990). In these studies, the earliest clinical sign of cisplatin neuropathy was decreased vibratory sense, with diminished ankle jerks following shortly thereafter. Patients may infrequently experience dysesthetic pain, which may occur late in the course of their peripheral neuropathy or even during recovery. More severe sensory disturbances result in sensory ataxia and can be debilitating. Signs and symptoms of peripheral neuropathy commonly worsen for as long as 6 months following treatment cessation (LoMonaco et al., 1992; Hovestadt et al., 1992). They significantly improve at 12 months, with continued gradual improvement occurring for as long as 48 months (Ostchega et al., 1988). The theoretical concern that cisplatin neurotoxicity may be irreversible (Krarup-Hansen et al., 1993) has not proved true for the majority of patients despite the fact that platinum concentrates in dorsal root ganglia and its level in neural tissue diminishes little with time (Gregg et al., 1992).

Lhermitte's sign, in which patients complain of electric shock sensations on neck flexion, occurs in patients with platinum neuropathy (Inbar et al., 1992) and is believed to be due to myelin loss in the dorsal columns, similar to that occurring in multiple sclerosis or radiation myelopathy. Scant pathologic evidence exists to support this contention, however. The concomitant marked proprioceptive loss observed in these cases (Dewar et al., 1986) suggests involvement of either posterior columns or large fibers, consistent with the finding that somatosensory evoked potentials are the most sensitive physiologic means of detecting cisplatin changes (Boogerd et al., 1990). Development of Lhermitte's sign may be delayed for as long as 5 months following cisplatin treatment. Cautious therapy may be continued without adverse side effects even after patients demonstrate Lhermitte's sign (Siegal and Haim, 1990). Clinicians should bear in mind, however, that a case has been reported (List and Kummet, 1990) of cervical myelopathy following cisplatin and etoposide chemotherapy of small cell lung cancer. The myelopathy affected cervical dorsal columns and sensory and motor neurons but not pyramidal tracts and was heralded by Lhermitte's sign.

Motor symptoms have been reported far less frequently than for vincristine neuropathy. Weakness with electrophysiologic evidence of denervation may be found later in the clinical course; cramps, however, are not rare (Siegal and Haim, 1990) and may be present early. Even more than with vincristine neuropathy, motor deficits contribute less to the incapacitation of patients than do sensory ataxia. Patients with early objective severe weakness should be evaluated for other causes, such as thiamine and B_{12} deficiency, paraprotein neuropathy, and thyroid disorders.

In the early studies of platinum neuropathy, the autonomic nervous system was thought to be spared injury. Autonomic symptoms may be overlooked or may be mistakenly considered due to other causes (Rosenfeld and Broder, 1984). While not as prominently in patients undergoing treatment with the Vinca alkaloids or taxanes, autonomic dysfunction does occur in cisplatin neurotoxicity (Boogerd et al., 1990) and particularly affects cardiovascular reflexes. This is especially important given the marked emetogenic nature of platinum chemotherapy, which increases the risk for orthostatic hypotension because of the synergistic effects of hypovolemia, anticholinergic therapy, and vagal stimulation.

Risk factors for developing platinum neuropathy include pre-existing neuropathy, but it is uncertain whether patient age, history of alcohol use, or diabetes mellitus increases risk (Mollman et al., 1988). Increased age positively correlated with the severity of neuropathy symptoms in one series (Ostchega et al., 1988; Pirovano et al., 1992), and diabetes mellitus has been found to be a risk factor in another (Rowinsky et al., 1993b). The dosage schedule may play a critical role; dosing schemes that use more frequent schedules or continuous infusion cause less neuropathy for a given dose than schedules that use a high-dose bolus of cisplatin (Cavaletti et al., 1992; Sebille et al., 1990).

Low serum magnesium levels may be a risk factor for cisplatin neuropathy. In a prospective study, 54% of patients developed clinically evident peripheral neuropathy, and a significant association between the development of hypomagnesemia and neuropathy was observed (Ashraf et al., 1983). In this study, 71% of patients given 50 to 100 mg/m^2 of cisplatin with a saline diuresis on an every-4-week basis, alone or in combination with cyclophosphamide, bleomycin, and doxorubicin, developed hypomagnesemia (serum magnesium less than 1.5 mEq/L) during the course of their therapy. Hypomagnesemic patients received significantly higher doses of cisplatin, weighed more, and had greater body surface area than patients who maintained normal serum magnesium levels. In this series, none of the normomagnesemic patients developed peripheral neuropathy, whereas 75% of the patients with hypomagnesemia did. Another study of 12 patients noted hypomagnesemia in 63% of their chemotherapy cycles. Six of these patients developed clinically significant peripheral neuropathy, and five patients had ototoxicity (Trump and Hortvet, 1985). Whether maintaining normal serum magnesium levels in patients during treatment lessens peripheral neuropathy is unknown.

How cisplatin, whose presumed mechanism of action is through impairing DNA synthesis, causes damage to nonmitotic peripheral nerve remains unknown, but damage likely results from cisplatin's deleterious effects on the synthetic mechanisms of the axonal perikaryon. Platinum comes from the same elemental family of the heavy metal neurotoxins arsenic and lead, sharing with them a propensity to concentrate in nervous system tissue. The prominence of sensory signs and symptoms reflects the vulnerability of the dorsal root ganglion, site of the sensory axon's soma, which bears the brunt of injury from cisplatin (Krarup-Hansen et al., 1993). In an important autopsy study (Gregg et al., 1992) of 21 patients who had been treated with cisplatin, elemental platinum was found in highest concentration in the dorsal root ganglion, which lies outside the blood–brain barrier. Platinum concentration directly correlated with cumulative dose and did not appear to diminish over time. This study argues for setting a limit to the amount of cisplatin that can be safely used, much like the therapeutic limits set for doxorubicin and irradiation.

TREATMENT OF NEUROPATHIES

Limit Exposure

The best treatment of iatrogenic neuropathy is avoidance. Once the neuropathy has become symptomatic, the clinician must decide whether to continue therapy and risk a debilitating toxicity or switch to a less neuropathic program. Measures to control neuropathic pain with low-dose tricyclic antidepressants (amitriptyline, desipramine, or doxepin) helps many patients. The tricyclics should be used at the lowest possible effective dose; for some patients 10 mg of amitriptyline before sleep will suffice.

Gabapentin, developed as an adjuvant anticonvulsant, has probably found more use as a remedy for neuropathic pain. Although it is significantly more expensive than amitriptyline (Morello et al., 1999), gabapentin has a more favorable toxicity profile (Rosner et al., 1996). The effective dose from most studies is between 900 and 1500 mg per day in three divided doses; significant benefit can be gained with much lower doses. Patients, particularly the elderly, should be started at a dose of 100 mg three times a day with the dose gradually advanced until an acceptable benefit is achieved.

Narcotics are sometimes needed as well. Braces, splints, walkers, household aids, and the benefits of physical and occupational therapy to neuropathy patients should not be discounted (O'Connell and Levinson, 1991). A healthy and varied diet, rich in the B, C, and E vitamins, should be encouraged whenever possible, as this general health measure will speed recovery.

Neuroprotection

Efforts to protect peripheral nerves from chemotherapy toxicity may permit use of higher doses of chemotherapy and help to avoid significant treatment-related morbidity. Encouraged by a desire to avoid morbidity and increase the therapeutic margin, particularly for cisplatin, clinicians have attempted many strategies. The hope of application to other neuropathies (particularly diabetic) also motivates interest in neuroprotection from chemotherapeutic agents (de Wied, 1990). Two broad strategies have been adopted: *(1)* efforts to promote peripheral nerve regeneration and *(2)* attempts to block the chemotherapy's noxious effects while not effacing its efficacy as an antineoplastic agent.

The pyrimidine isaxonine (2-[isopropylamino] pyrimidine) enhances the rate of regeneration of peripheral nerve following various experimental axonal injuries, and in one double-blind, controlled study it was demonstrated to decrease vincristine-induced neuropathy (Duhamel and Parlier, 1982). Unfortunately, isaxonine has significant hepatic toxicity, and further clinical studies with it have been stopped (Le Quesne et al., 1985).

A mixture of bovine brain gangliosides has been reported to promote peripheral nerve regeneration, and at least one animal study (Favaro et al., 1988) demonstrated a protective effect for vincristine neuropathy without any loss of antineoplastic efficacy. A human clinical trial of gangliosides (DeAngelis et al., 1991) failed to prevent vincristine-induced neuropathy during intensive chemotherapy for lymphoma. European investigations with diabetic neuropathy are still ongoing, but the drug has not gained wide acceptance.

Peptides derived from the melanocyte-stimulating hormone portion of the adrenocorticotrophic hormone (ACTH) polypeptide have generalized neurotrophic effects, serving to both protect and promote regeneration of neurons during a host of injuries, including the noxious effects of cisplatin (Windebank et al., 1994; Hamers et al., 1991, 1993b; Gispen et al., 1992; de Wied, 1990; Gerritsen van der Hoop et al., 1988), vincristine (Kiburg et al., 1994), and paclitaxel (Hamers et al., 1993c). They may facilitate repair of pre-existing disease as well (Gispen et al., 1992). Early reports of protection with the ACTH-derived peptide ORG 2766 (H-Met[O2]-Glu-His-Phe-D-Lys-Phe-OH) (van Kooten et al., 1992) were promising, but wider enthusiasm was tempered by the drug's parenteral delivery requirement. ORG 2766 may act by promoting reinnervation and thus ought not to interfere with chemotherapeutic antitumor effects; however, for at least two lymphoma cell lines, ORG 2766 has been shown to enhance the tumoricidal effects of vincristine (Kiburg et al., 1994).

A number of neurotrophic factors have been identified and manufactured using recombinant DNA technology, which has opened new horizons of therapy for central as well as peripheral nervous system diseases (Cuello, 1989). These factors, which have been characterized in recent years and which are increasing in numbers, selectively stimulate different subsets of neurons, share effector pathways, and overlap in function. Identified factors with neurotrophic activity include nerve growth factor, ciliary neurotrophic factor, brain-derived neurotrophic factor, neurotrophin 3 and neurotrophin 4/5 (Wong et al., 1993), interleukins 6 and 11, oncostatin M (Boulton et al., 1994; Yang, 1993), leukemia inhibitory factor (Thaler et al., 1994), fibroblast growth factor-5, and insulin-like growth factor-1 (Apfel et al., 1993; Hughes et al., 1993). Other trophic factors are being uncovered.

Nerve growth factor selectively promotes growth of sensory neurons and has experimentally protected against the development of cisplatin (Apfel et al., 1992) and paclitaxel (Apfel et al., 1991) neurotoxicity. This benefit has not been observed in all experimental model systems (Windebank et al., 1994). Ciliary neurotrophic factor is critical to sympathetic neuron survival (Burnham et al., 1994) and is one of a host of factors that support motor neurons (Hughes et al., 1993). Clinical trials with ciliary neurotrophic factor have been undertaken for motor neuron disease. Given the complexity of interactions between these growth factors and their functional overlap with cytokines, mixtures of the agents or pharmacologic manipulation of their peptide structures may eventually permit the development of neurologic tonics that can protect peripheral nerves from toxic injury and possibly promote recovery once damage has occurred.

The thiols have well-established neuroprotective qualities due to their ability to stabilize both DNA and proteins and act as antioxidants (Yim et al., 1994). A number of thiol compounds have been considered as antidotes for chemotherapy toxicity, including glutathione, diethylthiolcarbamate, metallothionein, alpha lipoic acid, and amifostine (S-2-[3-aminopropylamino]ethyl phosphorothioic acid) (Treskes and van der Vijgh, 1993). Reduced glutathione has been shown to prevent cisplatin toxicity in at least three European clinical trials (Hamers et al., 1993a; Bogliun et al., 1992; Pirovano et al., 1992), but, as with all thiol compounds, concerns have been raised that the tumor may be protected from the effects of the treatment as well.

Amifostine (WR 2721, ethiofos) may preferentially protect healthy tissues (Bergstrom et al., 1999), and clinical investigation with this compound has accelerated. Inactive in its native form, amifostine must be dephosphorylated into an active thiol compound to produce its beneficial effects. Healthy, as opposed to tumor, cells dephosphorylate the drug more efficiently (Treskes et al 1992a,b), affording a potential therapeutic advantage. An experimental trial (Treskes et al., 1994) of carboplatin toxicity modulation using amifostine demonstrated myeloprotection and actual potentiation of carboplatin's tumoricidal effects.

In an important early study (Mollman et al., 1988) of neuropathy protection, 69 patients received six different chemotherapy programs, including cisplatin, with 28 patients also receiving amifostine. The patients given amifostine developed less neuropathy, but all the patients except two, who were not given the antioxidant, were given regimens consisting of other chemotherapeutic agents. In this study, tumor control was decreased for the amifostine group. Nineteen percent of the patients who did not receive the radioprotector died, whereas more than 54% died in the group that received amifostine. A phase I clinical trial found toxicities to include hypotension, anaphylaxis, and hypocalcemia (Wadler et al., 1993). Numerous subsequent studies have demonstrated that amifostine provided hematologic, renal, and, to a lesser extent, neuroprotection from platinum intoxication.

Alpha lipoic acid (2-dithiolane-3 pentanoic acid; 1,2-dithiolane-3 valeric acid; thioctic acid) is a naturally occurring disulfide catalyst important in pyruvate metabolism (Reed et al., 1951), which has both antioxidant and chelating benefits. It has proved effective in human diabetic neuropathy trials (Ziegler et al., 1999) and in experimental lead intoxication (Gurer et al., 1999) in doses that should be well tolerated in humans. Because of its chelating effects, it may prove therapeutic for established heavy metal neuropathy such as that caused by cisplatin.

Nimodipine, a calcium channel blocker, was shown to protect rats against peripheral neuropathy from cisplatin (Hamers et al., 1991). The possibility that calcium channel drugs may block the multidrug resistance gene enough to improve chemotherapy efficacy (Pasman and Schouten, 1993; Lum et al., 1993) makes this strategy of neuropathy prevention particularly worthy of pursuit for xenobiotic neurotoxins such as the Vinca alkaloids and the taxanes, which are influenced by this gene. Hypotension limits the use of presently available drugs, but, fortuitously, some calcium channel blocker enantiomers lose blocking ability without any loss of multidrug resistance gene inhibition (Hollt et al., 1992), perhaps permitting development of more specific therapeutic agents.

The ototoxicity and optic neuropathy seen with platinum therapy are not, strictly speaking, peripheral neuropathies, affecting specialized sensory end organ systems. Optic neuropathy or retinopathy is rare unless the platinum is given intra-arterially. In a prospective study of six patients with malignant glioma treated with intra-arterial cisplatin, five patients developed progressive optic neurotoxicity (Maiese et al., 1992). Ototoxicity from platinum is common and can result in severe tinnitus. Risk factors include reduced serum albumin and hemoglobin levels and dark eye color (Barr-Hamilton et al., 1991). Cisplatin, in an experimental model (Delb et al., 1993), was ninefold more ototoxic than carboplatin, paralleling their relative peripheral neurotoxicities. Efforts to abrogate ototoxicity with amifostine have not, however, been encouraging (Markman et al., 1991; Planting et al., 1999).

Study of specialized sensory neurotoxic effects, along with the hypophyseal dysfunction due to cisplatin therapy, may provide clues to the etiology of the more widespread and troubling side effects of peripheral neuropathy. Similarly, careful study of the neuropathies caused by oncologic neurotoxins can yield clues to the pathogenesis and treatment of other neurologic disorders that remain shrouded in mystery.

REFERENCES

Anderson RJ, Robertson DG, Henderson JD, Wilson BW. 1988. DFP-induced elevation of strength–duration threshold in hen peripheral nerve. Neurotoxicology 9:47–52.

Annino DJ Jr, MacArthur CJ, Friedman EM. 1992. Vincristine-induced recurrent laryngeal nerve paralysis. Laryngoscope 102:1260–1262.

Apfel SC, Arezzo JC, Lewis ME , Kessler JA. 1993. The use of insulin-like growth factor I in the prevention of vincristine neuropathy in mice. Ann N Y Acad Sci 692:243–245.

Apfel SC, Arezzo JC, Lipson L , Kessler JA. 1992. Nerve growth factor prevents experimental cisplatin neuropathy. Ann Neurol 31:76–80.

Apfel SC, Lipton RB, Arezzo JC, Kessler JA.1991. Nerve growth factor prevents toxic neuropathy in mice. Ann Neurol 29:87–90.

Ashraf M, Scothel PL, Krall JM, Flink EB. 1983. Cis-platinum–induced hypomagnesemia and peripheral neuropathy. Gynecol Oncol 16:309–318.

Back H, Jagenburg R, Rodjer S, Westin J. 1993. Serum deoxythymidine kinase: no help in the diagnosis and prognosis of monoclonal gammopathy. Br J Haematol 84:746–748.

Bady B, Vial C, Brudon F, Lapras J, Kopp N, Trillet M.1988. [Peripheral neuropathies simulating amyotrophic lateral sclerosis in gammopathies]. Rev Neurol (Paris) 144: 710–715.

Bannister R, Mathias C. 1988. Testing autonomic reflexes. In: Bannister R (ed), Autonomic Failure: A Textbook of Clinical Disorders of the Autonomic Nervous System. Oxford: Oxford University Press, pp 289–307.

Barr-Hamilton RM, Matheson LM, Keay DG. 1991. Ototoxicity of cis-platinum and its relationship to eye colour. J Laryngol Otol 105:7–11.

Bergstrom P, Johnsson A, Bergenheim T, Henriksson R. 1999. Effects of amifostine on cisplatin induced DNA adduct formation and toxicity in malignant glioma and normal tissues in rat. J Neurooncol 42:13–21.

Bertelsmann FW, Heimans JJ, Weber EJ, van der Veen EA, Schouten JA.1985. Thermal discrimination thresholds in normal subjects and in patients with diabetic neuropathy. J Neurol Neurosurg Psychiatry 48:686–690.

Bleasel AF, Hawke SH, Pollard JD, McLeod JG. 1993. IgG monoclonal paraproteinaemia and peripheral neuropathy. Neurol Neurosurg Psychiatry 56:52–57.

Boccadoro M, Battaglio S, Omede P, et al. 1991. Increased serum neopterin concentration as indicator of disease severity and poor survival in multiple myeloma. Eur J Haematol 47:305–309.

Bogliun G, Marzorati L, Cavaletti G, Frattola L. 1992. Evaluation by somatosensory evoked potentials of the neurotoxicity of cisplatin alone or in combination with glutathione. Ital J Neurol Sci 13:643–647.

Boogerd W, ten Bokkel Huinink WW, Dalesio O, Hoppenbrouwers WJ, van der Sande JJ. 1990. Cisplatin induced neuropathy: central, peripheral and autonomic nerve involvement. J Neurooncol 9:255–263.

Boulton TG, Stahl N, Yancopoulos GD. 1994. Ciliary neurotrophic factor/leukemia inhibitory factor/interleukin 6/oncostatin M family of cytokines induces tyrosine phosphorylation of a common set of proteins overlapping those induced by other cytokines and growth factors. J Biol Chem 269:11648–11655.

Bradley WG. 1970. The neuromyopathy of vincristine in the guinea pig. An electrophysiologic and pathological study. J Neurol Sci 10:133–162.

Bradley WG, Lassman LP, Pearce GW, Walton JN. 1970. The neuromyopathy of vincristine in man. Clinical, electrophysiological and pathologic studies. J Neurol Sci 10: 107–131.

Burnham P, Louis JC, Magal E, Varon S. 1994. Effects of ciliary neurotrophic factor on the survival and response to nerve growth factor of cultured rat sympathetic neurons. Dev Biol 161:96–106.

Bussel A. 1993. [Indications of plasma extraction during the treatment of monoclonal gammopathies]. Rev Prat 43: 326–329.

Cavaletti G, Marzorati L, Bogliun G, et al. 1992. Cisplatin-induced peripheral neurotoxicity is dependent on total-dose intensity and single-dose intensity. Cancer 69:203–207.

Chaudhry V, Rowinsky EK, Sartorius SE, Donehower RC, Cornblath DR. 1994. Peripheral neuropathy from taxol and cisplatin combination chemotherapy: clinical and electrophysiological studies. Ann Neurol 35:304–311.

Cuello AC. 1989. Towards trophic factor pharmacology? Neurobiol Aging 10:539–540.

DeAngelis LM, Gnecco C, Taylor L, Warrell RP Jr. 1991). Evolution of neuropathy and myopathy during intensive vincristine/corticosteroid chemotherapy for non-Hodgkin's lymphoma. Cancer 67:2241–2246.

Delb W, Feilen S, Koch A, Federspil P. 1993. [Comparative studies of the ototoxicity of cisplatin and carboplatin]. Laryngorhinootologie 72:24–27.

Dewar J, Lunt H, Abernethy DA, Dady P, Haas LF. 1986. Cisplatin neuropathy with Lhermitte's sign. J Neurol Neurosurg Psychiatry 49:96–99.

de Wied D. 1990. Neurotrophic effects of ACTH/MSH neuropeptides. Acta Neurobiol Exp (Warsz) 50:353–366.

Dimopoulos MA, Moulopoulos A, Delasalle K, Alexanian R. 1992. Solitary plasmacytoma of bone and asymptomatic multiple myeloma. Hematol Oncol Clin North Am 6:359–369.

Duhamel G, Parlier Y. 1982. [Protective effect of isaxonine against vincristine-induced neuropathy]. Nouv Presse Med 11:1254–1256.

Egan GF, Lewis SC, Scala RA. 1980. Experimental design for animal toxicity studies. In: Spencer PS (ed), Experimental and Clinical Neurotoxicology, 2nd ed. Baltimore: Williams & Wilkins, pp 708–725.

Favaro G, Di Gregorio F, Panozzo C, Fiori MG. 1988. Ganglioside treatment of vincristine-induced neuropathy. An electrophysiologic study. Toxicology 49:325–329.

Garcia-Bragado F, Fernandez JM, Navarro C, Villar M, Bonaventura I. 1988. Peripheral neuropathy in essential mixed cryoglobulinemia. Arch Neurol 45:1210–1214.

Gerritsen van der Hoop R, de Koning P, Boven E, Neijt JP, Jennekens FG, Gispen WH, et al. 1988. Efficacy of the neuropeptide ORG.2766 in the prevention and treatment of cisplatin-induced neurotoxicity in rats. Eur J Cancer Clin Oncol 24:637–642.

Gherardi R, Zuber M, Viard JP. 1988. [Dysglobulinemic neuropathies]. Rev Neurol (Paris) 144:391–408.

Gispen WH, Hamers FP, Vecht CJ, Jennekens FG, Neyt JP. 1992. ACTH/MSH like peptides in the treatment of cisplatin neuropathy. J Steroid Biochem Mol Biol 43:179–183.

Green LS, Donoso JA, Heller-Bettinger IE, Samson FE. 1977. Axonal transport disturbances in vincristine-induced peripheral neuropathy. Ann Neurol 1:255–262.

Gregg RW, Molepo JM, Monpetit VJ, et al. 1992. Cisplatin neurotoxicity: the relationship between dosage, time, and platinum concentration in neurologic tissues, and morphologic evidence of toxicity. J Clin Oncol 10:795–803.

Griffin JW, Watson DF. 1988. Axonal transport in neurological disease. Ann Neurol 23:3–13.

Griffiths JD, Stark RJ, Ding JC, Cooper IA. 1986. Vincristine neurotoxicity enhanced in combination chemotherapy including both teniposide and vincristine. Cancer Treat Rep 70:519–521.

Gurer H, Ozgunes H, Oztezcan S, Ercal N. 1999. Antioxidant role of alpha-lipoic acid in lead toxicity. Free Rad Biol Med 27:75–81.

Haim N, Barron SA, Robinson E. 1991. Muscle cramps associated with vincristine therapy. Acta Oncol 30:707–711.

Hamers FP, Brakkee JH, Cavalletti E, et al. 1993a. Reduced glutathione protects against cisplatin-induced neurotoxicity in rats. Cancer Res 53:544–549.

Hamers FP, Pette C, Bravenboer B, Vecht CJ, Neijt JP, Gispen WH. 1993b. Cisplatin-induced neuropathy in mature rats: effects of the melanocortin-derived peptide ORG 2766. Cancer Chemother Pharmacol 32:162–166.

Hamers FP, Pette C, Neijt JP, Gispen WH. 1993c. The ACTH-(4-9) analog, ORG 2766, prevents taxol-induced neuropathy in rats. Eur J Pharmacol 233:177–178.

Hamers FP, van der Hoop RG, Steerenburg PA, Neijt JP, Gispen WH. 1991. Putative neurotrophic factors in the protection of cisplatin-induced peripheral neuropathy in rats. Toxicol Appl Pharmacol 111:514–522.

Hanson P, Schumacker P, Debugne T, Clerin M. 1992. Evaluation of somatic and autonomic small fibers neuropathy in diabetes. Am J Phys Med Rehabil 71:44–47.

Hirvonen HE, Salmi TT, Heinonen E, Antila KJ, Valimaki IA. 1989. Vincristine treatment of acute lymphoblastic leukemia induces transient autonomic cardioneuropathy. Cancer 64:801–805.

Hollt V, Kouba M, Dietel M, Vogt G. 1992. Stereoisomers of calcium antagonists which differ markedly in their potencies as calcium blockers are equally effective in modulating drug transport by P-glycoprotein. Biochem Pharmacol 43:2601–2608.

Horiguchi J, Inami Y, Sasaki A, Nishimatsu O, Sikegawa T. 1992. Periodic leg movements in sleep with restless legs syndrome: effect of clonazepam treatment. Jpn J Psychiatry Neurol 46:727–732.

Hovestadt A, van der Burg ME, Verbiest HB, van Putten WL, Vecht CJ. 1992. The course of neuropathy after cessation of cisplatin treatment, combined with Org 2766 or placebo. J Neurol 239:143–146.

Hughes RA, Sendtner M, Thoenen H. 1993. Members of several gene families influence survival of rat motoneurons in vitro and in vivo. J Neurosci Res 36:663–671.

Inbar M, Merimsky O, Wigler N, Chaitchik S. 1992. Cisplatin-related Lhermitte's sign. Anticancer Drugs 3:375–377.

Jerian SM, Sarosy GA, Link CJ Jr, Fingert HJ, Reed E, Kohn EC. 1993. Incapacitating autonomic neuropathy precipitated by taxol. Gynecol Oncol 51:277–280.

Johnson MK, Willems JL, De Bisschop HC, Read DJ, Benschop HP. 1988. High doses of soman protect against organophosphorus-induced delayed polyneuropathy but tabun does not. Toxicol Appl Pharmacol 92:34–41.

Kiburg B, van de Loosdrecht AA, Schweitzer KM, et al. 1994. Effects of the ACTH(4-9) analogue, ORG 2766, on vincristine cytotoxicity in two human lymphoma cell lines, U937 and U715. Br J Cancer 69:497–501.

Krarup-Hansen A, Fugleholm K, Helweg-Larsen S, et al. 1993. Examination of distal involvement in cisplatin-induced neuropathy in man. An electrophysiological and histological study with particular reference to touch receptor function. Brain 116:1017–1041.

Latov N, Hays AP, Sherman WH. 1988. Peripheral neuropathy and anti-MAG antibodies. Crit Rev Neurobiol 3:301–332.

Legha SS. 1986. Vincristine neurotoxicity. Pathophysiology and management Med Toxicol 1:421–427.

Legha SS, Dimery JW. 1985. High-dose cisplatin administration without hypertonic saline: observation of disabling neurotoxicity. J Clin Oncol 3:1373–1378.

Le Quesne PM, Fowler CJ, Harding AE. 1985. A study of the effects of isaxonine on vincristine-induced peripheral neuropathy in man and regeneration following peripheral nerve crush in the rat. J Neurol Neurosurg Psychiatry 48:933–935.

Li K, Kyle RA, Dyck PJ. 1992. Immunohistochemical characterization of amyloid proteins in sural nerves and clinical associations in amyloid neuropathy. Am J Pathol 141: 217–226.

Lipton RB, Apfel SC, Dutcher JP, et al. 1989. Taxol produces a predominantly sensory neuropathy. Neurology 39:368–373.

List AF, Kummet TD. 1990. Spinal cord toxicity complicating treatment with cisplatin and etoposide. Am J Clin Oncol 13:256–258.

LoMonaco M, Milone M, Batocchi AP, Padua L, Restuccia D, Tonali P. 1992. Cisplatin neuropathy: clinical course and neurophysiological findings. J Neurol 239:199–204.

Lum BL, Gosland MP, Kaubisch S, Sikic BI. 1993. Molecular targets in oncology: implications of the multidrug resistance gene. Pharmacotherapy 13:88–109.

Maiese K, Walker RW, Gargan R, Victor JD. 1992. Intra-arterial cisplatin-associated optic and otic toxicity. Arch Neurol 49:83–86.

Markman M, D'Acquisto R, Iannotti N, et al. 1991. Phase-1 trial of high-dose intravenous cisplatin with simultaneous intravenous sodium thiosulfate. J Cancer Res Clin Oncol 117:151–155.

McGinnis S, Kohriyama T, Yu RK, Pesce MA, Latov N. 1988. Antibodies to sulfated glucuronic acid containing glycosphingolipids in neuropathy associated with anti-MAG antibodies and in normal subjects. J Neuroimmunol 17:119–126.

McGuire SA, Gospe SM Jr, Dahl G. 1989. Acute vincristine neurotoxicity in the presence of hereditary motor and sensory neuropathy type I. Med Pediatr Oncol 17:520–523.

Mollman JE, Glover DJ, Hogan WM, Furman RE. 1988. Cisplatin neuropathy. Risk factors, prognosis and protection by WR-2721. Cancer 61:2192–2195.

Morello CM, Leckband SG, Stoner CP, Moorhouse DF, Sahagian GA. 1999. Randomized double-blind study comparing the efficacy of gabapentin with amitriptyline on diabetic peripheral neuropathy pain. Arch Int Med 159:1931–1937.

Moretto A, Capodicasa E, Peraica M, Lotti M. 1991. Age sensitivity to organophosphate-induced delayed polyneuropathy. Biochemical and toxicological studies in developing chicks. Biochem Pharmacol 41:1497–1504.

Nachbaur DM, Herold M, Maneschg A, Huber H, et al. 1991. Serum levels of interleukin-6 in multiple myeloma and other hematological disorders: correlation with disease activity and other prognostic parameters. Ann Hematol 62:54–58.

Nobile-Orazio E, Marmiroli P, Baldini L, et al. 1987. Peripheral neuropathy in macroglobulinemia: incidence and antigen-specificity of M proteins. Neurology 37:1506–1514.

Norman M, Elinder G, Finkel Y. 1987. Vincristine neuropathy and a Guillain-Barre syndrome: a case with acute lymphatic leukemia and quadriparesis. Eur J Haematol 39:75–76.

O'Connell PG, Levinson SF. 1991. Experience with rehabilitation in the acquired immunodeficiency syndrome. Am J Phys Med Rehabil 70:195–200.

Ostchega Y, Donohue M, Fox N. 1988. High-dose cisplatin-related peripheral neuropathy. Cancer Nurs 11:23–32.

Pasman PC, Schouten HC. 1993. Multidrug resistance mediated by P-glycoprotein in haematological malignancies. Neth J Med 42:218–231.

Paul T, Katiyar BC, Misra S, Pant GC. 1978. Carcinomatous neuromuscular syndromes. A clinical and quantitative electrophysiological study. Brain 101:53–63.

Pazdur R, Kudelka AP, Kavanagh JJ, Cohen PR, Raber MN. 1993. The taxoids: paclitaxel (Taxol) and docetaxel (Taxotere). Cancer Treat Rev 19:351–386.

Pestronk A, Li F, Griffin J, et al. 1991. Polyneuropathy syndromes associated with serum antibodies to sulfatide and myelin-associated glycoprotein. Neurology 41:357–362.

Pirovano C, Balzarini A, Bohm S, Oriana S, Spatti GB, Zunino F. 1992. Peripheral neurotoxicity following high-dose cisplatin with glutathione: clinical and neurophysiological assessment. Tumori 78:253–257.

Planting AS, Catimel G, de Mulder PH, et al. 1999. Randomized study of a short course of weekly cisplatin with or without amifostine in advanced head and neck cancer. EORTC Head and Neck Cooperative Group. Ann Oncol 10:693–700.

Postma TJ, Benard BA, Huijgens PC, Ossenkoppele GJ, Heimans JJ, et al. 1993. Long-term effects of vincristine on the peripheral nervous system. J Neurooncol 15:23–27.

Reed LJ, DeBusk BG, Gunsalus IC, et al. 1951. Crystalline alpha-lipoic acid: a catalytic agent associated with pyruvate dehydrogenase. Science 114:93–94.

Roca E, Bruera E, Politi PM, et al. 1985. Vinca alkaloid–induced cardiovascular autonomic neuropathy. Cancer Treat Rep 69:149–151.

Roelofs RI, Hrushesky W, Rogin J, Rosenberg L. 1984. Peripheral sensory neuropathy and cisplatin chemotherapy. Neurology 34:934–938.

Rosenfeld CS, Broder LE. 1984. Cisplatin-induced autonomic neuropathy. Cancer Treat Rep 68:659–660.

Rosenthal S, Kaufman S. 1974. Vincristine neurotoxicity. Ann Intern Med 80:733–737.

Rosner H, Rubin L, Kestenbaum A. 1996. Gabapentin adjunctive therapy in neuropathic pain states. Clin J Pain 12:56–58.

Rowinsky EK, Chaudhry V, Forastiere AA, et al. 1993a. Phase I and pharmacologic study of paclitaxel and cisplatin with granulocyte colony-stimulating factor: neuromuscular toxicity is dose-limiting. J Clin Oncol 11:2010–2020.

Rowinsky EK, Eisenhauer EA, Chaudhry V, Arbuck SG, Donehower RC. 1993b. Clinical toxicities encountered with paclitaxel (Taxol). Semin Oncol 20:1–15.

Rowland LP. 1985. Cramps, spasms and muscle stiffness. Rev Neurol (Paris) 141:261–273.

Sahenk Z, Brady ST, Mendell JR. 1987. Studies on the pathogenesis of vincristine-induced neuropathy. Muscle Nerve 10:80–84.

Schilder RJ, LaCreta FP, Perez RP, et al. 1994. Phase I and pharmacokinetic study of ormaplatin (tetraplatin, NSC 363812) administered on a day 1 and day 8 schedule. Cancer Res 54:709–717.

Sebille A, St-Guily JL, Angelard B, de Stabenrath A. 1990. Low prevalence of cisplatin-induced neuropathy after 4-day continuous infusion in head and neck cancer. Cancer 65:2644–2647.

Siegal T, Haim N. 1990. Cisplatin-induced peripheral neuropathy. Frequent off-therapy deterioration, demyelinating syndromes, and muscle cramps. Cancer 66:1117–1123.

Simmons Z, Albers JW, Bromberg MB, Feldman EL. 1993. Presentation and initial clinical course in patients with chronic inflammatory demyelinating polyradiculoneuropathy: comparison of patients without and with monoclonal gammopathy. Neurology 43:2202–2209.

Tada S, Iida M, Yao T, Kitamoto T, Yao T, Fujishima M. 1993. Intestinal pseudo-obstruction in patients with amyloidosis: clinicopathologic differences between chemical types of amyloid protein. Gut 34:1412–1417.

Teräväinen H, Larsen A. 1977. Some features of the neuromuscular complications of pulmonary carcinoma. Ann Neurol 2:495–502.

Thaler CD, Suhr L, Ip N, Katz DM. 1994. Leukemia inhibitory factor and neurotrophins support overlapping populations of rat nodose sensory neurons in culture. Dev Biol 161:338–344.

Thompson SW, Davis LE, Kornfeld M, Hilgers RD, Standefer JC. 1984. Cisplatin neuropathy. Clinical, electrophysiologic, morphologic, and toxicologic studies. Cancer 54:1269–1275.

Treskes M, Boven E, van de Loosdrecht AA, et al. 1994. Effects of the modulating agent WR2721 on myelotoxicity and antitumour activity in carboplatin-treated mice. Eur J Cancer 30A:183–187.

Treskes M, Nijtmans L, Fichtinger-Schepman AM, van der Vijgh WJ. 1992a. Cytostatic activity of cisplatin in the presence of WR2721 and its thiol metabolite WR1065 in OVCAR-3 human ovarian cancer cells as compared to V79 fibroblasts. Anticancer Res 12:2261–2265.

Treskes M, Nijtmans LG, Fichtinger-Schepman AM, van der Vijgh WJ. 1992b. Effects of the modulating agent WR2721 and its main metabolites on the formation and stability of cisplatin-DNA adducts in vitro in comparison to the effects of thiosulphate and diethyldithiocarbamate. Biochem Pharmacol 43:1013–1019.

Treskes M, van der Vijgh WJ. 1993. WR2721 as a modulator of cisplatin- and carboplatin-induced side effects in comparison with other chemoprotective agents: a molecular approach. Cancer Chemother Pharmacol 33:93–106.

Trump DL, Hortvet L. 1985. Etoposide and very high dose cisplatin: salvage therapy for patients with advanced germ cell neoplasms. Cancer Treat Rep 69:259–261.

van der Hoop GR, van der Burg ME, ten Bokkel Huinink WW, van Houwelingen C, Neijt JP. 1990. Incidence of neuropathy in 395 patients with ovarian cancer treated with or without cisplatin. Cancer 66:1697–1702.

van Glabbeke M, Renard J, Pinedo HM, et al. 1988. Iproplatin and carboplatin induced toxicities: overview of phase II clinical trial conducted by the EORTC Early Clinical Trials Cooperative Group (ECTG). Eur J Cancer Clin Oncol 24:255–262.

van Kooten B, van Diemen HA, Groenhout KM, et al. 1992. A pilot study on the influence of a corticotropin (4-9) analogue on Vinca alkaloid-induced neuropathy. Arch Neurol 49:1027–1031.

Wadler S, Beitler JJ, Rubin JS, et al. 1993. Pilot trial of cisplatin, radiation, and WR2721 in carcinoma of the uterine cervix: a New York Gynecologic Oncology Group study. J Clin Oncol 11:1511–1516.

Waller AV. 1852. A new method for the study of the nervous system. Lond J Med 43:609–625.

Walters AS, Hening WA, Kavey N, Chokroverty S, Gidro-Frank S. 1988. A double-blind randomized crossover trial of bromocriptine and placebo in restless legs syndrome. Ann Neurol 24:455–458.

Walters AS, Wagner ML, Hening WA, et al. 1993. Successful treatment of the idiopathic restless legs syndrome in a randomized double-blind trial of oxycodone versus placebo. Sleep 16:327–332.

Walton T, Kolb KW. 1991. Treatment of nocturnal leg cramps and restless leg syndrome. Clin Pharm 10:427–428.

Wieman TJ, Huang KC, Tsueda K, Thomas MH, Lucas LF, Simpson P. 1989. Peripheral somatic sensory neuropathy and skin galvanic response in the feet of patients with diabetes. Surg Gynecol Obstet 168:501–506.

Windebank AJ, Smith AG, Russell JW. 1994. The effect of nerve growth factor, ciliary neurotrophic factor, and ACTH analogs on cisplatin neurotoxicity in vitro. Neurology 44:488–494.

Wong V, Arriaga R, Ip NY, Lindsay RM. 1993. The neurotrophins BDNF, NT-3 and NT-4/5, but not NGF, up-regulate the cholinergic phenotype of developing motor neurons. Eur J Neurosci 5:466–474.

Yamamoto T, Iwasaki Y, Konno H. 1984. Retrograde axoplasmic transport of adriamycin: an experimental form of motor neuron disease? Neurology 34:1299–1304.

Yang YC. 1993. Interleukin 11: an overview. Stem Cells 11:474–486.

Yim MB, Chae HZ, Rhee SG, Chock PB, Stadtman ER. 1994. On the protective mechanism of the thiol-specific antioxidant enzyme against the oxidative damage of biomacromolecules. J Biol Chem 269:1621–1626.

Zanusso GL, Moretto G, Bonetti B, Monaco S, Rizzuto N. 1992. Complement neoantigen and vitronectin are components of plaques in amyloid AL neuropathy. Ital J Neurol Sci 13:493–499.

Ziegler D, Hanefeld M, Ruhnau KJ, et al. 1999. Treatment of symptomatic diabetic polyneuropathy with the antioxidant alpha-lipoic acid: a 7-month multicenter randomized controlled trial (ALADIN III Study). ALADIN III Study Group. Alpha-Lipoic Acid in Diabetic Neuropathy. Diabetes Care 22:1296–1301.

18

Plexopathies

KURT A. JAECKLE

Tumors may invade the cervical, brachial, and lumbosacral plexus by direct extension from primary tumors in regional organs or by secondary invasion following metastases to regional lymph nodes. Occasionally, tumor tracks along the epineurium surrounding the trunks of the nerve plexuses. In the previously treated cancer patient, the major differential diagnostic consideration is radiation-induced plexopathy. Less frequently, the plexopathy results as a complication of regional (usually intra-arterial) chemotherapy or is due to fibrosis following surgical resection of primary tumor within the region.

Tumor plexopathy is a symptomatic complication in approximately 1 of 100 patients with cancer. In two retrospective reviews from cancer hospitals, based on 12,000 patient visits per year, the prevalence of brachial plexopathy resulting from tumor invasion was 0.43%, and the prevalence of lumbosacral plexopathy was 0.71% (Kori et al., 1981; Jaeckle et al., 1985). The actual prevalence may be higher, as not all patients with plexopathy accompanying terminal malignancy are reported. The best estimates have been obtained from breast cancer patients treated with conventional radiotherapy in whom the prevalence of brachial plexopathy at 5 years was 1.8% to 4.9%; however, this study likely included some patients with radiation-induced plexopathy (discussed below) (Pierce et al., 1992; Powell et al., 1990; Sheldon et al., 1987).

Familiarity with plexus neuroanatomy is necessary to correctly interpret the clinical findings and to distinguish between plexopathies and neurologic dysfunction due to epidural compression by tumor, neoplastic meningitis, and other disorders of peripheral nerves. In clinical practice, physicians usually encounter patients with brachial or lumbosacral plexopathy. Cervical plexopathy is also discussed as its clinical presentation, tumor histologies, and therapeutic implications differ somewhat, although there is considerable overlap with brachial plexopathy. Finally, one must be able to distinguish between those patients with plexopathies due to radiation or other causes, which is discussed separately.

CERVICAL PLEXOPATHY

Anatomy

The *cervical plexus* is formed from the ventral rami of the four upper cervical nerve roots (C1–C4). Afferent sensory fibers from the skin and soft tissues of the neck travel via the greater and lesser occipital nerves (posterior occiput and postauricular area); the great auricular and transverse cervical nerves (preauricular area, mandibular angle, anterosuperior neck, and submandibular area); and the medial and lateral supraclavicular nerves (inferior anterolateral neck) through the cervical plexus. The cervical plexus supplies motor innervation to the diaphragm and, deep cervical and hyoid muscles and via the spinal accessory nerve to the sternocleidomastoid and trapezius muscles (Truex and Carpenter, 1969).

Pathophysiology

The cervical plexus is usually invaded by tumor from neighboring soft tissue or bony structures (Fig. 18–1). The neoplasm may invade the plexus directly or indirectly by metastatic spread to regional lymph nodes, ribs, or vertebral bodies. The most commonly associated tumors of the cervical plexus include squamous cell carcinoma of the head and neck, lymphoma, and adenocarcinomas of the lung and breast.

Clinical Presentation

Patients with cervical plexopathy usually present with pain located in the neck, shoulder, or throat, which is often exacerbated by neck movement, swallowing, and coughing. The pain is often deep, boring, and constant, but may have intermittent sharp components or caulsalgic features. On examination, the cervical musculature may be tender to palpation. One should suspect tumor plexopathy from tumor invasion if large palpable tumors or firm anterior or posterior cervical chain or supraclavicular nodes are present. Local sensory loss may be demonstrable, but is often incomplete due to overlap of root zones. Often, one must distinguish postsurgical sensory loss from that due to tumor recurrence. The timing and location of sensory loss are useful points of distinction. Most commonly, surgical dissection transects superficial branches of the greater auricular nerve over the preauricular area and mandibular angle, or the transverse cervical branches, producing numbness in the skin of the upper anterior neck and submandibular area.

Tumor may involve the phrenic nerve producing a paralyzed hemidiaphragm, which can be confirmed by chest radiograph or fluoroscopy. Patients may have dyspnea and paradoxical diaphragmatic excursions. Motor dysfunction of branches to the deep cervical and hyoid muscles are usually asymptomatic. Involvement of the spinal accessory XIth cranial nerve may produce shoulder weakness and instability. Sternocleidomastoid weakness may produce head deviation or tilt. Head and neck tumors and lymphomas

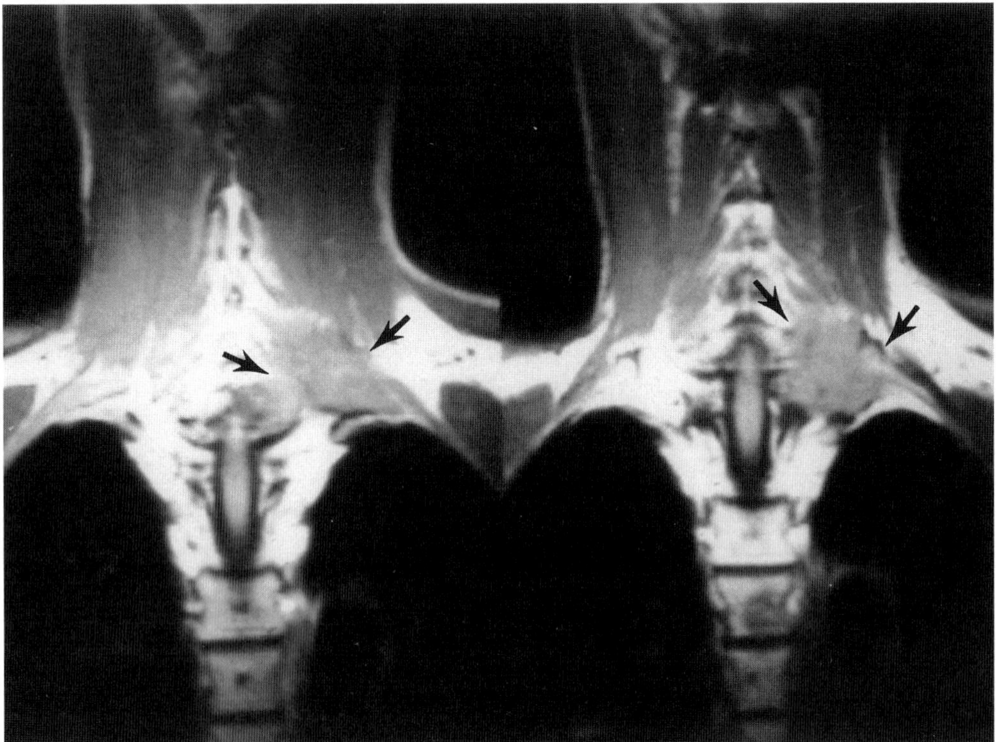

Figure 18–1. Cervical plexopathy. Magnetic resonance imaging scan of metastatic adenocarcinoma from submandibular primary tumor to lower left cervical plexus (arrows), producing C4–C5 pain, tingling, hoarseness, and Horner's syndrome.

involving the anterior cervical lymphatic chain may grow inferiorly, producing additional involvement of the upper brachial plexus.

By definition, involvement of the cervical plexus implies a close proximity of the tumor to the cervical spine. If sharp and severe pain occurs with neck movements, or pain is elicited with percussion over the spine, there may be associated involvement of the cervical spine or impending epidural extension.

BRACHIAL PLEXOPATHY

Anatomy

The brachial plexus originates from ventral rami of the lower four cervical (C5–C8) and the first thoracic roots and forms three *trunks:* a superior trunk (C5–C6); a medial trunk (C7); and an inferior trunk (C8–T1). These trunks each divide into *dorsal* and *ventral divisions.* The three dorsal divisions join together to form the *posterior cord,* which then splits into *(1)* the thoracodorsal nerve, to the latissimus dorsi; *(2)* the subscapular nerve, which innervates the subscapularis; *(3)* the axillary nerve, which supplies the deltoid; and *(4)* the radial nerve, which innervates the triceps, brachioradialis, wrist, and finger extensors and provides sensory supply to the posterior arm and forearm. The ventral division forms two cords: the *lateral cord,* which receives contributions from the superior and medial trunks, and the *medial cord,* which is a direct continuation of the inferior trunk. The lateral cord then divides into two branches: one becomes the *musculocutaneous nerve* (C5–C7, motor to biceps, brachialis, coracobrachialis and sensory innervation of the radial forearm); and the other joins a similar branch from the medial cord to form the *median nerve* (C8–T1, forearm flexors and pronators, medial hand flexor, and lumbrical muscles; and sensation to medial palm, first three fingers, and radial one-half of the fourth finger). The remaining portion of the medial cord forms *(1)* the *medial brachial cutaneous nerve* (T1, sensory to medial arm); *(2)* the *medial antebrachial cutaneous nerve* (C8–T1, sensory to medial forearm) and; *(3)* the *ulnar nerve* (C8–T1, ulnar forearm flexor muscles, interossei, and lumbricals; and sensation to the ulnar aspect of hand the hand and fifth finger) (Truex and Carpenter, 1969).

Pathophysiology

More than two-thirds of tumors involving the brachial plexus originate from the lung or breast and generally spread to the plexus directly from the lung or from regional metastases to the axillary lymph nodes or lung apex (Kori et al., 1981) (Fig. 18–2). Early in the disease process, the tumor often invades the lower plexus, particularly the inferior trunk and medial cord, a pattern that was part of the original description of the superior sulcus syndrome (Pancoast, 1932). Conversely, tumors of the head and neck usually invade the superior trunk or posterior cord from above. Often, the clinical pattern of plexus involvement is patchy, due to irregular involvement of the plexus by growth from the relatively random arrangement of lymph node metastases. Patchy involvement is most commonly identified when formal electrophysiologic investigations are performed.

Clinical Presentation

In a large series of patients with cancer and brachial plexopathy, pain was the most common presenting symptom (75%), followed by dysesthesias (25%) (Kori et al., 1981). The pain was typically located in the shoulder and axilla and often radiated along the medial aspect of the arm and forearm into the fourth and fifth fingers. Initially, pain was often incorrectly attributed to other potential causes, such as arthritis and fibromyalgia. Pain, reflex changes, and atrophy were concentrated in the lower plexus (C8–T1) distribution in 75% of patients, whereas the remaining 25% of patients had global signs of involvement of the entire (C5–T1) plexus.

When brachial plexopathy is due to tumor, lymphedema is relatively infrequent (15%). It is most often seen in the setting of prior radiotherapy or axillary lymph node dissection. Involvement of the sympathetic trunk or ganglia near the upper thoracic (particularly T1) vertebrae may produce unilateral Horner's syndrome, which has been identified in approximately 23% of patients. When Horner's syndrome is present, concomitant epidural disease can be identified in 32% of patients. In general, the presence of Horner's syndrome, serratus anterior or rhomboid muscle weakness, or pain consistent with vertebral involvement should raise the clinical suspicion of epidural extension.

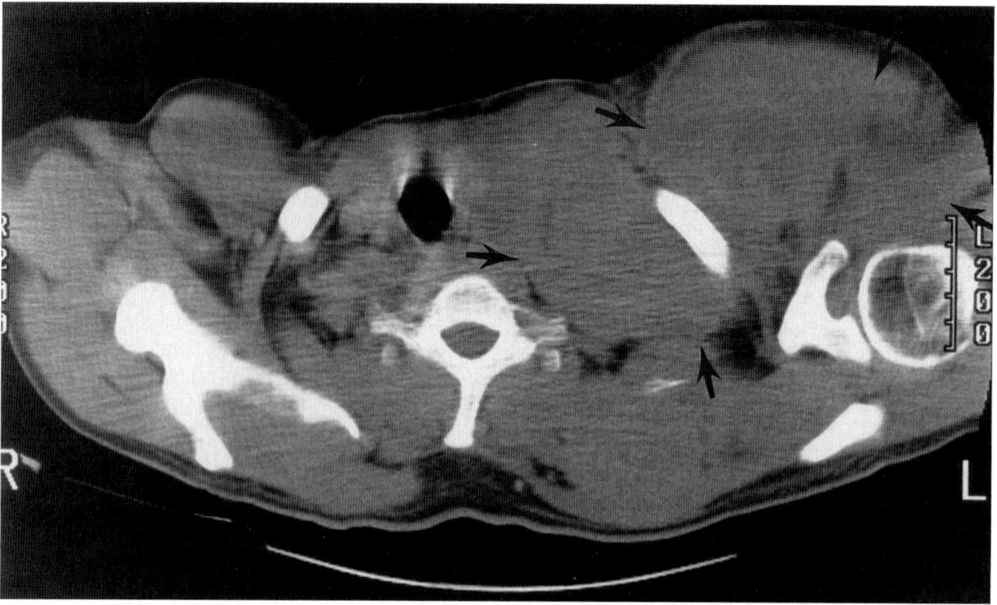

Figure 18–2. Brachial plexopathy. Computed tomography scan of patient with non-Hodgkin's lymphoma showing a huge shoulder and chest wall mass displacing mediastinal structures and invading the left brachial plexus (arrows).

LUMBOSACRAL PLEXOPATHY

Anatomy

The lumbosacral plexus forms from the ventral rami of the L1–S2 nerve roots and is anatomically divided into lumbar and sacral portions. The lumbar plexus forms within the iliacus muscle lateral to the L1–L4 vertebrae and then courses posterolaterally, just anterior to the iliac wing.

The *lumbar plexus* consists of *anterior* and *posterior divisions.* The anterior division gives rise to the *iliohypogastric, ilioinguinal,* and *genitofemoral nerves* (L1–L2), which carry sensory fibers from the skin of the lower abdomen, upper thigh, and lateral genitalia, and the *obturator nerve* (L2–L4), which provides motor supply to the adductors and gracilis muscles. The posterior division of the lumbar plexus divides into the *iliohypogastric* and *lateral femoral cutaneous nerves* (L2–L3), which provide sensation to the lateral hip and thigh, and to the *femoral nerve* (L2–L3), which carries motor fibers to the psoas, iliacus, sartorius, and quadriceps muscles and provides sensory fibers to the skin of the anterior thigh and medial upper leg.

The *sacral plexus* arises from the ventral rami of S1–S4 and runs lateral to the border of the sacrum, penetrating the sciatic notch. A portion of the lower lumbar plexus (L4–L5) connects to the sacral plexus via the lumbosacral trunk, which runs over the sacral ala to join the upper sacral plexus within the true pelvis. The *anterior division* of the sacral plexus provides motor supply to the gemelli, quadratus femoris, obturator internus, and hamstrings; the remaining components continue as the *tibial nerve* (L4–S3), which provides motor supply to the foot plantar flexors and intrinsic muscles and sensation to the heel and sole. The *posterior division* continues as the *common peroneal nerve* (L4–S2) to the peroneal muscles, the tibialis anterior, extensor digitorum, and extensor hallucis muscles and carries sensory fingers from the lateral leg and dorsal foot and toes. The posterior division also gives rise to the *superior* (L4–S1) and *inferior* (L5–S2) *gluteal nerves,* which supply the gluteus muscles. The *sciatic nerve,* which contains components of the common peroneal and tibial nerves, is part of the posterior division; the *posterior femoral cutaneous nerve* (S1–S3), which follows the course of the sciatic nerve as a separate bundle, carries sensory fibers from skin of the posterior thigh from the buttock to the knee. The *pudendal nerve* (S2–S4), along with many smaller nerve bundles, supplies the pelvic floor and genital musculature, as well as the external anal and urethral sphincters. This nerve also carries afferent sensory fibers from the perineum (Truex and Carpenter, 1969).

Pathophysiology

Tumors commonly invade the lumbosacral plexus by direct extension from pelvic primary neoplasms and less frequently by secondary extension from metastases to regional pelvic lymph nodes, the sacrum or iliac wings, or lumbar vertebrae (Fig. 18–3). The most commonly reported tumors producing lumbosacral plexopathy include carcinomas of the colon and rectosigmoid, gynecologic malignancies, retroperitoneal sarcomas, and lymphomas (Jaeckle et al., 1985; Pettigrew et al., 1984). Plexopathy is part of the original tumor presentation in approximately 15% of patients. In general, bulky tumors within the pelvis compress and invade the plexus directly. On occasion, tumor tracks along the connective tissue and epineurium of the nerve trunks (Ebner et al., 1990). This tendency to infiltrate along the nerve may explain why some patients with findings of diffuse plexopathy do not have radiographically demonstrable mass lesions and why in some circumstances the location of the pelvic tumor seems unrelated to the principal site of neurologic involvement.

Clinical Presentation

Tumors invading the lumbosacral plexus typically produce clinical syndromes based on their level of involvement. Clinical patterns of plexus involvement include the upper plexus (L1–L4), the lumbosacral trunk (L4–L5), and the lower plexus (S1–S4). Plexopathy is usually unilateral, although bilateral findings are present in 25% of patients. Patients typically present with leg pain, which is often followed weeks to months later by progressive leg numbness and weakness. The pain is typically severe, constant, dull, and aching and may have sharp or cramping superimposed local, referred, or radicular components. Pain is often worse when the patient becomes supine; usually the patient has difficulty finding a comfortable position. Additional pain that worsens with movement or weight bearing generally implies nearby bony invasion. Involvement of the iliopsoas muscle may force the patient to assume a position in bed with the hips and knees flexed, similar to that seen with meningeal inflammation. The pain may worsen following a bowel movement or be exacerbated by a rigorous neuro-

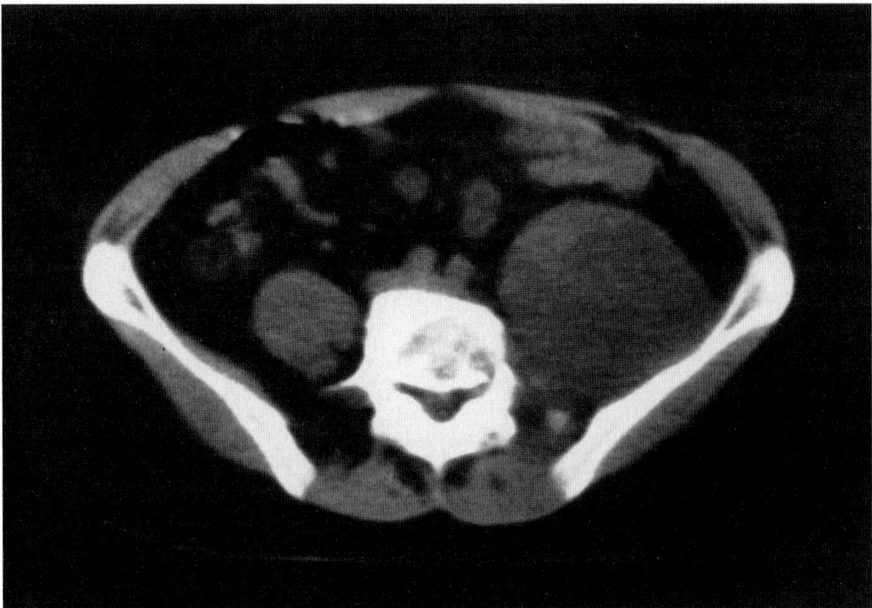

Figure 18–3. Lumbosacral plexopathy. Computed tomography scan showing large left pelvic node metastases from melanoma that caused severe pain and weakness in L4–L5 distribution.

logic examination. Pain is so common (98%) that its absence should raise a red flag regarding this diagnosis.

Symptomatic weakness and sensory complaints eventually develop in 60% of patients. In a series of 85 cancer patients with lumbosacral plexopathy and radiographic or surgical evidence of tumor in the region of the plexus (Jaeckle et al., 1985), objective leg weakness was identified in 86%, sensory loss in 73%, focal reflex loss in 64%, and ipsilateral leg edema in 47% of patients. Patients typically had tenderness over the sciatic notch, and straight leg raising tests often reproduced their pain. Clinical dysfunction of the lower plexus is most common and is most commonly seen with colorectal tumors. A dysesthetic syndrome ("hot dry foot") has been described in as many as one-third of patients (Dalmau et al., 1989) due to sympathetic plexus involvement within the pelvis. Incontinence and impotence are typically absent unless bilateral plexopathy is present.

Tumors deep in the pelvis, in particular those accompanying cervical carcinomas and tumors of the rectosigmoid region, present with numbness and dysesthesias in the perianal area and perineum. These patients may have a palpable rectal mass, decreased anal sphincter tone, and sensory loss of the perineum from involvement of the lower sacral plexus, located anterior to the piriformis muscle. The sensory symptoms often occur early and are followed later by lower extremity pain and weakness.

DIFFERENTIAL DIAGNOSIS: PLEXOPATHY IN THE CANCER PATIENT

Radiation Plexopathy

Because the timing of onset of tumor plexopathy following the original cancer diagnosis overlaps with the typical time frame for radiation plexopathy, the clinician is often confronted with the difficult task of distinguishing these two entities in previously treated patients. Complicating this issue, these conditions may coexist simultaneously in a given patient, which may in part explain why patients whose tumor responds to treatment may not have clinical improvement. The single most valuable diagnostic clinical parameter suggestive of tumor plexopathy is the demonstration of persistent or recurrent tumor in the general region of the plexus (e.g., in the axilla or lung apex), as determined by clinical examination, magnetic resonance imaging (MRI), and/or computed tomography imaging (CT) (Thyagarajan et al., 1995). Radiation plexopathy is implicated if there is evidence of radiation-induced changes in skin, bone or soft tissues and if myokymic discharges are found on electromyography (EMG), which are unusual findings in tumor plexopathy.

The syndromes of brachial and lumbosacral plexopathy due to irradiation have been reasonably well described (Kori et al., 1981; Pierce et al., 1992; Powell et al., 1990; Sheldon et al., 1987; Basso-Ricci et al., 1980; Bagley et al., 1978; Harper et al., 1989; Killer and Hess, 1990; Mondrup et al., 1990; Thomas et al., 1985; Olsen et al., 1990; Ashenhurst et al., 1977). The incidence was probably higher in patients treated in the 1960s with telecobalt therapy. Recently, a long-term (34 years) follow-up study of 71 breast cancer patients who received a calculated dose of 57 Gy in 16 to 17 fractions over 3 to 4 weeks to the axilla, supraclavicular area, and parasternal lymph nodes, reported that late-stage progressive plexopathy was common. Eleven of the 12 patients alive at the time of follow-up had paralysis of the limb (Johansson et al., 2000).

The frequency of radiation plexopathy in treated patients is approximately 1.8% to 4.9% (Pierce et al., 1992; Powell et al., 1990; Sheldon et al., 1987). Sheldon et al. (1987) reported this complication in 2% of patients with stage III breast cancer treated with 4.5 to 5 Gy to the breast and regional lymphatics at a median follow-up period of 65 months (5 years). In other series, the interval between administration of radiotherapy and the development of plexopathy ranged from 3 months to 14 years, with a median of 1.5 years, and was most frequent at tissue doses greater than 50 Gy (Kori et al., 1981; Killer and Hess, 1990).

Radiation plexopathy probably has a multifactorial etiology. Cavanaugh (1968) studied the effects of radiation and crush injury of rat sciatic nerve at doses between 200 and 2000 R. At doses above 1000 R, there was failure of cellular proliferation and development of pathologic changes in Schwann cells, endoneurial fibroblasts, and vascular and perineural cells. In another physiologic study, severe delayed damage of the anterior and posterior nerve roots was observed following 35 Gy administered to the lumbar region in rodents (Bradley et al., 1977). In humans, radiation plexopathy is presumably caused by tissue fibrosis with retraction of nerve trunks, direct toxic effects on axons, and radiologic effects involving the vasa nervorum, producing microinfarction of nerve axons (Greenfield and Stark, 1948).

In the clinical setting, several points can help to distinguish radiation-induced from tumor-induced plexopathy (Table 18–1). Radiation plexopathy usually presents with causalgic dysesthesias in the arm, often accompanied by lymphedema. In contrast, only a small percentage of patients with tumor plexopathy will present with dysesthesias, and lymphedema is less frequent. In tumor plexopathy, the presenting feature is often severe unrelenting pain; in contrast, pain usually develops late in the course of radiation plexopathy and is less often the major symptom. These two entities can sometimes be distinguished by the level of plexus involvement: Radiation plexopathy usually affects the upper (77%) or entire (23%) plexus; in tumor plexopathy, the lower plexus (75%) or the entire plexus (25%) appears to be more frequently affected (Kori et al., 1981; Mondrup et al., 1990). However, recent studies have shown that the neurologic level of plexus involvement can be more variable than noticed in these earlier reports (Boyaciyan et al., 1996). Sparing of the lower plexus from radiation damage afforded by intervening bony and soft tissues has been postulated as a reason for the more frequent occurrence of upper plexus involvement with radiation, but seems questionable based on studies of tissue dosimetry and observations of associated radionecrosis of the clavicle or ribs in these patients (Pierce et al., 1992). Many patients with radiation-induced plexopathy also have skin changes, including telangiectasia, atrophy, and diffuse induration; radiographs may show other associated radiation changes, including typical changes in the apex of the lung, radionecrosis of regional bony structures, and pericardial fibrosis.

The lumbosacral plexus is also subject to radiation-induced injury. The median onset of this complication is approximately 5 years (range, 1 month to 31 years) (Thomas et al., 1985). Another series found an earlier onset of 12 months (range, 1 month to 156 months) (Ashenhurst et al., 1977). The incidence appears to be higher with larger doses of radiation, but has been reported at doses as low as 17 Gy.

The clinical features of radiation plexopathy overlap with tumor plexopathy. Patients with radiation plexopathy usually present with weakness (60%), numbness, or paresthesias (50%) (Thomas et al., 1985). As in radiation brachial plexopathy, pain at presentation is also uncommon (10%) in patients with radiation lumbosacral plexopathy and frequent (98%) in patients with recurrent tumor. Later in the course of lumbosacral plexopathy due to radiation, pain develops in 50% of patients. Weakness is often bilateral in radiation plexopathy in contrast to tumor plexopathy, in which more than 75% of patients primarily have unilateral involvement. The distribution of plexopathy is not as useful a distinguishing point as it is in brachial plexopathy; both conditions most commonly affect the lower (L5–S1) portion. The presence of a rectal mass supports tumor

Table 18–1. Differential Diagnosis of Radiation Plexopathy Versus Recurrent Tumor Plexopathy

	Tumor	*Radiation*
Presentation	Pain	Paresthesias, weakness
Pain	Common, severe	Occasional
Edema	Occasional	Common
Plexus involvement		
Brachial	Usually lower plexus	Upper or whole plexus
Lumbrosacral	Lower plexus, unilateral	Commonly bilateral
Horner's syndrome	Common	Infrequent
Local tissue necrosis	Infrequent	Common
Rectal mass lumbosacral plexopathy (LSP)	Common	Unusual
Myokymia (EMG)	Unusual	Common
Nerve enhancement (MRI)	Common	Unusual

recurrence; sphincteric dysfunction is slightly more common with radiation-induced plexopathy. Leg edema occurs with approximately equal frequency in the two conditions. The progression of neurologic dysfunction is generally slower in radiation plexopathy than with tumor recurrence.

Electromyography appears to be helpful in distinguishing between these two entities. Approximately 60% of patients with radiation-induced plexopathy will exhibit myokymia, which is rarely seen in metastatic plexopathy (Roth et al., 1988). Neuroimaging with CT (Moskovic et al., 1992) or with MRI can be of help in distinguishing tumor recurrence from radiation injury. Magnetic resonance imaging appears to be more sensitive than CT in detecting tumor recurrence (Taylor et al., 1997).

The treatment of radiation-induced plexopathy is symptomatic. Most patients have a slow but steady progressive loss of motor function and require supportive therapy.

Additional Causes of Plexopathy in Cancer Patients

Plexopathy following chemotherapy appears to be associated primarily with regional intra-arterial administration (Kahn et al., 1989). Although rare, plexopathy has been reported as a paraneoplastic disorder and on occasion may be steroid responsive (Lachance et al., 1991). When making a diagnosis, the physician must also consider conditions affecting the plexus that occur in noncancer patients, including aortic aneurysms (Chapman et al., 1964); diabetic amyotrophy (Chokroverty et al., 1977), vasculitis, and other rare conditions (Chad and Bradley, 1987). Idiopathic or postinfectious brachial neuritis can produce symptoms very similar to those of metastatic plexopathy, although the onset is usually more acute and often follows a history of viral infection or immunization. Because patients with metastatic systemic cancer often have more than one site of nervous system involvement, the possibility of concomitant leptomeningeal or epidural metastases must be considered, which can have a similar clinical appearance.

DIAGNOSIS

The clinical diagnosis of metastatic plexopathy is best confirmed by MRI or CT scanning of the appropriate areas. Magnetic resonance imaging provides the best anatomic detail and is usually a preferred procedure, when available. MRI has been shown to be more sensitive than CT in the identification of tumor plexopathy (Taylor et al., 1997; Qayyum et al., 2000; Thyagarajan et al., 1995). Diagnosis can be difficult if the scan does not show a mass lesion. In these instances, one must maintain a high clinical suspicion of tumor recurrence and consider repeating the imaging procedures at further neurologic progression. Although CT or MRI scans may identify tumor recurrence, the radiographic appearance can be difficult to interpret. Increased T_2 intensity within nerve trunks with or without enhancement has been identified in patients meeting clinical criteria for radiation plexopathy, findings considered more typical for tumor plexopathy; and fibrotic masses may also mimic local tumor recurrence (Wouter van Es et al., 1997). A careful evaluation by an experienced radiologist may be helpful, as detection of a pattern of T_2 abnormalities and enhancement and an associated mass effect may provide provisional bias toward one of these diagnoses.

The presence of a local or regional tumor recurrence, by clinical examination or imaging, supports the diagnosis of tumor plexopathy. In one study, the absence of a palpable axillary mass was inversely diagnostic as 95% of patients with CT evidence of brachial plexus tumor have a palpable axillary mass (Moskovic et al., 1992). In a recent study, positron emission tomography (PET) was utilized to evaluate the brachial plexopathy in 19 breast carcinoma patients with plexopathy; 14 had abnormal 18-fluorodeoxyglucose uptake within the involved plexus. However, the specificity and sensitivity of PET for tumor plexopathy have not been elucidated (Ahmad et al., 1999).

Electromyography can be useful in delineating the distribution and extent of denervation. It occasionally reveals more extensive findings than would have been predicted clinically. The main clinical usefulness appears to be in distinguishing radiation plexopathy from neoplastic involvement, as stated above, and occasionally in supplementing the radiographic findings when planning treatment fields. Electromyography in experienced hands can be used to differentiate plexopathy from other entities, such as neoplastic meningitis, radiculopathy from epidural tumor, and neuropathy.

TREATMENT

Treatment of cancer-related plexopathy is largely palliative and symptom directed. Treatment generally involves radiation to the involved field and pain control measures. Consultation with pain management specialists is recommended. Studies have shown that pain is often poorly controlled in patients with plexopathy. Proper pain control often requires multimodality approaches, including a clear understanding of the proper use of opiate analgesics, continuous infusion pumps, local and regional blocks, sympathectomy, rhizotomy, or other specialized procedures that are generally outside the normal experience of radiation and medical oncologists. In appropriate settings, specific chemotherapy for the underlying neoplasm is warranted, and tumor response may be associated with improvement of pain and other symptoms (particularly in responsive tumors such as lymphomas). Occasional relief of chronic pain has been achieved with plexus dissection and neurolysis (Sundaresan and DiGiacinto, 1987). Dysesthesias and causalgia are resistant to therapy, but may respond to transcutaneous nerve stimulation, tricyclic antidepressants, anticonvulsants such as gabapentin, carbamazepine or phenytoin, or regional nerve or sympathetic ganglion blocks. Often, opiate analgesics are required. Lymphedema may be treated with compressive devices and elevation.

Unfortunately, the reported results of treatment are largely disappointing. In brachial plexopathy, radiation therapy to the involved plexus relieved pain in only 46% of cases (Kori et al., 1981). Treatment of tumor in the lumbosacral plexus produced improvement in pain in only 15% of patients reassessed at 1 month from treatment; objective improvement in strength occurred in only 17% and objective reduction in tumor size in only 28% (Jaeckle et al., 1985). In another study of 28 patients with carcinomatous lumbosacral plexus neuropathy, radiation produced improvement in 85% but only a 29% objective response rate (Ampil, 1986). The best subjective/objective treatment result was observed with a total dose of at least 30 Gy. In most cases, the duration of response has been brief, and the relatively short survival of patients with tumor plexopathy suggests that its occurrence represents a late-stage complication of malignancy.

Plexopathy patients are particularly prone to painful contractures, compressive neuropathies, pressure ulcerations, respiratory and urinary tract infections, joint subluxations, and deep venous thromboses. Preventative measures, including adequate pain management, initiation of physical rehabilitation, and assessment of home equipment needs may have a significant impact on preservation of quality of life in these patients.

REFERENCES

Ahmad A, Barrington S, Maisey M, Rubens RD. 1999. Use of positron emission tomography in evaluation of brachial plexopathy in breast cancer patients. Br J Cancer 79:478–482.

Ampil FL. 1986. Palliative irradiation of carcinomatous lumbosacral plexus neuropathy. Int J Radiation Oncol Biol Phys 12:1681–1686.

Ashenhurst EM, Quartey GR, Starreveld A. 1977. Lumbo-sacral radiculopathy induced by radiation. Can J Neurol Sci 4:259–263.

Basso-Ricci S, della Costa C, Viganotti G, Ventafridda V, Zanolla R. 1980. Report on 42 cases of postirradiation lesions of the brachial plexus and their treatment. Tumori 66:117–122.

Bagley FH, Walsh JW, Cady B, Salzman FA, Oberfield RA, Pazianos AG. 1978. Carcinomatous versus radiation-induced brachial plexus neuropathy in breast cancer. Cancer 41:2154–2157.

Boyaciyan A, Oge AE, Yazici J, Aslay I, Baslo A. 1996. Electrophysiological findings in patients who received radiation therapy over the brachial plexus: a magnetic stimulation study. Electroencephalogr Clin Neurophysiol 101:483–490.

Bradley WG, Fewings JD, Cumming WJ, Harrison RM. 1977. Delayed myeloradiculopathy produced by spinal X-irradiation in the rat. J Neurol Sci 31:63–82.

Cavanaugh JB. 1968. Prior X-irradiation and the cellular response to nerve crush: duration of effect. Exp Neurol 22:253–258.

Chad DA, Bradley WG. 1987. Lumbosacral plexopathy. Semin Neurol 7:97–107.

Chapman EM, Shaw RS, Kubik CS. 1964. Sciatic pain from arterioscleriotic aneurysm of pelvic arteries. N Engl J Med 271:1410–1411.

Chokroverty S, Reyes MG, Rubino FA, Tonaki H. 1977. The syndrome of diabetic amyotrophy. Ann Neurol 2:181–194.

Dalmau J, Graus F, Marco M. 1989. "Hot and dry foot" as initial manifestation of neoplastic lumbosacral plexopathy. Neurology 39:871–872.

Ebner I, Anderl H, Mikuz G, Frommhold H. 1990. [Plexus neuropathy: tumor infiltration or radiation damage]. ROFO Fortschr Geb Rontgenstr Neuen Bildgreb Verfahr 152:662–666.

Greenfield MM, Stark FM. 1948. Post-irradiation neuropathy. Am J Roentgen 60:617–619.

Harper CM Jr, Thomas JE, Cascino TL, Litchy WJ. 1989. Distinction between neoplastic and radiation-induced brachial plexopathy, with emphasis on the role of EMG. Neurology 39:502–506.

Jaeckle KA, Young DF, Foley KM. 1985. The natural history of lumbosacral plexopathy in cancer. Neurology 35:8–15.

Johansson S, Svensson H, Larsson LG, Denekamp J. 2000. Brachial plexopathy after postoperative radiotherapy of breast cancer patients—a long-term follow-up. Acta Oncol 39:373–382.

Kahn CE Jr, Messersmith RN, Samuels BL. 1989. Brachial plexopathy as a complication of intraarterial cisplatin chemotherapy. Cardiovasc Intervent Radiol 12:47–49.

Killer HE, Hess K. 1990. Natural history of radiation-induced brachial plexopathy compared with surgically treated patients. J Neurol 237:247–250.

Kori SH, Foley KM, Posner JB. 1981. Brachial plexus lesions in patients with cancer: 100 cases. Neurology 31:45–50.

Lachance DH, O'Neill BP, Harper CM Jr, Banks PM, Cascino TL. 1991. Paraneoplastic brachial plexopathy in a patient with Hodgkin's disease. Mayo Clin Proc 66:97–101.

Mondrup K, Olsen NK, Pfeiffer P, Rose C. 1990. Clinical and electrodiagnostic findings in breast cancer patients with radiation-induced brachial plexus neuropathy. Acta Neurol Scand 81:153–158.

Moskovic E, Curtis S, A'Hern RP, Harmer CL, Parsons C. 1992. The role of diagnostic CT scanning of the brachial plexus and axilla in the follow-up of patients with breast cancer. Clin Oncol (R Coll Radiol) 4:74–77.

Olsen NK, Pfeiffer P, Mondrup K, Rose C. 1990. Radiation-induced brachial plexus neuropathy in breast cancer patients. Acta Oncol 29:885–890.

Pancoast HK. 1932. Superior pulmonary sulcus tumor. J Am Med Assoc 99:1391–1393.

Pettigrew LC, Glass JP, Maor M, Zornoza J. 1984. Diagnosis and treatment of lumbosacral plexopathies in patients with cancer. Arch Neurol 41:1282–1285.

Pierce SM, Recht A, Lingos TI, et al. 1992. Long-term radiation complications following conservative surgery (CS) and radiation therapy (RT) in patients with early stage breast cancer. Int J Radiat Oncol Biol Phys 23:915–923.

Powell S, Cooke J, Parsons C. 1990. Radiation-induced brachial plexus injury: follow-up of two different fractionation schedules. Radiother Oncol 18:213–220.

Qayyum A, MacVicar AD, Padhani AR, Revell P, Husband JE. 2000. Symptomatic brachial plexopathy following treatment for breast cancer: utility of MR imaging with surface-coil techniques. Radiology 214:837–842.

Roth G, Magistris MR, Le Fort D, Desjacques P, Della Santa D. 1988. [Postradiation brachial plexopathy. Persistent conduction block. Myokymic discharges and cramps]. Rev Neurol (Paris) 144:173–180.

Sheldon T, Hayes DF, Cady B, et al. 1987. Primary radiation therapy for locally advanced breast cancer. Cancer 60:1219–1225.

Sundaresan N, DiGiacinto GV. 1987. Antitumor and antinociceptive approaches to control cancer pain. Med Clin North Am 71:329–348.

Taylor BV, Kimmel DW, Krecke KN, Cascino TL. 1997. Magnetic resonance imaging in cancer-related lumbosacral plexopathy. Mayo Clin Proc 72:823–829.

Thomas JE, Cascino TL, Earle JD. 1985. Differential diagnosis between radiation and tumor plexopathy of the pelvis. Neurology 35:1–7.

Thyagarajan D, Cascino T, Harms G. 1995. Magnetic resonance imaging in brachial plexopathy of cancer. Neurology 45:421–427.

Truex RC, Carpenter MB. 1969. Segmental and peripheral innervation. In: Human Neuroanatomy, 6th ed. Baltimore: Williams & Wilkins, 194 pp.

Wouter van Es H, Engelen AM, Witkamp TD, Ramos LM, Feldberg MA. 1997. Radiation induced brachial plexopathy: MR imaging. Skeletal Radiol 26:284–288.

19

Paraneoplastic Neurologic Disease

KURT A. JAECKLE

The term *paraneoplastic neurologic disease* (PND) encompasses several degenerative central or peripheral nervous system disorders that result from indirect effects of systemic cancer on elements of the nervous system. By definition, the dysfunction does not result from invasion or metastasis by tumor. The concept of a remote or indirect effect of cancer on the nervous system arose in the latter nineteenth century by empiric association between peripheral neuropathy and lung cancer (Oppenheim, 1888). During the first half of the twentieth century, the term *paraneoplastic disease* was applied to nearly any neurologic dysfunction in a cancer patient for which an etiology was not readily apparent. As a result, the category included a variety of metabolic, nutritional, vascular, and infectious disorders. In the latter half of the twentieth century, the autoimmune etiology of many paraneoplastic disorders evolved, beginning with the discovery of antineuronal antibodies in patients with small cell lung cancer (SCLC) (Croft and Wilkinson, 1965). Several different serum autoantibody markers have now been associated with the paraneoplastic neurologic clinical syndromes, which has allowed the clinician to confirm the diagnosis in suspect cases.

However, the pathogenetic relationship between PND antibodies, clinical syndromes, and neuropathologic abnormalities has not been entirely clarified. Furthermore, not all patients with such autoantibodies have syndromes consistent with PND. Additional etiologies may be involved, such as infectious or parainfectious processes, nutritional deficiencies, or direct neurotoxicity from proteins and other substances elaborated by the tumor. Nonetheless, the description of specific autoantibodies in PND has resulted in separation of a group of patients with PND from others without antibodies. Many PND autoantibodies have now been associated with specific tumors, particularly those from lung, breast, gynecologic, and testicular neoplasms. In some circumstances, this has allowed the clinician to expedite the discovery of the primary cancer in suspect patients and designate the complicated neurologic illness in given patients as a paraneoplastic condition. A major future challenge still remains—the identification of effective therapies for these largely unresponsive conditions. Such therapies are likely to result from elucidation of the pathogenetic mechanisms involved in the production of these disorders.

INCIDENCE

Overall, PND is rare. The reported incidence of PND is higher if all peripheral nerve and neuromuscular disorders are included. In one study, more than 50% of patients with ovarian epithelial neoplasms had evidence of peripheral neuropathy (Cavalleti et al., 1991). In patients with SCLC, peripheral nerve disease has been clinically observed in as many as 45% of patients. At autopsy, changes in dorsal root ganglia were observed in 70% and in anterior horn cell neurons in 45% of patients (Kida et al., 1992). However, in many of these patients, peripheral neuropathy was likely due to other causes, such as effects from neurotoxic medications and metabolic or nutritional disorders. In a series of 1476 cancer patients, "true" paraneoplastic neuromyopathy was reported in 7% (Croft and Wilkinson, 1965). The myasthenic (Lambert-Eaton) syndrome occurs in approximately 3% of patients with SCLC (Elrington et al., 1991).

If one excludes the neuromyopathies, clinically recognizable central nervous system (CNS) PND occurs in <1 % of patients with cancer (Anderson et al., 1987).

HISTORIC CONSIDERATIONS

The first report of a paraneoplastic syndrome was probably the description of peripheral neuropathy in a lung cancer patient at the end of the nineteenth century (Oppenheim, 1888). A series of reports followed that clearly defined the clinical syndromes and associated cancers. Several paraneoplastic conditions were described, including myasthenia gravis in association with thymic tumor (Weigert, 1901); dermatomyositis with gastric carcinoma (Stertz, 1916); subacute cerebellar degeneration (Brouwer, 1919), later associated with ovarian and SCLC (Brain et al., 1951); sensory neuronopathy with lung cancer (Denny-Brown, 1948); myasthenic syndrome with SCLC (Lambert et al., 1956); encephalomyelitis (Henson et al., 1965); and cancer-associated retinopathy (Sawyer et al., 1976).

Investigators during the last 40 years have explored the pathogenesis of PND. This effort began in earnest in the mid-1960s with the discovery of serum autoantibodies that reacted with neurons (Wilkinson, 1964). Several investigators later described serum and cerebrospinal fluid (CSF) autoantibodies with affinity for central or peripheral nervous system protein antigens (Trotter et al., 1976; Kornguth et al., 1982; Greenlee and Brashear, 1983; Jaeckle et al., 1985; Graus et al., 1985; Voltz et al., 1999; Honnorat et al., 1996). The antibodies have been used to identify and characterize corresponding protein antigens and also to clone cDNA for production and characterization of recombinant protein antigens (Dropcho et al., 1987; Szabo et al., 1991; Fathallah-Shaykh et al., 1991; Thirkill et al., 1992; Sakai et al., 1992; Buckanovich et al., 1993) (Table 19–1).

In some cases, PND antibodies show relative affinity for sites of pathologic nervous system involvement (Dalmau et al., 1991). In addition, the antineuronal antibodies are also reactive with autologous tumor (Furneaux et al., 1990). Finally, cytotoxic T cells have been shown to transform in response to specific paraneoplastic antigens, and these cells are capable of inducing tumor cell cytotoxicity (Albert et al., 2000).

PATHOGENESIS

Several etiologies have been proposed for the paraneoplastic diseases (Brain and Norris, 1965), including toxins (e.g., proteins, lipids, and soluble neurotoxins and their products); viruses (e.g., the JC polyomavirus in progressive multifocal leukoencephalopathy); nutritional deficiencies (e.g., vitamins B_1, B_6, B_{12}, amino acids); and autoimmunity. By definition, many of these potential etiologies (nutritional, progressive multifocal leukoencephalopathy, viral encephalitis) are generally not considered part of the modern definition of PND. To date, there has not been a definitive animal model for most manifestations of PND.

It is possible that several separate pathogenetic mechanisms are responsible in different patients. For example, not all cancer patients with clinical PND have demonstrable autoantibodies (Posner and Furneaux, 1990). Undetected viral or other infectious etiologies, tumor-associated neurotoxins, and neuroendocrine influences have not been totally excluded.

An autoimmune disturbance involving "molecular mimicry" has been proposed. In this model, antibodies react with shared protein antigens in tumor and in the CNS or peripheral nervous system. Some patients have identifiable serum and CSF complement-fixing antineuronal antibodies of the pathogenic IgG subtype (Dalmau et al., 1991; Jean et al., 1994) that cross react with autologous tumor antigens. Local synthesis of paraneoplastic autoantibodies can be identified in the CNS (Furneaux et al., 1990). Occasional patients show improvement and reduction of antibody titers after tumor removal or therapy (Greenlee et al., 1986; Tsukamoto et al., 1993). Plasmapheresis, which removes autoantibody, has also resulted in disease stabilization in rare patients; unfortunately, this treatment is usually unsuccessful (Jaeckle et al., 1985; Graus et al., 1992). Other immune suppressive therapies and intravenous immunoglobulin have been tried but are also largely ineffective (Grisold et al., 1995; Keime-Guibert et al., 2000).

Table 19–1. Paraneoplastic Neurologic Antibodies

Clinical Syndrome	*Tumor Type*	*Antibody*	*Western Blot Antigen (kD)*	*Recombinant Antigen*	*Reference*
Encephalomyelitis	SCLC, breast	Anti-Hu	37–42	HuD; PLE21/HuC	Szabo et al., 1991
	SCLC, breast,	Anti-Hel-N1	37–42	Hel-N1	Levine et al., 1993
	other	Anti-CV2	66	Ulip/CRMP	Honnorat et al., 1999
Limbic encephalitis	Testicular, breast	Anti-Ma 2 (Ta)	40	Ma2	Sutton et al., 2000
Cerebellar degeneration	Breast, Gyn	Anti-Yo	62	Cdr2	Fathallah-Shaykh et al., 1991
	Breast, Gyn	Anti-Yo	34	pCDR13	Dropcho et al., 1987
	Breast, Gyn	Anti-PCA-1	52	p52	Sakai et al., 1992
	SCLC, breast, colon, other	Anti-Ma 1	40	Ma 1	Voltz et al., 1999
	—	—	58	p58	Sato et al., 1991
Opsoclonus-Myoclonus-ataxia	Breast, lung, GI	Anti-Ri	55	Nova 1, 2	Buckanovich et al., 1993
Cancer-associated retinopathy	Lung, melanoma	Anti-CAR	23–26	CAR	Thirkill et al., 1992
Lambert-Eaton	SCLC	Anti-P/Q VGCC	(Bioassay)	—	Leys et al., 1991

kD, kiloDaltons; SCLC, small cell lung cancer; Gyn, gynecologic malignancies; GI, gastroenteric malignancies; VGCC, voltage-gated calcium channel.

Theoretically, quiescent memory T cells, which were transiently exposed in the fetus to developmental antigens, might escape thymic deletion and reside in the periphery until tumor-associated antigens are again expressed and processed by antigen-presenting dendritic cells. T-cell–facilitated B-cell proliferation might then result in secretion of autoantibody, which cross reacts with similar antigenic epitopes expressed within nervous system components or neurons. Presumably, complement-mediated antibody-dependent cytotoxicity or a separate process involving antigen-dependent, T-cell–mediated neuronal lysis would ensue. There is preliminary in vitro evidence that complement-mediated neuronal lysis occurs with paraneoplastic antibody (Greenlee et al., 1993). In addition, recent data suggest that cytotoxic T cells may play a role in the pathogenesis (Albert et al., 2000).

CLINICAL USE OF PND ANTIBODIES

Several PND autoantibodies and their associated antigens have now been characterized (Table 19–1). These markers have significant clinical value as they can be given to appropriate patients to confirm the diagnosis of a paraneoplastic syndrome and allow earlier detection of an associated systemic malignancy. Several of the antibodies are relatively specific for certain PND and neoplasm types.

Most of the available assays for the PND antibodies are of two general types: immunochemical detection methods, in which serum or CSF is screened for antineuronal antibodies using immunohistochemistry or Western blotting, with human or rodent tissues as antigenic sources; or by ELISA or immunoblots, using recombinant PND antigen prepared from cloned DNA. Immunohistochemical methods have the advantage of detection of uncommon or previously not described antineuronal antibodies that are not detected with cloned protein antigens; for example, antibody-positive patients are identified who have the neurologic syndrome but no cancer (Greenlee et al., 1992) or a cancer and no neurologic disorder (Brashear et al., 1989). However, the specificity of antibody reactivity for antigens in tissue sections is probably less than that obtained utilizing cloned proteins as the antigen source. There has been a difference of opinion regarding the relative merits and shortcomings of both immunochemical and molecular methods for detection of PND (King et al., 1999). Nonetheless, commercial laboratories have been established that offer "clinical panels" for antibody detection by a variety of different methods.

The best characterized PND antibodies and associated neoplasms are listed in Table 19–1. At least two different antibodies have been described in patients with *paraneoplastic encephalomyelitis:* the anti-Hu (ANNA-1, type IIa) antibody in patients with small cell carcinoma, and the Ma and Ta antibodies in patients with limbic encephalitis and testicular carcinoma. An additional antibody in patients with encephalomyelitis reactive with oligodendroglia has been identified (Honnorat et al., 1996). In *paraneoplastic cerebellar degeneration* (PCD), the most common antibody subtype in gynecologic malignancies has been the anti-Yo antibody (also known as PCA-1 or APCA). It should be mentioned that in some patients the anti-Hu antibody is also associated with PCD and small cell carcinoma. The primary antibody in the *paraneoplastic opsoclonus-ataxia-myoclonus* syndrome is the anti-Ri antibody, also known as ANNA-2 or type IIb. The antibody associated with *paraneoplastic retinopathy* is the anti-CAR (cancer-associated retinopathy) or anti-recoverin antibody. In *Lambert-Eaton myasthenic syndrome* (LEMS) the most common antibodies identified are antivoltage-gated calcium channel (VGCC) antibodies. In *paraneoplastic polymyositis,* antibody to the extractable nuclear antigen Jo-1 can occasionally be identified.

As mentioned above, paraneoplastic autoantibodies are often reactive with antigens in the autologous tumor of PND patients (Furneaux et al., 1990; Szabo et al., 1991) and cultured tumor cell lines (Sakai et al., 1992; Jaeckle et al., 1992; Winter et al., 1993). Several of the antibodies are relatively specific for certain tumor types, allowing clinicians to focus on testing for specific systemic cancers.

CLINICAL SYNDROMES

General Considerations

A descriptive classification of the paraneoplastic neurologic disorders is given in Table 19–2. The association of clinical syndromes with specific autoantibodies has redefined these disorders, and discovery of additional markers may result in future refinement

Table 19–2. Classification of Paraneoplastic Neurologic Diseases

I. Disorders of the cerebrum, brain stem, and cerebellum
  A. Encephalomyelitis
  B. Limbic encephalitis
  C. Bulbar encephalitis
  D. Subacute cerebellar degeneration

II. Disorders of the optic and oculomotor pathways
  A. Retinal degeneration (CAR)
  B. Optic neuritis
  C. Opsoclonus-myoclonus-ataxia

III. Disorders of the spinal cord
  A. Subacute necrotizing myelopathy
  B. Myelitis
  C. Anterior horn cell disease
    1. Atypical motor neuron disease
    2. Subacute motor neuronopathy

IV. Disorders of peripheral nerve ganglia
  A. Sensory neuronopathy
  B. Autonomic neuronopathy

V. Disorders of peripheral nerve
  A. Acute inflammatory demyelinating polyneuropathy
  B. Chronic inflammatory demyelinating polyneuropathy
  C. Sensorimotor neuropathy
  D. Mononeuritis multiplex
  E. Plexopathy

VI. Disorders of muscle and neuromuscular junction
  A. Polymyositis/dermatomyositis
  B. Lambert-Eaton myasthenic syndrome
  C. Myasthenia gravis
  D. Neuromyopathy
  E. Neuromuscular hyperexcitability syndrome

VII. Other possible paraneoplastic neurologic disorders
  A. Dementia
  B. Progressive supranuclear palsy

of this classification. Such a revised classification has been suggested, grouping disorders into four categories, based on the reactivity of the PND antibody with the target antigen: *(1)* neuromuscular junction proteins, *(2)* nerve terminal/vesicle proteins, *(3)* neuronal RNA binding proteins, or *(4)* neuronal signal transduction proteins (Darnell, 1996).

The symptoms and signs of some paraneoplastic syndromes are so striking that the clinician encountering such a patient should suspect an underlying malignancy. Syndromes that should prompt evaluation include cancer-associated retinopathy, limbic encephalitis, cerebellar degeneration, and subacute sensory neuropathy.

Many different neoplasms have been associated with PND (Table 19–3). The most common underlying tumors have been SCLC, breast and gynecologic malignancies, gastrointestinal carcinomas, Hodgkin's disease, and non-Hodgkin's lymphomas.

The diagnosis of the paraneoplastic syndromes is based primarily on the clinical presentation and the absence of identifiable alternative diagnoses. In addition to performing antibody studies, other ancillary analyses can be helpful. In the myasthenic syndrome, the characteristic electromyographic findings of an incremental increase in compound motor nerve action potential with repetitive stimulation at high frequencies can aid in diagnosis. Muscle biopsy is the most definitive way to make the diagnosis of paraneoplastic polymyositis. Although neuroradiologic findings are often normal or nonspecific in most CNS

Table 19–3. Tumors Associated with Paraneoplastic Neurologic Disease

A. Carcinomas
  1. Lung
    a. Small cell
    b. Non-small cell
  2. Gynecologic
    a. Ovarian
    b. Fallopian tube
    c. Endometrial
    d. Breast
  3. Gastrointestinal
    a. Colon
    b. Gastric
    c. Esophageal
    d. Pancreas
  4. Genitourinary
    a. Prostate
    b. Renal cell
    c. Testicular

B. Lymphomas
  1. Hodgkin's disease
  2. Non-Hodgkin's disease
  3. Thymoma

C. Miscellaneous tumors
  1. Sarcoma
  2. Carcinoid
  3. Melanoma

PND, some patients with limbic encephalitis show areas of increased intensity on T_2-weighted or FLAIR sequences or enhancement in limbic structures, particularly in the hippocampus. Occasional patients with paraneoplastic myelopathy will also demonstrate intramedullary signal intensities on T_2-weighted images. Electroretinograms may be helpful in screening patients for paraneoplastic retinopathy; and loss of light adaptation reflexes with night blindness may be observed.

In general, treatment of the paraneoplastic syndromes, except the opsoclonus-myoclonus syndrome, polymyositis, and Lambert-Eaton myasthenic syndrome, has been largely ineffective. In other paraneoplastic disorders, treatment with corticosteroids, chemotherapeutic agents, intravenous immunoglobulin, and plasmapheresis has been mostly unsuccessful (Graus et al., 1992). However, occasional patients have responded to tumor removal or treatment (Greenlee et al., 1986; Tsukamoto et al., 1993).

Encephalomyelitis

The concept of an encephalomyelitis syndrome or spectrum (Table 19–4) was first proposed by Henson and Urich (see Henson et al., 1965). Patients with encephalomyelitis typically exhibit dysfunction of more than one area of the neuraxis. Subacute sensory neuronopathy, in association with variable degrees of dorsal column and motor neuron abnormalities, and limbic encephalitis may be the most common clinical presentations encountered. Often, one or more areas of the nervous system are predominantly affected. Some patients will present with cerebellar degeneration, ascending myelitis, sensory neuronopathy, and motor neuronopathy. The term *encephalomyelitis* is utilized when more than one area of involvement occurs in a given patient.

The pathologic findings in encephalomyelitis include neuronal loss, scattered lymphocytic perivascular infiltrates, proliferation of microglia, degeneration of ascending and descending tracts, and gliosis (Henson and Urich, 1982a). The degree of lymphocytic infiltration may vary considerably, probably due to differential timing of pathologic examination from the onset of the disease process. Involvement is often irregular and patchy and often corresponds incompletely with areas of clinical involvement. Most patients with encephalomyelitis have evidence of mild CSF lymphocytic pleocytosis, elevated IgG synthesis, and oligoclonal bands (Posner and Furneaux, 1990).

In many patients, the onset of the neurologic disease process predates finding the causative neoplasm. Syndromes are generally subacute at onset, typically progressing over a period of weeks to months. The conditions may stabilize, with or without severe neurologic disability, or progress to death, which is usually due to the neurologic illness and intercurrent illness precipitated by the debilitated state.

The original clinical description of encephalomyelitis by Henson and Urich (see Henson et al., 1965) was later supported by finding a similar spectrum of neurologic syndromes in patients with the anti-Hu antibody. This antibody binds to a 37 kD neuronal protein antigen that has also been identified in tumor tissue (Dalmau et al., 1992). The antibody has been used to clone a gene encoding a protein (HuD) that bears significant homology to ELAV, an RNA-binding protein in *Drosophila* (Szabo et al., 1991). HuD belongs to a family of RNA-binding proteins (including HuD, HuC/ple21, Hel-N1, and others) that have a putative role in neuronal development and maintenance (Liu et al., 1995). In paraneoplastic encephalomyelitis, intrathecal synthesis of anti-Hu antibody is common, but is infrequent in patients presenting primarily with subacute sensory neuronopathy (see below) as the main manifestation (Vega et al., 1994).

An additional antibody has been described, called anti-CV2, that reacts with a 66 kD rat brain protein

Table 19–4. Spectrum of Paraneoplastic Encephalomyelitis

Limbic encephalitis	Bulbar encephalitis	Cerebellitis	Opsoclonus-myoclonus-ataxia
Retinal degeneration			Lambert-Eaton Syndrome
Myelitis	Motor neuronopathy	Sensory neuronopathy	Autonomic neuronopathy

(After Henson and Urich, 1982,ab,c.)

(POP66) present in oligodendrocytes and Ulip4/CRMP3, a member of a protein family involved in developmental axonal guidance (Honnorat et al., 1999). This antibody has been detected in PND patients with various clinical presentations of paraneoplastic encephalomyelitis and other PND (Honnorat et al., 1996).

Limbic Encephalitis

Limbic encephalitis is often characterized by a subacute progressive onset of anxiety, depression, confusion, hallucinations, recent memory loss, or seizures. The course is often variable, with many patients eventually stabilizing. Pathologic findings include gliosis and inflammatory infiltrates in the medial temporal lobes, Somner's sector, the amygdaloid nucleus, caudate, putamen, globus pallidus, thalamus, hypothalamus, and subthalamus. In cortical regions, abnormalities may be identified in cingulate, pyriform, parahippocampal, and orbital frontal cortex (Henson and Urich, 1982a). Limbic encephalitis may be accompanied by myelopathy or sensory ganglionitis. This syndrome most commonly occurs in patients with SCLC, and many have anti-Hu antibodies (Jaeckle et al., 1988). Patients may have T_2 hyperintensity on MRI scans within the medial temporal lobes (Sutton et al., 1993).

In one study, symptoms of limbic encephalitis preceded the discovery of tumor in 60% of 50 patients (Gultekin et al., 2000). Associated tumor types were lung (50%), testicular (20%), and breast (8%). Thirty patients (60%) had antineuronal antibodies, which were type anti-Hu (60%), anti-Ma (33%), or anti-Ma2 (Ta) (7%). A considerable number of patients (44%) showed clinical improvement at 8 months median follow up, particularly if tumor treatment was received and if antibody studies were negative. The association of limbic encephalitis with anti-Ma and anti-Ma2 (Ta) antibodies has recently been described in patients with testicular neoplasms (Voltz et al., 1999) and medullary breast carcinoma (Sutton et al., 2000).

Treatment is largely supportive; occasional patients have stabilized following tumor removal. Plasmapheresis, immunosuppression with corticosteroids or chemotherapeutic agents (cyclophosphamide, azathioprine), and intravenous immunoglobulin therapy have been largely ineffective.

Bulbar Encephalitis

A bulbar encephalitis syndrome was described in the older literature. Symptoms of bulbar encephalitis include nystagmus, vomiting, cranial nerve palsies, intranuclear ophthalmoplegia, opsoclonus, corticospinal tract findings, and rigidity. Pathologically, lesions are present in the medulla, particularly in the inferior olives and in the nuclei of cranial nerves XIII, X, and XII. Wallerian degeneration of ascending and descending fiber tracts are common. Many of these patients have associated cerebellar signs and often have anti-Hu antibodies and SCLC. This condition is rare without other signs of encephalomyelitis, and often some clinical aspects of bulbar encephalitis are observed in patients with paraneoplastic encephalomyelitis and anti-Hu antibodies. Response to treatment is unusual.

Cerebellitis

Although described as part of encephalomyelitis in the older literature, cerebellitis is essentially indistinguishable from paraneoplastic cerebellar degeneration, which is described below. It is now primarily used as a descriptive term for patients who demonstrate a prominent cerebellar component in addition to other signs of paraneoplastic encephalomyelitis.

Myelitis

Paraneoplastic myelitis usually presents with rapidly progressive weakness and lower motor neuron signs, including atrophy and fasciculations. Patients may have associated corticospinal and posterior column signs and often have evidence of sensory autonomic neuronopathy. Upper cervical cord or bulbar dysfunction may develop terminally, producing respiratory and pharyngeal insufficiency. This syndrome is most commonly seen in patients with SCLC and breast carcinoma and occasionally Hodgkin's disease. Pathologically, inflammatory cells, demyelination, spongiform changes, and neuronal loss are identified in the spinal cord, with secondary degenerative changes in ascending and descending tracts and in peripheral nerve roots. Magnetic resonance imaging scans may show intramedullary T_2 abnormalities. As in other encephalomyelitis conditions, patients often have serum and CSF anti-Hu antibodies.

Subacute Sensory Neuronopathy (Dorsal Root Ganglionitis)

Approximately one-third of patients with sensory neuronopathy (SSN) are found to have SCLC (Henson and Urich, 1982b; Dalmau et al., 1992). In more than any other PND syndrome, neurologic dysfunction in SSN usually precedes the discovery of neoplasm. The onset is characterized by a subacute progressive loss of sensory modalities, often accompanied by dysesthetic distal extremity pain. Within a matter of weeks to months, the symptoms spread to proximal limbs and the trunk. Sensory ataxia ultimately prevails and may be sufficiently severe to prevent the patient from sitting up in bed.

Associated dysautonomic function may result in cardiopulmonary complications or gastrointestinal dysfunction, including pseudo-obstruction (Kusunoki and Kanazawa, 1992) or dysphagia. Motor function is usually spared unless myelitis with motor neuronopathy accompanies the disorder. The disease usually progresses over several weeks to months, but may stabilize (Posner and Furneaux, 1990). Pathologically, dense inflammatory infiltrates, neuronal loss, and nodules of Nageotte are identified within dorsal root ganglia (Henson and Urich, 1982b). In occasional patients, evidence of in situ antibody within dorsal root ganglia neurons has been observed (Graus et al., 1985). Nerve conduction studies show delayed sensory nerve latencies with relative preservation of motor nerve function.

This syndrome has also been most commonly associated with the anti-Hu antibody and SCLC. Despite the suggestion of an immunologic pathogenesis, therapies with immunosuppressants, steroids, and plasmapheresis have not proved effective.

Autonomic Neuropathy

Occasional patients with cancer present with a dysautonomia syndrome, usually characterized by gastroenteric dysmotility, particularly constipation or dysphagia. Other findings of dysautonomia may be present, including neurogenic bladder dysfunction, orthostatic hypotension, pupillary and sudomotor dysfunction, or cardiac dysrhythmias (Dalmau et al., 1992; Lennon et al., 1991). Approximately one-fourth of anti-Hu–positive patients, usually with sensory neuronopathy, exhibit signs of autonomic neuropathy. Interestingly, the anti-Hu antibody has been shown to bind to neurons in the myenteric plexus of the intestinal wall (Lennon et al., 1991). Antibodies that bind to and block acetylcholine ganglionic receptors can also be identified in nearly one-half of patients with idiopathic or paraneoplastic autonomic neuropathy (Vernino et al., 2000).

PARANEOPLASTIC CEREBELLAR DEGENERATION

Paraneoplastic cerebellar degneration (PCD) accounts for approximately 9% of paraneoplastic syndromes (Henson and Urich, 1982c). Early descriptions indicated an equal incidence between men and women. However, the correlation between serum anti-Purkinje cell antibody (anti-Yo) with PCD has shown that the disorder is primarily a disease of women, as the anti-Yo antibody occurs almost exclusively in association with gynecologic malignancies (Anderson et al., 1988b). The most frequently observed associated tumors include adenocarcinoma of the ovary, adnexa, endometrium, and breast. Occasional patients with adenocarcinomas of the prostate and gastrointestinal tract, or with sarcomas, are included. Patients with Hodgkin's and non-Hodgkin's lymphomas may also develop this clinical syndrome, but are often negative for anti-Purkinje cell antibodies (Hammack et al., 1992). Most males with PCD have either SCLC (and are anti-Hu positive) or lymphoma as underlying malignancies.

Patients may develop neurologic evidence of PCD before or at the time of discovery of the neoplasm or during apparent remission. The onset may mimic labyrinthitis, with initial dizziness, vertigo, nausea and vomiting, and imbalance. However, in days to weeks, dysmetria, truncal and appendicular ataxia, tremor of the extremities and head, and dysarthria develop. Most patients also have nystagmus. The tremor may be so marked as to mimic intention myoclonus. Occasionally, signs of dysfunction of other areas of the neuraxis may occur, including corticospinal abnormalities, bulbar symptoms, and opsoclonus. Alteration in mental status has been described, but usually is mild or difficult to evaluate because of the presence of dysarthria and ataxia.

Pathologically, there is nearly total loss of cerebellar Purkinje neurons, thinning of the granular neuronal layer, perivascular lymphocytic infiltrates, and secondary changes in related brain stem nuclei and tracts (Henson and Urich, 1982c).

Patients with PCD often have serum and CSF anti-Purkinje cell antibodies, designated anti-Yo (type I, APCA, or PCA-1) reactive with a 62 kD (cdr2) protein; the antibody also reacts with 52 and 34 kD cloned neuronal protein antigens (Sakai et al., 1992; Dropcho et al., 1987; Fathallah-Shaykh et al., 1991). The cdr2 antigen is a DNA-binding protein. Cytotoxic T cells specific for cdr2 have been identified in the peripheral blood and CSF of patients with PCD, suggesting that an autoimmune T-cell–mediated response may be involved in the pathogenesis of PCD (Albert et al., 2000).

Almost all PCD patients are women with breast or gynecologic cancers, with limited local or regional tumor spread (Peterson et al., 1992). In nearly two-thirds of the anti-Yo–positive PCD patients, the neurologic syndrome precedes the cancer diagnosis, and in many instances the neurologic signs and the presence of the anti-Yo antibody lead to an evaluation for malignancy.

Patients with PCD and small cell carcinoma of the lung or breast may alternatively have anti-Hu antibodies. It has been shown that prominent cerebellar involvement is present in approximately 15% of patients overall who have demonstrable anti-Hu antibodies (Dalmau et al., 1992). In addition, some patients with the anti-Ri antibody will have a syndrome of PCD without prominent opsoclonus or myoclonus. As a result, it may be helpful in clinical evaluation to screen patients with suspected PCD for any of these three antibody subtypes, depending on the tumor and clinical presentation.

Treatment has been largely ineffective, although occasional patients have stabilized or improved with tumor removal, chemotherapy, plasmapheresis, or intravenous IgG. However, most reports of treatment have been negative.

PARANEOPLASTIC OPSOCLONUS-MYOCLONUS-ATAXIA

Best known for its association with childhood neuroblastoma, paraneoplastic opsoclonus-myoclonus-ataxia (POMA) is a rare syndrome that may also occur in adults. Approximately one-fifth of patients with opsoclonus-myoclonus have underlying neoplasms (Digre, 1986). Patients with POMA often present subacutely with evidence of brain stem dysfunction. Usually with imbalance, vertigo, or nausea and vomiting at onset, the syndrome progresses to produce frank ataxia and cerebellar tremor, which may be associated with true opsoclonus ("dancing eyes") and systemic myoclonus. The eye movements include rapid, chaotic, direction-changing oscillatory nystagmus that is usually conjugate. Although present in the primary position, it is worsened with volitional eye movements. There also may be systemic myoclonus, which can be symmetric or asymmetric. Ataxia is often severe, limits ambulation and functional daily activities, and is similar to that observed in paraneoplastic cerebellar degeneration. Mental status abnormalities are occasionally prominent. Patients may vary in the amount and degree of ataxia, opsoclonus, and myoclonus, respectively.

The paraneoplastic antibody anti-Ri (ANNA-2, type IIb), reactive with neuronal nuclear and cytoplasmic protein, has been associated with POMA and breast carcinoma (Luque et al., 1991), although gynecologic and bronchogenic carcinomas may be present. Few neuropathologic data are available: Usually the findings are similar to those of patients with cerebellar degeneration (Anderson et al., 1988a). The Ri antigen is a 55 kD neuronal protein antigen identified on Western immunoblots. The anti-Ri antibody has been used to clone a cDNA encoding a target antigen (Buckanovitch et al., 1993). This antibody binds to a group of nuclear RNA binding proteins (Nova-1 and Nova-2), which may be important neuron-specific regulatory proteins involved in neuronal development. Absence of Nova in null mice results in death from apoptosis of brain stem and spinal neurons (Buckanovich et al., 1996; Jensen et al., 2000).

The disorder is usually progressive, although spontaneous response or long-term remissions have occurred with administration of corticosteroids or ACTH (Dropcho et al., 1993).

RETINAL DEGENERATION (CANCER-ASSOCIATED RETINOPATHY)

Clinically, patients with cancer-associated retinopathy (CAR) develop progressive and painless loss of visual acuity and night blindness. Initially, the visual obscurations may be episodic, but the deficit quickly becomes more persistent. On examination, ring and central scotomata and color loss are observed. The syndrome may start unilaterally but rapidly becomes bilateral, and visual loss may progress to blindness within months (Posner and Furneaux, 1990; Thirkill et al., 1993a). Electroretinograms are flat or markedly abnormal. Most patients have an underlying SCLC.

Pathologically, there is loss of photoreceptor cells, with secondary degeneration, demyelination, and axonal loss in the optic nerves and tracts (Kornguth et al., 1986). A serum antibody reactive with a 23 to 26 kD calcium-binding protein (recoverin) has been identified in some patients (Thirkill et al., 1993b). Recoverin is a calcium-binding protein from the EF family that is involved in transduction of light by vertebrate photoreceptors (Polans et al., 1995). Recoverin proteins are thought to activate guanylate cyclase to synthesize cGMP, resulting in opening of calcium ion channels in the rod outer segments. This process is important in light-to-dark adaptation mechanisms (Lambrecht and Koch, 1991).

Recoverin has been identified in tumor tissue of patients with CAR (Polans et al., 1995). Intravitreous injection of anti-CAR antibody in rodents produces apoptosis and thinning of the retinal outer nuclear layer, which can be partially blocked with corticosteroid or cyclosporin A (Ohguro et al., 1999). Similarly, occasional patients have responded to steroid treatment or intravenous immunoglobulin, suggesting that CAR may be one of the more responsive PNDs to treatment if identified before visual loss is advanced (Guy and Aptsiauri, 1999).

SUBACUTE MOTOR NEURONOPATHY

Subacute motor neuronopathy is clinically distinguishable from myelitis in paraneoplastic encephalomyelitis (Schold et al., 1979). Typically, patients have Hodgkin's or non-Hodgkin's lymphomas and present with an almost pure motor neuron disease of the spinal cord. A distinguishing feature of subacute motor neuronopathy is sparing of the lateral corticospinal tract, and thus upper motor neuron signs are generally not present. Patients often develop a subacute, progressive, painless weakness that begins in the legs and may later affect the upper extremities. Often the disease is slightly asymmetric, but is usually bilateral.

Sensory loss is mild or absent. Electromyogram and nerve conduction studies are consistent with neuronopathy. Cerebrospinal fluid is generally normal except for mild increased protein content, and the MRI scan is also usually normal. Although it has been postulated that the neuronopathy results from radiotherapy, some patients have developed typical motor neuron signs outside the radiation ports, suggesting another cause (Schold et al., 1979). Pathologically, neuronal loss in the anterior horns of the spinal cord and mild dorsal column demyelination are noted, without significant inflammatory infiltrates. Antibodies in the serum of patients have not been consistently identified. In contrast to many of the progressive paraneoplastic diseases, patients often show spontaneous stabilization or improvement, usually after a period of several months to years, which does not appear to be hastened by anti-inflammatory therapy.

LAMBERT-EATON MYASTHENIC SYNDROME

Lambert-Eaton myastheic syndrome (LEMS) arises in the absence of cancer in about 30% to 50% of patients (Gutmann and Phillips, 1992). When associated with an underlying neoplasm, nearly two-thirds have SCLC (O'Neill et al., 1988). The syndrome appears in approximately 3% of SCLC patients overall (Zenone et al., 1992). Commonly, the primary symptom is subacute progressive weakness, which may improve with increasing effort. Bulbar and cranial nerve distribution weakness is unusual, but difficulties with respiration may occur in advanced cases; the incidence of respiratory failure is lower than in patients with myasthenia gravis (Barr et al., 1993; Laroche et al., 1989). Because many of these patients are receiving radiation and chemotherapy and have significant cachectic weight loss and anorexia, nonspecific weakness may be falsely attributed to other causes. The diagnosis should be considered in any SCLC patient who is having significant impairment of ambulation. Many patients will also have associated autonomic findings, including dysmotility, xerostomia, xerophthalmus, and impotence (Bady et al., 1992; Chalk et al., 1990). Neurologic examination will demonstrate hyporeflexia and weakness, which may improve with effort.

Electromyography initially reveals compound muscle action potentials of low amplitude. Repetitive stimulation at 50 Hz shows a characteristic increase in compound muscle-action potential amplitude (Bady et al., 1992). Concurrent axonal neuropathy may be associated with LEMS, complicating the clinical picture.

The myasthenic syndrome is a disorder of quantal release of acetylcholine at the presynaptic motor axon bulb, similar to that which occurs in botulinum intoxication. IgG from LEMS patients binds to voltage-gated calcium channels (VGCCs) (Leys et al., 1991; Lennon et al., 1982), which are distinct from those blocked by nifedipine (Johnston et al., 1994), but identical to those blocked by a 27-peptide toxin from a fish-hunting marine snail, *Conus geographus* (Olivera et al., 1984). IgG may bind the synaptic vesicle protein synaptotagmin (p65) (Martin-Moutot et al., 1993), also a target for the black widow spider venom α-latrotoxin (Petrenko et al., 1991). Synaptotagmin, using a mechanism dependent on a calcium-calmodulin protein kinase, appears to be responsible for docking presynaptic vesicles containing acetylcholine at the synaptic membrane (Popoli, 1993). In LEMS, antibodies bind, in particular, to the P/Q type VGCCs (Takamori et al., 2000).

Passive transfer of LEMS IgG to mice produces a defect similar to that in humans in neuromuscular junction transmission (Prior et al., 1985). The antibody has also been used to clone cDNA encoding a recombinant protein that is structurally similar to the β-subunit of the calcium channel (Rosenfeld et al., 1993).

Lambert-Eaton myasthenic syndrome may respond to treatment or removal of tumor. Other therapies have included immunosuppression (Chalk et al., 1990), immunoglobulin infusion (Bird, 1992), and 3,4-diaminopyridine (McEvoy et al., 1989; Molgo and Guglielmi, 1996). Use of 3,4-diaminopyridine has to be carefully individualized (Lundh et al., 1993) by following the neurophysiologic effect on compound muscle-action potential amplitudes and clinical response. Plasmapheresis has also been utilized in refractory cases with varying degrees of success.

DERMATOMYOSITIS AND POLYMYOSITIS

There has been debate in the literature as to whether dermatomyositis and polymyositis occur more frequently in patients with an underlying cancer, as opposed to their occurrence in the normal population. It is generally believed that dermatomyositis is most likely to occur in patients with an underlying malignancy, particularly of the lung, and that males (particularly smokers) over the age of 50 years who develop polymyositis or dermatomyositis should be carefully evaluated for an occult malignancy. This disorder occurs with equal frequency in men and women. Adenocarcinomas of the lung, breast, ovary, and gastrointestinal tract are present in approximately 10% to 20% of patients (Brooke, 1977).

Although the cardinal feature is proximal muscle weakness, other symptoms may alert the clinician to the diagnosis. In dermatomyositis, nonspecific systemic symptoms such as fever, irritability, fatigue, and gastrointestinal symptoms may occur. An erythematous or violaceous rash may appear before the onset of weakness, affecting the face, upper trunk, and extremities. The rash is particularly prominent in sun-exposed areas; skin may become thickened over the joints, including the elbows, knees, and knuckles. Muscular aches are present in two-thirds of patients and may be accompanied by mild muscle edema. Weakness usually develops over a period of days to weeks, producing difficulty in arising from a chair and with ambulation. Bulbar symptoms are unusual. The disease course may be one of steady progression or may exhibit relapsing and remitting episodes. Long-term, severe cases typically are complicated by intercurrent life-threatening illness.

The diagnosis is made by finding a high serum creatine phosphokinase level, the characteristic EMG findings of an inflammatory myopathy, and muscle biopsy, which shows inflammatory cells and perifascicular atrophy. This disease may be associated with antibodies directed against transfer-RNA synthetases (Mathews et al., 1984), particularly Jo-1 histidyl-tRNA synthetase (Marguerie et al., 1990). Although deposition of immunoglobulins within vessels and inflammatory infiltrates has been identified pathologically, the etiology is unclear (Whitaker and Engel, 1972). Many patients improve with immunosuppressant therapy, including corticosteroids, methotrexate, azathioprine, or cyclophosphamide.

CONCLUSION

Paraneoplastic neurologic disorders are rare but fascinating illnesses, as they provide unique opportunities to study the relationship between the host immune system and associated neoplasms. Although originally characterized on the basis of clinical presentations and neuropathologic areas of involvement, the finding of related autoantibodies and subsequent cloning and characterization of associated antigens has prompted a reclassification of these disorders. This process continues to evolve as the structure and function of the antigens is made known. The categorization of antibodies has allowed a better understanding of the clinical disorders and in some cases earlier detection of neoplasms. However, treatment has largely been ineffective, with the possible exception of the paraneoplastic opsoclonus-myoclonus-ataxia syndrome, cancer-associated retinopathy, Lambert-Eaton myasthenic syndrome, and polymyositis. It is hoped that clarification of their pathogenesis will lead to a better understanding of host immune response to neoplasm and effective treatments for these devastating disorders.

REFERENCES

Albert ML, Austin LM, Darnell RB. 2000. Detection and treatment of activated T cells in the cerebrospinal fluid of patients with paraneoplastic cerebellar degeneration. Ann Neurol 47:9–17.

Anderson NE, Budde-Steffen C, Rosenblum MK, et al. 1988a. Opsoclonus, myoclonus, ataxia, and encephalopathy in adults with cancer: a distinct paraneoplastic syndrome. Medicine (Baltimore) 67:100–109.

Anderson NE, Cunningham JM, Posner JB. 1987. Autoimmune pathogenesis of paraneoplastic neurologic syndromes. Crit Rev Neurobiol 3:245–299.

Anderson NE, Rosenblum MK, Posner JB. 1988b. Paraneoplastic cerebellar degeneration: clinical–immunologic correlations. Ann Neurol 24:559–567.

Bady B, Vial C, Chauplannaz G. 1992. [Lambert-Eaton syndrome: clinical and electrophysiological study of 18 cases associated with lung cancer]. Rev Neurol (Paris) 148:513–519.

Barr CW, Claussen G, Thomas D, Fesenmeier JT, Pearlman RL, Oh SJ. 1993. Primary respiratory failure as the presenting symptom in Lambert-Eaton myasthenic syndrome. Muscle Nerve 16:712–715.

Bird SJ. 1992. Clinical and electrophysiologic improvement in Lambert-Eaton syndrome with intravenous immunoglobulin therapy. Neurology 42:1422–1423.

Brain WR, Daniel PM, Greenfield JG. 1951. Sub-acute cortical cerebellar degeneration in relation to carcinoma. J Neurol Neurosurg Psychiatry 14:59–75.

Brain WR, Norris FH Jr. 1965. The Remote Effects of Cancer on the Nervous System: The Proceedings of a Symposium. New York: Grune & Stratton, pp 104–221.

Brashear HR, Greenlee JE, Jaeckle KA, Rose JW. 1989. Anticerebellar antibodies in neurologicly normal patients with ovarian neoplasms. Neurology 39:1605–1609.

Brouwer B. 1919. Beitrag zur kenntnis der chronischen diffusen kleinhirner krankungen. Mendels Neurol Zbl 38:674–682.

Brooke MH. 1977. A Clinician's View of Neuromuscular Diseases. Baltimore: Williams & Wilkins, 225 pp.

Buckanovich RJ, Posner JB, Darnell RB. 1993. Nova, the paraneoplastic Ri antigen, is homologous to an RNA-binding protein and is specifically expressed in the developing motor system. Neuron 11:657–672.

Buckanovich RJ, Yang YY, Darnell RB. 1996. The onconeural antigen Nova-1 is a neuron-specific RNA-binding protein, the activity of which is inhibited by paraneoplastic antibodies. J Neurosci 16:1114–1122.

Cavaletti G, Bogliun G, Marzorati L, Marzola M, Pittelli MR, Tredici G. 1991. The incidence and course of paraneoplastic neuropathy in women with epithelial ovarian cancer. J Neurol 238:371–374.

Chalk CH, Murray NM, Newsom-Davis J, O'Neill JH, Spiro SG. 1990. Response of the Lambert-Eaton myasthenic syndrome to treatment of associated small-cell lung carcinoma. Neurology 40:1552–1556.

Croft PB, Wilkinson M. 1965. The incidence of carcinomatous neuromyopathy in patients with various types of carcinoma. Brain 88:427–434.

Dalmau J, Furneaux HM, Rosenblum MK, Graus F, Posner JB. 1991. Detection of the anti-Hu antibody in specific regions of the nervous system and tumor from patients with paraneoplastic encephalomyelitis/sensory neuronopathy. Neurology 41:1757–1764.

Dalmau J, Graus F, Rosenblum MK, Posner JB. 1992. Anti-Hu-associated paraneoplastic encephalomyelitis/sensory neuronopathy. A clinical study of 71 patients. Medicine (Baltimore) 71:59–72.

Darnell R. 1996. Onconeural antigens and the paraneoplastic neurologic disorders: at the intersection of cancer, immunity, and the brain. Proc Natl Acad Sci USA 93:4529–4536.

Denny-Brown D. 1948. Primary sensory neuropathy with muscular changes associated with carcinoma. J Neurol Neurosurg Psychiatry 11:73–87.

Digre KB. 1986. Opsoclonus in adults. Report of 3 cases and review of the literature. Arch Neurol 43:1165–1175.

Dropcho EJ, Chen YT, Posner JB, Old LJ. 1987. Cloning of a brain protein identified by autoantibodies from a patient with paraneoplastic cerebellar degeneration. Proc Natl Acad Sci USA 84:4552–4556.

Dropcho EJ, Kline LB, Riser J. 1993. Antineuronal (anti-Ri) antibodies in a patient with steroid-responsive opsoclonus-myoclonus. Neurology 43:207–211.

Elrington GM, Murray NM, Spiro SG, Newsom-Davis J. 1991. Neurological paraneoplastic syndromes in patients with small cell lung cancer. A prospective survey of 150 patients. J Neurol Neurosurg Psychiatry 54:764–767.

Fathallah-Shaykh H, Wolf S, Wong E, Posner JB, Furneaux HM. 1991. Cloning of a leucine-zipper protein recognized by the sera of patients with antibody-associated paraneoplastic cerebellar degeneration. Proc Natl Acad Sci USA 88:3451–3454.

Furneaux HM, Rosenblum MK, Dalmau J, et al. 1990. Selective expression of Purkinje-cell antigens in tumor tissue from patients with paraneoplastic cerebellar degeneration. N Engl J Med 322:1844–1851.

Graus F, Cordon-Cardo C, Posner JB. 1985. Neuronal antinuclear antibody in sensory neuronopathy from lung cancer. Neurology 35:538–543.

Graus F, Vega F, Delattre JY, et al. 1992. Plasmapheresis and antineoplastic treatment in CNS paraneoplastic syndromes with antineuronal autoantibodies. Neurology 42:536–540.

Greenlee JE, Brashear HR. 1983. Antibodies to cerebellar Purkinje cells in patients with paraneoplastic cerebellar degeneration and ovarian carcinoma. Ann Neurol 14: 609–613.

Greenlee JE, Brashear HR, Jaeckle KA, Geleris A, Jordan K. 1992. Pursuing an occult carcinoma in a patient with subacute cerebellar degeneration and anticerebellar antibodies. Need for a vigorous follow-up. West J Med 156: 199–202.

Greenlee JE, Brashear HR, Rodnitzy RL, et al. 1986. Fall in antineuronal antibody titers and improvement of neurologic deficit following tumor removal in paraneoplastic cerebellar degeneration. Neurology 36:334A.

Greenlee JE, Parks TN, Jaeckle KA. 1993. Type IIa ("anti-Hu") antineuronal antibodies produce destruction of rat cerebellar granule neurons in vitro. Neurology 43:2049–2054.

Grisold W, Drlicek M, Liszka-Setinek U, Wondrusch E. 1995. Anti-tumour therapy in paraneoplastic neurological disease. Clin Neurol Neurosurg 97:106–111.

Gultekin SH, Rosenfeld MR, Voltz R, Eichen J, Posner JB, Dalmau J. 2000. Paraneoplastic limbic encephalitis: neurological symptoms, immunological findings and tumour association in 50 patients. Brain 123:1481–1494.

Gutmann L, Phillips LH 2nd. 1992. Trends in the association of Lambert-Eaton myasthenic syndrome with carcinoma. Neurology 42:848–850.

Guy J, Aptsiauri N. 1999. Treatment of paraneoplastic visual loss with intravenous immunoglobulin: report of 3 cases. Arch Ophthalmol 117:471–477.

Hammack J, Kotanides H, Rosenblum MK, Posner JB. 1992. Paraneoplastic cerebellar degeneration. II. Clinical and immunologic findings in 21 patients with Hodgkin's disease. Neurology 42:1938–1943.

Henson RA, Hoffman HL, Urich H. 1965. Encephalomyelitis with carcinoma. Brain 88:449–464.

Henson RA, Urich H. 1982a. Cancer in the Nervous System, 1st ed. London: Blackwell Scientific, pp 315–319.

Henson RA, Urich H. 1982b. Cancer in the Nervous System, 1st ed. London: Blackwell Scientific, pp 324–329.

Henson RA, Urich H. 1982c. Cancer in the Nervous System, 1st ed. London: Blackwell Scientific, pp 346–358.

Honnorat J, Antoine JC, Derrington E, Aguera M, Belin MF. 1996. Antibodies to a subpopulation of glial cells and a 66 kDa developmental protein in patients with paraneoplastic neurological syndromes. J Neurol Neurosurg Psychiatry 61:270–278.

Honnorat J, Byk T, Kusters I, et al. 1999. Ulip/CRMP proteins are recognized by autoantibodies in paraneoplastic neurological syndromes. Eur J Neurosci 11:4226–4232.

Jaeckle KA, Graus F, Houghton A. 1985. Autoimmune response of patients with paraneoplastic cerebellar degeneration to a Purkinje cell cytoplasmic protein antigen. Ann Neurol 18:592–600.

Jaeckle KA, Rogers L, Wong M. 1988. Autoimmune paraneoplastic limbic encephalitis. Neurology 38:390A.

Jaeckle KA, Shaw MV, Greenlee JE. 1992. Allogenic tumor lines express paraneoplastic neurologic diseases (PND) antigens. Neurology 42:389A.

Jean WC, Dalmau J, Ho A, Posner JB. 1994. Analysis of the IgG subclass distribution and inflammatory infiltrates in patients with anti-Hu–associated paraneoplastic encephalomyelitis. Neurology 41:140–147.

Jensen KB, Dredge BK, Stefani G. 2000. Nova-1 regulates neuron-specific alternative splicing and is essential for neuronal viability. Neuron 25:359–371.

Johnston I, Lang B, Leys K, Newsom-Davis J. 1994. Heterogeneity of calcium channel autoantibodies detected using a small-cell lung cancer line derived from a Lambert-Eaton myasthenic syndrome patient. Neurology 44:334–338.

Keime-Guibert F, Graus F, Fleury A, et al. 2000. Treatment of paraneoplastic neurological syndromes with antineuronal antibodies (Anti-Hu, anti-Yo) with a combination of immunoglobulins, cyclophosphamide, and methylprednisonlone. J Neurol Neurosurg Psychiatry 68:479–482.

Kida E, Barcikowska M, Michalska T, Joachimowicz E, Siekierzynska A. 1992. Peripheral nervous system alterations in small cell lung cancer. Clinical–pathologic study. Neuropathol Pol 30:43–56.

King PH, Redden D, Palmgren JS, Nabors LB, Lennon VA. 1999. Hu antigen specificities of ANNA-I autoantibodies in paraneoplastic neurological disease. J Autoimmun 13:435–443.

Kornguth SE, Kalinke T, Grunwald GB, Schutta H, Dahl D. 1986. Antineurofilament antibodies in the sera of patients with small cell carcinoma of the lung and with visual paraneoplastic syndrome. Cancer Res 46:2588–2595.

Kornguth SE, Klein R, Appen R, Choate J. 1982. Occurrence of anti-retinal ganglion cell antibodies in patients with small cell carcinoma of the lung. Cancer 50:1289–1293.

Kusunoki S, Kanazawa I. 1992. [Carcinomatous autonomic neuropathy and the autoantibodies in paraneoplastic neuropathy]. Nippon Rinsho 50:834–839.

Lambert EH, Eaton LM, Rooke ED. 1956. Defect of neuromuscular conduction associated with malignant neoplasms. Am J Physiol 187:612–613.

Lambrecht HG, Koch KW. 1991. A 26 kd calcium binding protein from bovine rod outer segments as modulator of photoreceptor guanylate cyclase. EMBO J 10:793–798.

Laroche CM, Mier AK, Spiro SG, Newsom-Davis J, Moxham J, Green M. 1989. Respiratory muscle weakness in the Lambert-Eaton myasthenic syndrome. Thorax 44:913–918.

Lennon VA, Lambert EH, Whittingham S, Fairbanks V. 1982. Autoimmunity in the Lambert-Eaton myasthenic syndrome. Muscle Nerve 5:S21–S25.

Lennon VA, Sas DF, Busk MF, et al. 1991. Enteric neuronal autoantibodies in pseudoobstruction with small-cell lung carcinoma. Gastroenterology 100:137–142.

Levine TD, Gao F, King PH, Andrews LG, Keene JD. 1993. Hel-N1: an autoimmune RNA-binding protein with specificity for 3′uridylate-rich untranslated regions of growth factor mRNAs. Mol Cell Biol 13:3494–3504.

Leys K, Lang B, Johnston I, Newsom-Davis J. 1991. Calcium channel autoantibodies in the Lambert-Eaton myasthenic syndrome. Ann Neurol 29:307–314.

Liu J, Dalmau J, Szabo A, Rosenfeld M, Huber J, Furneaux H. 1995. Paraneoplastic encephalomyelitis antigens bind to the AU-rich elements of mRNA. Neurology 45: 544–550.

Lundh H, Nilsson O, Rosen I, Johansson S. 1993. Practical aspects of 3,4-diaminopyridine treatment of the Lambert-Eaton myasthenic syndrome. Acta Neurol Scand 88:136–140.

Luque FA, Furneaux HM, Wray SH, Ferziger R. 1991. Anti-Ri: an antibody associated with paraneoplastic opsoclonus in breast cancer. Ann Neurol 29:241–251.

Marguerie C, Bunn CC, Beynon HL, et al. 1990. Polymyositis, pulmonary fibrosis and autoantibodies to aminoacyl-tRNA synthetase enzymes. Q J Med 77: 1019–1038.

Martin-Moutot N, el Far O, Leveque C, et al. 1993. Synaptotagmin: a Lambert-Eaton myasthenic syndrome antigen that associates with presynaptic calcium channels. J Physiol Paris 87:37–41.

Mathews MB, Reichlin M, Hughes GR, Bernstein RM. 1984. Anti-threonyl-tRNA synthetase, a second myositis-related autoantibody. J Exp Med 160:420–434.

McEvoy KM, Windebank AJ, Daube JR, Low PA. 1989. 3,4-Diaminopyridine in the treatment of the Lambert-Eaton myasthenic syndrome. N Engl J Med 321:1567–1571.

Molgo J, Guglielmi JM. 1996. 3,4-Diaminopyridine, an orphan drug, in the symptomatic treatment of Lambert-Eaton myasthenic syndrome. Pflugers Arch 431:R295–R296.

Ohguro H, Ogawa K, Maeda T, Maeda A, Maruyama I. 1999. Cancer-associated retinopathy induced by both anti-recoverin and anti-hsc70 antibodies in vivo. Invest Ophthalmol Vis Sci 40:3160–3167.

Olivera BM, McIntosh JM, Cruz LJ, Luque FA, Gray WR. 1984. Purification and sequence of a presynaptic peptide toxin from *Conus geographus* venom. Biochemistry 23: 5087–5090.

O'Neill JH, Murray NMF, Newsom-Davis J. 1988. The Lambert-Eaton myasthenic syndrome. A review of 50 cases. Brain 111:577–596.

Oppenheim H. 1888. Uber hirnsymptome gei carcinomatose ohne nachweibare veranderungen um gehirm. Charite-Ann Berlin 13:335–344.

Peterson K, Rosenblum MK, Kotanides H, Posner JB. 1992. Paraneoplastic cerebellar degeneration. I. A clinical analysis of 55 anti-Yo antibody-positive patients. Neurology 42:1931–1937.

Petrenko AG, Perin MS, Davletov BA, Ushkaryov YA, Geppert M, Sudhof TC. 1991. Binding of synaptotagmin to the alpha-latrotoxin receptor implicates both in synaptic vesicle exocytosis. Nature 353:65–68.

Polans AS, Witkowska D, Haley TL, Amundson D, Baizer L, Adamus G. 1995. Recoverin, a photoreceptor-specific calcium-binding protein, is expressed by the tumor of a patient with cancer-associated retinopathy. Proc Natl Acad Sci USA 92:9176–9180.

Popoli M. 1993. Synaptotagmin is endogenously phosphorylated by Ca^{++}/calmodulin protein kinase II in synaptic vesicles. FEBS Lett 317:85–88.

Posner JB, Furneaux HM. 1990. Paraneoplastic syndromes. In: Waksman BH (ed), Immunologic Mechanisms and Neurologic and Psychiatric Disease. New York: Raven Press, p 187.

Prior C, Lang B, Wray D, Newsom-Davis J. 1985. Action of Lambert-Eaton myasthenic syndrome IgG at mouse motor nerve terminals. Ann Neurol 17:587–592.

Rosenfeld MR, Wong E, Dalmau J, et al. 1993. Cloning and characterization of a Lambert-Eaton myasthenic syndrome antigen. Ann Neurol 33:113–120.

Sakai K, Negami T, Yoshioka A, Hirose G. 1992. The expression of a cerebellar degeneration-associated neural antigen in human tumor cell lines. Neurology 42:361–366.

Sato S, Inuzuka T, Nakano R, et al. 1991. Antibody to a zincfinger protein in a patient with paraneoplastic cerebellar degeneration. Biochem Biophys Res Commun 178:198–206.

Sawyer RA, Selhorst JB, Zimmerman LE, Hoyt WF. 1976. Blindness caused by photoreceptor degeneration as a remote effect of cancer. Am J Ophthalmol 81:606–613.

Schold SC, Cho ES, Somasundaram M, Posner JB. 1979. Subacute motor neuronopathy: a remote effect of lymphoma. Ann Neurol 5:271–287.

Stertz G. 1916. Polymyositis. Berl Klin Wochenschr 53:489.

Sutton I, Winer J, Rowlands D, Dalmau J. 2000. Limbic encephalitis and antibodies to Ma2: a paraneoplastic presentation of breast cancer. J Neurol Neurosurg Psychiatry 69:266–268.

Sutton RC, Lipper MH, Brashear HR. 1993. Limbic encephalitis occurring in association with Alzheimer's disease. J Neurol Neurosurg Psychiatry 56:808–811.

Szabo A, Dalmau J, Manley G, et al. 1991. HuD, a paraneoplastic encephalomyelitis antigen contains RNA-binding domains and is homologous to Elav and Sex-lethal. Cell 67:325–333.

Takamori M, Komai K, Iwasa K. 2000. Antibodies to calcium channel and synaptotagmin in Lambert-Eaton myasthenic syndrome. Am J Med Sci 319:204–208.

Thirkill CE, Keltner JL, Tyler NK, Roth AM. 1993a. Antibody reactions with retina and cancer-associated antigens in 10 patients with cancer-associated retinopathy. Arch Ophthalmol 111:931–978.

Thirkill CE, Tait RC, Tyler NK, Roth AM, Keltner JL. 1993b. Intraperitoneal cultivation of small-cell carcinoma induces expression of the retinal cancer-associated retinopathy antigen. Arch Ophthalmol 111:974–978.

Thirkill CE, Tait RC, Tyler NK, Roth AM, Keltner JL. 1992. The cancer-associated retinopathy antigen is a recoverin-like protein. Invest Ophthalmol Vis Sci 33:2768–2772.

Trotter JL, Hendin BA, Osterland CK. 1976. Cerebellar degeneration with Hodgkin disease. An immunological study. Arch Neurol 33:660–661.

Tsukamoto T, Mochizuki R, Mochizuki H, et al. 1993. Paraneoplastic cerebellar degeneration and limbic encephalitis in a patient with adenocarcinoma of the colon. J Neurol Neurosurg Psychiatry 56:713–716.

Vega F, Graus F, Chen QM, Poisson M, Schuller E, Delattre JY. 1994. Intrathecal synthesis of the anti-Hu antibody in patients with paraneoplastic encephalomyelitis or sensory neruonopathy: clinical–immunologic correlation 44:2145–2147.

Vernino S, Low PA, Fealey RD, Stewart JD, Farrugia G, Lennon VA. 2000. Autoantibodies to ganglionic acetylcholine receptors in autoimmune autonomic neuropathies. N Engl J Med 343:847–855.

Voltz R, Gultekin SH, Rosenfeld MR, et al. 1999. A serologic marker of paraneoplastic limbic and brain-stem encephalitis in patients with testicular cancer. N Engl J Med 340:1788–1795.

Weigert C. 1901. Pathologisch-anatomischer Beitrag zur Erb'schen Krankheit (myasthenia gravis). Neurol Centralbl 20:597–601.

Whitaker JN, Engel WK. 1972. Vascular deposits of immunoglobulin and complement in idiopathic inflammatory myopathy. N Engl J Med 286:333–338.

Wilkinson PC. 1964. Serologic findings in carcinomatous neuromyopathy. Lancet 1:1301–1303.

Winter SF, Sekido Y, Minna JD, et al. 1993. Antibodies against autologous tumor cell proteins in patients with small-cell lung cancer—association with improved survival. J Natl Canc Inst 85:2012–2018.

Zenone T, Bady B, Souquet PJ, Bernard JP. 1992. [The Lambert-Eaton syndrome]. Rev Mal Respir 9:483–490.

20

Seizures and Syncope in the Cancer Patient

ALEXANDRA FLOWERS

Neurologic complications in cancer patients commonly involve altered levels of consciousness. This chapter discusses seizures and syncope, two problems in cancer patients that can have multiple causes. Whereas normally it is easy to distinguish between these two conditions, occasionally when there are no observers of the event, it can be difficult for the clinician to be certain whether a seizure or syncope has occurred. It is hoped that the sections that follow will help clarify the etiologies, presentations, and treatments for seizures and syncope in cancer patients, including those caused by drugs given for cancer therapy.

SEIZURES

Seizures are the first clinical manifestation in approximately 30% of patients with primary or metastatic brain tumors (Cascino, 1993; Stein and Chamberlain, 1991). In patients who have systemic cancer without brain metastases, the incidence of ictal phenomena is not well documented. In fact, there have been no prospective or retrospective studies of seizures in this group, and some seizures in these patients are not recognized as such (e.g., complex partial seizures). On occasion, non-ictal, abnormal movements may be confused with seizures.

Etiology

The etiology of seizures in cancer patients is presented in Table 20–1. More than one etiologic factor may be present in a patient, so an accurate evaluation will require a comprehensive work-up of each patient.

Primary and Metastatic Brain Tumors

Primary and metastatic brain tumors can present with focal or generalized seizures. Among infiltrating gliomas, low-grade gliomas, particularly those involving the temporal lobe, are the most likely to cause seizures, usually with onset in childhood or in the teenage years (Bartolomei et al., 1997; Britton et al., 1994; Rogers et al., 1993). Patients with seizures caused by brain tumors present with generalized tonic-clonic seizures or simple or complex partial seizures, with or without secondary generalization. Unfortunately, at times the seizures are difficult to treat. Additionally, an increased frequency of seizures in a patient with a known low-grade brain tumor may indicate tumor transformation to a more malignant histology.

In general, patients with primary brain tumors who present with seizures but do not have magnetic resonance imaging (MRI) or computerized tomography (CT) confirmation of tumor at their initial evaluation have a better prognosis. This fact may reflect an earlier diagnosis of tumor and/or lower grade of malignancy. Improvement in MRI scanning techniques allows these patients to be diagnosed with tumor at an earlier time.

Surgery, when feasible, is a desired therapeutic approach for both tumor removal and seizure control (Britton et al., 1994). Modern techniques, such as brain mapping and intraoperative electroen-

Table 20–1. Etiology of Seizures in Cancer Patients

Etiologic Factors	*Causes*
Intracranial tumors	
Parenchymal	Primary tumors (gliomas), metastatic tumors
Meningeal	
Mass lesions	Primary tumors (meningiomas), metastatic tumors
Diffuse	Primary tumors (meningeal gliomatosis), metastatic tumors (meningeal carcinomatosis, lymphomatosis)
Systemic cancer	
Treatment-related	
Radiation therapy	Increased edema, radiation necrosis
Chemotherapy	Platinum, methotrexate, cytarabine, busulfan, L-asparaginase, 5-fluorouracil, ifosfamide, paclitaxel Intratumoral chemotherapy
Biologic agents	IL-2, interferon, lymphokine-activated killer cells, granulocyte-macrophage colony-stimulating factor
Other drugs	
Narcotics	Meperidine, morphine, propoxyphene
Neuroleptics	Haloperidol, phenothiazine
Antidepressants	Tricyclics, Prozac, Wellbutrin
Antibiotics	Betalactams, quinolones
IV contrast media	Radiologic contrast media used for CT scanning
Metabolic	
Hyponatremia	Volume depletion, overhydration, syndrome of inappropriate antidiuretic hormone secretion
Hypoglycemia	Malnutrition, pancreatic tumors, total parenteral nutrition withdrawal
Hypocalcemia	Nutritional, secondary to chemotherapy (cisplatin)
Hypomagnesemia	Drug-related (chemotherapy—cisplatin, amphotericin B), hypoparathyroidism
Hypoxia	Pulmonary fibrosis (chemotherapy related), pulmonary embolism, lung cancer (primary or metastatic)
Vascular	Stroke (thrombotic, embolic), vasculitis (paraneoplastic, treatment induced)
Hemorrhagic	
Parenchymal	Tumor, mycotic aneurysms, aspergillomas
Subdural	Post-traumatic, due to thrombocytopenia, after spinal taps
Subarachnoid	Spontaneous, due to thrombocytopenia or coagulopathy
Infectious	
Viral	Herpes simplex, herpes zoster, cytomegalovirus
Bacterial	Common pathogens, *Listeria, Mycobacterium*
Fungal	*Aspergillus, Cryptococcus*
Parasitic	Toxoplasmosis

cephalography, allow accurate identification of the seizure focus (Lim et al., 1991; Cascino, 1990; Smith et al., 1991). When surgical resection is not feasible, radiation therapy (RT) can help control the seizures (Rogers et al., 1993).

Systemic cancers most likely to metastasize to the brain are melanoma, lung carcinoma, renal cell carcinoma, breast carcinoma, cancers of the gastrointestinal tract, and choriocarcinoma (Trillet and Biron, 1989; Flowers and Levin, 1993; Rosner et al.,

1986). As time of survival increases with the use of chemotherapy, other types of cancer are thus given more time to develop and can also metastasize to the brain. Seizures can also occur secondary to parenchymal brain metastases and with dural and leptomeningeal metastases (Wasserstrom et al., 1982; Blaney et al., 1991).

Seizures Related to Paraneoplastic Syndromes

Although rare, paraneoplastic encephalomyeloneuritis can manifest with complex partial or generalized seizures, and these occur most frequently with anti-Hu–associated paraneoplastic encephalomyeloneuritis in patients with small cell lung carcinoma. Occasionally seizures occur in patients with paraneoplastic encephalomyeloneuritis associated with prostate or renal cell carcinoma (Dalmau et al., 1992; Drislane, 1994; Franck et al., 1987; de Toffol et al., 1997). Paraneoplastic temporal lobe epilepsy has even been reported in a patient with testicular cancer (Ahern et al., 1994).

Seizures Related to Radiation Therapy

The frequency of preexisting seizures may increase acutely during RT because of increased cerebral edema. With the use of corticosteroids to control edema and careful monitoring of antiepileptic drug levels, this is a rather infrequent occurrence. Seizures may also occur as a result of radiation-induced brain necrosis or vasculopathy, which are delayed effects of RT (Ciaudo-Lacroix and Lapresle, 1985; Rider, 1963; Spencer, 1998). Positron emission tomography and single-photon emission computed tomography scans of the brain can help to distinguish brain tumors from radiation-induced necrosis, although active epileptogenic foci caused by radiation necrosis can demonstrate hyperperfusion and hypermetabolism (Sasaki et al., 1996).

Seizures have been reported as immediate side effects (occurring within the first 2 weeks) in patients treated with radiosurgery. This may be due to a direct effect of irradiation on cellular permeability and leakage of irritative chemical products; no connection has been made with prior external beam radiation, use of corticosteroids, target volume, isodose, or pretreatment edema (Werner-Wasik et al., 1999).

Seizures Related to Chemotherapy

Seizures occur in fewer than 1% of patients treated with systemic chemotherapy and can occur as a manifestation of the neurotoxicity of chemotherapeutic agents. In general, chemotherapy-associated neurotoxicity is related to specific drugs or drug combinations, dose intensity, and route of administration (Weiss et al., 1974). Because the early studies predated both the CT and MRI era, it is possible that small cerebral tumor metastases were present in the patient population reported. The chemotherapeutic agents most commonly reported to cause central nervous system (CNS) toxicity are cisplatin, methotrexate, L-asparaginase, and busulfan. Neurotoxicity is also caused by high doses of busulfan, which is administered to recipients of bone marrow transplants (Antonini et al., 1998; Kramer et al., 1997; Snider et al., 1994; Tahsildar et al., 1996).

The frequency of neurologic toxic effects increases with intra-arterial or intrathecal administration, and blood–brain barrier modification and also when chemotherapy (especially methotrexate) is administered in conjunction with RT (Weiss et al., 1974; Feun et al., 1991; Stewart et al., 1992; Newelt and Dahlborg, 1987). Seizures have also been induced by fat emboli during the intra-arterial administration of cisplatin (Menendez et al., 1990).

Methotrexate. Moderate and high doses of intravenous methotrexate can cause leukoencephalopathy with seizures and other neurologic symptoms (Genvresse et al., 1999). Methotrexate increases the concentration of homocysteine, which is oxidatively metabolized to the excitatory amino acid neurotransmitters homocisteic acid and cysteine sulfinic acid. Homocysteine also damages the vascular endothelium (Quinn et al., 1997). Seizures have been reported with intrathecal and intraventricular administration of methotrexate and cytosine arabinoside as well (Lee et al., 1997; Resar et al., 1993). Neuroimaging studies, particularly MRI scans of the brain, show diffuse white matter lesions, some of which may enhance, or may demonstrate a more focal pattern (Lovblad et al., 1998). Aminophylline has been reported to be an effective treatment for methotrexate-induced subacute neurotoxicity (Bernini et al., 1995).

Cisplatin. Seizures following intravenous cisplatin are mainly due to hypomagnesemia and hypocalcemia and thus are easily prevented by magnesium and, if necessary, calcium supplementation during the chemotherapy infusion (Bachmeyer et al., 1996; Fuse-Nagase et al., 1997).

5-Fluorouracil. Severe neurotoxicity with seizures, encephalopathy, syncope, ataxia, motor neuropathy, and demyelinating lesions evident on MRI scan has been reported in patients treated with 5-fluorouracil (5-FU). These patients had an underlying dihydropyrimidine dehydrogenase deficiency, an enzyme that is responsible for the rate-limiting step of 5-FU catabolism. This deficiency increased binding of 5-FU to thymidylate synthetase and incorporation into RNA (Shehata et al., 1999).

Pre-existing renal disease, which alters the clearance of chemotherapeutic agents, has been implicated in neurotoxicity, with seizures caused by treatment with *chlorambucil* and *cytosine arabinoside.* Decreasing the dose of the chemotherapeutic agent is recommended for such patients (Salloum et al., 1997; Smith et al., 1997).

Ifosphamide (ifosfamide). Ifosphamide, commonly used to treat sarcomas, medulloblastoma, and other pediatric and adult tumors, can cause severe neurotoxicity manifested by coma and seizures (Bhardwaj and Badesha, 1995; Gieron et al., 1988).

Paclitaxel (Taxol). Paclitaxel is highly active against ovarian, breast, and other cancers (lung, uterine). It is a mitotic spindle inhibitor, and it exerts its major neurotoxic effect on peripheral nerves. Recent reports link paclitaxel-induced encephalopathy with seizures, particularly in those patients treated with high doses (Nieto et al., 1999; Perry and Warner, 1996). Reversible encephalopathy and seizures have also been reported with vincristine. A brain biopsy specimen in one reported case revealed neurotubular dissociation (Hurwitz et al., 1988).

Cyclosporin. Immunosuppressant drugs such as cyclosporin are given to bone marrow transplant recipients to prevent rejection. These agents have been reported to induce seizures in patients pretreated with busulfan or platinum compounds (Ghany et al., 1991).

Biologic Response Modifiers. Encephalopathy and seizures have been reported after the administration of interferon, interleukin-2 (IL-2), lymphokine-activated killer cells, and some colony-stimulating factors (Dierckx et al., 1985; Karp et al., 1996; Meyers et al., 1991). Transient lesions in the occipital poles, cerebellum, and centrum semiovale have been described in patients treated with IL-2 who developed focal neurologic problems, including seizures (Karp et al., 1996).

Intratumoral Therapies. Intratumoral therapies seek to decrease systemic toxicity of a chemotherapeutic agent through a high level of regional drug delivery. However, the risk of causing seizures is higher in those patients with a prior history of tumor-related seizures. Increased frequency of seizures was noted in patients treated with intratumoral BCNU Wafers (Gliadel) (Brem et al., 1995); seizures typically occurred in the first 5 days after surgery, although they were also observed at 20 to 100 days after implantation.

Seizures Related to Other Drugs

Narcotics. Cancer patients often require narcotics for control of pain. Narcotics occasionally cause neurotoxicity and seizures. Specific drugs associated with the occurrence of seizures are meperidine (Demerol Hydrochloride), propoxyphene (Darvon), and, rarely, morphine sulfate. In the case of meperidine, the metabolite normeperidine has been implicated. Renal dysfunction may contribute to, but is not the determining factor for, the accumulation and neuroexcitatory effect of normeperidine (Goetting and Thirman, 1985; Kaiko et al., 1983; Szeto et al., 1977). Seizures have been reported in patients who have been treated with an intravenous morphine solution containing sodium bisulfate as a preservative (Meisel and Welford, 1992). An intrathecal or intraventricular morphine bolus can also cause seizures (Kronenborg et al., 1998). Propoxyphene has been reported to cause status epilepticus.

Antiemetics. Some neuroleptics used as antiemetics in conjunction with chemotherapy (phenothiazines, butyrophenones) have been reported to induce seizures. This phenomenon appears to be dose related. The newer antiemetics, such as ondansetron, cause less neurotoxicity.

Antibiotics. Many cancer patients with neutropenia and depressed immune systems due to malignancy and chemotherapy receive broad-spectrum antibiotics or multiple antibiotics. Some of these have been associated with encephalopathy and seizures. Most often implicated are the quinolones and betalactams.

The neurotoxicity of the quinolones is dose related. Experimental studies have shown that this is because gamma-aminobutyric acid–like substituents in the structure of quinolones act as antagonists at the gamma-aminobutyric acid receptors (Akahane et al., 1989). Renal failure and the presence or history of brain metastases are contributing factors (Walton et al., 1997).

Of the betalactams, imipenem/cilastatin (Primaxin) is the most neurotoxic. Betalactam neurotoxicity seems to be due to an increased concentration of the drug in brain tissue when it is given in high doses or given to patients with impaired renal function or caused by alterations in the blood–brain barrier due to infection or malignancy (Bodey et al., 1987). An impaired mechanism for clearance of the drug from brain tissue may be involved, but this has not yet been documented (Schliamser et al., 1991).

Methylphenidate (Ritalin). Patients with brain tumors or systemic cancer often experience fatigue, lethargy, depressed mood, and overall neurobehavioral slowing. These symptoms can be caused by the brain tumor itself or by the effects of RT and chemotherapy. Methylphenidate has been shown to improve patients' energy level and function (Meyers et al., 1998; Weitzner et al., 1995). There is some concern, however, that the drug may increase the frequency of seizures in patients who have a history of epilepsy or seizures due to the presence of brain tumor. This association has been demonstrated by results from studies of children with epilepsy and attention deficit hyperactivity disorder (Gross-Tsur et al., 1997). In contrast, a study of patients with brain injury and epilepsy suggests that methylphenidate may actually decrease the frequency of seizures (Wroblewski et al., 1992). In sum, the benefit of methylphenidate therapy for cancer patients with neurobehavioral slowing outweighs the remote risk of seizures.

Radiologic Contrast Medium. Intravenous contrast media used for CT scans of the brain have been reported to trigger either focal or generalized seizures (Avrahami et al., 1987), particularly in those patients who have primary or metastatic brain tumors. Contrast-induced seizures are caused by an increased susceptibility to seizures and increased permeability of the blood–brain barrier in these patients, and they are possibly a direct toxic effect of the agents used (Avrahami et al., 1989; Fischer, 1980).

Seizures with Metabolic Causes

Metabolic abnormalities are the most common cause of altered levels of consciousness in cancer patients. Hyponatremia, hypoglycemia, hypomagnesemia, hypocalcemia, and hypoxia lower the seizure threshold. Seizures caused by metabolic abnormalities tend to be generalized. The accompanying cerebral dysfunction is diffuse, even in the rare case of a focal or complex partial seizure (Cascino, 1993; Stein and Chamberlain, 1991).

Hyponatremia. Hyponatremia in cancer patients can be caused by volume depletion or volume overload, by drugs, or by a malignancy, such as occurs with paraneoplastic syndrome. Intravascular volume depletion occurs as a result of poor fluid intake, fluid loss with emesis, or retention of fluid in the abdominal cavity (ascites), either neoplastic or due to congestive heart failure. Aggressive hydration to enhance the renal clearance of some chemotherapeutic drugs (platinum, methotrexate) causes dilutional hyponatremia (McDonald and Dubose, 1993).

The syndrome of inappropriate antidiuretic hormone (SIADH) is another common cause of hyponatremia in patients with cancer. As in paraneoplastic syndrome, it occurs most commonly in patients with small cell lung carcinoma and also in those with Hodgkin's lymphoma, non–small cell lung carcinoma, and cancer of the pancreas, colon, prostate, or adrenal cortex. Small cell lung carcinoma cells produce arginine-vasopressin–like and atrial natriuretic–like factors, two hormones implicated in paraneoplastic SIADH (Franck et al., 1987; Vanhees et al., 2000). For other types of cancer, the production of ectopic hormones is less well documented.

SIADH also occurs in those patients with leptomeningeal metastases, tumors involving the hypothalamus, and basilar meningitis. Drugs that can cause the syndrome are carbamazepine, neuroleptics (haloperidol [Haldol]), tricyclic antidepressants, and cytotoxics (Vinca alkaloids, cyclophosphamide). Cisplatin can cause SIADH with secondary seizures (Ritch, 1988). Diagnosis is made on the basis of laboratory findings of hyponatremia, hypo-osmolality of the serum, and increased urine osmolality. Renal, hepatic, adrenal, and pituitary function are normal.

It is important to correctly diagnose the cause of hyponatremia to treat it appropriately. Hydration with normal saline solution corrects the problem of fluid depletion. Fluid restriction, sodium supplementation, and sometimes diuretics are indicated to treat fluid overload. The treatment of SIADH consists of restricting fluids, administering demeclocycline, and identifying and, if possible, removing the cause. Paraneoplastic SIADH usually resolves if the tumor can be removed or if it responds to radiation or chemotherapy. The syndrome may recur, indicating tumor recurrence (McDonald and Dubose, 1993; Richardson 1995; Ritch, 1988).

Hypoglycemia. Hypoglycemia occurs in cancer patients who receive total parenteral nutrition and results from either the insulin in the solution or withdrawal of total parenteral nutrition. Other causes are malnutrition and pancreatic tumors (insulinoma) (Daggett and Nabarro, 1984; Hazard et al., 1985). Seizures can occur with blood glucose levels below 40 mg/dL; they are usually preceded by diaphoresis, tremor, a sensation of hunger, and nervousness.

Hypocalcemia and Hypomagnesemia. Hypocalcemia and hypomagnesemia are two electrolyte abnormalities that have similar effects on the nervous system. Hypocalcemia and hypomagnesemia occur in patients who receive intensive chemotherapy, especially cisplatin, with overhydration (Bachmeyer et al., 1996; Fuse-Nagase et al., 1997). Hypocalcemia has also been reported in patients treated with amphotericin B. It occurs less commonly with malnutrition or in patients with secondary hypoparathyroidism following treatment for thyroid cancer. Seizures are a common manifestation of hypocalcemia because of the increased excitability of the cerebral cortex. Other clinical manifestations of hypocalcemia and hypomagnesemia, including tremor, carpopedal spasm (tetany), and myoclonus, can sometimes be confused with motor seizures.

Hypoxia. Hypoxia is another potential, although less common, cause of seizures in cancer patients. Acute hypoxia occurs with pulmonary embolism, prolonged syncope, massive pneumonitis, rapid progression of lung tumors, or metastatic lymphangitic spread. Patients with pulmonary fibrosis secondary to chemotherapy (bleomycin, nitrosoureas) or RT are also at risk.

Seizures with Infectious Causes

Cancer patients are very susceptible to infections, and seizures occur in those patients who have systemic infections or infectious processes in the CNS. Patients undergoing high-dose chemotherapy with bone marrow transplant are at particular risk. Central nervous system infections associated with seizures can be caused by viruses (herpes simplex virus, cytomegalovirus, herpes zoster virus); bacteria, including common pathogens and opportunistic agents (*Listeria, Mycobacterium*); fungi (*Aspergillus, Cryptococcus*); or parasites (*Toxoplasma*) (Bosi et al., 1998; Pruitt, 1991). Clinically, patients with seizures caused by infections present with confusion, altered level of consciousness (encephalitis), meningitic signs, or, in the case of abscess, focal findings.

Seizures with Vascular Causes

Cancer patients have both embolic and thrombotic strokes. The pathogenesis of cerebrovascular events in these patients includes cancer- and treatment-related causes (Graus et al., 1985).

Embolic Stroke. Embolic events can occur in the presence of cardiac arrhythmia, which occurs in patients treated with paclitaxel, in those with cardiomyopathy secondary to doxorubicin, and in cancer-associated marantic endocarditis (Rosen and Armstrong, 1973).

Thrombotic Stroke. Thrombotic strokes are observed in patients who have hypercoagulability syndromes, paraneoplastic phenomena associated with pancreatic cancer, breast carcinoma, and other malignancies (Collins et al., 1975; Patronas and Argyropoulou, 1992). Stroke in cancer patients can be caused by carotid artery stenosis following RT to the neck for treatment of head and neck tumors or by compression from neoplastic adenopathy. Radiotherapy to the brain can induce vasculopathy, another potential cause of ischemic stroke. Thrombotic and hemorrhagic strokes with secondary seizures have been reported in children whose leukemias were treated with L-asparaginase. L-asparaginase causes deficiencies of antithrombin, plasminogen, fibrinogen, and factors IX and XI (Priest et al., 1980). Chemotherapy-induced vascular events may be transient, and MRI scans may show areas of ischemia in the watershed distribution (Pihko et al., 1993).

Venous Sinus Thromboses. Venous sinus thromboses can occur with the secondary venous infarctions that can be caused by tumor invasion or metastatic or infectious meningitis. Venous infarctions are most often hemorrhagic.

Parenchymal and Intratumoral Hemorrhage. New-onset seizure or an increase in seizure frequency occurs in those patients with hemorrhage into a primary or metastatic brain tumor. Of the metastatic tumors, melanoma, renal cell carcinoma, and choriocarcinoma are most commonly associated with hemorrhages.

Spontaneous Subarachnoid Hemorrhage. While subarachnoid hemorrhage may occur in patients who have a malignancy, it may not always be possible to elucidate the pathogenesis of the process. One cause for subarachnoid hemorrhage or small cortical parenchymal hemorrhage is CNS aspergillosis. It is important to appreciate that subarachnoid hemorrhages can recur along with seizures as part of their clinical manifestation.

Traumatic Subdural or Subarachnoid Hemorrhage. These hemorrhages can occur in cancer patients who are thrombocytopenic or who develop a low-grade disseminated intravascular coagulation syndrome. In such cases, even minor trauma may cause hemorrhage.

Diagnosis

The diagnosis of seizures in cancer patients is made on the basis of a detailed history, physical and neurologic examinations, laboratory tests, neuroimaging results, and electroencephalographic findings. When taking the patient's history, the clinician must try to obtain an accurate description of the ictal event: timing of the event in relation to the diagnosis of tumor and the treatment for cancer, the presence or absence of aura, elements of focality, the behavior of the patient immediately before the seizure, the duration of the event and of the post-ictal period, and whether or not there are residual mental status changes or focal neurologic deficits. The clinician should also try to obtain information about the administration of all medications before the seizure and the presence of any signs of infection. It is important to elicit the past medical history, focusing on prior history of seizures, cardiac disease, pulmonary disease, diabetes, and head trauma. Common symptoms associated with seizures are headache, paresthesias, diaphoresis, difficulty breathing, gastric discomfort, and occasionally blurring of vision.

The physical and neurologic examinations will help to identify the cause(s) of the seizure. The presence of focal neurologic deficits suggests that the patient has a focal intracranial lesion (parenchymal or dural/meningeal), either neoplastic, infectious (abscess, empyema), hemorrhagic, or vascular. Focal leukoencephalopathy secondary to RT or chemotherapy can also present with focal deficits. Altered level of consciousness, myoclonus, and asterixis suggest metabolic disturbances.

The first seizure in a cancer patient should prompt laboratory tests, including complete blood cell count, with differential and platelet counts; chemistry profile; assay of magnesium level; blood and urine cultures; and blood levels for drugs such as cyclosporin, methotrexate, aminophylline, ethanol, and, if appropriate, street drugs.

Contrast-enhanced gadopentetic acid–enhanced MRI scan or CT scan of the brain can usually identify intracranial lesions, leptomeningeal disease, strokes, and hemorrhages. The extent of edema and mass effect can also be evaluated.

Lumbar puncture is indicated for the diagnosis of meningitis, leptomeningeal metastases, and subarachnoid hemorrhage. It must be performed with great caution in patients who have an intracerebral mass or thrombocytopenia. Platelet transfusion may be necessary during the procedure.

Electroencephalography helps to identify the seizure focus and differentiate between disease processes. Specific findings on electroencephalograms occur in herpesvirus encephalitis (periodic lateralized epileptiform discharges in the temporal lobes) and in some metabolic encephalopathies (triphasic waves).

The differential diagnosis must be made with other paroxysmal events, such as syncope, myoclonic jerks, tetany, transient encephalopathy, transient ischemic attacks, and panic attacks, which can all mimic seizures.

Treatment

An algorithm for the management of seizures in cancer patients is presented in Figure 21–1. To decide which therapy to use for ictal events, the neurologist must answer two important questions: whether the event was a seizure and whether anticonvulsants are indicated.

If the patient is in status epilepticus, efforts should focus on stopping the seizures. Airway patency must be established, and intravenous therapy with benzodiazepines (lorazepam, diazepam) and antiepileptic drugs (phenytoin, phenobarbital) must be initiated. If the work-up indicates a toxic or metabolic cause for the status epilepticus, antiepileptic drugs can be discontinued once the seizures have stopped and their cause has been eliminated. Any drugs known to be epileptogenic must be discontinued, the metabolic abnormalities must be corrected, and appropriate antibiotic therapy must be instituted for infection, avoiding quinolones and betalactams.

Long-term anticonvulsant treatment is indicated for patients with a pre-existing seizure disorder, primary or metastatic brain tumors, or other parenchymal lesions. The use of prophylactic antiepileptic drugs in patients with brain tumors who do not have seizures is controversial (Cohen et al., 1988). In such patients, antiepileptic drugs may cause adverse effects. Whether or not to use antiepileptic drugs is determined by the patient's condition and hepatic and renal function and by the concurrent administration of drugs that interfere with antiepileptic drugs' metabolism and excretion.

In patients with altered mental status, antiepileptic drugs must be administered parenterally. The drugs of choice are benzodiazepines, phenytoin, or phenobarbital.

For treatment of generalized seizures, phenytoin is usually the first drug administered. For complex partial seizures, carbamazepine may be the first-line drug. Phenobarbital is the drug of choice for children.

Phenytoin (Dilantin)

Phenytoin is the most widely used antiepileptic drug in the United States. A known effective anticonvulsant, it has several advantages: It can be administered by multiple routes (oral, intravenous, through a gastric tube in its elixir form); it has a long half-life, which allows once-a-day dosing; and it is inexpensive.

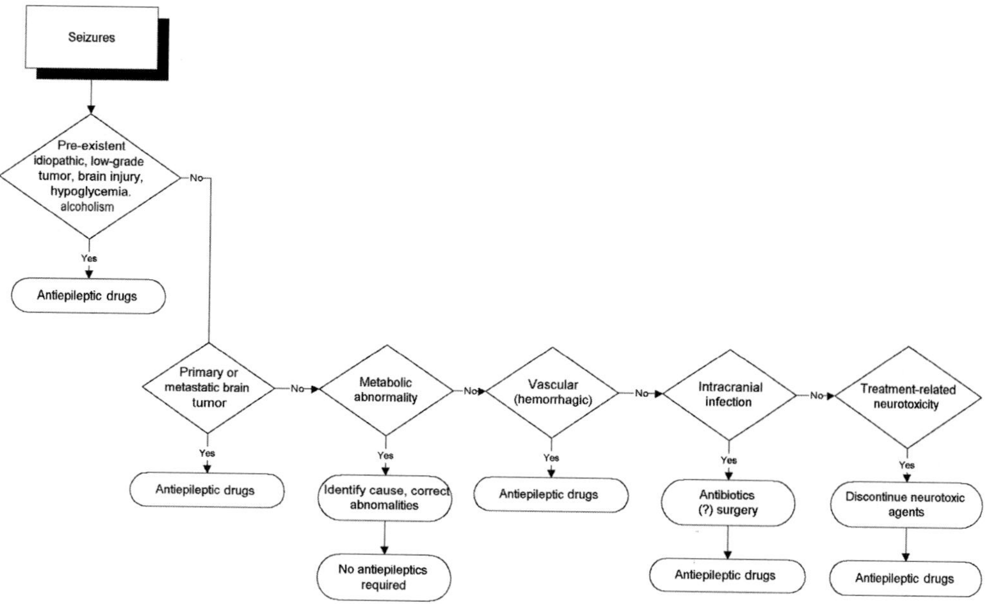

Figure 20–1. An algorithm for the management of seizures in the neuro-oncologic patient.

Problems associated with phenytoin are related to its pharmacokinetics. It is metabolized in the liver, and its serum levels are influenced by liver disease (metastatic or noncancer related) as well as by its multiple drug interactions (DeMonaco and Lawless, 1983; Gattis and May, 1996; Ghosh et al., 1992). Dexamethasone, commonly used in patients with primary and metastatic brain tumors as well as an adjuvant antiemetic in patients receiving chemotherapy, has been demonstrated to lower phenytoin levels (Gattis and May, 1996; Lackner, 1991). Platinum-containing chemotherapy regimens have been reported to decrease phenytoin levels to as low as 25% of the initial therapeutic level, with return to baseline after discontinuation of chemotherapy. Procarbazine, a chemotherapeutic agent related to disulfiram, can increase the level of phenytoin. Anticonvulsants also increase the risk of procarbazine hypersensitivity reactions (Lehmann et al., 1997). The phenytoin dose needs to be adjusted and the levels monitored closely in those patients receiving chemotherapy to avoid under dosing and toxic effects (Neef and de Voogd-van der Straaten, 1988; Grossman et al., 1989; Ghosh et al., 1992). Phenytoin also increases clearance and may thus decrease the efficacy of chemotherapeutic agents such as busulfan, paclitaxel, topotecan and related drugs (Grossman et al., 1998; Hassan et al., 1993; Zamboni et al., 1998). Because of decreased protein binding and increased free plasma drug levels, the dose must be decreased for patients who are being treated with warfarin or cimetidine.

Both total and free phenytoin levels should be monitored in patients who have impaired renal function because phenytoin excretion may be impaired. Seizures can occur in cancer patients receiving phenytoin when subtherapeutic levels of the drug are administered, and they can also occur as a manifestation of phenytoin toxicity. Phenytoin can cause allergic reactions, usually a cutaneous rash. Severe reactions, including Stevens-Johnson syndrome, have been described in patients being weaned from corticosteroids while receiving RT to the brain (Delattre et al., 1988).

In vitro, but not in vivo, studies indicated a possible radiosensitizing effect of phenytoin on astrocytoma cells (Lordo et al., 1987). Phenytoin and other enzyme inducers were reported to have a protective effect in patients receiving busulfan, reducing its neurotoxicity and myelotoxicity. Phenytoin is now used for seizure prophylaxis in patients receiving chemotherapy with busulfan (Fitzsimmons et al., 1990). Phenytoin was also shown to selectively enhance the cytotoxicity of microtubule inhibitors, such as Vinca alkaloids; this activity is presently under investigation for potential clinical use (Ganapathi et al., 1993).

Carbamazepine (Tegretol)

Carbamazepine and its newer derivative oxcarbazepine (Trileptal) is the anticonvulsant of choice for patients with complex partial seizures, and it is used as a second-line antiepileptic drug for patients with generalized seizures who either did not have adequate seizure control with phenytoin or developed allergic reactions to it. When administered together with phenytoin, carbamazepine decreases the phenytoin level. It can only be administered orally or through a gastrostomy tube and therefore cannot be used in emergency situations. The main difficulty with using carbamazepine in cancer patients is its myelotoxic effect, which causes neutropenia, lymphopenia, and aplastic anemia (Silverman and Chapron, 1995). These problems limit its use in patients who are receiving chemotherapy. Furthermore, carbamazepine levels are decreased by chemotherapeutic drugs such as platinum (Jain, 1993). Carbamazepine also causes SIADH. Like phenytoin, carbamazepine can cause allergic reactions, including Stevens-Johnson syndrome.

Valproic Acid

Valproic acid and its derivative divalproex sodium (Depakote) are used for patients with seizures that are not controlled by phenytoin. The drugs are administered orally and are metabolized in the liver. When administered together with phenytoin, valproate can either decrease or increase phenytoin levels. Methotrexate has been reported to cause an acute decline in the level of serum valproate (Schroeder and Ostergaard, 1994). Reported toxic effects that limit its use in cancer patients are hepatotoxicity, prolonged bleeding time, and dose-dependent thrombocytopenia.

Phenobarbital

Phenobarbital remains the drug of choice for controlling seizures in children. It is mainly used as an adjunct to phenytoin or for adult patients for whom other anticonvulsants have failed. Its main side effect is somnolence, although some patients experience arthralgias or allergic reactions.

Gabapentin (Neurontin)

A new class of antiepileptic drug, GABA agonists, has recently been released to the marketplace, and there is not much experience with their use by cancer patients. Neurontin is purported to cause fewer side effects than conventional antiepileptic drugs, but there have been no studies to evaluate its interactions, if any, with chemotherapeutic agents. Because it has so few side effects, it is commonly used in combination with phenytoin, carbamazepine, or valproate for brain tumor patients with refractory complex partial seizures.

Lamotrigine (Lamictal)

Lamotrigine is a new, structurally unique, anticonvulsant that acts on voltage-dependent sodium channels, resulting in decreased release of excitatory neurotransmitters. It is indicated for treatment of partial seizures but can cause severe dermatologic side effects and myelotoxicity. It has known interactions with other anticonvulsants, but to date there are no reports of interactions with chemotherapeutic drugs. Lamotrigine is a dehydrofolate reductase inhibitor and should not be used by patients treated with methotrexate and other antimetabolites.

Topiramate (Topamax)

Topiramate is another new anticonvulsant used as adjunctive therapy for partial seizures. It acts on sodium channels and as a GABA agonist. It produces no significant drug interactions, and its main side effect is psychomotor slowing. Topamax may cause leukopenia.

Gabitril (Tiagabine)

Gabitril is another new GABA-ergic anticonvulsant, which is indicated as an adjunctive treatment of complex partial seizures. It has no significant drug interactions, and it can be safely used with enzyme-inducing drugs. Rarely, it may cause anemia and thrombocytopenia. These new drugs can be used by patients with known allergy to the first-line anticonvulsants and as adjuncts for better seizure control by patients who fail anticonvulsant monotherapy.

Conclusions

Seizures are a common neurologic problem in patients with systemic and CNS malignancies and may have multiple etiologies. Examination should be aimed at identifying and treating all of its possible causes. The treatment of seizures in cancer patients must be individualized, and metabolic factors and drug interactions must be taken into consideration when anticonvulsant therapy is initiated.

SYNCOPE

Syncope is defined as a sudden transient loss of consciousness and postural tone with spontaneous recovery. The frequency of syncope in cancer patients is not well documented. Presyncope, with premonitory symptoms but without loss of consciousness ("faint feeling"), is probably even more common (Plum and Posner, 1982). Syncope occurs because of a transient interruption of cerebral blood flow. Common presyncopal symptoms are dizziness, lightheadedness, palpitations, diaphoresis, and, occasionally, paresthesias.

Etiology

The etiology of syncope in cancer patients is presented in Table 20–2. As in the case of seizures, several etiologic factors may contribute to syncope in cancer patients, the most common being orthostatic hypotension, with cardiac causes assuming a secondary role. Other causes are drugs, vasovagal reactions, and cerebrovascular disease (Kapoor, 1991, 1992; Manolis et al., 1990).

Orthostatic Hypotension

Orthostatic hypotension is commonly present in the terminal stages of cancer in those patients who are suffering from malnutrition and dehydration. It also occurs in those who become dehydrated from emesis caused by chemotherapy. Patients with severe anemia often present with syncope or presyncope caused by insufficient oxygenation of the brain rather than from volume depletion. The drop in blood pressure

Table 20-2. Etiology of Syncope in Patients with Malignancy

Etiologic Factors	*Causes*
Orthostatic hypotension	
Volume depletion	Dehydration, hemorrhage
Dysautonomia	Platinum compounds, Vinca alkaloids, taxanes, diabetes
Drug induced	Tricyclic antidepressants, vasodilators, diuretics
Neurotoxicity (drug induced)	Chemotherapeutic agents (fluorouracil, Vinca alkaloids, platinum compounds, taxanes), CNS depressants (barbiturates), biologic response modifiers
Hypoglycemia	Nutritional, pancreatic tumors (insulinoma)
Cardiac	
Reflex cardiogenic	Parapharyngeal tumors, radiation therapy to neck
Pump failure	Myocardial ischemia (mediastinal radiation, atherosclerosis), cardiomyopathy (adriamycin, graft-versus-host disease, viral)
Cardiac arrhythmia	Chemotherapy (paclitaxel, interleukin-2), mediastinal radiation, pre-existing cardiac disease
Pulmonary flow obstruction	Pulmonary embolism
Vasovagal	Micturition, coughing, swallowing, strong emotional stimuli
Cerebrovascular	Vertebrobasilar insufficiency

with change in position is accompanied by an increased heart rate. Chemotherapeutic agents such as cisplatin and Vinca alkaloids cause a peripheral neuropathy with dysautonomia. The heart rate does not increase significantly with the drop in blood pressure in patients who have this condition.

Another common cause of orthostatic hypotension in cancer patients is related to drugs such as diuretics and antidepressants. The pathogenetic mechanism of orthostasis in patients taking diuretics is intravascular volume depletion, whereas antidepressants, neuroleptics, and some antiemetics cause an anticholinergic effect. Hypotension with possible presyncope or syncope is a common side effect of biologic agents such as interferon, IL-2, and tumor necrosis factor. Orthostatic presyncope and syncope also occur in patients with severe infections that cause high fever and dehydration.

Drug Related

Syncope can be a side effect of medications, even in the absence of other etiologic factors. The mechanisms are orthostatic hypotension either through volume depletion (diuretics, mannitol), vasopressor effects (biologic response modifiers), anticholinergic effects (antidepressants), cardiac arrhythmia (paclitaxel, intravenous phenytoin), or peripheral neuropathy (vincristine, paclitaxel, platinum compounds).

Syncope is also part of the spectrum of direct neurotoxic effects of chemotherapeutic drugs such as fluorouracil (Hook et al., 1992; Shehata et al., 1999). Biologic response modifiers and colony-stimulating factors also cause hypotension with syncope or near-syncope (Lieschke et al., 1989).

Hypoglycemia

Syncope in hypoglycemic patients has a fairly typical clinical presentation, which suggests its diagnosis. It is preceded by a sensation of hunger. The patient becomes irritable, tremulous, and diaphoretic and may complain of dimming vision. The skin becomes pale. Loss of consciousness is brief and is usually not followed by confusion; however, with severe hypoglycemia, there may be associated seizure activity. Hypoglycemia occurs in patients who have insulinoma, malnutrition, and insulin-dependent diabetes and can be caused by insulin overdosing from total parenteral nutrition. The symptoms of patients with insulinoma typically occur in the morning, before breakfast, or between meals (Daggett and Nabarro, 1984; Hazard et al., 1985).

Cardiovascular Causes

Syncope is a common manifestation of cardiac disease. Cancer patients can experience the same problems that patients without malignancy do. The main pathogenetic mechanisms for syncope of cardiac origin are pump failure, heart blocks, and arrhythmias.

Pump failure occurs in myocardial infarction or cardiomyopathy. In cancer patients, cardiomyopathy can be caused by chemotherapy with anthracyclines, especially *daunorubicin,* which may be irreversible. Other cardiotoxic chemotherapeutic agents are *mitoxantrone* and *estramustin.* The risk for cardiac disease increases if such drugs are administered following RT to the chest and mediastinum. Viral myocarditis in the immunosuppressed patient and graft-versus-host disease following allogeneic bone marrow transplant are other causes of heart failure. Heart failure patients usually have symptoms suggestive of myocardial ischemia before syncope: chest pain, dyspnea, and signs of heart failure.

Heart blocks and cardiac arrhythmias in cancer patients are usually caused by a pre-existing cardiac condition. Arrhythmias do occasionally result from paclitaxel or IL-2 therapy. Several case reports of syncope describe cardiac arrhythmias, coronary artery stenosis, and defective cardiovascular reflexes in patients who were treated with RT to the mediastinum or neck (de Waard et al., 1996; Mary-Rabine et al., 1980; Shapiro et al., 1996). Syncope occasionally occurs after obstruction of pulmonary flow caused by pulmonary embolism.

Cerebrovascular Causes

Syncope can be a manifestation of cerebrovascular disease in the anterior or posterior circulation and may or may not be associated with focal neurologic deficits. Possible causes of altered cerebral blood flow in cancer patients include compression of the carotid artery by tumor, stenosis of the subclavian or carotid arteries following RT to the chest or neck, and thrombotic or embolic events. When syncope occurs after elevation or exertion of the left arm, a subclavian steal must be suspected, and blood pressure should be measured in both arms.

Tumor Related

Patients with head and neck tumors, thyroid tumors, and cervical lymphadenopathy can develop recurrent syncope related to carotid sinus hypersensitivity. Syncope in patients with head and neck tumors can occur through several mechanisms: glossopharyngeal neuralgia–asystole syndrome, carotid sinus syndrome, and glossopharyngeal-related reflex cardiogenic syncope without neuralgic pain (Cicogna et al., 1993; Dykman et al., 1981; Wang and Ng, 1995). Nasopharyngeal and parapharyngeal carcinomas cause these syndromes. In these patients, syncope does not respond to medical management or in some cases to pacemaker insertion. Syncope may resolve after treatment of the tumor or may require intracranial intervention to resect the glossopharyngeal nerve.

Vasovagal Response

Vasovagal syncope is one of the most common types of syncope in young adults, and patients usually present with a history of prior syncopal episodes. Vasovagal syncope occurs in response to stress, pain, fear, and heat and is preceded by symptoms such as palpitations, queasiness, nausea, diaphoresis, and abdominal discomfort. Incontinence is uncommon. The underlying pathophysiologic mechanism is thought to be a reflex withdrawal of sympathetic tone (Bezold-Jarisch reflex), indicated clinically by tachycardia, followed by bradycardia, pallor, and hypotension. Syncope that occurs during micturition or defecation (situational syncope), typically after a long period of bed rest, is more common in men than in women.

Diagnosis

The diagnosis of syncope is made primarily on the basis of the patient's clinical presentation (if the episode is witnessed) or an accurate and detailed history. The history should include data on the patient's complaints before the loss of consciousness, appearance of the patient (skin pale or flushed, diaphoresis, breathing pattern), duration of the episode, associated seizure activity, incontinence, and the presence or absence of confusion. Information should also be obtained about the patient's past medical history with regard to cardiac disease, hypertension or hypotension, diabetes and hypoglycemia, type of cancer, psychiatric history, medications, and circumstances of the event (micturition or defecation, crowded or overheated area, pain, stress). The physical and neurologic examinations, if feasible at or near the time of the event, can reveal the presence of hypotension, arrhythmia, or focal findings suggestive of a vascular or neoplastic brain lesion.

Examination should include measurement of blood pressure and heart rate in both supine and standing positions and in both arms to determine the presence of position hypotension or the subclavian steal syndrome. Auscultation of the heart can reveal arrhythmias and/or cardiac valve abnormalities. Cardiac monitoring, echocardiogram, and laboratory tests also help the clinician make the diagnosis. Laboratory tests should include hemoglobin, hematocrit, white blood cell count, differential count, and platelet count to rule out anemia and infection; electrolyte, glucose, calcium, and magnesium levels; drug levels when appropriate (psychotropics and antidepressants, opiates, barbiturates); and blood and urine cultures when infection is suspected.

When focal neurologic deficits are present, a CT or MRI scan of the brain is indicated. Electroencephalography is helpful in the differential diagnosis with seizures, especially in patients with focal neurologic deficits if seizure activity has been witnessed during syncope (Hoefnagels et al., 1991). Hypoglycemic syncope and the syncope in Adams-Stokes syndrome (third-degree heart block) can be associated with seizure activity.

Upright tilt-table testing is useful for diagnosing vasovagal syncope. It is performed by measuring blood pressure and heart rate (continuous electrocardiogram) in the supine position and then bringing the patient suddenly to an upright position on the tilt table and maintaining the upright position until presyncope or syncope occurs in association with hypotension and/or tachycardia. The test can be performed with or without infusion of isoproterenol (Kapoor, 1992). Lumbar puncture is usually not indicated except when meningitis or meningeal metastases are considered.

The differential diagnosis must be made taking into account all factors that can cause altered level of consciousness, including seizures, encephalopathy, cerebral ischemia, brain concussion, and drug or alcohol intoxication. In these cases, loss of consciousness is of longer duration, and the history and physical examinations establish the diagnosis. Psychiatric conditions such as conversion reactions, generalized anxiety disorder with hyperventilation, and panic attacks must also be considered. Information about psychotropic and antidepressant medications should be obtained from patients who have a psychiatric history.

Treatment

Syncope is a brief, usually fully reversible, episode of loss of consciousness that generally does not require specific treatment. However, when the cause of syncope is a life-threatening condition such as a heart block, malignant arrhythmia, or pulmonary embolus, close monitoring and urgent appropriate treatment must be instituted. Insertion of a cardiac pacemaker and, in some cases, intracranial section of the glossopharyngeal nerve are necessary. In simple syncope, the elimination of the causative agent(s) usually prevents further occurrences. Supportive therapy, maintenance of good nutritional status, hydration or blood transfusions to maintain adequate intravascular volume, correction of hypoglycemia and electrolyte abnormalities, and discontinuation of offending drugs can prevent the occurrence of syncope in cancer patients (Benitez del Rosario and Salinas Martin, 1997).

REFERENCES

Ahern GL, O'Connor M, Dalmau J, et al. 1994. Paraneoplastic temporal lobe epilepsy with testicular neoplasm and atypical amnesia. Neurology 44:1270–1274.

Akahane K, Sekiguchi M, Une T, Osada Y. 1989. Structure–epileptogenicity relationship of quinolones with special reference to their interaction with gamma-aminobutyric acid receptor sites. Antimicrob Agents Chemother 33:1704–1708.

Antonini G, Ceschin V, Morino S, et al. 1998. Early neurologic complications following allogeneic bone marrow transplant for leukemia: a prospective study. Neurology 50:1441–1445.

Avrahami E, Weiss-Peretz J, Cohn DF. 1987. Focal epileptic activity following intravenous contrast material injection in patients with metastatic brain disease. J Neurol Neurosurg Psychiatry 50:221–223.

Avrahami E, Weiss-Peretz J, Cohn DF. 1989. Epilepsy in patients with brain metastases triggered by intravenous contrast medium. Clin Radiol 40:422–423.

Bachmeyer C, Decroix Y, Medioni J, et al. 1996. [Hypomagnesemic and hypocalcemic coma, convulsions and ocular motility disorders after chemotherapy with platinum compounds]. Rev Med Interne (Paris) 17:467–469.

Bartolomei JC, Christopher S, Vives K, Spencer DD, Piepmeier JM. 1997. Low-grade glioma of chronic epilepsy: a distinct clinical and pathological entity. J Neurooncol 34:79–84.

Benitez del Rosario MA, Salinas Martin A. 1997. Hydration for control of syncope in palliative care. J Pain Symptom Manage 14:5–6.

Bernini JC, Fort DW, Griener JC, Kane BJ, Chappell WB, Kamen BA. 1995. Aminophylline for methotrexate-induced neurotoxicity. Lancet 345:544–547.

Bhardwaj A, Badesha PS. 1995. Ifosfamide-induced nonconvulsive status epilepticus. Ann Pharmacother 29:1237–1239.

Blaney SM, Balis FM, Poplack DG. 1991. Pharmacologic approaches to the treatment of meningeal malignancy. Oncology (Huntingt) 5:107–116.

Bodey GP, Elting L, Jones P, Alvarez ME, Rolston K, Fainstein V. 1987. Imipenem/cilastatin therapy of infections in cancer patients. Cancer 60:255–262.

Bosi A, Zazzi M, Amantini A, et al. 1998. Fatal herpesvirus 6 encephalitis after unrelated bone marrow transplant. Bone Marrow Transplant 22:285–288.

Brem H, Piantadosi S, Burger PC, et al. 1995. Placebo-controlled trial of safety and efficacy of intraoperative controlled delivery by biodegradable polymers of chemotherapy for recurrent gliomas. The Polymer-Brain Tumor Treatment Group. Lancet 345:1008–1012.

Britton JW, Cascino GD, Sharbrough FW, Kelly PJ. 1994. Low-grade glial neoplasms and intractable partial epilepsy: efficacy of surgical treatment. Epilepsia 35:1130–1135.

Cascino GD. 1990. Epilepsy and brain tumors: implications for treatment. Epilepsia 31[suppl 3]:S37–S44.

Cascino TL. 1993. Neurologic complications of systemic cancer. Med Clin North Am 77:256–278.

Ciaudo-Lacroix C, Lapresle J. 1985. [Pseudo-tumoral form of delayed radionecrosis of the brain]. Ann Med Interne (Paris) 136:137–141.

Cicogna R, Bonomi FG, Curnis A, et al. 1993. Parapharyngeal space lesions syncope-syndrome. A newly proposed reflexogenic cardiovascular syndrome. Eur Heart J 14:1476–1483.

Cohen N, Strauss G, Lew R, Silver D, Recht L. 1988. Should prophylactic anticonvulsants be administered to patients with newly diagnosed brain metastases? A retrospective analysis. J Clin Oncol 6:1621–1624.

Collins RC, Al-Mondhiry H, Chernik NL, Posner JB. 1975. Neurologic manifestations of intravascular coagulation in patients with cancer. A clinicopathologic analysis of 12 cases. Neurology 25:795–806.

Daggett P, Nabarro J. 1984. Neurological aspects of insulinomas. Postgrad Med J 60:577–581.

Dalmau J, Graus F, Rosenblum MK, Posner JB. 1992. Anti-Hu–associated paraneoplastic encephalomyelitis/sensory neuronopathy. A clinical study of 71 patients. Medicine (Baltimore) 71:59–72.

Delattre JY, Safai B, Posner JB. 1988. Erythema multiforme and Stevens-Johnson syndrome in patients receiving cranial irradiation and phenytoin. Neurology 38:194–198.

DeMonaco HJ, Lawless LM. 1983. Variability of phenytoin protein binding in epileptic patients. Arch Neurol 40:481–483.

de Toffol B, Uchuya M, Michalak S, Corcia P, Hommet C, Autret A. 1997. [Paraneoplastic encephalomyeloneuritis with anti-Hu antibodies and cancer of the rectum]. Rev Neurol (Paris) 153:135–137.

de Waard DE, Verhorst PM, Visser CA. 1996. Exercise-induced syncope as late consequence of radiotherapy. Int J Cardiol 13:289–291.

Dierckx RA, Michotte A, Schmedding E, Ebinger G, Degeeter T, van Camp B. 1985. Unilateral seizures in a patient with hairy cell leukemia treated with interferon. Clin Neurol Neurosurg 87:209–212.

Drislane FW. 1994. Nonconvulsive status epilepticus in patients with cancer. Clin Neurol Neurosurg 96:314–318.

Dykman TR, Montgomery EB Jr, Gerstenberger PD, Zeiger HE, Clutter WE, Cryer PE. 1981. Glossopharyngeal neuralgia with syncope secondary to tumor. Treatment and pathophysiology. Am J Med 71:165–170.

Feun LG, Savaraj N, Lee YY, et al. 1991. A pilot clinical and pharmacokinetic study of intracarotid cisplatin and bleomycin. Sel Cancer Ther 7:29–36.

Fischer HW. 1980. Occurrence of seizures during cranial computed tomography. Radiology 137:563–564.

Fitzsimmons WE, Ghalie R, Kaizer H. 1990. The effect of hepatic enzyme inducers on busulfan neurotoxicity and myelotoxicity. Cancer Chemother Pharmacol 27:226–228.

Flowers A, Levin VA. 1993. Management of brain metastases from breast carcinoma. Oncology (Huntingt) 7:21–26.

Franck G, Sadzot B, Salmon E, et al. 1987. [Paraneoplastic limbic encephalopathy, inappropriate ADH secretion and recurrent subclinical epileptic seizures. Clinical, anatomopathological and metabolic correlations by positron emission tomography]. Rev Neurol (Paris) 143:657–669.

Fuse-Nagase Y, Suwa K, Nagao Y. 1997. Partial seizures associated with cisplatin administration: a case report. Clin Electroencephalogr 28:55–56.

Ganapathi R, Hercberg A, Grabowski D, Ford J. 1993. Selective enhancement of vincristine cytotoxicity in multidrug-resistant tumor cells by dilantin. Cancer Res 35:3262–3265.

Gattis WA, May DB. 1996. Possible interaction involving phenytoin, dexamethasone and antineoplastic agents: a case report and review. Ann Pharmacother 30:520–526.

Genvresse I, Dietzmann A, Massenkeil G, Spath-Schwalbe E, Possinger K. 1999. Subacute encephalopathy after combination chemotherapy including moderate-dose methotrexate in a patient with gastric cancer. Anticancer Drugs 10:293–294.

Ghany AM, Tutschka PJ, McGhee RB Jr, et al. 1991. Cyclosporine-associated seizures in bone marrow transplant recipients given busulfan and cyclophosphamide preparative therapy. Transplantation 52:310–315.

Ghosh C, Lazarus HM, Hewlett JS, Creger RJ. 1992. Fluctuation of serum phenytoin concentrations during autologous bone marrow transplant for primary central nervous system tumors. J Neurooncol 12:25–32.

Gieron MA, Barak LS, Estrada J. 1988. Severe encephalopathy associated with ifosfamide administration in two children with metastatic tumors . J Neurooncol 6:29–30.

Goetting MG, Thirman MJ. 1985. Neurotoxicity of meperidine. Ann Emerg Med 14:1007–1009.

Graus F, Rogers LR, Posner JB. 1985. Cerebrovascular complications in patients with cancer. Cancer 64:16–35.

Grossman SA, Hochberg F, Fisher J, et al. 1998. Increased 9-aminocamptothecin dose requirements in patients on anticonvulsants. NABTT CNS Consortium. The New Approaches to Brain Tumor Therapy. Cancer Chemother Pharmacol 42:118–126.

Grossman SA, Sheidler VR, Gilbert MR. 1989. Decreased phenytoin levels in patients receiving chemotherapy. Am J Med 87:505–510.

Gross-Tsur V, Manor O, van der MJ, Meere J, Joseph A, Shalev RS. 1997. Epilepsy and attention deficit hyperactivity disorder: is methylphenidate safe and effective? J Pediatr 130:670–674.

Hassan M, Oberg G, Bjorkholm M, Wallin I, Lindgren M. 1993. Influence of prophylactic anticonvulsant therapy on high-dose busulfan kinetics. Cancer Chemother Pharmacol 33:181–186.

Hazard J, Simon D, Perlemuter L, et al. 1985. [Insulinoma: diagnostic elements. 13 cases]. Presse Med (Paris) 14:1775–1778.

Hoefnagels WA, Padberg GW, Overweg J, Roos RA, van Dijk JG, Kamphuisen HA. 1991. Syncope or seizure? The diagnostic value of the EEG and hyperventilation test in transient loss of consciousness. J Neurol Neurosurg Psychiatry 54:953–956.

Hook CC, Kimmel DW, Kvols LK, et al. 1992. Multifocal inflammatory leukoencephalopathy with 5-fluorouracil and levamisole. Ann Neurol 31:262–267.

Hurwitz RL, Mahoney DH Jr, Armstrong DL, Browder TM. 1988. Reversible encephalopathy and seizures as a result of conventional vincristine administration. Med Pediatr Oncol 16:216–219.

Jain KK. 1993. Investigation and management of loss of efficacy of an antiepileptic medication using carbamazepine as an example. J R Soc Med 86:133–136.

Kaiko RF, Foley KM, Grabinski PY, et al. 1983. Central nervous system excitatory effects of meperidine in cancer patients. Ann Neurol 13:180–185.

Kapoor WN. 1991. Diagnostic evaluation of syncope. Am J Med 90:91–106.

Kapoor WN. 1992. Evaluation and management of the patient with syncope, JAMA 268:2553–2560.

Karp BI, Yang JC, Khorsand M,, et al. 1996. Multiple cerebral lesions complicating therapy with interleukin-2. Neurology 47:417–424.

Kramer ED, Packer RJ, Ginsberg J, et al. 1997. Acute neurologic dysfunction associated with high-dose chemotherapy and autologous bone marrow rescue for primary malignant brain tumors. Pediatr Neurosurg 27:230–237.

Kronenberg MF, Laimer I, Rifici C,, et al. 1998. Epileptic seizures associated with intracerebroventricular and intrathecal morphine bolus. Pain 75:383–387.

Lackner TE. 1991. Interaction of dexamethasone with phenytoin. Pharmacotherapy 11:344–347.

Lee AC, Wong K W, Fong K W, So K T. 1997. Intrathecal methotrexate overdose. Acta Paediatr 86:434–437.

Lehmann DF, Hurteau TE, Newman N, Coyle TE. 1997. Anticonvulsant usage is associated with an increased risk of procarbazine hypersensitivity reactions in patients with brain tumors. Clin Pharmacol Ther 62:225–229.

Lieschke GJ, Cebon J, Morstyn G. 1989. Characterization of the clinical effects after the first dose of bacterially synthesized recombinant human granulocyte-macrophage colony-stimulating factor. Blood 74:2634–2643.

Lim SH, So NK, Luders H, Morris HH, Turnbull J. 1991. Etiologic factors for unitemporal vs bitemporal epileptiform discharges. Arch Neurol 48:1225–1228.

Lordo CD, Stroude EC, Del Maestro RF. 1987. The effects of diphenylhydantoin on murine astrocytoma radiosensitivity. J Neurooncol 5:339–350.

Lovblad K, Kelkar F, Ozdoba C, Ramelli G, Remonda L, Schroth G. 1998. Pure methotrexate encephalopathy presenting with seizures: CT and MRI features. Pediatr Radiol 28:86–91.

Manolis AS, Linzer M, Salem D, Estes NA 3rd. 1990. Syncope: current diagnostic evaluation and management. Ann Intern Med 112:850–863.

Mary-Rabine L, Waleffe A, Kulbertus HE. 1980. Severe conduction disturbances and ventricular arrhythmias complicating mediastinal irradiation for Hodgkin's disease: a case report. Pacing Clin Electrophysiol 3:612–617.

McDonald GA, Dubose TD Jr. 1993. Hyponatremia in the cancer patient. Oncology (Huntingt) 7:55–64.

Meisel SB, Welford PK. 1992. Seizures associated with high-dose intravenous morphine containing sodium bisulfite preservative. Ann Pharmacother 26:1515–1517.

Menendez LR, Bacon W, Kempf RA, Moore TM. 1990. Fat embolism syndrome complicating intraarterial chemotherapy with cis-platinum. Clin Orthop 254:294–297.

Meyers CA, Obbens EA, Scheibel RS, Moser RP. 1991. Neurotoxicity of intraventricularly administered alpha-interferon for leptomeningeal disease. Cancer 68:88–92.

Meyers CA, Weitzner MA, Valentine AD, Levin VA. 1998. Methylphenidate therapy improves cognition, mood, and function of brain tumor patients. J Clin Oncol 16:2522–2527.

Neef C, de Voogd-van der Straaten I. 1988. An interaction between cytostatic and anticonvulsant drugs. Clin Pharmacol Ther 43:372–375.

Newelt EA, Dahlborg SA. 1987. Chemotherapy administered in conjunction with osmotic blood–brain barrier modification in patients with brain metastases. J Neurooncol 4:195–207.

Nieto Y, Cagnoni PJ, Bearman SI, et al. 1999. Acute encephalopathy: a new toxicity associated with high-dose paclitaxel. Clin Cancer Res 5:501–506.

Patronas NJ, Argyropoulou M. 1992. Intravascular thrombosis as a possible cause of transient cortical brain lesions: CT and MRI. J Comput Assist Tomogr 16:849–855.

Perry JR, Warner E. 1996. Transient encephalopathy after paclitxel (Taxol) infusion. Neurology 46:1596–1599.

Pihko H, Tyni T, Virkola K, et al. 1993. Transient ioschemic cerebral lesions during induction chemotherapy for acute lymphoblastic leukemia. J Pediatr 123:718–724.

Plum F, Posner JB. 1982. The Diagnosis of Stupor and Coma, 3rd ed. Philadelphia: FA Davis, pp 210–211.

Priest JR, Ramsay NK, Latchaw RE,, et al. 1980. Thrombotic and hemorrhagic strokes complicating early therapy for childhood acute lymphoblastic leukemia. Cancer 46:1548–1554.

Pruitt AA. 1991. Central nervous system infections in cancer patients. Neurol Clin 9:867–888.

Quinn CT, Griener JC, Bottiglieri K, Hyland K, Farrow A, Kamen BA. 1997. Elevation of homocysteine and excitatory amino acid neurotransmitters in the CSF of children who receive methotrexate for the treatment of cancer. J Clin Oncol 15:2800–2806.

Resar LM, Phillips PC, Kastan MB, Leventhal BG, Bowman PW, Civin CI. 1993. Acute neurotoxicity after intrathecal cytosine arabinoside in two adolescents with acute lymphoblastic leukemia of B-cell type. Cancer 71:117–123.

Richardson GE. 1995. Hyponatremia of malignancy. Crit Rev Oncol Hematol 18:129–135.

Rider WD. 1963. Radiation damage to the brain—a new syndrome. J Can Assoc Radiol 14:67–69.

Ritch PS. 1988. Cis-dichlorodiammineplatinum II–induced syndrome of inappropriate secretion of antidiuretic hormone. Cancer 61:448–450.

Rogers LR, Morris HH, Lupica K. 1993. Effect of cranial irradiation on seizure frequency in adults with low-grade astrocytoma and medically intractable epilepsy. Neurology 43:1599–1601.

Rosen P, Armstrong D. 1973. Nonbacterial thrombotic endocarditis in patients with malignant aneoplastic diseases. Am J Med 54:23–29.

Rosner D, Nemoto T, Lane WW. 1986. Chemotherapy induces regression of brain metastases in breast carcinoma. Cancer 58:832–839.

Salloum E, Khan KK, Cooper DL. 1997. Chlorambucil-induced seizures. Cancer 79:1009–1013.

Sasaki M, Ichiya Y, Kuwabara Y, et al. 1996. Hyperperfusion and hypermetabolism in brain radiation necrosis with epileptic activity. J Nucl Med 37:1174–1176.

Schliamser SE, Cars O, Norrby SR. 1991. Neurotoxicity of betalactam antibiotics: predisposing factors and pathogenesis. J Antimicrob Chemother 27:405–425.

Schroeder H, Ostergaard JR. 1994. Interference of high-dose methotrexate in the metabolism of valproate? Pediatr Hematol Oncol 11:445–449.

Shapiro MH, Ruiz-Ramon P, Fainman C, Ziegler MG. 1996. Light-headedness and defective cardiovascular reflexes after neck radiotherapy. Biol Press Monit 1:81–85.

Shehata N, Pater A, Tang SC. 1999. Prolonged severe 5-fluorouracil–associated neurotoxicity in a patient with dihydropyrimidine dehydrogenase deficiency. Cancer Invest 17:201–205.

Silverman DA, Chapron DJ. 1995. Lymphopenic effect of carbamazepine in a patient with chronic lymphocytic leukemia. Ann Pharmacother 29:865–867.

Smith DF, Hutton JL, Sandemann D, et al. 1991. The prognosis of primary intracerebral tumours presenting with epilepsy: the outcome of medical and surgical management. J Neurol Neurosurg Psychiatry 54:915–920.

Smith GA, Damon LE, Rugo HS Ries CA, Linker CA. 1997. High-dose cytarabine dose modification reduces the incidence of neurotoxicity in patients with renal insufficiency. J Clin Oncol 15:833–839.

Snider S, Bashir R, Bierman P. 1994. Neurologic complications after high-dose chemotherapy and autologous bone marrow transplantation for Hodgkin's disease. Neurology 44:681–684.

Spencer MD. 1998. Leukoencephalopathy after CNS prophylaxis for acute lymphoblastic leukaemia. Pediatr Rehabil 2:33–39.

Stein DA, Chamberlain MC. 1991. Evaluation and management of seizures in the patient with cancer. Oncology (Huntingt) 5:33–39.

Stewart DJ, Belanger JM, Grahovac Z, et al. 1992. Phase I study of intracarotid administration of carboplatin. Neurosurgery 30:512–516.

Szeto HH, Inturrisi CE, Houde R, Saal S, Cheigh J, Reidenberg MM. 1977. Accumulation of normeperidine, an active metabolite of meperidine, in patients with renal failure of cancer. Ann Intern Med 86:738–741.

Tahsildar HI, Remler BF, Creger RJ, et al. 1996. Delayed, transient encephalopathy after marrow transplantation: case reports and MRI findings in four patients. J Neurooncol 27:241–250.

Trillet V, Biron P. 1989. [Brain metastases: diagnostic and therapeutic strategy]. Presse Med 18:1471–1475.

Vanhees SL, Raridaens K, Vansteenkiste JF. 2000. Syndrome of inappropriate antidiuretic hormone associated with chemotherapy-induced tumour lysis in small-cell lung cancer. Case report and literature review. Ann Oncol 11:1061–1065.

Walton GD, Hon JK, Mulpur TG. 1997. Ofloxacin-induced seizure. Ann Pharmacother 31:1475–1477.

Wang CH, Ng SH. 1995. Syncope as the initial presentation of nasopharyngeal carcinoma. J Neurooncol 25:73–75.

Wasserstrom WR, Glass JP, Posner JB. 1982. Diagnosis and treatment of leptomeningeal metastases from solid tumors: experience with 90 patients. Cancer 49:759–772.

Weiss HD, Walker MD, Wiernik PH. 1974. Neurotoxicity of commonly used antineoplastic agents (first of two parts). N Engl J Med 291:75–81.

Weitzner MA, Meyers CA, Valentine AD. 1995. Methylphenidate in the treatment of neurobehavioral slowing associated with cancer and cancer treatment. J Neuropsychiatry Clin Neurosci 7:347–350.

Werner-Wasik M, Rudoler S, Preston PE, et al. 1999. Immediate side effects of radiotherapy and radiosurgery. Int J Radiat Oncol Biol Phys 43:299–304.

Wroblewski BA, Leary JM, Phelan AM, et al. 1992. Methylphenidate and seizure frequency in brain injured patients with seizure disorders. J Clin Psychiatry 53:86–89.

Zamboni WC, Gajjar AJ, Heideman RL, et al. 1998. Phenytoin alters disposition of topotecan and N-desmethyl topotecan in a patient with medulloblastoma. Clin Cancer Res 4:783–789.

21

Cerebrovascular Disease

LISA R. ROGERS

Cerebrovascular disease is an important cause of neurologic morbidity and mortality in patients with cancer, and its presence must be considered in any cancer patient who experiences cerebral symptoms. It is the second most common cause of pathologically definable central nervous system (CNS) disease found in cancer patients at autopsy and is often symptomatic. An autopsy study from the Memorial Sloan-Kettering Cancer Center identified cerebrovascular disease in 500 (14.6%) of 3426 cancer patients at autopsy (Graus et al., 1985). Of those patients in whom cerebrovascular disease was identified, 51% had experienced clinical symptoms related to the disease.

Identifying cerebrovascular disease in the cancer patient is important because identification and treatment of the disorder can sometimes ameliorate neurologic symptoms and prevent subsequent episodes. Even when a stroke occurs in the setting of advanced cancer, treatment can improve the patient's quality of life. If a stroke occurs when cancer is limited, failure to identify and treat the cerebrovascular disease underlying the stroke may doom an otherwise successful outcome of the cancer treatment. In a small percentage of patients, stroke is the presenting sign of cancer, and identification of cerebrovascular disease in this subset may lead to the diagnosis of cancer.

Identifying cerebrovascular disease in the patient with cancer presents a challenge to the clinician, as the pathogenesis is often unique to this group of patients. In cancer patients, the common risk factors for stroke, such as systemic and cerebral atherosclerosis, hypertension, and advanced age, are overshadowed by the pathophysiologic effects of cancer and its treatment. Coagulation disorders, toxicity of antineoplastic treatment, and direct effects of cerebral tumor are the most common causes of stroke in this group. Neuroimaging studies are helpful in identifying the type and location of stroke, but the most important clues to its etiology in cancer patients are the type and extent of systemic cancer, the presence of CNS metastasis, and the type of antineoplastic therapy. This chapter reviews the cerebral hemorrhage and cerebral infarction syndromes that occur in cancer patients, with emphasis on the clinical settings in which they occur and current methods of diagnosis and treatment.

CEREBRAL HEMORRHAGE

Pathophysiology and Clinical Presentation

Table 21–1 lists the etiologies of the most common cerebral hemorrhage syndromes that occur in cancer patients. Hemorrhage is usually caused by coagulation abnormalities, brain metastasis, or a combination of the two. Hemorrhage typically occurs in the brain parenchyma, but associated intraventricular or subarachnoid hemorrhage may also occur, depending on the location of the primary hemorrhage. Primary subdural or subarachnoid hemorrhage is uncommon. Cerebral hemorrhage occurs more often in patients with leukemia than in those with lymphoma or solid tumors and is more common in acute than in chronic leukemias and in myelogenous rather than lymphocytic

Table 21–1. Pathophysiology of Cerebral Hemorrhage in Patients with Cancer

Etiology	*Pathology*	*Tumor Type and Setting*
Coagulopathy		
Disseminated intravascular coagulation	Intraparenchymal hemorrhage	Leukemia, especially early in the course of promyelocytic leukemia
Thrombocytopenia	Intraparenchymal hemorrhage	Leukemia, usually at relapse or the failure to induce remission
	Subdural or subarachnoid hemorrhage	Leukemia, often associated with disseminated intravascular coagulation or sepsis
Tumor related		
Hemorrhage into parenchymal brain metastases	Intraparenchymal hemorrhage	Melanoma, germ cell tumors, lung cancer
Ruptured neoplastic aneurysm	Intraparenchymal and subarachnoid hemorrhage	Cardiac myxoma, choriocarcinoma, lung cancer
Leukostasis, leukemic nodules	Intraparenchymal hemorrhage	Leukemia with hyperleukocytosis
Dural metastases	Subdural hemorrhage	Carcinoma, leukemia, lymphoma
Treatment related		
L-asparaginase	Intraparenchymal hemorrhage	Acute lymphocytic leukemia during induction therapy
Hemolytic uremic-like syndrome	Intraparenchymal hemorrhage	Adenocarcinoma treated with chemotherapy, especially mitomycin C
Miscellaneous		
Idiopathic thrombocytopenic purpura, platelet dysfunction, hyperviscosity, acquired von Willebrand's disease	Intraparenchymal hemorrhage	Lymphoma, multiple myeloma, or chronic myeloproliferative disorders
Hypertensive cerebrovascular disease	Intraparenchymal hemorrhage	Solid tumors

leukemias. The symptoms of intraparenchymal hemorrhage may be acute or gradual and include one or more of the following: headache, vomiting, reduced level of consciousness, seizures, focal neurologic signs, and confusion. The symptoms of subdural hematoma in cancer patients are typically confusion and lethargy, and these are usually acute. Rarely, there may be focal neurologic signs (e.g., hemiparesis, hemianopsia, monoparesis). Subdural hemorrhage is less often fatal than parenchymal hemorrhage (Graus et al., 1996). Subarachnoid or intraventricular hemorrhage usually produces rapid deterioration in the level of consciousness, resulting in coma.

Coagulopathy

In cancer patients, abnormal coagulation that predisposes to cerebral hemorrhage is typically due to *(1)* acute disseminated intravascular coagulation (DIC), *(2)* the presence of liver metastasis, *(3)* sepsis, and/or *(4)* thrombocytopenia induced by tumor invasion of the bone marrow or effects on the bone marrow of radiation or chemotherapy. Coagulation disorders are the most frequent cause of cerebral hemorrhage in patients with leukemia, and hemorrhages in these patients are usually symptomatic. In patients with acute promyelocytic leukemia, a subtype of acute myelogenous leukemia, DIC is triggered by release of procoagulant material from the granules in the progranulocytes. The coagulopathy worsens after the administration of chemotherapy. Cerebral hemorrhage occurs early in the course of this type of leukemia and is often fatal. In contrast, laboratory evidence of DIC is detected in as many as one-third of patients early in the course of acute lymphoblastic leukemia, but is rarely associated with clinically significant hemorrhage (Higuchi et al., 1998). Disseminated intravascular coagulopathy may become symptomatic in these patients during induction chemotherapy, especially in the presence of very low levels of fibrinogen (Sarris et al., 1996). Cerebral hemorrhage is usually a late complication of other types of leukemia and occurs at relapse or when remission cannot be induced. In the late stages of those leukemias, the pathogenesis of hemorrhage is multifactorial. Disseminated intravascular coagulopathy may be present, but is often accompanied by infection, liver disease, and/or hematologic complications of chemotherapy.

Primary subdural hemorrhage occurs in leukemia patients when there is severe and refractory thrombocytopenia. In some patients, DIC, sepsis, and meningeal leukemia are contributing factors to hemorrhage (Pitner and Johnson, 1973). Subdural hemorrhage is more common in patients with acute myelogenous leukemia after autologous rather than allogeneic bone marrow transplant (Graus et al., 1996). An unusual cause of brain hemorrhage is venous infarction due to cerebral sinus thrombosis associated with coagulopathy, typically occurring in patients who have leukemia (Raizer and DeAngelis, 2000). Figure 21–1 shows a postmortem example of fatal bilateral hemorrhagic infarctions caused by superior sagittal thrombosis in a patient with adenocarcinoma and coagulopathy. In patients with solid tumors, symptomatic parenchymal brain hemorrhage resulting from coagulopathy is rare and it is usually a terminal event.

Hemorrhage Associated with Cerebral Tumor

Hemorrhage into parenchymal metastatic brain tumor is the most common type of brain hemorrhage in patients with solid tumors. It occurs most frequently in patients with metastatic melanoma, germ cell tumors (especially choriocarcinoma), and carcinoma of the lung or kidney. It is caused by necrosis of tumor and the rupture of newly formed blood vessels or by invasion of blood vessels in the adjacent brain parenchyma (Kondziolka et al., 1987). In rare instances, especially with metastasis from malignant melanoma or choriocarcinoma, the metastasis underlying vascular invasion is microscopic. In more than one-half of patients, symptoms are acute and may be the first clinical sign of brain tumor metastasis

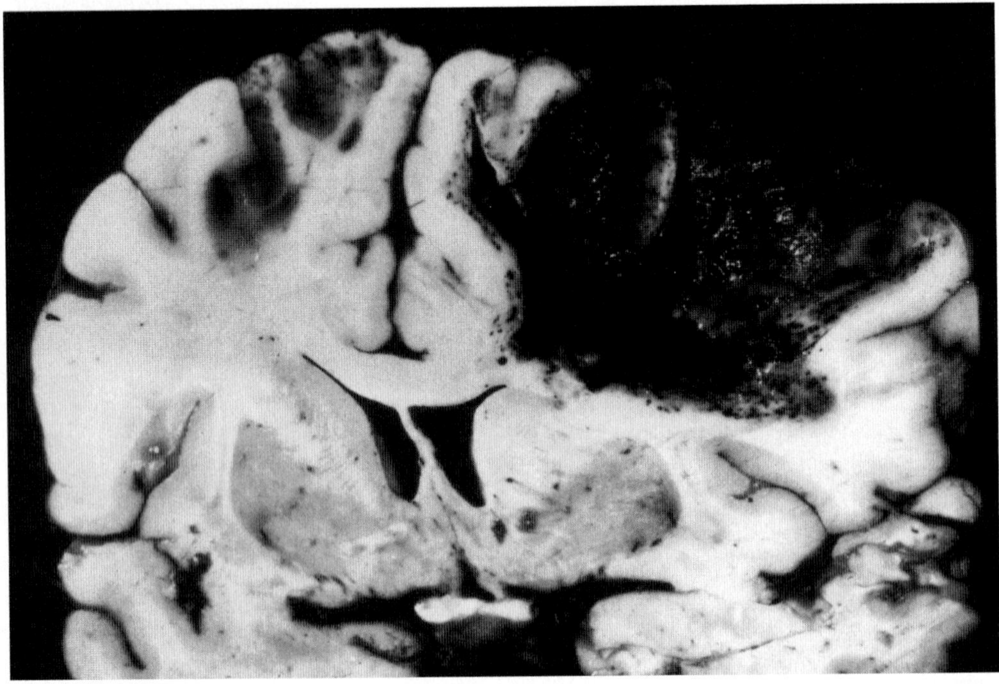

Figure 21–1. Bilateral cerebral hemorrhagic infarctions caused by nonmetastatic superior sagittal sinus thrombosis.

(Lieu et al., 1999). In other patients, the symptoms are superimposed on chronic or progressive symptoms of brain metastasis.

Ruptured neoplastic aneurysms are a rare cause of intracerebral hemorrhage and predominantly occur in patients who have cardiac myxoma, lung carcinoma, or choriocarcinoma (Kalafut et al., 1998). These aneurysms develop when tumor embolic material invades a cerebral vessel wall. After recanalization, the damaged wall dilates and ruptures (Murata et al., 1993). Rarely, aneurysms develop as a result of vascular invasion by a parenchymal metastasis. Neoplastic aneurysms are typically located in distal arterial branches, usually those of the middle cerebral artery.

Symptomatic subdural hemorrhage associated with tumor metastasis to the dura is uncommon. Dural metastasis develops from hematogenous spread of tumor to the dura or from skull metastasis that invades the dura. Figure 21–2 shows a subdural hematoma that was caused by dural metastasis of breast carcinoma. The subdural hemorrhage may be due to the rupture of vessels from vascular congestion by tumor or due to spontaneous hemorrhage of tumor. In some patients, there may be an effusion from tumor in the dura. The tumors that most commonly underlie subdural hemorrhage associated with dural metastasis are carcinomas (especially gastric, breast, or prostate); leukemia and lymphoma are less common (McKenzie et al., 1990). In some instances, a superimposed coagulopathy contributes to the hemorrhage (Minette and Kimmel, 1989). Signs of subdural hemorrhage usually develop gradually, and there may be focal neurologic signs in addition to headache. Epidural hematoma due to dural or skull metastasis is rare (McIver et al., 2001).

If DIC associated with acute promyelocytic leukemia is excluded, hyperleukocytosis (peripheral blast cell count in excess of 100,000/mm^3) is the most common cause of intracerebral hemorrhage at the time of diagnosis of leukemia. Hyperleukocytosis occurs most frequently in patients with acute myelogenous leukemia, especially the monocytic variant (Wurthner et al., 1999). Patients with hyperleukocytosis experience intracerebral hemorrhage in association with infiltration of cerebral capillaries by blast cells, but the pathogenesis of hemorrhage is controversial. In one series hemorrhage occurred while the white blood cell count was declining following chemotherapy administration (Wurthner et al., 1999). Postmortem studies reveal hemorrhage adjacent to dilated and thin-walled vessels that are filled with leukemic blasts (leukostasis) and adjacent to leukemic nodules (Freireich et al., 1960). Blast cells have less deformation than red blood cells; thus hyperviscosity, vascular endothelial damage, and competition with host cells to produce local hypoxia might result in hemorrhage.

Leukemic nodules enlarge and invade cerebral vessels. Leukostasis is more intense in the white matter, periventricular regions, and leptomeninges than in the cortex (Nowacki et al., 1995). Intracerebral hemorrhages associated with hyperleukocytosis are usually multiple and are located in the white matter. Intraventricular or subarachnoid hemorrhage may also occur. In contrast with patients who have hemorrhage caused by coagulopathy, only moderate thrombocytopenia is usually present, which would not be expected to cause spontaneous hemorrhage. A rare cause of intraparenchymal hemorrhage is cerebral perivascular infiltration of leukemic cells in leptomeningeal leukemia, resulting in the rupture of cerebral capillaries. Subarachnoid hemorrhage can also occur in patients with diffuse leptomeningeal tumor when there is thrombocytopenia.

Treatment-Related Hemorrhage

The use of L-asparaginase in induction therapy for acute lymphocytic leukemia results in cerebral hemorrhage or thrombosis in a small percentage of patients (Urban and Sager, 1981; Gugliotta et al., 1992). L-asparaginase is known to promote fibrinolysis and to deplete plasma proteins involved in coagulation, but the precise mechanism of thrombosis and hemorrhage is unknown. In some cases, cerebral hemorrhage is due to venous infarction from thrombosis of the superior sagittal sinus.

A hemolytic uremic–like syndrome is reported in patients with adenocarcinoma, sometimes developing after the administration of chemotherapy. The clinical manifestations are thought to be due to endothelial damage and include microangiopathic hemolytic anemia, thrombocytopenia, pulmonary edema, and renal insufficiency. Similar to the de novo hemolytic uremic syndrome, the neurologic signs include headache, confusion, hemiparesis, and coma. Originally reported as a complication of mitomycin C, it has now been associated with several antineoplastic agents, including bleomycin and cisplatin (Gordon and Kwaan, 1997). The onset after chemotherapy administration is highly variable and

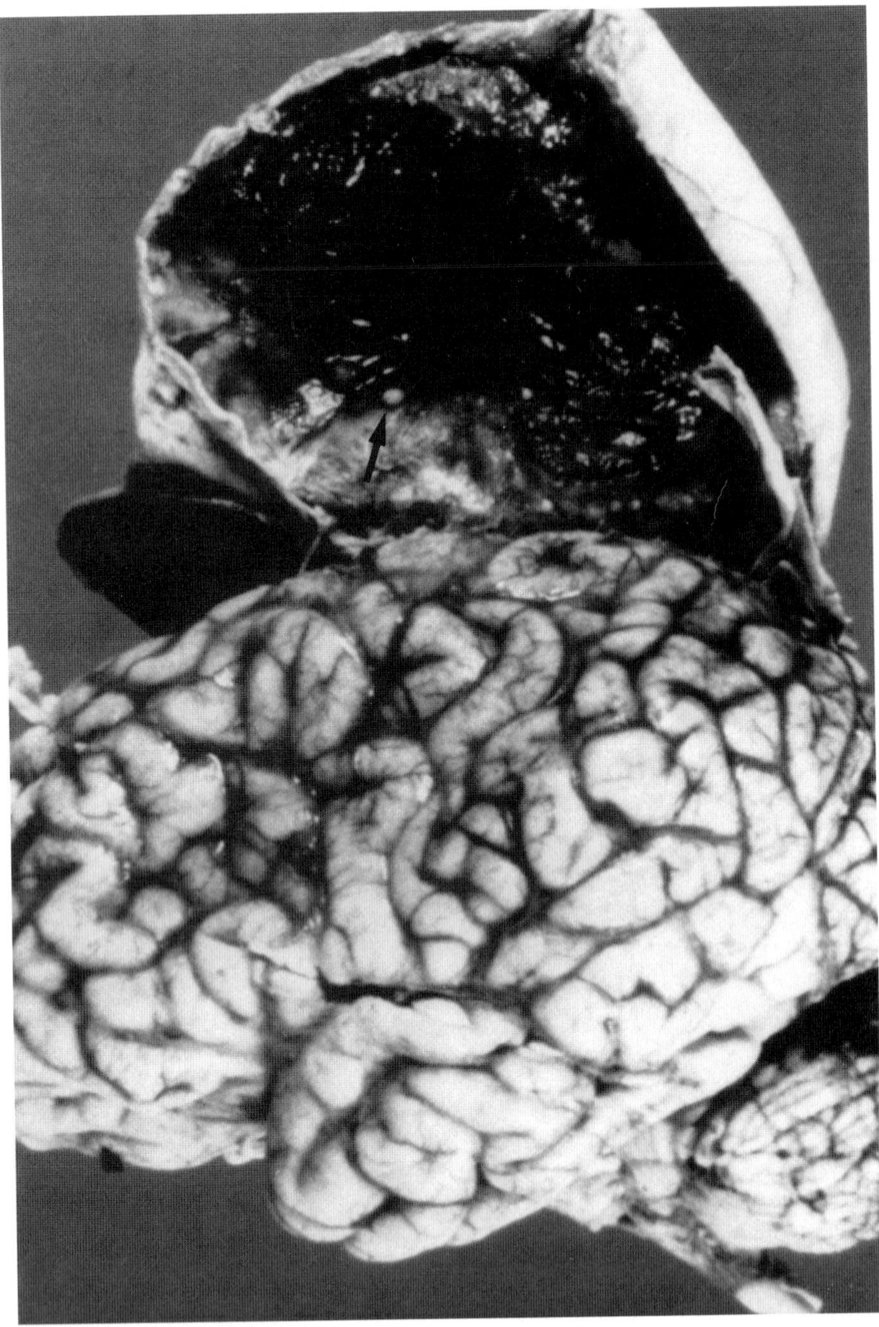

Figure 21–2. Postmortem examination of a subdural hematoma associated with nodular dural metastases (arrow) of breast carcinoma.

ranges from days to months. In other cancer patients, intracerebral hemorrhage occurs as a terminal event in the setting of severe thrombocytopenia induced by bone marrow failure from chemotherapy, radiation, or metastasis.

Miscellaneous

Hypertension is a rare cause of symptomatic intracerebral hemorrhage in cancer patients (Graus et al., 1985). It occurs primarily in patients with solid tumors. A high percentage of patients with chronic myeloproliferative disorders, especially chronic myelogenous leukemia and osteomyelofibrosis, experience intraparenchymal hemorrhage. Hemorrhage may coexist with intracerebral thromboses (Buss et al., 1985), and these tend to occur early in the disease (Wehmeier et al., 1991). In patients with lymphoma, intracerebral hemorrhage may be related to severe thrombocytopenia from idiopathic thrombocytopenic purpura or to an acquired form of von Willebrand's disease. In patients with myeloma, intracerebral hemorrhage may be related to thrombocytopenia and serum hyperviscosity. Primary subarachnoid hemorrhage is sufficiently rare in cancer patients so that congenital aneurysms should be considered. Among 24 patients with cancer and primary subarachnoid hemorrhage in the series by Graus et al. (1985), 4 had ruptured congenital aneurysms.

Diagnosis

Coagulopathy

The stage of the leukemia and associated clinical factors such as degree of thrombocytopenia and the presence of sepsis can suggest the cause of brain hemorrhage in patients with leukemia. The diagnosis of intracerebral hemorrhage is established by MRI or CT scans of the brain that reveal single or multiple hemorrhages. Patients who have acute DIC may also have systemic thrombosis, including deep vein thrombosis, pulmonary embolism, or myocardial infarction, and systemic hemorrhage, including hemorrhage in the mucosal surfaces, retinae, skin, genitourinary and gastrointestinal tracts, and at the site of venipuncture or bone marrow aspiration. Laboratory studies to confirm acute DIC include measurement of platelets, prothrombin time, activated partial thromboplastin time, fibrinogen, fibrin split products, fibrinopeptide A, the D-dimer assay, and the presence of schistocytes on the peripheral blood smear. In many patients with cancer, laboratory tests reveal evidence of chronic DIC, but this condition is rarely symptomatic; results of laboratory tests of coagulation function in all patients must be carefully interpreted in their clinical context.

Hemorrhage Associated with Cerebral Tumor

Computed tomography or MRI scans of the brain reveal single or multiple hemorrhages when there is hemorrhage into parenchymal brain metastasis. Clues to intratumoral hemorrhage include a multiplicity of hemorrhages, brain locations other than those usually found with hypertensive hemorrhage, and early edema and enhancement adjacent to the hemorrhage (Atlas et al., 1987). If an intratumoral brain hemorrhage is suspected but the patient is not known to have cancer, biopsy of the hematoma wall is indicated to establish the diagnosis. Parenchymal hemorrhages associated with ruptured neoplastic aneurysms may be single or multiple. Cerebral angiography in neoplastic aneurysms can reveal filling defects, fusiform and saccular aneurysms, and occluded vessels, but the sensitivity of angiography is unknown; in some instances, the hematoma obliterates the aneurysm and angiographic findings are normal.

In patients with subdural hematomas, CT and MRI brain scans can show acute or chronic subdural fluid collections. If dural metastasis is present, there may be evidence of adjacent skull metastasis and dural enhancement after injection of a contrast agent such as gadolinium. However, histologic examination of the dural membrane or subdural fluid may be necessary to establish the diagnosis of dural metastasis. Leptomeningeal metastasis is suggested by leptomeningeal enhancement on neuroimaging studies after injection of a contrast agent such as gadolinium and proven by identification of malignant cells in cerebrospinal fluid or in leptomeningeal biopsy specimens.

Treatment-Related Hemorrhage

Cerebral hemorrhage can occur during or immediately after induction therapy with L-asparaginase in patients with acute lymphocytic leukemia. Brain MRI and magnetic resonance venography can be diagnostic of venous occlusion. Systemic signs of a hemolytic uremic–like syndrome in conjunction with severe hemolytic anemia and thrombocytopenia associated with the administration of chemotherapy for adenocarcinoma suggest this diagnosis.

Miscellaneous

Laboratory tests that reveal evidence of extreme thrombocytosis, impaired platelet function, or hyperviscosity can be helpful in identifying the cause of cerebral hemorrhage in patients with chronic myeloproliferative disorders, lymphoma, and multiple myeloma.

Treatment

Coagulopathy

Successful therapy for acute DIC is multifaceted and controversial. Evacuation of an intracerebral hemorrhage in the setting of coagulopathy is difficult, and in patients with cancer who have cerebral hemorrhage caused by DIC treatment should be directed at controlling the systemic tumor and the associated medical conditions that contribute to the coagulopathy, such as sepsis. Treatment with heparin and fresh-frozen plasma can control DIC in some patients. Other therapies include replacement of clotting factors with blood products such as cryoprecipitate and platelet concentrations and antifibrinolytic agents. In patients with acute promyelocytic leukemia and DIC, it is controversial whether prophylactic heparin as an adjunct to induction chemotherapy can reduce the incidence of intracerebral hemorrhage. Chemotherapy, however, can increase the lysis of blast cells and aggravate DIC. All-*trans* retinoic acid administered for remission induction therapy of acute promyelocytic leukemia can differentiate abnormal promyelocytes into mature granulocytes, which improves coagulation function and results in a slight decrease of early brain hemorrhage (Tallman et al., 1997). Most patients with subdural hematoma caused by coagulopathy can be successfully managed without surgery (Graus et al., 1996).

Hemorrhage Associated with Cerebral Tumor

Survival of patients with massive intratumoral parenchymal brain hemorrhage or ruptured neoplastic aneurysms is poor, especially for those who have an acute onset of symptoms (Graus et al., 1985). These patients may die as a direct result of the hemorrhage. In some patients, resection of a single large hematoma is life saving (Little et al., 1979). The clinical course in patients with hemorrhage into brain metastasis who have a stable neurologic condition is no different from that of patients with nonhemorrhagic brain metastasis. These patients should receive radiation therapy directed to the underlying brain metastasis. For patients with ruptured neoplastic cerebral aneurysms, therapy should be directed to the systemic tumor (appropriate antineoplastic therapy in the case of systemic cancer and removal of the cardiac tumor in the case of cardiac myxoma). Brain irradiation is indicated for neoplastic aneurysms that arise from systemic carcinoma.

Therapy for subdural hemorrhage associated with dural metastasis is generally palliative and includes brain irradiation and drainage of subdural fluid. The use of antimetabolites and leukapheresis reduces the frequency of brain hemorrhage in acute leukemia patients presenting with hyperleukocytosis (Wurthner et al., 1999).

Treatment-Related Hemorrhage

The chances for neurologic recovery in patients experiencing L-asparaginase–induced thrombosis or hemorrhage are generally good (Feinberg and Swenson, 1988), and cerebrovascular events do not usually recur after re-treatment. Fresh-frozen plasma may be beneficial for patients with venous thrombosis, but it is not known if anticoagulation is necessary. The prognosis for patients with the hemolytic uremic–like syndrome induced by chemotherapy is poor, but steroids and plasma exchange may prolong survival (Gordon and Kwaan, 1997).

Miscellaneous

Conventional cytoreductive therapy reduces the incidence of cerebral ischemic or hemorrhagic events in patients with chronic myeloproliferative disorders (Wehmeier et al., 1991).

CEREBRAL INFARCTION

As is the case with cerebral hemorrhage, the risk factors for cerebral infarction in patients with cancer are usually different from those in patients without cancer. Table 21–2 lists the causes of cerebral infarction in cancer patients. Coagulation disorders, infection, the direct effects of CNS metastasis, and complications of antineoplastic treatment are the most common causes. Symptomatic cerebral infarction is more common in patients who have lymphoma and carcinoma than it is in those with leukemia, in whom cerebral hemorrhage predominates.

Two clinical factors make the identification of cerebral infarction in cancer patients and the determination of its cause difficult. First, cerebral infarctions in cancer patients are often multifocal, and the resulting multifocal neurologic signs are difficult to distinguish from those caused by encephalopathy. Therefore, the possibility of cerebral infarction must be considered for all cancer patients who experience

Table 21–2. Pathophysiology of Cerebral Infarction in Patients with Cancer

Etiology	*Pathology*	*Tumor Type and Setting*
Coagulopathy		
Nonbacterial thrombotic endocarditis	Cerebral infarction	Adenocarcinoma, usually widespread
Cerebral intravascular coagulation	Cerebral infarction, petechial hemorrhage	Lymphoma, leukemia, breast cancer, in advanced disease and sepsis
Coagulopathy, etiology undetermined	Superior sagittal sinus thrombosis with or without adjacent cerebral infarction	Lymphoma and solid tumors, usually in advanced disease
Infection		
Fungal sepsis	Cerebral infarction	Leukemia
Tumor-related		
Skull or dural metastases	Saggital sinus thrombosis with or without adjacent cerebral infarction	Lung cancer, neuroblastoma, lymphoma
Tumor embolism	Cerebral infarction	Lung and cardiac tumors
Leptomeningeal metastasis	Cerebral infarction	Solid tumors
Radiation-induced vasculopathy	Cerebral infarction	Head and neck cancer, lymphoma
Chemotherapy	Superior sagittal sinus occlusion	Leukemia, during induction therapy with L-asparaginase
Chemotherapy	Cerebral infarction	Breast cancer during multi-agent chemotherapy and hormonal therapy; other solid tumors during cisplatin-based chemotherapy
Miscellaneous		
Atherosclerosis	Cerebral infarction	Head and neck and lung cancer
Granulomatous angiitis	Cerebral infarction	Hodgkin's lymphoma, leukemia
Thrombocytosis	Cerebral infarction	Chronic myeloproliferative disorders, particularly essential thrombocytopenia

encephalopathy. Second, proving a link between coagulation abnormalities and cerebral infarction can be difficult because many cancer patients have abnormalities of coagulation function that are revealed by laboratory tests but are not clinically significant. The most important clues to the etiology of cerebral infarction are the type of cancer, the extent of systemic metastasis, the presence of CNS metastasis, and the type of antineoplastic treatment.

Pathophysiology and Clinical Presentation

Coagulopathy

The majority of patients with advanced solid tumors have laboratory evidence of clotting activation that is usually asymptomatic. In a small percentage of patients, however, the coagulopathy results in thrombosis of arteries or veins in the systemic or cerebral circulation. There are multiple risk factors for coagulopathy and thrombosis, including a complex interaction between tumor cells and their products with host cells, cancer treatment including single- or multiple-agent chemotherapy, hormonal therapy, and hematopoietic growth factors. Nonbacterial thrombotic endocarditis is the result of a hypercoagulable state and is characterized by the development of sterile platelet-fibrin vegetations on cardiac valves.

Nonbacterial thrombotic endocarditis is the most common cause of symptomatic cerebral infarction in cancer patients (Graus et al., 1985). Figure 21–3 shows cardiac nonbacterial thrombotic endocarditis in a patient with lung adenocarcinoma. Patients with cerebral infarction caused by nonbacterial thrombotic endocarditis usually experience focal neurologic signs, and angiography in these patients typically shows multiple branch occlusions of the middle

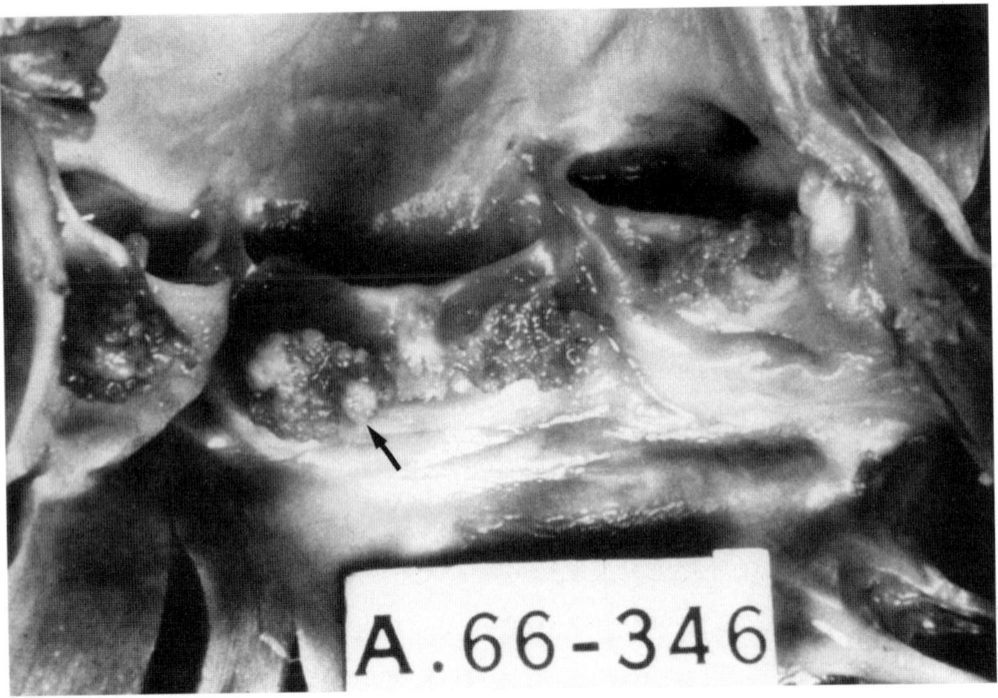

Figure 21–3. Postmortem examination demonstrating vegetations of nonbacterial thrombotic endocarditis attached to all cusps of the aortic valve. (The valve has been opened anteriorly.) The arrow indicates one area of vegetation.

cerebral artery. Focal signs may be preceded by transient ischemic attacks. Some patients also develop encephalopathy because of multifocal infarctions. Postmortem studies suggest that cerebral infarctions are caused by embolization of cardiac vegetations to the brain, cerebral intravascular thromboses that result from the associated coagulation disorder, or both (Reagan and Okazaki, 1974; Rogers et al., 1987). Nonbacterial thrombotic endocarditis occurs most commonly in patients with adenocarcinoma, especially mucin-producing carcinomas of the lung or gastrointestinal tract. It usually develops in patients with advanced cancer, but can occur in patients with early-stage cancer and can even be the presenting sign of cancer (Rogers et al., 1987). Evidence of systemic thrombosis or hemorrhage suggests the presence of nonbacterial thrombotic endocarditis.

Cerebral intravascular coagulation is due to thrombotic occlusion of small cerebral vessels caused by a coagulopathy unaccompanied by nonbacterial thrombotic endocarditis. It is the second most common cause of symptomatic cerebral infarction in patients with cancer (Graus et al., 1985). Patients with cerebral intravascular coagulation develop encephalopathy, and approximately one-half of patients have superimposed, sometimes transient, focal neurologic signs (Collins et al., 1975). The clinical course is progressive. Typically, multiple vessels in more than one major vessel territory of the brain and leptomeninges—usually small arteries, arterioles, capillaries, or venules—are occluded with fibrin. Figure 21–4 shows fibrin occlusions of leptomeningeal vessels in association with cerebral infarctions in a patient with breast cancer and cerebral intravascular coagulation. Cerebral intravascular coagulation is reported in patients with leukemia, breast cancer, and lymphoma, usually in the setting of advanced disease and sepsis. Amico et al. (1989) reported systemic and cerebral infarctions in six patients with mucinous cancers. At autopsy, mucin was present within vessels, macrophages, and areas of infarction. It is unknown whether mucin deposition results from metastasis or is associated with a cancer-related coagulopathy.

Nonmetastatic occlusion of large cerebral venous structures in cancer patients is caused by a coagulation disorder associated with cancer or with chemotherapy. The most common cerebral venous structure affected is the superior sagittal sinus, and the underlying tumor is usually leukemia (Raizer and DeAngelis, 2000). The incidence of this disorder is unknown

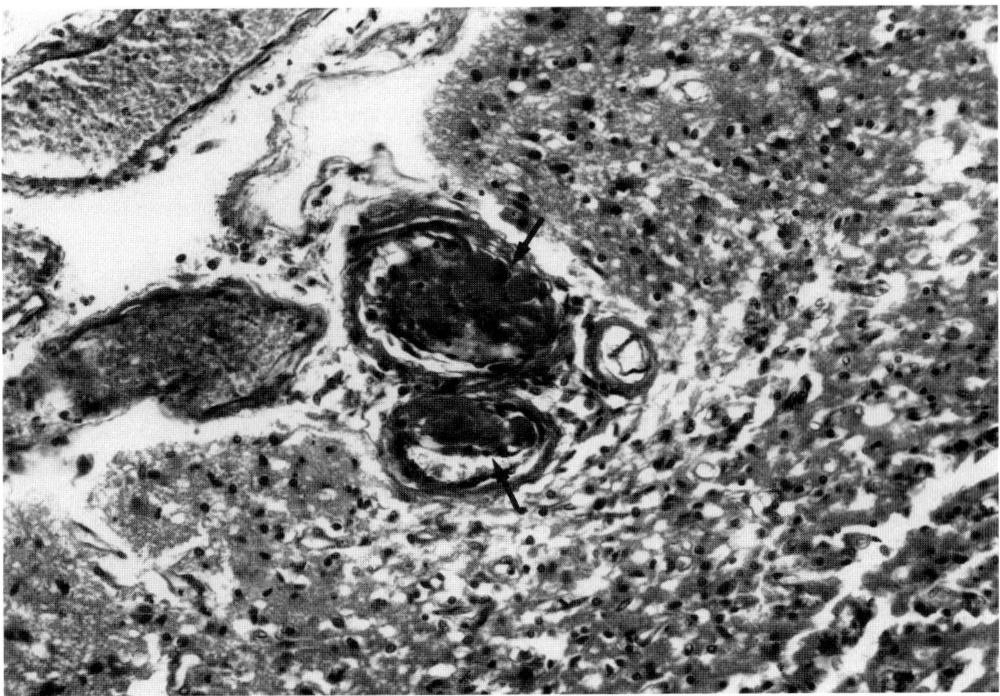

Figure 21–4. Organizing fibrin thrombi (arrows) in small leptomeningeal arteries overlying an area of cerebral infarction in a patient with disseminated breast carcinoma and cerebral intravascular coagulation. Hematoxylin and eosin; original magnification, ×50.

because the sinus occlusion can recanalize and is, therefore, underreported in autopsy series. The onset of symptoms from nonmetastatic superior sagittal sinus thrombosis is typically sudden headache; seizures, focal neurologic signs, or encephalopathy develop if there is brain hemorrhage or infarction. Superior sagittal sinus occlusion is associated with induction therapy that includes the administration of L-asparaginase to patients with acute lymphocytic leukemia (see "Treatment-Related Cerebral Infarction" in this chapter). In other patients with lymphoma or solid tumors, it usually occurs in the setting of widespread systemic metastatic disease.

Infarction Associated with Cerebral Infection

Cancer patients are predisposed to systemic infections because of immunosuppression caused by the tumor or by treatment with radiation, chemotherapy, broad-spectrum antibiotics, or immunosuppressants. Cerebral infarction associated with infection is most commonly caused by fungal septic emboli, typically of *Aspergillus* and *Candida* species. Fungal sepsis occurs more commonly in patients with leukemia than in those with lymphoma or carcinoma. Common sites of entry are the lower respiratory tract for *Aspergillus* and the gastrointestinal or genitourinary tracts or indwelling venous catheters for *Candida* species. Cerebral infarctions associated with cerebral infection are often multiple and may be hemorrhagic (Walsh et al., 1985). The neurologic signs usually consist of seizures, focal cerebral signs, or encephalopathy. Acute focal signs and seizures are more common in patients with *Aspergillus* infection, and encephalopathy is more common in patients with *Candida* infection. Meningitis is rarely present.

Infarction Associated with Cerebral Tumor

Skull or dural tumor that infiltrates or compresses the superior sagittal sinus can produce venous stasis and thrombosis. In contrast to patients with nonmetastatic superior sagittal sinus thrombosis, patients with the metastatic type of thrombosis develop subacute symptoms resulting from increased intracranial pressure (typically headache, vomiting, and papilledema). Focal neurologic signs or encephalopathy may be present if there is cerebral infarction. It occurs most commonly in patients with neuroblastoma, lung cancer, and lymphoma, but is reported in a variety of tumors.

Another mechanism for tumor-related cerebral infarction is embolism of a tumor fragment to the brain. This can produce focal or multifocal cerebral signs, sometimes preceded by transient ischemic attacks (O'Neill et al., 1987). Embolism of a tumor fragment to the brain is reported exclusively in patients with solid tumors, usually those with a primary or metastatic cardiac or lung tumor that is the source of the embolus. Cerebral embolism can occur at the time of manipulation of the lung in patients with lung tumor undergoing thoracotomy (Lefkovitz et al., 1986; O'Neill et al., 1987). It can be the presenting sign of cardiac tumor, especially cardiac myxoma. Leptomeningeal metastasis is a rare cause of cerebral infarction. Infarction may be the sole manifestation of this disorder, or there may be accompanying typical signs, including headache, cranial nerve palsies, and radiculopathies. Postmortem studies suggest that infarction occurs because tumor infiltrates the cerebral arteries in the Virchow-Robin spaces and causes vascular occlusion or spasm (Klein et al., 1989). The infarctions may be multifocal.

Treatment-Related Infarction

Neck radiation administered for head and neck cancer or lymphoma can produce delayed extracranial carotid stenosis or occlusion. In a prospective study of carotid duplex ultrasound performed in 240 patients with head and neck cancer who received radiation to the cervical region, a greater than 70% stenosis of the common and/or internal carotid artery was detected in 28 patients (11.7%) (Cheng et al., 1999). Histologic examination of the diseased artery suggests that radiation produces or accelerates atherosclerosis. Patients may develop transient ischemic attacks, including amaurosis fugax, or cerebral infarction. Murros and Toole (1989) reported a wide interval between radiation therapy and the development of this complication, with a mean interval of 19 years. Carotid artery rupture is a potentially fatal complication of head and neck tumor resection and neck irradiation. It is usually associated with orocutaneous fistulas, necrosis of the skin flap, and infection (McCready et al., 1983). Patients may die from exsanguination. If the carotid rupture is detected and the artery is ligated, there is a significant chance of cerebral infarction and death (Razack and Sako, 1982).

Potential mechanisms for abnormal coagulation function in patients receiving chemotherapy include alterations in coagulation factors or anticoagulant proteins and endothelial damage produced by these agents. Because of the small number of events occurring in individual treatment studies and the lack of uniform reporting of thromboembolism, including stroke, the evidence for a causal relationship with antineoplastic agents, regardless of other risk factors, is weak (Lee and Levine, 1999). The best-recognized cerebrovascular complication of chemotherapy is venous thrombosis caused by L-asparaginase used in combination induction chemotherapy for patients with acute lymphocytic leukemia (Lee and Levine, 1999; Gugliotta et al., 1992). L-asparaginase promotes fibrinolysis and causes a depletion of plasma proteins involved in coagulation. There may be promotion of thrombosis by a transient increase in unusually large plasma von Willebrand's factor multimers (Pui et al., 1987). There are also uncommon reports of systemic and cerebral venous and arterial thromboembolic complications in women with breast cancer receiving multiagent chemotherapy (Wall et al., 1989), especially when chemotherapy is combined with hormonal therapy (Saphner et al., 1991). Complications usually occur early in treatment.

A rare neurologic complication of chemotherapy is cerebral embolization from a ventricular mural thrombus that forms in association with cardiomyopathy resulting from chemotherapy with doxorubicin (Adriamycin) (Schachter and Freeman, 1982). Transient focal neurologic signs suggesting transient ischemic attacks can occur during interleukin-2 therapy (Bernard et al., 1990).

Miscellaneous

Atherosclerosis is the most common cause of cerebral infarction found at autopsy in patients with cancer, but it accounts for only 14% of symptomatic infarctions (Graus et al., 1985). The most common tumors associated with symptomatic cerebral infarction from atherosclerosis are head and neck cancers and lung cancer. A less common cause of symptomatic cerebral infarction is granulomatous angiitis occurring in patients with Hodgkin's disease or leukemia (Inwards et al., 1991; Lowe and Russell, 1987). Signs include headache, fever, confusion, seizures, obtundation, or hemiparesis. Patients with chronic myeloproliferative disorders who have extreme thrombocytosis can experience cerebral arterial or venous thromboembolic events (Randi et al., 1998). These complications are most common in patients with polycythemia vera and essential thrombocythemia and occur more often in older patients (Jabaily et al., 1983; Wehmeier et al., 1991). Platelet thromboembolism is likely caused by inherent alterations of platelet function in addition to the excessively high number of platelets. Neurologic symptoms are most common before and shortly after the diagnosis of chronic myeloproliferative disorders, probably because cytoreductive therapy administered after the diagnosis is effective (Michiels et al., 1993). In patients with essential thrombocythemia, symptoms are usually transient and are poorly localized; they include unsteadiness, dysarthria, and scotomas. Focal symptoms such as transient monocular blindness or limb weakness are less common. They are of sudden onset and are often accompanied by headache. Systemic arterial or venous thrombosis may also occur. Patients with Hodgkin's disease who are in remission or cured can experience episodic neurologic dysfunction that resembles transient ischemic attacks (Feldmann and Posner, 1986). The cause of these symptoms is unknown.

Diagnosis

Coagulopathy

Patients with stroke caused by coagulation disorders may have evidence of systemic thrombosis or hemorrhage. Particularly, patients with nonbacterial thrombotic endocarditis may have systemic bleeding, limb thrombophlebitis arterial occlusion, pulmonary embolism, or myocardial infarction (Reagan and Okazaki, 1974; Rogers et al., 1987). Laboratory tests may reveal evidence of DIC in some patients (Rogers et al., 1987), but in many patients abnormalities on coagulation function tests are indistinguishable from the abnormalities commonly associated with cancer. These abnormalities include markers of clotting activation, such as abnormal thrombin–antithrombin complex, prothrombin fragment F 1 + 2, and D-dimer.

Cardiac murmurs are rare, and transthoracic echocardiography is usually nondiagnostic because of the small size of the cardiac vegetations. Transesophageal echocardiography can be diagnostic (Blanchard et al., 1992). Computed tomography or MRI scans of the brain may reveal cerebral infarction. In patients who experience focal neurologic signs, cerebral angiography is a sensitive test for the diagnosis of cerebral infarction from nonbacterial thrombotic endocarditis. In these patients, cerebral angiography typically shows multiple branch occlusions of the middle cerebral artery (Rogers et al., 1987). Many patients with cerebral intravascular coagulation have systemic bleeding, but results of laboratory tests of coagulation function are nonspecific. In a study by Collins et al. (1975), neuroimaging studies performed in a small number of patients were normal. There is no method currently known to diagnose this syndrome aside from postmortem examination.

Magnetic resonance imaging of the brain is the imaging procedure of choice to detect superior sagittal sinus thrombosis caused by coagulopathy. It can document the lack of normal flow void within the occluded sinus and can reveal enlarged collateral veins (Sze et al., 1988). Adjacent cerebral hemorrhage or infarction can also be visualized. When MRI is nondiagnostic, magnetic resonance venography can be diagnostic (Fig. 21–5).

Infarction Associated with Infection

Computed tomography and MRI brain scans can reveal infarctions in patients with septic cerebral embolism. Focal enhancement may appear later if the infarctions evolve into abscesses. Cerebrospinal fluid examination is generally nondiagnostic because usually only mild pleocytosis and protein elevation are present. Cultures are typically negative. Hemorrhagic cerebrospinal fluid can be a clue to *Aspergillus* infection (Walsh et al., 1985). Blood cultures are often negative, but clinical or radiographic evidence of pulmonary infection suggests systemic *Aspergillus* infection. *Aspergillus* can be isolated from respiratory secretions or open lung biopsy specimens, but open lung biopsy is potentially hazardous in many cancer patients because of coexisting thrombocytopenia (Walsh et al., 1985).

Infarction Associated with Cerebral Tumor

Brain MRI and magnetic resonance venography are the methods of choice to diagnose metastatic superior sagittal sinus occlusion and to reveal associated cerebral infarction. In patients with superior sagittal sinus occlusion due to skull or dural tumor, MRI may also reveal evidence of adjacent skull or dural metastasis. Dural or leptomeningeal metastasis will usu-

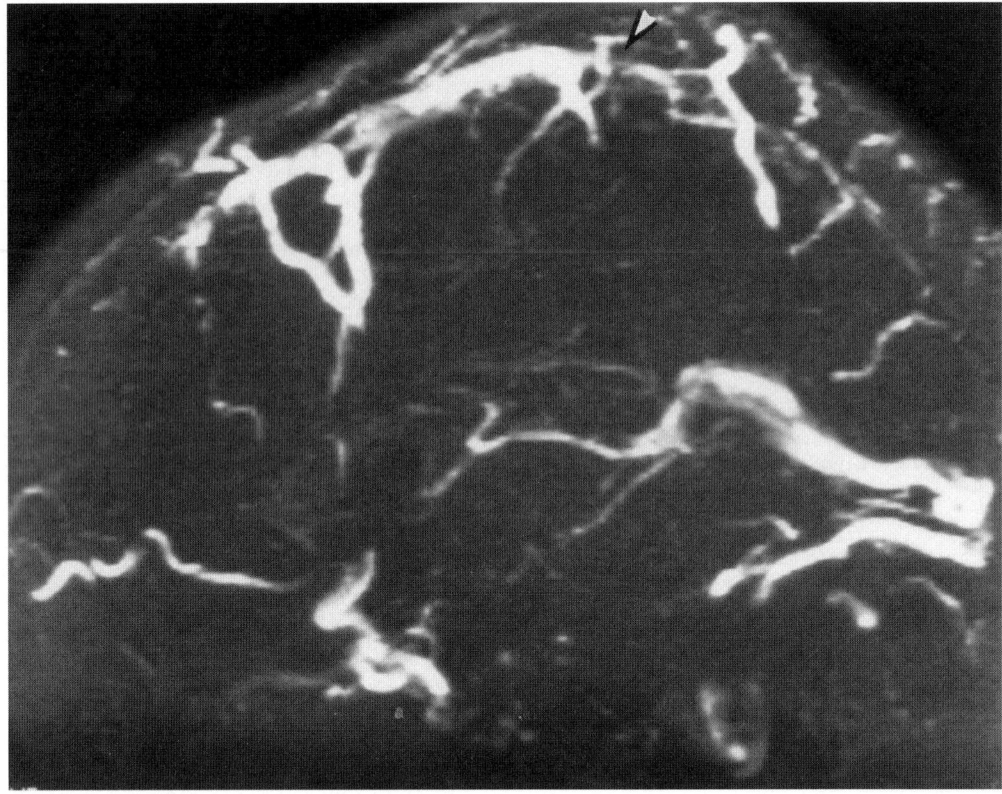

Figure 21–5. Nonmetastatic superior sagittal sinus occlusion (arrowhead) visible on two-dimensional time-of-flight magnetic resonance venogram.

ally enhance after injection of gadolinium. In patients with tumor embolic infarctions, the infarctions can be seen on CT or MRI scans, and angiography may reveal vascular occlusions (Marazuela et al., 1989; O'Neill et al., 1987); however, these findings are not specific, and a definitive diagnosis of tumor embolism can be established only if there is a simultaneous peripheral arterial embolism that can be examined histologically. Patients in whom tumor embolic infarction is suspected should undergo serial CT or MRI brain scans for evaluation of growth of the brain metastasis. Clinical clues to the presence of primary or metastatic cardiac tumor include a new onset of congestive heart failure, pericardial effusion, rapid cardiac enlargement, or arrhythmias that are difficult to control. Echocardiography is diagnostic.

Treatment-Related Infarction

Carotid angiography in patients with radiation-induced carotid artery disease usually reveals occlusion or extensive stenosis of the common carotid artery that is confined to the field of irradiation. The length of stenosis in these patients is typically greater than it is in patients with atherosclerosis not associated with irradiation (Fig. 21–6). Little information is available on neuroimaging abnormalities in patients who experience cerebral infarction related to chemotherapy administration except for patients with superior sagittal sinus occlusion. There are no laboratory tests that can diagnose chemotherapy-induced coagulation abnormalities.

Miscellaneous

Atherosclerotic brain infarction is suggested by the patient's age and the presence of typical risk factors for atherosclerosis. Granulomatous angiitis is suggested by the presence of cerebral infarctions, hemorrhages, or contrast-enhancing masses on CT or MRI brain scans in patients with lymphoma or leukemia. Angiography may show a classic beading pattern but

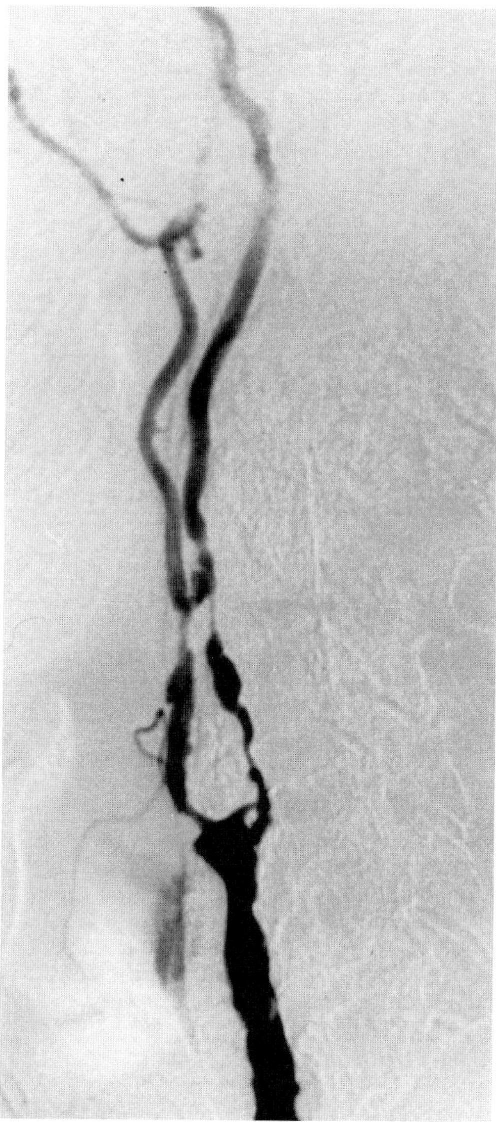

Figure 21–6. Cerebral angiography in a patient with laryngeal cancer and radiation-induced carotid atherosclerosis reveals irregularity and moderate stenosis of the distal left common carotid artery. There is a long segment of diffuse irregularity and severe stenosis alternating with zones of dilatation in the proximal internal and external carotid arteries. The area of involvement of the common, internal, and external carotid arteries corresponds to the field of radiation.

may be nonspecifically abnormal or normal. The most definitive method for diagnosis of granulomatous angiitis is biopsy, but its sensitivity is low (Inwards et al., 1991). The association of cerebral infarction with thrombocythemia can be determined by measuring the platelet count.

Treatment

Coagulopathy

Effective therapy for coagulation disorders must be directed to the underlying tumor, to associated medical conditions such as sepsis that predispose the patient to the disorder, and to the coagulation disorder itself. Management decisions for coagulopathy are still controversial, and therapy must be individualized. Low-molecular-weight heparin or low-dose warfarin can reduce the risk of systemic venous thromboembolism in cancer patients (Levine and Lee, 2001), but their role in the prophylaxis of stroke is unknown. Patients who experience cerebral infarction from nonbacterial thrombotic endocarditis may benefit from anticoagulation therapy. In the series by Rogers et al. (1987), heparin therapy was effective in reducing ischemic symptoms in some patients with cerebral infarction, and the incidence of hemorrhagic infarction and cerebral hemorrhage, possible side effects of this therapy, was no greater than in patients who were not anticoagulated. However, anticoagulation must be undertaken judiciously because of the risk of systemic and cerebral hemorrhage in patients with this disorder. Appropriate therapy for cerebral intravascular coagulation is not known. Heparin and urokinase are reported to be beneficial in reducing the morbidity of superior sagittal sinus thrombosis in patients without cancer (Einhaupl et al., 1991; De Bruijn and Stam, 1999; Philips et al., 1999), but no prospective studies have been performed in patients with cancer.

Infarction Associated with Infection

Patients with fungal septic cerebral infarction should be treated with antifungal therapy, but the prognosis for recovery and survival is poor (Walsh et al., 1985).

Infarction Associated with Cerebral Tumor

Patients with metastatic superior sagittal sinus occlusion should be treated with irradiation of the brain. It is not known whether anticoagulation therapy is effective in treating this disorder. In patients with embolic infarction from malignant tumors, the brain should also be irradiated. In those patients with cardiac tumors, removal of the cardiac tumor will prevent subsequent embolization. Patients with leptomeningeal metastasis should be treated with radiation to the symptomatic areas of the neuraxis and with systemic or intraventricular chemotherapy.

Treatment-Related Infarction

Patients with symptomatic or high-grade radiation-induced carotid stenosis can be effectively treated with endarterectomy; the long-term patency rates are similar to those in nonirradiated patients (Kashyup et al., 1999). Endovascular occlusion is a safe and effective method to avoid carotid artery ligation and prevent cerebral infarction in patients with carotid artery rupture (Citardi et al., 1995). If carotid ligation is required, low-dose heparin may reduce the risk of cerebral infarction (Leikensohn et al., 1978). There is no effective therapy known for the vascular complications of chemotherapy, although Feinberg and Swenson (1988) suggest that prophylactic fresh-frozen plasma be administered to patients receiving L-asparaginase. In other situations, the benefits of chemotherapy must be carefully weighed against the risk of recurrent thromboembolic events.

Miscellaneous

Granulomatous angiitis can respond to treatment directed to the underlying cancer (Hodgkin's disease or leukemia) or to steroids and cytotoxic drugs administered for vasculitis (Inwards et al., 1991). Aspirin and cytostatic reduction of the platelet count are effective in preventing recurrence of thrombotic events in patients with essential thrombocythemia (Michiels et al., 1993). The clinical course of patients with Hodgkin's disease who experience transient neurologic symptoms of unknown etiology is benign, and no treatment is indicated (Feldmann and Posner, 1986).

REFERENCES

Amico L, Caplan LR, Thomas C. 1989. Cerebrovascular complications of mucinous cancers. Neurology 39:522–526.

Atlas SW, Grossman RI, Gomori JM, et al. 1987. Hemorrhagic intracranial malignantneoplasms: spin-echo MR imaging. Radiology 164:71–77.

Bernard JT, Ameriso S, Kempf RA, Rosen P, Mitchell MS, Fisher M. 1990. Transient focal neurologic deficits complicating interleukin-2 therapy. Neurology 40:154–155.

Blanchard DG, Ross RS, Dittrich HC. 1992. Nonbacterial thrombotic endocarditis. Assessment by transesophageal echocardiography. Chest 102:954–956.

Buss DH, Stuart JJ, Lipscomb GE. 1985. The incidence of thrombotic and hemorrhagic disorders in association with extreme thrombocytosis: an analysis of 129 cases. Am J Hematol 20:365–372.

Cheng SW, Wu LL, Ting AC, Lau H, Lam LK, Wei WI. 1999. Irradiation-induced extracranial carotid stenosis in patients with head and neck malignancies. Am J Surg 178:323–328.

Citardi MJ, Chaloupka JC, Son YH, Ariyan S, Sasaki CT. 1995. Management of carotid artery rupture by monitored endovascular therapeutic occlusion (1988–1994). Laryngoscope 105:1086–1092.

Collins RC, Al-Mondhiry H, Chernik NL, Posner JB. 1975. Neurologic manifestations of intravascular coagulation in patients with cancer: a clinicopathologic analysis of 12 cases. Neurology 25:795–806.

De Bruijn SF, Stam J. 1999. Randomized, placebo-controlled trial of anticoagulant treatment with low-molecular-weight heparin for cerebral sinus thrombosis. Stroke 30:484–488.

Einhaupl KM, Villringer A, Meister W, et al. 1991. Heparin treatment in sinus venous thrombosis. Lancet 338:597–600.

Feinberg WM, Swenson MR. 1988. Cerebrovascular complications of L-asparaginase therapy. Neurology 38:127–133.

Feldmann E, Posner JB. 1986. Episodic neurologic dysfunction in patients with Hodgkin's Disease. Arch Neurol 43:1227–1233.

Freireich EJ, Thomas LB 3d, Frei E, Fritz RD Jr, Forhman CE. 1960. A distinctive type of intracerebral hemorrhage associated with blast crisis in patients with leukemia. Cancer 13:146–150.

Gordon LI, Kwaan HC. 1997. Cancer- and drug-associated thrombotic thrombocytopenic purpura and hemolytic uremic syndrome. Semin Hematol 34:140–147.

Graus F, Rogers LR, Posner JB. 1985. Cerebrovascular complications in patients with cancer. Medicine (Baltimore) 64:16–35.

Graus F, Saiz A, Sierra J, et al. 1996. Neurologic complications of autologus and allogeneic bone marrow transplantation in patients with leukemia: a comparative study. Neurology 46:1004–1009.

Gugliotta L, Mazzucconi MG, Leone G, et al. 1992. Incidence of thrombotic complications in adult patients with acute lymphoblastic leukaemia receiving L-asparaginase during induction therapy: a retrospective study. The GIMEMA Group. Eur J Haematol 49:63–66.

Higuchi T, Mori H, Niikura H, Omine M, Okada S, Terada H. 1998. Disseminated intravascular coagulation in acute lymphoblastic leukemia at presentation and in early phase of remission induction therapy. Ann Hematol 76:263–269.

Inwards DJ, Piepgras DG, Lie JT, O'Neill BP, Schiethauer BW, Habermann TM. 1991. Granulomatous angiitis of the spinal cord associated with Hodgkin's disease. Cancer 68:1318–1322.

Jabaily J, Iland HJ, Laszlo J, et al. 1983. Neurologic manifestations of essential thrombocythemia. Ann Intern Med 99:513–518.

Kalafut M, Vinuela F, Saver JL, Martin N, Vespa P, Verity MA. 1998. Multiple cerebral pseudoaneurysms and hemorrhages: the expanding spectrum of metastatic cerebral choriocarcinoma. J Neuroimaging 8:44–47.

Kashyap VS, Moore WS, Quinones-Baldrich WJ. 1999. Carotid artery repair for radiation-associated atherosclerosis is a safe and durable procedure. J Vasc Surg 29:90–96.

Klein P, Haley EC, Wooten GF, VandenBerg SR. 1989. Focal cerebral infarctions associated with perivascular tumor in-

filtrates in carcinomatous leptomeningeal metastases. Arch Neurol 46:1149–1152.
Kondziolka D, Bernstein M, Resch L, et al. 1987. Significance of hemorrhage into brain tumors: clinicopathological study. J Neurosurg 67:852–857.
Lee AY, Levine MN. 1999. The thrombophilic state induced by therapeutic agents in the cancer patient. Semin Thromb Hemost 25:137–145.
Lefkovitz NW, Roessmann U, Kori SH. 1986. Major cerebral infarction from tumor embolus. Stroke 17:555–557.
Leikensohn J, Milko D, Cotton R. 1978. Carotid artery rupture. Management and prevention of delayed neurologic sequelae with low-dose heparin. Arch Otolaryngol 104:307–310.
Levine MN, Lee AY. 2001. Treatment of venous thrombosis in the cancer patient. Acta Haematol 106:81–87.
Lieu AS, Hwang SL, Howng SL, Chai CY. 1999. Brain tumors with hemorrhage. J Formos Med Assoc 98:365–367.
Little JR, Dial B, Belanger G, Carpenter S. 1979. Brain hemorrhage from intracranial tumor. Stroke 10:283–288.
Lowe J, Russell NH. 1987. Cerebral vasculitis associated with hairy cell leukemia. Cancer 60:3025–3028.
Marazuela M, Garcia-Merino A, Yebra M, Brasa JM, Diego J, Durantez A. 1989. Magnetic resonance imaging and angiography of the brain in embolic left atrial myxoma. Neuroradiology 31:137–139.
McCready RA, Hyde GL, Bivins BA, Mattingly SS, Griffen WO Jr. 1983. Radiation-induced arterial injuries. Surgery 93: 306–312.
McIver JI, Scheithauer BW, Rydberg CH, Atkinson JL. 2001. Metastatic hepatocellular carcinoma presenting as epidural hematoma: case report. Neurosurgery 49:447–449.
McKenzie CR, Rengachary SS, McGregor DH, Dixon AY, Suskind DL. 1990. subdural hematoma associated with metastatic neoplasms. Neurosurgery 27:619–624.
Michiels JJ, Koudstaal PJ, Mulder AH, van Vliet HH. 1993. Transient neurologic and ocular manifestations in primary thrombocythemia. Neurology 43:1107–1110.
Minette SE, Kimmel DW. 1989. Subdural hematoma in patients with systemic cancer. Mayo Clin Proc 64:637–642.
Murata J, Sawamura Y, Takahashi A, Abe H, Saitoh H. 1993. Intracerebral hemorrhage caused by a neoplastic aneurysm from small-cell lung carcinoma: case report. Neurosurgery 32:124–126.
Murros KE, Toole JF. 1989. The effect of radiation on carotid arteries. A review article. Arch Neurol 46:449–455.
Nowacki P, Fryze C, Zdziarska B, Zyluk B, Grzelec H, Dudzik T. 1995. Central nervous system leukostasis in patients with leukemias and lymphomas. Folia Neuropathol 33:59–65.
O'Neill BP, Dinapoli RP, Okazaki H. 1987. Cerebral infarction as a result of tumor emboli. Cancer 60:90–95.
Philips MF, Bagley LJ, Sinson GP, et al. 1999. Endovascular thrombolysis for symptomatic cerebral venous thrombosis. J Neurosurg 90:65–71.
Pitner SE, Johnson WW. 1973. Chronic subdural hematoma in childhood acute leukemia. Cancer 32:185–190.
Pui CH, Jackson CW, Chesney CM, Abildgaard CF. 1987. Involvement of von Willebrand factor in thrombosis following asparaginase-prednisone-vincristine therapy for leukemia. Am J Hematol 25:299–298.
Raizer JJ, DeAngelis LM. 2000. Cerebral sinus thrombosis diagnosed by MRI and MR venography in cancer patients. Neurology 54:1222–1226.
Randi ML, Fabris F, Cella G, Rossi C, Girolami A. 1998. Cerebral vascular accidents in young patients with essential thrombocythemia: relation with other known cardiovascular risk factors. Angiology 49:477–481.
Razack MS, Sako K. 1982. Carotid artery hemorrhage and ligation in head and neck cancer. J Surg Oncol 19:189–192.
Reagan TJ, Okazaki H. 1974. The thrombotic syndrome associated with carcinoma. A clinical and neuropathologic study. Arch Neurol 31:390–395.
Rogers LR, Cho E, Kempin S, Posner JB. 1987. Cerebral infarction from nonbacterial thrombotic endocarditis. Clinical and pathological study including the effects of anticoagulation. Am J Med 83:746–756.
Saphner T, Tormey DC, Gray R. 1991. Venous and arterial thrombosis in patients who received adjuvant therapy for breast cancer. J Clin Oncol 9:286–294.
Sarris A, Cortes J, Kantarjian H, et al. 1996. Disseminated intravascular coagulation in adult acute lymphoblastic leukemia: frequent complications with fibrinogen levels less than 100 mg/dl. Leuk Lymphoma 21:85–92.
Schachter S, Freeman R. 1982. Transient ischemic attack and adriamycin cardiomyopathy. Neurology 32:1380–1381.
Sze G, Simmons B, Krol G, Walker R, Zimmerman RD, Deck MD. 1988. Dural sinus thrombosis: verification with spin-echo techniques. AJNR Am J Neuroradiol 9:679–686.
Tallman MS, Andersen JW, Schiffer CA, et al. 1997. All-trans-retinoic acid in acute promyelocytic leukemia. N Engl J Med 337:1021–1028.
Urban C, Sager WD. 1981. Intracranial bleeding during therapy with L-asparaginase in childhood acute lymphocytic leukemia. Eur J Pediatr 137:323–327.
Wall JG, Weiss RB, Norton L, et al. 1989. Arterial thrombosis associated with adjuvant chemotherapy for breast carcinoma: a Cancer and Leukemia Group B Study. Am J Med 87:501–504.
Walsh TJ, Hier DB, Caplan LR. 1985. Aspergillosis of the central nervous system: clinicopathological analysis of 17 patients. Ann Neurol 18:574–582.
Wehmeier A, Daum I, Jamin H, Schneider W. 1991. Incidence and clinical risk factors for bleeding and thrombotic complications in myeloproliferative disorders. A retrospective analysis of 260 patients. Ann Hematol 63:101–106.
Wurthner JU, Kohler G, Behringer D, Lindemann A, Mertelsmann R, Lubbert M. 1999. Leukostasis followed by hemorrhage complicating the initiation of chemotherapy in patients with acute myeloid leukemia and hyperleukocytosis: a clinicopathologic report of four cases. Cancer 85:368–374.

22

Rehabilitation of Patients with Neurologic Tumors and Cancer-Related Central Nervous System Disabilities

THERESA A. GILLIS, RAJESH YADAV, AND YING GUO

Neurologic tumors may involve the brain or spinal cord and are either primary or metastatic. Patients may become increasingly less independent as a result of direct injury of neural structures responsible for motor, sensory, cognitive, and speech functions. The indirect effects of chemotherapy and radiation therapy (RT) add to the functional deficits patients experience. The number of patients involved is quite large. More than 15,000 new cases of primary brain tumor and 4000 new spinal tumors are diagnosed every year (American Cancer Society, 1990). Approximately 2% of all cancer deaths are caused by brain tumors, which account for roughly 11,000 deaths per year (American Cancer Society, 1990). Metastatic lesions from various sites account for 20% to 40% of brain tumors (American Cancer Society, 1990), occur in approximately 15% of cancer patients (Black, 1991), and produce neurologic symptoms in approximately 85,000 patients each year. Most spinal tumors are extradural and are predominantly metastatic carcinomas, lymphomas, or sarcomas (Posner and Chernik, 1978).

Patients may undergo surgical resection, chemotherapy, and/or radiation to combat their tumors. It is important to note that significant functional deficits can exist even before treatments. The following signs were noted in 162 patients with cerebral metastases: impaired cognition (77%), hemiparesis (66%), unilateral sensory loss (27%), ataxia (24%), and aphasia (19%) (Caraceni and Martini, 1999a). Spinal cord compression can occur in 5% to 10% of cancer cases (Barron et al., 1959). Immediate functional consequences can include pain, sensory deficits, motor deficits, neurogenic bowel and bladder, and sexual dysfunction.

Rehabilitation management of impairments and disabilities is approached in the same manner as in noncancerous neurologic diseases. However, the pathology of the tumor and the anticipated course of disease progression must be considered carefully when developing rehabilitation goals as well as the time frame required to achieve these goals for an individual patient. The purpose of rehabilitation for cancer patients is similar to that for patients with other diseases; emphasis is placed on restoring or maximizing independence with activities of daily living (ADL), mobility, cognition, and communication. Rehabilitation interventions can be applied in all stages of the disease, although rehabilitation goals change as the stage of illness advances. Preventive rehabilitation maintains maximum functional independence in patients who undergo treatment and who have potential loss of function. When tumor progression causes a decline in functional skills, or the disease causes fluctuating abilities, rehabilitation assumes a supportive role, with goals adjusted to accommodate persistent anatomic and physiologic limitations. During terminal stages of illness, palliative rehabilitation can improve and maintain comfort and quality of life until the end of life. An optimal rehabilitation team consists of a physiatrist, primary physician, nurse, physical therapist, occupational therapist, speech-language therapist, recreational therapist, social worker, case manager, dietitian, and chaplain (Garden and Gillis, 1996). Benefits of rehabilitation are noted in Table 22–1.

REHABILITATION OF BRAIN TUMOR PATIENTS

It is important to understand that even a small low-grade malignant tumor may cause significant residual functional deficits if it resides in a critical location. Lesions located near the brain stem can be particularly damaging to motor functions, sensory functions, coordination, and cranial nerves. Primary malignant tumors in adults are mostly gliomas, which account for more than 90% of lesions (Bondy and Wrensch, 1993). Of these, glioblastoma multiforme has the worst prognosis and low-grade astrocytoma, the best (Black, 1991). The location of these tumors may or may not permit resection. Pituitary tumors may result in headaches, bilateral visual loss (due to their central location), and hormonal abnormalities (Black, 1991). With acoustic neuromas, hearing loss and/or vertigo may occur due to their proximity to the cranial nerve. Other symptoms associated with these tumors include facial palsy and numbness, dysphagia, and hydrocephalus. Visual loss and sexual dysfunction can be present with craniopharyngiomas in adults, and growth failure may occur in children with these tumors. Changes in behavior, appetite, memory, and endocrine function may be seen following radiation treatment (Black, 1991).

The lung and breast are the most frequent primary sources of metastatic CNS tumors. Other common primary sources are carcinomas from the colon/rectum, kidney, and pancreas, as well as malignant melanomas. These tumors tend to be highly invasive and destructive. Edema is often present and may extend for some distance beyond the tumor. Leptomeningeal metastases with multiple cranial nerve and spinal root involvement may also occur.

Table 22–1. Benefits of Rehabilitation

Training to maximize functional independence
Facilitation of psychosocial coping and adaptation by patient and family
Improved quality of life through community reintegration: includes resumption of prior home, family, recreational, and vocational activities
Recognition, management, and prevention of co-morbid illnesses that limit or impede function

Table 22–2. Common Complications of Brain Tumors and Their Treatments

Weakness
Sensory loss
Visuospatial deficits
Hemi-neglect or bilateral visual deficits
Ataxia
Cognitive deficits: thought processes, memory changes, apraxia, etc.
Speech difficulties
Dysphagia
Bowel and bladder dysfunction
Psychological issues
Behavioral abnormalities
Endocrine issues
Skin issues
Fatigue

General Considerations

It is essential to consider the fluctuant nature of disease progression for many of these patients and that the overall prognosis may not be very good when these tumors are present. Rehabilitation interventions should be guided by the evidence regarding the nature and behavior (aggressive or indolent) of each patient's tumor, the ongoing clinical course, and the patient's neurologic status. If the prognosis is very limited, or severe cognitive injury impedes patient learning and retention of new information, caregiver education and adaptation of the patient's environment become dominant components of the rehabilitation plan. In cases of expected survival of less than 2 months, primary goals usually shift to injury prevention, safety for patient and caregivers, and ease in performing tasks of hygiene and transfers into and out of bed. Common complications influencing the rehabilitation program for these patients are listed in Table 22–2.

With temporal lobe tumors, dysnomia, disturbance of comprehension, and defective hearing and memory may occur (Nelson et al., 1993). Loss of vision, spatial disorientation, memory loss, dressing apraxia, and proprioceptive agnosia may occur with parietal lobe tumors. Behavioral abnormalities can occur with frontal lobe tumors, and these may include personality or libido changes, with impulsive behavior, labile emotions, and excessive jocularity. Hyponatremia, as seen in the syndrome of inappropriate diuretic hormone (SIADH), may lead to mental status changes (Nelson et al., 1993). Fatigue may become an issue with radiation treatment. Steroid psychosis occasionally complicates the rehabilitation course.

With prolonged immobility in bed, supportive care is important. Measures should be taken to prevent pressure ulcers and deep venous thrombosis. Range of motion of all joints should be maintained with daily exercises or passive stretch if paralysis or altered mental status is present. Sensory stimulation should be provided, along with socialization.

Corticosteroids, which are commonly used to combat peritumoral edema, tend to improve diffuse neurologic dysfunction rather than focal deficits. Myopathy with proximal muscle weakness often ensues and is very difficult to reverse until steroid doses have been tapered or discontinued. Unfortunately, immobility and myopathy frequently create cumulative deficits in strength and endurance. Patients should receive strengthening therapies and exercise programs when steroid therapy is initiated.

Patients may have uninhibited bladder due to lack of cortical influence and may require frequent prompting. Behavioral training may be helpful in patients with unimpaired cognition. This involves progressively increasing the time between voiding, often by 10 to 15 minutes every 2 to 5 days until a reasonable interval between voiding is obtained. Drugs to inhibit bladder evacuations, such as anticholinergic and antispasmodic agents, should be judiciously used. External (condom) catheters may be an option for some male patients. If a diaper is used, it should be changed within 2 to 4 hours to avoid skin breakdown. Immobile or sedentary patients become constipated easily and may require a bowel program with higher fluid intake, stool softeners, and digital stimulation, along with suppositories, laxatives, and enemas.

Orthotic devices that support a limb or joint and assistive devices such as walkers and canes may be issued. Use of a wheelchair may be necessary for those with significant weakness and balance impairment. Occupational and physical therapists should be consulted early for evaluation and teaching of ADL, ambulation, and strengthening and stretching exercises. Speech therapists can assist with the assessment of cognition, linguistic, and communication deficits. They can also determine the presence of swallowing difficulties and recommend therapeutic exercises, compensatory maneuvers, and modified-consistency diets.

Seizures and hydrocephalus are complications of brain tumors that often negatively impact the course of rehabilitation through declining functional performance. Todd's paralysis and subclinical seizures may mimic other etiologies for declining neurologic status and prevent participation in a rehabilitation program. Hydrocephalus may also have a presentation suggestive of other diagnoses, may be acute or chronic in nature, and usually leads to a decline in functional status. It is classically described as a triad of subcortical dementia, incontinence, and gait disorder. Hydrocephalus should be suspected when changes in mentation occur, when a patient fails to make expected functional gains, or when spasticity, seizures, and emotional problems are present. Workup may include computed tomography (CT) scan, lumbar puncture, CT cisternography, and radionuclide cisternography. Neurosurgical consultation for shunt placement should be obtained.

Cranial Nerve Deficits

Cranial nerve function should be routinely assessed in patients with brain tumors, as appropriate intervention may greatly improve functional status. Visual and hearing deficits are frequently seen in meningiomas, acoustic neuromas, and pituitary adenomas. Ophthalmoplegia and facial pain may also present as symptoms of central nervous system (CNS) tumor (Rowland, 1995).

Suprasellar lesions can cause bitemporal hemianopsia, but can also cause diminished visual acuity, scotomata, quadrantic deficits, and blindness of one or both eyes. When treating patients with visual deficits, rehabilitation management should include an ophthalmology consultation to quantify the extent of the visual field loss. Training the patient to utilize compensatory techniques such as scanning will improve visual spatial awareness. Driving recommendations should be given before discharge, with plans for further evaluations as vision improves. Vision impairment typically leads to adverse effects on independent living and must be considered in discharge planning. Patients with double vision can be treated with alternating-eye patching.

Facial pain can be very debilitating and may be treated with tricyclic antidepressant, antiepileptic, or analgesic medications, alone or in combination or in combination with mild narcotic medications. Facial and eyelid paralysis may necessitate plastic surgery interventions for corneal protection or cosmesis. Hearing deficits may have a central or peripheral etiology. Audiology evaluations will differentiate sensorineural from conductive hearing loss. Speech pathology consultation is necessary to establish appropriate routes for communication.

Balance Abnormalities

The neurologic components of human balance are the visual, vestibular, and somatosensory systems. The brain stem and cerebellum process and integrate information about balance from various peripheral receptors, which is then sent onward through corticospinal and brain stem pathways. Balance abnormalities may include dizziness, unsteadiness, vertigo, muscle weakness, and proprioceptive sensory loss. Injuries of the posterior columns of the spinal cord or of the parasagittal or sensory cortex of the brain can lead to these difficulties. Many cancer-related problems and treatments contribute to imbalance, including poor nutrition, anemia, anxiety, postural hypotension, and dehydration. Medications such as antiemetics, tranquilizers, opiates, vestibulotoxic antibiotics (e.g., aminoglycosides), and diuretics may also cause loss of balance. Radiation therapy that includes the temporal bone and/or the posterior fossa can also lead to intermittent vertigo. While brain tumors at many different locations may lead to a sense of vertigo, nystagmus occurs with vestibular or posterior cranial fossa tumors. Patients frequently compensate by tilting their head to decrease the nystagmus. Acoustic neuromas can present as Ménière's disease, where vertigo is associated with hearing loss and tinnitus. Tumors affecting the cerebellum may lead to ataxia and dysdiadochokinesis.

Vestibular disturbance can be treated by habituation, which leads to decreased sensitivity of the vestibular response. The goals of rehabilitation are to resolve reversible deficits and to learn compensatory and adaptive techniques for irreversible deficits, thereby improving safety and increasing independence. Rehabilitation may include training patients to effectively use other sensory input and habituation to control symptoms provoked by activity. Spontaneous resolution can occur and is often related to the severity of the initial insult as well as the possible plasticity of the CNS.

The Balance Master System is a medical device (NeuroCom International, Clackamas, Oregon) used to quantify and treat balance abnormalities. It utilizes a partially enclosed environment with a monitor screen that changes visual orientation input. It has platforms on which a patient stands (both outside and inside the environment) to measure movements and/or provide tilts or weight shifts. Harnesses are available for safety. Parameters measured include *(1)* amount of weight bearing on either foot, *(2)* sway with upper body movement, *(3)* rhythmic weight shift with body movement in all planes, *(4)* limits of stability whereby patients are provided a mechanical force toward which they try to shift their weight to compensate to maintain balance, and *(5)* weight shifts during movements such as transfers from sitting to standing and walking. Visual feedback is then given regarding the patient's position while the therapist can give verbal cues. The results are stored for quantitative and graphic analysis. Vestibular and visual components can be isolated by the device's environment. A custom exercise program can then be developed based on the determined deficits. Proprioceptive responses may be improved via controlled mobility, improved anterior-posterior weight shifts, increasing trunk strength and range of motion, as well as increasing midline symmetry and transitional movements.

Pharmacologic treatments include meclizine and dimenhydrinate, which may cause sedation. Transdermal scopolamine patches can also be used and are believed to cause less sedation.

Cognition/Speech Deficits

Deficits in cognition and speech occur; they vary in type and severity by the location and type of tumor, anticancer treatment, pre-morbid cognitive baseline, and co-morbid medical conditions. Cognitive deficits arise from tissue injury caused by the tumor itself, surgical resection, and the acute effects of radiation and chemotherapy (Silberfarb, 1983). The neuropsychiatric side effects of both steroid and anticonvulsant therapy should also be considered in cognitive assessment (Lewis and Smith, 1983). Emotional sequelae such as depression and anxiety are common, may worsen cognitive functions, or are overlooked in the presence of cognitive deficits. Coexisting medical conditions such as hypothyroidism are treatable and should be considered in the differential diagnosis of cognitive impairment.

Cognitive deficits are most often seen in areas involving memory, attention, initiation, and psychomotor retardation. Primary interventions for memory impairment include memory aids and the use of visual imagery. Cognitive remediation programs teach patients adaptive strategies and compensatory techniques. Psychostimulants have been reported to be useful in treating psychomotor retardation, depression, and opioid-induced drowsiness (Bruera et al., 1989; Weitzner et al., 1996). Dopamine agonists and stimulating antidepressants improve attentional dysfunction, particularly distractibility and difficulty focusing, in higher level patients (Gualtieri et al., 1989). Bromocriptine can be effective for motor aphasias and neglect in some patients (Grujic et al., 1998). Carbamazepine, tricyclic antidepressants, trazodone, amantadine, and β-blockers have been prescribed to manage agitation in patients with traumatic brain injury (Brooke et al., 1992; Mysiw et al., 1988; Whyte, 1988).

Aphasia is a language disorder, whereas dysarthria is an articulation disorder. In contrast to aphasia, naming, fluency, repetition, and comprehension are normal in dysarthric conditions, and dysarthric patients can read and write without errors. The severity of aphasia correlates significantly with communication difficulty. Other disorders such as apraxia, visual constructive difficulties, and neglect need to be considered in the differential diagnosis of communication dysfunction.

REHABILITATION OF PATIENTS WITH SPINAL CORD TUMORS AND TREATMENT-INDUCED INJURY

Myelopathy with Tumors

Myelopathy may occur due to tumor involvement, irradiation, and intrathecal chemotherapy. Metastatic tumors may involve the spine or spinal cord. Back pain is a frequent symptom and in 10% of cases may be due to spinal instability (Gilbert et al., 1977; Portenoy et al., 1987; Rodichok et al., 1981). Any tumor can metastasize to the spine and cause sufficient destruction to produce spinal instability. The thoracic spine is the segment most commonly involved, followed by lumbosacral and then cervical vertebral levels (Casciato and Lowitz, 1983; Schlicht and Smelz, 1994).

Spinal cord compression eventually occurs in approximately 5% of patients with cancer (Casciato and Lowitz, 1983). Abrupt neurologic deterioration from spinal cord involvement may occur from rapidly growing lesions in the extradural space. Infarction of the vertebral blood supply can cause cord injury. Radiculopathy at any level is also possible (Gilbert et al., 1977; Rodichok et al., 1981). By the time treatment is pursued, as many as 50% of patients may not be able to ambulate, and 10% to 30% may be paraplegic (Shapiro and Posner, 1983; Shaw et al., 1980).

Symptoms include weakness, incoordination, gait abnormality, spinal or radicular pain, paresthesias, sensory disturbances, autonomic disturbances, as well as bowel or bladder problems. Pinprick and deep pain sensation is often retained until later in the course of the disease. Motor involvement typically occurs before sensory involvement with epidural extension (Galasko, 1999). With radiation treatment alone, ambulation is maintained in 79% of patients if they were ambulatory before treatment and in 42% with paraparesis. In 20% to 25% of patients, significant neurologic deterioration was noted during the course of treatment with radiation alone (Findlay, 1984).

Significant neurologic deterioration and progressive spinal instability require a neurosurgical consultation. High-dose steroids are used in the acute phase to control neurologic damage. Tetraplegia, whether complete or incomplete, occurs with spinal cord involvement at T1 or above. Below this level, injuries more commonly result in paraplegia, conus medullaris syndrome, or cauda equina syndrome. Local pain is typically described as constant and aching, whereas radicular pain is classically sharp and shooting. Referred pain can be either aching or sharp and at a location distant to the involved site. Pain can also occur with epidural involvement; this pain worsens with Valsalva maneuvers, coughing, and neck and back flexion (Gilbert et al., 1978; Gerber and Vargo, 1998). Functional prognostic factors are listed in (Tables 22–3 and 22–4).

Table 22–3. Findings Associated with Better Prognosis for Functional Recovery Following Cord Compression

- Diagnosis of myeloma, lymphoma, or breast cancer
- Slow evolution of symptoms or early neurologic signs
- Ambulatory status at time of diagnosis of spinal cord involvement

With use of radiation treatment and posterior laminectomy, the overall results were that complete paraplegia patients rarely recovered, but those who were ambulatory remained ambulatory and approximately one-half of patients with incomplete paraplegia regained ambulation (Posner, 1995). Recovery tends to occur first in the area of sensory disturbance, followed by motor abnormalities (Casciato and Lowitz, 1983; Schlicht and Smelz, 1994).

Radiation-Related Myelopathies

The detrimental effects of radiation are multifactorial and cannot be entirely attributed to dosage, site, or technique. Such myelopathy may be transient or delayed (Dropcho, 1991). With transient myelopathy, peak onset is at 4 to 6 months (Dropcho, 1991). Clinical onset may involve symmetric paresthesia or shock-like sensations in a nondermatomal pattern from spine to extremities (Leibel et al., 1991). Radiologic studies are usually normal. Symptoms typically resolve in 1 to 9 months (Dropcho, 1991). Conversely, delayed myelopathy is irreversible, has a latency period of 9 to 18 months, and generally occurs within 30 months (Dropcho, 1991). The incidence is reported at 1% to 12%. The latency period is decreased with increased radiation dose and in children (Leibel et al., 1991). The onset of symptoms begins with lower extremity paresthesias and is followed by sphincter disturbance. Partial Brown-Séquard syndrome (motor weakness on one side and some sensory changes on the contralateral side) may occur below the level of injury. Central pain syndrome may also occur, which is typically characterized by midback pain and dysesthetic pain in the lower extremities. Such pain is usually treated with steroids, anticonvulsants, and tricyclic antidepressants. Rehabilitation concerns are listed in Table 22–5.

Table 22–4. Findings Associated with a Poorer Prognosis for Functional Recovery Following Cord Compression

Sphincter incontinence
Complete paraplegia
Rapid evolution of symptoms (<72 hours)

Rehabilitation Considerations

In cases of myelopathy or significant radiculopathy, physical and occupational therapists should be consulted early to address ADLs and ambulation and to provide adaptive equipment and strengthening exercises. When spinal metastasis has occurred, other bony areas may also be affected, particularly the pelvis, femur, ribs, and skull. When there is skull involvement, compromise of adjacent neurologic structures can occur. Use of orthoses to limit spinal mobility, such as sternal-occipital-mandibular immobilization (SOMI), may be required for spinal stability for patients with tumors affecting the spine. Rigid thoracic-lumbar-sacral orthoses with a "clamshell" design can provide good external support but may not be tolerated by patients with painful rib or iliac crest bony involvement or by those with fragile skin due to steroids or chemotherapy (Garden and Gillis, 1996). The rehabilitation team must consider metastatic disease as a possible etiology for new pain or weaknesses that arise during the course of therapy. Adequate pain control is essential and enables patients to participate in therapy.

Table 22–5. Rehabilitation Issues in Cancer and Treatment-Related Myelopathy

Pain
Motor loss and difficulty with ambulation and transfers
Sensory loss
Autonomic dysreflexia (T6* or above)
Orthostatic hypotension
Neurogenic bowel and bladder
Spasticity
Pressure ulcers at sacrum, heel and trochanters
Spinal instability (with spinal column destruction)
Altered weight-bearing, limited lower extremity range of motion

*T6, The sixth thoracic spinal cord level.

Pain Management

Pain (see later in this chapter and Chapter 23) may be both acute and chronic. Pharmacologic options include opiates, nonsteroidal anti-inflammatory agents, tricyclic antidepressants, various antiepileptics, steroids, and other medications such as β-blockers and α-adrenergic agonists. Use of modalities such as heat, cold, and transcutaneous electrical nerve stimulation (TENS) should be considered. Nontraditional interventions such as acupuncture have also been used with success. In patients with spinal hardware, worsening pain could indicate malfunction or loosening of hardware or infection in the surrounding tissues.

Bladder Management

Patients with myelopathy can develop detrusor-sphincter-dyssynergia (DSD), a condition in which the bladder contracts but the bladder outlet (sphincters) fails to relax in a timely manner, leading to impaired emptying and increased bladder pressure. Patients may attempt to void on their own; however, postvoid residual volumes must be checked on multiple occasions to confirm complete emptying. If incomplete emptying occurs (i.e., residual volume >100 to 150 cc), intermittent catheterization should be performed every 4 hours. The goal is to have no more than 350 to 400 cc of urine in the bladder at any time to avoid overdistension, detrusor muscle injury, and retropropulsion of urine into the ureters. With chronically increased bladder volumes, bladder flaccidity may occur secondary to detrusor muscle injury.

The amount of urine produced is affected by the volume of fluid intake, medications, and hormonal abnormalities, such as SIADH, which may be seen particularly with lung malignancies and pituitary adenomas. Certain types of foods and drinks may also act as diuretics. Fluid intake should initially be restricted to 2 L per day if other medical concerns permit. The frequency of bladder catheterization may at first be kept at every 4 to 6 hours and can be adjusted so that bladder volumes do not exceed 400 cc. Patients should not restrict fluid intake simply to avoid catheterization. The intermittent catheterization program (ICP) should be taught to patients and caretakers. Patients with a cord injury at C7 or below can usually learn to independently perform such a program. Condom catheters may be used by men with hyperactive bladder (without dyssynergia) or those with normal bladder function but with incontinence due to impaired cognition or mobility. Indwelling catheters may be needed in women who cannot perform ICP and in men who cannot wear condom catheters or who have contraindications to ICP.

Bowel Management

A bowel program (more details follow in a later section) with fiber, stool softeners, and digital stimulation, along with judicious use of suppositories, laxatives, and enemas should be started. Warm fluids may be given after meals to supplement the gastrocolic reflex. Patients should be allowed to sit on a commode at regular times to facilitate bowel movements. Establishment of a set pattern (daily or every other day) for evacuation will minimize constipation and incontinence.

Management of Autonomic Dysreflexia

Autonomic dysreflexia is a medical emergency that occurs when a patient manifests a massive sympathetic discharge in response to a noxious stimulus. The clinical presentation is that of an anxious patient with paroxysmal hypertension, nasal congestion, sweating above the level of lesion, facial flushing, piloerection, and reflex bradycardia. Autonomic dysreflexia typically occurs with a spinal cord injury at the level of T6 or above. Most commonly, the noxious stimulus is a distended bladder or bowel. Other causes include enemas, tight clothing, infection, deep venous thrombosis, ingrown toenails, bladder catheterization, and pressure ulcers. Treatment focuses on eliminating the underlying noxious stimulus, such as emptying of the distended bladder or bowel. Such measures usually resolve the episode quickly; however, if a cause cannot be found promptly, treatment with antihypertensives must be initiated to prevent complications of rising blood pressure.

REHABILITATION OF PATIENTS WITH PLEXOPATHIES

A plexopathy may result from direct invasion by neoplasm or from radiation injury (see Chapter 18).

Table 22–6. Characteristic Differences Between Neoplastic and Post-radiation Brachial Plexopathies

Parameter	*Neoplastic*	*Post-radiation*
Incidence	10 times more common	Dose related
Initial symptom	Progressive pain 90% (preceding other symptoms by weeks/months)	Numbness, paresthesias, pain in <20%
		Pain stabilizes with onset of weakness
Signs	Lower trunk, Horner's syndrome	Upper trunk
Progression rate	Slow	Insidious, self-limiting
EMG	Denervation, no myokymia	Myokymia

Chemotherapy can enhance the radiation-induced injury in irradiated tissue and decrease the latency period for development of plexopathy. Predominant symptoms are pain and paresthesias. Clinical signs include sensory loss, decreased or absent reflexes, and weakness.

Brachial Plexopathy

Plexus lesions can result from compression or infiltration by tumor lying in contiguous tissues or may be seen after RT for breast and lung cancers. Characteristic differences between neoplastic and post-radiation plexopathies are listed in Table 22–6.

Pain typically occurs in the shoulder, elbows, hand, and fourth/fifth digits, whereas sensory disturbance occurs in the axilla with C8, T1, and T2 involvement. Breast cancer in particular may affect the upper brachial plexus, where pain referral is to the paraspinal region, shoulders, biceps, elbow, and hand. Burning dysesthesias in the index finger or thumb are common. A hallmark of this syndrome is the neuropathic character of the pain, with numbness, paresthesias, allodynia, and hyperesthesia complaints. All patients with brachial plexopathy should have a scan of the contiguous paravertebral region before RT because extension of disease is common in this area. Epidural invasion can occur in some patients with brachial plexopathy. Imaging of the epidural space is essential when a patient develops Horner's syndrome, panplexopathy, or vertebral body erosion or if a paraspinal mass is detected on CT scan. With radiation dosages exceeding 60 Gy, or large fractions of >190 cGy/day, fibrosis of the plexus can occur.

Lumbosacral Plexopathy

Pelvic malignancies, including bladder, uterus, prostate, and/or lung cancer or melanoma can lead to lumbosacral plexopathy. Retroperitoneal tumors, including sarcomas and metastatic nodal tumors, may affect the lumbosacral plexus or its roots more proximally (Table 22–7). The presenting symptom is usually pain in the buttocks or legs, and it often precedes other symptoms by weeks or months. Other symptoms include numbness, weakness, and later edema. Pain is usually of an aching or pressure-like quality, rarely burning (Caraceni and Martini, 1999b).

Table 22–7. Characteristic Differences Between Neoplastic and Post-radiation Lumbosacral Plexopathies

Parameter	*Neoplastic*	*Post-radiation*
Initial symptoms	Pain in 93%, paresthesia	Weakness in 50%
Signs	Bilateral in 10%–25%	Bilateral in 80%
Latency	Variable	Median 5 yr (1– 31 yr)
Tumor progression	Focal CT/MRI changes	No focal abnormality
EMG	Denervation	Myokymia

Lesions most commonly occur in the lower plexus (L4–S1) with an incidence of 50%, followed by upper lumbar plexus (L1–L4) at 33%. Panplexopathy involving two sites is less common at 20% (Jaeckle et al., 1985).

Pain management may require tricyclic antidepressants, antiepileptic agents such as gabapentin and carbamazepine, along with epidural catheters and neurosurgical approaches in more resistant cases. Neuropathic pain may also respond to radiation treatment. After acute inflammation and pain subside, low-resistance weight exercises and functional activities should be encouraged. Neck exercises and range of motion programs should be included in the treatment of brachial plexopathy, especially with injury to the upper portion of the plexus, to avoid functionally devastating contractures in that area. A sling should be given to prevent glenohumeral subluxation. With lower extremity involvement, assistive devices for ambulation, such as a cane, may be required by those patients with weakness and proprioceptive feedback loss. Orthoses and splints may be required for joint or limb support or to enable function and prevent injury.

REHABILITATION OF PATIENTS WITH NEUROPATHIES

Peripheral polyneuropathy may occur as a result of direct tumor invasion, as part of a paraneoplastic syndrome, or with chemotherapy (see Chapter 17). Paraneoplastic neuropathy may be related to an autoimmune process and may be sensorimotor in nature (see Chapter 19). Chemotherapy-associated peripheral neuropathies are generally distal and symmetric. Most frequently these neuropathies occur with Vinca alkaloid, taxane, or platinum-based therapies (Amato and Collins, 1998). Symptoms include numbness, paresthesias, and occasionally severe neuropathic pain.

Tricyclic antidepressants and antiepileptics should be given to manage pain. Adaptive strategies such as energy conservation, orthotics, and assistive and adaptive devices are prescribed. With sensory loss in the lower extremity, preventive measures such as those used for management of diabetic neuropathy and neuropathic ulcers should be instituted. Education, nonconstricting footwear, and daily inspection of feet are important in such cases. Patients with acute inflammatory demyelinating polyneuropathy benefit from a resistive exercise program.

REHABILITATION OF PATIENTS WITH LEPTOMENINGEAL DISEASE

Leptomeningeal disease is also known as carcinomatous meningitis or meningeal carcinomatosis (see Chapter 16). It is caused by dissemination of cancerous cells throughout the subarachnoid space. Life expectancy is usually very short, often only 3 to 6 months with treatment (Sause et al., 1988; Siegal et al., 1994). Both central and peripheral nervous system involvement can occur, along with cerebrospinal fluid flow obstruction leading to hydrocephalus. Symptoms can include mental status changes, polyradiculopathy with radicular pain, and cauda equina syndrome. Rehabilitation management is similar to that outlined earlier, based on the sites involved and the deficits encountered. The rehabilitation goals should include supportive and safety concerns and reflect the generally poor prognosis.

REHABILITATION OF PATIENTS WITH MUSCULOSKELETAL PROBLEMS

Primary and metastatic nervous system cancers and their treatments can cause multiple musculoskeletal problems. These problems can significantly compromise normal function. They require an accurate diagnosis, assessment of functional impairments, and implementation of appropriate rehabilitation interventions.

Corticosteroid-Induced Myopathy

Myopathies are a group of muscle diseases whose common principal symptom is weakness, usually in the proximal muscles of the shoulder and hip joints. Steroid myopathies most commonly occur in patients who undergo high-dose, long-term corticosteroid therapy. These patients generally show recovery after decreasing or discontinuing medication. Myopathy patients usually present with difficulty climbing stairs, rising from chairs, and performing transfers. Inpatient rehabilitation is sometimes necessary to regain strength, learn to perform ADLs safely, and use ambulatory aids. In the most severe cases, patients may require a wheelchair for all mobility and ADLs, but can achieve independence in those functions despite the use of a wheelchair. In such cases, adaptive equipment (e.g., transfer board, raised toilet seat, bathtub bench) is necessary for them to perform ADLs safely. As patient strength improves, gait training under the supervision of a physiatrist and physical therapist can continue on an outpatient basis.

Avascular Necrosis and Osteoporosis

Avascular necrosis and osteoporosis frequently occur in cancer patients. These problems are diagnosed radiographically and may be asymptomatic until the involved bone is subject to fracture or infection. Most avascular necrosis is attributable to the direct effects of RT or to the systemic effects of corticosteroids, although these effects appear to be dose dependent (Zizic, 1991). In addition to RT and steroids, avascular necrosis in cancer patients has been anecdotally associated with single-agent cyclophosphamide or methotrexate, as well as cyclophosphamide in combination with methotrexate and 5-fluorouracil (Pizzo and Poplack, 1997).

Like avascular necrosis, osteoporosis has been related to steroids and to RT (Duthie and Katz, 1998; Tefft et al., 1976). Glucocorticosteroids inhibit new bone formation and calcium absorption and increase bone resorption and renal calcium excretion. Steroid-induced hypogonadism contributes to the problem in both men and women. More than 50% of patients taking long-term steroids develop some degree of osteoporosis (Goroll et al., 1995). The risk of developing steroid-induced osteoporosis can be reduced by using a short-acting preparation at the lowest possible dose in an alternate-day regimen, by maintaining physical activity, and by ensuring adequate daily intake of calcium and vitamin D. Treatments for osteoporosis include

1. Therapies used to slow down bone involution and prevent contracture formation and postural deviations: weight-bearing exercises, upper and lower extremity muscle strengthening, balance training, back extension and chest expansion exercises, pectoralis muscle stretching, posture correction, and proper lifting techniques
2. Cessation or tapering of glucocorticoid intake
3. Hormone replacement therapy for men and women who do not have contraindications
4. Thiazide therapy for hypercalcemia
5. Vitamin D and calcium supplementation when appropriate
6. Bisphosphonate therapy
7. Environmental modification: proper footwear, adjustment of medications that may contribute to falling; assistive devices
8. Education of patients regarding risk factors such as smoking

Compression fractures may ensue with only minor trauma once sufficient structural integrity is lost. Pain may be managed with analgesic and anti-inflammatory medications and the use of spinal orthoses. Surgical fixation is sometimes necessary to attain stability. Early weight-bearing and limited immobilization should be encouraged to minimize continued bone loss.

Contracture of Joints

A limitation of passive joint range of motion, contracture commonly results from a restriction in connective tissue, tendons, ligaments, muscles, and joint elements. Contractures are most often related to spasticity, bed rest, localized heterotopic ossification, bleeding, infection, trauma, and edema. Prevention is achieved by minimizing the duration of bed rest and encouraging daily range of motion exercises.

Heterotopic Ossification

Heterotopic ossification is the formation of mature, lamellar bone in soft tissues. The variable incidence of heterotopic ossification has been reported in spinal cord injury patients (20% to 25%) and in head injury patients (10% to 20%) (An et al., 1987; Brooker et al., 1973; Evans, 1991; Garland, 1988; Ishikawa et al., 1982; Jensen et al., 1988; Stoikovic et al., 1955; Storey and Tegner, 1955; Stover et al., 1975). This condition has been observed in patients who require a prolonged ICU stay and is rarely seen in the cancer population. The chief symptoms of heterotopic ossification are joint and muscle pain and compromised range of motion. A triple-phase bone scan is able to detect heterotopic ossification at an early stage. Therapies include bisphosphonates, nonsteroidal anti-inflammatory drugs, RT, and physical therapy. Passive joint mobilization helps to maintain or increase joint mobility without promoting heterotopic ossication. Matured heterotopic ossification can be surgically excised.

Shoulder Pain

This problem often occurs in neurologically impaired populations. Shoulder pain may originate from rotator cuff tears, bicipital tendinitis, adhesive capsulitis, and subdeltoid bursitis. Other causes of shoulder pain in the hemiplegic population include excessive shoulder capsule stretch secondary to paresis of shoulder musculature, sympathetically maintained pain (reflex-sympathetic-dystrophy, shoulder-hand syndrome), and thalamic syndrome. Management is diagnosis dependent.

GENERAL REHABILITATION PATIENT CARE CONCERNS

Physiologic Deconditioning

Immobilization syndrome may occur during recovery from operative or other treatments, be caused by medical complications, or result from the neurologic sequelae of cancer. It negatively impacts multiple body systems and often causes a decline in the patient's functional status. Immobilization can contribute to intellectual, emotional, and behavioral disturbances, decreased muscle strength and endurance, poor coordination, and contracture of joints. Cardiovascular and pulmonary deconditioning may present with orthostatic hypotension, deep vein thrombosis, decreased vital capacity, and impairment of the cough mechanism. Anorexia, constipation, electrolyte disturbances, and pressure ulcers are also manifestations of immobilization (Hoffman et al., 1998). The best management of this syndrome is through prevention. Physical therapy should begin early, emphasizing progressive mobilization, starting with passive range of motion if necessary; progressing to assisted active range of motion; then to active range of motion. When postural hypotension is pronounced or when patients have been or are expected to be bed bound for more than one week, tilt-table use should begin as soon as the patient is stable. This device is beneficial for cardiovascular and respiratory reconditioning and can also help prevent osteoporosis. Once the patient tolerates a 70-degree angle for 30 minutes, standing and ambulation should begin. Signs and symptoms of hypercalcemia, pressure ulcer, urinary tract infection, and pneumonia should be watched for vigilantly.

Venous Thromboembolism

Deep venous thrombosis (DVT) has a high incidence in stroke patients (30% to 50%) (Gibberd et al., 1976), in spinal cord injury patients (Merli et al., 1993; Weinmann and Salzman, 1994), after hip arthroplasty (Imperiale and Speroff, 1994), in patients with cancer (Marik et al., 1997), and in immobilized patients (Giuntini et al., 1995). Elastic hosiery and sequential compression pumping of the calves should be continued until mobilization is underway. In spinal cord-injured and hemiplegic patients, administration of subcutaneous low-molecular-weight heparin is recommended. Exceptions are made for patients following intracranial surgery to avoid devastating hemorrhage. Patients with thrombocytopenia, especially those with hematologic malignancies and hemorrhagic tumors, require individualized assessment, and their anticoagulation risks should be addressed with the primary oncology team. A consensus on the optimal duration of prophylactic anticoagulation has not yet been reached.

A high index of suspicion for thrombosis should be maintained for patients with recent surgery or anesthesia, smoking history, current or recent prolonged bed rest, prior history of DVT, cardiac disease, obesity, extremity trauma, neoplasm, and in the elderly. If DVT is suspected, Doppler ultrasound and venography can be used to confirm the diagnosis. Once the clinical diagnosis of DVT is seriously considered or confirmed, intravenous heparin can be started, followed by oral anticoagulation therapy for a 3 month period. When a pulmonary embolism has occurred, 6 months of treatment is usually suggested (Bone et al., 1998).

Spasticity

Spasticity is a motor disorder characterized by a velocity-dependent resistance to movement associated with exaggerated phasic stretch reflexes (tendon jerks), representing one component of the upper motor neuron syndrome. Tone is the sensation of resistance felt by the examiner as passive range of motion is tested. Spasticity can be caused by a wide variety of disorders that damage descending motor tracts at the cortical, subcortical, brain stem, or spinal cord

Table 22–8. Clinical Scale for Spastic Hypertonia (Modified Ashworth Scale)

Scale	*Physical Findings*
0	No increase in tone
1	Slight increase in muscle tone manifested by a catch and release or by a minimal resistance at the end of the ROM when the affected part(s) are moved in flexion or extension
1+	Slight increase in muscle tone, manifested by a catch, followed by minimal resistance throughout the remainder (less than one-half) of the ROM
2	More marked increase in muscle tone through most of the ROM, but affected part(s) easily moved
3	Considerable increase in muscle tone and passive movement difficult
4	Affected part(s) rigid in flexion or extension

ROM, Range of motion of a joint.

levels. Examples include primary CNS tumors, metastatic CNS tumors, and radiation injury of the CNS.

Spasticity can be quantified by using the Modified Ashworth Scale (Table 22–8). Only those patients whose spasticity interferes with present function or potential future function, or whose condition is painful, should be treated. Spasticity treatment should begin with the least invasive techniques and advance as needed. Basic treatment includes a daily stretching program, use of proper positioning, and avoidance of noxious stimuli. Topical cold may provide short-term benefit. Casting and splinting techniques can improve the range of motion in hypertonic joint contractures. Oral medications (Table 22–9) to treat spasticity should be combined with basic treatment and are only effective in mild to moderate cases. Chemical neurolysis, such as phenol block, injections, epidural infusion of medications, botulinum toxin via an implantable pump, and surgery are options for severe spasicity management.

Skin and Wound Care

After Radiation Therapy

Radiation may impair wound healing and cause skin tightening. Persistent wound drainage with impaired wound healing, cutaneous fistulas, electrolyte imbalances, decreased protein reserves, and infections may also develop. Prior radiation and ongoing chemotherapy can disrupt normal wound healing, thus increasing the likelihood of postoperative wound infection and dehiscence (Alekhteyar et al., 1996; Springfield, 1993). Changes in skin integrity with radiation encompass local skin reactions, which may include epilation (loss of hair), erythema, and dry and wet desquamation. With a short course of cranial irradiation, mild scalp erythema may occur, especially around the external pinna. Complete alopecia is a more common problem with longer courses of cranial treatment; hair regrowth may take as long as 2 to 3 months. With larger dosages of radiation

Table 22–9. Oral Spasmolytic Medications

Agent	*Daily Dosage*	*Half-Life (Hours)*	*Mechanism of Action*
Baclofen	10 to >80 mg	3.5	Presynaptic inhibitor by activation of GABA B receptor
Diazepam	4 to >60 mg	27–37	Facilitates postsynaptic effects of GABA, resulting in increased presynaptic inhibition
Dantrolene	25 to >400 mg	8.7	Reduces calcium release, interfering with excitation-contraction coupling in skeletal muscles
Clonidine	0.1–0.4 mg (oral); 0.1–0.3 mg (patch)	12–16 (oral)	α_2-adrenergic agonist
Tizandine	4–36 mg	4	α_2-adrenergic agonist

GABA, Gamma-aminobutyric acid.

(>40 Gy) to the scalp, hair loss is usually permanent. Combination of irradiation with cytotoxic agents such as doxorubicin or actinomycin D may significantly increase skin toxicity (D'Angio et al., 1976).

For radiation-induced changes, skin should be kept dry and clean without use of lotions. Exposure to sunlight and temperature extremes must be avoided. Alterations in sweat glands may lead to drying, so petrolatum may be useful. Cornstarch may alleviate pruritus.

Pressure Ulcers

Pressure and shear forces are the two most important factors in ulcer formation. Risks are persistent pressure to the skin located above a bony prominence, shear forces, friction, and sensory deficits. Poor nutritional status and contact with moisture (such as urine, feces, or wound drainage) compound the problem. In bed-bound patients, the most common site for pressure ulcer formation is the sacrum, followed by the heels, ischium, scapula, and occiput. Prolonged pressure across a bony prominence initially causes damage to the overlying muscle. Prevention entails frequent turning (every 2 hours), daily skin checks, avoidance of friction and excessive moisture or dryness, and the use of specialized mattresses in high-risk situations. Understanding universal criteria like those listed in Table 22–10 can assist in treatment.

When ulcers develop, treatment requires complete pressure relief for healing to occur. Patients who cannot maintain positions of pressure relief and develop stage II ulcers should use low air-loss mattresses, whereas with stage III and IV ulcers, air-fluidized beds may be beneficial. Higher stage ulcers require plastic surgery consultation. Orthotic devices that elevate and disperse pressure over the heels will usually prevent pressure ulceration. Conditions that potentially aggravate wounds such as diabetes, hypoproteinemia, and infection, should be treated. Supplementation with zinc and vitamin C may be helpful.

Table 22–10. National Pressure Ulcer Advisory Panel Stages

Stage	*Characteristic*
I	Nonblanchable erythema
II	Partial skin loss (epidermis to dermis)
III	Full thickness
IV	Damage through level of deep fascia, muscle or bone

Bowel and Bladder Management

Constipation may result from prolonged immobilization or develop secondary to changes in metabolic demand, endocrine function, or decreased gastric and intestinal motility. Constipation in cancer patients is frequently related to narcotic medication. Some patients may present with diarrhea due to impaction rather than lack of bowel movements.

For patients with neurogenic bowel, establishing a consistent bowel program early in the course of treatment is extremely important. The management of a typical reflexic neurogenic bowel consists of a diet high in fiber to improve transit time, stool softeners, digital stimulation with or without suppositories, judicious use of laxatives, enemas in case of impaction and at the inception of the program, and performance of the bowel program 30 to 60 minutes after a meal to utilize the gastrocolic reflex to assist with peristalsis. This management can also be applied to the patient with constipation caused by prolonged bed rest and narcotic medication, omitting the digital stimulation component. Patients with thrombocytopenia (<10,000) or severe neutropenia should not be given suppositories or utilize digital stimulation.

Patients with lower motor neuron injuries, such as conus or cauda equina injuries or pudendal nerve injuries, have an areflexic bowel and a hypotonic external sphincter and are often more difficult to successfully manage. Excessive stool softeners may increase bowel accidents, and digital stimulation and cathartic suppositories are of limited use. Manual removal, straining, and enemas are often the only means of emptying the lower colon in this patient group.

Assuming an upright posture as frequently as possible, increasing ambulation, and maintaining an adequate fluid intake will help minimize difficulties initiating a urinary stream. An intermittent catheterization program (ICP) can be used in cases of urinary retention. Timed voiding is the management of choice for patients with an intracranial lesion and hyperreflexic bladder. Patients with spinal cord lesions may present with either a failure to store urine or a failure to empty the bladder.

The goals for neurogenic bladder management are to promote preservation of the upper urinary tract, maintain low storage and evacuation pressures in the bladder, and ensure patient compliance by choosing a technique appropriate for his or her lifestyle. A basic evaluation should include a clear history for difficulty or inability to void and a neurologic examination. The examination should include perianal sensation (touch and pinprick), anal tone and voluntary contraction of the anal sphincter, and bulbocavernosus reflex. Evaluating the prostate size during rectal examination is important for assessing obstruction.

Urodynamic studies should be performed for patients with spinal cord lesions whose survival is expected to exceed 1 year. Postvoid residual (PVR) measurements should be routinely done for all patients with known or suspected spinal cord injuries. A PVR >100 ml or more than 20% of the total voided urine is considered abnormal, and catheterization with a straight catheter (14 French) should be continued every 4 hours with a bladder volume goal of no more than 500 cc. These patients should later be objectively evaluated by urodynamic study and treated accordingly.

Failure of the bladder to store urine is treated with anticholinergic medications, such as oxybutynin chloride (5 mg orally two to three times/day), or propantheline bromide (5 to 30 mg orally three to four times/day), or dicyclomine hydrochloride (10 to 20 mg orally four times/day). Failure of the bladder to empty secondary to a hyperreflexic sphincter in male patients can be treated with a combination of external sphincterotomy and use of an external collecting device.

Nutrition

Proper nutrition is an important aspect of rehabilitation. Cancer and its associated treatments can adversely affect nutritional status. Weight loss may be due to an increase in energy requirements and/or decrease in oral intake, directly or indirectly related to the cancer. Some of the direct nutritional effects include the physical location of a tumor leading to obstruction of the alimentary canal and the type of surgical treatment rendered. Indirect effects occur with decreases in appetite related to the release of cytokines and with the nausea and vomiting associated with chemotherapy.

Rapidly reproducing cells of the gastrointestinal tract are vulnerable to the effects of chemotherapy. Acutely, nausea, vomiting, and anorexia are the most common gastrointestinal side effects. Delayed side effects may include stomatitis, mucosal ulceration, pharyngitis, gastroenteritis, glossitis, and malabsorption. Nutritional deficiencies may also occur with chemotherapy.

Surgical cancer interventions may interfere with the ability to eat. Radiation treatment of the head and neck region may lead to alterations in taste and saliva production. Changes to the oral mucosa cause distortion of temperature and texture sensations. Other post-radiation changes adversely affecting nutrition include nausea, vomiting, anorexia, and esophagitis.

Medical treatment should be given as necessary to prevent or reduce nausea, vomiting, hyposalivation, and decreased appetite. Antiemetics include phenothiazines such as prochlorperazine, promethazine, and chlorpromazine. Selective 5-HT3 receptor antagonists for treatment of nausea and vomiting include ondansetron, dolasetron, and granisetron. Cannabinoid medications (dronabinol) and trimethobenzamide may also be used. To prevent dry mouth and hyposalivation, anticholinergic medications should be avoided and lubricating mouth products should be used as necessary. Agents for appetite stimulation are dronabinol, megestrol, and cyproheptadine.

Patients often reject specific foods or certain flavors during the course of cancer treatment. Such behavior may be associated with side effects following consumption of certain foods, such as meats, vegetables, and caffeinated beverages (Mattes et al., 1987). To avoid this aversion to familiar food items, consumption should occur 24 hours before nausea-producing therapy (Gerber and Vargo, 1998). Intake of other high protein sources should be encouraged, such as dairy products, eggs, and liquid nutritional supplements. Cold foods and foods with little odor and less seasoning may be better tolerated.

In order to speed recovery after anticancer treatments and for general improvement in functional status, optimal nutritional status should be maintained. Caloric intake should range from 115% to 130% of the patient's resting metabolic rate. Protein requirements range from 1.5 to 2.5 g/kg per day (Burgess, 1989; Maillet, 1987). Vitamin and mineral supplementation should be given as needed. Fluid and electrolyte balance should be verified in the presence of malabsorption, diarrhea, and large wounds with associated fluid losses. Enteral or parenteral feeding supplementation should be considered without delay in nutritionally compromised patients who are not eating well. Nutritional status may be followed with albumin, pre-albumin, serial weights, lymphocyte count, and calorie count.

Pain

Distinguishing whether pain (see Chapter 23) is acute or chronic in nature can assist in selecting appropriate management. Pain tends to be less prominent in patients with brain tumors, but may be significant with spinal column and cord involvement. In patients with spinal stabilization using hardware, increasing pain should prompt an evaluation of the construct's integrity. Headaches occur in 48% to 71% of patients with brain tumors. These are usually mild to moderate and can resemble tension headaches but may increase with changes in position (Forsyth and Posner, 1993; Suwanwela et al., 1994; Caraceni and Martini, 1999b). Increasing severity or accompanying nausea and vomiting may signify increasing intracranial pressure, which often responds to steroids (Caraceni and Martini, 1999b).

Medical management typically includes nonsteroidal anti-inflammatory agents (NSAIDS) and non-narcotic and narcotic analgesics. Neuropathic pain, which may be seen with spinal cord involvement, can be managed with tricyclic antidepressants, anticonvulsants, steroids, and occasionally opiates. Tricyclic agents may potentiate opiate analgesia. Antihistamine agents such as hydroxyzine may help with analgesia and provide antiemetic effects, but these usually occur only with relatively high parenteral dosages (Beaver and Feise, 1976). Benzodiazepines may be helpful in managing anxiety or muscle spasms but are not useful for analgesia (Beaver et al., 1966). Short-term administration of high-dose corticosteroids can provide significant pain relief in patients with bony or neural structure involvement. Dosage of steroids should be tapered as alternative means are implemented (Ettinger and Portenoy, 1988; Bruera et al., 1985). Bisphosphonates should be considered for patients with refractory bone pain (Payne, 1989). Anticholinergic drugs like scopolamine should be considered for refractory pain from bowel obstruction. Neurostimulants such as methylphenidate and dextroamphetamine can be analgesic in low doses (Bruera et al., 1987).

Physical medicine modalities for pain control can serve as an adjunct to cancer pain management (U.S. Department of Health and Human Services, 1994). Cold modalities are generally safe. Heat modalities can be superficial or deep (usually ultrasound) and may increase circulation to the involved area. However, this method may increase the potential for metastatic spread, and application of ultrasound over malignant tissues is generally contraindicated. Transcutaneous electrical stimulation (TENS) is particularly helpful in the management of radiculopathy or incisional pain. Conventional high-frequency settings are usually effective, but expertise in electrode placement may be required to attain pain relief. Trigger point injections can help myofascial pain. Nerve blocks, epidural injections, and ablative surgical procedures may also be useful for treating acute pain.

Appropriate use of orthotics can be invaluable. Examples include shoulder support with a sling in patients with malignant brachial plexopathy or glenohumeral subluxation with brain tumor; or use of cervical, thoracic, and lumbosacral orthoses for patients with metastatic spinal involvement. Psychological approaches including hypnosis, relaxation training, and distraction techniques may be considered. Acupuncture has also been useful in acute pain management.

Delirium and Dementia

Alterations in consciousness may occur during the rehabilitation evaluation or treatment course and require accurate diagnoses and intervention to maximize functional outcome. Delirium (see Chapter 27) is a confusional state with an acute onset, manifesting as a global impairment of mental function. It occurs frequently in elderly cancer patients (Breitbart and Cohen, 1998). The causes of delirium include a variety of drugs, primary intracranial diseases, systemic diseases secondarily affecting the brain, withdrawal from alcohol or sedative-hypnotic medications, metabolic disorders such as hyponatremia and hypoglycemia, infections, and seizures. Determination of the causative agent or factor and removal or correction of the cause is the primary treatment.

Detecting dementia is important for rehabilitation decision-making. Rehabilitation is based on a patient's ability to learn and retain information. Moderately or severely demented patients have limited rehabilitation potential due to their difficulty retaining new information. A brief trial of rehabilitation may still be justified in such situations to train caregivers and to clarify learning abilities. Too often, mental status observations in the acute hospital setting underestimate the patient's cognitive function in a more supportive and stimulating environment and their function following resolution of acute illness. Discharge planning for patients with dementia needs to include caregiver education to ensure awareness of the individual's cognitive strengths and weaknesses and instructions for how to handle potential behavioral problems. Community resources and educational materials can be very helpful to caregivers. The incidence of dementia is higher in the cancer patient population for the following reasons:

1. Occurrence of leukoencephalopathy secondary to chemotherapy such as intrathecal chemotherapy, especially the combination of irradiation and methotrexate (Abrey et al., 1998)
2. Slowly progressing viral infections (Manuelidis et al., 1988)
3. Radiation-related dementia characterized either by dementia alone or by dementia with gait abnormalities and incontinence. A small number of patients will also have hydrocephalus and benefit by ventricular-abdominal shunting (Asai et al., 1989)

Parkinsonism

The major clinical features of Parkinson's disease are recognized as a symptom complex manifested by any combination of six cardinal features: tremor at rest, rigidity, bradykinesia-hypokinesia, flexed posture, loss of postural reflexes, and the freezing phenomenon. At least two of these features, with at least one being either tremor at rest or bradykinesia, must be present for a diagnosis of Parkinson's disease. The biochemical pathology in this disorder is decreased dopaminergic neurotransmission in the basal ganglia. Parkinsonism can occur in cancer patients for the following reasons:

1. Use of dopamine antagonists and depleting agents
2. Radiation injury, including radiation necrosis
3. Hydrocephalus/normal pressure hydrocephalus
4. CNS hypoxia
5. Following encephalitis
6. Parathyroid dysfunction
7. Tumor
8. Multi-infarct state
9. Idiopathic Parkinson's disease co-existing in the cancer population

The clinical features of tremor, rigidity, and flexed posture are referred to as positive phenomena; bradykinesia, loss of postural reflexes, and freezing are negative phenomena. In general, the negative phenomena are more disabling. Bradykinesia results in difficulty with speech, swallowing, ADL, and mobility. Walking, transferring, and even bed mobility can be affected. Severe bradykinesia prevents these patients from driving due to slowed foot movement between the accelerator and the brake pedal. Loss of postural reflexes leads to increased risk of falls and a high incidence of hip fractures in parkinsonian patients. Affected patients also have cognitive and behavioral signs such as decreased attention span, visuospatial impairment, and personality changes. They are often more fearful, indecisive, and passive, as well as depressed, than is normal (Dropcho, 1991). Autonomic disturbances are also encountered. Patients may experience constipation, urinary retention, hypotension, and/or erectile dysfunction.

Treatment is aimed at controlling symptoms through use of standard antiparkinsonian medications and rehabilitation interventions. Physical and occupational therapies play an important role in maintaining ADL and muscle strength and slowing development of contractures and the accompanying characteristically stooped posture. Functional deficits often worsen disproportionately with periods of immobility; thus mobility should be preserved as much as possible despite intercurrent illnesses. Rehabilitation also involves treatment of dysphagia, management of bowel and bladder problems, and assistance with psychosocial difficulties caused by declining cognition.

Psychological Issues

Psychological symptoms can include reactive anxiety and depression, major depression, and organic brain disorder. The incidence of these disorders is generally greater with higher levels of disability and advanced illness (Breitbart et al., 1998). Symptoms of depression may include anorexia, insomnia, fatigue, weight loss, dysphoric mood, hopelessness, worthlessness, excessive guilt, and suicidal ideation (Massie and Holland, 1990). Symptoms are initially likely to be reactive to the diagnosis of a malignancy and then depressive as the functional deficits caused by neurologic impairments are manifested. Endicott (1984) suggested substitution criteria for making the diagnosis of depression, as somatic symptoms of depression might be unreliable and nonspecific in cancer patients.

Anxiety is frequently encountered during the course of rehabilitation. Recognition of anxiety can be challenging in the face of neurologic disease, use of corticosteroids, and other medications. Common signs and symptoms include restlessness, jitteriness, vigilance, insomnia, distractibility, dyspnea, numbness, apprehension, autonomic hyperactivity, and worry. Physical symptoms may be more prevalent than psychological or cognitive ones.

Sexual Dysfunction

Sexual dysfunction may be due to a malignancy or its related treatments. It can be affected by changes in nervous, vascular, endocrine, as well as psychological function. Along with depression, patients may feel less sexually attractive. Frontal lobe brain tumors can cause libido changes. Endocrine changes may occur with pituitary involvement and with hormonal treatments for prostate cancer. Hormonal treatments reduce sexual desire and function in most cases. Chemotherapy can cause changes in testosterone production, spermatogenesis, and premature menopause with associated symptoms. Problems include low sexual drive, dry orgasm, vaginal mucosal changes leading to dyspareunia, erectile dysfunction, and decreased pleasure with orgasm (Schover et al., 1993; Gerber and Vargo, 1998). Neuropathies can amplify all of these problems.

Because psychological adjustment is an important determinant of sexual function, counseling should be provided. Patients should be encouraged to pursue intimacy and physical closeness, focusing on various aspects of an intimate relationship. Hormonal replacement therapy should be given for premature menopause when no contraindications are present, along with water-based lubricants. Regular douching should be encouraged to avoid odor. A peer-support system can also be of benefit (Gerber and Vargo, 1998; Garden and Gillis, 1996).

Family Interaction

Lack of an adequate support system can be a barrier to successful rehabilitation. Family interventions include counseling, education, and identifying additional support frameworks for the caregiver. Both education and counseling interventions significantly improve caregiver knowledge. Specific techniques for care should be taught, including

1. Performing physical functions such as transfers, mobility, and other ADL
2. Encouraging patients to perform any activity that he or she is capable of doing
3. Coping and compensatory strategies to deal with cognitive deficits
4. Preventing complications

Common teaching points can include maintaining bowel and bladder function, administering medications, swallow training with appropriate dietary modifications, maintenance of nutrition and hydration, safety training, and a home exercise program.

Equipment/Orthosis Needs

Patient equipment needs are usually assessed when they approach discharge or experience a sudden decline in function. Equipment available for in-home medical management includes ventilators, suctioning devices, supplemental oxygen, and tube feeding devices. Mobility equipment includes wheelchairs, walkers, crutches, and canes. Rehabilitation professionals choose devices according to the patient's functional level. Assistive devices help to achieve an improved level of independence in ADLs and include transfer boards, tub/shower chairs, raised toilet seats, long-handled reachers, sock-aids, elastic shoelaces, dressing sticks, modified eating utensils, and bath and grooming aids.

Orthoses are prescribed for support, alignment, and protection. Four important functions of the upper limb—reaching, carrying, prehension, and release—should be taken into account when considering an orthosis for the upper extremity. Lower extremity orthoses are primarily to assist with safety in weight bearing.

Discharge Planning/Family Training

The following factors are considered when planning discharge: architectural barriers, available assistance,

Table 22–11. Karnofsky Performance Status Scale

Activity Level	*Scale %*	*Criteria*
Able to carry on normal activity and to work; no special care needed	100	Normal; no complaints; no evidence of disease
	90	Able to carry on normal activity; minor signs or symptoms of disease
	80	Normal activity with effort; some signs or symptoms of disease
Unable to work; able to live at home and care for most personal needs; varying amount of assistance needed	70	Able to care for self; unable to carry on normal activity or to do active work
	60	Requires occasional assistance, but is able to care for most of own needs
	50	Requires considerable assistance and frequent medical care
Unable to care for self; requires equivalent of institutional or hospital care; disease may be progressing rapidly	40	Disabled; requires special care and assistance
	30	Severely disabled; hospitalization indicated; although death is not imminent
	20	Very sick; hospitalization is necessary; active supportive treatment is necessary
	10	Moribund; fatal process progressing rapidly
	0	Dead

availability of home therapy, and quality of life. A suitable caregiver, either a family member or a hired provider, needs to be adequately trained before discharge. If a patient is not safe cognitively or physically and there is no assistance at home, a nursing home or assisted living facility must be considered. If a patient's prognosis is poor, hospice care can provide tremendous support for the family and patient and may improve the patient's quality of life.

PATIENT OUTCOME GOALS

Functional/Social Outcomes

The most widely used scale for clinical and research outcome measurement in the oncologic literature is the Karnofsky Performance Scale (KPS) (Table 22–11). In the absence of any medical treatment, the KPS was found to be the best determinant of ultimate

Table 22–12. Eastern Cooperative Oncology Group (ECOG) Scale Performance Status

Grade	*Definition*
0	Fully active, able to carry on all pre-disease performance without restriction
1	Restricted in physically strenuous activity; ambulatory; able to perform light or sedentary work
2	Capable of all self-care; ambulatory; unable to perform work activities; up and about more than 50% of waking hours
3	Only capable of limited self-care; confined to bed more than 50% of waking hours
4	Completely disabled; cannot carry out any self-care activity; totally confined to bed or chair

patient survival in a national hospice study. With a score of 40, patients lived on the average less than 50 days; with a score of 20, they lived only 10 to 20 days (Reuben et al., 1988).

The KPS does not address cognitive function or quality of life. Additional limitations of this scale, which hinder its use as a functional outcomes measure, are its inability to objectively quantify the amount of assistance needed and its linkage of physical function with medical status. These criteria fail to accommodate severely disabled but otherwise healthy patients. Its linkage of medical status with

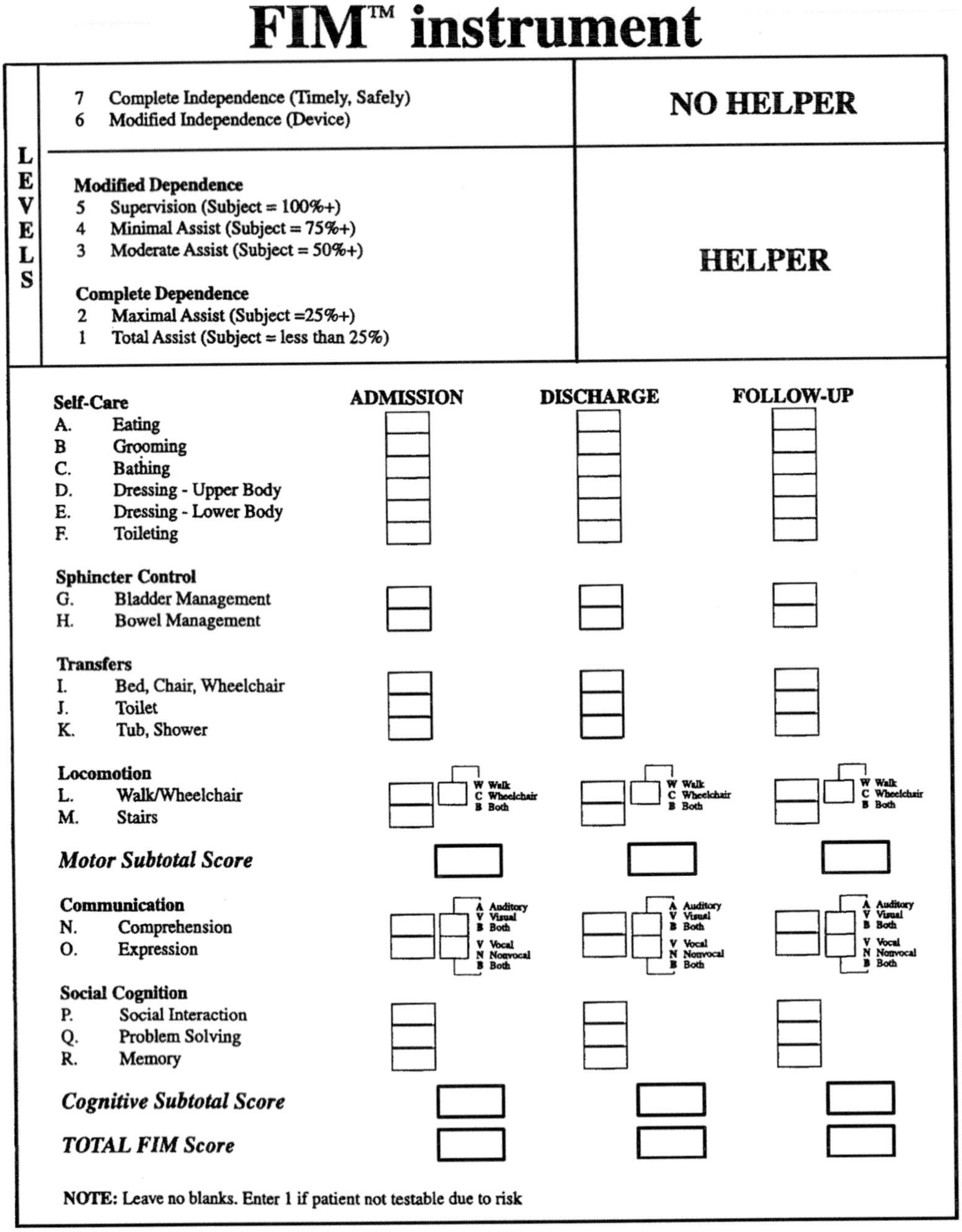

FIM™ instrument

LEVELS		
	7 Complete Independence (Timely, Safely) 6 Modified Independence (Device)	**NO HELPER**
	Modified Dependence 5 Supervision (Subject = 100%+) 4 Minimal Assist (Subject = 75%+) 3 Moderate Assist (Subject = 50%+) **Complete Dependence** 2 Maximal Assist (Subject =25%+) 1 Total Assist (Subject = less than 25%)	**HELPER**

	ADMISSION	DISCHARGE	FOLLOW-UP
Self-Care			
A. Eating			
B Grooming			
C. Bathing			
D. Dressing - Upper Body			
E. Dressing - Lower Body			
F. Toileting			
Sphincter Control			
G. Bladder Management			
H. Bowel Management			
Transfers			
I. Bed, Chair, Wheelchair			
J. Toilet			
K. Tub, Shower			
Locomotion			
L. Walk/Wheelchair	W Walk C Wheelchair B Both	W Walk C Wheelchair B Both	W Walk C Wheelchair B Both
M. Stairs			
Motor Subtotal Score			
Communication			
N. Comprehension	A Auditory V Visual B Both	A Auditory V Visual B Both	A Auditory V Visual B Both
O. Expression	V Vocal N Nonvocal B Both	V Vocal N Nonvocal B Both	V Vocal N Nonvocal B Both
Social Cognition			
P. Social Interaction			
Q. Problem Solving			
R. Memory			
Cognitive Subtotal Score			
TOTAL FIM Score			

NOTE: Leave no blanks. Enter 1 if patient not testable due to risk

Figure 22–1. Function Independence Measure (FIM). Copyright 1990 by the Research Foundation of the State University of New York.

work status is often heavily influenced by completely nonmedical factors (insurance, family support, type of work done, and so forth). These criticisms also hold true for the ECOG and similar performance status scales (Table 22–12).

Functional status at presentation was the most important outcome predictor in a study on mortality and functional decline in a group of 92 patients with malignant glioma receiving radiotherapy (Davies et al., 1996). In this study, 13% of predominantly bedbound patients had functional improvement, whereas 80% of patients presenting with no disability continued to have no deficits at 6 months (Davies et al., 1996). In patients with spinal cord tumor involvement, research suggests a better 1-year survival rate among those who remained ambulatory (66% vs. 10%) (Hill et al., 1993). Bell et al. (1998) found that a population of tumor patients admitted to inpatient rehabilitation units had a generally poorer functional prognosis than did noncancer patients.

Among rehabilitation professionals, one of the most commonly used scales has been the Functional Independence Measure (FIM) (Fig. 22–1). This may also be inadequate to assess brain tumor patients, who have fewer persisting motor and communication disorders than for patients with other neurologic disorders such as stroke (Meyers, 1994).

Quality of Life

General quality of life (see Chapter 26) questionnaires for patients with cancer are listed in Table 22–13. Quality of life status may be more strongly predictive of survival than performance status (Coates et al., 1992; Kaasa et al., 1989; Osoba and MacDonald, 1999; Ruckdeschel and Piantadosi, 1991). Factors associated with a better quality of life include absence of depression, good social involvement, greater energy, and fewer symptoms. Age has not been demonstrated to be a significant factor (Bell et al., 1998; Giovagnoli et al., 1996; Mackworth et al., 1992; Weitzner et al., 1996).

Employment

Work is identified in many studies as a significant factor in quality of life. There is little literature regarding employment among patients with neurologic tumors specifically, although in one study of cancer patients only 56% were working (Bell et al., 1998; Rothstein et al., 1995). Cognitive impairment, which would prevent return to work, is more likely among patients with brain tumors compared with other tumors. Kleinberg and associates reported in a study that of 30 primary glioma patients who underwent resection and irradiation, 68% returned to work after treatment, 62% remained at work 1 year later, and 58% were still working 2 to 4 years later (Bell et al., 1998; Kleinberg et al., 1993).

CONCLUSION

Successful rehabilitation of patients with neurologic tumors requires understanding the behavior of tumor pathology, flexibility in determining functional goals and timelines for achievement of goals, and awareness of the complications of cancer and its treatments, which negatively impact patient function. The ultimate goals of rehabilitation interventions are to maximize

Table 22–13. General Quality of Life Questionnaires for Patients with Cancer

Name	*Acronym*
Cancer Rehabilitation Evaluation System Short Form	CARES-SF
European Organization for Research and Treatment of Cancer Core Quality of Life Questionnaire	EORTC QLQ-C-30
Functional Assessment of Cancer Therapy	FACT
Functional Living Index for Cancer	FLIC
Linear Analog Self-Assessment Scale	LASA
Medical Outcomes Study Short Form	MOS SF-36
McGill Quality of Life Questionnaire	MQOL
Quality of Life Index	QLI
Rotterdam Symptom Checklist	RSCL

function, promote adaptive and compensatory strategies when full function cannot be restored, and enhance quality of life for cancer patients.

REFERENCES

Abrey LE, DeAngelis LM, Yahalom J. 1998. Long-term survival in primary CNS lymphoma. J Clin Oncol 16:859–863.

Alekhteyar KM, Leung DH, Brennan MF, Harrison LB. 1996. The effect of combined external beam radiotherapy and brachytherapy on local control and wound complications in patients with high-grade soft tissue sarcomas of the extremity with positive microscopic margin. Int J Radiat Oncol Biol Phys 36:321–324.

Amato AA, Collins MP. 1998. Neuropathies associated with malignancy. Semin Neurol 18:125–144.

American Cancer Society. 1990. Cancer Facts and Figures. New York: American Cancer Society.

An HS, Ebraheim N, Kim K, Jackson WT, Kane JT. 1987. Heterotopic ossification and pseudoarthrosis in the shoulder following encephalitis. A case report and review of the literature. Clin Orthop 219:291–298.

Asai A, Matsutani M, Kohno T, et al. 1989. Subacute brain atrophy after radiation therapy for malignant brain tumor. Cancer 63:1962–1974.

Barron KD, Hirano A, Araki S, et al. 1959. Experience with metastatic neoplasms involving the spinal cord. Neurology 9:91–106.

Beaver WT, Feise G. 1976. Comparison of the analgesic effects of morphine, hydroxyzine and their combination in patients with postoperative pain. In: Bonica JJ (ed), Advances in Pain Research and Therapy, vol 1. New York: Raven Press.

Beaver WT, Wallenstein SL, Houde RW, Rogers A. 1966. A comparison of the analgesic effects of methotrimeprazine and morphine in patients with cancer. Clin Pharmacol Ther 7:436–446.

Bell KR, O'Dell MW, Barr K, et al. 1998. Rehabilitation of the patient with brain tumor. Arch Phys Med Rehabil 79:S37–S46.

Black PM. 1991. Brain tumors. Part 1 and part 2. N Engl J Med 324:1471–1476, 1555–1564.

Bondy ML, Wrensch M. 1993. Update on brain cancer epidemiology. Cancer Bull 45:365–369.

Bone RC, et al. 1999. Bone's Atlas of Pulmonary and Critical Care Medicine, Baltimore: Williams & Wilkins.

Breitbart W, Chochinov HM, Passik S. 1998. Psychiatric aspects of palliative care. In: Doyle D, Hanks GWC, MacDonald N (eds), Oxford Textbook of Palliative Medicine, 2nd ed. New York: Oxford University Press, pp 933–947.

Breitbart W, Cohen KR. 1998. Delirium. In: Holland JC, Breitbart W, et al. (eds), Psycho-oncology. New York: Oxford University Press, pp 564–575.

Brooke MM, Patterson DR, Questad KA, Cardenas D, Farrel-Roberts L. 1992. The treatment of agitation during initial hospitalization after traumatic brain injury. Arch Phys Med Rehabil 73:917–921.

Brooker AF, Boweran JW, Robinson RA, Riley LH Jr. 1973. Ectopic ossification following total hip replacement. Incidence and method of classification. J Bone Joint Surg Am 55:1629–1632.

Bruera E, Brenneis C, Paterson AH, MacDonald RN. 1989. Use of methylphenidate as an adjuvant to narcotic analgesics in patients with advanced cancer. J Pain Symptom Manage 4:3–6.

Bruera E, Chadwick S, Brenneis C, Hanson J, MacDonald RN. 1987. Methylphenidate associated with narcotics for the treatment of cancer pain. Cancer Treat Rep 71:67–70.

Bruera E, Roca E, Cedaro L, Carraro S, Chacon R. 1985. Action of oral methylprednisolone in terminal cancer patients: a prospective randomized double-blind study. Cancer Treat Rep 69:751–754.

Burgess J. 1989. Cancer therapy. In: Skipper A (ed), Dietitians' Handbook of Enteral and Parenteral Nutrition. Rockville, MD: Aspen Publishers, 121 pp

Caraceni A, Martini C. 1999a. Neurological problems. In: Doyle D, Hanks GWC, MacDonald N (eds), Oxford Textbook of Palliative Medicine, 2nd ed. New York: Oxford University Press, pp 727–749.

Caraceni A, Martini C. 1999b. Neurological problems. In: Doyle D, Hanks GWC, MacDonald N (eds), Oxford Textbook of Palliative Medicine, 2nd ed. New York: Oxford University Press, pp 733–734.

Casciato DA, Lowitz BB. 1983. Manual of Bedside Oncology, 1st ed. Boston: Little, Brown, 699 pp.

Coates A, Gebski V, Signorini D, et al. 1992. Prognostic value of quality-of-life scores during chemotherapy for advanced breast cancer. Australian New Zealand Breast Cancer Trials Group. J Clin Oncol 10:1833–1838.

Cope DN. 1987. Ed. Psychopharmacologic considerations in the treatment of traumatic brain injury. J Head Trauma Rehab 2(4):1–5.

D'Angio GJ, Meadows A, Mike V, et al. 1976. Decreased risk of radiation-associated second malignant neoplasms in actinomycin-D–treated patients. Cancer 37:1177–1185.

Davies E, Clarke C, Hopkins A. 1996. Malignant cerebral glioma—I: Survival, disability, and morbidity after radiotherapy. BMJ 313:1507–1512.

Dropcho EJ. 1991. Central nervous system injury by therapeutic irradiation. Neurol Clin 9:969–988.

Duthie EH Jr, Katz PR. 1998. Practice of Geriatrics, 3rd ed. Philadelphia: WB Saunders, 599 pp.

Endicott J. 1984. Measurement of depression in patients with cancer. Cancer 53:2243–2249.

Ettinger AB, Portenoy RK. 1988. The use of corticosteroids in the treatment of symptoms associated with cancer. J Pain Symptom Manage 3:99–104.

Evans EB. 1991. Heterotopic bone formation in thermal burns. Clin Orthop 263:94–101.

Findlay GF. 1984. Adverse effects of the management of malignant spinal cord compression. J Neurol Neurosurg Psychiatry 47:761–768.

Forsyth PA, Posner JB. 1993. Headaches in patients with brain tumors: a study of 111 patients. Neurology 43:1678–1683.

Galasko CSB. 1999. Orthopedic principles and management. In: Doyle D, Hanks GWC, MacDonald N (eds), Oxford Textbook of Palliative Medicine, 2nd ed. Oxford: Oxford University Press, pp 482–485.

Garden FH, Gillis TA. 1996. Principles of cancer rehabilitation. In: Braddom RL (ed), Physical Medicine and Rehabilitation, 1st ed. Philadelphia: WB Saunders, pp 1199–1214.

Garland DE. 1988. Clinical observations on fractures and heterotopic ossification in the spinal cord and traumatic brain injured population. Clin Orthop 233:86–101.

Gerber LH, Vargo M. 1998. Rehabilitation for patients with cancer diagnoses. In: Delisa JA, Gans BM, Bockenek WL, et al. (eds), Rehabilitation Medicine: Principles and Practice, 3rd ed. Philadelphia: Lippincott Raven, pp 1293–1315.

Gibberd FB, Gould SR, Marks P. 1976. Incidence of deep vein thrombosis and leg oedema in patients with strokes. J Neurol Neurosurg Psychiatry 39:1222–1225.

Gilbert HA, Kagan AR, Nussbaum H,, et al. 1977. Evaluation of radiation therapy for bone metastases: pain relief and quality of life. AJR Am J Roentgenol 129:1095–1096.

Gilbert RW, Kim JH, Posner JB. 1978. Epidural spinal cord compression from metastatic tumor: diagnosis and treatment. Ann Neurol 3:40–51.

Giovagnoli AR, Tamburini M, Boiardi A. 1996. Quality of life in brain tumor patients. J Neurooncol 30:71–80.

Giuntini C, Di Ricco G, Marini C, Melillo E, Palla A. 1995. Pulmonary emoblism: epidemiology. Chest 107:3S–9S.

Goroll AH, May LA, Mulley AG Jr. 1995. Primary Care Medicine: Office Evaluation and Management of the Adult Patient, 3rd ed. Philadelphia: Lippincott, 1162 p.

Grujic Z, Mapstone M, Gitelman DR, et al. 1998. Dopamine agonists reorient visual exploration away from the neglected hemispace. Neurology 51:1395–1398.

Gualtieri T, Chandler M, Coons TB, Brown LT. 1989. Amantadine: a new clinical profile for traumatic brain injury. Clin Neuropharmacol 12:258–270.

Hill ME, Richards MA, Gregory WM, Smith P, Rubens RD. 1993. Spinal cord compression in breast cancer: a review of 70 cases. Br J Cancer 68:969–973.

Hoffman MD, Sheldahl LM, Kraemer WJ, et al. 1998. Therapeutic exercise. In: Delisa JA, Gans BM, Bockenek WL, et al. (eds), Rehabilitation Medicine: Principles and Practice, 3rd ed. Philadelphia: Lippincott Raven pp 697–743.

Imperiale TF, Speroff T. 1994. A meta-analysis of methods to prevent venous thromboembolism following total hip replacement [published erratum appears in JAMA 1995, Jan 25;273(4):288]. JAMA 271:1780–1785.

Ishikawa K, Izumi K, Kitagawa T. 1982. Heterotopic ossification of the hip as a complication of tetanus. Clin Orthop 166:249–255.

Jaeckle KA, Young DF, Foley KM. 1985. The natural history of lumbosacral plexopathy in cancer. Neurology 35:8–15.

Jensen LL, Halar E, Little JW, Brooke MM. 1988. Neurogenic heterotopic ossification. Am J Phys Med: 66:351–363.

Kaasa S, Mastekaasa A, Lund E. 1989. Prognostic factors for patients with inoperable non-small cell lung cancer, limited disease. The importance of patients' subjective experience of disease and psychosocial well-being. Radiother Oncol 15:235–242.

Kleinberg L, Wallner K, Malkin MG. 1993. Good performance status of long-term disease-free survivors of intracranial gliomas. Int J Radiat Oncol Biol Phys 26:129–133.

Leibel SA, Guten PH, Davis RL. 1991. Tolerance of the brain and spinal cord. In Guten PH, Leibel SA, Sheline GE (eds), Radiation Injury to the Nervous System. New York: Raven Press, pp 239–256.

Lewis DA, Smith RE. 1983. Steroid-induced psychiatric syndromes: a report of 14 cases and a review of the literature. J Affect Disord 5:319–332.

Mackworth N, Fobair P, Prados MD. 1992. Quality of life self-reports from 200 brain tumor patients: comparisons with Karnofsky performance scores. J Neurooncol 14:243–253.

Maillet JO. 1987. The cancer patient. In: Lang CE (ed), Nutritional Support in Critical Care. Rockville, MD: Aspen Publishers, 250 pp.

Manuelidis L, Murdoch G, Manuelidis EE. 1988. Potential involvement of retroviral elements in human dementias. Ciba Found Symp 135:117–134.

Marik PE, Andrews L, Maini B. 1997. The incidence of deep venous thrombosis in ICU patients. Chest 111:661–664.

Massie MJ, Holland JC. 1990. Depression and the cancer patient. J Clin Psychiatry 51:12–19.

Mattes RD, Arnold C, Boraas M. 1987. Learned food aversions among cancer chemotherapy patients: incidence, nature, and clinical implications. Cancer 60:2576–2580.

Merli GJ, Crabbe S, Paluzzi RG, Fritz D. 1993. Etiology, incidence, and prevention of deep vein thrombosis in acute spinal cord injury. Arch Phys Med Rehabil 74:1199–1205.

Meyers CA. 1994. Neuropsychological aspects of cancer and cancer treatment. In: Garden FH, Grabois M (eds), Physical Medicine and Rehabilitation: State of the Art Reviews, vol 8. Philadelphia: Hanley & Belfus, pp 229–241.

Mysiw WJ, Jackson RD, Corrigan JD. 1988. Amitriptyline for post-traumatic agitation. Am J Phys Med Rehabil 67:29–33.

Nelson DF, McDonald JV, Lapham LW, et al. 1993. Central nervous system tumors. In: Rubin P, McDonald S, Qazi R (eds), Clinical Oncology: A Multidisciplinary Approach for Physicians and Students, 7th ed. Philadelphia: WB Saunders, pp 617–644.

Osoba D, MacDonald N. 1999. Disease-modifying management. In: Doyle D, Hanks GWC, MacDonald N (eds), Oxford Textbook of Palliative Medicine, 2d ed. New York: Oxford University Press, pp 933–947.

Payne R. 1989. Pharmacologic management of bone pain in the cancer patient. Clin J Pain 5(suppl 2):S43–S50.

Pizzo PA, Poplack DG. 1997. Principles and Practice of Pediatric Oncology, 3d ed. Philadelphia: Lippincott Raven, 1522 pp.

Portenoy RK, Lipton RB, Foley KM. 1987. Back pain in the cancer patient: an algorithm for evaluation and management. Neurology 37:134–138.

Posner JB. 1995. Neurologic complications of cancer. In: Contemporary Neurology Series, vol 45. Philadelphia: FA Davis, 482 pp.

Posner JB, Chernik NL. 1978. Intracranial metastases from systemic cancer. Adv Neurol 19:579–592.

Reuben DB, Mor V, Hiris J. 1988. Clinical symptoms and length of survival in patients with terminal cancer. Arch Intern Med 148:1586–1591.

Rodichok LD, Harper GR, Ruckdeschel JC, et al. 1981. Early diagnosis of spinal epidural metastases. Am J Med 70:1181–1188.

Rothstein MA, Kennedy K, Ritchie KJ, Pyle K. 1995. Are cancer patients subject to employment discrimination? Oncology (Huntingt) 9:1303–1306.

Rowland LP. 1995. Merritt's Textbook of Neurology, 9th ed. Baltimore: Williams & Wilkins, 1058 pp.

Ruckdeschel JC, Piantadosi S. 1991. Quality of life assessment. An independent prognostic variable for survival in lung cancer. J Thorac Surg 6:201–205.

Sause WT, Crowley J, Eyre HJ, et al. 1988. Whole brain irradiation and intrathecal methotrexate in the treatment of solid tumor leptomeningeal metastases—a Southwest Oncology Group study. J Neurooncol 6:107–112.

Schlicht LA, Smelz JK. 1994. Metastatic spinal cord compression. In: Garden FH, Grabois M (eds), Physical Medicine and Rehabilitation State of the Art Reviews. Philadelphia: Hanley & Belfus, pp 345–361.

Schover LR, Montague DK, Schain W. 1993. Sexual problems. In: DeVita VT Jr, Hellman S, Rosenber SA (eds), Cancer: Principles and Practice of Oncology, 4th ed. Philadelphia: Lippincott, pp 1464–2480.

Shapiro WR, Posner JB. 1983. Medical versus surgical treatment of metastatic spinal cord tumors. In: Thompson RA, Green JR (eds), Controversies in Neurology. New York: Raven Press, pp 57–65.

Shaw MD, Rose JE, Paterson A. 1980. Metastatic extradural malignancy of the spine. Acta Neurochir (Wien) 52: 113–120.

Siegal T, Lossos A, Pfeiffer MR. 1994. Leptomeningeal metastases. Analysis of 31 patients with sustained off-therapy response following combined-modality therapy. Neurology 44:1463–1469.

Silberfarb PM. 1983. Chemotherapy and cognitive defects in cancer patients. Annu Rev Med 34:35–46.

Springfield DS. 1993. Surgical wound healing. In: Verweij J, Pinedo HM, Suit HD (eds), Multidisciplinary Ttreatment of Soft Tissue Sarcomas. Boston: Kluwer Academic Publishers, pp 81–98.

Stoikovic JP, Bonfiglio M, Paul WD. 1955. Myositis ossificans complicating poliomyelitis. Arch Phys Med Rehabil 36:236–243.

Storey G, Tegner WS. 1955. Paraplegic para-articular calcification. Ann Rheum Dis 14:176–182.

Stover SL, Hataway CJ, Zeiger HE. 1975. Heterotopic ossification in spinal cord-injured patients. Arch Phys Med Rehabil 56:199–204.

Suwanwela N, Phanthumchinda K, Kaoropthum S. 1994. Headache in brain tumor: a cross-sectional study. Headache 34:435–438.

Tefft M, Lattin PB, Jereb B, et al. 1976. Acute and late effects on normal tissues following combined chemo- and radiotherapy for childhood rhabdomyosarcoma and Ewing's sarcoma. Cancer 37:1201–1217.

U.S. Department of Health and Human Services, PHS, Agency for Health Care Policy and Research. 1994. AHCPR Pub. No. 94-0592. Management of Cancer Pain Guideline Panel. Nonpharmacologic Management: Physical and Psychological Modalities. Management of Cancer Pain, Clinical Practice Guideline No. 9, pp 75–88.

Weinmann EE, Salzman EW. 1994. Deep-vein thrombosis. N Engl J Med 331:1630–1641.

Weitzner MA, Meyers CA, Byrne K. 1996. Psychosocial functioning and quality of life in patients with primary brain tumors. J Neurosurg 84:29–34.

Whyte J. 1988. Clinical drug evaluation. J Head Trauma Rehabil 3:95–99.

Zizic TM. 1991. Osteonecrosis. Curr Opin Rheumatol 3:481–489.

23

Assessment and Management of Cancer Pain

SURESH K. REDDY AND C. STRATTON HILL, JR.

PREVALENCE OF CANCER PAIN

It is estimated that from 30% to 50% of patients actively undergoing cancer therapy and from 60% to 90% of patients with advanced cancer have pain (Foley, 1979; Bonica, 1990; Twycross and Fairfield, 1982; World Health Organization, 1986; Levin et al., 1985). Approximately 50% of children in an inpatient pediatric cancer center and about 25% of outpatients experience pain (Miser et al., 1987). The World Health Organization Cancer Pain Relief Program indicates that approximately 5 million people worldwide suffer from cancer-related pain on a daily basis, and fully 25% of them die at home or in a hospital without relief (World Health Organization, 1990).

It is important to assess the effects of pain on the quality of life in multidimensional terms, and the development of valid and reliable measurement instruments for this purpose is currently an area of intense research (Aaronson, 1988). A number of validated tools have been used to track pain and other symptom intensity, such as the Edmonton Symptom Assessment System (ESAS) and The University of Texas M. D. Anderson Cancer Center Symptom Inventory (MDASI). It is useful to assess pain in conjunction with other symptoms so that appropriate treatment can be planned.

The loss of function, fear of death, and a multitude of other psychosocial ramifications of cancer and pain are intertwined. The term *suffering* has been used in this context to describe the overall negative impact of cancer on the life of the individual (Portenoy, 1990), and, while it must be recognized that pain is only one aspect of suffering, it is often a major one. Comprehensive management of the cancer patient with pain requires that all of the factors associated with the quality of life of the person as a whole be considered.

UNDERTREATMENT OF CANCER PAIN

It is a sad fact that pain is not satisfactorily managed for many cancer patients. For example, in one published study, 1308 patients were surveyed at 54 treatment sites participating in the Eastern Cooperative Oncology Group to evaluate the prevalence of pain and the adequacy of its treatment (Cleeland et al., 1994). In this study, 67% of patients reported daily pain and took analgesics daily. However, 42% of these patients had negative pain index scores, which are measures of the adequacy of analgesic therapy for pain. These scores match the severity of the patient's reported pain with the potency of the analgesic(s) prescribed. Not surprisingly, the patients who reported the most pain also reported the poorest function. At particular risk for undertreatment were patients of African-American, Hispanic American, and other minority ethnic groups, females, patients over the age of 70 years, and those who reported pain but had "good" performance status scores.

Results such as these and the significant variability in treatment outcomes for cancer pain management documented from a variety of sources led to the development of federal guidelines relating to the management of cancer pain published in the mid-1990s

(Jacox et al., 1994). The guidelines emphasize the need to adequately assess the causes of pain and to treat pain aggressively in an approach that individualizes therapy for each patient.

Barriers to Optimal Cancer Pain Management

Despite the increased knowledge of pain mechanisms, improved methods for treating generalized and specific pain syndromes, and an increased number of professional and government organizations dedicated to disseminating this information, an inordinate number of patients with pain experience inadequate relief. Reasons that account for this are *(1)* cultural and societal barriers to the adequate and appropriate use of opioids, *(2)* a general lack of awareness among healthcare providers of advances in opioid pharmacology culled from long-term studies in cancer patients experiencing chronic pain, and *(3)* the negative influence of state healthcare disciplinary boards and state and federal drug enforcement agencies on drug prescribing and dispensing practices (Hill, 1990). These situations alternately interdigitate to effect undertreatment of pain during the course of an individual's treatment. Each discrete reason, or a combination thereof, may exert a dominant influence at any given time during the course of a patient's pain treatment. For example, pain relief may initially be inadequate because of the physician's knowledge deficit about the pharmacology of opioids, but later in the course of treatment may be inadequate because of fear of regulatory sanctions.

All these difficulties specifically relate to the use of opioids. Yet, difficulty in achieving adequate pain control occurs most frequently with pain that is diffuse and of such intensity that it can be relieved only with these drugs. No similar limitations or restrictions are placed on other treatment modalities, nor are they associated with the same emotional milieu as found when opioids are a part of the treatment picture. Therefore, nonopioid treatment modalities are used with impunity to achieve the optimum benefit that can be attained with them.

Two of the above factors, cultural and societal barriers and government regulatory barriers, demonstrate how extramedical influences, by contributing to pain undertreatment, can be detrimental to providing quality medical care. The third reason, knowledge deficits about medical advances, demonstrates how difficult it is to replace information that has been ingrained into the accepted body of medical knowledge. This knowledge is, however, based on limited clinical studies and a restricted pain model, whereas the new information is based on more appropriate clinical studies carried out in an appropriate pain model—the cancer patient in pain.

This section explicates how the various interdictions to efficacious pain therapy interfere with adequate pain treatment and offers recommendations for overcoming this interference.

Cultural and Societal Barriers

The use of opioids by patients who take them for legitimate medical use is confused with the illegal abuse of them by individuals who take them for recreational nonmedical purposes. The dominance of the illegitimate image of these drugs in the minds of both healthcare professionals and the public is so pervasive that their effective use as drugs with a legitimate medical purpose is overshadowed. Patients have often been made to feel like criminals or morally inferior beings for taking these drugs. This general confusion frequently leads to physicians prescribing inappropriately low doses at intervals that exceed the effectiveness of the drugs. Patients who are undertreated in this manner become desperate for relief and often resort to behavior that mimics the drug seeker, prompting healthcare providers to label them as "addicts." Weissman and Haddox (1989) have coined the term "pseudoaddiction" for this iatrogenically created behavior.

Physicians' prescribing practices are strongly influenced by peer pressure. Despite an adequate knowledge of the pharmacokinetics and pharmacodynamics of opioid drugs, physicians often prescribe in the same manner as their peers even though this entails prescribing the wrong dose of the drug and for an interval that is inappropriately long, particularly for cancer patients. This widespread practice sets the standard for prescribing opioids in a given community, a practice that results in undertreatment and inadequately relieved pain. Drug regulatory agencies use a community standard to judge an individual physician's prescribing practices. Therefore, a physician who prescribes a proper dose of an opioid may be judged to be outside the normal standard of practice and subject to sanctions, including the loss of his or her license to practice medicine. Unfortunately, community standards often perpetuate undertreatment of pain.

Healthcare professionals have an irrational fear of causing psychological dependency (addiction) to drugs. Chronic use of opioids per se is, however, not synonymous with addiction. While patients who require chronic opioids for pain relief can become physiologically dependent on the opioid and experience an abstinence or withdrawal reaction if the drug is abruptly discontinued (reflecting the normal pharmacologic action of all opioids), addiction only results when a person becomes psychologically dependent on an opioid. Addiction is also a social condition, associated with a destructive life-style. The psychologically dependent individual has a compulsion to procure and take an opioid for mind-altering purposes for recreational, nonmedical reasons. The cancer patient in pain takes opioids for pain relief to restore a reasonably normal, functional life-style for the period of life remaining. Studies have shown that the number of individuals who become addicted to drugs by an introduction to them through medical use is extremely small (Portenoy and Payne, 1992).

It is unfortunate but common that physicians' unfamiliarity and discomfort with prescribing "strong" opioids chronically results in postponing their use far beyond the time indicated for good medical pain control practices. The global prejudice that opioid use is bad, no matter what the reason, inspires physicians when chronic use is contemplated or required to postpone treatment until a patient's survival is measured in only weeks or months. As a result, cancer patients often do not get adequate pain treatment until their agonal days because of this practice, although cancer pain may be severe for as long as years before death.

Knowledge Deficits

Information in modern pharmacology textbooks about the dosing of opioids is based on single-dose studies using a postoperative pain model (Twycross, 1988), and the pharmacodynamic action was studied in subjects who were not in pain. Dosing studies were also done in the only human pain model available at the time, which excluded cancer patients whose survival time was short and who had persistent complications that augmented their disease. Currently, cancer patients provide a new model for analgesic study, largely because their survival times have improved. Furthermore, cancer patients are suitable for meaningful pharmacodynamic studies because they represent a human model experiencing pain, in contrast to the earlier studies composed of a study population of volunteers who were former drug addicts and not experiencing pain.

Study results have demonstrated that pain itself alters the pharmacologic response to opiates by antagonizing the analgesic and respiratory depressant effects of the drugs (Hanks et al., 1981). Dose recommendations based on postoperative pain studies apply only to patients with this type of pain. Extrapolating these doses to patients with other types of pain, especially chronic cancer pain, is misleading. Postoperative pain rarely achieves the intensity of persistent, unrelieved cancer pain. Because of the antagonistic effects of pain on analgesia, doses of opioids must be tailored to whatever level is necessary to relieve the patient's pain. These doses almost always exceed recommended doses for postoperative pain in pharmacology textbooks. However, efficacious doses should not be viewed as "high," "large," or "excessive"; they are simply adequate to meet the patient's pain relief requirements.

ASSESSMENT OF PAIN IN THE CANCER PATIENT

Cancer patients with pain require a careful assessment to determine the nature of their pain and to design appropriate treatment. Painful manifestations of systemic cancer are often caused by damage to neurologic structures. The identification of neurologic dysfunction often helps to direct appropriate therapy. Gonzales et al. (1991), for example, after reviewing a large series of patients in a cancer referral center, found that neurologic consultation identified a previously undiagnosed etiology for pain in 64% of patients and resulted in adding antitumor therapies (radiotherapy, surgery, or chemotherapy) for 18% of patients evaluated. The importance of neurologic evaluation is underscored by the fact that pain is frequently the only manifestation of tumor involving critical neural structures. A complaint of back pain in a cancer patient, for example, may be the only apparent manifestation of epidural spinal cord compression and is, in fact, the only consistent sign or symptom (Byrne and Waxman, 1990). Similarly, pain was the only symptom of lumbosacral plexopathy in 24%

of patients in one series, and in 15% of these patients diagnosis resulted in the discovery of a primary pelvic tumor (Jaeckle et al., 1985).

In addition to the obvious difficulties of experiencing persistent pain, secondary consequences of unrelieved pain in the cancer patient include decreased functional activity and depressed appetite, which may negatively impact the course of the disease itself (Cleeland, 1984). Patients or families may also refuse palliative or potentially curative cancer treatment because of a perceived need to "end the suffering" of the patient (Foley, 1991). Despite our current level of sophistication in treating cancer pain, it is estimated that 29% of patients with cancer suffer from moderate to severe pain despite analgesic therapy (Ventafridda et al., 1987). This fact largely reflects errors in cancer pain treatment, such as inadequate dosing of analgesics in an attempt to avoid producing addiction (Hill and Fields, 1989; Foley, 1989).

The goal of the oncologist or any physician in evaluating and treating the painful manifestations of cancer is dual. The first and often understated task is diagnostic—to appropriately identify the source of pain. To accomplish this, knowledge of the natural history of specific cancer types as well as an appreciation of common pain syndromes occurring in the cancer patient are essential. The second task is therapeutic—to relieve or minimize pain using appropriate management techniques, thereby allowing the patient to be as active and pain-free as possible.

Mechanisms of Cancer Pain: Implications for Treatment

The majority of the pain in cancer is caused by direct tumor involvement of organic structures, notably neural structures. Pain associated with direct tumor involvement occurs in 65% to 85% of patients with advanced cancer (Foley, 1979). Cancer therapy accounts for pain in approximately 15% to 25% of patients receiving chemotherapy, surgery, or radiation therapy (Higginson, 1997). Between 3% and 10% of cancer patients have pain syndromes, which are most commonly observed in the general noncancer population (e.g., low back pain secondary to degenerative disc disease or diabetic neuropathy). Common clinical pain syndromes are listed in Table 23–1.

Cancer pain can occur after activation of peripheral nociceptors (somatic and visceral "nociceptive" pain) or as a result of direct injury to peripheral or central nervous structures (neuropathic or "deafferentation" pain). In addition, both nociceptive and neuropathic pain may be modified by involvement of

Table 23–1. Common Clinical Pain Syndromes and Their Causes

Pain due to tumor
- Bone pain due to metastasis (somatic pain) from breast, prostate, and other cancers
- Plexopathy pain (neuropathic pain) due to Pancoast's tumor/pelvic tumor
- Abdominal pain (visceral pain) due to pancreatic cancer and liver metastasis
- Chest wall pain due to mesothelioma (somatic and neuropathic pain)

Pain due to cancer treatment
- Postchemotherapy pain syndromes
  - Peripheral neuropathy due to cisplatin and paclitaxol
- Post-irradiation pain syndromes
  - Chronic throat pain due to radiation-induced mucositis
  - Chronic abdominal pain due to radiation-induced enteritis in fistulae
  - Radiation-induced plexopathy pain
- Post-surgical pain syndromes
  - Post-mastectomy pain syndrome
  - Post-radical neck dissection pain syndrome
  - Phantom limb pain syndrome

Pain syndrome unrelated to cancer
- Chronic low back pain due to degenerative process in the spine
- Pain secondary to osteoarthritis and rheumatoid arthritis
- Migraine headaches

the sympathetic nervous system (so-called reflex sympathetic dystrophy [RSD], currently called sympathetically maintained pain [SMP]. Each of these painful states has unique clinical characteristics, which may aid in identification and direct analgesic or antitumor therapies. A key step, therefore, in the evaluation of a cancer patient with pain is to elicit a careful history of the quality, nature, and location of perceived pain, which may provide valuable clues regarding the etiology of the complaint and may help direct investigative studies.

Somatic pain results from involvement of bone and muscle structures. Metastatic bone disease is the most common pain syndrome in patients with cancer. Myelinated and unmyelinated afferent fibers are present in bone, and their density is greatest in the periosteum. Prostaglandins (PGs) play a multifactorial role in the etiology of bone pain. Prostaglandin concentrations are increased at sites of bone metastasis (Galasko, 1976). In addition, PGs mediate osteolytic and osteoclastic metastatic bone changes. Prostaglandin E_2 sensitizes nociceptors and produces hyperalgesia. These observations have resulted in considerable interest in the use of steroidal and nonsteroidal anti-inflammatory medications as important therapies for metastatic bone pain (Stambaugh and Drew, 1988), although some have questioned their value in the treatment of bone pain (Mercadante, 1997).

Visceral pain is also common in the cancer patient and results from stretching or distending viscera or from the production of an inflammatory response and the release of analgesic substances in the vicinity of nociceptors. Visceral pain is commonly referred to cutaneous sites, which can mislead the examiner, particularly because those cutaneous sites may be tender to palpation. This phenomenon likely results from the convergence of visceral and somatic afferent information onto common neuronal pools in the dorsal horn of the spinal cord (Milne et al., 1981).

Neuropathic pain from neural injury, such as brachial plexus or lumbosacral plexus infiltration by tumor, is often severe. The hallmark of neuropathic pain is paroxysms of burning or electric shock sensations, which may result, at least in part, from spontaneous discharges in the peripheral and central nervous systems. By definition, the nervous system is not behaving normally in these painful states, and conventional analgesic therapies may not be efficacious. For example, Arner and Meyerson (1988) argued that opioids are ineffective for treating neuropathic pain. Although this view has been challenged (Portenoy et al., 1990), it was observed that larger doses of opioids were required to manage deafferentation pain compared with nociceptive pain. These clinical observations are consistent with recent experimental observations that report a fourfold decrease in the potency of morphine when primary afferent fibers are severed. However, recent studies support the use of opioids for severe neuropathic pain (Dellemijn, 1997; Cherny et al., 1994).

Somatic, visceral, and deafferentation pain may be modified by the sympathetic nervous system, as evidenced by the positive response of some patients to anesthetic and pharmacologic sympathetic blockade. Sympathetically maintained pain is often suspected when pain is severe in intensity (even after relatively trivial tissue insults) and is described as burning in quality, with associated features of allodynia, hyperpathia, brawny edema, and osteoporosis. Several mechanisms involving both the peripheral and central nervous systems have been postulated to explain SMP. One peripheral mechanism may be the development of ephaptic connections at sites of tissue injury whereby efferent sympathetic impulses produce activation of afferent nociceptive pathways. Other investigators have postulated that traumatic injury to peripheral tissues may produce sensitization of spinal cord nociceptive neurons, which may then be secondarily activated by efferent sympathetic activity. Despite debate concerning its physiological mechanisms, the clinical recognition of SMP is critical, as prompt sympathetic blockade and aggressive physical therapy and mobilization of the affected part(s) are vital for achieving a good clinical outcome.

It is common (indeed usual) for cancer patients to present with mixtures of the pain types, mandating initiation of multiple therapeutic approaches ("balanced analgesia") (Payne and Foley, 1984). Furthermore, the pattern of pain intensity is often not constant, but rather includes episodes of pain exacerbations, called *breakthrough pain,* which is defined as a "transitory exacerbation of pain that occurs on a background of otherwise stable persistent pain" (Reddy and Nguyen, 2000). Breakthrough pain is well recognized as the most intractable pain to manage and in some studies has been the reliable predictor of poor response to treatment with routine pharmacotherapy (Bruera et al., 1989c, 1995). This typical pattern suggests that continuous, or around-the-clock analgesic therapies are appropriate for the vast majority of cancer patients and that strategies for treating incident and breakthrough pain (Portenoy and Hagen, 1990) should be implemented to ensure adequate pain relief during periods of exacerbation.

As has been emphasized, the clinical assessment of pain may be critical in defining its etiology, and several principles have been delineated that are essential to this assessment. Table 23–2 lists the parameters involved in the assessment of cancer pain.

SPECIFIC PAIN SYNDROMES IN PATIENTS WITH CANCER

Neurologists and oncologists when evaluating the cancer patient with pain encounter several specific pain syndromes that present difficult diagnostic and therapeutic problems (Kelly and Payne, 1991). Clinical data comprising these syndromes are summarized below and listed in Table 23–3.

Invasion of bone by either primary or metastatic tumor causes pain in most patients with cancer. Important pain syndromes are often misdiagnosed because physicians are unfamiliar with their characteristic signs and symptoms, and plain X-rays of the involved areas may be (falsely) negative. Some of these syndromes are considered below.

Tumor Infiltration of Bone

The pathophysiology of metastatic bone pain is poorly understood. Although most patients with bone metastasis report pain, some patients with well-established lesions do not. Occasional patients report bone pain when radiographic lesions are not evident. This phenomenon has been best studied in breast cancer (Front et al., 1979), but also occurs in patients with prostate cancer. Tumor growth in bone may produce pain through several mechanisms: *(1)* Relatively rapid growth causes expansion of the marrow space and increases interosseal pressure (beyond 50 mm Hg). In theory, this may activate mechanoreceptive nociceptors in bone. Elevation or invasion of the periosteum may also activate nociceptors, which innervate this structure. *(2)* Weakening of the bone causes fractures. *(3)* Edema and inflammation associated with tumor growth in bone may liberate chemical mediators that activate nociceptors. *(4)* Finally, data regarding mechanisms of bone destruction postulate that osteoclasts may be stimulated by humoral factors associated with tumors. For example, carcinomas

Table 23–2. Assessment of Cancer Pain

History
1. Ask patient about pain and use a self-report form
   a. Use simple scales (e.g., 0–10 numerical scale or visual analog scale)
   b. Pain when patient is at rest and when moving
   c. Pattern of pain (i.e., the presence of continuous and/or breakthrough pain)
2. Evaluate psychosocial dimensions of pain and cancer experience
   a. Coexisting depression, anxiety, and psychological distress
   b. Meaning of pain to patient and family
   c. Attitudes about pain and drug use (especially opioid use) with patient and family

Physical and neurologic examinations
1. Evaluate site of pain and examine possible sites of referral
2. Evaluate presence of secondary myofascial pains, trigger points, or muscle spasms
3. Evaluate motor, sensory, and autonomic findings (especially for neuropathic pain syndromes)

Neuroimaging studies
1. Review radiographic studies to ensure that appropriate body parts were imaged
2. Be aware of false-negative bone scans in areas of prior irradiation
3. Know the limitations of plain radiographs in C7–T1 and base of skull areas
4. Pain may precede "objective" radiographic evidence of tumor recurrence

Reassess pain
1. Evaluate at frequent intervals
2. Evaluate at transition points in patient's care

Table 23–3 Intractable Pain Syndromes*

Pain Syndromes	*Clinical Characteristics*
Tumor-related infiltration of bone	Acute and chronic nociceptive pain
Skull-base metastasis	Severe head pain (usually referred to vertex or occiput) with associated cranial nerve deficits
	Bone scan and plain films of the skull may be negative
Vertebral metastasis	Significant risk of associated spinal cord compression†
Pelvis and long bone	Risk of pathologic fracture with weight-bearing activities; orthopedic consultation helpful
Tumor-related infiltration of nerve	Acute and chronic neuropathic pain
Brachial/lumbosacral plexopathy	May occur by contiguous spread of tumor or by hematogenous dissemination; radiographic studies helpful to distinguish from radiation-induced plexopathy
Spinal cord compression	Neurologic emergency requiring prompt treatment with corticosteroids, radiation therapy, and/or surgery
Meningeal carcinomatosis	Headache and meningeal signs cause significant pain in about 15% of patients
Visceral tumor infiltration‡	Acute and chronic visceral pain that is poorly localized and widely referred
Therapy related; post-surgical pain	Chronic pain that persists well beyond healing of the incision and may or may not be associated with recurrent disease
After thoracotomy	May be associated with recurrent tumor or may occur as a chronic intercostal neuralgia
After mastectomy	Occurs in 5% of women; more common in women undergoing modified radical procedure with axillary dissection; intercostal-brachioradial neuralgia is one etiology
After radical neck surgery	Mechanisms unclear; chronic infection may play a role
After amputation	Stump pain and phantom phenomena are common; role of preventive analgesic and anesthetic therapies under investigation

*List excludes significant but short-lived pain syndromes such as mucositis that complicate chemotherapy and radiation therapy and the acute pain associated with diagnostic and therapeutic procedures such as bone marrow aspiration.

†30% of patients with back pain and vertebral body metastases will eventually develop epidural spinal cord compression, and pain alone may precede root or spinal cord signs by many months.

‡Common examples include pancreatic carcinoma, liver metastasis, and pleural effusion.

may secrete PG (Galasko, 1982), which would have the dual role of activating osteoclasts and sensitizing nociceptors. These observations have provided a rationale for the use of corticosteroids and nonsteroidal anti-inflammatory analgesics such as naprosyn for the management of metastatic bone pain (Levick et al., 1988). Lymphomas and myelomas may secrete another chemical, osteoclast-activating factor. However, the effects of osteoclast-activating factor on bone nociceptors are not yet known.

Metastatic bone pain is often associated with neurologic dysfunction because of the close anatomic relationships between the brain and cranial nerves with the skull vault and spinal cord with the vertebral column. Therefore, characteristic clinical syndromes may be identified by the site of bony involvement, the co-existence of mechanical instability secondary to fractures, and neurologic dysfunction caused by tumor infiltration of contiguous neurologic structures. Bone metastases to the hip and pelvis often produce local pain, which is exacerbated by movement, especially during weight bearing. In addition to palliative radiotherapy, this type of "incident pain" may require specific orthopedic interventions for satisfactory control of pain, such as pinning and other mechanisms of mechanical stabilization. In fact, true incident pain is notoriously difficult to manage with conventional analgesic therapy alone. Unilateral incident pain at or below the waist, which has failed management with hormonal and radiation therapy in addition to analgesics, may require cordotomy as the ultimate means of treatment (Foley, 1993).

Spread of cancer to the vertebral bodies and calvarium, especially the skull base, often produces distinctive neurologic syndromes. It is important to recognize these early because prompt initiation of antitumor treatments (especially radiation) may prevent neurologic impairment. For example, local and radicular back or neck pain is the predominant symptom in epidural spinal cord compression, complicating vertebral body metastasis in these locations. Pain may be the only symptom of impending spinal cord compression and often precedes motor weakness and bowel or bladder incontinence by days or weeks. The spinal cord is compromised by growth of tumor in an anterior direction from the vertebral body. Irreversible spinal cord injury may occur when the vascular supply is compromised as a result of severe compression. Thoracic spine vertebral body metastases often produce bilateral radicular pain and sensory symptoms (a "band-like" squeezing sensation across the upper abdomen or chest) because of the close proximity of the thoracic nerve roots to the vertebral body. On the other hand, metastasis to the cervical or lumbar spine may produce unilateral pain and sensory loss as the vertebral bodies are wider in these areas and lateral extension of the tumor may compress only one root at the time.

Cervical Spine Metastasis

Metastatic disease involving the odontoid process of the axis (C1 vertebral body) results in a pathologic fracture. Secondary subluxation occurs and results in spinal cord or brain stem compression. The symptoms are usually severe neck pain radiating over the posterior aspect of the skull to the vertex, which is exacerbated by movement. Diagnostic evaluation may require tomography or computed tomography (CT) scanning as plain X-rays and bone scans may be negative. Imaging procedures must be done carefully and with neurosurgical consultation to ensure spinal stability.

Pain localized to the adjacent paraspinal area is characterized by a constant dull aching pain radiating bilaterally to both shoulders with tenderness to percussion over the spinous process. Radicular pain in a C7–8 distribution occurs most commonly unilaterally in the posterior arm, elbow, and ulnar aspect of the hand. Paresthesias and numbness in the fourth and fifth fingers and progressive hand and triceps weakness are the neurologic signs. Horner's syndrome suggests paraspinal involvement. The diagnostic evaluation must be done carefully. Plain X-rays are often negative because they visualize this area poorly and CT, or preferably magnetic resonance imaging (MRI), scans are necessary to define metastatic disease.

Lumbar Spine and Sacral Metastasis

Dull and aching mid-back pain exacerbated by lying or sitting and relieved by standing is the usual presenting complaint of L1 metastasis: Pain may be referred to the hip. Radicular pain occurs anteriorly to both paraspinal lumbosacral areas, and referred pain affects the sacroiliac joint or superior iliac crest.

Aching pain in the lower back or coccygeal region exacerbated by lying or sitting and relieved by walking is the common complaint associated with sacral metastases. Symptoms include perianal sensory loss, bowel and bladder dysfunction, and impotence (see section on lumbosacral plexopathy for a more complete discussion).

The onset of back pain in association with band-like tightening across the chest or upper abdominal area, or radicular arm or leg pain, may be the first sign of impending spinal cord compression. Motor and sensory losses occur later, and autonomic disturbances producing bladder and bowel incontinence occur later still. Thus, evaluation of the patient should begin at the onset of pain for the best chance to preserve motor and sphincteric function and should include plain X-rays of the entire spine, focused on the symptomatic area, and an MRI or CT myelogram, which image the entire spine. This is a necessary diagnostic step because there is an approximately 15% incidence of another (clinically silent) epidural lesion being present (Byrne and Waxman, 1990).

Corticosteroid therapy should be started before radiologic evaluation, which may decrease pain and protect the spinal cord from further compression caused by edema from tumor or radiotherapy. If metastatic disease is found on plain spine films, MRI or CT myelogram should be done to define the extent of tumor invasion into the epidural space. This information influences the size of radiation therapy ports and determines the dose and duration of corticosteroid therapy.

If anterior vertebral body subluxation has occurred and there is bony compression of the spinal cord, surgical decompression is indicated if the patient's medical condition is stable enough to withstand the procedure. Surgical decompression is usually followed by radiation therapy. Surgery is usually not attempted as the primary treatment modality because the results of radiation therapy and corticosteroid treatment together are usually equal to the results achieved from surgical decompression (Byrne and Waxman, 1990). This is especially true if a simple posterior decompressive laminectomy is performed. However, if patients have recurrent spinal cord compression in a previously irradiated port, then an anterior spinal approach with removal of tumor from the vertebral body, decompression of tumor from the spinal canal, and restructuring of the vertebral body with methylmethacrylate should be considered (Sundaresan et al., 1989). Recently vertebroplasty has gained popularity in vetebral metastasis causing pain due to fractures, without neurologic involvement (Cotten et al., 1996; Martin et al., 1999).

Local invasion of tumor from the pelvis into the sacrum may produce the syndrome of perineal pain, which is often difficult to manage. This syndrome is characterized by local pain in the buttocks and perirectal area, which is often accentuated by pressure on the perineal region such as that caused by sitting or lying prone. In its most extreme form, patients cannot sit to eat meals or lie flat to sleep and may spend much of their time standing. Because of the critical role of the parasympathetic sacral innervation to normal bladder and rectal sphincter function, continence is impaired early in the course of this syndrome (in distinction to spinal cord compression with more rostrally placed lesions), perhaps even before significant weakness can be discerned in the legs.

Skull Metastasis

Spread of tumor to the calvarium may produce neurologic symptoms via a number of mechanisms. Metastases to the skull vault, which compress the sagittal sinus, may produce a syndrome of severe headache with associated papilledema and seizures caused by elevated intracranial pressure. If untreated, focal neurologic deficits may occur secondary to (hemorrhagic) venous infarction of the brain. The cause of metastatic sagittal sinus occlusion is usually obvious and is easily confirmed by MRI imaging of the brain. Gadolinium-enhanced MRI demonstrates tumor metastasis as well as occlusion of the sagittal sinus. Nonmetastatic sagittal sinus occlusion may also occur as a complication of a hypercoagulable state induced by diethylstilbestrol treatment of prostate cancer or secondary to treatment with asparaginase for acute lymphoblastic leukemia.

Tumor metastasis to the base of the skull produces distinct neurologic syndromes (Greenberg et al., 1981). In general, bone metastasis to this portion of the skull often produces severe headache referred to the top of the head or occiput. Single or multiple cranial nerve palsies usually accompany basal skull metastasis. For example, clival metastases often compress the hypoglossal nerve, producing unilateral weakness of the tongue with deviation to the side of the lesion when protruded. Bone metastasis to the middle cranial fossa may compress and infiltrate the facial nerve, producing ipsilateral weakness of the upper and lower face. Tumor invasion of the jugular foramen will produce severe head pain with associated dysphagia, dysphonia, and hoarseness caused by dysfunction of the glossopharyngeal and vagal nerves that exit the skull base through this foramen.

Small lesions at the skull base may not be seen by plain films or bone scans of the skull. It is mandatory that CT scans with bone windows and 5 mm sections (so-called thin cuts) are done to demonstrate the tumor. It is sometimes desirable to image the base of the skull with MRI when CT scans are negative (Kelly and Payne, 1991). Radiation therapy directed to the base of the skull is the preferred treatment. Again, prompt recognition of these syndromes and aggressive treatment can prevent irreversible cranial nerve palsies, which often produce devastating neurologic impairments.

TUMOR INFILTRATION OR TRAUMA TO PERIPHERAL NERVE, PLEXUS, AND ROOT

These syndromes present with radicular pain in the neck, chest, or trunk. The differential diagnosis includes tumor infiltration of the peripheral nerves and surgical injury—either partial, complete, or secondary to direct surgical interruption or traction, nerve compression secondary to musculoskeletal imbalance, diabetic peripheral neuropathy, acute herpes zoster, and postherpetic neuralgia.

Managing pain in these syndromes is hindered in general by the lack of any well-established approach to treat neuropathic pain, characterized by constant burning pain with hypesthesias and dysesthesias in an area of sensory loss. The most common causes are tumor compression in the paravertebral or retroperitoneal area or metastatic tumor in the rib, which causes intercostal nerve infiltration.

Pain, either local, radicular, or referred, is usually the first sign that tumor has infiltrated nerve. Local and radicular pain occur when tumor infiltrates or compresses nerves peripheral to the paraspinal region, whereas referred pain with or without a radicular component occurs when tumor infiltrates the paraspinal region and more proximal areas. Associated autonomic dysfunction (i.e., loss of sweating and of axonal flair response to pin scratch) can help define the site of nerve compression or infiltration. Pain is initially characterized as a dull, aching sensation with tenderness to percussion in the distribution of the nerve. Mild paresthesiae or dysesthesiae may be the next sensory symptom, followed by the late appearance of motor symptoms and signs. As tumor invades the perineurium or compresses nerve externally, the nature of the pain changes to a burning, dysesthetic sensation. A careful neurologic examination followed by a CT scan to define the site of nerve compression are the diagnostic procedures of choice. Electromyography can help to define the site of nerve involvement, but is not diagnostic. Rib erosion and retroperitoneal and paraspinal soft tissue masses are the most common associated findings. For patients with paraspinal tumor, myelography (and/or MRI scanning) is often necessary to exclude epidural extension. Antitumor therapy is the first-line therapy when possible, but interim pain management with analgesics is almost always necessary.

Steroids may provide a useful diagnostic test while providing both anti-inflammatory and antitumor effects or may reduce local swelling and, secondarily, relieve pain. However, they are not an option for long-term management because of their toxicity. The sequelae of long-term steroid use are peripheral edema, weight gain, hyperglycemia, cataracts, osteoporosis with compression fractures, and an increased risk of infection from immunosuppression.

Brachial Plexopathy

In patients with cancer, brachial plexopathy may occur via

1. Metastatic spread of tumor to the plexus
2. Radiation injury producing transient sensory and motor symptoms and more prolonged neurologic dysfunction resulting from previous radiation therapy (RT) to a port that has included the plexus
3. Involvement of the plexus by radiation-induced tumor such as malignant schwannoma or fibrosarcoma
4. Trauma to the plexus during surgery and anesthesia

Tumor infiltration and radiation injury are the most common causes (Kori et al., 1981). A review of 100 cases suggested that reliable clinical signs and symptoms distinguish metastatic plexopathy from radiation injury. The characteristics of the pain are quite different from each cause and create useful distinguishing clinical signs.

Computed tomography is useful in diagnosing brachial plexus region pain, as described in the studies by Cascino et al. (1983). However, recently MRI scanning has been advocated as the optimal imaging technique for the brachial plexus region (Blair et al., 1987) and may be useful for diagnosing metastatic brachial plexopathy. Median nerve somatosensory evoked potentials (MSEP) is a useful neurodiagnostic tool to detect the site of nerve involvement in patients with pain of the upper extremity. This modality may detect brachial plexus lesions earlier than radiologic studies. Electrodiagnostic studies (electromyography [EMG]) are useful in distinguishing tumor infiltration of the brachial plexus from radiation injury. When present, myokymia is almost always associated with radiation injury of the plexus. However, in patients who present with neurologic symptoms in a C8–Tl distribution in a port of previous radiation, the presence of myokymia does not exclude tumor infiltration of the plexus. In fact, the authors have seen several patients with both radiation fibrosis and tumor occurring simultaneously in whom myokymia was present.

Rarely, biopsy of the brachial plexus may be necessary to distinguish (recurrent) tumor infiltration from radiation fibrosis or the occurrence of a new primary tumor (Payne and Foley, 1986). Biopsy is not, however, always definitive.

Metastases to the brachial plexus most commonly involve the lower cords of the brachial plexus, giving rise to neurologic signs and symptoms in the distribution of the C8, T1 roots. In contrast, radiation plexopathy most commonly involves the upper cords of the plexus, predominantly in the distribution of the

C5, C6, and C7 roots. Severe pain is most often associated with metastatic plexopathy, and Horner's syndrome is more frequently associated with metastatic plexopathy than with radiation plexopathy. A significant number of patients with metastatic plexopathy demonstrated epidural extension of disease. A primary tumor of the lung, the presence of Horner's syndrome, and involvement of the whole plexus should alert the physician to the possibility of epidural extension and warrants an immediate myelogram (or MRI scan). Neither a negative surgical biopsy nor observation for several years for other metastases rules out recurrence of tumor or a new primary tumor (Payne and Foley, 1986).

Brachial Plexopathy in Pancoast Tumors

Brachial plexopathy in Pancoast tumors, as described by Kanner et al. (1981), is an integral part of the disease. Pain in the distribution of C8–Tl is an early sign and is one aspect of the clinical diagnosis of Pancoast syndrome. Pain is the most reliable sign to follow as it closely reflects the progression of disease and may be the only sign of epidural cord compression. Plain X-rays and bone scans are not reliable diagnostic tests in assessing this disorder, whereas CT scans and myelograms yield the most important diagnostic information. As many as 50% of patients develop epidural cord compression, with pain being the earliest and most consistent clinical symptom. In patients who present with a Pancoast syndrome and involvement of the brachial plexus, the initial diagnostic work-up should include a CT scan, tomograms of the vertebral bodies, and myelography to determine the extent of tumor infiltration. Initial antitumor surgery should be directed at radial removal of all local tumor. Secondary treatment is composed of external radiation therapy and brachytherapy (Sundaresan et al., 1987).

The Pancoast syndrome is commonly misdiagnosed and confused with cervical disc disease, which appears in less than 5% of patients in a C8–Tl distribution. Early diagnosis of tumor is crucial to curative therapy, and neurologists often play an important role in the initial evaluation of these patients.

Lumbosacral Plexopathy

Lumbosacral plexus tumor infiltration most commonly occurs in genitourinary, gynecologic, and colonic cancers (Jaeckle et al., 1985). Pain varies with the site of plexus involvement. Radicular pain occurs in an L1 through L3 distribution (i.e., anterior thigh and groin) or down the posterior aspect of the leg to the heel with an L5/S1 distribution. In some instances, there is only referred pain without local pain over the plexus. Common referred points are the anterior thigh, knee, and lateral aspect of the calf. These areas are commonly painful, but the origin of the pain is in the plexus. Pain is the earliest symptom, followed later by complaints of paresthesiae, numbness, and dysesthesiae leading to motor and sensory loss.

The clinical symptoms and natural history of this disorder have been described by Jaeckle et al. (1985) in a review of 85 patients with lumbosacral plexopathy. Pain was noted to be of three types: local in 72 of 85 patients, radicular in 72 of 85 patients, and referred in 37 of 85 patients. Local pain in the sacrum or sciatic notch occurred in 59% of patients, followed by low back pain in 27% and pain in the groin or lower abdominal quadrant in 21%. Pain referred to the hip or flank occurred in patients who had upper plexus lesions, whereas pain in the ankle or the foot occurred in patients with a lower plexopathy. Typically, the pain precedes objective sensory, motor, and autonomic signs for weeks to months (mean of 3 months), and initially the CT scan may be negative. Unilateral and bilateral plexopathy with significant motor weakness is commonly associated with epidural extension, and both CT scan and myelography are necessary to define the extent of tumor infiltration and/or epidural compression. Plain X-rays are not often helpful because the lumbosacral plexus lies within the substance of the psoas muscle and is not radiodense. Specific antitumor therapy depends on the tumor type, and relief of pain symptomatology is directly related to tumor responsiveness. Patients with colorectal and cervical cancers and sarcomas have persistent pain and progressive plexopathy. Pain management for these patients is particularly difficult because selective analgesia cannot be provided without interfering with motor, sensory, and autonomic functions.

Overall, management of painful plexopathies is currently unsatisfactory, but a series of approaches have been tried with varying success. All patients should be managed with nonopioid and opioid analgesics. Steroids are helpful for those patients who have significant local swelling because they have anti-inflammatory and antitumor effects and provide additive analgesia. For patients with acute lancinating pain superimposed on dysesthetic pain, carbamazepine is sometimes helpful, as are tricyclic antidepressants (Wiffen et al., 2000; Swerdlow, 1984). Newer anticonvulsants like gabapentin, lamotrigine, and oxcarbazepine may offer advantages as far as their side effect profiles are concerned (Zakrzewska et al., 1997; McCleane, 2000; Remillard, 1994).

Specific anesthetic and neurosurgical pain management approaches vary with the site of tumor involvement. Epidural local anesthetics can provide local pain relief for lumbosacral plexopathy and can be appropriately titrated to provide only sensory loss. However, they cannot be maintained for long periods of time because a tolerance develops to their analgesic effects, along with infection of the catheter track and epidural space. Epidural or intrathecal phenol or alcohol are used to produce chemical neurolysis and can be titrated to produce predominant sensory changes. Recently, psoas compartment neurolysis has been shown to treat upper plexus pain (Calava et al., 1996). However, loss of motor function and in some cases bladder incontinence are limitations of these procedures. The patient's terminal status and the intractability of these pain syndromes may, however, provide a favorable risk/benefit ratio for taking these measures.

Subarachnoid administration of phenol and alcohol to block the cauda equina can produce bowel and bladder dysfunction with associated motor loss. No patient should undergo a subarachnoid lumbar block (or spinal opioid administration) with such agents until MRI has demonstrated the patency of the subarachnoid space (Cherry et al., 1986). The patient must understand the consequences of undergoing these procedures, which may involve loss of autonomic function and (mild) bilateral leg weakness.

Percutaneous or open cordotomy may be helpful for patients with unilateral lumbosacral plexopathy. However, for those with brachial plexopathy, the results are much less impressive because pain radiating to the neck and ears often escapes the cordotomy level. Bilateral pain from a bilateral lumbosacral plexopathy requires a bilateral cordotomy for effective pain control with a consequent risk to bowel and bladder function as well as bilateral corticospinal tract involvement. Epidural and intrathecal morphine infusions can provide analgesia that is selective without interfering with motor, sensory, and autonomic function (Payne, 1987). However, this technique is limited by the fact that escalation of drug doses as tolerance to the drug develops limits its usefulness for patients who have far advanced disease and a prior exposure to opioids. Epidural and intrathecal infusions are each associated with significant systemic uptake of the drugs and do not completely obviate the side effects of systemic drug administration (Max et al., 1987). Recently, epidural clonidine has been approved for cancer pain management and has been used successfully for neuropathic cancer pain (Eisenach et al., 1995). Neuronal-specific calcium channel blockers administered intrathecally may be used to treat such intractable neuropathic pain syndromes in the future (Bowersox et al., 1996). Although these techniques provide useful alternatives, they are not the sole techniques for treating these pain syndromes. In most cases, a multipronged approach provides optimal control of pain and other symptoms resulting from cancer.

Both dorsal column stimulation and periventricular brain stimulation have been of limited usefulness in this patient population. Behavioral techniques help patients cope with pain and control the associated symptoms of anxiety and depression, which occur with chronic pain and neurologic disability. These syndromes are particularly difficult to manage, and the effectiveness of the approaches used depends on the expertise available to the patient and his or her physician as well as a willingness on the part of the patient to undergo novel procedures in return for only partial relief.

Leptomeningeal Neoplasia

Pain occurs in 40% of patients with leptomeningeal metastases (Wasserstrom et al., 1982) and is of two types: headache with or without neck stiffness or back pain localized to the low back and buttocks. There may be associated confusion, delirium, cranial nerve palsies, radiculopathy, and myelopathy. Diagnostic work-up should include an MRI (with contrast) to determine enhancement in the basal subarachnoid cisterns and to rule out hydrocephalus. Magnetic resonance imaging can also rule out bulk disease on the nerve roots, which might require focal radiation therapy. A lumbar puncture should be performed to determine cerebrospinal fluid glucose, protein, cell count, cytology and biochemical markers (e.g., α-microglobulin, CEA, and LDH).

PAIN SYNDROMES ASSOCIATED WITH CANCER THERAPY

This category includes clinical pain syndromes that occur in the course of or subsequent to treatment of cancer patients with the common modalities of surgery, chemotherapy, or radiation therapy.

Post-Surgical Pain—Surgical Injury to Peripheral Nerves

Four distinct pain syndromes involving the peripheral nerves occur following surgery in patients who have cancer. These are outlined in the following sections.

Post-Thoracotomy Pain

Post-thoracotomy pain occurs in the distribution of an intercostal nerve following surgical interruption or injury. The intercostal neurovascular bundle (vein, artery, and nerve) courses along a groove in the inferior border of the rib. Traction on the ribs and rib resection are the common causes of nerve injury during a surgical procedure on the chest. Kanner et al. (1981) prospectively evaluated 126 consecutive patients undergoing thoracotomy and defined several groups of patients. In most (79 patients,) immediate postoperative pain was reduced at approximately 2 months, but 13 of the 79 patients had a recurrence of pain caused by recurrence of tumor in the distribution of the intercostal nerves. Immediate postoperative pain is characterized by an aching sensation in the distribution of the incision and sensory loss, with or without autonomic changes. There is often an exquisite point of tenderness at the most medial and apical point of the scar with a specific trigger point. In another group of patients, pain persisted in 16% (20/126) after thoracotomy and increased in intensity during the follow-up period. Local recurrences of disease and/or infection were the most common cause of increasing pain in this group of patients. In the third group, 14% (18/126) of patients had stable or decreasing pain, which resolved over time and did not represent a difficult management problem. Therefore, persistent or recurrent pain in the distribution of the thoracotomy scar in patients with cancer is commonly associated with recurrent tumor. The one caveat to this conclusion is that a small number of patients will have a traumatic neuroma at the site of a previous thoracotomy scar, but this should not be the initial consideration in their evaluation.

Chest X-rays are insufficient for evaluating recurrent disease. A CT scan (or MRI) through the chest with bone and soft tissue windows is the diagnostic procedure of choice. These imaging studies are also necessary before consideration of intercostal nerve blocks for pain management of these syndromes. If pain management is inadequate or the patient is not actively rehabilitated following surgery, a frozen shoulder and secondary reflex sympathetic dystrophy involving the arm can occur. This complication requires early and active mobilization of the arm and active physical therapy combined with analgesics, occasionally steroids, and occasionally sympathetic blocks of the stellate ganglion. The nature of the pain in patients with traumatic neuroma in contrast to tumor infiltration of the nerve is not sufficiently distinct clinically, and the ability to localize a specific trigger point and to provide dramatic pain relief with a local anesthetic blockade are strong indications to suggest traumatic neuroma as a possible etiology. Cryoprobes to freeze the peripheral nerve have also been used in the management of patients with post-thoracotomy pain (Katz et al., 1980) and may be useful in the other syndromes. The management of tumor infiltration depends on the type of cancer and the specific antitumor therapy available.

Post-Mastectomy Pain

Post-mastectomy pain occurs in the posterior arm, axilla, and anterior chest wall following any surgical procedure on the breast whether lumpectomy or radical mastectomy (Watson et al., 1989). It is especially likely to occur after axillary and lymph node dissection (Vecht et al., 1989). The marked anatomic variation in size and distribution of the intercostal brachial nerve accounts for the variable appearance of this syndrome in patients who are undergoing mastectomy. Pain results from interruption of the intercostal brachial nerve, a cutaneous sensory branch of Tl–T2. The pain may occur immediately after surgery and as long as 6 months later. It is characterized as a tight, constricting, burning pain in the posterior aspect of the arm and axilla radiating across the anterior chest wall. The pain is exacerbated by movement of the arm and relieved by its immobilization.

Patients often posture their arm in a flexed position close to the chest wall, placing them at risk of developing a frozen shoulder syndrome if adequate pain and post-surgical rehabilitation are not implemented early on. Approximately 5% of women undergoing surgical procedures on the breast develop this syndrome. The nature of the pain and the clinical symptomatology should readily distinguish it from tumor infiltration of the brachial plexus. The syndrome appears to occur most commonly in patients with postoperative complications who are at risk for local fibrosis in and about the nerve following surgery (e.g., following wound infection or seroma). Typically a trigger point in the axilla or on the anterior chest wall may be found, which is usually the site of the traumatic neuroma. Breast reconstruction does not alter the tight, constricting sensation in the anterior chest wall that is associated with this syndrome. The management of pain in this syndrome is similar to the management of pain for any patient with peripheral nerve injury and pain.

Post-Radical Neck Surgery

Prospective studies of post-radical neck dissection pain are lacking. In any patient in whom the pain occurs late (i.e., several months after the surgical procedure) and particularly any pain occurring several years following the surgical procedure, re-evaluation is necessary to exclude the recurrence of tumor. This is particularly true of adenocystic tumors involving the head and neck, which typically invade and metastasize locally along peripheral nerve, giving rise to sensory loss and several qualities of painful sensations, including burning dysesthesia and shock-like shooting and lancinating pains.

Post-Amputation Phenomena

Loss of a body part is often followed by a psychological adjustment period that may include a grief reaction (Bradway et al., 1984). The physiologic phenomena of nonpainful and painful phantom sensations (referred to the missing part), pain in the scar region (called a stump after limb amputation), and involuntary motor activity also occur.

Phantom sensations may be divided into three types. Kinetic sensations, the perception of movement, may be spontaneous or willed. Kinesthetic perceptions, those of size, shape, and position of the body part, may be normal or distorted. Exteroceptive perceptions of touch, temperature, pressure, itch, and vibration are frequently reported. Patients readily distinguish unpleasant or annoying sensations from those labeled as painful. Many patients note most sensations in the distal phantom limb or in the nipple of the phantom breast. A phantom visceral organ may be associated with functional sensations (e.g., the urge to urinate or defecate).

Phantom pains may be described as intense versions of normal exteroceptive sensations. Patients offer bizarre descriptors, such as "my foot is being crushed by a bar rolling over it, and my toes are twisted." The intensity, frequency, and duration of pain, as well as provocative and palliative factors, differ among individuals.

Stump pain may be associated with or occur independently of phantom pain. The usual postoperative wound pain is expected to resolve as healing takes place. Persistent stump pain may be due to a local pathologic process, for example, circulatory disturbance, infection, and tumor, or other lesions of skin, soft tissue, or bone. Neuromas, which develop at the severed end of peripheral nerve, may act as a trigger for phantom pain and contribute to stump pain (see "Pathophysiology", below).

The natural history of phantom limb pain has been best studied in trauma patients and those undergoing surgical amputation for nonmalignant conditions (Sherman et al., 1984). There is wide variation in the reported incidence of severe persistent phantom pain due to many factors. Many investigators fail to distinguish painful from nonpainful phantom sensations and phantom from stump pain. It is also known that patients may be reluctant to report their phantom sensations and pain. A thorough review of the literature supports the conclusion that virtually all patients have nonpainful phantom sensations and that the majority have unpleasant or painful phantoms even if only briefly (Jensen et al., 1984).

Painful and nonpainful phantoms change in character and location. Patients often describe "telescoping" or shortening of the phantom limb over time. They may perceive only the distal portion of the limb attached to the stump. Others have reported gradual fading of the phantom. A common course would be gradual reduction in the frequency and duration of painful episodes, generally over several weeks to 2 years. Late-appearing phantom pain has been reported, although most patients note the onset of phantom pain soon after amputation.

Although persistent phantom pain is unusual before age 8 years, patients as young as 4 years old have reported phantom limb pain (Simmel, 1962). Verbal children describe feelings in a limb that is no longer present and can distinguish phantom from stump pain.

The value of preoperative pain for predicting post-amputation pain is not well established. Some data support a positive predictive value of preoperative pain as a harbinger for postoperative pain (Wall et al., 1985; Jensen et al., 1985). One study has shown that preoperative pain predicted immediate postoperative pain that resembled preoperative pain in character and location. This implies a persistence of preoperative nociceptive paths, or memory of pain, which usually resolves in the subacute period (Katz and Melzack, 1990). Patients with significant preoperative pain have a similar risk as patients without preoperative pain of developing chronic phantom pain (different from their preoperative pain).

A few reports chart the course of post-amputation pain in malignant disease. In a study of 17 cancer patients who underwent forequarter amputation, after an average of 69 months follow up none of the 7 survivors experienced pain that required the use of analgesics (Steinke et al., 1991). Larger surveys of post-mastectomy patients reveal that at least 10% experience chronic phantom breast pain, a greater percentage than is generally believed (Kroner et al., 1989). Increasing pain in the cancer amputee may signify disease progression or recurrence (Sugarbaker et al., 1984; Boas et al., 1993).

Treatment Approaches for Phantom Limb Pain

Many treatment approaches have been tried to alleviate phantom pain, including medications, neurostimulation, ablation of peripheral and central nervous system structures, physical therapy, and psychological and behavioral methods. In 1984, Sherman reviewed phantom pain treatment methods in the United States. He noted that of the 68 treatment methods reported, none was uniformly successful. Subsequent reviews by Davis (1993) concluded similarly.

As for many other types of neuropathic pain, the efficacy of pharmacologic interventions varies between individuals. Thus, patients should be given sequential pharmacologic interventions, including opiates (Foley, 1993). The administration of intrathecal fentanyl reduced phantom limb pain and induced painless phantoms in a few cases of chronic phantom pain. Analgesia was not improved with concurrent administration of lidocaine (Jacobson et al., 1989, 1990). Anecdotal reports suggest that some patients benefit from carbamazepine (Patterson, 1988) and other anticonvulsants (Backonja, 2000). Amitriptyline may be efficacious for phantom pain in children (Rogers, 1989). In one randomized trial of topical application of capsaicin for general post-mastectomy pain, 62% of 13 patients reported 50% or better pain relief (Watson and Evans, 1992). Capsaicin has also been reported to relieve chronic stump pain (Rayner et al., 1989).

Physical stimulation of the stump by mechanical, thermal, and electrical means provides relief for some patients. In a randomized trial of 51 patients (Finsen, 1988), transcutaneous electrical nerve stimulation (TENS) resulted in faster stump healing, but did not affect postoperative pain or chronic phantom pain. Auricular TENS resulted in small but significant differences in painful and painless phantoms in a crossover study of 28 amputees (Katz and Melzack, 1991).

No specific recommendations can be offered to identify the operative procedures that are most likely to reduce the incidence of post-amputation pain. Postoperative compression bandaging or hard casting to reduce stump edema may facilitate rehabilitation. It is not certain if this contributes to pain relief.

In a small series of patients undergoing amputation for nonmalignant disease, a threefold reduction in the incidence of phantom pain 1 year after amputation was demonstrated after preoperative ("preemptive") treatment with an epidural infusion of opioid and local anesthetic (Bach, 1988).

Chemotherapy-Related Pain Syndromes

Painful dysesthesias follow treatment with several chemotherapeutic agents, in particular the Vinca alkaloid drugs (i.e., vincristine and vinblastine). Cisplatin and taxol are also toxic to peripheral nerve (Young and Posner, 1985; Asbury and Bird, 1992). These agents produce a symmetric polyneuropathy as a result of a subacute chronic axonopathy. Pain is usually localized to the hands and feet and is characterized as burning pain exacerbated by superficial stimuli, which improves as the drug is withdrawn.

Steroid pseudorheumatism (Rotstein and Good, 1957) is characterized by diffuse myalgias and arthralgias, with muscle and joint tenderness on palpation. It occurs from both rapid and slow withdrawal of steroid medication in patients taking these drugs for either short or long periods of time. The signs and symptoms revert with reconstitution of the steroid medication.

Aseptic necrosis of the humeral and, more commonly, femoral head is a known complication of chronic steroid therapy (Ihde and DeVita, 1975). Pain in the shoulder and knee or leg is the common presenting complaint, with X-ray changes occurring several weeks to months after the onset of pain. A bone scan and MRI scan are the most useful diagnostic procedures.

Post-herpetic neuralgia (Loeser, 1986) can be thought of as a postchemotherapy pain syndrome because immunocompromised patients are at risk for acute herpes zoster infection or a recurrence of latent zoster. Persisting pain after healing of the cutaneous eruption of herpes zoster infection usually has three components: *(1)* a continuous burning pain in the area of sensory loss, *(2)* painful dysesthesias, and *(3)* intermittent shock-like pain. Elderly patients are at greatest risk for developing this complication (Watson, 1982). Many anesthetic, surgical, and drug therapies have been proposed. The most consistently effective treatment is administration of tricyclic antidepressants such as amitriptyline and desipramine. Randomized controlled trials of substance P-depleting agents such as topical capsaicin are effective in some patients. Recently, a Japanese study suggested that intrathecal steroids might be used to effectively treat post-herpetic neuralgia (Kotani et al., 2000).

Post-Radiation Therapy Pain

Post-radiation therapy pain syndromes are occurring less frequently because of the increased sophistication by which radiation therapy portals are planned. Developments in this area have decreased radiation overdose to tissues, sparing the surrounding normal tissues. Nonetheless, radiation fibrosis of peripheral neural structures such as the brachial and lumbar plexus still occur, and radionecrosis of bone is occasionally seen.

Radiation fibrosis of the brachial plexus is discussed earlier in this chapter. Pain in the leg from radiation fibrosis of the lumbar plexus is characterized by its onset late in the course of progressive motor and sensory changes in the leg (Thomas et al., 1985). Lymphedema, a previous history of radiation therapy, myokymia on EMG, and X-ray changes demonstrating radiation necrosis of bone may help establish this diagnosis.

Pain is an early symptom in 15% of patients with radiation myelopathy (Jellinger and Sturm, 1971; Palmer, 1972). Some patients may demonstrate Lhermitte's sign, signifying transient demyelination in the posterior columns, which does not necessarily predict the development of myelopathy. Pain may be localized to the area of spinal cord damage or may be referred pain with dysesthesias below the level of injury. The neurologic symptoms and signs are often initially manifested as the Brown-Séquard syndrome (lateral hemi-"section" of the cord) whereby pain and temperature sensation are lost contralaterally to the side of weakness. Position and vibration sensation are lost ipsilaterally to the side of weakness. The incidence of myelopathy increases with increasing radiation exposure and approaches 50% with 1500 ret exposure. The latency from completion of radiation to the onset of symptoms of myelopathy ranges from 5 to 30 months, with an average of 14 months reported in most series.

A painful enlarging mass in an area of previous irradiation suggests the presence of a radiation-induced peripheral nerve tumor (Foley et al., 1980; Ducatman and Scheithauer, 1983; Thomas et al., 1983; Powers et al., 1983). In one study, seven of nine patients who developed radiation-induced nerve tumors presented with pain and progressive neurologic deficit with a palpable mass involving the brachial or lumbar plexus; these nine patients developed their tumors 4 to 20 years following radiation therapy. Neurofibromatosis is associated with an increased risk for radiation-induced peripheral nerve tumors (Foley et al, 1980).

MANAGEMENT OF CANCER PAIN

General Principles

Numerous approaches can be used to manage pain in cancer patients (Foley, 1993). These encompass multiple modalities of therapy, including pharmacologic, anesthetic, physical, behavioral/psychological, and neurosurgical approaches. In the mid-1990s, a comprehensive approach to the assessment of and guidelines for the management of pain in the patient with cancer was formulated by the Agency for Health Care Policy and Research (AHCPR) (Jacox et al., 1994). The guidelines emphasized the need to evaluate the extent of disease and use of appropriate antitumor therapies to treat the cancer whenever possible. Apart from humanistic considerations, treating cancer pain may be necessary for obtaining appropriate diagnostic studies to define the extent of disease or to allow the patient to complete radiotherapy or other treatments for cancer. For example, adequate titration of analgesics is often necessary to provide enough comfort for the patient to lie quietly so that CT or MR imaging may be completed to evaluate spinal cord compression or lumbosacral plexopathy. Guidelines established by the World Health Organization suggest using a three-step ladder approach, with titration of analgesic therapy following a continuum from mild pain, for which nonsteroidal anti-inflammatory analgesics and analgesic adjuvants are utilized, to moderate and severe pain, for which opioid drugs are added.

These and other guidelines regarding the appropriate use of opioid drugs for acute and chronic cancer pain advocate a basic knowledge of the clinical pharmacology of opioid analgesics, including the concepts of relative potency and dose titration to effect. Knowledge of these concepts permits selection of appropriate starting doses of opioids and provides a method for titration of the drugs. If unacceptable side effects intervene before pain relief is obtained (despite the use of adjuvant drugs to augment analgesia or to counteract side effects), another opioid drug should be used, or another route of administration or an alternative surgical or anesthetic approach should be considered. Although chronic opioid administration may produce physical dependence and tolerance, the need to augment opioid doses for a given patient is usually caused by increasing pain associated with progressive disease as opposed to tolerance caused by a change in opioid receptor responsiveness (Payne, 1989). Clearly, physical dependence and tolerance must be distinguished from psychological dependence. Fortunately, the occurrence of psychological dependence is rare in cancer patients who have not had a substance abuse disorder before the diagnosis of cancer. The fear of iatrogenic addiction should never be used as an excuse to withhold opioids for the treatment of pain.

Special Considerations in Bone Pain

As noted above, bone pain is a major cause of pain in many patients with cancer. Standard approaches for the treatment of bone pain include the use of nonsteroidal anti-inflammatory drugs (NSAIDs) in combination with opioids. NSAIDs are said to be uniquely efficacious for treating bone pain (Portenoy and Hagen, 1990). Several lines of data suggest that in lytic bone metastasis, as is typical of breast and lung cancer, NSAIDs may decrease pain and aid in the inhibition of bone destruction because they inhibit PG synthesis. It is now known that PGs enhance osteoclast function and activate and sensitize nociceptors. Several of the newer NSAID drugs such as ketoprofen (Stambaugh and Drew, 1988) and ketorolac (Buckley and Brogden, 1990) have analgesic potencies that are much greater than aspirin and that approach the effectiveness of 10 to 12 mg intramuscular morphine. It should be noted that NSAIDs appear to be as effective in treating osteoblastic metastasis from prostate cancer as they are for osteolytic metastasis. COX-2 inhibitors, recently approved by the FDA, offer the advantages of causing less gastric dyspepsia and a lesser incidence of peptic ulcer disease and inhibition of platelets (Hawkey, 1999), benefiting cancer patients in particular. Even the most potent, newer NSAIDs should not, however, be viewed as substitutes for morphine or other opioids in managing severe pain, as all drugs in this class have a ceiling to their analgesic efficacy.

The role of radiation and hormonal therapies in managing bone pain in prostate and other cancers is important. During the past 10 years or so, interest has focused on the role of intravenous administration of radiopharmaceuticals such as ^{32}Phosphorus, ^{90}Ytterium, and ^{89}Strontium to manage metastatic bone disease. Of the three nuclides, ^{89}Strontium may be less myelotoxic than the others by virtue of its relative selectivity for bone. Overall response rates for pain relief are reported to be as high as 80% (mean, 68%) (Bryne and Waxman, 1990). While these agents have been considered useful in treating bone pain from prostate metastases, in general all three agents have generally fallen out of use because they are myelosuppressive and frequently necessitate the postponement of cytotoxic chemotherapy.

Drugs in the bisphosphonate class are used to manage hypercalcemia associated with malignancy (Coleman, 1991) and may secondarily influence bone pain. Bisphosphonates such as etidronate and pamidronate have potent inhibitory effects on osteoclasts, thereby decreasing bone resorption. They are useful treatments for hypercalcemia and to promulgate bone remodeling in osteolytic metastasis. They do not appear, however, to be effective against bone pain in osteoblastic metastasis from prostate cancer (Smith, 1989). Bisphosphonates have been shown to reduce the incidence of fractures in breast cancer patients with bony metastasis and are administered monthly to breast cancer and multiple myeloma patients to reduce pain and osseous incidence (Hortobagyi et al., 1996; Berenson et al., 1996; Lahtinen et al., 1992).

Calcitonin also inhibits osteoclast function and is a treatment for hypercalcemia, as well as exerting antinociceptive effects in the central nervous system (Fraioli et al., 1984). Limited clinical trials have demonstrated analgesia when calcitonin is given intraspinally. Currently, this should be considered as experimental therapy for pain, as the FDA has not approved its use for this indication and the neurotoxicity of intrathecal calcitonin has not been fully studied. However, this therapy for bone pain is attractive for patients who do not obtain satisfactory relief from opioids because calcitonin provides a potential means of analgesia through nonopioid mechanisms. Thus, in theory, it provides a way to achieve pain relief in opioid tolerant or opioid nonresponsive patients. Conclusions await the results from future clinical trials.

Hypophysectomy has been used to manage generalized bone pain that has failed hormonal and systemic analgesic therapies (Waldman et al., 1987). Hypophysectomy is accomplished by alcohol injection and may produce immediate pain relief in 35% of patients, lasting as long as 20 weeks. Success rates as high as 90% have also been reported. The use of levodopa as a predictor of response to hypophysectomy and as a treatment in itself for metastatic bone pain is controversial. Earlier reports by Minton (1974) noted a 33% response rate in metastatic bone pain from breast cancer, but a more recent study reported a response rate in only 7% (1 of 14) of patients treated with levodopa-carbidopa for bone metastasis (Sjolin and Trykker, 1985).

Nonopioid Analgesics

Nonopioid analgesics (Table 23–4) constitute a heterogeneous group of substances differing in chemi-

Table 23–4. NSAIDs and COX-2 Inhibitors

NSAIDs	
Drug	*Usual Dosage*
Acetaminophen (Tylenol and others)	500–1000 mg orally every 4–6 hours
Acetylsalicylic acid (aspirin)	500–1000 mg orally every 4–6 hours
Diflunisal (Dolobid)	1000 mg (initially)
Naproxen (Naprosyn)	500 mg (initially); 250 mg orally every 6–8 hours
Ibuprofen (Motrin and others)	200–400 mg orally every 4–6 hours
Ketoprofen (Orudis)	25–50 mg orally every 4–8 hours
Flurbiprofen (Ansaid)	50 mg orally every 4–6 hours
Indomethacin (Indocin)	25 mg orally two or three times daily
Diclofenac sodium (Voltaren)	25–50 mg orally every 6–8 hours
Piroxicam (Feldene)	20 mg orally daily
Ketorolac (Toradol)	60 mg (initially) intramuscularly, then 30 mg intramuscularly every 6 hours; then 10 mg orally every 6 hours (limit 5 days)

COX-2 Inhibitors		
Drug	*Selectivity*	*Dose*
Celecoxib (SC 58635 Celebrix)	Specific	200–400 mg every 12 hours
Rofecoxib (MK 0966 Vioxx)	Specific	25–50 mg daily
Nimesulide (Mesulid)	Preferential	?
Meloxicam (Mobic)	Preferential	7.5–15 mg daily

cal structure and pharmacologic actions. With the probable exception of acetaminophen, these drugs vary in their roles as analgesic, anti-inflammatory, and antipyretic agents. Aspirin is the prototype of the group and is the most commonly used agent. As a group, these drugs are usually administered orally and are used to treat mild to moderate pain. In contrast to opioid analgesics, tolerance or physical dependence does not develop with these drugs. However, nonopioid analgesics have a ceiling to their effectiveness, and escalation of the dose of drug given beyond a certain level does not produce additive analgesic effects.

Increasing evidence suggests that nonopioid analgesics play a unique role in the management of pain for patients who have bone metastases. Because many of the nonopioid analgesics act as potent PG synthetase inhibitors, they appear to have specific analgesic, anti-inflammatory, and, in some instances, antitumor effects in cancer patients with bony disease.

The choice and use of nonopioid analgesic drugs must be individualized for each patient. Patients must be given an adequate trial of one drug before switching to an alternative agent. Such a trial should include administration of the drug to maximum levels at regular intervals. These drugs should be used judiciously because they may produce significant adverse effects in cancer patients—gastrointestinal (GI) hemorrhage, masking of fever in an immunocompromised host, and platelet dysfunction—that can each be a serious and potentially fatal complication of therapy.

This category is essentially limited to inhibitors of the enzyme cyclooxygenase (COX), thus inhibiting the synthesis of PGs and pain and inflammation mediators. The NSAIDs can be divided into COX-2–selective and COX-2–nonselective NSAID subgroups. These medications are only useful as step 1 drugs or adjuncts to opioid therapy in the most advanced cases. They have the advantage of a very low short-term side effect profile that does not affect the patient's lifestyle. In general, their use for cancer pain is limited due to a ceiling effect as well as a deleterious long-term side effect profile. Except for COX-2 inhibitors and nonacidic subgroups, they are contraindicated or, at best, controversial for all patients with thrombocytopenia, which constitutes a large sector of those receiving antineoplastic therapy.

Gastric and duodenal ulceration is another potential problem that could result from long-term use of aspirin and other nonselective NSAIDS. Several techniques used to limit this consequence include the concurrent administration of an H2-blocker or misoprostol, each of which has its own particular limitations. This is less of a problem with newer COX-2 inhibitors. It should be mentioned that, when appropriate, ketorolac offers the advantage of parenteral administration (including subcutaneous), making this agent unique. This advantage, however, does not affect concerns over maintaining the integrity of the gastric mucosa.

Finally, acetaminophen, with none of the above side effects, is used more often than other step 1 drugs, especially in combined preparations with opioids. The downside of acetaminophen use is a dose limitation at 3000 mg/day to avoid potential hepatotoxicity and its lack of peripheral anti-inflammatory properties.

The New Selective COX-2 Enzyme Inhibitors

COX-2 remains the predominant source of PGs in the human GI tract and platelets, the reason this group of drugs was developed. In preliminary trials, these agents exhibited a safety profile comparable with placebo in contrast with the non-selective group; however, they affect the kidney similarly. COX-2 inhibitors (Table 23–4) are equally as efficacious as the older agents so the promise they carry is mainly due to safety and elimination of the major NSAID contraindications, thus benefiting more cancer (and rheumatoid) patients. Celecoxib (Celebrex) with a recommended dose of 200 mg qd or 100 mg bid, and Rofecoxib (Vioxx) with a recommended dose of 25 to 50 mg qd, are commonly used. Other COX-2 inhibitors are in clinical trials.

Opioid Analgesics

Opioid analgesics are the mainstay of treatment for moderate to severe cancer-related pain. These drugs (Table 23–5) produce analgesia through binding to specific opiate receptors in the brain and spinal cord (Yaksh and Rudy, 1976) and are categorized by how they interact with the receptors: *(1)* opioid agonists (e.g., morphine) interact with the receptor to produce analgesia and *(2)* opioid antagonists reverse or block receptor effects but have analgesic properties. Opioid antagonists are divided into two drug classes and are distinguished as being either morphine-like or nalorphine-like on the basis of their pharmacologic effects and the character of their abstinence syndromes.

Table 23–5. Opioid Analgesics

Drug	*Usual Starting Dosages*
Full opioid agonists	
Morphine*	15 to 30 mg orally every 3 to 4 hours
	30 to 60 mg orally every 8 to 12 hours
Hydromorphone (Dilaudid)	2 to 4 mg orally every 4 to 6 hours
Levorphanol (Levo-Dromoran)	2 to 4 mg orally every 4 to 6 hours
Fentanyl (Duragesic)	25 to 50 μg/hr transdermally every 3 days
Codeine	15 to 30 mg orally every 3 to 4 hours
Oxycodone (Percodan and others)	5 to 10 mg orally every 3 to 4 hours
Meperedine (Demerol Hydrochloride)	75 to 100 mg intramuscularly every 3 to 4 hours
Methadone hydrochloride (Dolophine)	5 to 10 mg orally every 3 to 4 hours
Propoxyphene (Darvon and others)	100 mg orally every 4 to 6 hours
Partial agonists and mixed agonists/antagonists†	
Nalbuphine (Nubain)	10 mg intravenously every 3 to 4 hours
Butorphanol (Stadol)	0.5 to 2 mg intravenously every 3 to 4 hours
	1 to 2 mg sublingually three times a day
Dezocine (Dalgan)	10 mg intravenously every 3 to 4 hours
Pentazocine (Talwin)	50 mg orally every 4 to 6 hours

*Morphine can be given as an immediate-release formulation or as a sustained-release preparation. It is recommended that a relatively rapid onset, short-acting opioid preparation (such as immediate-release morphine) be available to patients who take sustained-release morphine to provide rescue medication for breakthrough pain.

†This class of drugs is *not* recommended for the management of chronic cancer pain because the drugs will reverse analgesia when co-administered with full opioid agonists and precipitate withdrawal in physically dependent individuals.

Opioids produce pharmacologic effects through binding to activated opioid receptors. Opioids that bind to receptors are classified as agonists (e.g., morphine) if they produce analgesia. Opioid antagonists (e.g., naloxone) block the action of an agonist: They have an affinity for opioid receptors but cannot activate the receptors to produce analgesia. Agonist–antagonist drugs (e.g., pentazocine and butorphanol) produce analgesia through their interaction with a specific receptor (e.g., kappa) but also bind to other receptors (e.g., mu) where they can block the action of an agonist. Partial agonists (e.g, buprenorphine) are opioid drugs that bind to receptors and produce analgesia, but, unlike morphine, they exhibit a ceiling effect: Increases in doses do not parallel increases in analgesia. The clinical use of mixed agonist–antagonists is limited by their ability to produce dysphoria and hallucinations; these effects are mediated by kappa receptors and possibly nonopioid sigma receptors. Mixed agonist–antagonists and partial agonists will each cause withdrawal syndromes when administered to a patient taking opiates chronically. Antagonists are used as an antidote for opiate overdose; they should be used judiciously because they will cause acute withdrawal in patients on chronic opioid therapy. Opioid overdose is an uncommon cause of encephalopathy in patients with cancer. Common causes of altered mental status changes should be sought before naloxone is administered. Sepsis in particular should be excluded, as this is one of the most common causes of delirium in cancer.

"Weak" Opioids: The Second Rung of the Analgesic Ladder

It is clinically useful to classify opioids as weak or strong, depending on their relative efficacy. Weak opioids are the second rung of the "analgesic ladder" and are used for less severe pain; their efficacy is limited by an increased incidence of side effects at higher doses (e.g., nausea and constipation with codeine, central nervous system excitation with propoxyphene). When weak opioids are given at a fixed oral dose mixed with a nonopioid analgesic their efficacy is limited by the maximal safe dose for nonopioid analgesics such as acetaminophen or aspirin. Strong opioids are used for more severe pain: They have a wide therapeutic window and no ceiling effect for analgesia. Higher doses produce an increasing level of analgesia; they are the third rung of the analgesic ladder. This is a simplistic but clinically useful approach once the decision to start opioid therapy has been made.

Codeine, an alkaloid of opium, is the prototype of the weak analgesics. Although a parenteral preparation is available, it is nearly always given by mouth, often in a fixed mixture with a nonopioid analgesic. A 200 mg dose is equipotent to 30 mg of morphine. The affinity of codeine for mu receptors is several thousand-fold less than morphine (Pasternak, 1993). The half-life of codeine is 2.5 to 3 hours; approximately 10% of orally administered codeine is demethylated to morphine; free and conjugated morphine can be found in the urine. The analgesic action of codeine may be due to its conversion to morphine (Millan, 1990), although analgesic structure–activity studies do not support this hypothesis (Beaver et al., 1978a,b). Constipation is the main side effect at the usual therapeutic doses (30 to 60 mg every 4 hours) and is thus used for some patients with chronic diarrhea.

Hydrocodone is a codeine derivative available in the United States only and is found in combination with acetaminophen or aspirin in doses of 2.5, 5, 7.5, and 10 mg. It is thought to be more potent than codeine, although convincing data are lacking. At the above doses its analgesic effect is very weak and probably only slightly superior to acetaminophen alone. Some pharmacists have started to formulate hydrocodone without acetaminophen.

Propoxyphene is a synthetic analgesic structurally related to methadone. It is approximately equipotent to codeine as an analgesic but lacks its antitussive properties; it binds to mu receptors. Its analgesic activity lasts 3 to 5 hours, and its half-life is 6 to 12 hours. Its major metabolite is norpropoxyphene, which has a half-life of 30 to 36 hours, which may be responsible for some of the toxicity observed (Chan and Matzke, 1987). Norpropoxyphene has local anesthetic effects similar to lidocaine, and high doses may cause arrhythmias. Seizures occur more often with propoxyphene intoxication than with opiate intoxication. Naloxone antagonizes the toxic effects of propoxyphene (Inturrisi and Foley, 1984), which is very irritating to vessels and soft tissues when used parenterally. Inadvertent injection into the brachial artery has resulted in amputation of digits. Because it is more difficult to manage and offers no advantage over other opioids, its usefulness is limited.

Meperidine, a synthetic phenylpiperidine derivative mu agonist with anticholinergic properties, is the analgesic most commonly prescribed for acute pain and is also widely used for chronic pain. The reasons for this enthusiasm are unclear and are likely irrational. A lesser rise in pressure in the common bile duct compared with morphine (Jaffe and Martin, 1990) has not been shown to be clinically advantageous. In contrast, the central nervous system (CNS) excitatory effects that appear after chronic use are instead well substantiated. The accumulation of its metabolite, normeperidine, causes multifocal myoclonus and grand mal seizures (Kaiko et al., 1983; Szeto et al., 1977), which are not reversed by naloxone. In this context dilated pupils and hyperactive reflexes are characteristic. The half-life of meperidine is 3 hours. It is, in part, demethylated to normeperidine, the only active metabolite, which has a half-life of 15 to 30 hours. Normeperidine accumulates only after chronic treatment, particularly in patients with renal dysfunction. Short-term treatment with meperidine has been associated with mild negative alterations in various elements of mood (Kaiko et al., 1983). When meperidine is given to patients being treated with monoamine oxidase inhibitors, two different patterns of toxicity have been observed: severe respiratory depression or excitation, delirium, hyperpyrexia, and convulsions. The dose equianalgesic to 10 mg of parenteral morphine is 75 to 100 mg. The oral to parenteral ratio is 1:4. Its use by either route is rarely justified.

Oxycodone is a semisynthetic derivative of the opium alkaloid thebaine. Because of its high bioavailability (>50%) it is suitable for oral administration and by this route is equipotent to morphine and 10-fold more potent than codeine (Beaver et al., 1978a,b) Parenterally, intensity and duration of analgesia are 25% less than morphine (Beaver et al., 1978b). It has a half-life of 2 to 3 hours and duration of action of 4 to 5 hours. It is metabolized like codeine: demethylated and conjugated in the liver and excreted in the urine (Beaver et al., 1978b). Its analgesic action is partially mediated by active metabolites. Oxycodone is considered a weak analgesic because of its use in a fixed combination with acetaminophen and aspirin. These combinations limit its dose to 10 mg every 4 hours. However, oxycodone is now available as a 5 mg tablet as well as 20 mg/ml liquid and should be classified as a strong opioid. Soon, even higher strength oxycodone tablets will be available. When oxycodone is used alone, like other opioid agonists it has no ceiling effect for analgesia. It has been reported to have fewer side effects than morphine (Kalso and Vainio, 1988, 1990). Its availability in 5 mg tablets permits careful titration for patients with a narrow therapeutic margin. Oxycodone is a versatile and flexible drug that can be used to treat pain of any intensity requiring an opiate analgesic (Beaver et al., 1978b; Glare and Walsh, 1993; Poyhia et al., 1993).

"Strong" Opioids: The Third "Rung" of the Analgesic Ladder

Morphine, a phenanthrene derivative, is the prototype opiate agonist. All other opiates are compared with morphine when determining their relative analgesic potency. It is the drug of choice for severe pain associated with cancer (World Health Organization, 1986). Like other "strong" opiates, there is no ceiling to morphine's analgesic effect, although side effects, particularly sedation and confusion, may intervene before optimal analgesia can be achieved. It is metabolized in the liver where it undergoes glucuronidation at positions 3 and 6.

Morphine-3-glucuronide (M3G) and morphine-6-glucuronide (M6G) accumulate with chronic administration of morphine (Sawe et al., 1983). M6G binds to mu receptors with an affinity similar to morphine (Pasternak et al., 1987), but also binds to delta receptors; this may account for its higher analgesic potency (Oguri et al., 1987). M6G is 3.7-fold more potent than morphine when administered subcutaneously and 45-fold more potent when administered in the cerebral ventricles (Pasternak et al., 1987); only 0.077% of this metabolite crosses the intact blood–cerebrospinal fluid barrier (Portenoy et al., 1991).

In single-dose morphine studies the relative parenteral/oral potency ratio has been shown to be 1:6 (Houde et al., 1966). After chronic use the ratio changes to 1:3 (Twycross, 1975); this is likely due to accumulation of active metabolites. There is experimental (Labella et al., 1979) and clinical (Morley et al., 1992) evidence that M3G, which has a negligible affinity for opioid receptors and does not produce analgesia, has an excitatory effect on neurons and can cause myoclonus and, rarely, a hyperalgesic state. These effects of M3G may be mediated by different receptor mechanisms (Smith et al., 1990). The half-life of morphine is about 2 hours; the half-life of M6G is somewhat longer (Jaffe and Martin, 1990). The duration of analgesia is 4 hours. Slow-release preparations, which permit a twice a day regimen, are safe and effective (Kaiko, 1990); they are generally best used after dose titration with morphine sulfate. Because morphine metabolites are eliminated by glomerular filtration and can accumulate in renal failure leading to an increased incidence of side effects (Osborne et al., 1986), morphine should be used with caution in renal failure. A useful strategy for patients with compromised renal function is to increase the interval of time between doses or use an alternative opioid.

Hydromorphone is another semisynthetic phenanthrene derivative opioid agonist commercially available as a highly water-soluble salt. When administered parenterally 1.3 mg of hydromorphone is equipotent to 10 mg of morphine; it is somewhat shorter acting but has a greater peak effect. Its bioavailability is 30% to 40% with an oral to parenteral ratio of 5:1 (Houde et al., 1986) and a half-life of 1.5 to 2 hours. Because of its high potency and water solubility, hydromorphone is the drug of choice via a subcutaneous route.

Levorphanol is a synthetic opioid agonist structurally related to the phenanthrene-derivative opiates. A potent mu agonist, it also binds to delta and kappa receptors (Pasternak, 1993; Tive et al., 1992). When administered parenterally, 2 mg of levorphanol is equianalgesic to 10 mg of morphine (Kaiko et al., 1981). The drug also has good oral efficacy with an intramuscular/oral ratio of 0.5. It has a half-life of 12 to 30 hours (Dixon, 1986), and its duration of analgesia is 4 to 6 hours. Therefore, repeated administration is associated with accumulation; a dose reduction may be required 2 to 4 days after starting the drug to avoid side effects from overdosage. For the same reason, it is best avoided by patients with impaired renal function or encephalopathy. It is sometimes useful as second-line drug for patients who cannot tolerate morphine.

Methadone is a synthetic diphenylheptane opioid mu agonist (Jaffee and Martin, 1990). The equianalgesic dose of 1 mg of methadone ranges from 4 to 10 mg of morphine sulfate (MSO6) (Ripamonte et al., 1998). An inexpensive and effective analgesic, its use is limited by the need for carefully individualized dosing and interval titration. Methadone is rapidly absorbed within 30 minutes of oral dosing, with bioavailability ranging from 41% to 99% (Meresaar et al., 1981). Plasma levels decline in a biexponential manner with a half-life of 2 to 3 hours during the initial phase and 15 to 60 hours during the terminal phase (Sawe, 1986); this biexponential decline accounts for its relatively short analgesic action of 4 to 6 hours (Beaver et al., 1967) and the tendency for drug accumulation with repeated dosing. A reduction of dose and interval of frequency are often needed during the first days of treatment to prevent side effects from overdosage. In addition, when urine pH exceeds 6, renal clearance of methadone is significantly decreased (Inturrisi and Foley, 1984); patients with cancer and patients 65 years of age or older have a decreased clearance; and plasma protein binding and rate of hepatic extraction also influence the highly variable half-life of this substance (Inturrisi et al., 1987).

Despite these and other factors that determine the need for a careful individual titration, it is an extremely effective second-line drug for patients who experience unrelieved pain and intolerable side effects with the use of morphine (Morley et al., 1992). Because of its low cost it could be excellent for use in developing countries or for patients requiring very high doses of opioids. The rare patient allergic to morphine might benefit from methadone because it has a different chemical structure (Morley et al., 1993). Methadone is excreted almost exclusively in the feces and has been proposed as a safe and effective analgesic for patients with chronic renal failure (Kreek et al., 1980). A possible mechanism for the action of methadone is the prevention of monoamine reuptake in the periaqueductal gray matter and presynaptic inhibition of *N*-methyl-D-aspartate (NMDA) receptors. Hence, methadone may offer advantages for patients with opioid tolerance and also for intractable neuropathic pain states (Gorman et al., 1997; Codd et al., 1995; Ebert et al., 1995; Davis and Inturrisi, 1999). Guidelines for methadone usage are now available (Davis and Walsh, 2001).

Fentanyl is a synthetic phenylpiperidine-derivative opioid agonist that interacts primarily with mu receptors (Jaffe and Martin, 1990). It is 80-fold more potent than morphine and is highly lipophilic; these properties render it as a suitable candidate when a transdermal route for opiate analgesia is desirable. Following results from the first clinical study in patients with cancer pain (Miser et al., 1989), the use of transdermal fentanyl became popular. Its use, however, should be limited to patients with chronic pain who are unable to take drugs by mouth and who do not require a rapid titration. The transdermal fentanyl therapeutic system delivers drug continuously to the systemic circulation for as long as 72 hours. The skin permeability constant of fentanyl is approximately 0.0021 ml/min/cm^2 (Michaels et al., 1975), a figure that is 60- to 120-fold lower than regional blood flow to the skin of the chest (Hwang et al., 1991). A special rate-controlling membrane provides additional control of drug release; only extreme conditions, such as the cutaneous blood supply being completely cut off, would therefore influence absorption.

The transdermal absorption of fentanyl is the same from chest, abdomen, and thigh (Roy and Flynn, 1990). A skin reaction at the application site occurs in 4% of patients (Hwang et al., 1991), although there is no skin sensitization. After application of the transdermal patch, systemic absorption is very low in a 0 to 4 hour period, increases in the 4 to 8 hour period, and remains relatively constant, with a coefficient of variation of 28%, from 8 to 24 hours (Varvel et al., 1989). The initial delay is likely due to the time required to establish a reservoir of fentanyl in the stratum corneum. Patients reach steady-state concentrations within 12 to 24 hours from application; adjustments in efficacy and toxicity can, therefore, be made on a daily basis. Following removal of the transdermal patch, serum fentanyl concentration falls about 50% in approximately 16 hours. This apparently long half-life is probably caused by the slow wash out of the cutaneous reservoir. These considerations translate clinically into a several hour delay in the onset of analgesia after an initial application and a persistence of analgesia and eventual side effects long after removal of the transdermal system. For patients with chronic pain, after a variable period of titration, it is possible to obtain relatively constant serum fentanyl concentrations comparable with continuous intravenous or subcutaneous infusions (Southam et al., 1991).

Fentanyl also has an important role via epidural and intrathecal routes. A more recent use of oral transmucosal fentanyl, which has been approved by the FDA, is for the treatment of breakthrough pain; initial pain relief was noted within a few minutes, with maximum effect occurring in 20 to 30 minutes (Fine et al., 1991).

Sufentanil, a synthetic derivative of fentanyl, is 5 to 10 times more potent, and it is generally reserved for anesthesia. As clinical familiarity with this agent increases and other routes of administration besides injection become available, it is expected that the use of sufentanil will increase for patients with cancer pain, especially those who are highly tolerant to opioids. Good results have been reported from intravenous use (including patient-controlled analgesia [PCA]) and in subcutaneous infusions in the context of palliative care (Paix et al., 1995). According to one report, sufentanil can be used successfully for breakthrough pain when applied sublingually (Paix et al., 1995; Kunz et al., 1993). In addition, neuraxial application is occasionally used for some patients.

ROUTES OF ANALGESIC DELIVERY

The onset, peak, and duration of analgesia vary with the drug used, the route of administration, and the individual patient. Recognition of this variability allows the appropriate choice of drug, route, and scheduling. When undertaking sequential trials of different opiates one-half of the calculated equianalgesic dose is recommended for initial titration (Foley, 1984).

For patients with acute severe pain, parenteral morphine is the opioid of choice. The drug should be titrated to effect, with boluses repeated every 15 minutes, if necessary, until either analgesia or intolerable side effects develop. The concomitant use of an anti-inflammatory drug is often warranted. An antiemetic might be needed. When the intensity of pain decreases to a bearable level, a continuous infusion of morphine should be started; the initial hourly dose can be obtained by dividing the total loading dose by three to four (the duration of analgesia after single morphine doses is 3 to 4 hours). Patients receiving chronic opioid therapy may require very high doses to control acute exacerbations of pain. An infusion pump with a device for self-administration of extra doses of medication every few minutes (PCA) should be used if available (Citron et al., 1986). The PCA dose can be as high as the hourly rate during the titration phase and when incident pain is a concern. The continuous basal rate should be adjusted frequently on the basis of the patient's self-reporting and the PCA usage.

When venous access is problematic the subcutaneous route should be used. It is good practice to avoid the intramuscular route. Once the exacerbation of the patient's acute pain abates, an oral route should be used. If the oral route is impractical, a transdermal system is available (Miser et al., 1989). An oral transmucosal route may be effective for rescue doses, but absorption is usually inadequate for more sustained relief; the same is true of the rectal route, which, in addition, is often uncomfortable for the patient and caregiver. Long-term intravenous opioid administration can be used for patients with central venous access who cannot take oral drugs (Portenoy et al., 1986). Long-term subcutaneous administration is a very effective alternative (Bruera et al., 1985).

For patients with mild to moderate pain, oral analgesics such as oxycodone or codeine are appropriate choices (World Health Organization, 1986). Fixed combinations with nonopioid analgesics are generally not advisable because they might limit the carefully individualized titration, which is the basis for therapeutic success.

Adjuvant analgesics (Table 23–6) should be given early in the pain treatment course (World Health Organization, 1986); like the opioids, they should be administered at regular intervals. Acetaminophen or NSAID medications should always be given unless contraindicated. Steroids can be highly effective in treating pain from direct tumor invasion of neural and somatic structures (Bruera et al., 1985); their side effects are numerous and well known but often without consequence in the terminal stages of life. Anticonvulsants are used for lancinating, paroxysmal pain. Antidepressants are used for dysesthetic pain, although no controlled studies of them in a cancer population are available. Neuroleptics and benzodiazepines are useful for some patients. Ketamine has been reported to be effective when the patient's pain does not respond to massive doses of opiates (Jaffe and Martin, 1990; Kanamaru et al., 1990). A putative mechanism is through reversing tolerance.

Table 23–6. Adjuvant Medications for Cancer Pain

Drug	*Therapeutic Effects*	*Comments*	*Dosage*
Antidepressants			
Amitriptyline	Analgesic, elevates mood, induces sleep	Effective for neuropathic pain	Start with 10–25 mg HS; increase gradually to 75–100 mg HS
Desipramine (Norpramin)	Analgesic, elevates mood	Effective for neuropathic pain	25–150 mg/day, orally
Doxepin	Analgesic, elevates mood, induces sleep	Effective for neuropathic pain	Start with 10–20 mg HS; increase gradually to 75–100 mg HS
Imipramine	Analgesic, elevates mood	Effective for neuropathic pain	200 mg HS for severe depression
Nortriptyline	Analgesic, elevates mood	Effective for neuropathic pain	Start with 10–25 mg HS; increase gradually to 75–100 mg HS
Venlafaxine	Analgesic, elevates mood	Effective for neuropathic pain	—
Anticonvulsants			
Carbamazepine	Anticonvulsant, decreases abnormal CNS neuronal activity	Useful for neuropathic pain; hematologic monitoring suggested	Start with 100 mg daily; increase by 100 mg q4d to 500–800 mg/d
Phenytoin	Anticonvulsant, decreases abnormal CNS neuronal activity	Useful for neuropathic pain; hematologic monitoring suggested	Start with 100 mg/d; increase by 25–50 mg q4d to 250–300 mg/day
Gabapentin	Anticonvulsant, decreases abnormal CNS neuronal activity	Useful for neuropathic pain; better toxicity profile	300 mg to 900 mg tid
Lamotrigine	Treatment of trigeminal neuralgia, migraine headaches, diabetic neuropathy	Inhibitor of voltage gated Na+ channels; suppresses glutamate release and inhibits serotonin reuptake	25–50 mg/day, increased by 50 mg/week, until max 900 mg bid or tid
Topirimate	Treatment of cluster headaches, diabetic neuropathy	Increases CNS GABA levels, blocks AMPA kainate excitatory receptors	200–400 mg/d with bid dosing. Start at 25 mg bid increasing 50 mg each week
Oxcarbazepine	Treatment of trigeminal neuralgia, neuropathic pain states	Blockade of voltage-gated Na^+ channels	300–600 mg/day, up to a max 1200–2400 mg/day
Zonisamide	Trials ongoing	Na^+ channel blockade; T-type Ca^{2+} channel blockade	
Tigabine	Neuropathic pain	GABA reuptake inhibitor	—
Corticosteroids			
Prednisolone	Potentiates analgesia, elevates mood	Effective for pain caused by compression of nerves, spinal cord, or intracranial contents; risk of GI bleeding	10 mg tid PO

(*Continued*)

Table 23–6. Adjuvant Medications for Cancer Pain (*Continued*)

Drug	*Therapeutic Effects*	*Comments*	*Dosage*
Dexamethasone	Improves appetite		≥4 mg PO q6h
Phenothiazines			
Methotrimeprazine	Produces moderate analgesia without risk of tolerance or physical dependence	Used as an alternative to narcotics if they are contraindicated	10–20 mg IM or 20–30 mg PO
Chlorpromazine	Reduces anxiety and psychotic behavior	Risk of orthostatic hypotension; rarely causes jaundice and neurologic reaction	10–25 mg q4–8h
Prochlorperazine	Antiemetic, no analgesic effect		5–10 mg q4–8h
Amphetamines			
Dextroamphetamine	Potentiates narcotic analgesia; elevates mood	For terminally ill patients with pain, depression, and lethargy	2.5 mg tid or 5 mg/day PO in morning
Methamphetamine	Potentiates narcotic analgesia; elevates mood	For terminally ill patients with pain, depression, and lethargy	5 mg in morning
Methylphenidate	Potentiates narcotic analgesia; elevates mood	For terminally ill patients with pain, depression, and lethargy	5–10 mg bid; AM and midday
Anxiolytics			
Hydroxyzine	Potentiates opioid analgesia; reduces anxiety; antiemetic; sedative	Convulsions occur >500 mg/day	Start with 25 mg tid PO; increase to 50–100 mg q4–6h
Diazepam	Relieves acute anxiety and panic; antiemetic; sedative	More antiemetic and fewer sedative effects than chlorpromazine; risk of orthostatic hypotension and hypotonia	5–10 mg PO, IV, or rectally bid or tid

HS, at bedtime.

The epidural, intrathecal, and intracerebroventricular routes are reserved for the patient who fails a careful and sequential trial of different opiates and adjuvants.

GUIDELINES FOR THE USE OF OPIOID ANALGESICS

This section details a practical approach for individualizing treatment for each patient so as to provide optimal control of pain.

Start with a Specific Drug for a Specific Type of Pain

Parenteral morphine is the drug of choice for patients with acute severe pain. Oral analgesics such as codeine or hydrocodone are appropriate choices for patients with mild to moderate pain. Although meperidine is also used for this level of pain, its relatively poor oral potency and the stimulatory CNS effects of its metabolite normeperidine makes this a poor choice for chronic administration for most cancer patients (Kaiko et al., 1983).

Know the Pharmacology of the Drug Prescribed

Type of Drug

The opioid antagonist drugs produce psychotomimetic effects with increasing doses. Patients previously exposed to an opioid agonist are exquisitely sensitive to opioid antagonists. Administering an opioid antagonist such as pentazocine (Talwin) may precipitate an acute withdrawal state in such patients.

Duration of Analgesic Effects

The onset, peak, and duration of analgesic effect vary with each drug and its route of administration. Each drug has a specific time course of effectiveness. For example, methadone and levorphanol act for only 5 to 6 hours, whereas morphine (immediate release) and hydromorphone are effective for 3 to 4 hours. Sustained-release morphine may be active for 8 to 12 hours. In general, drugs administered by mouth have a slower onset of action and longer duration of effect, whereas drugs given parenterally have a rapid onset of action but a shorter duration of effect.

Pharmacokinetics of the Drug

Plasma levels of opioid analgesics do not correlate directly with their analgesic effect. More importantly, the plasma half-life of the drug, which reflects its route of elimination, does not correlate with its analgesic properties. Opioids such as methadone (half-life 17 to 50 hours) and levorphanol (half-life 12 to 16 hours) produce analgesic effects for only 5 to 6 hours and must be given at 4 to 6 hour intervals to maintain adequate analgesia. However, because of their long half-life, these drugs accumulate in plasma, which may account for their side effects with repeated administration. Adjustment of dose and dosing interval may be necessary during the initial use of these drugs. For this reason, they are generally not considered to be first-line agents for cancer pain management.

Equianalgesic Doses for the Opioid and its Route of Administration

Table 23–7 lists the equianalgesic doses of the commonly used opioid analgesics. These doses have been derived from double-blind relative potency studies by Houde and colleagues (1966) and provide a useful reference when switching from one opioid drug to another and from one route of administration to another. Unfamiliarity with these doses is one of the most common causes of undermedicating patients with pain. Special care should be exercised when switching to methadone, which is more potent, with a conversion ratio varying between 4 and 10 (Bruera et al., 1996; Lawlor et al., 1998; Ripamonti et al., 1998).

Administer Analgesics Regularly

Medication should be administered on an around-the-clock basis. This approach will keep pain at a tolerable level and limit the patient's anxiety about medication. It may also allow for a reduction in the total amount of drug given during a 24 hour period. Studies by Fordyce (1983) suggest that such an approach reduces abnormal pain behavior in hospitalized patients. The pharmacologic effect is to maintain plasma

Table 23–7. Equianalgesic Dosing and Conversion Table*

Opioid	*Parenteral Opioid to Parenteral Morphine*	*Parenteral Opioid to Oral Opioid*	*Oral Opioid to Oral Morphine*	*Oral Morphine to Oral Opioid*
Morphine	1	2.5	1	1
Hydromorphone	5	2	5	0.2
Meperidine	0.13	4	0.1	10
Levorphanol	5	2	5	0.2
Codeine	NA	NA	0.15	7
Oxycodone	NA	NA	1.5	0.7
Hydrocodone	NA	NA	0.15	7

NA, not applicable.

*Steps to use the table: *(1)* Take the total amount of opioid that effectively controls pain in 24 hours; *(2)* multiply by the conversion factor in the table and give 30% less of the new opioid to avoid partial cross tolerance; and *(3)* divide by the number of doses/day.

levels of the circulating drug in an effective dose range.

Use a Combination of Drugs

The additive effects of aspirin and acetaminophen when combined with morphine have been well demonstrated in clinical studies. Practically speaking, the addition on a regular basis of 650 mg of aspirin or acetaminophen to the standard opioid dose will often enhance analgesia without requiring escalation of the opioid drug dose. Antiemetic agents such as metoclopramide may be useful for suppressing nausea and vomiting, which can be caused by an opioid drug or underlying (GI or CNS) pathology. In special instances, the use of muscle relaxants and antianxiety drugs may be helpful, but these drugs often produce sedation. Both diazepam (Valium) and chlorpromazine (Thorazine) have been reported to have antianalgesic effects. The sedating effects of these drugs may limit the amount of opioid analgesic used. This practice is often a disservice to the patient who is oversedated with drugs that are not primarily analgesics. Appropriate treatment of pain will often lead to a marked reduction in anxiety, making the usefulness of antianxiety drugs specious. Amitriptyline used as a hypnotic drug for patients with pain may enhance analgesia, especially for neuropathic pain (Watson et al., 1982). In bedtime doses as low as 25 to 50 mg, it can be a useful adjunctive medication.

Gear the Route of Administration to the Patient's Needs

Oral administration has a slower onset of action than parenteral administration. Parenteral administration is the route of choice for patients who require immediate relief. For patients who cannot take oral drugs or for whom parenteral administration is contraindicated, the rectal route should be considered. Oxymorphone (Numorphan) and hydromorphone (Dilaudid) suppositories are available. Intravenous administration of an opioid produces the most rapid onset of action, with analgesia occurring 10 to 15 minutes following its administration. However, the duration of analgesia is also markedly reduced, requiring frequent dosing at 1 to 2 hour intervals. Continuous intravenous infusion of drugs is important for some hospitalized patients (Portenoy et al., 1986; Miser et al., 1980). Infusions can maintain therapeutic plasma levels and obviate difficulties inherent to erratic absorption. The starting intravenous dose is usually one-half the parenteral dose, but must be adjusted to the needs of the patient. Subcutaneous infusions using portable pumps have also been effective (Bruera et al., 1985).

Side Effects of Opioids

Diminution or elimination of side effects is an important aspect of effective opioid therapy. With few exceptions, dose readjustment should be the first measure taken to manage adverse reactions.

Constipation. Constipation is one of the most common side effects and tends to be refractory to treatment. Because tolerance develops very slowly if it develops, patients will likely require regular laxative treatment for the duration of opioid therapy. A bowel stimulant (e.g., Senna) and a softening agent (e.g., Docusate) is the combination most commonly used. Single-agent prophylaxis with gradual increments may be necessary to reach the desired effect, which is assessed by the patient's subjective reports as well as by clinical examination, sometimes necessitating imaging of the abdomen. Resorting to an osmotic laxative such as lactulose or bowel preparations is reserved for severe cases and might produce diarrhea. As a back-up measure, bowel lavage can be used in refractory cases until regular bowel movements are restored. Caution should be exercised with patients in whom constipation could be due to ileus or intestinal obstruction, which is not uncommon in cases of abdominal and pelvic malignancies. Occasionally, oral naloxone or methylnaltrexone has been tried to manage particularly severe cases of constipation (Chater et al., 1998; Ellison et al., 1997).

Nausea and Vomiting. Nausea and vomiting are the second most common side effects. Tolerance usually occurs within the first few days of opioid administration. It is useful to attempt to determine the dominant mechanism (central versus peripheral) to guide therapy with neuroleptics versus motility agents, respectively. Metoclopramide is frequently used because of its multiple mechanisms of action that antagonize opioids both at the chemoreceptor trigger zone and in the GI tract. Other agents include prochlorperazine, diphenhydramine, butyrophenones, serotonin antagonists such as ondansetron, benzodiazepines, and steroids. A more aggressive approach should be taken for patients who are also receiving a chemotherapy regimen.

Sedation. Sedation is a commonly encountered side effect often signifying excessive dosing. Downward titration of the dose to the level of analgesia is recommended. Drug combinations of opioids and other adjuvant medications create an opioid sparing effect, thereby minimizing a sedative side effect. If the sedation tends to be refractory, the addition of a CNS stimulant (e.g., methylphenidate or dextroamphetamine) with upward titration might help (Bruera et al., 1989a). Methylphenidate is started with an initial dose of 5 mg on awakening and 5 mg at noon and can be titrated up until a response is achieved.

Cognitive Impairment. Patients who undergo a significant increase in the dose of intermittent narcotics experience significant cognitive impairment for approximately 1 week after dose escalation (Bruera et al., 1989b). At other times, alternative sources for cognitive impairment should be aggressively sought before opioid medications are implicated as the cause. Delirium, hallucinations, agitation, or somnolence can occur with sepsis, leptomeningeal disease, brain metastases, metabolic derangements (especially hypercalcemia), ifosfamide therapy (Merimsky et al., 1992), radiation-induced encephalopathy (Crossen et al., 1994), and hepatic encephalopathy.

Cancer patients often take a variety of psychotropic medications for depression and other conditions. Alone or in conjunction with opioids, these may produce mental status changes. Benzodiazepines, in combination with opioids and other psychotropic drugs, tend to produce sedation, dizziness, and cognitive impairment. If opioids are causing cognitive impairment, the initial step should be to lower the dose, the results of which can also be diagnostic. It is highly recommended that other medications to treat agitation or other symptoms should not be added. If manipulation of the analgesic regimen, including rotation of the opioids used, is not effective, haloperidol or a drug from the same class may be considered.

Respiratory Depression. Respiratory depression is a rare occurrence in patients receiving chronic opioid therapy as tolerance to this action of opioid drugs usually develops after a short period of time. However, this adverse effect has been known to result from accidental administration of a very large dose of drugs due to miscommunication about the concentration and unit set on the PCA pumps. As long as respiratory function is not significantly impaired, temporary discontinuation and recommencement at a lower dose when recovery becomes evident are recommended. Opioids taken in combination with benzodiapines is a common cause of respiratory problems. When respiration is compromised and causes derangements in blood gas values, the opioid antagonist naloxone should be titrated to response in 40 μg increments. This action can help avoid inducing a withdrawal syndrome. Cases of tachyarrhythmias leading to myocardial compromise as well as pulmonary edema have been observed with a bolus dose of 400 μg of naloxone, as commonly recommended in most major textbooks on pain management. Occasionally, a continuous infusion of naloxone is required to prevent recurrence of respiratory depression because of its short half-life.

Myoclonus. Myoclonus is a dose-dependent phenomenon presumably related to opioid metabolites, mainly those of meperidine, which cause central motor excitability and might indicate that the patient's level of tolerance is being overwhelmed. A simple dose adjustment may abate the symptoms, but occasionally rotation of opioids or addition of a benzodiazepine, specifically clonazepam, becomes necessary.

Urinary Retention. Urinary retention is a relatively rare adverse reaction usually observed in very old and very young patients and is most likely to occur when concomitantly administered with medications having anticholinergic properties. Tolerance occurs rapidly and occasionally requires temporary catheterization.

Watch for the Development of Tolerance

Tolerance occurs in all patients taking opioids chronically. "Tolerance" describes the inevitable resistance to the analgesic effect of a drug, necessitating increasing doses of the drug to maintain analgesia. Tolerance develops to all of the effects of opioid drugs, but at varying rates. The earliest sign of developing tolerance is the patient's complaint that the duration of effective analgesia has decreased so that increasing the frequency of administration or the amount of drug at each dose is necessary to overcome tolerance. Cross-tolerance among the opioid drugs occurs, but it is not complete, and, therefore, switching from one opioid drug to another in an individual patient can provide more adequate pain control. This is best accomplished by switching to an alternative opioid drug but using a dose one-half the equianalgesic dose as the starting dose and slowly escalating the dose.

Withdraw the Medication Slowly

Abrupt withdrawal of opioid analgesics after their chronic use produces agitation, tremors, insomnia, fever, and marked autonomic nervous system hyperexcitability. Slowly tapering the dose prevents such symptomatology. The appearance of abstinence symptoms after drug withdrawal is related to the elimination curve of the particular drug. The nature of abstinence symptoms similarly varies with the individual drug; for example, with morphine, withdrawal symptoms will occur within 6 to 12 hours following cessation. Reinstituting administration of the drug in doses of approximately 25% of the previous daily dose suppresses these symptoms.

Respect Individual Differences Among Patients

The metabolism of opioid drugs is variable. Individual variations in analgesia and side effects commonly have a pharmacologic basis rather than being caused by the "psychological" state of the patient. All attempts should be made to optimize therapy for each patient.

Do Not Use Placebos to Assess the Nature of the Pain

The placebo response is a potent phenomenon in clinical medicine, but its appropriate use is not widely recognized (Lasagna et al., 1954; Goodwin et al., 1979). For a patient with pain, a positive analgesic effect from intramuscular saline suggests that the patient is a placebo responder. It does not suggest that the patient's pain is "unreal" or less severe than reported. Such misuse of placebos tends to create mistrust between patient and physician, which can interfere with adequate pain control.

COMPLICATIONS OF OPIOID ANALGESICS

In general, there are no demonstrable long-term effects on intellectual function of the chronic use of opioids; no definable deterioration in personality testing; and no important long-term metabolic derangements (although transient endocrine abnormalities occur with disruption of the normal hypothalamic-pituitary axis, which reverts to normal with continued use of the drug). Chronic opioid use may produce sustained elevation of albumin with increased albumin synthesis, although this is almost never clinically significant. The major complications of the opioid analgesics are as follows.

Tolerance

The development of tolerance results in escalation of the dose of drug necessary to provide adequate analgesia, which has been previously discussed. For the cancer patient, a rapid escalation of opioid requirements is often associated with increased pain from progressive tumor growth.

Physical Dependence

"Physical dependence" describes the phenomenon of withdrawal with acute discontinuance of the opioid drug or with administration of an opioid antagonist.

Addiction

Tolerance and physical dependence are both predictable pharmacologic effects of chronic opioid administration. These states are distinct from psychological dependence (addiction) in which there is a concomitant behavioral pattern of drug abuse by an individual who craves a drug for other than pain relief. Fear of addiction limits the use of opioid analgesics in clinical practice; however, there are few available published data that delineate the degree of addiction in patients receiving opioid analgesics for cancer and pain.

Many of the studies before 1954 present a biased view by using opioid addicts admitted to a treatment facility as the subjects of their studies. In another prospective study, Porter and Jick (1980) monitored the incidence of opioid addiction in 11,882 hospitalized medical patients who received at least one opioid preparation. There were only four cases of reasonably well-documented addiction in patients who had no history of addiction. Analysis of the patterns of drug intake in a series of cancer patients receiving opioid analgesics chronically suggests that drug abuse and psychological dependence did not occur in the population of patients with cancer (Kanner et al., 1981). The dearth of clinical studies offers limited support to the belief that chronic opioid use for analgesia is associated with a high risk of addiction.

Overdose

Escalating the dose of a drug to maintain adequate analgesia may lead to excessive sedation and respiratory depression. Respiratory depression in patients receiving opioids on a chronic basis is rare, however. Use of naloxone to reverse the effect of sedation and respiratory depression should be undertaken with extreme caution. Thorough evaluation of respiratory status, which involves respiratory rate, oxygen saturation, and sedation intensity, should be assessed before routinely giving an ampoule of naloxone. Generally, only close observation is required while the effects of the opioids slowly subside.

For patients chronically receiving opioids, diluted doses of naloxone (0.4 mg in 10 cc saline) should be titrated carefully to prevent severe withdrawal symptoms while reversing respiratory depression. For the comatose patient, an endotracheal tube should be placed before naloxone administration to prevent aspiration-associated respiratory compromise with excessive salivation and bronchial spasm. For patients with cancer who take opioid analgesics chronically and who develop the side effects of excessive sedation or respiratory depression, excessive drug intake is rarely the cause of stupor. More commonly, the cause is medical deterioration of the patient with a superimposed metabolic encephalopathy. Reducing the dose of the opioid drug with careful assessment of the patient's metabolic status will usually provide the diagnosis.

Inappropriate Antidiuretic Hormone Syndrome

Inappropriate antidiuretic hormone syndrome occurs rarely and is usually transient. It occurs most commonly with morphine and methadone.

Drug Interactions Involving Opioids

Examples of drug interactions with meperidine, methadone, and propoxyphene are as follows (Inturrisi and Foley, 1984).

1. Meperidine with phenobarbital: Phenobarbital enhances *N*-demethylation of meperidine. Increasing the metabolite normeperidine produces CNS toxic effects without added analgesia.
2. Meperidine with monoamine oxidase inhibitors: This combination may produce malignant hyperthermia, which may be fatal.
3. Methadone with rifampin: Rifampin induces opioid withdrawal by lowering plasma concentrations of the drugs and increasing urinary excretion of its major metabolite.

4. Propoxyphene with phenytoin: Propoxyphene interferes with Dilantin metabolism by inhibiting hydroxylating enzymes.

ANALGESIC ADJUVANT DRUGS

Clinical interest in the use of analgesic adjuvant drugs (Table 23–6) in pain management has developed from understanding the neuropharmacology of pain. Recognition of the important role of neurotransmitters in central pain modulation and the ability of these analgesic adjuvant drugs to enhance or block neurotransmitter function has led to clinical trials in painful states.

The analgesic effects of some of these drugs have been well established in controlled clinical trials (i.e., phenytoin or carbamazepine for trigeminal neuralgia; methotrimeprazine for postoperative pain. [Swerdlow, 1984; Lasagna and Kornfield, 1961]), but anecdotal data or clinical surveys provide the rationale for the use of others. Recently, gabapentin in diabetic neuropathy and post-herpetic neuralgia (Backonja et al., 1998; Rowbotham et al., 1998) has been shown to be effective. A number of anecdotal reports show gabapentin to be safe and effective for neuropathic pain. Newer generation anticonvulsants may offer a better side-effect profile (Backonja et al., 1998; Rowbotham et al., 1998).

The clinical use of these drugs to manage cancer pain has not been well established. They have been used primarily as "co-analgesics," intended to increase the analgesic effects of the opioid analgesics either additively or synergistically or to counteract the undesirable side effects of these agents. Therefore, any attempt to develop guidelines for the use of adjuvant drugs in clinical cancer pain management must be prefaced with certain caveats:

1. Appropriate use of the drugs to enhance analgesia or to treat side effects depends on careful assessment of clinical signs and symptoms.
2. The drugs have been developed and released for clinical indications other than analgesia. A partial list of these indications includes nausea, vomiting, anxiety, mania, depression, psychosis, delirium, and epilepsy.
3. The drugs are not as effective in relieving pain as the opioid analgesics, except in certain instances such as methotrimeprazine and amitriptyline (Lasagna and De Kornfield, 1961).
4. There are no efficacy studies for their co-analgesic properties in cancer patients.
5. The choice of adjuvants should be individualized, using the simplest and most potent combination of drugs.

These caveats notwithstanding, attention to and inclusion of these drugs in the management of pain must be at least considered, but caution must be used when designing guidelines based on anecdotal information.

Tricyclic Antidepressants

Tricyclic antidepressants (TCAs) are the main group of antidepressants currently being used for the purpose of treating neuropathic pain syndromes. Several theories have been suggested to explain their analgesic properties, yet none has yet been proved (Magni, 1991). They probably act by inhibiting serotonin and norepinephrine reuptake by nerve endings in the spinal cord and brain. Their pharmacologic action is independent of their mood-altering effects, and they either exert an inherent influence over the nervous system or modulate opioid pathways by an unknown mechanism (Haddox, 1992). These agents, because of their nonanalgesic properties, are particularly useful for patients who are depressed or have insomnia, conditions that are frequently encountered in the cancer pain patient population.

Tricyclic antidepressants are not universally tolerated especially at the initiation of therapy and often have to be discontinued or decreased due to dose-limiting side effects, most commonly anticholinergic and sedative effects. Amitriptyline and nortriptyline (lower cardiovascular side-effect profile) are thought to be the most efficacious agents and are the most often used. The dose should be gradually escalated from 10 mg, and patients should be told that the full benefit does not occur until after the first week or two of therapy.

Anticonvulsants

Anticonvulsants have been traditionally used with good results to treat diabetic neuropathy, post-herpetic neuralgia, trigeminal neuralgia, and similar syndromes (Kloke et al., 1991), which has encouraged researchers to conduct trials of these drugs with other types of pain with variable outcomes. Although the conditions listed above can co-exist in cancer patients, space-occupying lesions cause the most significant pain secondary to brachial and lumbosacral plexopathies. Phantom pain is also commonly seen in our practice and can be treated with anticonvulsants.

Phenytoin, valproate, carbamazepine, and clonazepam have been used. Because of issues regarding their safety and side effects, their use has been strictly limited to pain control to situations when they are most needed, namely, neuropathic pain.

Gabapentin can be considered a breakthrough drug in this regard. Despite its lack of domination in the field of seizure control, the opposite can be said for its place in pain management. With its wide therapeutic window and similar (or better) efficacy compared with other anticonvulsants, gabapentin was very beneficial for clinicians prescribing anticonvulsants because there is no need to monitor blood levels or perform other clinical testing during its administration. Sedation is a side effect, which can be reduced by starting therapy at 100 mg tid and adding 100 mg to each dose every second or third day until the desired effect is acquired. If necessary, dose escalation up to 3600 mg/day is recommended.

Lidocaine

Analgesia from the sodium channel blocking activity of lidocaine can be derived from systemic administration, as evidenced by several case reports. Like gabapentin, the greatest benefit is acquired in neuropathic pain syndromes and in phantom pain with mainly central features (Nagaro et al., 1995; Brose and Cousins, 1991). Slow-rate infusions have been used as a third or fourth line of treatment, especially for opioid-tolerant patients. Incremental rate infusions over 20 to 30 minutes can, on the other hand, be used as a therapeutic test before starting the oral form of mexiletine in patients where anticonvulsants are not effective. Cardiac monitoring is mandatory.

Ketamine

The analgesic properties of ketamine, an anesthetic agent (NMDA receptor antagonist), have been well documented. Over the past 10 years, a large series of reports of its use as an analgesic in subanesthetic doses, mainly in cancer patients, have been published (Mercadante et al., 1995; Clark and Kalan, 1995; Yang et al., 1996). Ketamine can be used in cases of extreme opioid tolerance and for long-term palliative care. Starting doses of 150 mg/day by subcutaneous infusion or 1 mg every 12 hours intrathecally have been suggested (Yang et al., 1996). It is also available in oral and rectal forms. In the authors' experience, ketamine is particularly beneficial for counteracting opioid tolerance in patients taking chronic high-dose opioids and undergoing surgery. Additional investigations and clinical trials are needed before ketamine is used routinely.

Capsaicin

Due to its high toxicity profile, capsaicin is used only as a topical cream to treat neuropathic pain (Ellison et al., 1997). It acts by inhibiting substance P formation at the skin. It is effective in only 50% to 60% of patients.

Miscellaneous Drugs

In refractory pain situations, drugs from other classes have been tried, some with potentially good responses and others with only a minimal response. They include psychotropic drugs (Breitbart, 1998; Patt et al., 1994), benzodiazepines (Reddy and Patt, 1994), bisphosphonates (Bruera et al., 1996), steroids, radiopharmaceuticals (^{89}Strontium, Sumarium), antibiotics in infection, and occasionally in head and neck cancer patients (Bruera et al., 1996). Recent studies have concluded that pamidronate or a drug from that class can be used routinely for metastatic bone disease, especially in breast cancer.

PHYSICAL MEDICINE APPROACHES: NONPHARMACOLOGIC, NONINVASIVE TREATMENTS

There has been only limited scientific research into the analgesic benefits of many commonly used treatments, especially in the cancer population. A random survey of American adults was reported in the *New England Journal of Medicine* (Eisenberg et al., 1993) and confirmed that one out of three American adults pays out of pocket to obtain treatment from "alternative" healthcare providers. The two most commonly used therapies were chiropractic manipulation and massage therapy. The leading medical diagnosis for which such treatments were obtained was chronic back pain. Chiropractic bony adjustments of the skeleton and massage therapy (soft-tissue manipulation) are part of a spectrum of manipulative interventions that also includes orthopedic and osteopathic manipulation and physical treatment modalities usually delivered by physical therapists.

Physical Therapy

The true incidence of musculoskeletal conditions in cancer patients is unknown. Major deforming surgical procedures of the neck, trunk, and extremities may result in musculoskeletal imbalances. Physical treatments such as massage, ultrasound, hydrotherapy, electroacupuncture, and trigger point injection are clinically indicated for musculoskeletal pain. Skillful soft tissue manipulation is probably underutilized in the traditional medical setting. Exercises for strength, general conditioning, and ambulation training are necessary components of an overall rehabilitation program (see Chapter 22).

The use of "passive" modalities of treatment has been criticized in the setting of chronic nonmalignant pain, due to the potential reinforcement of dependency on caregivers. However, cancer patients often feel stigmatized and socially isolated. A physical demonstration of caring through a "hands-on" method, if it alleviates this, might offset the possible negative outcome of reinforced dependency.

Physiologic and Psychological Effects of Massage

Massage may be studied in terms of the physiologic basis of its effects; the psychological effects; the effects of different techniques; effects on tissue, organ or system; or its application as a treatment for a specific condition. Massage therapy has been shown to reduce pain intensity in nonmalignant chronic pain and headache (Konrad et al., 1992; Koes et al., 1992; Jensen et al., 1990; Puustjarvi et al., 1990). Limited data suggest that massage might serve as a useful adjunctive therapy for cancer pain. One study has demonstrated that patient acceptance of this type of treatment is high (Engel et al., 1987); complications are unusual (Tachi et al., 1990).

Other Physical Therapy Modalities

The application of thermal agents produces analgesia through the physiologic responses of the tissues treated. Heat may be applied superficially or deeply. Counterirritation with topical salves may act through the depletion of analgesic mediators such as substance P.

Electrical stimulation of surface tissues may produce analgesia via amplification of non-noxious inputs that interfere with nociceptive transmission of sensation at the level of the dorsal horn. Stimulation of spinal cord or brain stem structures is thought to activate segmental or descending modulating influences, which inhibit ascending nociceptive transmission.

Traction may be applied manually by a therapist or with various devices. This is effective for stretching soft tissue contractures and mobilizing stiff joints and may be useful when these conditions contribute to painful limitation of motion.

Psychological Interventions

Providing analgesia through pharmacologic methods helps to mitigate the stress of ongoing pain. Many patients would also like to utilize methods that enhance their sense of personal control and thus assist them in regaining a sense of personal integrity. Psychological strategies are widely employed in the treatment of chronic pain of nonmalignant origin. The psychological treatment of cancer patients has been reviewed elsewhere (Trijsburg et al., 1992). New cognitive strategies for coping may need to be learned. Supportive psychotherapy is indicated at times of particular psychological stress on coping mechanisms (Breitbart, 1989) (see Chapter 26.)

Simple relaxation methods can be used for acute and chronic pain. More complex relaxation techniques, such as those that utilize music, imagery, or biofeedback, have also been shown to be effective analgesic methods (ACHPR Acute Pain Guidelines).

NEUROSURGICAL AND ANESTHETIC APPROACHES

A major challenge to the oncologist in managing the patient with intractable pain relates to the timing and selection of alternative therapies. The alternative therapies are often costly and invasive, thereby posing a significant risk of morbidity to the patient, and often are not as convincingly efficacious as first-line treatments.

Standard analgesic therapies such as oral morphine in combination with NSAIDs and adjuvant drugs used in accordance with World Health Organization guidelines should almost always be exhausted before alternative approaches are tried. In addition, the decision to initiate alternative analgesic therapies also implies that no further antitumor treatments will be effective for the management of the primary tumor. As stated before and repeated for emphasis here, treatment failure with conventional analgesic therapies implies titration of all drug therapies to maximum doses, such that the patient reaches dose-limiting side effects, until adequate pain relief is achieved. For most patients with cancer pain, this also means that alternative routes of opioid administration, such as subcutaneous or intravenous infusion and patient-controlled administration (PCA), have been tried and failed.

Both neurosurgical and anesthetic procedures play a small but significant role in the management of cancer pain. According to the AHCPR guidelines, approximately 10% of all cancer patients could benefit from some of these procedures. They are, however, best regarded as complimentary to other therapies, which include primary treatment for cancer, pharmacotherapy, and behavioral and psychiatric approaches.

Principles of anesthetic procedures are as follows:

1. They are useful and/or needed in 10% to 15% of patients.
2. They are not a panacea, but useful when complimentary to other therapies.
3. They are usually reserved for patients with intractable pain, experiencing dose-limiting side effects.
4. Local anesthetic blocks have limited value, but can act as diagnostic tools.
5. Neurolytic blocks have a favorable risk/benefit ratio when given in terminal situations, except for sympathetic blocks like celiac and hypogastric, which some physicians believe are best administered early in the course of treatment.
6. Intrathecal therapy is reserved for pain of the lower body and for patients with a prognosis of at least 6 months or more. Clonidine may help patients with neuropathic pain syndromes.
7. Epidural therapy is preferable for patients with thoracic and lower body pain, especially neuropathic, and for patients with a prognosis of 1 to 3 months. Infection and cost are the limiting factors.
8. Neurosurgical procedures have a limited role secondary to complications and the wider use of pharmacotherapy. Useful neurosurgical procedures include cordotomy and myelotomy.

Types of Anesthetic Nerve Blocks

Somatic Nerve Blocks

Somatic nerve blocks (Table 23–8) may be diagnostic (i.e., to determine an indication for permanent neurolysis of somatic nerves), facilitative, prophylactic, or therapeutic and are indicated for pain that is well characterized, well localized, and somatic in origin. Somatic nerve blocks include paravertebral block for localized chest pain and brachial plexus block for upper extremity pain. Unless a neurolytic agent is used to neurolyze somatic nerves, the local anesthetic block lasts for the duration of local anesthetic effect. However, the neurolytic blocks, which are aimed at chemical destruction of the nerve, may be limited in use secondary to neurologic deficits that may result from the block. Somatic neurolytic blocks may also result in post-block dysesthesias, pain that can be worse than the original pain being treated.

Sympathetic Nerve Blocks

Sympathetic nerve blocks (Table 23–8) are indicated for SMP as well as for visceral pain (e.g., complex regional pain syndrome type 1), or reflex sympathetic dystrophy, visceral pain as in pancreatic cancer, and pelvic pain. A stellate ganglion block is indicated for SMP of the upper extremity (Warfield, 1984). Celiac ganglion blocks are used for pancreatic cancer pain (Bridenbaugh et al, 1964) and hypogastric blocks for pelvic pain (Plancarte et al., 1990). The effects from blocks used with local anesthesia are short lived and are used only for diagnostic and prognostic purposes. If a block with local anesthetic is successful, a neurolytic block with either alcohol or phenol is given to achieve longer lasting relief.

Table 23–8. Anesthetic Approaches for Cancer Pain

*Procedures**	*Usual Indication(s)*	*Examples*
Local anesthetic blocks with or without steroids	Diagnostic blocks. Used to diagnose source of pain and to diagnose type of pain	Stellate ganglion blocks
	Prognostic blocks. Used as a prelude to paravertebral block or neurolytic block	Celiac plexus block
		Epidural steroid injection
		Brachial plexus and lumbar plexus block
Neurolytic blocks† (with alcohol or phenol)	Localized refractory pain that is expected to persist, usually in the presence of a short life expectancy; pain localized to a region that is associated with a low risk of neurologic complications	Alcohol celiac plexus block
		Phenol intercostals saddle block
Thoracic subarachnoid neurolysis	Focal chest wall pain	
Intercostal neurolysis	Focal chest wall pain	
Lumbar subarachnoid neurolysis	Unilateral leg pain in bed-bound patients	
Psoas compartment block	Unilateral pain in upper lumbar dermatomes	
Celiac plexus/splanchnic/neurolysis	Abdominal pain, back pain	
Superior hypogastric plexus neurolysis	Pelvic pain	
Phenol saddle block	Perineal pain with urinary diversion	
Gasserian ganglion	Facial pain	Trigeminal nerve block branches
Spinal analgesics‡	Refractory pain, usually in lower body, but may be widespread or diffuse	Externalized epidural catheter (useful when large volume infusion is needed, e.g., local anesthesia)
		Intrathecal catheter with fully implanted pump (useful when prognosis is expected to be >6 months)

*These blocks are temporary and usually last for the duration of local anesthetic.

†These blocks can cause temporary or permanent neurologic deficits. Hence, they are done if the risk/benefit ratio is favorable (e.g., in terminal cancer situation and localized pain).

‡These procedures are useful if pain is intractable and refractory to other modalities. They offer better risk/benefit ratio versus neurolytic procedures; most helpful for patients with a prognosis of 3 months or more.

Intrathecal/Epidural Analgesia

Administration of opioids and other medications into the neural axis is well documented and widely practiced (Bennett et al., 2000). It is a routine practice in acute pain management as well as for labor pain. However, long-term use of these medications requires special expertise in patient selection and techniques for implantation of devices. The principle underlying this therapy is that a drug can be administered at close proximity to opioid and other receptors, requiring minute quantities while achieving superior analgesia. This assumption has been recently questioned, but for a selected patient population this method may prove to be quite effective. The CNS can be accessed by an epidural, intrathecal, or intraventricular route.

Epidurals are useful for patients who have intractable neuropathic pain that has not responded to either oral or parenteral therapy, and who most likely need a moderate amount of local anesthetic in the epidural space, e.g., lumbosacral plexopathy resulting from a pelvic tumor. But their long-term use is associated with tolerance, infection, and expense. Hence, epidural use is limited to patients whose prognosis is likely to be from 1 to 3 months (Bedder et al., 1991; Hassenbusch et al., 1992).

Intrathecal opioids are indicated for patients with diffuse somatic pain syndromes that do not respond to either oral or parenteral opioid therapy or for patients with dose-limiting side effects from other routes. Intrathecal administration is useful for patients who have bilateral or midline pain below the level of the midthorax (Payne, 1987). However, the pharmacokinetics of spinally administered morphine are such that supraspinal effects such as sedation and nausea/vomiting might not be avoided (Max et al., 1987). Of interest, one study showed that epidural morphine was indistinguishable from systemic morphine in its effect on cognitive function (Sjogren and Banning, 1989). Therefore, spinal morphine administration should not be considered as a first line of therapy for most patients with intractable cancer pain

Administration of opioids by this route requires implantation of a special pump that delivers opioid continuously into the cerebrospinal fluid. Minor surgery is required for implantation. The infection rate is low compared with epidurals because of internalization of the delivery system. In addition to opioids, other medications like clonidine, local anesthetic, and neuronal-specific calcium channel blockers (ziconotide) may be used. Cost is an issue, but may be justified if the pain control provided is stable and the patient's prognosis is expected to be more than 6 months (Bedder et al., 1991; Hassenbusch et al., 1992). This method is best suited for cancer survivors who have intractable chronic pain syndromes resulting from treatment of cancer (e.g., peripheral neuropathy from chemotherapy, post-surgical pain syndromes, and radiation-induced pain).

Neurosurgical Procedures

Neurosurgical procedures (Table 23–9) are infrequently used because of their lack of efficacy, high complication rate, and the wide availability and effective use of opioids and adjuvant medications. Moreover, intrathecal techniques and infusion of various opioids and nonopioids have resulted in a decreased need for neuroablative procedures. Some of the neurosurgical procedures that are still used effectively include pituitary adenolysis (Levin, 1980), percutaneous cordotomy for unilateral lower extremity pain (Rosomoff et al., 1965; Sanders and Zuurmond, 1995), and myelotomy for midline pain (Hassenbusch et al., 1997). Surgical ablation may also be accomplished by rhizotomy (section of nerve root) (Broager, 1974) or dorsal root entry-zone lesions (Nashold and Nashold, 1996). Spinal anterolateral tractotomy, mesencephalotomy, medullary tractotomy, and cingulotomy are rarely performed and should be reserved for carefully selected patients.

Cordotomy may be an alternative for patients with midline sacral or perineal pain who have failed systemic and spinal opioid therapy. This can be accomplished safely by an experienced neurosurgeon using a percutaneous approach to produce a destructive lesion in the spinothalamic tract in the cervical cord. Most patients obtain immediate pain relief, and as

Table 23–9. Neurosurgical Procedures for the Control of Cancer Pain

Operation	*Target Site*	*Method*
Peripheral neurotomy	Sensory or mixed nerve, greater occipital nerve, glossopharyngeal nerves, intercostal nerves, trigeminal divisions, trigeminal spinal	Radiofrequency—thermal, chemical, surgical
Rhizotomy		Radiofrequency—thermal, chemical, surgical
Stereotactic thalamotomy	VPM/VPL basal thalamus	Radiofrequency—thermal
DREZ lesion	Spinal	Radiofrequency—thermal
Cordotomy	C1–2, T2, lower cervical	Radiofrequency—thermal, microsurgical; anterior approach to low cervical
Commisural myelotomy	Segmental, conus medullaris	Microsurgical ± laser
Trigeminal glycerol rhizolysis	Gasserian ganglion	Radiofrequency—thermal, chemical
Hypophysectomy	Pituitary	Open or stereotactic radiofrequency—thermal, chemical, or radiosurgery

many as 60% maintain pain relief for 6 months. Transient urinary retention and ipsilateral paralysis are the most common side effects. Fewer than 1% of patients develop uncomfortable post-cordotomy paresthesia, generally occurring more than 18 months after the procedure. Percutaneous cordotomy should be considered early in the course for a patient with incident pain because the rapid increase in pain with movement does not usually allow adequate treatment with opioids, even when PCA is attempted. However, new pain sites are unmasked in many patients after a unilateral cordotomy, and bilateral procedures are required for the management of midline or bilateral pain.

REFERENCES

Aaronson NK. 1988. Quality of life: what is it? How should it be measured? Oncology (Huintingt) 2:69–76.

Arner S, Meyerson BA. 1988. Lack of analgesic effect of opioids on neuropathic and idiopathic forms of pain. Pain 33:11–23.

Asbury AK, Bird SJ. 1992. Disorders of peripheral nerve. In: Asbury AK, McKhann GM, McDonald WI (eds), Diseases of the Nervous System: Clinical Neurobiology, 2nd ed, vol 1. Philadelphia: WB Saunders, p 252.

Bach S, Noreng MF, Tjellden NU. 1988. Phantom limb pain in amputees during the first 12 months following limb amputation, after preoperative lumbar epidural blockade. Pain 33:297–301.

Backonja MM. 2000. Anticonvulsants (antineuropathics) for neuropathic pain syndromes. Clin J Pain 16(suppl): S67–72.

Backonja M, Beydoun A, Edwards KR, et al. 1998. Gabapentin for the symptomatic treatment of painful neuropathy in patients with diabetes mellitus: a randomized controlled trial. JAMA 280:1831–1836.

Beaver WT, Wallenstein SL, Houde RW, Rogers A. 1967. A clinical comparison of the analgesic effects of methadone and morphine administered intramuscularly, and of orally and parenterally administered methadone. Clin Pharmacol Ther 8:415–426.

Beaver WT, Wallenstein SL, Rogers A, Houde RW. 1978a. Analgesic studies of codeine and oxycodone in patients with cancer. I. Comparisons of oral with intramuscular codeine and of oral with intramuscular oxycodone. J Pharmacol Exp Ther 207:92–100.

Beaver WT, Wallenstein SL, Rogers A, Houde RW. 1978b. Analgesic studies of codeine and oxycodone in patients with cancer. II. Comparisons of intramuscular oxycodone with intramuscular morphine and codeine. J Pharmacol Exp Ther 207:101–108.

Bedder MD, Burchiel K, Larson A. 1991. Cost analysis of two implantable narcotic delivery systems. J Pain Symptom Manage 6:368–373.

Bennett G, Sefrani M, Burchiel K, et al. 2000. Evidence-based review of the literature on intrathecal delivery of pain medication. J Pain Symptom Manage 20:S12–S36.

Berenson JR, Lichtenstein A, Porter L, et al. 1996. Efficacy of pamidronate in reducing skeletal events in patients with advanced multiple myeloma. Myeloma Aredia Study Group. N Engl J Med 334:488–493.

Blair DN, Rapoport S, Sostman HD, Blair OC. 1987. Normal brachial plexus: MR imaging. Radiology 165:763–767.

Boas RA, Schug SA, Acland RH. 1993. Perineal pain after rectal amputation: a 5-year follow-up. Pain 52:67–70.

Bonica JJ. 1990. Cancer Pain. In: Bonica JJ (ed), The Management of Pain, 2nd ed. Philadelphia: Lea & Febiger, p 400.

Bowersox SS, Gadbois T, Singh T, Pettus M, Wang XX, Luter RR. 1996. Selective N-type neuronal voltage-sensitive calcium channel blocker, SNX-111, produces spinal antinociception in rat models of acute, persistent and neuropathic pain. J Pharmacol Exp Ther 279:1243–1249.

Bradway JK, Malone JM, Racy J, et al. 1984. Psychological adaptation to amputation—an overview. Orthot Prosthet 38:46–50.

Breitbart W. 1989. Psychiatric management of cancer pain. Cancer 63(suppl):S2336.

Breitbart W. 1998. Psychotropic adjuvant analgesics for pain in cancer and AIDS. Psychooncology 7:333–345.

Bridenbaugh LD, Moore DC, Campbell DD. 1964. Management of upper abdominal cancer pain. JAMA 190:877–890.

Broager B. 1974. Commissural myelotomy. Surg Neurol 2:71–74.

Brose WG, Cousins MJ. 1991. Subcutaneous lidocaine for treatment of neuropathic cancer pain. Pain 45:145–148.

Bruera E, Brenneis C, Paterson AH, MacDonald RN. 1989a. Use of methylphenidate as an adjuvant to narcotic analgesics in patients with advanced cancer 1989. J Pain Symptom Manage 4:3–6.

Bruera ED, Chadwick S, Bacovsky R, Macdonald N. 1985. Continuous subcutaneous infusion of narcotics using a portable disposable pump. J Palliat Care 1:46–47.

Bruera E, MacMillan K, Hanson J, MacDonald RN. 1989b. The cognitive effects of the administration of narcotic analgesics in patients with cancer pain. Pain 39:13–16.

Bruera E, MacMillan K, Hanson J, MacDonald RN. 1989c. The Edmonton staging system for cancer pain: preliminary report. Pain 37:203–209.

Bruera E, Pereira J, Watanabe S, Belzile M, Kuehn N, Hanson J. 1996. Opioid rotation in patients with cancer pain. A retrospective comparison of dose ratios between methadone, hydromorphone, and morphine. Cancer 78:852–857.

Bruera E, Schoeller T, Wenk R, et al. 1995. A prospective multicenter assessment of the Edmonton staging system for cancer pain 1995. J Pain Symptom Manage 10:348–355.

Bryne TN, Waxman SG. 1990. Spinal Cord Compression: Diagnosis and Principals of Management. Contemporary Neurology Series, Vol. 33. Philadelphia: FA Davis, 278 pp.

Buckley MM, Brogden RN. 1990. Ketorolac. A review of its pharmacodynamic and pharmacokinetic properties, and therapeutic potential. Drugs 39:86–109.

Calava JM, Patt RB, Passik SD, Reddy S, Lefkowitz M. 1996. Pain in AIDS: a call for action. Pain Clin Updates IV 1:1–4.

Cascino TL, Kori S, Krol G, Foley KM. 1983. CT of the brachial plexus in patients with cancer. Neurology 33:1553–1557.

Chan GL, Matzke GR. 1987. Effects of renal insufficiency on the pharmacokinetics and pharmacodynamics of opioid analgesics. Drug Intell Clin Pharm 21:773–783.

Chater S, Viola R, Paterson J, Jarvis V. 1998. Sedation for intractable distress in the dying—a survey of experts. Palliat Med 12:255–269.

Cherny NI, Thaler HT, Friedlander-Klar H, et al. 1994. Opioid responsiveness of cancer pain syndromes caused by neuropathic or nociceptive mechanisms: a combined analysis of controlled, single-dose studies. Neurology 44:857–861.

Cherry DA, Gourlay GK, Cousins MJ. 1986. Epidural mass associated with lack of efficacy of epidural morphine and undetectable CSF morphine concentrations. Pain 25:69–73.

Citron ML, Johnston-Early A, Boyer M, Krasnow SH, Hood M, Cohen MH. 1986. Patient-controlled analgesia for severe cancer pain. Arch Intern Med 146:734–736.

Clark JL, Kalan GE. 1995. Effective treatment of severe cancer pain of the head using low-dose ketamine. J Pain Symptom Manage 10:310–314.

Cleeland CS. 1984. The impact of pain of the patient with cancer. Cancer 54:2635–2641.

Cleeland CS, Gonin R, Hatfield AK, Edmonson JH, Blum RH, Stewart JA, Pandya KJ. 1994. Pain and its treatment in outpatients with metastatic cancer. N Engl J Med 330:592–596.

Codd EE, Shank RP, Schupsky JJ, Raffia RB. 1995. Serotonin and norepinephrine uptake inhibiting activity of centrally acting analgesics: structural determinants and role in antinociception. J Pharmacol Exp Ther 274:1263–1270.

Coleman RE. 1991. Bisphosphonate treatment of bone metastases and hypercalcemia of malignancy. Oncology 5:55–60.

Cotten A, Dewatre F, Cortet B, Assaker R, Leblond D, Duquesnoy B, Chastanet P, Clarisse J. 1996. Percutaneous vertebroplasty for osteolytic metastases and myeloma: effects of the percentage of lesion filling and the leakage of methyl methacrylate at clinical follow-up. Radiology 200:525–530.

Crossen JR, Garwood D, Glatstein E, Neuwelt EA. 1994. Neurobehavioral sequelae of cranial irradiation in adults: a review of radiation-induced encephalopathy. J Clin Oncol 12:627–642.

Davis RW. 1993. Phantom sensation, phantom pain, and stump pain. Arch Phys Med Rehabil 74:79–91.

Davis AM, Inturrisi CE. 1999. d-Methadone blocks morphine tolerance and *N*-methyl-D-aspartate-induced hyperalgesia. J Pharmacol Exp Ther 289:1048–1053.

Davis MP, Walsh D. 2001. Methadone for relief of cancer pain: a review of pharmacokinetics, pharmacodynamics, drug interactions and protocols of administration. Support Care Cancer 9:73–83.

Dellemijn PL, Vanneste JA. 1997. Randomised double-blind active-placebo–controlled crossover trial of intravenous fentanyl in neuropathic pain. Lancet 349:753–758.

Dixon R. 1986. Pharmacokinetics of levorphanol. Adv Pain Res Ther 8:217–224.

Ducatman BS, Scheithauer BW. 1983. Postirradiation neurofibrosarcoma. Cancer 51:1028–1033.

Ebert B, Andersen S, Krogsgaard-Larsen P. 1995. Ketobemidone, methadone and pethidine are non-competitive *N*-methyl-D-aspartate (NMDA) antagonists in the rat cortex and spinal cord. Neurosci Lett 187:165–168.

Eisenach JC, DuPen S, Dubois M, Miguel R, Allin D. 1995. Epidural clonidine analgesia for intractable cancer pain. The Epidural Clonidine Study Group. Pain 61:391–399.

Eisenberg DM, Kessler RC, Foster C, Norlock FE, Calkins DR. 1993. Unconventional medicine in the United States. Prevalence, costs, and patterns of use. N Engl J Med 328: 246–252.

Ellison N, Loprinzi CL, Kugler J, et al. 1997. Phase III placebo-controlled trial of capsaicin cream in the management of surgical neuropathic pain in cancer patients. J Clin Oncol 15:2974–2980.

Engel JM, Josenhans G, Hoder J, Binzus G. 1987. [Value of physical therapy from the viewpoint of the patient. Results of a questionnaire]. Z Rheumatol 46:250–255.

Fine PG, Marcus M, De Boer AJ, Van der Oord B. 1991. An open label study of oral transmucosal fentanyl citrate (OTFC) for the treatment of breakthrough cancer pain. Pain 45:149–153.

Finsen V, Persen L, Lovlien M, et al. 1988. Transcutaneous electrical nerve stimulation after major amputation. J Bone Joint Surg Br 70:109–112.

Foley KM. 1979. Pain syndromes in patients with cancer. In: Bonica JJ, Bentafridda V (eds), Advances in Pain Research and Therapy. New York: Raven Press, pp 59–75.

Foley KM. 1984. The treatment of cancer pain. N Engl J Med 313:84–95.

Foley KM. 1989. Controversies in cancer pain. Medical perspectives. Cancer 63:2257–2265.

Foley KM. 1991. The relationship of pain and symptom management to patient requests for physician-assisted suicide. J Pain Symptom Manage 6:289–297.

Foley KM. 1993. Management of cancer pain. In: DeVita VT Jr, Hellman S, Rosenberg SA (eds), Cancer: Principles and Practice of Oncology, 4th ed. Philadelphia: JB Lippincott, p 2417.

Foley KM, Woodruff JM, Ellis FT, Posner JB. 1980. Radiation-induced malignant and atypical peripheral nerve sheath tumors. Arch Neurol 7:311–318.

Fordyce WE. 1983. The validity of pain behavior measurement. In: Melzack R (ed), Pain Measurement and Assessment. New York: Raven Press, p 145.

Fraioli F, Fabbri A, Gnessi L, et al. 1984. Calcitonin and analgesia. In: Benedetti C, Chapman CR, Morrica G (eds), Recent Advances in the Management of Pain, vol 7. New York: Raven Press, p 237.

Front D, Schneck SO, Frankel A, Robinson E. 1979. Bone metastases and bone pain in breast cancer. Are they closely associated? JAMA 242:1747–1748.

Galasko CSB. 1976. Mechanisms of bone destruction in the development of skeletal metastases. Nature 263:507–508.

Galasko CS. 1982. Mechanisms of lytic and blastic metastatic disease of bone. Clin Orthop 169:20–27.

Glare PA, Walsh TD. 1993. Dose-ranging study of oxycodone for chronic pain in advanced cancer. J Clin Oncol 11: 973–978.

Gonzales GR, Elliot KJ, Portenoy RK, Foley KM. 1991. Impact of a comprehensive evaluation in the management of cancer pain. Pain 47:141–144.

Goodwin JS, Goodwin JM, Vogel AV. 1979. Knowledge and use of placebos by house officers and nurses. Ann Intern Med 91:106–110.

Gorman AL, Elliott KJ, Inturrsi CE. 1997. The d-and l-isomers of methadone bind to the non-competitive site on the *N*-methyl-D-asparate (NMDA) receptor in rat forebrain and spinal cord. Neurosci Lett 223:5–8.

Greenberg HS, Deck MD, Vikram B, Chu Fc, Posner JB. 1981. Metastasis to the base of the skull: clinical findings in 43 patients. Neurology 31:530–537.

Haddox JD. 1992. Neuropsychiatric drug use in management of pain. In: Raj PP (ed), Practical Management of Pain, 2nd ed. St. Louis: Mosby, 1096 pp.

Hanks GW, Twycross RG, Lloyd JW. 1981. Unexpected complication of successful nerve block. Morphine induced respiratory depression precipitated by removal of severe pain. Anesthesia 36:37–39.

Hassenbusch SJ, Paice PJ, Patt RB, Bedder MD, Bell GK. 1997. Clinical realities and economic considerations: economics of intrathecal therapy. J Pain Symptom Manage 14:S36–S48.

Hawkey CJ. 1999. Cox-2 inhibitors. Lancet 353:307–314.

Higginson IJ. 1997. Innovations in assessment: epidemiology and assessment of pain in advanced cancer. In: Jenson TS, Turner JA, Wiesenfeld-Hallin Z (eds), Proceeding of the 8th World Congress on Pain, Progress in Pain Research and Therapy, vol 8. Seattle: IASP Press, pp 707–716.

Hill CS Jr. 1990. Relationship among cultural, educational, and regulatory agency influences on optimum cancer pain treatment. J Pain Symptom Manage 5:S37–S45.

Hill CS Jr, Fields WS. 1989. Advances in Pain Research and Therapy, vol 11. Treatment of Cancer Pain in a Drug-Oriented Society. New York: Raven Press.

Hortobagyi GN, Proter L, Blayney D, et al. 1996. Reduction of skeletal related complications in breast cancer patients with osteolytic bone metastasis receiving chemotherapy by monthly pamidronate sodium infusion. ASCO Proc15:103.

Houde RW, Wallenstein SL, Beaver WT. 1966. Evaluation of analgesics in patients with cancer pain. In: Lasagna L (ed), Clinical Pharmacology. International Encyclopedia of Pharmacology and Therapeutics. New York: Pregamon Press, p 59.

Hwang SS, Nichols KC, Southam MA. 1991. Transdermal permeation: physiological and physiochemical asoects. In: Lehmann KA, Zech D (eds), Transdermal Fentanyl: A New Approach to Prolonged Pain Control. New York: Springer-Verlag, p 1.

Ihde DC, DeVita VT. 1975. Osteonecrosis of the femoral head in patients with lymphoma treated with intermittent combination chemotherapy (including corticosteroids). Cancer 36:1585–1588.

Inturrisi CE, Colburn WN, Kaiko RF, Houde RW, Foley KM. 1987. Pharmacokinetics and pharmacodynamics of methadone in patients with chronic pain. Clin Pharmacol Ther 41:392–401.

Inturrisi CE, Foley KM. 1984. Narcotic analgesics in the management of pain. In: Kuhar MJ, Pasternak GW (eds), Analgesics: Neurochemical, Behavioral and Clinical Perspectives. New York: Raven Press, p 257.

Jacobson L, Chabal C, Brody MC. 1989. Relief of persistent postamputation stump and phantom limb pain with intrathecal fentanyl. Pain 37:317–322.

Jacobson L, Chabal C, Brody MC, Mariano AJ, Chaney EF. 1990. A comparison of the effects of intrathecal fentanyl and lidocaine on established postamputation stump pain. Pain 40:137–141.

Jacox A, Carr DB, Payne R 1994. New clinical-practice guidelines for the management of pain in patients with cancer. N Engl J Med 330:651–655.

Jaeckle KA, Young DF, Foley KM. 1985. The natural history of lumbosacral plexopathy in cancer patients. Neurology 35:8–15.

Jaffe JH, Martin WR. 1990. Opioid analgesics and antagonists. In: Gilman AG, Rall TW, Nies AS, Taylor P (eds), Goodman and Gilman's the Pharmacologic Basis of Therapeutics, 8 ed. New York: Pergamon Press, p 485.

Jellinger K, Sturm KW. 1971. Delayed radiation myelopathy in man. Report of twelve necropsy cases. J Neurol Sci 14: 389–408.

Jensen TS, Krebs B, Nielsen J, Rasmussen P. 1984. Non-painful phantom limb phenomena in amputees: incidence, clinical characteristics and temporal course. Acta Neurol Scand 70:407–414.

Jensen TS, Krebs B, Nielsen J, Rasmussen P. 1985. Immediate and long-term phantom limb pain in amputees: incidence, clinical characteristics and relationship to pre-amputation limb pain. Pain 21:267–278.

Jensen OK, Nielsen FF, Vosmar L. 1990. An open study comparing manual therapy with the use of cold packs in the treatment of post-traumatic headache. Cephalalgia 10: 241–250.

Kaiko RF. 1990. Controlled-release oral morphine for cancer-related pain. The European and North-American experiences. Adv Pain Res Ther 16:171–189.

Kaiko RF, Wallenstein SL, Rogers A, Grabinski P, Houde RW. 1981. Relative analgesic potency of intramuscular heroin and morphine in cancer patients with postoperative pain and chronic pain due to cancer. NIDA Res Monogr 34: 213–219.

Kaiko RF, Wallenstein SL, Rogers AG, Houde RW. 1983. Sources of variation in analgesic responses in cancer patients with chronic pain receiving morphine. Pain 15:191–200.

Kalso E, Vainio A. 1988. Hallucinations during morphine but not during oxycodone treatment [letter]. Lancet 2:912.

Kalso E, Vainio A. 1990. Morphine and oxycodone hydrochloride in the management of cancer pain. Clin Pharmacol Ther 47:636–646.

Kanamaru T, Saeki S, Katsumata N, Mizuno K, Ogawa S, Suzuki H. 1990. [Ketamine infusion for control of pain in patients with advanced cancer.] Masui 39:1368–1371.

Kanner RM, Martini N, Foley KM. 1981. Epidural spinal-cord compression in Pancoast syndrome (superior pulmonary sulcus tumor): clinical presentation and outcome. Ann Neurol 10:77.

Katz J, Melzack R. 1990. Pain "memories" in phantom limbs: review and clinical observations. Pain 43:319–336.

Katz J, Melzack R. 1991. Auricular transcutaneous electrical nerve stimulation (TENS) reduces phantom limb pain. J Pain Symptom Manage 6:73–83.

Katz J, Nelson W, Forest R, Bruce DL. 1980. Cryoanalgesia for post-thoracotomy pain. Lancet 1:512–513.

Kelly JB, Payne R. 1991. Pain syndromes in the cancer patient. Neurol Clin 9:937–953.

Kloke M, Hoffken K, Olbrich H, Schmidt CG. 1991. Anti-depressants and anticonvulsants for the treatment of neuropathic pain syndromes in cancer patients 1991. Onkologie 14:40–43.

Koes BW, Bouter LM, van Mameren H, et al. 1992. Randomised clinical trial of manipulative therapy and physiotherapy for persistent back and neck complaints: results of one year follow up. BMJ 304:601–605.

Konrad K, Tatrai T, Hunka A, Vereckei E, Korondi I. 1992. Controlled trial of balneotherapy in treatment of low back pain. Ann Rheum Dis 51:820–822.

Kori SH, Foley KM, Posner JB. 1981. Brachial plexus lesions in patients with cancer in 100 cases. Neurology 31:45–50.

Kotani N, Kushikata T, Hashimoto H,, et al. 2000. Intrathecal methylprednisolone for intractable postherpetic neuralgia. N Engl J Med 343:1563–1565.

Kreek MJ, Schecter AJ, Gutjahr CL, Hecht M. 1980. Methadone use in patients with chronic renal disease. Drug Alcohol Depend 5:197–205.

Kroner K, Krebs B, Skov J, Jorgensen HS. 1989. Immediate and long-term phantom breast syndrome after mastectomy: incidence, clinical characteristics and relationship to pre-mastectomy breast pain. Pain 36:327–334.

Kunz KM, Theisen JA, Schroder ME. 1993. Severe episodic pain: management with sublingual sufentanil [letter]. J Pain Symptom Manage 8:189–190.

Labella FS, Pinsky C, Havlicek V. 1979. Morphine derivatives with diminished opiate receptor potency show enhanced central excitatory activity. Brain Res 174:263–271.

Lahtinen R, Laakso M, Palva I, Virkkunen P, Elomaa I. 1992. Randomised, placebo-controlled multicenter trial of clodronate in multiple myeloma. Finnish Leukaemia Group. Lancet 340:1049–1052.

Lasagna L, De Kornfield TJ. 1961. Methotrimeprazine: a new phenothiazine derivative with analgesic properties. JAMA 178:887–890.

Lasagna L, Mosteller F, Von Felsinger JM, Beecher HK. 1954. A study of placebo response. Am J Med 16:770–779.

Lawlor PG, Turner KS, Hanson J, Bruera ED. 1998. Dose ratio between morphine and methadone in patients with cancer pain: a retrospective study. Cancer 82:1167–1173.

Levick S, Jacobs C, Loukas DF, Gordon DH, Meyskens FL, Uhm K. 1988. Naproxen sodium in the treatment of bone pain due to metastatic cancer. Pain 35:253–258.

Levin AB, Katz J, Benson RC, Jones AG. 1980. Treatment of pain of diffuse metastatic cancer by stereotactic chemical hypophysectomy: long term results and observations on mechanism of action. Neurosurgery 6:258–262.

Levin DN, Cleeland CS, Dar R. 1985. Public attitudes toward cancer pain. Cancer 56:2337–2339.

Loeser JD. 1986. Herpes zoster and postherpetic neuralgia. Pain 25:149–164.

Magni G. 1991. The use of antidepressants in the treatment of chronic pain. A review of the current evidence. Drugs 42:730–748.

Martin JB, Jean B, Sugiu K, et al. 1999. Vertebroplasty: clinical experience and follow-up results. Bone 25:11S–15S.

Max MB, Culnane M, Schafer SC, et al. 1987. Amitriptyline relieves diabetic neuropathy pain in patients with normal or depressed mood. Neurology 37:589–596.

McCleane GJ. 2000. Lamotrigine in the management of neuropathic pain: a review of the literature. Clin J Pain 16:321–326.

Mercadante S. 1997. Malignant bone pain: pathophysiology and treatment. Pain 69:1–18.

Mercadante S, Lodi F, Sapio M, Calligara M, Serretta R. 1995. Long-term ketamine subcutaneous continuous infusion in neuropathic cancer pain. J Pain Symptom Manage 10:564–568.

Meresaar U, Nilsson MI, Holmstrand J, Anggard E. 1981. Single dose pharmacokinetics and bioavailability of methadone in man studied with a stable isotope method. Eur J Clin Pharmacol 20:473–478.

Merimsky O, Reider-Groswasser I, Wigler N, Chaitchik S. 1992. Encephalopathy in ifosfamide-treated patients. Acta Neurol Scand 86:521–525.

Michaels AS, Chandrasekaran SK, Shaw JE. 1975. Drug permeation through human skin—theory and in vitro experimental measurement. Aiche J 21:985–996.

Millan MJ. 1990. Kappa-opioid receptors and analgesia. Trends Pharmacol Sci 11:70–76.

Milne RJ, Foreman RD, Giesler GJ Jr, Willis WD. 1981. Convergence of cutaneous and pelvic visceral nociceptive inputs onto primate spinothalamic neurons. Pain 11:163–183.

Minton JP. 1974. Proceedings: the response of breast cancer patients with bone pain to L-dopa. Cancer 33:358–363.

Miser AW, Dothage JA, Miser JS. 1987. Continuous intravenous fentanyl for pain control in children and young adults with cancer. Clin J Pain 3:152–157.

Miser AW, Miser JS, Clark BS. 1980. Continuous intravenous infusion of morphine sulfate for control of severe pain in children with terminal malignancy. J Pediatr 96:930–932.

Miser AW, Narang PK, Dothage JA, Young RC, Sindelar W, Miser JS. 1989. Transdermal fentanyl for pain control in patients with cancer. Pain 37:15–21.

Morley JS, Miles JB, Wells JC, Bowsher D. 1992. Paradoxical pain [letter]. Lancet 340:1045.

Morley JS, Watt JW, Wells JC, Miles JB, Finnegan MJ, Leng G. 1993. Methadone in pain uncontrolled by morphine [letter]. Lancet 342:1243.

Nagaro T, Shimizu C, Inoue H, et al. 1995. [The efficacy of intravenous lidocaine on various types of neuropathic pain]. Masui 44:862–867.

Nashold BS, Nashold JRB. 1966. The DREZ operation. In: Tindall GT, Cooper PR, Barrow DL (eds), The Practice of Neurosurgery. Baltimore: Williams & Wilkins, pp 3129–3151.

Oguri K, Yamada-Mori I, Shigezane J, Hirano T, Yoshimura H. 1987. Enhanced binding of morphine and nalorphine to opioid delta receptor by glucuronate and sulfate conjugations at the 6-position. Life Sci 41:1457–1464.

Osborne RJ, Joel SP, Slevin ML. 1986. Morphine intoxication in renal failure: the role of morphine-6-glucuronide. BMJ (Clin Res Ed) 292:1548–1549.

Paix A, Coleman A, Lees J, et al. 1995. Subcutaneous fentanyl and sufentanil infusion substitution for morphine intolerance in cancer pain management. Pain 63:263–269.

Palmer JJ. 1972. Radiation myelopathy. Brain 95:109–122.

Pasternak GW. 1993. Pharmacological mechanisms of opioid analgesia. Clin Neuropharmacol 16:1–18.

Pasternak GW, Bodnar RJ, Clarck JA, Inturrisi CE. 1987. Morphine-6-glucuronide, a potent mu agonist. Life Sci 41: 2845–2849.

Patt RB, Proper G, Reddy S. 1994. The neuroleptics as adjuvant analgesics. J Pain Symptom Manage 9:446–453.

Patterson JF. 1988. Carbamazepine in the treatment of phantom limb pain. South Med J 81:1100–1102.

Payne R. 1987. Role of epidural and intrathecal narcotics and peptides in the management of cancer pain. Med Clin North Am 71:313–327.

Payne R. 1989. Cancer pain. Anatomy, physiology and pharmacology. Cancer 63:2266–2274.

Payne R, Foley KM. 1984. Advances in the management of cancer pain. Cancer Treat Rep 68:173–183.

Payne R, Foley K. 1986. Exploration of the brachial-plexus in patients with cancer. Neurology 36:S329.

Plancarte R, Amescua C, Patt RB, Aldrete JA. 1990. Superior hypogastric plexus block for pelvic cancer pain. 73:236–239.

Portenoy RK. 1990. Pain and quality of life: clinical issues and implications for research. Oncology (Huntingt.) 4:172–178.

Portenoy RK, Foley KM, Inturrisi CE. 1990. The nature of opioid responsiveness and implications for neuropathic pain: new hypothesis derived from studies of opioid infusions. Pain 43:273–286.

Portenoy RK, Hagen NA. 1990. Breakthrough pain: definition, prevalence and characteristics. Pain 41:273–281.

Portenoy RK, Khan E, Layman M, et al. 1991. Chronic morphine therapy for cancer pain: plasma an cerebrospinal fluid morphine and morphine-6-glucuronide concentrations. Neurology 41:1457–1461.

Portenoy RK, Moulin DE, Rogers A, Inturrisi CE, Foley KM. 1986. I.V. infusion of opioids for cancer pain: clinical review and guidelines for use. Cancer Treat Rep 70:575–581.

Portenoy RK, Payne R. 1992. Acute and chronic pain. In: Lowinson JH, Ruiz P, Millman R, Langrod JG (eds), Substance Abuse: A Comprehensive Textbook, 2nd ed. Baltimore: Williams & Williams, p 691.

Porter J, Jick H. 1980. Addiction rare in patients treated with narcotics. N Engl J Med 302:123.

Powers SK, Norman D, Edwards MSB. 1983. Computerized tomography of peripheral nerve lesions. J Neurosurg 59:131–136.

Poyhia R, Vainio A, Kalso E. 1993. A review of oxycodone's clinical pharmacokinetics and pharmocodynamis. J Pain Symptom Manage 8:63–67.

Puustjarvi K, Airaksinen O, Pontinen PJ. 1990. The effects of massage in patients with chronic tension headache. Acupunct Electrother Res 15:159–162.

Rayner HC, Atkins RC, Westerman RA. 1989. Relief of local stump pain by capsaicin cream. Lancet 2:1276–1277.

Reddy SK, Nguyen P. 2000. Breakthrough pain in cancer patients: new therapeutic approaches to an old challenge. Curr Rev Pain 4:242–247.

Reddy S, Patt RB. 1994. Benzodiazepines as adjuvant analgesics. J Pain Symptom Manage 9:510–514.

Remillard G. 1994. Oxcarbezepine in the treatment of trigeminal neuralgia. Epilepsia 35(S3):587–929.

Ripamonti C, Groff L, Brunelli C, Polastri D, Stavrakis A, De Conno F. 1998. Switching from morphine to oral methadone in treating cancer pain: what is the equianalgesic dose ratio? J Clin Oncol 16:3216–3221.

Rogers AG. 1989. Use of amitriptyline (Elavil) for phantom limb pain in younger children. J Pain Symptom Manag 4:96.

Rosomoff HL, Brown CJ, Sheptak P. 1965. Percutaneous radiofrequency cervical cordotomy: technique. J Neurosurg 23:639–644.

Rotstein J, Good RA. 1957. Steroid pseudorheumatism. Arch Intern Med 99:545.

Rowbotham M, Harden N, Stacey B, Bernstein P, Magnus-Miller L. 1998. Gabapentin for the treatment of postherpetic neuralgia: a randomized controlled trial. JAMA 280:1837–1842.

Roy SD, Flynn GL. 1990. Transdermal delivery of narcotic analgesics: pH, anatomical and subject influences of cutaneous permeability of fentanyl and sulfentanil. Pharmacol Res 7:842–847.

Sanders M, Zuurmond W. 1995. Safety of unilateral and bilateral percutaneous cervical cordotomy in 80 terminally ill cancer patients. J Clin Oncol 13:1509–1512.

Sawe J. 1986. High-dose morphine and methadone in cancer patients. Clinical pharmacokinetic considerations of oral treatment. Clin Pharmacokinet 11:87–106.

Sawe J, Svensson JO, Rane A. 1983. Morphine metabolism in cancer patients on increasing oral doses—no evidence of autoinduction or dose-dependence. Br J Clin Pharmacol 16:85–93.

Sherman RA, Sherman CJ, Parker L. 1984. Chronic phantom and stump pain among American veterans: results of a survey. Pain 18:83–95.

Simmel ML. 1962. Phantom experiences following amputation in childhood. J Neurol Neurosurg Psychiatry 25:69–78.

Sjogren P, Banning A. 1989. Pain, sedation and reaction time during long-term treatment of cancer patients with oral and epidural opioids. Pain 39:5–11.

Sjolin SU, Trykker H. 1985. Unsuccessful treatment of severe pain from bone metastases with Sinemet 25/100. N Engl J Med 312:650–651.

Smith JA Jr. 1989. Palliation of painful bone metastases from prostate cancer using sodium etidronate: results of a randomized, prospective, double-blind, placebo-controlled study. J Urol 141:85–87.

Smith MT, Watt JA, Cramond T. 1990. Morphine-3-glucuronide—a potent antagonist of morphine analgesia. Life Sci 47:579–585.

Southam M, Gupta B, Knowles N, Hwang SS. 1991. Transdermal fentanyl: an overview of pharmacokinetics, efficacy and safety. In: Lehmann KA, Zech D (eds), Transdermal Fentanyl: A New Approach to Prolonged Pain Control. New York: Springer-Verlag, p 107.

Stambaugh J, Drew J. 1988. A double-blind parallel evaluation of the efficacy and safety of a single dose of ketoprofen in cancer pain. J Clin Pharmacol 28:S34–S39.

Steinke NM, Ostgard SE, Jensen OM, Nordentoft AM, Sneppen O. 1991. [Thoraco-scapular amputation in sarcomas of the shoulder girdle]. Ugeskr Laeger 153:2555–2557.

Sugarbaker PH, Weiss CM, Davidson DD, Roth YF. 1984. Increasing phantom limb pain as a symptom of cancer recurrence. Cancer 54:373–375.

Sundaresan N, DiGiacinto GV, Krol G, Hughes JE. 1989. Spondylectomy for malignant tumors of the spine. J Clin Oncol 7:1485–1491.

Swerdlow M. 1984. Anticonvulsant drugs and chronic pain. Clin Neuropharmacol 7:51–82.

Szeto HH, Inturrisi CE, Houde R, Saal S, Cheigh J, Reidenberg MM. 1977. Accumulation of normeperidine, an active metabolite of meperidine, in patients with renal failure of cancer. Ann Intern Med 86:738–741.

Tachi J, Amino N, Miyai K. 1990. Massage therapy on neck: a contributing factor for destructive thyrotoxicosis? Thyroidology 2:25–27.

Thomas JE, Cascino TL, Earle JD. 1985. Differential diagnosis between radiation and tumor plexopathy of the pelvis. Neurology 35:1–7.

Thomas JE, Piepgras DG, Scheithauer B, Onofrio BM, Shives TC. 1983. Neurogenic tumors of the sciatic nerve. A clinicopathologic study of 35 cases. Mayo Clin Proc 58:640–647.

Tive L, Ginsberg K, Pick CG, Pasternak GW. 1992. Kappa 3 receptors and levorphanol-induced analgesia. Neuropharmacology 9:851–856.

Trijsburg RW, van Knippenberg FC, Rijpma SE. 1992. Effects of psychological treatment on cancer patients: a critical review. Psychosom Med 54:489–517.

Twycross RG. 1975. The use of narcotic analgesics in terminal illness. J Med Ethics 1:10–17.

Twycross RG. 1988. The management of pain in cancer: a guide to drug and dosages. Oncology (Huntingt.) 2:35–44.

Twycross RG, Fairfield S. 1982. Pain in far-advanced cancer. Pain 14:303–310.

Varvel JR, Shafer SL, Hwang SS, Coen PA, Stanski DR. 1989. Absorption characteristic of transdermally administered fentanyl. Anesthesiology 70:928–934.

Vecht CJ, Van de Brand HJ, Wajer OJ. 1989. Post-axillary dissection pain in breast cancer due to a lesion of the intercostobrachial nerve. Pain 38:171–176.

Ventafridda V, Tamburini M, Caraceni A, De Conmo F, Naldi F., et al 1987. A validation study of the WHO method for cancer pain relief. Cancer 59:850–856.

Waldman SD, Feldstein GS, Allen ML 1987. Neuroadenolysis of the pituitary: description of a modified technique. J Pain Symptom Manage 2:45–49.

Wall R, Novotny-Joseph P, Macnamara TE. 1985. Does preamputation pain influence phantom limb pain in cancer patients? South Med J 78:34–36.

Warfield CA. 1984. The sympathetic dystrophies. Hosp Pract (Off Ed) 19:52C–52J.

Wasserstrom WR, Glass JP, Posner JB. 1982. Diagnosis and treatment of leptomeningeal metastases from solid tumors: experience with 90 patients. Cancer 49:759–772.

Watson CP, Evans RJ. 1992. The postmastectomy pain syndrome and topical capsaicin: a randomized trial. Pain 51:375–379.

Watson CP, Evans RJ, Reed K, Merskey H, Goldsmith L, Warsh J. 1982. Amitriptyline versus placebo in postherpetic neuralgia. Neurology 32:671–673.

Watson CP, Evans RJ, Watt VR. 1989. The post-mastectomy pain syndrome and the effect of topical capsaicin. Pain 38:177–186.

Weissman DE, Haddox JD. 1989. Opioid pseudoaddiction: an iatrogenic syndrome. Pain 36:363–366.

Wiffen P, Collins S, McQuay H, Carroll D, Jadad A, Moore A. 2000. Anticonvulsant drugs for acute and chronic pain (Cochrane review). Cochrane Database Syst Rev 3.

World Health Organization. 1986. Cancer Pain Relief. Geneva: World Health Organization, 74 pp.

World Health Organization.1990. Cancer Pain Relief and Palliative Care: Report of a WHO Expert Committee. Geneva: World Health Organization, 75 pp.

Yaksh TL, Rudy TA. 1976. Analgesia mediated by a direct spinal action of narcotics. Science 192:1357–1358.

Yang CY, Wong CS, Chang JY, Ho ST. 1996. Intrathecal ketamine reduces morphine requirements in patients with terminal cancer pain. Can J Anaesth 43:379–383.

Young DF, Posner JB. 1985. Nervous system toxicity of chemotherapeutic agents. In: Vinken PJ, Bruyn GW, Klawans H, Frederiks JAM (eds), Handbook of Clinical Neurology. New York: Elsevier Science, p 91.

Zakrzewska JM, Chaudrey Z, Nurmikko TJ, Patton DW, Mullens EL. 1997. Lamotrigine (Lamictal) in refractory trigeminal neuralgia: results from a double-blind placebo controlled crossover trial. Pain 73:223–230.

24

Neuroendocrine Function

RENA VASSILOPOULOU-SELLIN

Cancer therapies have become increasingly complex and frequently include many antineoplastic modalities together or in sequence, often separated by the passage of many years. Neuroendocrine dysfunction is generally caused by particular systemic treatments, interventions that are directed at the central nervous system (CNS), or products of the tumors themselves. Hormonal and metabolic abnormalities can profoundly affect the well being of patients or directly prove to be life threatening. If uncorrected, they may alter the toxicity profile of other cancer treatments and complicate the overall care of patients.

Often the neuroendocrine abnormalities last only for the duration of a particular treatment (e.g., exogenous hypercortisolism in patients with hematologic malignancies). In other cases their impact may be prolonged either because an indolent tumor may continue to contribute to certain abnormalities (e.g., hypercalcemia in some patients with islet cell tumors) or because the impact of treatment may evolve over several years and linger thereafter (e.g., hypothalamic or pituitary dysfunction after cranial irradiation; Table 24–1) (Blackman et al., 1978; Odell, 1997).

EFFECTS OF SYSTEMIC THERAPY ON NEUROENDOCRINE FUNCTION

Neuroendocrine dysfunction may compromise patient welfare even when the malignancy is outside the CNS. Some tumors are associated with paraneoplastic syndromes; ectopic hormone secretion in this case may, for example, cause activation of osteoclasts in the skeleton (resulting in hypercalcemia) or stimulation of cortisol secretion from the adrenal glands (resulting in Cushing's syndrome). In other patients, antineoplastic therapy (including medical, radiation, or surgical treatments) may directly affect the normal function of endocrine glands and cause a cascade of hormone deficiencies (outlined in the discussion of hypothalamic/pituitary dysfunction, below). These metabolic abnormalities may increase the morbidity of the patients' disease as well as interfere with their ability to tolerate appropriate cancer treatment. Surveillance for the early detection and correction of such side effects is needed to optimize the oncologic outcome.

Hypercalcemia

The most common endocrine complication of malignancy, hypercalcemia (Mundy and Guise, 1997; Coleman, 1997; Harvey, 1995), not infrequently compromises the health of patients with cancer (especially breast, non–small cell lung cancer, myeloma). Depending on its severity, hypercalcemia can cause neuromuscular morbidity (e.g., weakness, fatigue, obtundation, and even coma); cardiac complications (e.g., bradycardia or arrhythmias); in addition to constipation, anorexia, nausea, vomiting, and dehydration, which may lead to renal insufficiency.

Among several implicated mechanisms, the most prominent etiologies include

1. Paraneoplastic secretion of parathyroid hormone (PTH)-related protein (a peptide that shares similarity with the bioactive N-terminus region of PTH), especially in patients with solid tumors

Table 24–1. Annual Surveillance of Hypothalamic/Pituitary Integrity After Cranial Irradiation Is Suggested for First Decade and Biannual Surveillance Is Suggested for Second Decade After Irradiation

1. Growth hormone
   a. Monitor growth curve (children)
   b. Serum IGF-1 level
2. Gonadotropins
   a. Pubertal maturation (adolescents)
   b. Menstrual regularity (premenopausal women)
   c. Serum FSH level (postmenopausal women)
   d. Serum testosterone level (adult men)
3. Prolactin
   a. Serum level

If any abnormalities in 1 through 3, then add thyroid and adrenal evaluation

2. Destruction of the bone or release of cytokines with osteoclastic activity such as transforming growth factor (TGF) or tumor necrosis factor (TNF) by the tumor, especially in patients with skeletal metastases
3. Increased enzymatic conversion of vitamin D to its biologically active form in some hematologic malignancies (as observed in patients with granulomatous diseases)

The treatment of hypercalcemia depends, in part, on how high the calcium level is and how curable the underlying disease is.

Acutely, therapy usually includes hydration and inhibitors of bone resorption (such as bisphosphonates, calcitonin, plicamycin, or gallium). Many patients with hematologic malignancies may promptly respond to glucocorticoids, in part because of their antitumor efficacy. Numerous patients require chronic management for hypercalcemia, which may include periodic administration of fluids and bisphosphonates. Whereas the progression of the underlying disease generally determines the patient's prognosis, hypercalcemia may itself become lethal in some patients with oncologically indolent neuroendocrine cancers. Clearly, control of the malignancy corrects the problem.

Hyponatremia

Severe hyponatremia may develop as a result of renal, cardiac, or liver disease or overhydration or hypovolemia in patients who are already compromised from their illness. Another possible cause is paraneoplastic secretion of antidiuretic hormone or atrial natriuretic peptide, especially in patients with small cell lung cancer. Patients with brain or lung involvement may also be affected. Hyponatremia can result in altered mental status, including confusion, seizures, and coma; the severity of symptoms is tempered by the rate of fall of the sodium level and the underlying CNS integrity of the patient (Shapiro and Richardson, 1995; McDonald and Dubose, 1993; Berghmans, 1996).

Acutely, treatment should include fluid restriction and judicious use of lasix or hypertonic saline; this regimen may be problematic for patients who otherwise need chemotherapy with hydration and may necessitate delay of cancer treatment. Chronically, demeclocycline may be helpful for patients with relatively stable disease and mild to modest hyponatremia. Co-existing thyroid or adrenal insufficiency will also impair free water clearance and should be excluded as clinically appropriate.

Hypoglycemia

Hypoglycemia is an expected presenting symptom in patients with insulinoma; surgical resection is generally curative as these are usually benign tumors. In patients with malignant insulinomas, repeated and prolonged episodes of severe hypoglycemia may become a major, if not lethal, morbidity. Infrequently reported are cases of paraneoplastic secretion of insulin-like products (Phillips and Robertson, 1993; Marks and Teale, 1991). These occur most frequently in patients who have mesenchymal tumors; insulin-like growth factor 2 (IGF-2) has been identified in several such cases, presumably causing hypoglycemia by cross-reacting with insulin receptors. Acutely, treatment involves administration of intravenous glucose. Because the underlying disease may pursue a relatively indolent course, chronic management may be needed; glucocorticoids, growth hormone, glucagon, and even glucose infusion have been used successfully.

In other patients, hypoglycemia may be caused by excessive glucose utilization by the tumor coupled with relative liver insufficiency or by glycogen depletion due to destruction of liver parenchyma by the tumor. Infusion of glucagon acutely (1 mg IV) may help distinguish paraneoplastic hypoglycemia (the glucose rises promptly) from liver failure hypoglycemia (no glucose response). In the latter cases glucose infusion is the mainstay of therapy.

Hypercortisolism

Prolonged hypercortisolism, regardless of etiology, exerts significant morbidity in most clinical settings. Increased weight with a characteristic centripetal distribution, moon facies, and buffalo hump are accompanied by muscle weakness and thinning and easy bruising of the skin. Personality changes, diabetes mellitus, or hypertension may develop or become exacerbated. In addition, suppression of the patients' immune function places them at increased risk for serious and difficult to overcome infections. In patients with malignant diseases, hypercortisolism is rarely the result of functioning adrenocortical cancer; more commonly, however, it results from paraneoplastic secretion of adrenocorticotropic hormone (ACTH) or corticotropin-releasing factor (CRF) and from therapeutic administration of glucocorticoids in high doses.

Paraneoplastic Hypercortisolism

Ectopic ACTH secretion may occur in patients with small cell lung cancer, medullary thyroid cancer, carcinoid tumors, or pheochromocytoma. These tumors may secrete ACTH (Dimopoulos et al., 1992) and, occasionally, ACTH-releasing factor. Because the underlying diseases may have an indolent course, the evolution of Cushing's syndrome is chronic and the clinical features more typical. At the same time, such patients frequently live for many years with stable or slowly progressive disease. The morbidity from hypercortisolism may become the leading medical priority; occasionally, bilateral adrenalectomy is performed, followed by physiologic adrenal replacement therapy (Becker and Aron, 1994).

Therapeutic Administration of High-dose Glucocorticoids:

Glucocorticoids (Walsh and Avashia, 1992; Coleman, 1992) are powerful antineoplastic agents for a number of malignancies that are primarily hematologic. They are also used in various oncology settings: to prevent nausea after chemotherapy, for cerebral edema when brain metastases are a problem, or for chronic graft-versus-host disease after bone marrow transplantation. Prolonged administration of exogenous glucocorticoids exposes patients to complications similar to those seen with endogenous hypercortisolism. In addition, pharmacologic glucocorticoid administration may suppress the hypothalamic-pituitary (HP)-adrenal axis and cause severe secondary adrenal insufficiency if abruptly interrupted. Such patients must, therefore, be closely monitored when taking glucocorticoids and carefully tapered off when the therapeutic indication has ended. Diabetic patients may experience deterioration of blood glucose control during the period of glucocorticoid treatment; this becomes particularly problematic if high-dose glucocorticoids are used intermittently, as they are in several multiple myeloma regimens.

HYPOTHALAMIC / PITUITARY DYSFUNCTION AFTER SUPRASELLAR SURGERY OR CRANIAL IRRADIATION

The most frequent and important neuroendocrine morbidity of treatment for CNS tumors is the development of hypothalamic and/or pituitary (HP) dysfunction. The extent of injury and its health repercussions depend on the location of the tumor, type of therapy, age of the patient, and compounding effect of other antineoplastic therapies that may be added to achieve tumor control.

Surgery for pituitary tumors directly affects the pituitary gland and may produce pituitary insufficiency (see Chapter 8). Surgery for tumors at or about the suprasellar area may also result in HP dysfunction through direct damage of the hypothalamus or pituitary glands or interruption of the neural pathways that regulate HP physiology. Postoperative HP damage generally occurs relatively soon after treatment and may affect any of the HP/peripheral axes with similar frequency depending on the anatomic location of the surgical interruption.

Cranial irradiation, on the other hand, frequently used to treat CNS tumors and CNS metastases or for CNS prophylaxis, may create HP dysfunction gradually and insidiously several years after its application (Samaan et al., 1987; Shalet et al., 1988; Lam et al., 1991; Constine et al., 1993; Sklar and Constine, 1995; Shalet, 1983; Rappaport and Brauner, 1989; Oberfield et al., 1997a,b; Heikens et al., 1998; Arlt et al., 1997). Radiation-induced HP damage varies depending on the dose to the HP region, the age at time of treatment, and the lag time since therapy. Its overall health impact is often determined by the age and life situation of the patient. Induction of secondary hypogonadism due to gonadotropin deficiency, for example, is a much more serious complication for children who have not yet entered puberty (who face both physical maldevelopment and infertility). It is less serious for young adults who have matured normally but have not yet had their own family (and face infertility); it is least critical for mature adults or elderly individuals past their reproductive years who also have an overall more limited life expectancy. The secretion of growth hormone (GH) and gonadotropins is most frequently affected, whereas HP-thyroid and HP-adrenal axes appear more resistant.

Growth Hormone Deficiency

Growth hormone deficiency develops in most patients who receive cranial irradiation either for leukemia prophylaxis (lower dose) or brain tumor treatment (higher dose). Hypothalamic damage affecting the production of GH-releasing hormone appears more frequent than pituitary hyposecretion of GH, per se. The health implications of GH deficiency are quite different for children, who are still growing physically, than for adults. Because normal GH secretion is required to achieve normal adult height, untreated GH-deficient children are at risk for extreme short stature, which is associated with psychosocial morbidity (McGauley et al., 1996; Burman et al., 1995). Growth hormone deficiency also contributes to decreased skeletal (Vassilopoulou-Sellin et al., 1999) and lean body mass, increased cardiovascular morbidity, and, perhaps, impaired quality of life.

Because of these nonstatural morbidities of GH deficiency, GH replacement is approved and generally considered appropriate regardless of the patient's age. For patients with cancer, the decision to begin GH replacement is often tempered by concerns that it might induce tumor recurrence; this does not appear to be a problem in children (Ilveskoski et al., 1997; Vassilopoulou-Sellin et al., 1995), whereas no data are available for adults. Growth hormone replacement therapy should be considered for patients (especially children) who have been treated successfully and have a good prognosis for disease-free survival.

Hypogonadism

Ovarian and testicular integrity and fertility rely on a precise interplay between hypothalamic and pituitary rhythm periodicity under the influence of the pineal gland and higher CNS centers; cranial irradiation frequently disturbs these circuits and results in gonadal dysfunction. It should be noted that abdominal irradiation and several cytotoxic chemotherapy agents might directly damage the gonads and create premature testicular failure or ovarian dysfunction.

In adults, abnormalities may be limited to fertility impairment (irregular menstrual cycles or anovulation in women and decreased sperm count in men); for patients who have completed their family these defects do not pose a significant problem. For patients who have HP-gonadal dysfunction wishing to have children, stimulation of the target gonads with gonadotropin infusions can theoretically restore fertility but remains relatively cumbersome. When HP damage also causes impaired sex steroid production, additional problems ensue (e.g., accelerated bone loss, increased adipose tissue, and decreased muscle mass). Unlike primary gonadal failure, climacteric symptoms are not likely to develop with HP dysfunction. Estrogen and testosterone replacement therapy are appropriate for such patients unless they have been treated for a hormone-responsive tumor (e.g., breast or prostate cancer).

The impact of HP-hypogonadism is far more serious for prepubertal children. In this group, normal growth and development rely on the timely stimulation of the gonads, which allows the development of secondary sex characteristics, pubertal growth spurt, skeletal maturation, and initiation of ovarian cycles in girls and spermatogenesis in boys. Because GH, an important participant in normal pubertal development, is also almost always deficient in this group of children, the problem is compounded. Careful and coordinated sex hormone (and GH, if appropriate) replacement is needed to achieve a smooth progression of puberty without accelerating epiphysial closure of the growth plates that might compromise final adult height. Infertility is almost always permanent in these patients. In a minority of patients cranial irradiation may, instead, induce precocious puberty, perhaps due to pineal gland dysfunction (Quigley et al., 1989; Brauner et al., 1984).

Because GH and sex steroids participate critically in the development of normal peak bone mass, especially during the second and third decades of life, careful monitoring of skeletal health should include periodic measurements of bone mineral density and counseling about proper nutrition and physical fitness. Adjustment of the hormone replacement schedule for these children may be needed to avoid the development of osteopenia, or even osteoporosis, both becoming recognized as other clinically important sequelae of cancer therapies.

Hyperprolactinemia

Prolactin secretion by the pituitary is under the influence of hypothalamic inhibition and is easily disturbed by various drugs and by cranial irradiation. Mild to moderate hyperprolactinemia is a fairly frequent occurrence. Although no direct morbidity has been attributed to prolactin elevation in people, it may disrupt HP-gonadal function and cause galactorrhea, amenorrhea, or infertility. Medical therapy (e.g., bromocryptine or cabergoline) is quite effective and may be sufficient to restore normal gonadal function, including fertility, in affected individuals.

Hypothalamic-Pituitary Thyroid Dysfunction

Irradiation-induced pituitary or hypothalamic deficiency of thyroid-stimulating hormone (TSH) or TSH-releasing hormone occurs infrequently. Although it is possible to demonstrate some impairment of TSH secretion using dynamic endocrine testing, clinically significant hypothyroidism occurs in fewer than 15% of patients. When the radiation field abuts the neck or after total-body irradiation for bone marrow transplantation, however, primary hypothyroidism may develop from direct damage of the thyroid gland. Thyroid hormone replacement is readily available and should be used to treat affected patients.

Hypothalamic-Pituitary Adrenal Dysfunction

The HP-adrenal axis, like the HP-thyroid axis, is also relatively resistant to damage from irradiation, and clinically significant adrenal insufficiency is uncommon. More often, HP-adrenal suppression in patients with malignant diseases is due to pharmacologic administration of glucocorticoids, which are used frequently and often for prolonged periods of time to prevent edema (e.g., CNS tumors) or chemotherapy-induced nausea and to treat steroid-responsive diseases (e.g., multiple myeloma or hematologic malignancies). This practice may result in prolonged, although reversible, HP-adrenal suppression, which may be difficult to distinguish from direct and irreversible irradiation damage in patients who have received both interventions. Careful tapering of steroids should be followed by dynamic endocrine testing to avoid the life-threatening sequelae of untreated adrenal insufficiency. Parenthetically, high-dose Megace (Mann et al., 1997), a progestational agent frequently used to improve appetite, may also interact with glucocorticoid receptors and contribute to HP-adrenal suppression.

Diabetes Insipidus

Interruption of the pituitary stalk or destruction of the supraoptic and paraventricular nuclei of the hypothalamus may disrupt the HP tract and cause vasopressin deficiency (i.e., central diabetes insipidus). This problem may develop after sellar or suprasellar surgery but does not generally ensue from irradiation alone. Metastatic deposits (e.g., breast cancer) may also disrupt the HP tract and cause diabetes insipidus. Intranasal and oral vasopressin are effective for preventing dehydration. Because some patients with hypothalamic damage may also have abnormalities of thirst perception, they may become severely dehydrated (or accidentally overmedicated and water overloaded) unless a careful therapeutic regimen is developed for them.

Hypothalamic Obesity

Patients whose hypothalamic region has been disrupted by neoplasms or surgery tend to gain weight relentlessly until they become obese. This has generally been attributed to destruction of the satiety center (in the ventromedial nucleus) and resetting of the weight set point. Whether additional abnormalities of leptin regulation are also involved is not clear at this time. In adults, long-learned eating behavior patterns can be used to control caloric intake. Children, however, cannot easily restrict themselves and are more likely to become morbidly obese. Their obesity is compounded by the reduced lean body mass and increased adipose mass that characterize gonadotropin and GH deficiency (which frequently co-exist in such patients), creating a unique phenotype.

Weight loss is extremely difficult if not unachievable. It is, therefore, important to recognize the potential for obesity early and to intervene with rigorous education and behavior modification before the obesity becomes established. In addition, careful replacement of the other deficient hormones can be used to improve cardiovascular, skeletal, and overall health.

SURVEILLANCE OF NEUROENDOCRINE INTEGRITY AFTER CANCER TREATMENT

Patients who have been treated with cranial irradiation in particular require prolonged surveillance because the deleterious effects of irradiation may not become apparent for many years. Although it is generally true that GH and HP-gonadal axes are most susceptible to radiation-induced HP damage, whereas the HP-adrenal and HP-thyroid axes are most resistant, exceptions do occur especially if additional therapies (with potential independent toxicities) have been applied. A comprehensive review of the patient's oncologic history is needed at completion of therapy to design an appropriate surveillance strategy. Irradiation-induced HP dysfunction usually manifests itself within the first 5 years, and the incidence tends to plateau after the first decade. Accordingly, surveillance tailored to the anticipated potential abnormalities should continue annually for at least 5 years and preferably for 10 years or longer.

For children who have received cranial irradiation, growth velocity should be monitored closely, and an updated growth curve should be maintained; foot size is also a reliable measure of growth that is less subject to posture or measuring error. For children who fail to meet expected growth standards more detailed evaluation should include a GH secretion assessment using standard biochemical dynamic and radiologic testing. If GH deficiency is detected, replacement therapy is effective in correcting growth failure and allowing patients to achieve their genetic height potentials. Around the age of 8 to 10 years, particular attention should focus on the detection of delayed or precocious puberty, combining physical examination and Tanner staging with biochemical screening tests as needed. For children with documented GH or HP-gonadal dysregulation, bone mineral density should also be evaluated to appropriately manage potential osteopenia.

Detection of HP abnormalities is more challenging in adults because growth and development, very sensitive and easily detected features in children, are not useful parameters for adults. Although not foolproof, one reasonable strategy is to routinely screen for the integrity of the GH axis (serum IGF-1 level) and HP-gonadal axis (menstrual and sexual history or hormone levels), the most sensitive of HP axes. Physical examination should focus on signs of pituitary dysfunction, such as loss of axillary or pubic hair, fine wrinkling of the skin, and adipose tissue redistribution. If HP dysfunction is suspected, more thorough evaluation can be performed with standard biochemical basal or dynamic tests to diagnose and accurately treat prolactin, HP-adrenal, or HP-thyroid abnormalities. Advancing age and hypopituitarism both constitute additional risk factors for the development of osteoporosis in adults of either gender; periodic bone mineral density measurement, nutritional counseling, and life-style education are very important for this group of patients.

CONCLUSION

Neuroendocrine dysfunction is frequently seen in patients who are treated for cancer. It may develop due to secreted tumor products, as a result of systemic treatments, or more directly after therapy to the CNS. The severity of these changes is related to patient age, treatment dose intensity or agent combinations, the underlying health of the patient, and the presence of co-morbid conditions. The appropriate interventions and the therapeutic priorities to correct neuroendocrine dysfunction can vary depending on the age and prognoses of the involved patients. Careful surveillance for the early detection of potential problems is particularly important because both accurate diagnosis and effective treatment are generally available for most neuroendocrine abnormalities.

REFERENCES

Arlt W, Hove U, Muller B, et al. 1997. Frequent and frequently overlooked: treatment-induced endocrine dysfunction in adult long-term survivors of primary brain tumors. Neurology 49:498–506.

Becker M, Aron DC. 1994. Ectopic ACTH syndrome and CRH-mediated Cushing's syndrome. Endocrinol Metab Clin North Am 23:585–606.

Berghmans T. 1996. Hyponatremia related to medical anticancer treatment. Support Care Cancer 4:341–350.

Blackman MR, Rosen SW, Weintraub BD. 1978. Ectopic hormones. Adv Intern Med 23:85–113.

Brauner R, Czernichow P, Rappaport R. 1984. Precocious puberty after hypothalamic and pituitary irradiation in young children. N Engl J Med 311:920.

Burman P, Broman JE, Hetta J, et al. 1995. Quality of life in adults with growth hormone (GH) deficiency: response to treatment with recombinant human GH in a placebo-controlled 21-month trial. J Clin Endocrinol Metab 80: 3585–3590.

Coleman RE. 1992. Glucocorticoids in cancer therapy. Biotherapy 4:37–44.

Coleman RE. 1997. Skeletal complications of malignancy. Cancer 80:1588–1594.

Constine LS, Woolf PD, Cann D, et al. 1993. Hypothalamic-pituitary dysfunction after radiation for brain tumors. N Engl J Med 328:87–94.

Dimopoulos MA, Fernandez JF, Samaan NA, Holoye PY, Vassilopoulou-Sellin R. 1992. Paraneoplastic Cushing's syndrome as an adverse prognostic factor in patients who die early with small cell lung cancer. Cancer 69:66–71.

Harvey HA. 1995. The management of hypercalcemia of malignancy. Support Care Cancer 3:123–129.

Heikens J, Michiels EM, Behrendt H, Endert E, Bakker PJ, Fliers E. 1998. Long-term neuro-endocrine sequelae after treatment for childhood medulloblastoma. Eur J Cancer 34:1592–1571.

Iveskoski I, Saarinen UM, Wiklund T, et al. 1997. Growth impairment and growth hormone therapy in children treated for malignant brain tumours. Eur J Pediatr 156:764–769.

Lam KS, Tse VK, Wang C, Yeung RT, Ho JH. 1991. Effects of cranial irradiation on hypothlamic-pituitary function—a 5-year longitudinal study in patients with nasopharyngeal carcinoma. Q J Med 78:165–176.

Mann M, Koller E, Murgo A, Malozowski S, Bacsanyi J, Leinung M. 1997. Glucocorticoidlike activity of megestrol. A summary of Food and Drug Administration experience and a review of the literature. Arch Intern Med 157:1651–1656.

Marks V, Teale JD. 1991. Tumours producing hypoglycaemia. Diabetes Metab Rev 7:79–91.

McDonald GA, Dubose TD Jr. 1993. Hyponatremia in the cancer patient. Oncology (Huntingt) 7:55–64.

McGauley G, Cuneo R, Salomon F, Soksen PH. 1996. Growth hormone deficiency and quality of life. Horm Res 45:34–37.

Mundy GR, Guise TA. 1997. Hypercalcemia of malignancy. Am J Med 103:134–145.

Oberfield SE, Chin D, Uli N, David R, Sklar C. 1997a. Endocrine late effects of childhood cancers. J Pediatr 131:37–41.

Oberfield SE, Nirenberg A, Allen JC, et al. 1997b. Hypothalamic-pituitary-adrenal function following cranial irradiation. Horm Res 47:9–16.

Odell WD. 1997. Endocrine/metabolic syndromes of cancer. Semin Oncol 24:299–317.

Phillips LS, Robertson DG. 1993. Insulin-like growth factors and non-islet cell tumor hypoglycemia. Metabolism 42: 1093–1101.

Quigley C, Cowell C, Jimenez M, et al. 1989. Normal or early development of puberty despite gonadal damage in children treated for acute lymphoblastic leukemia. N Engl J Med 321:143–151.

Rappaport R, Brauner R. 1989. Growth and endocrine disorders secondary to cranial irradiation Pediatr Res 25: 561–567.

Samaan NA, Schultz PN, Yang KP, et al. 1987. Endocrine complications after radiotherapy for tumors of the head and neck. J Lab Clin Med 109:364–372.

Shalet SM. 1983. Disorders of the endocrine system due to radiation and cytotoxic chemotherapy. Clin Endocrinol (Oxf) 19:637–659.

Shalet SM, Clayton PE, Price DA. 1988. Growth and pituitary function in children treated for brain tumours or acute lymphoblastic leukaemia. Horm Res 30:53–61.

Shapiro J, Richardson GE. 1995. Hyponatremia of malignancy. Crit Rev Oncol Hematol 18:129–135.

Sklar CA, Constine LS. 1995. Chronic neuroendocrinological sequelae of radiation therapy. Int J Radiat Oncol Biol Phys 31:1113–1121.

Vassilopoulou-Sellin R, Brosnan P, Delpassand A, Zietz H, Klein MJ, Jaffe N. 1999. Osteopenia in young adults survivors of childhood cancer. Med Pediatr Oncol 32:272–278.

Vassilopoulou-Sellin R, Klein MJ, Moore 3rd BD, Reid HL, Ater J, Zietz HA. 1995. Efficacy of growth hormone replacement therapy in children with organic growth hormone deficiency after cranial irradiation. Horm Res 43:188–193.

Walsh D, Avashia J. 1992. Glucocorticoids in clinical oncology. Cleve Clin J Med 59:505–515.

25

Altered Mental Status

ARTHUR FORMAN

Although the majority of alterations in sensorium in cancer patients are caused by endogenous or exogenous intoxication, the clinician must be alert to the possibility of structural disease in any patient who experiences a change in mental status. Accurate diagnosis of structural disease and prompt intervention can significantly improve the outcome of cancer treatments.

Mogami et al. (1983) note five causes of increased intracranial pressure due to structural lesions in cancer patients: *(1)* intracranial space-occupying lesions, especially malignant tumors; *(2)* leptomeningeal tumors; *(3)* hemorrhage into brain tumors; *(4)* intracranial hemorrhage due to hemorrhagic diathesis related to malignant tumors; and *(5)* cerebral thrombosis or embolism due to an increase in blood coagulability caused by malignancy. Raised intracranial pressure may also occur as a complication of nonstructural conditions such as chronic infectious meningitis (Wilhelm and Ellner, 1986) the encephalitides, and severe metabolic disturbances such as hepatic encephalopathy, respiratory failure, and exogenous intoxications.

Ironically, severe intracranial hypertension may accompany treatment of intracranial metastases, especially tumors that are sensitive to therapy. This commonly occurs with radiotherapy, including radioisotope therapy (Datz, 1986) for sensitive tumors. Cerebral herniation, which leads to increased intracranial pressure, is a possible, but uncommon complication of systemic chemotherapy (Walker et al., 1988) and cytokine treatment (Goey et al., 1988). Herniation has also been described as a complication of photodynamic therapy (Ji et al., 1992) for experimental gliomas. Patients with occult brain metastasis are in particular danger during the initiation of cytoreductive therapy. When the malignant cells are injured by therapy, they swell and induce edema in the surrounding tissues, thereby increasing intracranial pressure.

PATHOPHYSIOLOGY

Altered consciousness is caused by dysfunction in cerebral hemispheres, the diencephalon, or the tegmentum. The most minimal lesions producing altered consciousness are those affecting the posterior hypothalamus, midbrain, or cephalad brain stem. The pace with which a lesion develops influences the degree of altered function produced. Rapidly developing lesions such as arterial hemorrhage or embolic stroke produce greater deficits for the same volume of injury than more slowly evolving pathologies such as subdural hematoma or tumor (Plum and Posner, 1982).

Unilateral hemispheric disease alone does not alter consciousness (Haerer, 1992), but it may do so by *(1)* increasing intracranial pressure enough to cause dysfunction to both cerebral hemispheres; *(2)* causing sufficient inequalities in intracranial compartment pressures to provoke ischemia and herniation of vital neuronal arousal systems; or *(3)* blocking cerebrospinal fluid pathways, which leads to acute hydrocephalus, brain edema, diminished arterial flow, and, ultimately, bihemispheral dysfunction. In any one instance of altered consciousness due to a mass lesion, multiple mechanisms are almost always in effect.

EXAMINATION

Lundberg's literature review of case reports of intracranial space-occupying lesions and increased intracranial pressure lists 50 associated signs and symptoms (Lundberg, 1960). Many of these symptoms are nondescript, such as headache or dizziness, and can challenge diagnostic acumen. Symptoms such as visual obscurations, neck pain, or restlessness are liable to be overlooked by clinicians, particularly if intracerebral lesions are not expected.

The neurologic examination of the comatose patient allows the clinician to chart central nervous system (CNS) physiology from moment to moment. Computerized tomography and magnetic resonance imaging (MRI) scans or neurophysiologic monitoring cannot replace skilled observation by the caretakers of comatose patients. The patient's eye movements and pupils tell a great deal about the integrity of diencephalic and brain stem structures critical to the maintenance of consciousness (Fisher, 1969) and are briefly reviewed.

Pupillary light reaction should be checked in a darkened room for the rate of constriction and symmetry of reaction between the two eyes. Asymmetric, sluggish reaction of a pupil before dilation can alert the clinician to early tentorial herniation. Examination of the extraocular movements by oculocephalic reflex or caloric testing establishes whether diencephalic and brain stem structures adjacent to the alerting network of the reticular activating system are functioning normally. Oculocephalic (doll's eyes maneuver) testing is performed by slowly turning the patient's head from side to side and observing how the eyes respond. Normally, the eyes move conjugately in a direction opposite to that in which the head is turned. The eye movements in response to head turning should be unambiguously recorded.

A more reliable bedside examination of mesial rhombencephalic physiology is caloric testing, which is performed by placing the patient's head at approximately 30 degrees and gently irrigating the external auditory meatus with approximately 50 ml of ice-cold water over a span of a few minutes. The ear canals and tympanic membranes should be examined with an otoscope before irrigation to ensure that the tympanic membrane is intact and that there is no evidence of infection. Cerumen impaction should be cleared if it obstructs the external auditory meatus. Ice-water irrigation should be avoided if the patient is conscious, as it will precipitate unpleasant vertigo. The normal response is bilateral conjugate deviation of both eyes toward the ear receiving the ice water after a latent period of a few seconds. Pupillary and caloric testing are extremely resistant to metabolic disturbance, and abnormalities of these examinations argue strongly for structural disease in the midbrain or brain stem, although focal brain stem findings may rarely occur in patients with severe metabolic derangement.

Posturing of the limbs, either decorticate (arms flexed, legs extended) or decerebrate (arms and legs extended), is an ominous sign seen in severe midbrain dysfunction. Paroxysmal posturing is often mistaken for seizure, even, at times, by experienced clinicians. Abnormalities of tone, posturing, and Babinski's reflex may be seen in metabolic disturbance and on occasion asymmetrically in patients with underlying cerebrovascular disease or diabetes mellitus. When these symptoms are found, the patient should be urgently evaluated for the presence of an expanding intracranial mass. These signs implicate structural disease as the cause of altered consciousness, particularly when they are asymmetric or occur in association with abnormalities of ocular motility or pupillary reflexes.

BRAIN EDEMA

The presence of a mass lesion in the cranial vault increases intracranial pressure because of the incompliant nature of the skull to an expanding space-occupying lesion. The edema such a mass may induce in the surrounding brain can contribute to increased intracranial pressure to a much greater extent than the volume added by the tumor itself. Small tumors may cause massive edema (Fig. 25–1), and large tumors may cause only slight edema. On occasion, the tumor induces edema rapidly after a period of relatively harmonious co-existence, as if the relationship between the tumor and the surrounding normal brain tissue had suddenly been disturbed. Metastatic renal cell carcinoma and melanoma seem particularly capricious in this regard.

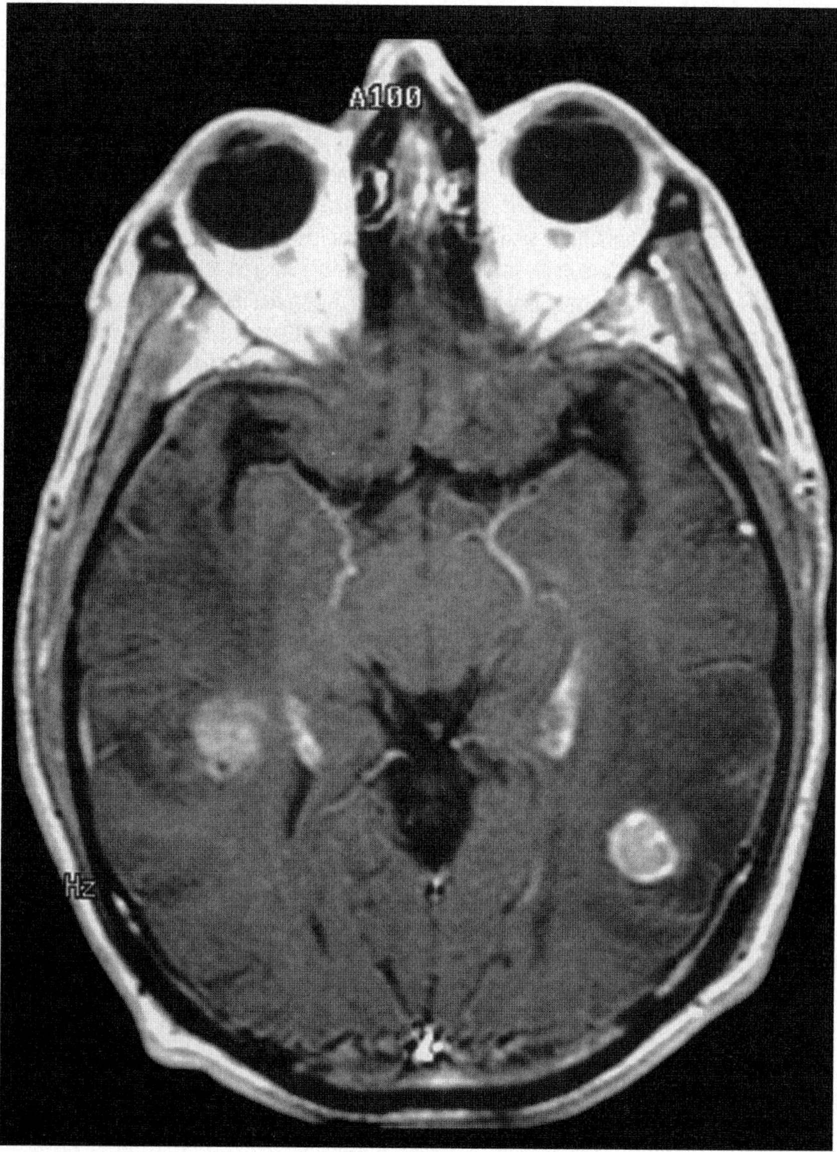

Figure 25–1. Magnetic resonance imaging scan of patient with bilateral brain metastasis from non–small cell lung cancer who presented with progressive headache and somnolence. Note the relative sizes of the tumors and the surrounding edema. Both metastatic deposits were resected, and the patient enjoyed improved function as a result.

Pathophysiologic Considerations

Brain edema is defined as an increase in water content per unit volume of brain parenchyma. Brain edema mechanisms are classically divided into three categories: cytotoxic, vasogenic, and interstitial (Klatzo, 1967). Cytotoxic edema is caused by noxious injury that produces cellular swelling and subsequent water increase in the intracellular compartment. Vasogenic edema is due to the release of water and solute from the intravascular compartment into the brain's interstitial space. Interstitial edema occurs when a hindrance to cerebrospinal fluid reabsorption increases intraventricular pressure enough to result in transependymal reabsorption of water and sodium into the brain's periventricular interstitial space (Fishman, 1975). In most clinical situations, more than one mechanism contributes to brain edema.

Understanding the relationship between a lesion and the surrounding normal brain parenchyma is critical to any appreciation of the forces at play in producing intracerebral edema. The blood–brain barrier's integrity, dependent on the dynamic interaction of astrocytes, cerebral endothelium, and cerebral interstitium, plays a major but not exclusive role in the development of brain edema. Instances of relatively pure cytotoxic edema, such as may be seen following anoxic injury, produce swelling despite a closed blood–brain barrier. In anoxia the brain suffers swelling of all cellular components with resultant shrinkage of the extracellular space (Tommasino, 1992). In contradistinction, vasogenic edema results from an open (or leaky) blood–brain barrier that is associated with extravasation of plasma water, crystalloid, and colloid.

Factors at play in the production of brain edema can be better understood by applying the principles expressed by the Starling equation for fluid flow into interstitial tissues across a capillary vessel wall (Klatzo 1987). In this special case,

$$\mathit{flow} = K_f(\Delta P - \Delta \pi)$$

where K_f is the water conductivity of the capillary membrane and ΔP and $\Delta \pi$ are the differences between plasma and interstitial tissue hydrostatic pressure and plasma and interstitial tissue oncotic pressure, respectively. The differences between plasma and interstitial tissue hydrostatic pressure and between plasma and interstitial tissue oncotic pressure provide the motive force for fluid flow. This equation reveals that water conductivity of the capillary endothelial membrane, which is directly related to capillary permeability, is the greatest determinant of fluid flow when hydrostatic pressure and oncotic pressure remain relatively constant, as is the case in most acute clinical situations.

That the water conductivity of capillary endothelium does not depend exclusively on interruption of the blood–brain barrier is demonstrated by the fact that the area of brain edema surrounding tumor deposits frequently exceeds the nidus of contrast enhancement associated with the mass. Some of the edema may reflect locally increased oncotic pressure due to fractionation of proteins and peptides leaked from the region of blood–brain barrier breakdown (Rasmussen and Klatzo, 1969). Diffusion of these protein fragments and the resultant shift in oncotic forces likely plays a particularly important role in edema formation around tumors, especially those lesions associated with necrosis.

In addition to the increase in interstitial oncotic pressure from peptide leakage, brain edema surrounding tumor is affected by a host of vasoactive substances released from injured adjacent parenchymal tissue or from the tumor itself. Important among these substances may be the arachidonic acid metabolites (Yen and Lee, 1987), especially leukotrienes and prostaglandins, which are formed by the action of phospholipases from the tumor, and inflammatory cells (Aktan et al., 1991) on the rich lipid stores of the CNS. Elevated levels of leukotriene C4 are found in glioblastoma multiforme lesions as well as in the surrounding edematous tissue (Black et al., 1986). Corticosteroids suppress this edema mechanism through induction of a phospholipase inhibitor (Flower and Blackwell, 1979).

Brain tumors promote the production of numerous other factors that increase vascular permeability (Bruce et al., 1987). Inflammatory substances thought to be involved in brain tumor edema formation include histamine (Kolb, 1991), serotonin (Makarov et al., 1991), prostacyclin (Butti et al., 1991), thromboxanes (Gaetani et al., 1991), kallikrein-kinin (Maier-Hauff et al., 1984), glutamate (Baethmann et al., 1989), and other permeability factors (Ohnishi et al., 1990; Bruce et al., 1987) whose roles are as yet incompletely defined. The large number of inflammatory factors implicated in brain edema reflects the brain's enormous inherent inflammatory capability, particularly once the blood–brain barrier has been breached or when the inflammatory stimulus resides in the interstitial or subarachnoid space.

The brain has no inherent lymphatic drainage system, but the subarachnoid space serves as an efficient conduit for local wastes and nutrients. The free flow of fluid through the Virchow-Robin spaces, investitures of subarachnoid space that surround small arterioles for a short distance as they enter the brain, permits such rapid movement of even large protein molecules that it can be considered the "third circulation" (Cushing, 1926) for the CNS. Horseradish peroxidase injected into the subarachnoid space rapidly disperses throughout the cerebral interstitium but is largely excluded from regions of vasogenic edema (Blaumanis et al., 1990). Ironically, regions where the blood–brain barrier is disturbed release vasoactive substances into the interstitium but flush out fewer of these noxious substances than the normal parenchyma does, reinforcing the development of edema.

Vasogenic edema mostly spares gray matter, with white matter bearing the brunt of the increased water and sodium content. The brain's white matter is largely composed of axons running parallel to one another that serve as orderly conduits for edema fluid. In contrast, the gray matter's neuropil forms a feltwork mesh that presents a relative impediment to interstitial fluid flow (Klatzo, 1987). Thus, vasogenic edema typically affects gray matter less than white matter. In a cat plasma-infusion model of vasogenic edema, cerebral blood flow did not change in edematous white matter, but the cerebral metabolic rate for glucose was significantly increased (Sutton et al., 1989). Vasogenic edema induces local anaerobic metabolism and local lactate production.

HYDROCEPHALUS

Cerebrospinal fluid is continuously formed, primarily by the choroid plexus in the lateral and fourth ventricles. Cerebrospinal fluid is secreted at a rate of about 0.35 ml/minute or 500 ml/day. The combined ventricular and subarachnoid cerebrospinal spaces have a capacity of about 150 ml, so the cerebral spinal fluid is turned over about three times a day (Rowland et al., 1991). Cerebrospinal fluid reabsorption occurs at the pacchionian granulations that are located over the cerebral convexities adjacent to the superior sagittal sinus, into which they drain. The pacchionian granulations, also called the *arachnoid villi,* function as valves that allow for unidirectional flow of cerebrospinal fluid from the subarachnoid space into the venous system. All components of the cerebrospinal fluid, including red blood cells and even microbes, can clear the cerebrospinal fluid and enter the blood stream through this bulk-flow drainage system.

Intracranial volume remains constant within the confines of the rigid outer skull. The intracranial volume is equal to the combined volumes of the brain, the intracranial blood, and the cerebrospinal fluid. When cerebrospinal fluid production exceeds cerebrospinal fluid absorption (removal), hydrocephalus results with consequent increases in intraventricular volume and intracranial pressure. Magnetic resonance imaging has shown that, under normal circumstances, caudal movements of the basal ganglia and pons as great as 1.5 mm may be seen during each normal systolic addition of about 100 ml of arterial blood to the closed system (Greitz et al., 1992). When transependymal flow of fluid occurs during hydrocephalus, these physiologic excursions may become exaggerated and contribute to the risk of herniation, particularly if there is an associated mass lesion.

Cerebrospinal fluid rarely causes hydrocephalus in cases of choroid plexus papilloma; the vast majority of hydrocephalus cases are due to impediment of cerebrospinal fluid drainage. Blockage of flow through this system produces progressive enlargement of the proximal ventricles because of the continual production of cerebrospinal fluid. Obstruction to flow can occur at the level of the pacchionian granulations, in which case all of the ventricles are in communication with one another and all are enlarged. The causes of communicating hydrocephalus include subarachnoid hemorrhage, meningitis, and grossly elevated cerebrospinal fluid protein.

INCREASED INTRACRANIAL PRESSURE

Whether the cranial vault pressure increases because of the growth of a mass within it (tumor, hemorrhage, or abscess), the development of hydrocephalus, or brain edema, the consequences are similar (Cushing, 1902). Although for over 200 years experimental evidence has demonstrated that elevated intracranial pressure alone is sufficient to cause coma, the mechanisms by which physiologic dysfunction arises are still being elicited. Table 25–1 summarizes many of the factors affecting intracranial pressure. The history of studies on cerebral dysfunction caused by elevated intracranial pressure has been admirably reviewed by Lundberg (1960) in his important monograph on human ventricular pressure monitoring.

If intracranial pressure increases above arterial pressure, tachycardia ensues, and the respiratory rate decreases. The brain consumes 15% of the cardiac output, and it is exquisitely sensitive to ischemia. White matter is more sensitive to ischemic damage, probably because white matter receives about 25%

Table 25–1. Factors Affecting Intracranial Pressure

Increased intracranial pressure
Hypercapnia (any degree)
Hypoxia (Pao_2 <50 mm Hg)
Hyperthermia
REM sleep
Halothane
Nitrous oxide
Decreased intracranial pressure
Hypocapnia (any degree)
Hyperoxia (Pao_2 >1000 mm Hg)
Hypothermia
Barbiturates
Narcotics
Muscle relaxants

Source: Modified from North and Reilly (1990).

less blood flow per unit volume of brain than the more metabolically active gray matter.

The cerebral arterioles are the main resistance vessels, rapidly responding to alterations in systemic blood pressure, pH, and Pco_2. Cerebral arterioles constrict when systemic blood pressure increases and dilate when it decreases, serving to maintain a relatively constant rate of cerebral blood flow. The cerebral arterioles are profoundly affected by changes in arterial CO_2 tension. Breathing 5% CO_2 increases cerebral blood flow by 50%, and breathing 7% CO_2 doubles it (Brust, 1991). A series of animal experiments have demonstrated that cerebral blood flow changes by 2% to 4% for each 1 mm Hg change in arterial CO_2 pressure (Harper and Glass, 1965). Similarly, acidosis increases cerebral blood flow and alkalosis decreases it.

Hypothermia lowers intracranial pressure by diminishing cerebral blood flow and protects neurons from ischemic injury by simultaneously lowering neuronal oxygen requirements. Unfortunately, rebound-raised intracranial pressure during rewarming limits hypothermia's clinical benefit.

Hyperthermia, on the other hand, increases intracranial pressure (Malkinson et al., 1985, 1990), with the chill phase causing the greatest rise in pressure. Heating experiments with normal rhesus monkeys, cats, and rats (Meyer and Handa, 1967) demonstrated a steady increase in cerebral blood flow, expired CO_2 content, and rate of cerebral metabolism of oxygen up to a temperature of 42°C, at which point metabolic activity and blood flow rapidly decline. In these experiments, the cerebral blood flow increased by 50% and the cerebral oxygen consumption by 33%. In an injured brain, the effects are even more profound. In one experiment, monkeys with cold-induced edematous brain lesions were warmed on heating blankets to 40°C. After only 2 hours at this temperature, they suffered 40% edema increases in the lesions (Clasen et al., 1974). On the basis of results of these and other experiments, it should not be surprising that hyperthermia can be catastrophic for patients with increased intracranial pressure. These patients should be aggressively treated with antipyretics and cooling blankets if necessary.

Critical to understanding the mechanisms by which tumors cause increased intracranial pressure is an understanding of the changes in local autoregulation wrought by pathologic tumor arterioles. In a cat xenotransplantation tumor model (Okada et al., 1992), clear correlation was noted between tumor pH decline and increased water content, whereas in peritumoral edema pH increased because of the efflux of alkaline lactate salts from the tumor into surrounding tissues. Such alterations in regional metabolism favor decreased peritumoral blood flow and diminished clearance of edema-associated molecules from peritumoral tissues by the circulation. This serves to maintain edema if the offending lesion is not removed.

Of the intracranial components, blood is the most labile. Under normal conditions, there is about 100 ml of blood in the cranium. Seventy percent of this volume resides in the venous system and its plexi, forming a high-capacity volume buffer against the vagaries of alterations in cerebral venous return to the systemic circulation. Change in venous return from the skull, which can be caused by respiratory fluctuations in thoracic pressure and their consequent effect on jugular venous pressure, congestive heart failure, or the superior vena cava syndrome, may have profound effects on intracranial pressure. Once venous capacity mechanisms are overwhelmed, intracranial pressure may rise dramatically.

When he monitored direct intracranial pressure in brain tumor patients, Lundberg (1960) observed waves of pressure increase that could be used to predict functional decompensation and herniation. These pressure waves ranged from 50 to 100 mm Hg and lasted 5 to 20 minutes. The waves reflect changes in cerebral compliance and cerebrovascular capacity associated with increased intracranial pressure. Common signs and symptoms during sustained pressure waves include headache, neck pain, head noises, disordered consciousness, confusion, restlessness, rigidity of the arms, legs, or neck, clonic movements of the arms, bradycardia and hypertension (the Cushing response), hyperpnea, air hunger, nausea and vomiting, flushing of the face, sweating, urge to micturate, and itching of the nose. Unfortunately, the clinical syndrome is highly variable, and detection demands diligent observation by all who care for patients with increased intracranial pressure.

HERNIATION SYNDROMES

The brain's delicate structure and functional integrity are based on precise architectural relationships. Herniation disturbs these relationships and produces severe dysfunction. Table 25–2 summarizes symptoms commonly seen with cerebral herniation.

The commonly encountered herniation sites are *(1)* the mesial temporal lobes at the tentorial notch (uncal herniation), *(2)* the cerebellar tonsils through the foramen magnum, and *(3)* the cingulate gyrus of the frontal lobes underneath the cerebral falx. Less frequently, a central herniation syndrome may occur in which both mesial temporal lobes compress diencephalic structures. This syndrome is heralded by the midbrain tectal signs of bilateral ptosis and paresis of upward gaze (North and Reilly, 1990). Brain may herniate through a craniotomy site.

Table 25–2. Symptoms Associated with Cerebral Herniation

Headache, neck ache
Blurring of vision, amaurosis
Abducens paresis
Restlessness
Confusion
Rigidity of the neck
Opisthotonos, trismus
Rigidity and tonic extension or flexion of arms and legs
Bilateral extensor responses of plantar reflexes and other signs of spinal automatism
Cardiovascular disturbances
Respiratory disturbances
Rise in temperature
Nausea, vomiting
Hiccups

Table 25–3. Signs and Symptoms of Temporal Lobe Herniation from Supratentorial Tumor

Fluctuations in state of consciousness
Anisocoria
Nuchal rigidity
Imbalances of extraocular muscles
Cardiopulmonary and thermoregulatory disturbances
Pyramidal tract signs
Decerebrate rigidity

Source: From Schwartz and Rosner (1941).

A detailed clinicopathologic study of mesial temporal lobe herniations due to supratentorial tumors found that seven signs and symptoms occur regularly (Schwartz and Rosner, 1941) (see Table 25–3). The syndrome arises when an expanding supratentorial mass lesion displaces the uncus against the tentorial notch and thus compresses the ipsilateral third nerve, causing venous engorgement of the diencephalon, hippocampus, and brain stem. Consequent compression of the ipsilateral cerebral peduncle produces contralateral pyramidal tract dysfunction manifested by hemiparesis, hyperreflexia, and Babinski's sign. Infrequently, the cerebral peduncle contralateral to the mass may be caught against the tentorial notch and produce hemiparesis ipsilateral to the tumor. This is known as *Kernohan's notch phenomenon* (Kernohan and Woltman, 1929). Symptoms of herniation of the mesial temporal lobe usually progress from ipsilateral third nerve paresis, altered consciousness, and hemiparesis to vasomotor and respiratory instability over a course of hours, so prompt recognition and expedient intervention are essential if catastrophe is to be averted.

The tonsil of the cerebellum or the gyri of the flocculonodular lobe may herniate against the medulla oblongata when a mass in the posterior fossa expands. These attacks can be confused as a seizure unless a careful history is taken and neurologic examination performed. Respiratory arrest and autonomic dysfunction can rapidly ensue with little premonitory warning other than intermittent spells of the kind well described by Jackson (1871) in a report of a patient with a midline cerebellar tumor:

> His hands were clenched; his forearms were flexed on the arms which were generally kept to the sides. The head was drawn back and the back was curved. His legs were always extended to the fullest possible degree, the feet being arched backwards. Sometimes he passed feces and urine in an attack. The seizures generally lasted three or four minutes, and, when passing off, they returned if he were moved about. He was not unconscious. . . .

A posterior fossa mass must be considered in any cancer patient who experiences vague symptoms of dizziness, tinnitus, vertigo, and blurred vision accompanied by nausea, vomiting, nuchal rigidity, or abnormal eye movements. Keen awareness of the possibility of an expanding posterior fossa lesion is critical, as surgical evacuation of a posterior fossa mass can restore normal function provided that irreversible damage to rhombencephalic structures has not occurred.

Frontal lobe masses can cause displacement of the cingulate gyrus and the anterior cerebral arteries under the falx cerebri, producing compressive ischemic injury of this important limbic system structure. Patients with subfalcine herniation demonstrate varying degrees of abulia or lack of interest in their surroundings. They become apathetic, withdraw, and have slow, minimal responses. Grasp (unilateral or bilateral) and suck reflexes may be released. Subfalcine herniation proceeds to coma at a more leisurely pace than the other herniation syndromes do and can even be compatible with long, albeit neurologically reduced, survival.

TREATMENT CONSIDERATIONS

Alterations in consciousness due to structural disease must be recognized so that treatment can be instituted promptly and irreparable damage to the brain can be avoided. Few endeavors in medicine require equal clinical tenacity. Alterations in consciousness due to structural disease often occur in patients with advanced stages of cancer, and the clinician must exercise considerable judgement when designing a treatment plan. The best plan is one that seeks to provide the highest possible quality of life for the patient while taking into account overall prognosis and the patient's wishes for aggressive or palliative therapy.

Monitoring

Except in the perioperative setting, invasive and expensive continuous intracranial pressure monitoring is not justified in the management of cerebral edema due to CNS neoplasm. Physiologic testing, including electroencephalography and the measurement of brain stem auditory and somatosensory evoked potentials, has improved the understanding of how intracranial catastrophe occurs (Stone et al., 1990, Lindsay et al., 1990). Noninvasive transcranial Doppler monitoring is an indirect measure of intracranial pressure (Trieb et al., 1998), and many invasive probes are presently used clinically to monitor intracranial pressure as well as regional oxygen saturation, jugular bulb oxygen saturation, and cerebral perfusion pressure (Nara et al., 1998). While useful for understanding the pathophysiology of increased intracranial pressure, these techniques are of limited value for oncologic patients, for whom the etiology of raised intracranial pressure is the greatest determinant of outcome. Except for patients who are paralyzed or in pharmacologically induced comas, careful and frequent neurologic examination remains the most practical and cost-effective means of examining patients with coma due to tumors.

General Measures

Pain can greatly increase intracranial pressure, and reluctance to treat pain because of concerns about confounding the neurologic examination is not only cruel but foolish, particularly as both narcotics and barbiturates lower intracranial pressure (Williams and Hanley, 1993). Muscle relaxants are widely used in intensive care units, especially to contend with patients who resist ventilatory support. These should be used only when critical to patient management and then only with assurance that the patient is adequately sedated so that he or she will not experience the horror of being paralyzed on a ventilator and in pain.

Changes in thoracic venous return during Valsalva's maneuver, coughing, positive pressure ventilation, and endotracheal suctioning can dangerously elevate intracranial pressure, but the elevation can be minimized by gently sedating the patient (Ersson et al., 1990) and using prophylactic hyperventilation. For similar reasons, neck constriction by bandages and endotracheal tube ties must be avoided. A stool softener should be given to patients who are inclined to strain. If possible, the head should be elevated to an angle of 30 degrees, which serves to lower intracranial pressure without unduly diminishing carotid and vertebral artery pressures (North and Reilly, 1990).

Fever must be treated aggressively with antipyretics and, if ineffective, a cooling blanket. Hypotension can be disastrous in a patient with increased intracranial pressure, as it triggers autoregulatory mechanisms to induce cerebral arteriolar dilatation, promoting further elevation of intracranial pressure and potentially diminishing cerebral perfusion pressure. Free water (hypotonic fluids such as 5% dextrose in water) must be avoided, even as a vehicle for delivering medication. Hyponatremia promotes migration of free water from the intravascular space into the cerebral interstitium and must be scrupulously avoided. Furosemide and acetazolamide may be used for a short time to maintain osmolality at 300 to 310 mOsm, but the clinician should not allow hypovolemia to develop (North and Reilly, 1990). Clinicians should bear in mind a prospective study of 244 patients with subarachnoid hemorrhage that demonstrated less cerebral ischemia and improved survival for patients not treated with fluid restriction or antihypertensive therapy (Hasan et al., 1989).

Acute Increased Intracranial Pressure and Herniation

A number of methods including hyperventilation, osmotic agents, and corticosteroids can be used to reduce acute increased intracranial pressure.

Hyperventilation

Hyperventilation can lower intracranial pressure within minutes. This technique is typically utilized for operative and perioperative patients who suddenly develop increased intracranial pressure. Typically, an acutely decompensated patient is intubated and hyperventilated to a $Paco_2$ of 25 mm Hg; once the patient has responded, the $Paco_2$ should be allowed to drift gradually up to 35 mm Hg over 1 or 2 days while the patient is carefully monitored (Williams and Hanley, 1993). Protracted hyperventilation produces hypochloremia, which can be countered with KCl infusions. In at least one study of traumatic increased intracranial pressure, hyperventilation was found to diminish brain tissue oxygenation (Kiening et al., 1997), so caution must be exercised in its use.

Osmotic Diuretics

Osmotic diuretics work by establishing an osmotic gradient between the intravascular compartment and the cerebral parenchyma, promoting the movement of water out of brain tissue. Adequate urine flow is essential for osmotic diuretic therapy to succeed. One of the most popular osmotic agents is mannitol, a freely filterable isomer of the inert sugar sorbitol that is widely used to reduce intracranial pressure. Mannitol crosses the blood–brain barrier poorly, which increases its efficacy as a cerebral dehydrating drug. Unfortunately, the relative lack of a blood–brain barrier in tumor deposits causes a greater dehydration effect in the contralateral normal brain than in the lesion (Reichenthal et al., 1990).

Intravenous mannitol is available as a 10% to 25% solution and is given in a dose of approximately 1 gm/kg of body weight. The solution should be given over about 20 to 45 minutes; this time frame lessens the risk of hemolysis while establishing a swift osmotic gradient between the blood and cerebral parenchymal compartments to effect cerebral dehydration. Mannitol is generally given acutely once or twice a day. While it can be given multiple times per day for several days, chronic dosing can precipitate hypovolemia and electrolyte disturbance, while accumulation of mannitol in edematous white matter can produce a reverse osmotic gradient and exacerbation of edema (Kauffman and Cardoso, 1992). Mannitol depletes intravascular volume and produces hypernatremia, so careful attention must be paid to the patient's state of hydration and electrolyte balance. Mannitol may have additional benefits for patients with elevated intracranial pressure, such as free radical scavenging and improved blood flow dynamics (Paczynski, 1997).

For as long as 80 years, hypertonic saline solutions have been known to dehydrate the brain (Weed and McKibben, 1919), but their clinical use has only recently been championed. Solutions of between 3% and 29% saline have been used to treat refractory increased intracranial pressure both in animal experiments (Scheller et al., 1991) and in limited clinical trials (Suarez et al., 1998; Schatzmann et al., 1998). Hypertonic saline augments rather than depletes intravascular volume, which consequently supports cerebral perfusion pressure. Hypertonic saline solution's role in increased intracranial pressure management has yet to be determined (Prough and Zornow, 1998); likely it will be an important one.

Glycerol and urea (Beks and Weeme, 1967) are orally absorbed osmotic diuretics that have been used to treat brain edema. As is the case with mannitol, rebound edema is a problem in their use unless concomitant glucocorticoids are administered. Neither glycerol nor urea is excluded from the cerebrospinal fluid, which lessens their potency as cerebral dehydrating agents. Urea's clinical utility is limited because it causes gastrointestinal upset. Glycerol's effects on brain edema are more gradual in onset and more sustained than those of mannitol (Garcia-Sola et al., 1991), but a reverse osmotic gradient may be established with chronic use (Rottenberg et al., 1977) with consequent worsening of edema formation. An oral dose of 1.5 gm/kg a day given in six divided doses (every 4 hours) significantly reduces cerebral edema (Meyer et al., 1971). We have used it in an every 4 hour schedule for 3 days followed by more chronic scheduling of every 6 to 8 hours for patients intolerant of or unwilling to take enough glucocorticoid to control their brain tumor–induced cerebral edema. Glycerol must be used cautiously by patients with diabetes mellitus.

The loop diuretics like furosemide reduce cerebral edema in experimental settings (Albright et al., 1984), but they are prone to produce hypotension and thus decrease cerebral perfusion pressure. In one study of patients with cerebral edema from tumor, furosemide produced no significant reduction in edema visible on the computerized tomography scan while mannitol did (Cascino et al., 1983). Loop diuretics contribute to the electrolyte disturbances associated with osmotic diuresis, but their effect on cerebral edema is not as great as that of the other diuretics, so their routine use is best avoided. They do have a place in reducing fluid retention in patients receiving chronic glucocorticoid therapy for brain tumor edema.

Corticosteroids and Vasogenic Edema

Corticosteroids, especially dexamethasone, have been the mainstay of treatment for brain tumor edema for more than 30 years and are one of the most effective therapies for vasogenic edema, which so frequently accompanies primary or secondary tumors or abscesses. Dexamethasone remains the favored corticosteroid for treating vasogenic cerebral edema because of its potent anti-inflammatory effects, lack of mineralocorticoid activity, and relatively low binding to plasma proteins, which allows for greater availability of the drug for the brain. Despite the efficacy and widespread use of corticosteroids, the mechanisms of their beneficial action in vasogenic cerebral edema are still not fully understood.

The clinical response to steroids varies greatly and is related to differences in tumor steroid responsiveness, tissue corticosteroid receptor concentration (Yu et al., 1981), and constitutional factors. Patients with low serum albumin and cachexia may have a greater response to corticosteroids than patients with normal levels. The optimal dose of steroid depends on the individual, but, for patients with neurologic emergencies, erring on the high side of steroid dosage seems prudent. Patients with acute increases in intracranial pressure or recent decompensation in neurologic status require a loading dose of 10 to 20 mg of dexamethasone intravenously. This can quickly be reduced to 8 to 16 mg of dexamethasone a day in two to four divided doses. Dosage must be regularly adjusted based on careful clinical observation, with occasional patients requiring much higher doses. In extreme instances, boluses of 100 mg of dexamethasone may be life saving. If given over 5 to 10 minutes, these large boluses will not produce the unpleasant perineal sensations associated with more rapid infusions.

Whereas in experimental models of cerebral vasogenic edema a significant effect of steroids was noted at 1 hour (Shapiro et al., 1990), their benefit in clinical settings may not be seen for 4 to 12 hours and may not reach maximum benefit for 72 hours. For cases of life-threatening cerebral vasogenic edema, more rapidly acting measures such as osmotic diuresis or, rarely, hyperventilation should be initiated during this period before steroids take effect.

Corticosteroid Toxicities. The systemic toxicities of corticosteroids limit their use. In a retrospective series of steroid-dependent neuro-oncology patients, corticosteroid toxicity correlated with duration of use and total dose. In addition, patients with low serum albumin levels had increased steroid toxicity. More than 50% of the patients in this study had significant steroid toxicity, and almost 20% required hospitalization to manage these complications (Weissman et al., 1987). The less serious, although certainly annoying, side effects of corticosteroids include insomnia (which may be minimized by giving the drug in two divided doses; giving about two thirds of the dexamethasone dose in the morning and the remainder in the early afternoon to mimic the natural steroid rhythm), tremor, hiccups, systemic edema, blurred vision, and euphoria.

Unfortunately, corticosteroids also produce disabling and potentially fatal complications. They induce a catabolic state and, with chronic use, may cause muscular atrophy. Chronic use may infrequently cause a severe myopathy that some clinicians feel can be remedied by switching to nonfluorinated steroids when patients must be maintained on anti-inflammatory therapy (Dropcho and Soong, 1991). Infection with opportunistic organisms occurs during chronic steroid therapy, and *Pneumocystis carinii* pneumonia typically develops during a steroid wean (Henson et al., 1991).

Gastrointestinal bleeding and bowel perforation are particularly treacherous complications of steroid therapy, although extremely rare in brain tumor patients. Glucocorticoids may mask the symptoms of intra-abdominal catastrophe until late, so any gastrointestinal symptoms in patients on glucocorticoids must be evaluated diligently. All patients taking glucocorticoids should be placed on antiulcer therapy and a bowel regularity program. The dosage must be weaned as rapidly as clinically possible, as toxicity relates to both total dose and duration of therapy. Avascular necrosis of the femoral head may complicate steroid use.

Modifying schedules to twice daily dosing with lower doses of steroid can decrease the incidence of toxicity (Weissman et al., 1991), although the prolonged half-life of dexamethasone means that a steady state may not be achieved for days. Corticosteroids should be given with caution to patients with glaucoma, diabetes mellitus, and pre-existing tuberculosis infection. Hypothalamic-pituitary-adrenal axis suppression can arise after a few weeks of steroid treatment, so patients being weaned must be checked for addisonian symptoms and signs. Hydrocortisone replacement at 20 mg in the morning and 10 mg in the afternoon may be needed for selected patients. Patients experiencing physiologic stress who are hypothalamic-pituitary-adrenal axis suppressed should be given 100 mg of hydrocortisone parenterally every 8 hours.

Corticosteroids' anti-inflammatory effects are likely responsible for most, but not all, of their salubrious effects in treating cerebral vasogenic edema. Steroids suppress leukocyte migration and their ability to elaborate lymphokines. They inhibit production, function, and release of the leukotrienes, interleukin-1, tumor necrosis factor, interferon-α, prostaglandins, phospholipase A_2, platelet-activating factor, macrophage migration inhibition factor, and neutrophil-derived tissue plasminogen activator (Haynes, 1990). Such broad effects speak for the fundamental role for steroids in moderating inflammation.

Corticosteroids improve brain compliance (Kose et al., 1989), even in patients without vasogenic edema. Other non–anti-inflammatory benefits of steroids for patients with brain edema include restoration of noradrenaline and dopamine levels in regions adjacent to tumor (Bayens-Simmonds et al., 1989; Chang, 1989) and moderation of the effects of the capillary permeability factors expressed by tumors (Ohnishi et al., 1991).

The use of more specific anti-inflammatory drugs is on the horizon. Indomethacin, given intravenously to severe head trauma patients in bolus doses of 30 to 50 mg, lowered intracranial pressure and reduced cerebral blood flow while increasing cerebral perfusion pressure (Slavik and Rhoney, 1999) and likely produces less toxicity than corticosteroids. Drugs that block discrete inflammatory processes may be attractive in the management of tumoral edema. Two tumor necrosis factor inhibitors (Bass et al., 1996; Megyeri et al., 1999) have recently demonstrated efficacy in reducing experimental brain edema, offering hope for more specific drugs with less deleterious side effects.

Hydrocephalus

Recognition of hydrocephalus as the cause of altered neurologic function demands a high level of clinical suspicion. Progressive deficits in ambulation or level of consciousness, especially if accompanied by nausea, headache, or intrascapular pain, should alert the clinician to the possibility of acute hydrocephalus. The pace of neurologic deterioration largely determines therapeutic decisions for patients with acute hydrocephalus. Rapid progression of symptoms may occur more commonly when the brain is inflamed; and the risk of cerebral herniation is far greater when hydrocephalus is unevenly distributed within the ventricular system (i.e., noncommunicating hydrocephalus).

Computerized tomography or MRI scanning demonstrates characteristic ballooning of the frontal and temporal horns, rostral to caudal ventricular enlargement, and a band of periventricular edema. Surgical intervention with the placement of a burr hole and ventricular drain is necessary only for the acutely hydrocephalic patient who is in severe pain and/or experiences neurologic decompensation over a short period of time. External ventricular drainage may be required but carries a risk of infection and should be used for the minimum amount of time needed. Using an electrical pump to control the rate of cerebrospinal fluid drainage may lessen the patient's discomfort and ensure that excessive drainage does not occur. Upward herniation following drainage is a risk for patients who have a posterior fossa mass (Pillay et al., 1989; Rappaport and Shalit, 1989). This life-threatening complication may be avoided by removing the infratentorial lesion before shunting.

Occasionally, surgical intervention may be postponed or avoided altogether by draining cerebrospinal fluid by serial lumbar puncture (Hasan et al., 1991), provided that the hydrocephalus is communicating. Less pressing hydrocephalus may respond to corticosteroid or acetazolamide therapy. These nonsurgical measures for hydrocephalus can postpone more definitive treatment and, in some cancer patients, can obviate surgery altogether, although the side effects of medical therapy often prove intolerable over long periods of time.

CONCLUSION

The diagnosis and management of altered mental status due to structural disease is one of the most challenging tasks in clinical oncology. The physician must intervene swiftly if disaster is to be avoided, yet must act in a manner consistent with the overall prognosis and stage of the patient's underlying condition. Reviving a comatose patient with advanced bone metastasis or pulmonary disease may result in a prolonged survival but one marked by extreme discomfort.

REFERENCES

Aktan S, Aykut C, Oktay S, et al. 1991. The alterations of leukotriene C_4 and prostaglandin E_2 levels following different ischemic periods in rat brain tissue. Prostaglandins Leukot Essent Fatty Acids 42:67–71.

Albright AL, Latchaw RE, Robinson AG. 1984. Intracranial and systemic effects of osmotic and oncotic therapy in experimental cerebral edema. J Neurosurg 60:481–489.

Baethmann A, Maier-Hauff K, Schurer L, et al. 1989. Release of glutamate and of free fatty acids in vasogenic brain edema. J Neurosurg 70:578–591.

Bass R, Engelhard D, Trembovler V, Shohami E. 1996. A novel nonpsychotropic cannabinoid, HU-211, in the treatment of experimental pneumococcal meningitis J Infect Dis 173:735–738.

Bayens-Simmonds J, Boisvert DP, Baker GB. 1989. Effect of dexamethasone on monoamine and metabolite levels in a brain-tumor model. Brain Res Bull 22:187–190.

Beks JW, ter Weeme C. 1967. The influence of urea and mannitol on increased intraventricular pressure in cold-induced cerebral oedema. Acta Neurochir (Wien) 16:97–107.

Black KL, Hoff JT, McGillicuddy JE, Gebarski SS. 1986. Increased leukotriene C_4 and vasogenic edema surrounding brain tumors in humans. Ann Neurol 19:592–595.

Blaumanis OR, Rennels ML, Grady PA. 1990. Focal cerebral edema impedes convective fluid/tracer movement through paravascular pathways in cat brain. Adv Neurol 52:385–389.

Bruce JN, Criscuolo GR, Merrill MJ, Moquin RR, Blacklock JB, Oldfield EH. 1987. Vascular permeability induced by protein product of malignant brain tumors: inhibition by dexamethasone. J Neurosurg 67:880–884.

Brust JC. 1991. Cerebral circulation: stroke. In: Kandel ER, Schwartz JH, Jessell TM (eds), Principles of Neural Science, 3rd ed. New York: Elsevier, 1041 pp.

Butti G, Gaetani P, Chiabrando C, et al. 1991. A study on the biological behavior of human brain tumors. Part II: steroid receptors and arachidonic acid metabolism. J Neurooncol 10:241–246.

Cascino T, Baglivo J, Conti J, Szewczykowski J, Posner JB, Rottenberg DA. 1983. Quantitative CT assessment of furosemide- and mannitol-induced changes in brain water content. Neurology 33:898–903.

Chang CC. 1989. Neurotransmitter amines in brain edema of a rat glioma model. Neurol Med Chir (Tokyo) 29:187–191.

Clasen RA, Pandolfi S, Laing I, Casey D Jr. 1974. Experimental study of relation of fever to cerebral edema. J Neurosurg 41:576–581.

Cushing H. 1902. Some experimental and clinical observations concerning states of increased intracranial tension. Am J Med Sci 124:375–400.

Cushing H. 1926. Studies in Intracranial Physiology and Surgery: The Third Circulation, the Hypophysics, the Gliomas. London: Humphrey Milford, pp 1–50.

Datz FL. 1986. Cerebral edema following iodine-131 therapy for thyroid carcinoma metastatic to the brain. J Nucl Med 27:637–640.

Dropcho EJ, Soong SJ. 1991. Steroid-induced weakness in patients with primary brain tumors. Neurology 41:1235–1239.

Ersson U, Carlson H, Mellstrom A, Ponten U, Hedstrand U, Jakobsson S. 1990. Observations on intracranial dynamics during respiratory physiotherapy in unconscious neurosurgical patients. Acta Anaesthesiol Scand 34:99–103.

Fisher CM. 1969. The neurological examination of the comatose patient. Acta Neurol Scand 45(suppl 36):1–56.

Fishman RA. 1975. Brain edema. N Engl J Med 293:706–711.

Flower RJ, Blackwell GJ. 1979. Anti-inflammatory steroids induce biosynthesis of a phospholipase A_2 inhibitor which prevents prostaglandin generation. Nature 278:456–459.

Gaetani P, Butti G, Chiabrando C, et al. 1991. A study on the biological behavior of human brain tumors. Part I. Arachidonic acid metabolism and DNA content. J Neurooncol 10:233–140.

Garcia-Sola R, Pulido P, Capilla P. 1991. The immediate and long-term effects of mannitol and glycerol. A comparative experimental study. Acta Neurochir (Wien) 109:114–121.

Goey SH, Voerman HJ, Strack van Schijndel RJ, et al. 1988. Swelling of metastatic tumors with high-dose interleukin therapy. N Engl J Med 318:643–644.

Greitz D, Wirestam R, Franck A, Nordell B, Thomsen C, Stahlberg F. 1992. Pulsatile brain movement and associated hydrodynamics studied by magnetic resonance phase imaging. The Monroe-Kellie doctrine revisited. Neuroradiology 34:370–380.

Haerer AF. 1992. DeJong's, The Neurologic Examination. Revised by A.F. Haerer. Philadelphia: JB Lippincott, p 709.

Harper AM, Glass HI. 1965. Effect of alterations in the arterial carbon dioxide tension on the blood flow through the cerebral cortex at normal and low arterial blood pressures. J Neurol Neurosurg Psychiatry 28:449–452.

Hasan D, Lindsay KW, Vermeulen M. 1991. Treatment of acute hydrocephalus after subarachnoid hemorrhage with serial lumbar puncture. Stroke 22:190–194.

Hasan D, Vermeulen M, Wijdicks EF, Hijdra A, van Gijn J. 1989. Effect of fluid intake and antihypertensive treatment on cerebral ischemia after subarachnoid hemorrhage. Stroke 20:1511–1515.

Haynes RC Jr. 1990. Adrenocorticotrophic hormone; adrenocortical steroids and their synthetic analogs; inhibitors of the synthesis and actions of adrenocortical hormones. In: Goodman AG (ed), Goodman and Gilman's The Pharmacological Basis of Therapeutics, 8th ed. New York: Pergamon Press, pp 1431–1462.

Henson JW, Jalaj JK, Walker RW, Stover DE, Fels AO. 1991. *Pneumocystis carinii* pneumonia in patients with primary brain tumors. Arch Neurol 48:406–409.

Jackson JH. 1871. Case of tumour of the middle lobe of the cerebellum. BMJ 2:528–529.

Ji Y, Walstad D, Brown JT, Powers SK. 1992. Improved survival from intracavitary photodynamic therapy of rat glioma. Photochem Photobiol 56:385–390.

Kauffman AM, Cardoso ER. 1992. Aggravation of vasogenic cerebral edema by multiple-dose mannitol. J Neurosurg 77: 584–589.

Kernohan JW, Woltman HW. 1929. Incisura of the crus due to contralateral brain tumor. Arch of Neurol Psychiatry 21:274–287.

Kiening KL, Hartl R, Unterberg AW, Schneider GH, Bardt T, Lanksch WR. 1997. Brain tissue pO2-monitoring in comatose patients: implications for therapy. Neurol Res 19: 233–240.

Klatzo I. 1967. Presidential address. Neuropathological aspects of brain edema. J Neuropathol Exp Neurol 26:1–14.

Klatzo I. 1987. Pathophysiological aspects of brain edema. Acta Neuropathol (Berl) 72:236–239.

Kolb E. 1991. [Current knowledge on the formation of nitric oxide in endothelial cells of blood vessels, in nerve cells and macrophages as well as its significance in vascular dilatation, information transmission and damage of tumor cells]. Z Gesamte Inn Med 46:431–436.

Kose S, Tamaki N, Kimura M, Matsumoto S. 1989. [Effect of steroids on intracranial pressure and pressure-volume index in patients with hydrocephalus]. No To Shinkei 41: 185–191.

Lindsay K, Pasaoglu A, Hirst D, Allaroyce G, Kennedy I, Teasdale G. 1990. Somatosensory and auditory brain stem conduction after head injury: a comparison with clinical features in prediction of outcome. Neurosurgery 26:278–285.

Lundberg N. 1960. Continuous recording and control of ventricular fluid pressure in neurosurgical practice. Acta Psych Neurol Scand 36(suppl 149):1–193.

Maier-Hauff K, Baethmann AJ Lange M, Schurer L, Unterberg A. 1984. The kallikrein-kinin system as mediator in vasogenic brain edema. Part 2: studies on kinin formation in focal and perifocal brain tissue. J Neurosurg 61:97–106.

Makarov A, Pomnikov VG, Sheludchenko FI, Lodoba EB, Goncharova VA.1991. [Serotonin and kinins in the cerebrospinal fluid in brain tumors]. Vopr Onkol 37:437–440.

Malkinson TJ, Cooper KE, Veale WL. 1990. Cerebrospinal fluid pressure in conscious rats during prostaglandin E1 fever. Am J Physiol 258:R783–787.

Malkinson TJ, Veale WL, Cooper KE. 1985. Fever and intracranial pressures. Brain Res Bull 15:315–319.

Megyeri P, Nemeth L, Pabst KM, Pabst MJ, Deli MA, Abraham CS.1999. 4-(2-Aminoethyl)benzenesulfonyl fluoride attenuates tumor-necrosis-factor-alpha-induced blood–brain barrier opening. Eur J Pharmacol 374:207–211.

Meyer JS, Charney JZ, Rivera VM, Mathew NT. 1971. Treatment with glycerol of cerebral oedema due to acute cerebral infarction. Lancet 2:993–997.

Meyer JS, Handa J. 1967. Cerebral blood flow and metabolism during experimental hyperthermia (fever). Minn Med 50:37–44.

Mogami H, Ushio Y, Hayakawa T, Yamada K.1983. [Intracranial hypertension]. Gan To Kagaku Ryoho 10:165–170.

Nara I, Shiogai T, Hara M, Saito I. 1998. Comparative effects of hypothermia, barbiturate, and osmotherapy for cerebral oxygen metabolism, intracranial pressure, and cerebral perfusion pressure in patients with severe head injury. Acta Neurochir Suppl (Wien) 71:22–26.

North B, Reilly P. 1990. Raised Intracranial Pressure: A Clinical Guide, Oxford: Heinemann Medical, pp 1–109.

Ohnishi T, Sher PB, Posner JB, et al. 1990. Capillary permeability factor secreted by malignant brain tumor. Role in peritumoral brain edema and possible mechanism for anti-edema effect of glucocorticoids. J Neurosurg 72:245–251.

Ohnishi T, Sher PB, Posner JB, Shapiro WR.1991. Increased capillary permeability in rat brain induced by factors secreted by cultured C6 glioma cells: role in peritumoral brain edema. J Neurooncol 10:13–25.

Okada Y, Kloiber O, Hossmann KA. 1992. Regional metabolism in experimental brain tumors in cats: relationship with acid/base, water, and electrolyte homeostasis. J Neurosurg 77:917–926.

Paczynski RP. 1997. Osmotherapy. Basic concepts and controversies. Crit Care Clin 13:105–129.

Pillay P, Barnett GH, Lanzeiri C, Cruse R. 1989. Dandy-Walker cyst upward herniation: the role of magnetic resonance imaging and double shunts. Pediatr Neurosci 15:74–79.

Plum F, Posner JB. 1982. The Diagnosis of Stupor and Coma. Philadelphia: FA Davis, pp 4–6.

Prough DS, Zornow, MH. 1998. Mannitol: an old friend on the skids? Crit Care Med 26:997–998.

Rappaport ZH, Shalit MN. 1989. Perioperative external ventricular drainage in obstructive hydrocephalus secondary to infratentorial brain tumours. Acta Neurochir (Wien) 96:118–121.

Rasmussen LE, Klatzo I. 1969. Protein and enzyme changes in cold injury edema. Acta Neuropathol (Berl) 13:12–28.

Reichenthal E, Kaspi T, Cohen ML, et al. 1990. The ambivalent effects of early and late administration of mannitol in cold-induced brain oedema. Acta Neurochir Suppl (Wien) 51:110–112.

Rottenberg DA, Hurwitz BJ, Posner JB. 1977. The effect of oral glycerol on intraventricular pressure in man. Neurology 27:600–608.

Rowland LP, Fink ME, Rubin L. 1991. Cerebrospinal fluid: blood–brain barrier, brain edema and hydrocephalus. In: Kandel ER, Schwartz JH, Jessell TM (eds), Principles of Neural Science, 3rd ed. New York: Elsevier, pp 1050–1060.

Schatzmann C, Heissler HE, Konig K, et al. 1998. Treatment of elevated intracranial pressure by infusions of 10% saline in severely head injured patients. Acta Neurochir Suppl 71:31–33.

Schwartz GA, Rosner AA. 1941. Displacement and herniation of the hippocampal gyrus through the incisura tentorii. Arch Neurol Psychiat 46:297–321.

Shapiro WR, Hiesiger EM, Cooney GA, Basler GA, Lipschutz LE, Posner JB. 1990. Temporal effects of dexamethasone on blood-to-brain and blood-to-tumor transport of 14C-alpha-aminoisobutyric acid in rat C6 glioma. J Neurooncol 8:197–204.

Slavik RS, Rhoney DH. 1999. Indomethacin: a review of its cerebral blood flow effects and potential use for controlling intracranial pressure in traumatic brain injury patients. Neurol Res 21:491–499.

Stone JL, Ghaly RF, Subramanian KD, Roccaforte P, Kane J. 1990. Transtentorial brain herniation in the monkey: analysis of brain stem auditory and somatosensory evoked potentials. Neurosurgery 26:26–31.

Suarez, JI, Qureshi AI, Bhardwaj A, et al. 1998. Treatment of refractory intracranial hypertension with 23.4% saline. Crit Care Med 26:1118–1122.

Sutton LN, Barranco D, Greenberg J, Dante S, Florin S, Welsh F. 1989. Cerebral blood flow and glucose metabolism in experimental brain edema. J Neurosurg 71:868–874.

Tommasino C. 1992. [Postoperative cerebral edema. Pathophysiology of the edema and medical therapy]. Min Anestesiol 58:35–42.

Treib J, Becker SC, Grauer M, Haass A. 1998. Transcranial doppler monitoring of intracranial pressure therapy with mannitol, sorbitol and glycerol in patients with acute stroke. Eur Neurol 40:212–219.

Walker RW, Cairncross JG, Posner JB. 1988. Cerebral herniation in patients receiving cisplatin. J Neurooncol 6:61–65.

Weed LH, McKibben PS. 1919. Experimental alteration of brain bulk. Am J Physiol 48:531–555.

Weissman DE, Dufer D, Vogel V, Abeloff MD. 1987. Corticosteroid toxicity in neuro-oncology patients. J Neurooncol 5:125–128.

Weissman DE, Janjan NA, Erickson B, et al. 1991. Twice-daily tapering dexamethasone treatment during cranial radiation for newly diagnosed brain metastases. J Neurooncol 11:235–239.

Wilhelm C, Ellner JJ. 1986. Chronic meningitis. Neurol Clin 4:115–141.

Williams MA, Hanley DF. 1993. Intracranial pressure monitoring and cerebral resuscitation. In: Grotta JC (ed), Management of the Acutely Ill Neurological Patient. New York: Churchill Livingstone, pp 49–74.

Yen MH, Lee SH. 1987. Effects of cyclooxygenase and lipoxygenase inhibitors on cerebral edema induced by freezing lesions in rats. Eur J Pharmacol 144:369–373.

Yu ZY, Wrange O, Boethius J, Hatam A, Granholm L, Gustafsson JA. 1981. A study of glucocorticoid receptors in intracranial tumors. J Neurosurg 55:757–760.

Zornow MH, Oh YS, Scheller MS. 1990. A comparison of the cerebral and haemodynamic effects of mannitol and hypertonic saline in an animal model of brain injury. Acta Neurochir Suppl 51:324–325.

26

Neurocognitive Function

CHRISTINA A. MEYERS AND ANNE E. KAYL

Cancers of the nervous system, particularly primary malignant brain tumors, can be devastating illnesses, characterized by a very low cure rate, short survival time, and significant morbidity as the disease progresses. Malignant primary brain tumors cause profound changes in cognitive function, personality, psychological well being, and ability to perform daily activities. These changes negatively affect the productivity and independence of brain tumor patients, impacting their social functioning, financial status, and self-esteem (Sherer et al., 1997).

The effects of the tumor, tumor treatment, and other factors that have the potential to impact brain functioning and the patient's life can be differentiated by appropriate evaluation methods, which can then guide the institution of therapeutic and palliative intervention strategies. In fact, quality of life may be one of the few areas where the health care provider can have a significant impact. An appreciation of the cognitive deficits and behavioral changes that may occur in brain tumor patients can aid in the design of intervention strategies, improve the quality of patient care, and ultimately improve the overall quality of life for brain tumor patients and their families.

NEUROBEHAVIORAL CHANGES ASSOCIATED WITH BRAIN TUMORS

Various factors contribute to the neurobehavioral changes associated with brain tumors. While manifestations of this disease vary substantially between patients, some general comments regarding tumor-related and patient-related factors and their impact on cognition are warranted.

Location

Brain tumors, whether primary or metastatic, almost always cause deficits of cognitive function. The type of impairment observed is in part related to the site of the lesion. For instance, left hemisphere tumors may produce language disorders that impair the patient's ability to communicate with others and comprehend spoken or written language (Haas et al., 1982). Tumors in the right hemisphere of the brain may cause deficits in visual perception and visual scanning, resulting in impaired driving skills or the inability to navigate in familiar places (Scheibel et al., 1996). Memory loss is often seen in association with tumors of either hemisphere. Impairments of frontal lobe function (executive deficits manifested by impairments of cognitive flexibility, abstraction, motivation, planning and organizational skills, ability to benefit from experience, personality changes, and so forth) are ubiquitous in brain tumor patients (Vilkki, 1992; Goldstein et al., 1993; Ackermann et al., 1996). One obvious reason is that the frontal lobes comprise one-third of the cerebrum, and a large proportion of patients has frontal tumors. However, many patients with nonfrontal tumors also exhibit executive deficits (Lilja et al., 1992). This is due in part to the fact that the frontal lobes have rich afferent and efferent connections with all other brain regions. Thus, a lesion in a nonfrontal location will disconnect the frontal lobe from information from that region and also interrupt modulatory frontal influences on its function. In addition, marked personality changes can occur following removal of tumors in certain regions of the brain, causing impairment in social functioning, motivation, and judgment (Meyers et al., 1992a).

Pathologic Type

Individuals diagnosed with low-grade tumors that have been present for many years may have no detectable changes in brain function due to cerebral plasticity and reorganization (Meyers et al., 1992b). In contrast, patients with very rapidly growing tumors may have widespread impairment due to mass effect on adjacent brain regions (Hom and Reitan, 1984). Despite the initial differences, the cognitive functioning of patients with anaplastic astrocytoma and patients with glioblastoma multiforme do not vary appreciably following surgery (Scheibel et al., 1996). This finding illustrates the potentially beneficial effects of surgery on mass effect, intracranial pressure, and other adverse effects on distal brain regions (diaschisis).

Patient Characteristics

The age of the patient also contributes to the manifestation and severity of neurobehavioral deficits. For example, older patients tend to have more malignant brain tumors, and even histologically less malignant tumors behave more aggressively in the older patient (Cohaden et al., 1985). Older patients are also at higher risk for having other concurrent neurodegenerative illnesses, such as Parkinson's disease or vascular disease. Finally, older patients may be more sensitive to the toxic side effects of treatment.

NEUROBEHAVIORAL CHANGES DUE TO TREATMENT

Cognitive dysfunction in brain tumor patients is often more generalized than expected for a focal lesion. This may be due to microscopic tumor infiltration, a high rate of tumor growth causing diaschisis, or the adverse effects of treatment (Meyers, 1986). Hochberg and Slotnick (1980) found diffuse cognitive difficulties in patients who were long-term survivors of malignant astrocytomas that were unrelated to tumor type, location, other medical factors, or psychiatric factors and were thought to be due to aggressive treatment. LeBaron et al. (1988) found that more than 50% of children treated for posterior fossa tumors had significant intellectual, motor, and academic problems 20 months after treatment cessation. Different adverse effects are likely attributable to radiation, chemotherapy, immunotherapy, and adjunctive medications.

Adverse Effects of Radiation Therapy

Brain irradiation may be associated with delayed brain injury and related cognitive deficits. The damage from radiation treatments is generally evident several years following treatment (Leibel and Sheline, 1987) and may be progressive and irreversible. Research with monkeys has shown that brain radiation in the therapeutic range (60 Gy) causes focal areas of necrosis within 6 months (Nakagaki et al., 1976). The area of injury may present as an expanding mass of necrosis that is virtually indistinguishable from recurrent tumor or as diffuse progressive white matter disease (leukoencephalopathy). Older patients, young children, and individuals who receive concomitant high-dose chemotherapy are at greatest risk for suffering from the adverse effects of radiation. Symptoms in adults generally include memory loss, gait disturbance, weakness, and tremor. In children, dementia and severe learning disabilities may be seen following aggressive treatment (Duffner et al., 1983).

Irradiation causes injury to subcortical white matter, with larger treatment volumes causing more impairment (Gregor et al., 1996). Most studies that include neuropsychological assessment of brain tumor patients before and after radiation therapy reveal significant impairments of information-processing speed, executive functions, memory, sustained attention, and motor coordination in those with no evidence of disease recurrence (Scheibel et al., 1996; Salander et al., 1995; Archibald et al., 1994; Taphoorn et al., 1994; Imperato et al., 1990; Lieberman et al., 1982; Hochberg and Slotnick, 1980). These deficits are correlated with reduced cerebral blood flow seen on single-photon emission computed tomography imaging (Ebmeier et al., 1994).

Many studies have focused on memory deficits as the primary adverse effect of therapy in brain tumor patients. Salander et al. (1995) found that patients with malignant gliomas (grade III–IV) who were disease free and without neurologic deficits developed impairments of verbal learning and memory but did not differ from their spouses on tests of verbal comprehension, visuospatial skills, or abstract reasoning 5 months after their initial treatment. Archibald et al. (1994) found that memory and concentration tended to be most impaired 18 months after treatment, with further declines in frontal lobe executive functions and new learning ability during the ensuing 2 years. Kleinberg et al. (1993) reported, in contrast, that 65% of their glioma patients had only mild memory deficits that did not prevent them from returning to work. However, memory impairment was rated by patient self-report and not formally tested, and it could not be determined if the patients required any assistance or compensation techniques to maintain their level of function. An excellent review of the neurobehavioral effects of radiation therapy in brain tumor patients can be found in Crossen et al. (1994).

Even radiation not directed at the brain can cause cognitive impairment. For example, a substantial percentage of patients who receive therapeutic radiation for tumors of the anterior skull base have cognitive deficits. Memory impairment was detected in 80% of patients with paranasal sinus tumors, even though the brain was not the target of irradiation (Meyers et al., 2000). The neuropsychological effects of treatment do not appear to be tightly correlated with the appearance of white matter changes on neuroimaging, although the development of white matter changes is closely correlated with radiation dose (Corn et al., 1994). This is due to both the resolution of anatomic changes on magnetic resonance imaging and the fact that many changes in brain function are caused by biochemical alterations that occur before structural abnormalities may be visualized (Ebmeier et al., 1994; van der Knaap et al., 1992).

Adverse Effects of Chemotherapy

Cognitive and emotional changes reported during and after chemotherapy include memory loss, decreased information-processing speed, reduced attention, anxiety, depression, and fatigue (Meyers and Abbruzzese, 1992). Most of the older literature suggests that neurotoxic side effects of chemotherapy are acute and reversible (Weiss et al., 1974), generally resolving within 48 to 72 hours after treatment. The risk of severe delayed effects, such as leukoencephalopathy, is primarily seen following administration of higher doses (van Dam et al., 1998), intra-arterial (Glass et al., 1986) or intraventricular administration, and concomitant radiation therapy. The neurobehavioral effects of most cancer therapy agents tend to be nonspecific and diffuse, except for those that have a mechanism of action that is expected to affect focal brain regions (Meyers et al., 1997) or biologic response modifiers that are known to affect particular proinflammatory cytokines, neurotransmitters, and neuroendocrine hormones (Valentine et al., 1998). Although cognitive changes following chemotherapy have been well documented, there have been very few prospective studies investigating the long-term effects of chemotherapeutic agents on cognition.

Adverse Effects of Immunotherapy

Cytokines such as interferon-alpha (IFN-α) and interleukin-2 (IL-2) have been used in a number of therapeutic trials for primary brain tumors and leptomeningeal disease (LMD). These agents are known to have both acute and persistent neurotoxic side effects. Acute toxicity is characterized by fever, headache, and myalgia, which generally resolve over several days. Subacute neurotoxicity, evident within a week of starting therapy, is characterized by inattention, slowed thinking, and lack of motivation. After several months of treatment, more than two-thirds of patients develop difficulty with memory, frontal lobe executive functions (e.g., problem solving, planning, sequencing), motor coordination, and mood (Pavol et al., 1995). These neurotoxic side effects are not always reversible following treatment cessation (Meyers et al., 1991b). The route of administration is also an important consideration. Intraventricular administration of IFN-α has caused a reversible vegetative state in patients with LMD (Meyers et al., 1991a), and intraventricularly administered IL-2 may produce a progressive dementia in otherwise "cured" patients treated for LMD (Meyers and Yung, 1993).

Adverse Effects of Adjunctive Medications

Steroids

Glucocorticoid treatment for mass effect and raised intracranial pressure is ubiquitous among brain tumor patients. However, steroids may also have adverse effects on mental and emotional functioning.

The incidence of steroid-induced psychiatric syndromes ranges from 5.7% to 50% (Lewis and Smith, 1983). These side effects include euphoria, mania, insomnia, restlessness, and increased motor activity. Some patients become anxious and depressed. Steroids are also known to have adverse effects on memory, even in normal control subjects (Wolkowitz et al., 1990), and have been implicated in the pathophysiology of major depression and Alzheimer's disease (Martignoni et al., 1992). Treatment with glucocorticoids may also potentiate the neurotoxic side effects of other agents (Sapolsky, 1985).

Anticonvulsants

For many patients, seizures are the initial symptom of a brain tumor. The overall incidence of epilepsy among brain tumor patients is estimated at 35% (Keles and Berger, 2000). When the dosages of anticonvulsant drugs such as phenytoin (Dilantin) and carbamazepine (Tegretol) are carefully monitored, their cognitive effects are minimal (Drane and Meador, 1996). Use of phenobarbital, however, has been associated with greater adverse cognitive effects (Devinsky, 1995; Drane and Meador, 1996). Regardless of the specific medication used, too rapid an introduction of the anticonvulsant, polypharmacy, or excessive concentrations may result in changes in arousal, attention, memory, and psychomotor functioning (Kaufman, 1995). It should be noted, however, that the majority of children and adults who take these drugs experience few (if any) side effects (Bourgeois, 1998; Devinsky, 1995). In fact, at least one antiepileptic drug appears to have favorable effects on psychological well being (Meador and Baker, 1997).

Medical Complications

Endocrine dysfunction due to hypothalamic/pituitary injury is also very common following radiation therapy. Thyroid dysfunction, loss of libido, and erectile dysfunction are present in a large proportion of patients. In fact, one study found that only 23% of brain tumor patients had normal thyroid, gonadal, and adrenal hormone levels following treatment (Arlt et al., 1997). Endocrine replacement therapy has the potential to improve cognition and mood in patients who have subnormal hormone levels due to hypothalamic injury related to treatment (Arlt et al., 1997).

Seizures occur in 50% to 70% of patients at some time during their illness and have a significant impact on neurobehavioral functioning and quality of life. Persistent, poorly controlled seizures reduce cognitive efficiency and exacerbate underlying cognitive deficits. Patients with seizures are often fearful of having them and may become socially isolated because of the possibility of having one in a public place or around people they know.

Anemia is a side effect of some chemotherapy regimens. For children and adults, research suggests that treatment with cisplatin (Petersdorf et al., 1993), etoposide (Chamberlain and Kormanik, 1997; Chamberlain, 1997), and high-dose carboplatin/etoposide combination therapy (Castello et al., 1990) may be complicated by anemia. Among anemic patients, the cognitive problems observed on neuropsychological testing include deficits in attention, perceptual-motor speed, memory, and verbal fluency (Brown et al., 1991; Marsh et al., 1991; Temple et al., 1995). Neurophysiological assessment of auditory evoked potentials also revealed increased latency of certain components (Brown et al., 1991; Marsh et al., 1991). These cognitive deficits and slowed evoked potentials often improve following reversal of anemia with erythropoietin (Brown et al., 1991; Marsh et al., 1991; Nissenson, 1989; Temple et al., 1995). For most patients receiving chemotherapy for a brain tumor, anemia and other treatment-related complications are medically manageable.

Quality of Life Issues

Comprehensive studies of quality of life (QOL) of brain tumor patients have revealed increased emotional reactivity, lowered frustration tolerance, and reduced family functioning (Giovagnoli et al., 1996; Weitzner et al., 1996; Aiken, 1994; Taphoorn et al., 1992). Brain tumor patients at risk for poorer QOL are female, are divorced, have bilateral tumor involvement, have received chemotherapy, and have a poor performance status (Weitzner et al., 1996; Irle et al., 1994). Age, surprisingly, is not a factor in QOL or well being despite being an extremely important prognostic factor (Sneed et al., 1995). The site of the lesion also has an impact on mood. Patients with tumors in ventromedial frontal or parietal association areas are more likely to experience anxiety, irritability, and fatigue than are patients with lesions in other locations. Patients with lesions in dorsolateral frontal and somatosensory regions tend to exhibit emotional indifference and even euphoria (Irle et al., 1994). In addition, tumor patients have been found to mimic nearly every psychiatric illness, such as obsessive-compulsive disorder (Paradis et al., 1992) and personality disorder (Meyers et al., 1992b).

Overall QOL is not as related to histopathologic diagnosis, prognosis, or age as much as it is to social support systems, personality characteristics, and access to services (Weitzner and Meyers, 1997; Lyons, 1996). The disease causes changes in life-style and roles for family members as well as for patients (Newton and Mateo, 1994). Uncertainty regarding the disease history and outcome is a source of stress for the family. Uncertainty can also be positive, however, allowing patients and their families some hope for a better-than-anticipated course (Newton and Mateo, 1994).

DIAGNOSTIC CONSIDERATIONS

Differential Diagnosis

Accurate diagnosis of cognitive impairment versus emotional reactions to illness and stress is important for a number of reasons. Brain tumor patients frequently have complicated treatment regimens, and compliance may be adversely affected by cognitive deficits. Problems with memory or the inability to initiate activity can negatively impact adherence to treatment regimens. Patients may be offered experimental treatments, and the decision to participate and give informed consent requires intact reasoning, the ability to weigh risks and benefits, and the appreciation of long-term consequences. Differential diagnosis of observable behavior changes may be difficult. A patient who is apathetic, withdrawn, and lacks motivation may be depressed or may have an organic brain syndrome. Levine et al. (1978) reported that 64% of general cancer patients with delirium were misdiagnosed as depressed. This number may be even greater for patients with primary brain involvement. The distinction is an important one, however, because misdiagnosis and subsequent treatment of depression in a patient with an organic brain syndrome might worsen the condition.

Many patients with brain tumors, at least early in their course, do not have overt evidence of impaired cognitive functioning on casual observation or during routine medical examinations and yet have cognitive deficits that limit their ability to function in their normal activities. Standard assessments of performance status, such as the Karnofsky and Zubrod scales, which globally measure the patient's ability for self-care and ambulation, do not address cognitive impairments in brain tumor patients and have questionable reliability and validity (Orr and Aisner, 1986). For example, a patient who is able to walk and perform basic activities of daily living may be rated as having a good performance status even though he or she may be unreliable in following treatment regimens, lack judgement, be unable to perform his or her usual work, or have temper outbursts that compromise family function.

An informal survey of the problems and incidents reported by inpatient and outpatient neuro-oncology nurses sheds light on how these various deficits adversely affect healthcare provider–patient–family–relationships. These include

1. Inadequate insight and self-appraisal on the part of the patient. For instance, the patient may overrate his or her ability to be independent, refuse assistance in activities of daily living, and have an accident.
2. Memory problems with confabulation that may appear to represent noncompliance. For instance, the patient may inaccurately report the type, frequency, and amount of medication he or she has been taking, leading to subtherapeutic or toxic medication levels.
3. Subtle problems with language comprehension that limit the amount and type of information the patient can process and retain. Although this type of problem may not be readily identified in the hospital or clinic setting because of the high level of structure, the patient may have great difficulty following multistep, complicated instructions at home.
4. Poor initiation and maintenance of activity that may resemble a "bad attitude" or depression. This patient may have difficulty initiating and following through personal hygiene routines, performing usual work and leisure activities, and so forth.
5. Hemispatial inattention that may be manifested as "paranoia" when people approach from the unattended side or as problems in dressing and eating.

6. Subtle visuospatial problems that are manifested by the patient becoming easily lost and confused, even in familiar settings.

Deficit Versus Handicap

The impact of a primary brain tumor on the individual is best conceptualized by the three-tiered system developed by the World Health Organization (1980). *Impairment* is the deficit of brain function caused by the disease and is assessed by neurologic and neuropsychological evaluations. *Disability* is the impact of the deficit on the patient's ability to perform activities and is assessed by performance status and functional status measures. *Handicap* is the impact of the disability on the patient's subjective well being, which includes the patient's overall comfort level and satisfaction, and is generally assessed by QOL questionnaires.

A specific cognitive deficit may or may not be handicapping to a given individual. The impact of a given impairment needs to be considered in the entire social context of the patient. Each person carries with himself or herself a unique array of environmental variables, such as education level, type of occupation, degree of social support, and access to services. These multiple factors determine the degree of handicap the brain tumor patient experiences in rejoining the mainstream of community activities and the work environment. Because of this dynamic relationship between neurologic impairment and environment, individuals with the same type and severity of deficit may experience different degrees of disability. For instance, a person who has sustained a severe verbal memory impairment may find it difficult to remain in college, but may experience few problems working in a well-established routine environment.

Neuropsychological Assessment

Often these problems, if unrecognized, lead to inaccurate judgment on the part of the staff regarding the patient's ability for self-care, requirements for supervision or special safety measures, and reliability in following his or her therapeutic regimen. Formal neuropsychological assessment of brain function is often helpful in determining the nature and extent of cognitive impairments that are not detected in routine medical evaluations.

Neuropsychological assessment involves the administration of standardized psychometric tests that comprehensively evaluate brain functioning. These functions include attention, ability to acquire new memories, recall of stored memories, expressive speech, language comprehension, visual-perception, reasoning, emotional behavior, interpersonal behavior, and executive functions. This detailed description of intellectual status and personality characteristics allows for more rational management and planning postoperatively.

Knowledge of the patient's capabilities and limitations should be incorporated into conferences held with the patient, family members, and the healthcare team. Such information is helpful as the participants work to set realistic goals, determine the patient's capacity for independent self-care (including the ability to drive, manage finances, and handle emergencies), and determine what types of compensation and management techniques might be most useful.

Quality of Life Assessment

The current standard of QOL assessment is multidimensional and addresses concerns that are unique to patients with brain tumors. There are several subjective QOL instruments that have been developed for patients with brain tumors, including the Functional Assessment of Cancer Therapy—Brain (FACT-Br) (Weitzner et al., 1995) and the European Organization for Research and Treatment of Cancer Quality of Life Questionnaire—Brain module (EORTC QLQ-BCM) (Osoba et al., 1996). These scales differ slightly in their development methods. The core FACT and EORTC QLQ questionnaires address physical, family, social, emotional, and functional well being. The QLQ-BCM items were obtained from interviews of patients and caregivers participating in a brain cancer support group. The items for the FACT Brain module were initially developed from interviews with patients in a neuro-oncology outpatient clinic. Additional items for both of these brain tumor modules were obtained from the input of healthcare professionals, and the methods for determining reliability, validity, and internal consistency were similar.

A thorough listing of QOL tools used in general cancer settings can be found in Cella and Bonomi (1995). The PRESTON Profile (Lyons, 1996) is another tool designed for brain tumor patients and addresses several different domains, including physical, emotional, and social functioning, relationship with family, tomorrow and the future, ongoing needs, and limited neurologic deficits. It does not address cognitive impairments and has not undergone validity or reliability assessments.

Some groups are defining QOL in clinical trials as a combination of survival and the amount of time patients have adverse effects of disease and treatment (Murray et al., 1995). This approach (quality-adjusted survival analysis) provides more information on patient function than the Karnofsky performance score (KPS). However, brain tumor patients are less likely to be free of symptoms than other cancer patients. In addition, censoring is assumed to be random and uninformative (Scott, 1997). In fact, censoring of brain tumor QOL assessments is informative when the information is missing because the patient can no longer read or understand the questions. Many cognitively impaired patients cannot complete QOL instruments, so there may be substantial amounts of missing data. If questionnaires are only given to patients who are cognitively most intact, the interpretation of the outcome of the trial may be biased.

Some investigators have caregivers assess the QOL of the patient (proxy assessment) and have reported modest correlations between patient and proxy results (Sneeuw et al., 1997). However, the similarity between the patient and proxy assessment is lower for the more cognitively impaired patients, which is exactly when the proxy assessments are most likely to be done. Patients with brain tumors, particularly in the frontal lobe, often have diminished appreciation of their disabilities and limitations and report a level of function that is not realistic. They may report a good QOL in the face of substantial mental impairment because of their lack of insight. In clinical trials, at least, subjective QOL questionnaires should be supplemented by other objective assessments of patient function.

INTERVENTIONS AND MANAGEMENT STRATEGIES

Most individuals with brain tumors develop behavioral, emotional, and intellectual difficulties that compromise their ability to live independently and return to work. In fact, few brain tumor patients return to their usual work and activities. One study reported that only 18% of patients return to work full-time, and 10% return to work part-time (Fobair et al., 1990). The costs to the patient, family, and society include loss of self-esteem, lost income, and the necessity for disability payments. Cognitive and vocational rehabilitation have the potential to reduce the morbidity associated with this disease and its treatment, improve recovery of cognitive and emotional function, and reduce the financial costs and losses to patients, their families, and society. However, rehabilitation of brain tumor patients is in the beginning stages of development. At this time there is little established knowledge about the major rehabilitation problem areas of brain tumor patients, and no rehabilitation approaches exist to address the problems that have been specifically validated in this clinical population. Rehabilitation of brain tumor patients is given little emphasis in major reviews of rehabilitation for non-brain cancers (Hersh et al., 1988; LaBan, 1990; McGarvey, 1990; Raven, 1992). Nevertheless, there is increasing interest in the possibility of rehabilitating brain tumor patients, and initial steps toward a specialty of brain tumor rehabilitation are being taken. The goal of this section is to describe current rehabilitation methods used with brain tumor patients and to identify trends in new programs designed for this population.

Rehabilitation Problems of Brain Tumor Patients

One obstacle to the development of specialized brain tumor rehabilitation services is identification of the major rehabilitation problems within this patient population. It has often been assumed that the rehabilitation problems of brain tumor patients are similar to those of stroke patients, survivors of traumatic brain injury (TBI), and other groups of persons receiving rehabilitation services. In fact, available data support a different and more complex picture of brain tumor patients' needs (Lehmann et al., 1978; Taphoorn et al., 1992; Marciniak et al., 1996). Brain tumor patients not only have different types of problems, but the progressive nature of their disease complicates treatment planning and decisions. Although the goals of treatment and the duration of intervention programs need to be flexible for all rehabilitation patients (Gamble et al., 1990), this is especially true for patients diagnosed with brain tumors.

It is undoubtedly true that patients with brain tumors may benefit from many of the same types of services that are helpful for other rehabilitation populations such as stroke or TBI survivors. For example, physical therapy can improve strength and mobility; occupational therapy improves self-care skills; and speech and language therapy may help patients overcome various aphasic conditions. This group of patients, however, varies in terms of the types of problems that most frequently present for remediation. One large-scale survey found that the most frequent category of rehabilitation problem among patients with nervous system cancers was "psychological" (Lehmann et al., 1978). Problems in this category were more common than problems with ambulation, transfers, and general weakness. It is noteworthy that problems with return to work occurred at the same frequency among cancer patients as did physical disabilities. These general findings were confirmed in a study in the Netherlands of patients with slow-growing gliomas (Taphoorn et al., 1992).

In a survey of 30 caregivers of brain tumor patients, we found that the problems facing this group of patients were very different from the concerns of other medically ill populations. Using the Sickness Impact Profile (Bergner, 1977), we found that the most salient problems facing brain tumor patients were lack of energy, inability to perform usual activities around the home (i.e., paying bills, making repairs), social isolation, lack of sexual activity, generalized slowing of behavior, and problems with reasoning, memory, and concentration. In contrast to other medically ill populations, some problems were not endorsed by brain tumor caregivers as being of concern. These "nonproblems" included depression, ability to perform basic activities of daily living such as dressing and eating, ambulation, and ability to speak and be understood. Although the rehabilitation needs of brain tumor patients are becoming more widely known, there are few facilities with experience in treating this population.

Approximately 5 years ago, we surveyed acute and post-acute rehabilitation facilities across the United States to determine current clinical practice. Of the 262 questionnaires mailed out, 108 replied (41%), 77 of which were acute care facilities. Of the total group, 62% treated fewer than 10 brain tumor patients per year and 72% did not provide any specialized rehabilitation services or staff training for brain tumor patients. Problems frequently identified by these facilities included poor judgment on the part of the patient, side effects of cancer treatment, uncertain medical prognosis attached to brain cancer, and emotional adjustment to cancer.

Despite similarities in the types of therapies employed, the nature of the problems faced by cancer patients necessitates an adjustment in the approach to rehabilitation and the goals of services. For many patients, especially those diagnosed with a malignant brain tumor, deterioration of function over time is the most likely course of the disease. Even if gains achieved in physical, occupational, or speech therapy are temporary, however, they may significantly improve the patient's QOL (Haut et al., 1991) by improving productivity and independence (Sherer et al., 1997). Although we have not completed a follow-up survey to the one described above, anecdotal evidence suggests that brain tumor patients remain woefully underserved.

Traditional Rehabilitation Approaches

Dietz (1984) and others have described four different rehabilitation approaches applicable to cancer patients in general. In the *preventive* approach, the goal is to prevent complications that are anticipated to result from disease or treatment. An example of this approach is having mastectomy patients begin an exercise program to prevent postoperative lymphedema and deconditioning. The goal of the *restorative* approach is to return patients' functioning to the pre-disease level, which is not generally appropriate for brain tumor patients. The *supportive* approach attempts to improve a patient's functioning within the limits set by neurologic deficits, which are assumed to be permanent. In the *palliative* approach, the goal is to relieve suffering and maintain functioning during periods of disease progression. Examples of this approach are pain management and the use of exercises to preserve range of motion. Most of the rehabilitation methods used with brain tumor patients follow the supportive approach as defined above, but our experience suggests that a model that includes the preventive approach may also be useful for this population.

Implementing traditional cognitive and vocational rehabilitation for brain tumor patients is complicated by the fact that existing programs are not entirely appropriate. First, brain tumor patients have different patterns and types of cognitive deficits than do stroke or trauma patients. One study found that patients with brain tumors have milder cognitive deficits and greater variability in the nature and extent of their deficits than people with strokes in the same neuroanatomic site (Anderson et al., 1990). Second, the natural history of the disease process differs from cerebrovascular disease or TBI. The latter two conditions are usually characterized by an acute onset and gradual recovery. In the case of brain tumors, the onset of the disease is relatively insidious, and although some recovery of function may be seen following surgery or other therapy, most patients experience a gradual deterioration of function as the tumor progresses. Hence, the goals of rehabilitation may be different from those in stroke or brain trauma rehabilitation. Finally, most existing rehabilitation programs take at least 6 months to complete and are costly (frequently more than $20,000). Complicating the cost, funding agencies and insurance carriers may be reluctant to provide or reimburse services for brain tumor patients.

Inpatient Rehabilitation Programs

Inpatient rehabilitation is indicated for those brain tumor patients who are disabled in ambulation and self-care because of neurologic deficits but who have the potential to improve. The reader is referred to comprehensive reviews of inpatient rehabilitation for stroke (Goldberg, 1991) and head injury patients (Berrol, 1992) for detailed information. The specific therapy activities used with a given patient are tailored to the patient's physical and neurobehavioral deficits and are upgraded as the patient recovers. During early stages of recovery, basic physical activities (e.g., feeding) are emphasized, whereas in later stages more advanced activities (e.g., ambulation) can be addressed. The specific therapy techniques used are based on each patient's neurologic and functional problems so that a particular problem might be treated using similar techniques regardless of whether the deficit was caused by brain tumor or stroke (Blossom and Barnhart, 1985).

In contrast to the large body of outcome research data on the inpatient rehabilitation of other neurologically impaired patient groups, there are few data reported for brain tumor patients. Feder et al. (1989) reviewed their 10 year experience with 76 patients who had undergone surgical removal of meningiomas. Despite the fact that 72% of the patients were graded on admission as having "severe" or "very severe" disabilities (criteria not stated), the majority had marked functional improvement and virtually all surviving patients were discharged home. The average length of stay was 106 days, similar to the typical length of stay for stroke patients at the same hospital. The major single predictor of outcome was whether the tumor resection was total or subtotal. The authors note that this predictor could have represented a proxy effect of other clinical features (i.e., surgically inaccessible tumor) that are independently associated with outcome. It would be valuable to replicate this type of study with patients who have primary gliomas.

In a retrospective study of 159 cancer patients admitted to an inpatient rehabilitation program (Marciniak et al., 1996), deconditioning was the most common impairment or problem identified. Of these 159 patients, 72 had a diagnosis of primary brain tumor and the frequency of cognitive impairments was 49%. While the length of stay in the program across patient types ranged from 5 to 93 days (mean = 32, SD = 19), patients diagnosed with brain tumors remained in the program for an average of 34 days (SD = 20), with 75% eventually being discharged home. The authors concluded that inpatient rehabilitation services are beneficial for patients with a variety of cancer diagnoses, including those with primary brain tumors.

It is not currently known what proportion of brain tumor patients would benefit from acute, inpatient rehabilitation. A survey of more than 800 cancer patients in university hospitals (Lehmann et al., 1978) found that most primary physicians were not aware of rehabilitation problems in their patients or did not know what rehabilitation might offer. Because there is no established model for inpatient rehabilitation of brain tumor patients, even the predictors of length of stay and rehabilitation outcome in this population are unknown. Thus, there is a strong need for research on predictors of outcome, typical problem areas, rate of progress, utilization of different services, amount of spontaneous recovery, and complications experienced by brain tumor patients in inpatient rehabilitation.

Cognitive Rehabilitation

With the establishment of postacute day-treatment rehabilitation programs in the late 1970s and early 1980s, the needs of patients with moderate to severe TBI began to be more formally addressed (Ben-Yishay et al., 1982; Prigatano et al., 1986). Many of these programs adopted a holistic approach to rehabilitation, incorporating various activities designed to facilitate patient progress and adaptation (Prigatano and Ben-Yishay, 1999). As reviewed in depth by Prigatano (1999), the major components of a holistic neuropsychological rehabilitation program include the establishment of a therapeutic milieu, cognitive rehabilitation or retraining sessions, psychotherapy, involvement and education of family members, and a protected work trial. Whereas the early aim of such activities was to restore cerebral functioning to the highest degree possible, more contemporary cognitive remediation programs strive to manage the individual's disability rather than treat the underlying impairment (Wilson, 1997). Although there is little evidence that cognitive retraining (the restorative approach) directly improves higher cerebral functioning in adults after acquired brain injury (Prigatano, 1999), there are benefits to participation in cognitive rehabilitation programs. Initially, cognitive retraining sessions may help patients better understand the nature and degree of their impairment or disability and, as they progress through the program, cognitive rehabilitation helps them use residual skills to improve their abilities to problem solve and adapt.

Modification of special programs dedicated to rehabilitating the neurobehavioral problems of TBI patients are being developed for brain tumor patients (e.g., Sherer et al., 1997). The most common type of neurobehavioral-oriented program is the day-treatment program with emphasis on cognitive and vocational rehabilitation. Although these programs are frequently affiliated with an inpatient rehabilitation program, many are located in the community to provide better access to resources.

The first step in cognitive and vocational rehabilitation is to identify realistic goals for the patient, often through formal neuropsychological and vocational testing to identify preserved skills. The major therapeutic strategy is to train patients to compensate for their neurobehavioral deficits at home and on the job. Brain tumor patients would appear to be excellent candidates for cognitive rehabilitation because patients with focal lesions and relatively restricted cognitive deficits may be in a better position than persons with more diffuse impairments to recognize the need to use compensatory strategies (Prigatano, 1999). Typical areas targeted for retraining include memory, problem solving, and social behavior. In examining the efficacy of cognitive remediation, the greatest success has been in compensating for memory disorders (Baddeley et al., 1995). For instance, patients with memory deficits may compensate by using written reminders, alarm watches, pagers, and other devices. Unfortunately, the efficacy of compensation strategies in addressing deficits in other areas of functioning (i.e., judgment and problem solving) has not been conclusively demonstrated (von Cramon and Matthes-von Cramen, 1992). For some patients, a major treatment goal may be to improve the appropriateness of behavior. This may include teaching the patient to inhibit socially inappropriate remarks or to improve frustration tolerance. Patients and family members often need counseling about the need to accept less demanding jobs, which are not as financially rewarding and prestigious.

The majority of the brain tumor patients seen in our clinic are experiencing cognitive difficulties. Feelings of confusion and frustration often accompany cognitive changes and can affect not only the patient but also those persons close to him or her. For many patients, whether they are newly diagnosed or already in treatment, a neuropsychological assessment can be helpful in delineating the individual patient's cognitive strengths and weaknesses as well as validating the concerns of patients and their families. In some instances, the neuropsychological evaluation provides concrete evidence of impairment for the patient who is unable or unwilling to acknowledge that impact of the disease and/or their treatment on cognition.

Many of our patients reside out of state or at a distance from the facility, which prohibits frequent visits for cognitive remediation. Although referrals to accredited rehabilitation facilities are provided when appropriate, some patients benefit from an intensive "problem-solving" approach that can be completed in conjunction with scheduled clinic visits. Maintaining a strong therapeutic alliance with the patient and close professional relationships with speech and language pathologists, physical therapists, occupational therapists, psychiatrists, and primary care physicians are crucial to the success of this approach.

Vocational Rehabilitation

In our needs assessment survey of brain tumor patients, we found that more than 40% were unable to work. Not all of these individuals are candidates for vocational rehabilitation, but there are those who could benefit greatly. Modification of programs dedicated to vocational rehabilitation of TBI patients may prove beneficial for brain tumor patients.

A newer vocational rehabilitation approach that has been successful and cost-effective with TBI patients is *supported employment.* In this approach, patients who are capable of holding employment are placed directly in jobs and are initially assisted by a job coach who trains the patient to perform the work and acts as the patient's direct supervisor. As the patient becomes more independent on the job, the job coach decreases the amount of supervision until job coaching is unnecessary. The supported employment approach can be modified for patients returning to a position in which a job coach may not be appropriate by assigning a co-worker to act as a mentor to the patient as he or she resumes the job responsibilities. These vocational rehabilitation approaches are reviewed by Wehman and Kreutzer (1990).

Pharmacologic Strategies

Neurobehavioral slowing is the hallmark of frontal lobe dysfunction and treatment-related adverse effects in brain tumor patients. The syndrome of neurobehavioral slowing is generally due to involvement of the monamine pathways of the frontal–brain stem reticular system. In addition, catecholamines have an important role in the modulation of attention and working memory.

The use of neurostimulants in the brain-injured population has been shown to increase participation in therapy by improving arousal and attention (Kaelin et al., 1996). Methylphenidate (Table 26–1) has proven efficacious in improving the cognitive and emotional symptoms of human immunodeficiency virus (Brown, 1995), alleviating apathy in a patient with multiple subcortical infarcts (Watanabe et al., 1995), improving attention and functional outcome in brain-injured adults (Kaelin et al., 1996), and enhancing recovery rates in moderately severe brain-injured patients (Plenger et al., 1996). Stimulant treatment also has been useful for concentration difficulties, psychomotor retardation, and fatigue frequently seen in brain tumor patients and helped to elevate mood (Meyers et al., 1998). A conservative dose of 10 mg bid significantly improved cognitive function as assessed by objective tests, and doses in excess of 30 mg bid were well tolerated. Subjective improvements included improved gait, increased stamina and motivation to perform activities, and improved bladder control. There were no significant side effects, and many patients taking steroids were able to decrease their dose (Meyers et al., 1998). Long-term experience with this agent is lacking to determine if tolerance to therapeutic effects can develop.

Table 26–1. Neurocognitive Functions Improved by the Use of Methylphenidate

Speed of information processing
Memory
Word retrieval
Executive function
Fine motor speed

Education, Support, and Strategies for Caregivers

Family involvement is an important component of the patient's rehabilitation. Prigatano (1999) offers some guidelines for the establishment of a good working alliance with family members. These guidelines include listening carefully to the perspective of the family member, viewing family members as consultants, providing clear expectations of their role and level of involvement, incorporating educational materials and discussions, and recognizing that part of the therapist's job is to engage family members.

In addition to providing rehabilitation to appropriate brain tumor patients, patients' family members should be offered education and emotional support. Problems of brain tumor patients' spouses and caregivers are receiving increasing attention (Haut et al., 1991). In our experience, families of brain tumor patients are burdened by the patients' cognitive and behavioral changes in addition to the typical psychological problems of coping with cancer in a family member. They may have particular difficulty dealing with neurologically caused personality changes such as loss of initiative, quick mood changes, loss of control over emotions, and lack of insight into limitations. Support groups for brain tumor patients and their family members may be of great benefit. In our support group, one meeting each month is devoted to a topic discussion or lecture on an area of interest such as seizure medications. The other meeting each month is for open discussion and is more supportive in nature. Similar programs are available at other cancer centers, partly through the advocacy efforts of the National Brain Tumor Foundation (www.braintumor.org) and support from the American Brain Tumor Association (www.abta.org).

National Brain Tumor Foundation
414 Thirteenth Street, Suite 700
Oakland, CA 94612-2603
www.braintumor.org
800-934-2873

American Brain Tumor Association
2720 River Road
Des Plaines, IL 60018
www.abta.org
800-886-2282

CONCLUSION

At the present time, rehabilitation efforts for brain tumor patients and, indeed, for cancer patients in general have focused on symptom management (i.e., pain control), psychological support, nutritional support, and management of the medical complications of treatment (McLaughlin, 1984). There are increasing numbers of services available for the totally disabled and terminally ill, but not for those individuals who may have milder, yet incapacitating deficits. A "good outcome" for brain tumor patients is often considered by medical personnel to be preservation of life and possibly rehabilitation of motor deficits by physical therapy. However, there has been little or no effort to offer cognitive and vocational rehabilitation to brain tumor patients who may have the ability and desire to return to work following the acute phase of their illness (Conti, 1990). According to the former commissioner of the Rehabilitation Services Administration of the U.S. Department of Education, "It is RSA's position that persons disabled by cancer may be eligible for vocational rehabilitation services and that such services should be provided if the individual wants to work and can work even if for a limited period of time" (U.S. D.H.E.W., 1980).

The current lack of sophisticated rehabilitation effort is due to several factors. One reason is a lack of awareness on the part of rehabilitation professionals, patients, and medical caregivers about services that are available. Second, many brain tumor patients may not be encouraged to seek rehabilitation because they may not have marked sensory, linguistic, or motor deficits such as those seen in stroke patients even though most experience problems in executing work-related activities. Finally, there may be concern about expending resources on individuals who may eventually die from their disease. However, the resources expended on brain tumor patients may compare favorably with those expended on patients with heart disease, diabetic complications, mental disorders, and other chronic disabling conditions. In addition, these disorders share the possibility that the condition will progress or recur.

Along with formal rehabilitation, helping brain tumor patients attain an acceptable QOL may include helping them to accept the permanent changes, both cognitive and social, that having brain cancer might cause. Among the most disturbing losses sustained by the brain tumor patient are the loss of self-esteem, the loss of work and working relationships, and the loss of self-confidence. Brain tumor patients and their families may need to invest their efforts in new activities and interests and learn to enjoy leisure. Families may need to have occasional respite from their caretaking responsibilities. Quality of life needs to be defined on a highly individualized basis, requiring a great deal of flexibility on the part of the healthcare team, consultative services, and the patients and families. The need for continued psychosocial and neuropsychological assessment, rehabilitation, and counseling services will continue to grow as brain tumor patients survive for increasingly longer periods of time.

REFERENCES

Ackermann H, Dau I, Schugens MM, Grodd W. 1996. Impaired procedural learning after damage to the left supplementary motor area (SMA). J Neurol Neurosurg Psychiatry 60:94–97.

Aiken RD. 1994. Quality-of-life issues in patients with malignant gliomas. Semin Oncol 21:273–275.

Anderson SW, Damasio H, Tranel D. 1990. Neuropsychological impairments associated with lesions caused by tumor or stroke. Arch Neurol 47:397–405.

Archibald YM, Lunn D, Ruttan LA, et al. 1994. Cognitive functioning in long-term survivors of high-grade glioma. J Neurosurg 80:247–253.

Arlt W, Hove U, Muller B, et al. 1997. Frequent and frequently overlooked: treatment-induced endocrine dysfunction in adult long-term survivors of primary brain tumors. Neurology 49:498–506.

Baddeley AD, Wilson BA, Watts FN. 1995. Handbook of Memory Disorders. Chichester, England: Wiley and Sons.

Ben-Yishay Y, Rattok J, Ross B, et al. 1982. A rehabilitation-relevant system for cognitive, interpersonal and vocational rehabilitation of traumatically head injured persons. In: Rehabilitation Monograph No. 64: Working Approaches to Remediation of Cognitive Deficits in Brain Damaged Persons. New York: New York University Medical Center of Rehabilitation Medicine, pp 1–15.

Bergner M. 1977. Sickness Impact Profile. Seattle: University of Washington.

Berrol S. 1992. Traumatic brain injury rehabilitation [issue]. Phys Med Rehabil Clin North Am 3:1.

Blossom B, Barnhart L. 1985. Brain tumors. In: DA Umphred (ed), Neurological Rehabilitation. St Louis: Mosby.

Bourgeois BF. 1998. Antiepileptic drugs, learning, and behavior in childhood epilepsy. Epilepsia 39:913–921.

Brown G. 1995. The use of methyphenidate for cognitive decline associated with HIV disease. Int J Psychiatry Med 25:21–37.

Brown WE, Marsh JT, Wolcott D, et al. 1991. Cognitive function, mood and P3 latency: effects of the amelioration of anemia in dialysis patients. Neuropsychologia 29:35–45.

Castello MA, Clerico A, Deb G, Dominici C, Fidani P, Donfrancesco A. 1990. High-dose carboplatin in combination with etoposide (JET regimen) for childhood brain tumors. Am J Pediatr Hematol Oncol 12:297–300.

Cella DF, Bonomi AE. 1995. Measuring quality of life: 1995 update. Oncology 9:47–60.

Chamberlain MC. 1997. Recurrent supratentorial malignant gliomas in children. Long-term salvage therapy with oral etoposide. Arch Neurol 54:554–558.

Chamberlain MC, Kormanik PA. 1997. Chronic oral VP-16 for recurrent medulloblastoma. Pediatr Neurol 17:230–234.

Cohaden F, Aouad N, Rougier A, Vital C, Rivel J, Dartigues JF. 1985. Histologic and non-histologic factors correlated with survival time in supratentorial astrocytic tumors. J Neurooncol 3:105–111.

Conti JV. 1990. Cancer rehabilitation: why can't we get out of first gear? J Rehabil 56:19.

Corn BW, Yousem DM, Scott CB, et al. 1994. White matter changes are correlated significantly with radiation dose. Observations from a randomized dose-escalation trial for malignant glioma (Radiation Therapy Oncology Group 83-02). Cancer 74:2828–2835.

Crossen JR, Garwood D, Glatstein E, Neuwelt EA. 1994. Neurobehavioral sequelae of cranial irradiation in adults: a review of radiation-induced encephalopathy. J Clin Oncol 12:627–642.

Devinsky O. 1995. Cognitive and behavioral effects of antiepileptic drugs. Epilepsia 36:S46–65.

Dietz JH. 1984. Rehabilitation and reconstruction for the cancer patient. In: Pilch YH (eds), Surgical Oncology. New York: McGraw-Hill, p 1041.

Drane DL, Meador KJ. 1996. Epilepsy, anticonvulsant drugs and cognition. Baillieres Clin Neurol 5:877–885.

Duffner PK, Cohen ME, Thomas P. 1983. Late effects of treatment on the intelligence of children with posterior fossa tumors. Cancer 51:233–237.

Ebmeier KP, Booker K, Gregor A, Cull A, Dougall N, Sellar R, Goodwin GM. 1994. Single photon emission computed tomography in long-term survivors of adult brain tumours. J Neurol Neurosurg Psychiatry 57:729–733.

Feder M, Ring H, Solzi P, Eldar R. 1989. Rehabilitation outcomes following craniotomy for intracranial meningiomas. J Neurol Rehabil 3:15.

Fobair P, Mackworth N, Varghese A, Prados M. 1990. Quality of life issues among 200 brain tumor patients treated at the University of California in San Francisco, interviewed 1988. Presented at the Brain Tumor Conference: A Living Resource Guide, San Francisco, CA.

Gamble GL, Brown PS, Kinney CL, Maloney FP. 1990. Cardiovascular, pulmonary, and cancer rehabilitation. 4. Cancer rehabilitation: principles and psychosocial aspects. Arch Phys Med Rehabil 71:S244–S247.

Giovagnoli AR, Tamburini M, Boiardi A. 1996. Quality of life in brain tumor patients. J Neurooncol 30:71–80.

Glass JP, Lee YY, Bruner J, Fields WS. 1986. Treatment-related leukoencephalopathy. Medicine 65:154–162.

Goldberg G. 1991. Stroke rehabilitation [issue]. Phys Med Rehabil Clin North Am 2:1.

Goldstein LH, Bernard S, Fenwick PB, Burgess PW, McNeil J. 1993. Unilateral frontal lobectomy can produce strategy application disorder. J Neurol Neurosurg Psychiatry 56:274–276.

Gregor A, Cull A, Traynor E, Stewart M, Lander F, Love S. 1996. Neuropsychometric evaluation of long-term survivors of adult brain tumours: relationship with tumour and treatment parameters. Radiother Oncolo41:55–59.

Haas J, Vogt G, Schiemann M, Patzold U. 1982. Aphasia and non-verbal intelligence in brain tumour patients. J Neurol 227:209–218.

Haut MW, Haut JS, Bloomfield SS. 1991. Family issues in rehabilitation of patients with malignant brain tumors. NeuroRehabilitation 1:39.

Hersh D, Grabois M, Decker N. 1988. Rehabilitation of the cancer patient. In: Delisa J (ed), Rehabilitation Medicine: Principles and Practice. Philadelphia: JB Lippincott, 660 pp.

Hochberg FH, Slotnick B. 1980. Neuropsychologic impairment in astrocytoma survivors. Neurology 30:172–177.

Hom J, Reitan RM. 1984. Neuropsychological correlates of rapidly vs. slowly growing intrinsic cerebral neoplasms. J Clin Neuropsychol 6:309–324.

Imperato JP, Paleologos NE, Vick NA. 1990. Effects of treatment on long-term survivors with malignant astrocytomas. Ann Neurol 28:818–822.

Irle E, Peper M, Wowra B, Kunze S. 1994. Mood changes after surgery for tumors of the cerebral cortex. Arch Neurol 51:164–174.

Kaelin DL, Cifu DX, Matthies B. 1996. Methylphenidate effect on attention deficit in the acutely brain-injured adult. Arch Phys Med Rehabil 77:6–9.

Kaufman DM. 1995. Clinical Neurology for Psychiatrists, 4th ed. Philadelphia: WB Saunders, pp 239–241.

Keles GE, Berger MS. 2000. Seizures associated with brain tumors. In: Bernstein M, Berger MS (ed), Neuro-oncology:

The Essentials. New York: Thieme Medical Publishers, pp 473–477.

Kleinberg L, Wallner K, Malkin MG. 1993. Good performance status of long-term disease-free survivors of intracranial gliomas. Int J Radiat Oncol Biol Phys 26:129–133.

LaBan M. 1990. Rehabilitation of patients with cancer. In: Kottke FJ, Lehmann JF (eds), Krusen's Handbook of Physical Medicine and Rehabilitation, 4th Ed. Philadelphia: Saunders.

LeBaron S, Zeltzer PM, Zeltzer LK, Scott SE, Marlin AE. 1988. Assessment of quality of survival in children with medulloblastoma and cerebellar astrocytoma. Cancer 62:1215–1222.

Lehmann JF, DeLisa JA, Warren CG, deLateur BJ, Bryant PL, Nicholson CG. 1978. Cancer rehabilitation: assessment of need, development, and evaluation of a model of care. Arch Phys Med Rehabil 59:410–419.

Leibel SA, Sheline GE. 1987. Radiation therapy for neoplasms of the brain. J Neurosurg 66:1–22.

Levine PM, Silberfarb PM, Lipowski ZJ. 1978. Mental disorders in cancer patients: a study of 100 psychiatric referrals. Cancer 42:1385–1391.

Lewis DA, Smith RE. 1983. Steroid induced psychiatric syndromes. A report of 14 cases and a review of the literature. J Affect Disord 5:319–332.

Lieberman AN, Foo SH, Ransohoff J, et al. 1982. Long term survival among patients with malignant brain tumors. Neurosurgery 10:450–453.

Lilja Å, Brun A, Salford LG, et al. 1992. Neuropsychological indexes of a partial frontal syndrome in patients with nonfrontal gliomas. Neuropsychology 6:315–326.

Lyons GJ. 1996. The "PRESTON Profile"—the first disease-specific tool for assessing quality of life in patients with malignant glioma. Disabil Rehabil 18:460–468.

Marciniak CM, Sliwa JA, Spill G, Heinemann AW, Semik PE. 1996. Functional outcome following rehabilitation of the cancer patient. Arch Phys Med Rehabil 77:54–57.

Marsh JT, Brown WS, Wolcott D, et al. 1991. rHuEPO treatment improves brain and cognitive function of anemic dialysis patients. Kidney Int39:155–163.

Martignoni E, Costa A, Sinforiani E, et al. 1992. The brain as a target for adrenocortical steroids: cognitive implications. Psychoneuroendocrinology 17:343–354.

McGarvey CL III. 1990. Physical Therapy for the Cancer Patient. New York: Churchill Livingstone.

McLaughlin WJ. 1984. Cancer rehabilitation: people investing in people. J Rehabil 50:57.

Meador KJ, Baker GA. 1997. Behavioral and cognitive effects of lamotrigine. J Child Neurol 12:S44–47.

Meyers CA. 1986. Neuropsychological deficits in brain tumor patients: effects of location, chronicity, and treatment. Cancer Bull 38:30.

Meyers CA, Abbruzzese JL. 1992. Cognitive functioning in cancer patients: effect of previous treatment. Neurology 42: 434–436.

Meyers CA, Berman SA, Scheibel RS, Hayman A. 1992a. Case report: acquired antisocial personality disorder associated with unilateral left orbital frontal damage. J Psychiatr Neurosci 17:121–125.

Meyers CA, Berman SA, Hayman A, Evankovich K. 1992b. Pathological left-handedness and preserved function associated with a slowly evolving brain tumor. Dev Med Child Neurol 34:1110–1116.

Meyers CA, Geara F, Wong PF, Morrison WH. 2000. Neurocognitive effects of therapeutiuc irradiation for base of skull tumors. Int J Radiation Oncol Biol Phys 46:51–55.

Meyers CA, Kudelka AP, Conrad CA, Gelke CK, Grove W, Pazdur R. 1997. Neurotoxicity of CI-980, a novel mitotic inhibitor. Clin Cancer Res 3:419–422.

Meyers CA, Obbens EA, Scheibel RS, Moser RP. 1991a. Neurotoxicity of intraventricularly administered alpha-interferon for leptomeningeal disease. Cancer 68:88–92.

Meyers CA, Scheibel RS, Forman AD. 1991b. Persistent neurotoxicity of systemically administered interferon-alpha. Neurology 41:672–676.

Meyers CA, Weitzner MA, Valentine AD, Levin VA. 1998. Methylphenidate therapy improves cognition, mood, and function of brain tumor patients. J Clin Oncol 16: 2522–2527.

Meyers CA, Yung WK. 1993. Delayed neurotoxicity of intraventricular interleukin-2: a case report. J Neurooncol 15:265–267.

Murray KJ, Nelson DF, Scott C, et al. 1995. Quality-adjusted survival analysis of malignant glioma. Patients treated with twice-daily radiation (RT) and carmustine: a report of Radiation Therapy Oncology Group (RTOG) 83-02. Int J Radiat Oncol Biol Phys 31:453–459.

Nakagaki H, Brunhart G, Kemper TL, Caveness WF. 1976. Monkey brain damage from radiation in the therapeutic range. J Neurosurg 44:3–11.

Newton C, Mateo MA. 1994. Uncertainty: strategies for patients with brain tumor and their family. Cancer Nurs 17:137–140.

Nissenson AR. 1989. Recombinant human erythropoietin: impact on brain and cognitive function, exercise tolerance, sexual potency, and quality of life. Semin Nephrol 9(suppl 2):25–31.

Orr ST, Aisner J. 1986. Performance status assessment among oncology patients: a review. Cancer Treat Rep 70:1423.

Osoba D, Aaronson NK, Muller M, et al. 1996. The development and psychometric validation of a brain cancer quality-of-life questionnaire for use in combination with general cancer-specific questionnaires. Qual Life Res 5: 139–150.

Paradis CM, Friedman S, Hatch M, Lazar RM. 1992. Obsessive-compulsive disorder onset after removal of a brain tumor. J Nerv Ment Dis 180:535–536.

Pavol MA, Meyers CA, Rexer JL, Valentine AD, Mattis PJ, Talpaz M. 1995. Pattern of neruobehavioral deficits associated with interferon-alpha therapy for leukemia. Neurology 45:947–950.

Petersdorf S, Upchurch C, Eyre H, et al. 1993. A Phase II study of external beam radiation and chemotherapy with cisplatin/BCNU followed by BCNU alone for the treatment of incompletely resected high-grade brain tumors. Proc Annu Meet Am Soc Clin Oncol. 12:A501.

Plenger PM, Dixon CE, Castillo RM, Frankowski RF, Yablon SA, Levin HS. 1996. Subacute methylphenidate treatment for moderate to moderately severe traumatic brain injury: a preliminary double-blind placebo-controlled study. Arch Phys Med Rehabil 77:536–540.

Prigatano GP. 1999. Principles of Neuropsychological Rehabilitation. New York: Oxford University Press.

Prigatano GP, Ben-Yishay Y. 1999. Psychotherapy and psychotherapeutic interventions in brain injury rehabilitation. In: Rosenthal M (ed), Rehabilitation of the Adult and Child with Traumatic Brain Injury, 3rd ed. Philadelphia: FA Davis.

Prigatano GP, et al. 1986. Neuropsychological Rehabilitation after Brain Injury. Baltimore: Johns Hopkins University Press.

Raven RW. 1992. A Practical Guide to Rehabilitation Oncology. Park Ridge, NJ: Parthenon.

Salandar P, Karlsson T, Bergenheim T, Henriksson R. 1995. Long-term memory deficits in patients with malignant gliomas. J Neurooncol 25:227–238.

Sapolsky RM. 1985. A mechanism for glucocorticoid toxicity in the hippocampus: increased neuronal vulnerability to metabolic insults. J Neurosci 5:1228–1232.

Scheibel RS, Meyers CA, Levin VA. 1996. Cognitive dysfunction following surgery for intracerebral glioma: influence of histopathology, lesion location, and treatment. J Neurooncol 30:61–69.

Scott CB. 1997. Quality-adjusted survival analysis of malignant glioma patients. Control Clin Trials 18:277–285.

Sherer M, Meyers CA, Bergloff P. 1997. Efficacy of postacute brain injury rehabilitation for patients with primary malignant brain tumors. Cancer 80:250–257.

Sneed PK, Prados MD, McDermott MW, et al. 1995. Large effect of age on the survival of patients with glioblastoma treated with radiotherapy and brachytherapy boost. Neurosurgery 36:898–904.

Sneeuw KC, Aaronson NK, Osoba D, et al. 1997. The use of significant others as proxy raters of the quality of life of patients with brain cancer. Med Care 35:490–506.

Taphoorn MJ, Heimans JJ, Snoek FJ,, et al. 1992. Assessment of quality of life in patients treated for low-grade glioma: a preliminary report. J Neurol Neurosurg Psychiatry 55:372–376.

Taphoorn MJ, Schiphorst AK, Snoek JF, et al. 1994. Cognitive functions and quality of life in patients with low-grade gliomas: the impact of radiotherapy. Ann Neurol 36:48–54.

Temple RM, Deary IJ, Winney RJ. 1995. Recombinant erythropoietin improves cognitive function in patients maintained on chronic ambulatory peritoneal dialysis. Nephrol Dial Transplant 10:1733–1738.

U.S. D.H.E.W. 1980. O.H.D., R.S.A. Memorandum from the commissioner Robert R. Humphreys to the RSA regional program director. Seattle, Washington, March 28.

Valentine AD, Meyers CA, Kling M, Richelson E, Hauser P. 1998. Mood and cognitive side effects of interferon-α therapy. Semin Oncol 25(suppl 1):39–47.

van Dam FS, Schagen SB, Muller MJ, et al. 1998. Impairment of cognitive function in women receiving adjuvant treatment for high-risk breast cancer: high-dose versus standard-dose chemotherapy. J Natl Cancer Inst 90:210–218.

van der Knaap MS, van der Grond J, Luyten PR, den Hollander JA, Nauta JJ, Valk J. 1992. ^{1}H and ^{31}P magnetic resonance spectroscopy of the brain in degenerative cerebral disorders. Ann Neurol 31:202–211.

Vilkki J. 1992. Cognitive flexibility and mental programming after closed head injury and anterior or posterior cerebral excisions. Neuropsychologia 30:807–814.

von Cramen DY, Matthes-von Cramen G. 1992. Reflections on the treatment of brain-injured patients suffering from problem-solving disorders. Neuropsychol Rehabil 2:207–229.

Watanabe MD, Martin EM, DeLeon OA, Gaviria M, Pavel DG, Trepashko DW. 1995. Successful methylpheniate treatment of apathy after subcortical infarcts. J Neuropsychiatry Clin Neurosci 7:502–504.

Wehman P, Kreutzer JS. 1990. Vocational Rehabilitation of Persons with Traumatic Brain Injury. Rockville MD: Aspen.

Weiss HD, Walker MD, Wiernik PH. 1974. Neurotoxicity of commonly used antineoplastic agents. N Engl J Med 291:127–133.

Weitzner MA, Meyers CA. 1997. Cognitive functioning and quality of life in malignant glioma patients: a review of the literature. Psychooncology 6:169–177.

Weitzner MA, Meyers CA, Byrne K. 1996. Psychosocial functioning and quality of life in patients with primary brain tumors. J Neurosurg 84(1):29–34.

Weitzner MA, Meyers CA, Gelke CK, Byrne KS, Cella DF, Levin VA. 1995. The Functional Assessment of Cancer Therapy (FACT) Scale: development of a brain subscale and revalidation of the general version (FACT–G) in patients with primary brain tumors. Cancer 75:1151–1161.

Wilson BA. 1997. Cognitive rehabilitation: how it is and how it might be. J Int Neuropsychol Soc 3:487–496.

Wolkowitz OM, Reus VI, Weingartner H, et al. 1990. Cognitive effects of corticosteroids. Am J Psychiatry 147:1297–1303.

World Health Organization. 1980. International Classification of Impairments, Disabilities, and Handicaps: a Manual of Classification Relating to the Consequences of Disease. Geneva: World Health Organization.

27

Psychiatric and Psychosocial Issues

ALAN D. VALENTINE, STEVEN D. PASSIK, AND MARY JANE MASSIE

Central nervous system (CNS) cancer, including primary brain tumors, CNS metastases, and nonmetastatic effects of cancer on the CNS, often has serious psychiatric and psychosocial consequences for the patient and for caregivers (Passik and Ricketts, 1998). The psychiatric impact of CNS cancer and associated treatment is unique because of direct effects on the brain and, thus, on mind, personality, memory, and self-concept. Patients often experience dramatic changes in mood and cognition, as well as decreased ability to function independently. Patients and family members are often unprepared for the neurologic sequelae of systemic cancer (Patchell and Posner, 1989). The same is true of behavioral consequences of primary or metastatic CNS cancer, possibly because of associated stigma or because of difficulties interpreting implications of the clinical presentations. The social impact of these diseases affect the spouse or significant other, as well as family members and caregivers, all of whom may be called on to provide a greater level of support than is typically required for cancer patients. Understanding the psychiatric and psychosocial impacts of neuro-oncologic illnesses on patients, families, and healthcare providers is essential to effectively treat cancer in this setting. Comprehensive treatment of CNS cancer entails use of appropriate psychopharmacologic, psychotherapeutic, cognitive, and behavioral interventions for the patient, as well as group and individual interventions for caregivers and staff.

The psychiatric and psychosocial effects of CNS cancer may be modest or subtle in initial stages of involvement. Long-term sequelae are often complex and severe. Patients are particularly vulnerable to such difficulties because a progressive disease course is generally characterized by an incipient cognitive and functional decline, along with multiple neurologic deficits. Coping with issues such as loss of independence is made more difficult by the effects of organic mental syndromes, including delirium, dementia, and mood disorders. Because most forms of CNS cancer have a poor prognosis, grief and mourning are central issues for the patient and close supporters (Passik et al., 1994).

We describe in this chapter the common psychiatric disorders (and some uncommon neuropsychiatric syndromes) encountered in neuro-oncology, as well as psychosocial problems facing patients and caregivers. Psychopharmacologic and psychotherapeutic interventions for the patient are discussed, as are individual and group psychotherapeutic interventions for caregivers and staff. In all cases, the intent is to improve quality of life, palliate distressing symptoms, and minimize adverse effects on treatment or end-of-life care.

PREVALENCE OF PSYCHIATRIC DISORDERS AND PSYCHOSOCIAL ISSUES IN ONCOLOGY AND NEURO-ONCOLOGY

Cancer patients in general are at high risk for psychiatric disorders. In a major epidemiologic study of mental disorders in cancer, almost 50% of randomly assessed outpatients and inpatients had psychiatric disorders detectable by standardized interview, using

DSM-III criteria (Derogatis et al., 1983). Adjustment disorders (with anxious and/or depressed features) and major depression accounted for the majority of these diagnoses (68% and 13%, respectively). Organic mental syndromes (including delirium and dementia) accounted for 8% of the detected disorders. Adjustment disorders by definition are psychological reactions with symptomatology severe enough to interfere with daily function. Depending on the criteria used, the rate of major depression detected by Derogatis and colleagues (1983) is perhaps twice as prevalent as in the general population. The rate of detected psychiatric disorders in cancer patients may be expected to increase for at least two reasons. First, with greater importance assigned to quality of life as a valid treatment endpoint, more attention is being directed at specific ways to detect and treat psychological and psychosocial distress at all points in the disease process. Second, as the American population ages, a higher percentage of individuals vulnerable to cancer will also be at risk for psychiatric disorders associated with increased age (e.g., dementia, delirium).

Patients with CNS cancer are at even higher risk of behavioral difficulties because of direct effects of disease on the brain and direct and indirect effects of cancer therapies. However, the actual prevalence of psychiatric disorders in neuro-oncology patients is unknown. Large studies from the first half of the twentieth century report psychiatric symptoms in 50% to 80% of brain tumor patients who came to autopsy (Price et al., 1997). Massie et al. (1991) reviewed the psychiatric diagnoses of patients admitted to the neuro-oncology service at the Memorial Sloan–Kettering Cancer Center and referred for psychiatric consultation. In this sample, 41% of patients had organic mental disorders, 11% had major depression, and 26% had adjustment disorders.

NEUROPSYCHIATRIC EFFECTS OF CANCER IN THE CENTRAL NERVOUS SYSTEM

Cancer in the CNS (and its treatment) has been associated with myriad neurobehavioral symptoms and disorders. The literature abounds with case reports and small series of unusual presentations of cognitive, perceptual, personality, and mood disorders associated with brain tumors (Manes and Robinson, 2000; Lishman, 1998a) and paraneoplastic syndromes (Dropcho, 1998; Lishman, 1998b). As mentioned, initial behavioral presentations of CNS malignancy can be subtle. Most often they will be accompanied by frank neurologic signs and symptoms (e.g., headache, nausea, seizures). However, behavioral or mood disturbance alone may be the first indication of the presence of a brain tumor or other cancer in the nervous system (Manes and Robinson, 2000).

In the case of brain tumors, lesion location and its relationship to particular behavioral syndromes has received considerable attention (Lishman, 1998a; Price et al., 1997). Before the availability of neuroimaging as the primary diagnostic modality in neuro-oncology, the potential to predict the presence or location of a tumor based on behavior had greater importance. In addition, it is well recognized that behavioral syndromes associated with a disease in a particular region of the brain may be caused by lesions in others because of diaschisis or disconnection effects (Price et al., 1997).

While cancer in the CNS is always associated with the possibility of a very complex or idiosyncratic behavioral presentation, the clinician caring for neuro-oncology patients will often encounter and should be prepared to address several common neuropsychiatric syndromes.

Delirium (Encephalopathy)

Delirium is a disorder of generalized CNS dysfunction characterized by an altered level of consciousness and abnormal attention, perception, memory, motor behavior, and sleep–wake cycle. A common problem in all seriously ill patients, it affects as many as 85% of those with advanced cancer (Massie et al., 1983). Those with delirium may demonstrate a variable level of arousal, ranging from stupor to hyperalertness and hypervigilance. Motor activity similarly ranges from profound psychomotor retardation to severe hyperactivity. Delirious patients are unable to pay attention; consequently short-term memory is usually impaired, as are other cognitive functions. Delirious patients are often disoriented. Sensory misperceptions (illusions) are common, as are frank hallucinations; these are most often visual, but can be auditory, tactile, or somatic. The patient may experience paranoid delusions. Disrupted sleep–wake cycles may precede onset of delirium or may be a function of it.

The disorder is of acute onset, usually hours to days. If the underlying cause or causes can be addressed, delirium will resolve quickly. It may also evolve into a more stable, but persistent, state of impaired consciousness and cognition and may be a preterminal event. Patients who recover from a delirium or persistent encephalopathic state often have no memory of the time during which they were impaired. Family members frequently find the acute behavioral and personality changes associated with delirium to be extremely frightening and more difficult to deal with than even the implications and neurologic sequelae of advancing or terminal disease.

Causes of acute altered mental status in neuro-oncology may be direct, indirect, or iatrogenic. In the case of primary and metastatic tumors and leptomeningeal disease, increased intracranial pressure may present with an acute or gradual decrease in level of arousal. The same is true of generalized and complex partial seizures due to tumor or post-treatment seizure focus. In most cases, CNS malignancy directly causes mental status changes along with focal neurologic signs or symptoms. The presentation may, however, be strictly behavioral.

Metabolic abnormalities are the most common cause of delirium in cancer and include severe electrolyte disturbances, hypercalcemia, and hypoxia. Other common causes include systemic or CNS infection and nutritional derangements (Breitbart and Cohen, 1998). Patients with advancing CNS malignancy and associated impairment, like those with other serious brain disorders (e.g., dementia, cerebrovascular accidents) are also vulnerable to systemic insults.

As a whole, pharmacologic agents used in supportive care are more likely to cause acute altered sensorium than are antineoplastics. Patients with compromised CNS function are sensitive to the effects of opioid analgesics, benzodiazepines, corticosteroids, and sympathomimetics, including bronchodilators and vasopressors (Slaby and Erle, 1993; Stiefel et al., 1989). The list of antineoplastics *commonly* associated with acute altered mental status is relatively small and includes methotrexate, ifosphamide, and cytosine arabinoside (Fleishman and Kalash, 1998). These agents will most often cause a delirium or dementia with behavioral disinhibition, as will biologic response modifiers (e.g., interleukin-2) used alone or in combination therapy (Denicoff et al., 1987; Meyers and Valentine, 1995). Assessment of delirium in the neuro-oncology patient should always include a review of all drugs the patient is taking. Radiation therapy to the brain infrequently causes an acute toxicity syndrome characterized by delirium or rapid cognitive decline (Posner, 1995). This can occur during or shortly after treatment, and is thought to be due to edema and increased intracranial pressure. It is controlled (and usually prevented) by administration of corticosteroids before/during radiation therapy.

Dementia

The hallmark of dementia is progressive cognitive impairment in the face of a clear sensorium. Associated mood, personality, and behavioral disturbances often accompany dementia. In the day-to-day care of patients with cancer in the nervous system, these associated problems may require the most attention. Prominent symptoms of dementia include short-term and long-term memory impairment, altered judgment and abstract reasoning, and disturbance of higher cortical function. The onset and progression of dementia is usually gradual and can be quite subtle. In the setting of progressive CNS disease, cognitive decline can be rapid. Patients may be competent in some areas of cognitive function and severely impaired in others. Patients with dementia, regardless of etiology, are at high risk for other psychiatric disorders such as delirium and depression (Liptzin, 1996; Alexopoulos, 1996) and are vulnerable to metabolic derangements and side effects from medications that others might easily tolerate.

Malignant disease in the nervous system causes dementia in several ways. Direct invasion of the brain by primary or metastatic tumor is the most obvious cause. Disconnection syndromes may occur as a result of tumor, surgical resection, or progressive radiation injury. In such cases disrupted neurotransmitter pathways may lead to cognitive impairment caused by lesions in areas not primarily associated with cognitive function. Chronic increased intracranial pressure may have diffuse effects on level of arousal with subsequent impairment of cognitive ability.

Organic mental syndromes caused by whole-brain radiation therapy are well described. An *acute radiation syndrome* is associated with acute change in mental status, headache, and nausea. Associated cognitive impairment resolves quickly if the underlying problem is treated. *Late delayed radiation toxicity* usually causes a dementing syndrome, which is progressive, permanent, and may be fatal (Posner, 1995; DeAngelis et al., 1989). While dementia is intuitively associated with progression of CNS malignancy, few patients or families are actually prepared for the consequences of impairment. It is also difficult to accept the fact that some aspects of treatment (i.e., progressive necrosis after radiation therapy) may produce deleterious side effects even in the face of stable disease. As is the case with primary dementias (i.e., Alzheimer's disease), caretakers are often under great strain and are themselves at high risk for physical and psychological morbidity.

It is often problematic to differentiate between dementia and cognitive dysfunction associated with depression (pseudodementia). Early in the course of the disease, cognitive deficits may be suspected, but are difficult to actually detect at clinical examination. Formal neuropsychological testing (see Chapter 26) can be extremely useful in such situations. Testing also provides objective measures of cognitive status over time, which is important in treatment planning. Identifying cognitive strengths and weaknesses assists with counseling about vocational choices and in deciding whether or not to refer a patient for cognitive rehabilitation.

Personality and Behavioral Changes

Patients with CNS cancer may demonstrate changes in personality and behavior as an initial sign of the presence of disease and as disease and treatment progress. Such changes can pose a significant management problem for caretakers, and, in the worst cases, can place the patient and others in physical danger. Tumor involvement or other involvement of the frontal lobes, temporal lobes, corpus callosum, and diencephalon may lead to irritability, paroxysmal anger and rage, affective lability, facetiousness, impulsivity, and, especially with diencephalic tumors, inappropriate eating, sleeping, and sexual behaviors (Lishman, 1999a). Accompanying progressive CNS dysfunction, one may encounter "coarsening" of personality, where more objectionable personality and behavior traits become increasingly prominent, similar to the behavior exhibited in primary dementing illnesses. Patients may or may not be aware of these behaviors and in any case may not be able to control them.

Disinhibition and aggression may be functions of structural damage or represent physiologic alterations of critical neurotransmitter pathways. When behaviors are caused by these events, they are likely to become chronic management issues. Adverse drug reactions should also be considered. As noted above, corticosteroids can produce manic or psychotic behaviors. Neuroleptic antiemetics can cause akathisia, which can lead to aggressive behavior as an inexpressive patient is frustrated by attempts to convey discomfort. Psychostimulants used to treat cognitive decline can cause anxiety and agitation. Behavioral disinhibition is a common adverse effect associated with benzodiazepine anxiolytics in patients with cognitive impairment. Unrelieved pain is also a possible cause of agitation in cognitively impaired or aphasic patients.

MANAGEMENT OF DELIRIUM, DEMENTIA, AND BEHAVIORAL SYMPTOMS

Managing cognitive and behavioral syndromes in patients with CNS cancer should ideally begin with identification and treatment of the etiology of the patient's medical problems, if possible. This approach is most likely to be successful in managing delirium, but more problematic for managing dementing illnesses and paroxysmal aggression due to fixed CNS lesions. During the search for a reversible cause, or in the face of a chronic structural or physiologic insult that cannot be reversed, medications and behavioral approaches are indicated for treatment.

Pharmacotherapy

Antipsychotic Medications

Antipsychotic drugs are useful not only against hallucinations and perceptual disturbances but also for anxiolysis and management of disinhibition caused by CNS disease. Some antipsychotics are also effective antiemetics. Several new antipsychotic drugs have recently become available (Table 27–1). Because patients with CNS malignancy may be ultrasusceptible to both the positive and negative effects of antipsychotics, the well-known recommendation to "start low and go slow" applies.

Haloperidol is a high-potency antipsychotic drug that is effective in reducing confusion and agitation without causing undue sedation. It can be given orally,

Table 27–1. Selected Neuroleptic Medications for Patients with Neuro-oncologic Illness

Drug Name	*Starting Daily Dosage (PO or IV)*
Haloperidol*	0.5 mg (mild symptoms)
	2–4 mg (severe symptoms)
Risperidone	1 mg bid
Olanzapine	2.5–5 mg
Chlorpromazine*	10–50 mg qd to tid
Thioridazine	10–25 mg qd to tid

*Parenteral forms available.

in tablet or liquid concentrate form, or by parental injection. Although not formally approved for intravenous (IV) administration, haloperidol is commonly, rapidly, and safely delivered by this route to patients experiencing agitation or who are unable to take oral medications. It is thought that haloperidol's potency is effectively doubled by IV administration. Like other high-potency antipsychotics, haloperidol is associated with the risk of akathisia and parkinsonian side effects (as well as relatively less severe anticholinergic effects and α-adrenergic blockade than are low-potency neuroleptics), although this risk appears to be reduced with IV administration. If necessary, these side effects can also be treated with benzotropine, benzodiazepines, and other medications. Dosing requirements vary greatly and are governed in part by the severity of the symptoms in question and stage of illness. Severely ill, end-stage, or elderly patients may require very modest doses (0.5 to 1.0 mg per OS [PO] or IV once or twice per day or every few hours as needed until symptom control is achieved). In the case of persistent or severe agitation (e.g., hyperactive delirium), significantly higher doses may be given to sedate the patient.

Chlorpromazine is a lower potency antipsychotic drug that is more sedating than haloperidol and may be administered by the same routes (including continuous IV infusion in extreme cases). Typical doses are in the range of 25 to 50 mg PO or IVPB every 6 to 12 hours. Because of anticholinergic and α-adrenergic blockade effects, there is a significant risk of hypotension when chlorpromazine is given at high doses or administered intravenously.

Thioridazine is a low-potency antipsychotic. At low doses (25 to 100 mg) it is also an effective primary anxiolytic, particularly for patients who are vulnerable to the side effects of benzodiazepines.

Risperidone and olanzapine are newer agents, which are administered orally and with exceptions appear to be well tolerated (i.e., are less likely to cause akathisia). In the setting of CNS cancer, they can be used to treat low-intensity delirium or chronic behavioral symptoms. They may be only relatively useful in emergency situations when parental dosing is not possible.

Anticonvulsants

Anticonvulsant medications have been used to treat agitation and other behavioral disorders associated with senile dementia (Roane et al., 2000; Grossman, 1998), developmental disorders, and traumatic brain injury. The medications also have recognized utility in managing some primary psychiatric disorders. Whereas there are, to date, no reported trials employing these medications in neuro-oncology, they are used when other medications have not been effective or as adjuncts to behavioral therapy. Anticonvulsants employed in this setting include carbamazepine, valproic acid, and gabapentin.

Psychostimulants

Psychostimulant medications that have a role in the treatment of depression in the medically ill have additional efficacy as palliative agents against psychomotor slowing and dementia associated with CNS cancer (Weitzner et al., 1995; DeLong et al., 1992). In one open-label trial using methylphenidate, cognitive and functional performance improved over time, even in the face of progressive disease or radiation necrosis (Meyers et al., 1998). These drugs, including d-amphetamine, methylphenidate, and pemoline, appear to work as direct or indirect dopamine agonists.

Common side effects include anxiety, insomnia, gastrointestinal distress, and autonomic disturbance (hypertension). These drugs inhibit metabolism of tricyclic antidepressants, coumadin anticoagulants, and some anticonvulsants, including phenobarbital and phenytoin (Meyers et al., 1998). Despite these potential problems, patients with primary brain tumor appear to tolerate psychostimulants very well. When used to treat cognitive decline or psychomotor slowing, typical starting doses are 5 mg of methylphenidate or d-amphetamine two times per day, but the doses can be titrated up. In severely impaired patients, doses of methylphenidate approaching 100 mg/day have been safely and effectively employed.

MOOD AND ANXIETY DISORDERS

Depression and adjustment disorders are the most common psychiatric disorders in the general oncology population; it is not surprising that they are typically encountered when malignant disease involves the CNS. The cause may be due to pre-existing or recurrent mood disorders (primary mood disorders), direct effects of disease or side effects of treatment (secondary mood disorders), or psychological reactions to severe stress (adjustment disorders).

Depression

Mood disorders exist on a continuum from severe depression (major depression) to frank mania. Patients with depressive disorders experience psychological and physical symptoms. The former may include dysphoria (sadness), anhedonia, feelings of guilt, and suicidal thoughts. Somatic symptoms include fatigue, impaired concentration, altered sleep and appetite, and decreased libido. Anxiety is increasingly recognized as a symptom of mood disorders as well.

Diagnosis of depression in the medically ill is complicated by problems inherent in distinguishing vegetative symptoms caused by mood disorder from those caused by disease and treatment. In the setting of other brain disorders (e.g., cerebrovascular accident) there is even disagreement over the clinical utility of vegetative symptoms (Robinson, 2000; Erban et al., 2000). In psycho-oncology, some clinicians and researchers recommend that emphasis be placed on psychological symptoms when establishing a diagnosis (Massie and Popkin, 1998). Additional psychological symptoms have been proposed and successfully employed as substitute criteria in place of vegetative symptoms on a standard depression rating scale (Endicott, 1984).

All patients with depressive symptoms should be evaluated for possible suicidal intent. Assessing suicidal ideation requires careful determination of whether it reflects depressive illness or is a function of a wish to exert control over intolerable circumstances. Breitbart and Krivo (1998) have outlined factors that place a cancer patient at high risk for suicide: poor prognosis and advanced disease; current or past depression; uncontrolled pain, delirium, past history of suicide attempts; family history of suicide and alcohol abuse; and feelings of isolation or helplessness.

Pathology in particular areas of the brain is most likely to be associated with depressive syndromes. This includes damage (e.g., tumor, radiation necrosis) to the dorsolateral frontal lobes or their anatomic/physiologic circuits, producing executive dysfunction consistent with subcortical dementia (Chow and Cummings, 1999; Starkstein and Robinson, 1999), as well as dominant temporal lobe lesions (Lishman, 1998a). Patients with pituitary or hypophyseal lesions and associated neuroendocrine dyscrasias are subject to mood and vegetative symptoms that appear in primary depression.

Few drugs used to treat CNS malignancy are associated with depressive disorders. Of these, corticosteroids are the most problematic (Stiefel et al., 1989) and are associated with symptoms ranging the spectrum of mood disorders. Patients may become anxious with psychomotor agitation and racing thoughts consistent with mania. They may also become dysphoric with negative or nihilistic ruminative thoughts, sometimes escalating to the point of psychosis. Because reactions are idiosyncratic, it is difficult to predict which patients will have adverse reactions to steroids. It is sometimes possible to minimize depressive reactions by changing agents or by decreasing dose. The interferons are associated with depressive reactions, usually at high doses or over long treatment periods. On rare occasions, acute depressive reactions occur shortly after treatment begins. Interferon-α is most likely to cause neuropsychiatric side effects. Interferon-β, which is used more often in neuro-oncology, is generally less problematic (Valentine et al., 1998).

Central nervous system depressants may cause depressive syndromes in sensitive individuals. These drugs include opioid analgesics, benzodiazepine anxiolytics, hypnotics, and some anticonvulsants (e.g., phenobarbital, phenytoin). These presentations usually resolve or decrease in intensity with dose reduction or discontinuation of medication.

Anxiety

Persistent and incapacitating anxiety symptoms in cancer patients may be an exacerbation of pre-existing primary psychiatric disorders (e.g., generalized anxiety disorder, panic disorder) or may be a function of the disease process. Patients typically experience fear, worry, and irritability. They have intrusive, ruminative, unpleasant thoughts and are often hyperalert or hypervigilant. If anxiety becomes severe, physical symptoms may be encountered, including palpitations, diaphoresis, dyspnea, and numerous gastrointestinal complaints. Sleep becomes difficult. If anxiety proceeds to panic, the patient may experience feelings of impending death and severe pain. In fact, panic attacks are in the differential diagnosis of myocardial infarction.

Primary anxiety and panic disorders are relatively common in the general population. They tend to be persistent or recurrent over time, which aids in establishing the diagnosis and emphasizes the need for taking an adequate history. Predisposed patients are at some risk for exacerbation of these disorders when subjected to the physical processes of cancer diagnosis and treatment, including use of magnetic resonance imaging scanners, immobilization for radiation therapy or surgery, or placement of indwelling catheters.

Several secondary causes of anxiety and panic are encountered in neuro-oncology patients. Anxiety is a recognized prodromal and post-event symptom associated with seizures. Other physical causes of anxiety symptoms are similar to those considered in the etiology of delirium: hypoxia of any cause (including anemia or evolving pulmonary embolus), electrolyte and endocrine abnormalities, sepsis, and unrelieved pain.

Many drugs (i.e., corticosteroids) used in primary or supportive treatment of cancer in the nervous system often cause anxiety symptoms. Various phenothiazine antiemetics and other neuroleptics (e.g., haloperidol) can cause akathisia that is described by patients as "anxiety." Drugs of any class with significant anticholinergic effects can cause anxiety and agitation, as can benzodiazepine anxiolytics and opioid analgesics.

Adjustment Disorder with Depressed or Anxious Features

Not all etiologies of depression or anxiety in this setting are "organic." Patients with clear sensorium react emotionally to the diagnosis of CNS cancer in a manner similar to patients diagnosed with other malignancies. Psychological reactions to this severe stress most often include depression and/or anxiety. These reactions may be mild or severe, with major disruption of daily life. Whether neuro-oncology patients are at higher risk than other cancer patients for such symptoms is not known. Recent studies of primary brain tumor patients treated with surgery have found lower rates of anxiety and depression than those reported in the general oncology population (Anderson et al., 1999).

The initial reactions to a cancer diagnosis may include shock and disbelief followed by dysphoria, despair, anger, and anxiety. The ability to concentrate and carry out activities of daily living is impaired; there are intrusive thoughts about the diagnosis and worry about a future that cannot be controlled (Massie and Holland, 1992). Vegetative or somatic symptoms (i.e., insomnia, anorexia, fatigue) may be experienced; the syndrome can be identical to that involving secondary or primary mental disorders.

Emotional turmoil at times of great stress in cancer patients is normal, and patients benefit from reassurance and support provided by the neuro-oncology staff. Psychiatric intervention is generally not required unless the symptoms interfere with function or when they are highly distressing or prolonged. Patients with symptoms in excess of those "expected" receive a diagnosis of adjustment disorder with depressed or anxious features, or both.

Psychiatric interventions are aimed at helping the individual resume successful coping. Several modalities are used. Individual psychotherapy focuses on clarifying the medical situation and the meaning of the illness to the patient and on reinforcing the patient's positive coping strategies. It is often desirable to include a spouse or family member in the sessions to enhance support at home. Couples and family therapy are particularly useful when interpersonal issues are prominent. Group therapy, with a focus on illness, can also be helpful, as can behavioral interventions such as hypnosis or relaxation training (Passik and Massie, 1996).

The decision to prescribe psychotropic medications to treat adjustment disorders requires the presence of a persistent level of distress that interferes with treatment or ability to carry out activities of daily living. Benzodiazepine anxiolytics can be very helpful for managing acute anxiety, although caution is required in the setting of significant cognitive impairment or with the use of other CNS depressant medications. Dependence and abuse are usually not an issue for psychologically healthy individuals.

Pharmacotherapy of Depression

Antidepressants are effective for treating primary and secondary mood disorders. Antidepressants with several different mechanisms of action are available and are thought to be equally efficacious in treating depression. There is no "gold standard" antidepressant for use in general psychiatry or oncology. The choice of antidepressant depends on several factors, including the side effect profile of the drug in question, the patient's particular symptoms and medical status, and cost. Antidepressants usually take 2 to 4 weeks to achieve antidepressant effect. Beneficial effects on insomnia can occur sooner. Ambulatory patients with normal metabolic function can be started on antidepressants at doses consistent with those used in the general population. In the face of hepatic or renal impairment, and for the elderly, it is best to start at half or even quarter doses and titrate up, if tolerated. Antidepressant therapy often is continued for at least 6 months after antidepressant response is achieved. Selected antidepressants for use in neuro-oncology are listed in Table 27–2.

Selective Serotonin Reuptake Inhibitors

Selective serotonin reuptake inhibitors (SSRIs) are the first line of therapy for treating depression because of their excellent safety and side effect profile, if not superior efficacy. Several of the SSRIs now have indications for treatment of panic and phobic disorders. These include fluoxetine, sertraline, paroxetine, and citalopram. Their relative lack of anticholinergic

Table 27–2. Selected Antidepressant Medications Used by Patients with Neuro-oncologic Illnesses

Drug Name	*Starting Daily Dosage (mg PO)*	*Therapeutic Daily Dosage (mg PO)*
Selective serotonin inhibitors		
Fluoxetine*	10–20	20–60
Sertraline*	25–50	50–200
Paroxetine*	10–20	10–60
Citalopram	10–20	20–60
Atypical antidepressants		
Bupropion	100 bid	200–450
Trazodone	50–100	150–400
Venlafaxine	37.5–75	75–350
Nefazodone	100 bid	300–600
Mirtazapine	15 qh	15–45
Tricyclic antidepressants		
Amitriptyline	25–50	75–150
Imipramine	25–50	75–200
Desipramine	25–50	75–200
Nortriptyline	25–50	50–150
Psychostimulants		
Methylphenidate	2.5 at 8 AM and noon	5–30
D-amphetamine	2.5 at 8 AM and noon	5–30
Pemoline	18.75 in AM and noon	37.5–150

*SSRIs maybe used at high end of dose range for anxiety/panic.

and α-adrenergic blocking properties makes them good choices for patients with a serious medical illness. Unlike tricyclic antidepressants, SSRIs have not proven lethal in overdose, making them a good choice for use by severely ill or unstable, depressed patients.

Common side effects of SSRIs include anxiety and nausea; these effects are usually short lasting. Weight loss and sexual dysfunction are potentially problematic with fluoxetine, although its "activating" effects are a potential advantage. Some individuals become sedated on paroxetine and citalopram, a problem that can be minimized with nighttime dosing. Sexual side effects (anorgasmia) can also occur with these drugs. Usual starting doses of fluoxetine are 10 to 20 mg every morning; sertraline, 20 to 25 mg every morning; paroxetine, 10 to 20 mg every morning or at bedtime; and citalopram 10 to 20 mg at bedtime.

Tricyclic Antidepressants

Use of the tricyclic antidepressants (TCAs) is now secondary to use of SSRIs and newer "third-generation" agents. However, their advantages include cost and the ability (in the healthy adult population) to obtain accurate therapeutic blood levels. Tricyclic antidepresssants are also useful for treatment of neuropathic pain and, in some cases, are effective antiemetics. Antihistaminic, anticholinergic, and α-adrenergic blockade effects (sedation, dry mouth, constipation, orthostatic hypotension) are more serious with tertiary amines (e.g., amitriptyline, imipramine) than secondary amines (e.g., nortriptyline, desipramine). These side effects may be problematic in patients with CNS impairment or in the elderly. They are, however, successfully employed to treat depressive syndromes associated with Parkinson's disease and cerebrovascular accidents.

Tricyclic antidepressants are potentially lethal in overdose, especially in combination with alcohol or CNS depressants, and must be used cautiously by patients with cardiac conduction abnormalities. Weight gain is an unacceptable side effect for some patients. Sedation, which is a disabling side effect for others, may actually be advantageous to patients with insomnia. In the setting of CNS cancer, initial dosing of TCAs should be conservative (25 to 50 mg at bedtime) with dose escalation in 25 to 50 mg increments every few days until effective. Determination of therapeutic blood levels requires that the drugs be at steady-state metabolism, achieved after 5 to 7 days at a given dose.

"Third-Generation" Antidepressants

The newer antidepressants were developed in response to advances in understanding the neurochemistry mood disorders. These agents, which affect norepinephrine and/or serotonin metabolism, include venlafaxine, mirtazapine, and nefazodone. Their efficacy in the oncology setting has not yet been determined by clinical studies. As with other antidepressants, side effect profiles may dictate which drug is chosen. This generation of antidepressants causes less difficulty with sexual dysfunction, sedation, and weight change associated with SSRIs and TCAs.

Psychostimulants

Stimulants (e.g., methylphenidate, d-amphetamine, pemoline) have an established role in treating depression in the medically ill (Masand and Tesar, 1996; Rosenberg, 1992) and are also used to counteract opioid-induced sedation (Bruera et al., 1992). These drugs appear to have a more rapid onset of antidepressant action than other agents. Improvements in mood, level of physical activity, and appetite are sometimes seen within 2 to 3 days after initiating treatment. In the setting of medical depression, as with cognitive decline, it is possible to maintain psychostimulant therapy for 1 year or longer. Psychostimulants have occasionally been employed in conjunction with standard antidepressants to achieve an immediate improvement in energy and mood until the SSRI or TCA becomes effective. The stimulant is then tapered and discontinued. Initial dosing should be conservative—2.5 mg every morning and noon for d-amphetamine and methylphenidate. A sustained-release form of methylphenidate is now available. Doses can be titrated upward if tolerated, but it is usually not necessary to increase the dosage beyond 20 to 30 mg/day. Side effects of psychostimulants include anxiety, insomnia, gastrointestinal upset, and hypertension or hypotension. At high doses patients may develop involuntary motor movements, paradoxical sedation, and delirium. If such effects do occur, the stimulant can be discontinued and the symptoms will likely resolve.

Atypical and Other Antidepressants

Other antidepressants have utility and are prescribed if a patient has been successfully treated with a given antidepressant in the past. Bupropion has "activating" effects, which make it attractive in the setting of depression with psychomotor slowing. There is also less risk of sexual dysfunction with use of this antidepressant, and the slow-release formulation is currently utilized as adjunctive therapy for smoking cessation. Use of bupropion is associated with a modest increased risk of seizures that may make its use problematic in patients with CNS disease.

Monoamine oxidase inhibitors (MAOIs) are effective antidepressants whose use is made more difficult because of the need for patient compliance with dietary restrictions to avoid tyramine-associated hypertensive crises. Those requirements along with the potential for interaction with other drugs used in oncology (i.e., procarbazine, meperidine) make MAOIs less useful for treating depression in this setting.

Lithium

Patients who have been receiving lithium before development of cancer should be maintained on it through treatment, if possible. Close monitoring may be required in preoperative or postoperative periods when fluid intake may be restricted. Dose reduction may be necessary for seriously ill patients.

Pharmacotherapy of Anxiety

Several different classes of psychotropic drugs are useful for managing anxiety. In the face of CNS cancer, the clinician must carefully consider drug side effects and the possibility that anxiety is a function of an underlying neurologic, metabolic, or iatrogenic disturbance that requires attention. Advances in the pharmacotherapy of general anxiety and panic disorders may change prescribing practices in oncology.

Benzodiazepines

Benzodiazepines (BZPs) are currently the drugs of choice for managing acute and chronic anxiety states in oncology patients (Table 27–3). Used appropriately, these medications are safe and effective. In addition to anxiolysis, BZPs have variable hypnotic, antiemetic, anticonvulsant, and muscle-relaxant effects that are of benefit. Unease about dependence or abuse is usually not a significant concern in the oncology setting. These medications may add to sedation caused by other drugs, and patients with CNS compromise must be treated carefully because of risk of behavioral disinhibition or precipitation of delirium. Tolerance develops more quickly with short-acting BZPs than with longer acting agents. If used regularly, they should be tapered to avoid withdrawal syndromes.

Short-acting BZPs such as lorazepam, alprazolam, and oxazepam have a relatively rapid onset and short duration of action, making them useful for treating acute-onset anxiety or panic. Their metabolic profiles make them better tolerated by patients with impaired hepatic or renal function. Lorazepam and oxazepam

Table 27–3. Selected Benzodiazepines Commonly Prescribed for Patients with Neuro-oncologic Illnesses

Drug	*Approximate Dose Equivalent*	*Initial PO Dosage (mg)*	*Half-Life (Hours)*	*Active Metabolite*
Short half-life				
Alprazolam	0.5	0.25–0.5 tid	10–15	No
Lorazepam*	1.0	0.5–2.0 tid	10–20	No
Oxazepam	10.0	10–15 tid	5–15	No
Temazepam†	5.0	15–30 qh	10–15	No
Intermediate/long half-life				
Clonazepam	0.5	0.5 bid	18–50	No
Diazepam	5.0	5–10 bid	20–70	Yes

*Lorazepam can also be administered intramuscularly; other benzodiazepines are erratically absorbed when given intramuscularly.

†Hypnotic agent.

are conjugated and eliminated, whereas alprazolam's metabolite is inactive. These medications are typically given two to four times per day as needed for anxiety. They can be given on a regular schedule if necessary. In cases of extremely severe anxiety or panic, lorazepam may be administered by intramuscular or IV injection.

Longer acting BZPs such as diazepam and clonazepam are useful for persistent anxiety states, and clonazepam is appropriate for managing some aggressive behavioral syndromes as well. The longer duration of action of these drugs is potentially problematic for the elderly or severely ill.

Alternative Anxiolytics

Used at low doses, neuroleptics (haloperidol, risperidone, olanzapine, and especially thioridazine) may be safer and more effective than BZPs for managing acute and chronic anxiety in patients with CNS compromise or those with a history of adverse reactions to standard antianxiety drugs. Buspirone is effective for treatment of anxiety in some patients naïve to benzodiazepines.

Selective serotonin reuptake inhibitor antidepressants (paroxetine, sertraline, fluoxetine) are a first line of therapy for chronic anxiety and panic disorders. Their favorable side-effect profiles, especially their effect on sensorium and cognitive function, make them attractive candidates for use in oncology and neuro-oncology. Typically SSRIs are given at moderate to high doses (paroxetine 40 to 60 mg/day, sertraline 100 to 150 mg/day) to effectively treat anxiety and panic. Benzodiazepines can be given for acute anxiety control while waiting for the SSRI to take effect.

PSYCHOTHERAPEUTIC INTERVENTIONS

Psychotherapy can help patients with neuro-oncologic illnesses cope with the many realities of their disease and its treatment. Neuro-oncology patients struggle to make difficult adjustments common to all cancer patients, but have the added burden of damage to the brain. The loss of cognitive abilities, motor control and strength, language abilities, and control of bodily functions can disrupt relationships and life plans, ultimately resulting in inevitable disability and dependency. In addition, the effects of disease, surgery, and medication side effects (e.g., from corticosteroids) can cause drastic changes in appearance, which can seriously compromise body image and the patient's and/or partner's interest in sex.

Many patients with systemic cancers adjust well before the development of brain metastases. These patients may have adjusted to increased dependency and disruption of life plans and may have learned to cope with changes in appearance and existential issues. Upon development of neurologic symptoms (and, possibly, behavioral symptoms), previously effective coping strategies may become ineffective. The fear of loss of control and of "losing one's mind" is significant for patients who find that they can no longer achieve the same sense of mastery over their illness that they once enjoyed. Awareness of cognitive deficits for patients with primary or metastatic neurologic disease can be frightening and frustrating.

For example, a patient who has expressive or receptive aphasia caused by disease affecting Broca's or Wernicke's area of the brain often struggles to speak and communicate. The resulting isolation can be profound, as the illness decreases the patient's ability to interact with family members. The direct effects of the tumor on the brain combined with vulnerability to organic mental syndrome cause the patient to have to adjust to loss of control of behavior. In cases of transient behavioral changes, such as those caused by delirium, the resolution of an episode is often accompanied by bewilderment and embarrassment. It is common for neuro-oncology patients to feel they have become burdens to their families, a realization that can be so intolerable that it is sometimes accompanied by suicidal thoughts. For families, the stigma associated with mental illness as well as fear about the implications of neurologic or psychiatric impairment may make the development of CNS disease far more difficult to tolerate than other systemic involvement.

Psychotherapy for neuro-oncology patients is supportive in nature, drawing upon crisis intervention and psychoeducational techniques (Massie et al., 1989; Sourkes et al., 1998). The therapist utilizes the principles of crisis intervention therapy when helping a patient confront the overwhelming nature of a neuro-oncologic illness. These principles involve *(1)* an adoption of an active and involved stance on the part of the therapist, *(2)* an emphasis on providing information and techniques for coping with specific and solvable problems, *(3)* the goal of restoring the patient to baseline function (as opposed to a goal for personal change or growth), and *(4)* the importance of stressing symptom control as an aid to adaptation. As in all crisis intervention work, the therapist must be available to assist the patient and must assume an active consultative role.

Coping is generally facilitated by the acquisition of accurate and useful information. Teaching patients and their caregivers about the effects of the illness and its treatments is reassuring, especially when the patient or caregivers misinterpret the meaning or consequences of emerging symptoms. The therapist normalizes and validates the patient's reactions to his or her illness and helps the patient prepare for the "typical" disease course. Information is provided at a rate that is comfortable for the patient, utilizing jargon-free language and a manner that invites questions and exploration. Information and support can help the patient define problems at various points in the disease course that can be solved and then, in turn, engender a sense of accomplishment.

Neuro-oncology patients, if not too impaired in attention and concentration, can benefit from relaxation therapy and other cognitive behavioral techniques with a family member acting as a co-therapist. The co-therapist helps augment the patient's memory and assists with the practice and application of techniques learned with the therapist outside of sessions. Keeping a diary is another technique for augmenting failing memory and cognitive abilities. It can be useful for patients with memory problems to write down one or two key points during each session. Ideally, the diary should be kept in a book that is small enough for patients to keep with them at all times. The diary can help the patient recall important aspects of the therapy and can evoke a sense of support and decreased isolation. The scheduling of sessions is altered to accommodate neuro-oncology patients. Sessions should be short, generally no longer than 20 to 30 minutes, so as not to overwhelm or fatigue the patient, and are scheduled frequently to provide a sense of continuity and connection.

Anticipatory bereavement and preparation for death is one focus of psychotherapy with neuro-oncology patients. Patients who are slowly watching their independent function decrease as they lose cognitive function and other abilities have much to mourn. For some patients, there is often a sense of urgency to accomplish certain goals, not before death but before abilities are lost. We have found it helpful to encourage patients to give advance directives regarding treatment alternatives and resuscitation early in the course of illness. Making these wishes known can decrease the burden the patient feels he or she is imposing on the family and give a sense of control over an illness course that can be overwhelming. Some individuals "postpone" talk of advance directives because such talk is inconsistent with their need to maintain hope. Others are not troubled by simultaneously entertaining seemingly contradictory aspects of their situation.

Family members sometimes support the patient's need to hold off thoughts of death and dying. The process of death and its aftermath can be made more difficult for those individuals, who may need their own forum to confront these issues. Nonverbal techniques, such as music and art therapy, can help the patient learn to communicate and express himself or herself when the illness has made verbal expression difficult or impossible. We know of several patients with brain tumors who realized their artistic abilities only after their diagnosis of cancer. One patient, a talented sculptor, filled his home with extraordinary works of art during the course of his illness. The patient felt that the art would leave behind a tangible reminder of him that would help his wife cope with his death. Another patient, a talented artist who could no longer paint because of his tumor, sought self-expression by arranging and re-arranging the books on his bookshelves (Passik and Massie, 1996).

At times, speech disorders induced by neuro-oncologic illnesses may affect second and third languages the patient had learned but that were not his or her primary language or "mother tongue." Thus, the degree of ability of the patient to speak his or her first language should be investigated, as this factor can be used in the service of the therapy and to increase quality of life. Physical and cognitive rehabilitation techniques developed during work with brain-injured and stroke patients can also be applied to and benefit neuro-oncology patients. Referral of patients to rehabilitation centers continues to be an obstacle, as some centers seem slow to accept brain tumor patients.

Cognitive rehabilitation strategies can teach patients how to improve their concentration and aid their memory. Small gains in these areas can pay big dividends in psychotherapy. Decreased perception of dependency can increase self-esteem and quality of life.

PSYCHOSOCIAL IMPACT ON SPOUSES AND FAMILIES

Interactions with Family Members

The families of patients with neuro-oncologic illnesses face the typical stressors that affect families of patients with non-neurologic cancer. These stressors have prompted mental health professionals who work with cancer patients to recognize family members as "second-order patients" (Lederberg, 1998). Family members face a different and ongoing process of adjustment throughout all stages of the patient's illness; they confront the onerous tasks of providing emotional support as well as basic care-taking, sharing responsibility for making medical decisions, weathering financial and social costs, and maintaining stability in the midst of change. The unique nature of the symptomatology of neuro-oncologic illness, both primary and treatment related, amplifies the difficulty of making these adjustments. By rendering the patient less capable of interacting with staff and family and by compromising his or her cognitive capacities, this illness produces a shift in the responsibility to the grieving family members.

Feelings of loss, of being overwhelmed, and anger at the patient for behavior that cannot be controlled are often followed by feelings of guilt. Family members may experience conflict after assuming care-taking and medical decision-making burdens that they may feel ill prepared to handle. The medical team must give the family attention to help prepare them for often intense and conflicted emotional responses to the patient's disease and treatment course. Ambivalent feelings about providing high levels of care while watching loved ones suffer with loss of dignity and poor quality of life are difficult to endure. It is not unusual for family members to wish that the disease would quickly run its course and take the life of the patient. Such feelings, while common, are not easily entertained. These feelings are often accompanied by loneliness and exhaustion. Often motivated by the desire to hide the patient from children or friends in an attempt to protect the patient's waning sense of dignity, spouses will take on complete 24 hour care to avoid exposing others to the stark realities of the illness.

Family members of neuro-oncology patients face a set of unique stressors, including an almost universally poor prognosis and complicated disease course. This complex, downward course is marked by the accumulation of multiple irreversible neurologic deficits, which cause patients to lose the ability to function independently, creating a burdensome caregiving responsibility. The families of neuro-oncology patients find themselves in a state of mourning (anticipatory bereavement) long before the actual death of the patient. The multiple losses they face include *(1)* the loss of the patient's cognitive function and emotional state; *(2)* the loss of the characteristic marital, sexual, and family relationships; and *(3)* the loss of the spouse's self-image due to changes in his or her relationship with the patient. If the patient can no longer engage in sexual activity, for example, the well spouses (if they are to remain faithful, as most do) must adapt to view themselves as not sexually active. The following case illustrates appropriate referral for family therapy of a patient at odds with her support system because of her decreasing autonomy.

A 39-year-old woman with a history of ovarian cancer was admitted to the neuro-oncology service for progressive difficulty with coordination and ambulation, problems that progressed from incoordination to complete inability to walk in a 2 month period of time. After a lumbar puncture, the diagnosis of paraneoplastic cerebellar degeneration was made. Her cognitive functioning was unaffected, but she appeared depressed. The patient described how she had been able to resume her role as a single working parent shortly after completing cancer treatment. Her boyfriend had helped her cope with the sexual problems caused by the treatment; once the neurologic symptoms began to appear, however, the patient felt completely devastated and helpless about the loss of autonomy caused by these symptoms. In particular, she blamed herself for parenting difficulties with her increasingly rebellious adolescent daughter. Family meetings were helpful in bringing out their collective grief over the patient's loss of autonomy.

A role reversal often occurs in families of cancer patients. For example, if the breadwinner of the family becomes ill, the well spouse, by necessity, often adopts this role. The patient, in turn, assumes a dependent position, often needing family members to perform intimate physical care. The well spouse, in particular, is called on to adopt a parental-like role vis-à-vis the patient, assuming responsibility for the total well-being of the patient. The mode of communication between the patient and family changes dramatically, and family members must rely heavily on nonverbal cues to determine the patient's needs, which can be exhausting and frustrating for all.

Dementia or withdrawal caused by destruction of the brain is often interpreted by family members as a psychological event, depression, or loss of the desire to "fight the illness." The patient's waxing and waning behaviors caused by organic factors are thus sometimes viewed as volitional. Patients may have moments of extraordinary clarity, providing heartbreaking glimpses characteristic of pre-morbid individuals and highlighting their degree of suffering. Helping the family understand that the effects of the illness are more distressing when viewed by an observer with intact cognitive ability than may be experienced by the patient offers solace to many distressed families.

The principles of assessment of sexual dysfunction and sex therapy have been applied successfully to cancer patients and cancer survivors (Auchincloss, 1989; Schover, 1998). Sex therapy techniques can be valuable for neuro-oncology patients and their spouses who present with sexual disorders or alterations in sexual functioning stemming from the disease and its treatment. For example, women taking antiestrogen therapies for primary brain tumors can experience premature menopause with drying of the vaginal mucosa, which can lead to painful intercourse. Pain, in turn, can cause avoidance of sexual intercourse and decreased desire. Such problems can compound feelings of lost femininity and attractiveness and increase feelings of isolation.

Men can develop hypoactive desire as a result of the emotional and physical strains of treatment. Such problems can compound erectile difficulties caused by diminished physical state and medications. Often, if intercourse becomes untenable, male patients will avoid sexual intimacy nearly completely, increasing their sense of isolation and loss of control and compounding their feelings of diminished masculinity and personal power.

Behavioral techniques are an important aspect of sexual therapy and can help a couple to systematically increase intimacy. Such approaches often deemphasize intercourse until the couple has learned new ways to express intimacy while, in some instances, simultaneously unlearning problematic patterns of sexual behavior and avoidance set in motion by the cancer experience.

Couples are often unsure about the safety of intimacy during treatment for CNS cancer. The resulting loss of physical contact is isolating for both the patient and the partner. Intimate touching is safe and pleasurable and is often a fulfilling replacement for intercourse for patients with catheters or sexual dysfunction due to medications. Referral for sexual counseling can significantly improve quality of life for the cancer patient and spouse.

Group Interventions for Patients and Families

The neuro-oncology treatment team at Memorial Sloan–Kettering Cancer Center maintains a psychoeducational support program for the spouses of CNS cancer patients. The group was established to enhance spouses' adjustment to the illness and to facilitate improved family/staff communication in order to improve inpatient and outpatient care. Goals are met by providing information, education, and emotional support; decreasing isolation and alienation through creation of a spouses' support network; and sharing concrete care-taking ideas and suggestions. Better family and staff communication results in timely planning of respite admissions, identification of relief caretakers, or organizing home visits by medical professionals, with intent to improve home care and reduce unnecessary admissions. Led by the interdisciplinary treatment team psychiatrist or psychologist, the oncology treatment team meets with family members twice monthly for 90 minutes, the first third of which is devoted to information and education on topics, including psychiatric effects of disease and treatment, social work services, and practical care-taking suggestions. The remainder of the session is devoted to supportive psychotherapy. The group averages 5 to 10 members each session and is attended by spouses of patients at all stages of disease course, as well as widows of brain tumor patients whose presence helps new group members prepare for the inevitable state of grieving.

A similar program at the M. D. Anderson Cancer Center actively encourages patients to participate with family members. Led by a neuro-oncology social worker and a psychiatric nurse specialist, the group meets monthly. Internal and external experts on primary and supportive aspects of care of the neuro-oncology patient are invited to discuss issues of interest and concern to group members. Following questions and discussion of the educational topic, the group continues to meet in a supportive psychotherapy session. The group focuses on strategies for enhancing the health of patients and family members and of the family itself throughout the treatment process.

PSYCHOSOCIAL IMPACT ON THE MEDICAL STAFF

The nursing and medical care of patients with neuro-oncologic illnesses are demanding and complex and are accompanied by frustrations not encountered by staff working with patients who have non-neurologic cancers. The inability to communicate easily with patients while administering high levels of custodial care is exhausting. The psychological reactions of staff members mirror those of family members, but staff members must also care for the grief-stricken family members. Patients' volatility and/or potentially physically assaultive behavior heighten the stress. Patients have a uniformly poor prognosis; treatment options are of limited benefit and can leave the patient more neurologically impaired than before treatment. Staff members often care for patients with high levels of suffering, many of whom require, but have not accepted, their need for hospice-type palliative care. Additionally, staff members are often provided less emotional support on a diverse and busy neurology service than they might encounter in the hospice setting where group support is a routine aspect of unit function.

Such problems are often reflected in some of the ethical dilemmas encountered in neuro-oncology, such as the application of resuscitation efforts. Patients whose disease affects their ability to communicate may never have had the opportunity to indicate their wishes regarding resuscitation and other aspects of treatment. Family members and staff often become divided over their understanding of the patient's wishes. Staff, wanting to avoid futile efforts to revive a dying patient who is unlikely to survive for long or who is not assured a substantive quality of life following a resuscitation effort, may pressure families to have "Do Not Resuscitate" orders written. Such pressure can put families and staff at odds and worsen the family's feelings of isolation.

Another dilemma is whether a patient without cognitive capacity would choose to have a potentially treatable medical complication (such as pneumonia) go untreated while he is slowly dying of a brain tumor. The issues inherent in administering treatments that essentially extend the life of dying patients can be very divisive for the staff. Physicians often see their role as requiring them to treat a potentially dangerous complication; the nursing staff, who generally spend more time with the patient, often observe the limitations in the patient's quality of life and more often are against extending the patient's life. Family members called on to act as surrogate decision makers are often conflicted, and their stress is transmitted to the staff.

In the psychology of the medical staff, the poor prognosis of patients with CNS tumors moves bereavement and grief issues to center stage. Grief has a tremendous impact on staff members in oncology units generally and is even more problematic on a neuro-oncology service. Patients with primary cancers that are outside the CNS are often admitted to the neuro-oncology service with CNS complications that mark the beginning of the terminal stage of illness. Additionally, the first appearance of neurologic symptoms are devastating losses for the patient and his or her family as the patient, for the first time, is struggling with cognitive changes that threaten independent functioning. Thus, patients and families on neuro-oncology services are likely to be more bereft than those encountered on other services where cure is still a viable possibility and where the patients are healthier and more capable of independent functioning.

Patients with primary CNS cancers and their families are in a near-constant state of mourning for the patient's loss of cognitive, motor, or speech functioning. Each admission seems to culminate in increasing neurologic deficits and the piecemeal loss of the patient's personality, sadly affecting the family and staff. "Professionalism" limits the extent to which the staff can express their feelings; overwhelming and unexpressed grief can render the clinician ineffective, but the complete denial of sadness precludes the empathic stance necessary to meet the emotional needs of the bereft. The mental health professional working on a neuro-oncology service must know how to detect pathologic grief reactions (Lindemann, 1944) in staff members. A high degree of somatic distress, preoccupation with images of a recently deceased patient, guilt about actions during the care of the patient, hostile reactions to the actions of other staff members, and even the adoption of traits of the deceased patient are signs of pathologic behavior that should prompt a referral for individual counseling. Such symptoms of difficult or problematic grief mirror those of burnout and even post-traumatic stress disorder and can be managed through psychotherapy, altered forms of coping and self-expression, and work rotations.

Less pathologic forms of grief and mourning can be seen in the staff's reaction to the death of a "special patient." Various factors may facilitate a staff member's identification with a given patient, such as closeness in age or the patient's having been a healthcare provider. When special patients die the staff may participate in rituals such as attending the patient's funeral. The grief work that staff needs to accomplish for all the losses they suffer may be embodied in this process.

A Group Intervention for Staff Members on a Neuro-Oncology Service

There are various ways in which the stresses experienced when working on a neuro-oncology service can be mitigated. For nurses, rotating demanding patients or difficult families is essential. Physicians-in-training benefit from close supervision and brief rotations. At Memorial Sloan–Kettering Cancer Center, in recognition of the high level of stress encountered on the neuro-oncology service, the psychiatry service started a weekly multidisciplinary support group for staff members called "Psychosocial Rounds." The structured, task-oriented group is co-led by a social worker, head nurse, and psychiatrist or psychologist.

Patients or family members who have been difficult to manage are discussed. The discussion emphasizes medical, nursing, social, psychological, administrative, spiritual, and ethical perspectives. Staff reactions to working in neuro-oncology are discussed, as are thoughts about palliative versus curative modes of patient care, coping with loss, and ethical beliefs. The group attempts to derive concrete plans for managing patients and their families. Staff members are encouraged to express themselves, but by staying focused on clinical issues they can maintain dignity and emotional control so they can remain professional in their interactions and prevent emotional reactions from becoming too personal. It is not unusual for staff members who are most affected by the topics discussed to approach group leaders for further private discussion. The group has been enormously successful in generating a sense of unity among the staff working in this high-pressure environment.

ISSUES FOR SURVIVORS OF NEURO-ONCOLOGIC ILLNESSES

The poor prognosis of neuro-oncologic illnesses for most patients can lead healthcare providers to overlook issues relevant to the small subset of patients who survive free of disease for significant periods of time. While only approximately 5% of glioblastoma patients can expect a 5 year disease-free survival, depending on histology, 30% to 50% of anaplastic glioma patients can expect to be alive at 8 years after diagnosis (Levin et al., 2001). These patients often find it difficult to re-enter normal life.

The growing number of cancer survivors face many difficulties beyond living with the physical and emotional effects of their cancer experience, including discrimination by employers, the inability to secure health insurance, and changes in personal relationships. For survivors of neuro-oncologic illnesses, these issues can be complicated by the loss of cognitive and other functions that can render former occupations and interests impossible to pursue. For younger patients, those most likely to enjoy a lengthy period of survival from neuro-oncologic illness, this can cause a derailment of career plans and a return to dependency on parents and others that had been relinquished earlier in their development. Cognitive rehabilitation techniques that have been used for patients with head injuries and stroke can be a useful part of the recovery for brain tumor patients and are a valuable adjunct to supportive psychotherapy.

CONCLUSION

The psychiatric and psychosocial issues in neuro-oncology are highly complex. The nature of the issues faced test the clinician's flexibility and understanding of organic and psychological disorders and require that the focus of treatment go beyond patients to include those around them. Despite the poor prognosis often associated with cancer in the nervous system, associated primary and secondary psychiatric disorders can be successfully treated with consequent improvement in quality of life for patients and families.

REFERENCES

Alexopoulos GS. 1996. Affective disorders. In: Sadavoy J, Lazarus LW, Jarvik LF, Grossberg GT (eds), Comprehensive Review of Geriatric Psychiatry–II, 2nd ed. Washington, DC: American Psychiatric Press, pp 563–592.

Anderson SI, Taylor R, Whittle IR. 1999. Mood disorders in patients after treatment for primary intracranial tumors. Br J Neurosurg 13:480–485.

Auchincloss SS. 1989. Sexual dysfunction in cancer patients: issues in evaluation and treatment. In: Holland JC, Rowland JH (eds), Psycho-oncology. New York: Oxford University Press, pp 383–413.

Breitbart W, Cohen KR. 1998. Delirium. In: Holland JC (ed), Psycho-oncology. New York: Oxford University Press, pp 564–565.

Breitbart W, Krivo S. 1998. Suicide. In: Holand JC (ed), Psycho-oncology. New York: Oxford University Press, pp 541–547.

Bruera E, Miller MJ, Macmillan K, Kuehn N. 1992. Neuropsychological effects of methylphenidate in patients receiving a continuous infusion of narcotics for cancer pain. Pain 48:163–166.

Chow TW, Cummings JL. 1999. Frontal-subcortical circuits. In: Miller BL, Cummings JL (eds), The Human Frontal Lobes: Functions and Disorders. New York: Guilford Press, pp 3–26.

DeAngelis LM, Delattre JY, Posner JB. 1989. Radiation-induced dementia in patients cured of brain metastases. Neurology 39:789–796.

DeLong R, Friedman H, Friedman N, Gustafson K, Oakes J. 1992. Methylphenidate in neuropsychological sequelae of radiotherapy and chemotherapy of childhood brain tumors and leukemia [letter]. J Child Neurol 7:462–463.

Denicoff KD, Rubinow DR, Papa MZ, et al. 1987. The neuropsychiatric effects of treatment with interleukin-1–2 and lymphocyte-activated killer cells. Ann Intern Med 107: 293–300.

Derogatis LR, Morrow GR, Fetting J, et al. 1983. The prevalence of psychiatric disorders among cancer patients. JAMA 249:751–757.

Dropcho EJ. 1998. Neurologic paraneoplastic syndromes. J Neurol Sci 153:264–278.

Endicott J. 1984. Measurement of depression in patients with cancer. Cancer 53:2243–2249.

Erban H, Ochoa E, Borod J, Feinberg T. 2000. Consequences of right cerebrovascular accident on emotional functioning: diagnostic and treatment implications. CNS Spectrums 3:25–38.

Fleishman SB, Kalash GR. 1998. Chemotherapeutic agents and neuropsychiatric side effects. In: Holland JC (ed), Psycho-oncology. New York: Oxford University Press, pp 630–638.

Grossman F. 1998. A review of anticonvulsants in treating agitated demented elderly patients. Pharmacotherapy 18:600–606.

Lederberg MS. 1998. The family of the cancer patient. In: Holland JC (ed), Psycho-oncology. New York: Oxford University Press, pp 981–993.

Levin VA, Leibel SA, Gutin PH. 2001. Neoplasms of the central nervous system. In: DeVita VTJ, Hellman S, Rosenberg SA (eds), Cancer: Principles and Practice of Oncology, 6th ed. Philadelphia: Lippincott-Raven, pp 2100–2160.

Lindemann E. 1944. Symptomatology and management of acute grief in 1944. Am J Psychiatry 101:141–148.

Liptzin, B. 1996. Delirium. In: Sadavoy J, Lazarus LW, Jarvik LF, Grossberg GT (eds), Comprehensive Review of Geriatric Psychiatry–II, 2nd ed. Washington, DC: American Psychiatric Press, pp 479–495.

Lishman WA. 1998a. Organic Psychiatry: The Psychological Consequences of Cerebral Disorder, 3rd ed. Oxford: Blackwell Science, pp 218–236.

Lishman WA. 1998b. Organic Psychiatry: The Psychological Consequences of Cerebral Disorder, 3rd ed. Oxford: Blackwell Science, pp 668–770.

Manes FF, Robinson RG. 2000. Neuropsychiatric aspects of brain tumors. In: Sadock BJ, Sadock VA (eds), Kaplan & Sadok's Comprehensive Textbook of Psychiatry, 7th ed. Philadelphia: Lippincott, pp 253–261.

Masand PS, Tesar GE. 1996. Use of stimulants in the medically ill. Psychiatr Clin North Am 19:515–547.

Massie MJ, Breibart W, Butler RW. 1991. Psychiatric diagnoses and neuropsychological evaluation of patients with neuro-oncologic illness. In: Neuro-Oncology IV: Recent Developments in the Management of Neuro-Oncologic Illnesses. New York: Syllabus of the Post-Graduate Course, Memorial Sloan–Kettering Cancer Center, 231 pp.

Massie MJ, Holland JC. 1992. The cancer patient with pain: psychiatric complications and their management. J Pain Symptom Manage 7:99–109.

Massie MJ, Holland JC, Slaker N. 1989. Pyschotherapeutic interventions. In: Holland JC, Rowland JH (eds), Handbook of Psychooncology. New York: Oxford University Press, pp 455–469.

Massie MJ, Holland J, Glass E. 1983. Delirium in terminally ill cancer patients. Am J Psychiatry 140:1048–1050.

Massie MJ, Popkin MK. 1998. Depressive disorders. In: Holland JC (ed), Psycho-oncology. New York: Oxford University Press, pp 518–540.

Meyers CA, Valentine AD. 1995. Neurological and psychiatric adverse effects of immunological therapy. CNS Drugs 3:56–68.

Meyers CA, Weitzner MA, Valentine AD, Levin VA. 1998. Methylphenidate therapy improves cognition, mood, and function of brain tumor patients. J Clin Oncology 16:2522–2527.

Passik S, Breitbart W, Malkin M, Horowitz S. 1994. Psychosocial aspects of neuro-oncologic illness. J Psychosoc Oncol 12:101–122.

Passik S, Massie MJ. 1996. Psychiatric and psychosocial issues. In: Levin VA (ed), Cancer in the Nervous System. New York: Churchill Livingstone, pp 389–410.

Passik SD, Ricketts PL. 1998. Central nervous system tumors. In: Holland JC (ed), Psycho-oncology. New York: Oxford University Press, pp 303–313.

Patchell RA, Posner JB. 1989. Neurologic complications of systemic cancer. In: Holland JC, Rowland JH (eds), The Handbook of Psychooncology. New York: Oxford University Press, pp 327–341.

Posner JB. 1995. Side Effects of Radiation Therapy. Neurologic

Complications of Cancer. Philadelphia: FA Davis, pp 311–337.

Price TR, Goetz KL, Lovell MR. 1997. Neuropsychiatric aspects of brain tumors. In: Yudofsky SC, Hales RE (eds), The American Psychiatric Press Textbook of Neuropsychiatry, 3rd ed. Washington, DC: American Psychiatric Press, pp 635–662.

Roane DM, Feinberg TE, Meckler L, Miner CR, Scicutella A, Rosenthal RN. 2000. Treatment of dementia-associated agitation with gabapentin. J Neuropsychiatry Clin Neurosci 12:40–43.

Robinson RG. 2000. An 82-year-old woman with mood changes following a stroke. JAMA 283:1607–1614.

Rosenberg PB, Ahmed I, Hurwitz S. 1992. Methylphenidate in depressed medically ill patients. J Clin Psychiatry 52:263–267.

Schover LR. 1998. Sexual dysfunction. In: Holland JC (ed), Psycho-oncology. New York: Oxford University Press, pp 494–499.

Slaby AE, Erle SR. 1993. Dementia and delirium. In: Stoudemire A, Fogel BS (eds), Psychiatric Care of the Medical Patient. New York: Oxford University Press, pp 415–453.

Sourkes BM, Massie MJ, Holland JC. 1998. Psychotherapeutic issues. In: Holland JC (ed), Psycho-oncology. New York: Oxford University Press, pp 694–700.

Starkstein SE, Robinson RG. 1999. Depression and frontal lobe disorders. In: Miller BL, Cummings JL (eds), The Human Frontal Lobes: Functions and Disorders. New York: Guilford Press, pp 537–546.

Stiefel FC, Breitbart WS, Holland JC. 1989. Corticosteroids in cancer: neuropsychiatric complications. Cancer Invest 7:479–491.

Valentine AD, Meyers CA, Kling MA, Richelson E. Hauser P. 1998. Mood and cognitive side effects of interferon-α therapy. Semin Oncol 25(supp 1):39–47.

Weitzner MA, Meyers CA, Valentine AD. 1995. Methylphenidate in the treatment of neurobehavioral slowing associated with cancer and cancer treatment. J Neuropsychiatry Clin Neurosci 7:347–350.

Index

Page numbers followed by "f" indicate figures; numbers followed by "t" indicate tables; "CF" indicates color figures.